Advances in Obesity and Lipid Management in CVD
(Cutting Edge Strategies by Multispeciality Lens)
A Textbook of Cardiology

Message

डॉ. जितेन्द्र सिंह
राज्य मंत्री (स्वतंत्र प्रभार),
विज्ञान और प्रौद्योगिकी मंत्रालय,
पृथ्वी विज्ञान मंत्रालय,
राज्य मंत्री प्रधान मंत्री कार्यालय,
कार्मिक, लोक शिकायत तथा पेंशन मंत्रालय,
परमाणु उर्जा विभाग तथा अंतरिक्ष विभाग,
भारत सरकार

सत्यमेव जयते

DR. JITENDRA SINGH
Minister of State (Independent Charge),
Ministry of Science & Technology,
Ministry of Earth Sciences,
Minister of State, Prime Minister's Office,
Ministry of Personnel, Public Grievances and Pensions,
Department of Atomic Energy & Department of Space,
Government of India

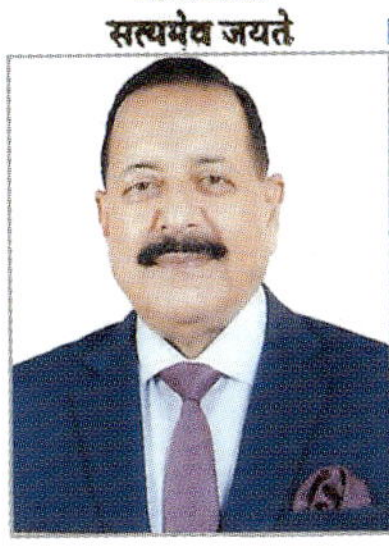

Advances in Obesity and Lipid Management in CVD (Cutting Edge Strategies by Multispeciality Lens): A Textbook of Cardiology deals with an important contemporary subject.

The theme attempts to underscore the transition from conventional risk factor control to precision prevention leveraging advances in molecular biology, innovative metabolic modulation, lipid-lowering therapies, and digital health solutions.

Obesity and dyslipidemia have emerged as major public health challenges, contributing substantially to the growing burden of cardiovascular morbidity and mortality in India and across the globe. Rapid advances in pathophysiological understanding, preventive strategies, pharmacotherapy, and evidence-based interventions particularly in the domains of metabolic medicine and lipid management have transformed contemporary cardiovascular care.

This textbook aptly captures these developments including the implications of advances in management of obesity inflicted morbidity and mortality such as CVD, CKD, DM, HF and Cardiometabolic modulation by GLP-1 RA such as Semaglutide and Tirzepatide and lipid management with statins, ezetimibe, bempedoic acid, PCSK9i, inclisiran apheresis and gene therapy.

The growing burden of obesity ideally needs preventive healthcare, an area repeatedly highlighted by Hon'ble Prime Minister Shri Narendra Modi Ji as essential for national well-being.

Our Hon'ble Prime Minister highlighted the rising obesity menace in India and quoted Lancet report, projecting 44 crores obese Indians by 2050, which is a dangerous prediction, posing economic and health risks. Enhancing awareness on obesity management is, therefore, the need of the hour. This book could serve as an effort in this direction.

I extend my best wishes to Dr HK Chopra and the entire team led by him for this academic endeavor.

(Dr. Jitendra Singh)
MBBS (Stanley, Chennai)
MD Medicine, Fellowship Diabetes (AIIMS, New Delhi)
MNAMS Diabetes & Endocrinology
FICP (Fellow, Indian College of Physicians)

Anusandhan Bhawan, 2, Rafi Marg
New Delhi - 110001
Tel. : 011-23316766, 23714230
Fax : 011-23316745

South Block, New Delhi - 110011
Tel. : 011-23010191, Fax : 23016857
Kartavya Bhavan-03, New Delhi - 110001
Tel. : 011-24010700, 011-24010555

Advances in Obesity and Lipid Management in CVD (Cutting Edge Strategies by Multispeciality Lens)

A Textbook of Cardiology

Editors-in-Chief

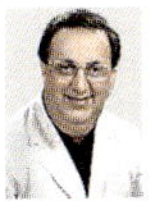

HK Chopra
Chief Cardiologist
Medanta Moolchand Heart Institute, New Delhi, India
Chairman, CME, Moolchand Medcity, New Delhi
Dean, Moolchand Medical Education Institute, New Delhi
Trustee, Moolchand Hospital, New Delhi
National Awardee, DST, Government of India
Chairman, World Wellness Foundation, WHA
Country Head, American Heart Association (AHA)
Former National President, CSI and IAE
Former National Editor-in-Chief, IHJ, JIAE
Editor-in-Chief, Top 14 Textbooks of Cardiology
Chief Advisor, Health Committee SCOPE

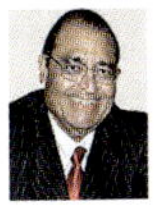

Navin C Nanda
Distinguished Professor
Department of Medicine and Cardiovascular Disease
University of Alabama at Birmingham
Birmingham, Alabama, USA
Editor-in-Chief, Echocardiography: A Journal of Cardiovascular Ultrasound and Allied Techniques
President, International Society of Cardiovascular Ultrasound (ISCU)

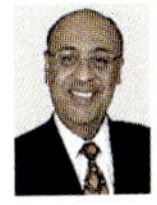

Jagat Narula
Executive Vice President
Chief Academic Officer
UTHealth Houston
Houston, Texas, USA
President, World Heart Federation

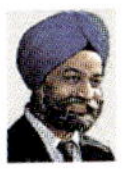

GS Wander
Professor and Head
Department of Cardiology
Dayanand Medical College and Hospital
Unit of Hero DMC Heart Institute
Ludhiana, Punjab, India
Past President, API

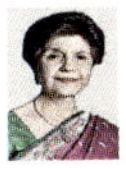

Sarita Bajaj
Senior Consultant Endocrinologist
Former Director-Professor and Head
Department of Medicine
MLN Medical College
Prayagraj, Uttar Pradesh, India

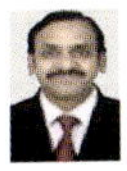

Satyendra Tewari
Professor
Department of Cardiology
Sanjay Gandhi Postgraduate Institute of Medical Sciences
Lucknow, Uttar Pradesh, India

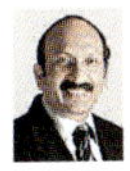

Praveen Chandra
Chairman
Institute of Cardiac Sciences
Medanta—The Medicity
Gurugram, Haryana, India

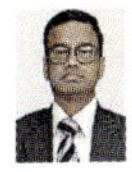

Viveka Kumar
Chairman
Department of Cardiology
Max Heart and Vascular Institute
Saket, New Delhi, India

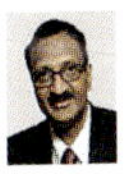

Tiny Nair
Head
Department of Cardiology
PRS Hospital
Thiruvananthapuram
Kerala, India

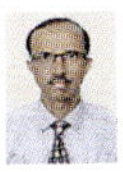

CK Ponde
Head
Department of Cardiology
PD Hinduja National Hospital and Medical Research Centre
Mumbai, Maharashtra, India
Past President, IAE

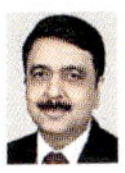

Dinesh Khullar
Chairman and Head
Department of Nephrology and Renal Transplant Medicine
Max Super Speciality Hospital
Saket, New Delhi, India

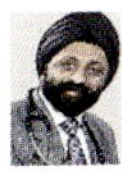

JPS Sawhney
Chairperson
Department of Cardiology
Dharma Vira Heart Center
Sir Ganga Ram Hospital
New Delhi, India

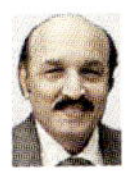

AK Pancholia
Head
Department of Medicine
Clinical and Preventive Cardiology
Arihant Hospital
Indore, Madhya Pradesh, India

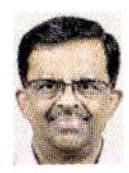

S Shanmugasundaram
Senior Consultant Cardiologist
Billroth Hospitals
Chennai, Tamil Nadu, India

National Principal Editors

- U Kaul, New Delhi
- KK Talwar, New Delhi
- G Vijayaraghavan, Kerala
- Debabarat Roy, Kolkata
- P Krishnam Raju, Hyderabad
- Anita Saxena, New Delhi
- Sandeep Bansal, New Delhi
- Saumitra Ray, Kolkata
- Rakesh Gupta, New Delhi
- Ravi R Kasliwal, Gurugram
- Poonam Malhotra Kapoor, New Delhi
- KK Kapur, New Delhi
- Vinod Sharma, New Delhi
- NN Khanna, New Delhi
- Rajeev Gupta, Jaipur
- Nitin Burkule, Mumbai
- Sameer Srivastava, New Delhi
- SC Govind, Bengaluru
- Ajay Sinha, Patna
- OP Yadava, New Delhi
- V Amuthan, Madurai
- Aditya Kapoor, Lucknow
- SS Mishra, Cuttack
- IB Vijayalakshmi, Bengaluru
- Asha Moorthy, Chennai
- Priya Jagia, New Delhi
- Mona Bhatia, New Delhi
- Roopali Khanna, Lucknow
- Sarita Rao, Indore
- SN Routray, Cuttack
- Harshwardhan, New Delhi
- Sanjay Mittal, Gurugram
- Ashwin Mehta, New Delhi
- Manish Bansal, Gurugram
- S Ramakrishan, New Delhi
- Prafulla Kerkar, Mumbai
- Sadanand Shetty, Mumbai
- Rajeev Agarwala, Meerut
- Mangesh Tiwaskar, Mumbai
- Ashok Kirpalani, Mumbai
- Yugal K Mishra, New Delhi
- Yatin Mehta, Gurugram
- Anil Bhan, New Delhi
- Rajneesh Malhotra, New Delhi
- Vanita Arora, New Delhi
- Aparna Jaswal, New Delhi
- SK Wangnoo, New Delhi
- Vishal Rastogi, New Delhi
- Vidyut Jain, Indore
- Shibha Takkar Chabra, Ludhiana
- Atul Mathur, New Delhi
- Mohit Gupta, New Delhi
- G Justin Paul, Chennai
- AK Oma, New Delhi
- Tripti Deb, Hyderabad
- Rajiv Passey, New Delhi
- Anuj Maheshwari, Lucknow
- Vivudh Pratap Singh, New Delhi
- Rohit Mody, Bathinda
- Kavita Tyagi, New Delhi

JAYPEE

JAYPEE BROTHERS MEDICAL PUBLISHERS
The Health Sciences Publisher
New Delhi | London

Jaypee Brothers Medical Publishers (P) Ltd

Headquarters
EMCA House, 23/23-B
Ansari Road, Daryaganj
New Delhi 110 002, India
Landline: +91-11-23272143, +91-11-23272703
+91-11-23282021, +91-11-23245672
e-mail: jaypee@jaypeebrothers.com

Corporate Office
4838/24, Ansari Road, Daryaganj
New Delhi 110 002, India
Phone: +91-11-43574357
Fax: +91-11-43574314
e-mail: jaypee@jaypeebrothers.com

Overseas Office
JP Medical Ltd.
83, Victoria Street, London
SW1H 0HW (UK)
Phone: +44-20 3170 8910
e-mail: info@jpmedpub.com

EU GPSR Authorised Representative
Logos Europe, 9 rue Nicolas Poussin
17000, La Rochelle, France
Phone: +33 (0) 6 67 93 73 78
e-mail: contact@logoseurope.eu

Website: www.jaypeebrothers.com
Website: www.jaypeedigital.com

Inquiries for bulk sales may be solicited at: jaypee@jaypeebrothers.com

Advances in Obesity and Lipid Management in CVD (Cutting Edge Strategies by Multispeciality Lens): A Textbook of Cardiology

First Edition: **2026**

ISBN: 978-93-7202-043-4

Printed at: Samrat Offset Pvt. Ltd.

Dedicated to

Cardiological Society of India (CSI)
our parents, our teachers, all the members of CSI
our colleagues, patients, students, and our families.

Contributors

A George Koshy
Senior Consultant
Department of Cardiology
Cosmopolitan Hospital, Thiruvananthapuram
Former Professor and Head
Department of Cardiology
Government Medical College
Thiruvananthapuram, Kerala, India

Abbas Ali Khatai
Head
Department of Emergency and Urgent Care
Moolchand Hospital
New Delhi, India

Abdirahman Wardhere
Division of Cardiovascular Medicine
University of Texas Medical Branch
Galveston, TX, USA

Abhishek
Consultant
Department of Nephrology and
Renal Transplant Medicine
Max Super Specialty Hospital
New Delhi, India

Abhishek Garg
Resident
Department of Cardiology
Dayanand Medical College and Hospital
Hero DMC Heart Institute
Ludhiana, Punjab, India

Abhishek Kumar Tiwari
Associate Consultant
Department of Cardiology
Medanta—The Medicity
Gurugram, Haryana, India

Abhishek Nagar
Consultant and Interventional Cardiologist
Department of Cardiology
Apollo Hospitals
Indore, Madhya Pradesh, India

Abhishek Rathore
Consultant, Interventional Cardiologist
and Electrophysiologist
Department of Cardiology
Apollo Hospitals
Indore, Madhya Pradesh, India

Abraham Oomman
Senior Consultant
and Interventional Cardiologist
Apollo Main Hospital
Chennai, Tamil Nadu, India

Achukatla Kumar
Senior Research Consultant
Department of Cardiology
Apollo Hospitals
Indore, Madhya Pradesh, India

Aditya Kapoor
Professor and Head
Department of Cardiology
Sanjay Gandhi Postgraduate Institute
of Medical Sciences
Lucknow, Uttar Pradesh, India

Aditya Porwal
Intern in Medicine
Jawaharlal Nehru Medical College
KLE Academy of Higher Education
and Research
Belagavi, Karnataka, India

Ajay K Sinha
Director
Clinical Cardiology and Research
Jaiprabha Medanta Super Speciality Hospital
Patna, Bihar, India

Ajaykumar U Mahajan
Head
Department of Cardiology
Seth GS Medical College
and KEM Hospital
Mumbai, Maharashtra, India

AK Bali
Department of Medicine
Moolchand Medcity
New Delhi, India

AK Pancholia
Head
Department of Clinical and
Preventive Cardiology
Arihant Hospital and Research Centre
Indore, Madhya Pradesh, India

Akash Batta
Associate Professor
Department of Cardiology
Dayanand Medical College and Hospital
Hero DMC Heart Institute
Ludhiana, Punjab, India

Akriti Rastogi
Senior Consultant
Head and Neck Surgery and Oncology
Moolchand Medcity
New Delhi, India

Alamelu Alagappan
Senior Resident (DM)
Cardiovascular Radiology and
Endovascular Interventions
All India Institute of Medical Sciences
New Delhi, India

Alok Modi
Senior Consultant and Physician
Kevalya Hospital, Jupiter Hospital
Mumbai, Maharashtra, India

Ameet G Sattur
Director (Cath Lab)
HCG Suchirayu Hospital and Sattur Heart Care
Hubballi, Karnataka, India

Amit Jaiswal
Senior Resident
Department of Cardiology
Sanjay Gandhi Postgraduate Institute
of Medical Sciences
Lucknow, Uttar Pradesh, India

Amrish Agrawal
Senior Consultant and Cardiologist
Associate Professor of Medicine
Fujairah Hospital, EHS
Fujairah, UAE

Andru Krishna Vamsi
Resident
Department of Cardiology
Maharishi Markandeshwar Medical College
Ambala, Haryana, India

Anil Bhoraskar
Senior Consultant
Department of Diabetology
and Endocrinology
Asian Heart Institute
Mumbai, Maharashtra, India

Anil Dhall
Senior Consultant and Cardiologist
The Heart Clinic
Gurugram, Haryana, India

Anil Nanda
Asthma and Allergy Center
Lewisville and Flower Mound, TX, USA
Adjunct Professor of Medicine
Division of Allergy and Immunology
University of Texas Southwestern
Medical Center
Dallas, TX, USA

Anil Pareek
President
Medical Affairs and Clinical Research
Ipca Laboratories Limited
Mumbai, Maharashtra, India

Aniruddha De
Consultant
Suraksha Diagnostics Private Limited
Kolkata, West Bengal, India

Anish Kumar Gupta
Senior Research Officer
Department of Nephrology and Renal
Transplant Medicine
Max Super Speciality Hospital
New Delhi, India

Anita N Wasan
Allergy and Asthma Center, McLean, VA
Clinical Instructor of Medicine
The John Hopkins University School of Medicine, Baltimore, MD
Assistant Professor of Medicine
Department of Pediatrics
Georgetown School of Medicine
Washington, DC, USA

Ankit Agarwal
Department of Cardiology
Atal Bihari Vajpayee Institute of Medical Sciences and
Dr Ram Manohar Lohia Hospital
New Delhi, India

Ankit Kumar Choudhury
Senior Resident
Department of Cardiology
Rajiv Gandhi Superspeciality Hospital
New Delhi, India

Ankit Sahu
Addl Professor
Department of Cardiology
Sanjay Gandhi Postgraduate Institute of Medical Sciences
Lucknow, Uttar Pradesh, India

Anshul Jain
Visiting Senior Consultant
Fortis Hospital and Jaipur Golden Hospital
New Delhi, India

Anu Gaur
Consultant
US and Global Regulatory Affairs for Medical Devices
Boston, MA, USA

Anu Grover
Director (Scientific Communication)
Mangrove Creations
New Delhi, India

Anuj Maheshwari
Professor
Department of Medicine
Hind Institute of Medical Sciences
Sitapur, Uttar Pradesh, India

Aparajita Kumar
Associate Consultant Cardiology
Medanta—The Medicity
Gurugram, Haryana, India

Arati Dave Lalchandani
Former Principal and Dean
GSVM Medical College
Kanpur, Uttar Pradesh, India
Member Board of Governors
AIIMS, Gorakhpur

Archit Dahiya
Senior Interventional Cardiologist
Holy Heart Hospital
Rohtak, Haryana, India

Arjun Tandon
Senior Resident (Cardiology)
Institute of Medical Sciences
Banaras Hindu University
Varanasi, Uttar Pradesh, India

Arup Das Biswas
Emeritus Professor
Department of Cardiology
PKG Medical College and Hospital, Kolkata
Former Director, Head and Professor
Department of Cardiology
The Institute of Cardiovascular Sciences
Postgraduate Medical Education and Research
Kolkata, West Bengal, India

Arvind Gupta
Senior Consultant and Head
Department of Internal Medicine and Diabetes
Rajasthan Hospital Limited
Jaipur, Rajasthan, India

Arvind Kumar
Senior Consultant and Interventional Cardiologist
Jeevak Heart Hospital
Patna, Bihar, India

Arvind Sharma
C/o Rohit Tandon
Consultant Physician
Dayanand Medical College and Hospital
Hero DMC Heart Institute
Ludhiana, Punjab, India

Asha Mahilmaran
Senior Consultant and Cardiologist
Apollo Hospitals
Chennai, Tamil Nadu, India

Asha Moorthy
Senior Consultant and Cardiologist
Professor and Head
Sri Ramachandra Medical College and Saveetha Medical College (Emeritus)
Chennai, Tamil Nadu, India

Asharam Panda
Assistant Professor
Department of Cardiology
Dreams University and institute of Health Sciences
and Padmini Care Hospital
Cuttack, Odisha, India

Ashima Gosai
Third Year MBBS Student
Amrita School of Medicine
Faridabad, Haryana, India

Asim Siddiqui
Apollo Centre for Obesity, Diabetes and Endocrinology
Apollo Hospitals
New Delhi, India

Atul Kaushik
Fortis Escorts Heart Institute
New Delhi, India

Avani Jain
Physician
DNS Hospitals
Indore, Madhya Pradesh, India

B Hilbert Sahoo
Department of Cardiology
Sanjay Gandhi Postgraduate Institute of Medical Sciences
Lucknow, Uttar Pradesh, India

Bhavik S Shah
Assistant Professor
Department of Cardiology
Seth GS Medical College and KEM Hospital
Mumbai, Maharashtra, India

Bhawani Pathak
Department of Surgical Oncology
All India Institute of Medical Sciences
New Delhi, India

Bhuban Majhi
Professor
Department of Cardiology
RG Kar Medical College
Kolkata, West Bengal, India

Bijender Singh
Head (Medicine) and Senior Consultant
Positron Multi Speciality Hospital
Rohtak, Haryana, India

Biswaranjan Mishra
Senior Consultant and Cardiologist
Max Diagnostics
Cuttack, Odisha, India

Chandi Garg
Assistant Professor
Department of Medicine
Penn State College of Medicine, USA
Core Faculty
IM Residency Programme, Harrisburg, Pennsylvania

Chandramukhi Sunehra
Senior Consultant and Cardiologist
AIG Hospital
Hyderabad, Telangana, India

CK Ponde
Head
Department of Cardiology
PD Hinduja National Hospital
Mumbai, Maharashtra, India
Past President, IAE

D Santosh
Department of Cardiology
Sir Ganga Ram Hospital
New Delhi, India

Daran Amini
C/o Deepika Misra
Attending, Clinical Cardiology
Columbia University
Division of Cardiology
Mount Sinai Medical Center, USA

Dayasagar Rao Vala
Senior Consultant and Cardiologist
KIMS
Secunderabad, Telangana, India

Debabrata Roy
Senior Consultant, Interventional Cardiologist
and Academic Co-ordinator
Department of Cardiology
Rabindranath Tagore International Institute
of Cardiac Sciences
Kolkata, West Bengal, India

Debasish Das
DrNB Trainee
Department of Cardiology
Rabindranath Tagore International Institute
of Cardiac Sciences
Kolkata, West Bengal, India

Deepak K Jumani
Senior Sexual Health Physician
and Counsellor
Sir JJ Group of Government Hospitals
and Grant Medical College
Mumbai, Maharashtra, India

Deepak Kumar Panigrahi
Senior Consultant
Department of Nephrology and
Renal Transplant Medicine
Max Super Specialty Hospital
New Delhi, India

Deepika Misra
Attending, Clinical Cardiology
Columbia University
Division of Cardiology
Mount Sinai Medical Center, USA

Deepinder Singh
Assistant Professor
Kalpana Chawla Government Medical
College and Hospital
Karnal, Haryana, India

Deepti Yadav
Consultant and Interventional Cardiologist
Medanta—The Medicity
Gurugram, Haryana, India

Dharmendra Jain
Professor
Department of Cardiology
Institute of Medical Sciences
Banaras Hindu University
Varanasi, Uttar Pradesh, India

Dhiman Kahali
Director (Interventional Cardiology)
BM Birla Heart Hospital
Kolkata, West Bengal, India
National President, CSI

Dikshant Jain
Assistant Professor
Department of Cardiology
Vardhman Mahavir Medical College
and Safdarjung Hospital
New Delhi, India

Dinesh Khullar
Group Chairman
Nephrology and Renal Transplant Medicine
Max Healthcare Institute Limited
New Delhi, India

Divya Bajpai
Professor (Add)
Department of Nephrology
Seth GS Medical Collage and KEM Hospital
Mumbai, Maharashtra, India

Dushyant Singh Gaur
Professor and Head
Immunohematology and Blood Transfusion
Himalayan Institute of Medical Sciences
Dehradun, Uttarakhand, India

Geeta S Sheth
Professor and Head
Department of Nephrology
Grant Government Medical College and
Sir JJ Group of Hospitals
Mumbai, Maharashtra, India

Geetha Subramaniam
Former Head and Professor
Department of Cardiology
Rajiv Gandhi Government General Hospital
Chennai, Tamil Nadu, India

Gottipati Divya Chowdary
NRI Medical College
Guntur, Andhra Pradesh, India

Guhan Senthilkumaran
Consultant Nephrologist
CURI Hospitals
Chennai, Tamil Nadu, India

Gurpreet Singh Wander
Professor
Department of Cardiology
Dayanand Medical College and Hospital
Hero DMC Heart Institute
Ludhiana, Punjab, India

Hala Elmarsafawy
Professor
Department of Pediatrics and Pediatric
Cardiology
Director, Cardiac Catheterization Laboratory
Children Hospital
Mansoura University, Egypt

Hanumanth K Reddy
Clinical Adjunct Professor
Department of Internal Medicine
St Louis University Medical School, St Louis, MO
Medical Director
Cardiovascular Institute of Southern
Missouri Poplar Bluff, USA

Harinder K Bali
Chairman (Cardiac Sciences) and
Dean (Academics and Research)
Livasa Hospital
Mohali, Punjab, India

Harmesh Aggarwal
Senior Physician and Cardiologist
Aggarwal Centre for Diabetes and Cancer Care
Gurugram, Haryana, India

Harsh Chaudhary
Apollo CVHF Heart Institute
Ahmedabad, Gujarat, India

Harsh Wardhan
Principal Director (Cardiac Sciences)
Supreme Hospital
Faridabad, Haryana, India

Harshit Khare
Assistant Professor
Department of Cardiology
Sanjay Gandhi Postgraduate Institute
of Medical Sciences
Lucknow, Uttar Pradesh, India

Himanshu Garg
Resident
Department of Cardiology
Dayanand Medical College and Hospital
Hero DMC Heart Institute
Ludhiana, Punjab, India

Himanshu Jain
Clinical Assistant
Indraprastha Apollo Hospital
New Delhi, India

HK Chopra
Chief Cardiologist
Medanta Moolchand Heart Institute
New Delhi, India
Chairman, CME, Moolchand Medcity, New Delhi
Dean, Moolchand Medical Education Institute
New Delhi
Trustee, Moolchand Hospital, New Delhi
National Awardee, DST, Government of India
Chairman, World Wellness Foundation, WHA
Country Head, American Heart Association (AHA)
Former National President, CSI and IAE
Former National Editor-in-Chief, IHJ, JIAE
Editor-in-Chief, Top 14 Textbooks of Cardiology
Chief Advisor, Health Committee SCOPE

I Sathyamurthy
Senior Interventional Cardiologist
Apollo Main Hospitals
Chennai, Tamil Nadu, India

IB Vijayalakshmi
Professor Emeritus, Former Professor and Head (Pediatric Cardiology)
Shri Jayadeva Institute of Cardiovascular Sciences and Research
Bengaluru Medical College and Research Institute
Bengaluru, Karnataka, India

Indu Bansal Aggarwal
Group Director and Head
Radiation Oncology
Paras Hospital
Gurugram, Haryana, India

Isha Nandal
Consultant
Yellow Fertility and IVF Centre
Rohtak, Haryana, India

J Cecily Mary Majella
Head and Professor
Department of Cardiology
Government Multi Super Specialty Hospital
Chennai, Tamil Nadu, India

Jabir Abdullakutty
Senior Consultant, Cardiologist and Director of Cardiovascular Clinical Research
Lisie Hospital
Kochi, Kerala, India

Jayagopal PB
Director and Senior Interventional Cardiologist
Lakshmi Hospital
Palakkad, Kerala, India

Jayakrishan Pillai
Assistant Professor
Department of Medicine
Armed Forces Medical College
Pune, Maharashtra, India

Jhanja Mohapatra
Senior Resident
Department of Radiotherapy
Dharamshila Narayana Super Specialty Hospital
New Delhi, India

Jostol Pinto
Professor
Department of Cardiology
Father Muller Medical College
Mangaluru, Karnataka, India

Joy Dev Mukherji
Vice Chairman and Head
Department of Neurology
Institute of Neurosciences
Max Super Speciality Hospital
New Delhi, India

JPS Sawhney
Chairperson
Department of Cardiology
Dharma Vira Heart Center
Sir Ganga Ram Hospital
New Delhi, India

Jugal Kishor Sharma
Senior Consultant and Medical Director
Central Delhi Diabetes and Obesity Centre
New Delhi, India

Juhi Singh
Senior Resident
Department of Cardiology
Dharma Vira Heart Center
Sir Ganga Ram Hospital
New Delhi, India

Juliana Spanova
Resident (Internal Medicine)
Department of Medicine
University of Alabama at Birmingham
Birmingham, Alabama, USA

Jyotirmoy Pal
Department of Medicine
Sagar Dutta Medical College and Hospital
Kamarhati, West Bengal, India

K Roshan Rao
Senior Interventional Cardiologist and Head
Department of Cardiology
Apollo Hospitals
Indore, Madhya Pradesh, India

Kamlesh Raut
Consultant (Cardiology)
Max Super Specialty Hospital
New Delhi, India

Kanhai Lalani
Associate Professor
Department of Cardiology
Kasturba Medical College, Manipal
Manipal Academy of Higher Education
Manipal, Karnataka, India

Kanika Sood Sharma
Director and Clinical Lead
Department of Radiotherapy
Dharamshila Narayana Superspeciality Hospital
New Delhi, India

Kaushik Manna
Interventional Cardiologist
Department of Cardiology
Rabindranath Tagore International Institute of Cardiac Sciences
Kolkata, West Bengal, India

Kavita Tyagi
Department of Cardiology
Sir Gangaram Hospital
New Delhi, India

Khizer Anees
C/o Dr Hanumanth K Reddy
Clinical Adjunct Professor
Department of Internal Medicine
St Louis University Medical School, St Louis, MO
Medical Director, Cardiovascular Institute of Southern Missouri
Poplar Bluff, USA

Kiron Varghese
Professor
Department of Cardiology
St John's Medical College
Bengaluru, Karnataka, India

KK Kapur
Chief Consultant (Noninvasive Lab)
Apollo Hospital
New Delhi, India

KM Vivek
Senior Resident
Department of Cardiology
Dharma Vira Heart Center
Sir Ganga Ram Hospital
New Delhi, India

KN Srinivasan
Senior Interventional Cardiologist
Apollo Main Hospitals
Chennai, Tamil Nadu, India

Krishna Rao
Professor of Cardiology and Clinical Medicine
University of Rochester
Strong Memorial Hospital
Rochester, NY, USA

Krishna Vaitheeswaran
Department of Ophthalmology
Moolchand Medcity
New Delhi, India

Kulwant Singh
Principal Consultant
Department of Nephrology and Renal Transplant Medicine
Max Super Specialty Hospital
New Delhi, India

Lovelina Singh
Director
Department of Neurology
Moolchand Medcity
New Delhi, India

M Bharathkumaran
C/o R Manivasagam
Interventional and Echo Cardiologist
Director, Heart Care and Cure Centre
Tiruchirappalli, Tamil Nadu, India

Madhupada Kiran Kumar
Associate Cardiology Consultant
Apollo Hospital
Hyderabad, Telangana, India

Mahpaekar Mashhadi
Apollo CVHF Heart Institute
Ahmedabad, Gujarat, India

Mainak Mandal
Resident
Department of Medicine
KPC Medical College
Kolkata, West Bengal, India

Mainak Mukhopadhyay
Consultant
Department of Cardiology
Manipal Hospitals
Kolkata, West Bengal, India

Manasmukul Dutta
C/o Yugal Mishra
Chief of Clinical Services
Chairman, Manipal Institute
of Cardiac Sciences
Chief Cardiovascular Surgeon
Manipal Hospitals
New Delhi, India

Mangesh Tiwaskar
Senior Consultant, Physician
and Diabetologist
Shilpa Medical Research Centre
Mumbai, Maharashtra, India

Manikanth Vivek
Sir Ganga Ram Hospital
New Delhi, India

Manish Bansal
Senior Director
Clinical and Preventive Cardiology
Medanta—The Medicity
Gurugram, Haryana, India

Manisha Arora
Director
Department of Internal Medicine
CK Birla Hospital
New Delhi, India

Manisha Sahay
Professor and Head
Department of Nephrology
Osmania Medical College and General Hospital
Hyderabad, Telangana, India

Manoranjan Mandal
Professor and Head
Department of Cardiology
NRS Medical College
Kolkata, West Bengal, India

Manotosh Panja
Director
Department of Cardiology
Belle Vue Clinic
Kolkata, West Bengal, India

Manpreet Singh Brar
PG Resident
Department of ENT
Krishna Mohan Medical College
Mathura, Uttar Pradesh, India

Mansi Kaushik
Senior Consultant (Clinical and Preventive
Cardiology)
Medanta—The Medicity
Gurugram, Haryana, India

Manu Prakash
Senior Consultant
Department of Nephrology and Renal
Transplant Medicine
Max Super Specialty Hospital
New Delhi, India

Manu Sabu
Senior Resident
Department of Nephrology
Grant Government Medical College
and Sir JJ Group of Hospitals
Mumbai, Maharashtra, India

Manuhaar
DM Resident
Department of Cardiology
Dayanand Medical College and Hospital
Hero DMC Heart Institute
Ludhiana, Punjab, India

Manvika Tiwari
Moolchand Medcity
New Delhi, India

Masood Ahmad
Department of Cardiovascular Medicine
University of Texas Medical Branch
Galveston, TX, USA

Mayank Butola
Department of Cardiology
Artemis Hospital
Gurugram, Haryana, India

Md Inamul Haque
Department of ICU
Moolchand Medcity
New Delhi, India

Meghna Gupta
Consultant
Department of Psychiatry
City Institute of Medical Sciences
Mathura, Uttar Pradesh, India

Milan Bhardwaj
Visiting Consultant
Department of Cardiology
PSRI Hospital
New Delhi, India

Mitendra Singh Yadav
Department of Cardiology
Max Super Specialty Hospital
New Delhi, India

Moaz Ahmad
C/o Dr Hanumanth K Reddy
Clinical Adjunct Professor
Department of Internal Medicine
St Louis University Medical School
St Louis, MO
Medical Director
Cardiovascular Institute of Southern Missouri
Poplar Bluff, USA

Mohamed Nor
Stamford Hospital
Columbia University Vagelos College
of Physicians and Surgeons
Stamford, CT, USA

Mohan Bhargava
Director (Cardiology)
Max Superspecialty Hospital
New Delhi, India

Mohan Deepa
Dr Mohan's Diabetes Specialties Centre and
Madras Diabetes Research Foundation
Chennai, Tamil Nadu, India

Monika Nadar
Department of Ophthalmology
Moolchand Medcity
New Delhi, India

Mrinal Kanti Das
Past President, CSI and Asian Heart Society
Former Member of the Assembly of
International Governors of ACC
Kolkata, West Bengal, India

Mukesh Kumar
Department of Neurosciences
Max Super Specialty Hospital
New Delhi, India

Muthu Jayaraman
Former Professor
Department of Nephrology
Stanley Medical College
Chennai, Tamil Nadu, India

Nagendra Chauhan
Senior Director
Institute of Cardiac Sciences
Medanta—The Medicity
Gurugram, Haryana, India

Namrata Gaur
Additional Professor and Head Unit-2
Department of Cardiothoracic and
Vascular Surgery
All India Institute of Medical Sciences
Rishikesh, Uttarakhand, India

Narayan Prasad
Professor and Head
Department of Nephrology
Sanjay Gandhi Postgraduate Institute
of Medical Sciences
Lucknow, Uttar Pradesh, India

Narinder Pal Singh
Consultant (Academics)
Department of Nephrology and
Renal Transplant Medicine
Max Super Specialty Hospital
New Delhi, India

Narra Lavanya
Consultant and Interventional Cardiologist
KIMS Hospitals
Hyderabad, Telangana, India

Navdeep S Sidhu
Assistant Professor
Department of Cardiology
All India Institute of Medical Sciences
Bilaspur, Himachal Pradesh, India

Naveen Garg
Senior Consultant
Department of Cardiology
Civil Hospital, Govt of Haryana, India
Palwal, Haryana, India

Navin C Nanda
Distinguished Professor
Department of Medicine and
Cardiovascular Disease, Cardiology Division
University of Alabama at Birmingham
Birmingham, Alabama, USA

Nayna Nanda
Plano West Senior School
Plano, Texas, USA

Neeraj Pandit
Professor and Head
Department of Cardiology
Rajiv Gandhi Super Speciality Hospital
New Delhi, India

Neha Chopra
Senior Resident
Department of Cardiology
Vardhman Mahavir Medical College
and Safdarjung Hospital
New Delhi, India

Nikhil Chaudhari
Institute of Vascular and Endovascular Sciences
Sir Ganga Ram Hospital
New Delhi, India

Nikhila Sri Rao
State University of New York Upstate
Medical University
750 E Adams St, Syracuse
NY 13210, USA

Nilesh Jadhao
Department of Neurosciences
Max Superspeciality Hospital
New Delhi, India

Nilesh Sai Rao
State University of New York
Upstate Medical University
Syracuse, NY, USA

Nilufar Fatema
Assistant Professor
Department of Cardiology
Bangladesh Medical University
Dhaka, Bangladesh

Nirmal Ghati
Assistant Professor
Department of Cardiology
All India Institute of Medical Sciences
New Delhi, India

Nitin Saini
Senior Resident
Department of Cardiology
Dharma Vira Heart Center
Sir Ganga Ram Hospital
New Delhi, India

Nitish Naik
Professor
Department of Cardiology
All India Institute of Medical Sciences
New Delhi, India

NK Singh
Director
Diabetes and Heart Centre
Dhanbad, Jharkhand, India
Founder and Editor-in-Chief, CME India

Ojas Jain
Second Year DM Student
Department of Cardiology
Atal Bihari Vajpayee Institute of Medical
Sciences and Dr Ram Manohar Lohia Hospital
New Delhi, India

Omar Hallak
Consultant and Cardiologist
Al Zahra Hospital
Dubai, UAE

Pallavi Prasad
Associate Professor
Department of Nephrology
Vardhman Mahavir Medical College
and Safdarjung Hospital
New Delhi, India

Pankti Parikh
Assistant Professor
Department of Endocrinology
Kasturba Medical College, Manipal
Manipal Academy of Higher Education
Manipal, Karnataka, India

Parneesh Arora
Director
Department of Cardiology
Medanta Hospital
Noida, Uttar Pradesh, India

Parv Kamra
C/o Vitull K Gupta
Senior Consultant
Kishori Ram Hospital and Diabetes Care Centre
Bathinda, Punjab, India

PK Asokan
Senior Consultant and Cardiologist
Director, Cardio Life Care
Fathima Heart Foundation
Kozhikode, Kerala, India

Pooja Khosla
Senior Consultant and Co-Chairperson
Department of Internal Medicine
Sir Ganga Ram Hospital
New Delhi, India

Poonam Malhotra Kapoor
Professor
Department of Cardiac Anesthesiology
and Critical Care
Cardio Thoracic Centre
All India Institute of Medical Sciences
New Delhi, India

Poonam Singla
Senior Consultant
Department of ENT
Moolchand Medcity
New Delhi, India

Prachi Gupta
Moolchand Medcity
New Delhi, India

Pradeep Jain
Senior Interventional Cardiologist
Indraprastha Apollo Hospital
New Delhi, India

Prakas Chandra Mondal
Head
Department of Cardiology
Director, Apollo Heart Institute
Apollo Multispecialty Hospital
Kolkata, West Bengal, India

Prashant Gautam
Assistant Professor
Department of Cardiology
Sanjay Gandhi Postgraduate Institute
of Medical Sciences
Lucknow, Uttar Pradesh, India

Prashant Moorthy
Senior Consultant and Radiologist
MGM Hospital
Chennai, Tamil Nadu, India

Prasun Sagar
Associate Consultant
Max Super Specialty Hospital
New Delhi, India

Pratap Chandra Rath
Director and Head
Department of Cardiology
Apollo Hospitals
Hyderabad, Telangana, India
President, Cardiological Society of India
Past President, Indian College of Cardiology

Pratap Kumar
DM Scholar
Department of Cardiology
Institute of Medical Sciences
Banaras Hindu University
Varanasi, Uttar Pradesh, India

Praveen Chandra
Chairman
Institute of Cardiac Sciences
Medanta—The Medicity
Gurugram, Haryana, India

Praveen Jaswal
Consultant and Interventional Cardiologist
Department of Cardiology
Apollo Hospitals
Indore, Madhya Pradesh, India

Prayaag Kini
Department of Cardiology
Sri Sathya Sai Institute of Higher Medical Sciences Whitefield
Bengaluru, Karnataka, India

Preeti Gupta
Professor
Department of Cardiology
Vardhman Mahavir Medical College and Safdarjung Hospital
New Delhi, India

Preetinder Kaur
Department of Ophthalmology
Moolchand Medcity
New Delhi, India

Prerna Goyal
Senior Consultant
RG Stone Urology and Laparoscopy Hospital
Ludhiana, Punjab, India

Priti Meena
Assistant Professor
Department of Nephrology
All India Institute of Medical Sciences
Bhubaneswar, Odisha, India

Priya Jagia
Professor and Head
Cardiovascular Radiology and Endovascular Interventions
All India Institute of Medical Sciences
New Delhi, India

Priyanka Gurram Reddy
C/o Dr Hanumanth K Reddy
Clinical Adjunct Professor
Department of Internal Medicine
St Louis University Medical School, St Louis, MO
Medical Director
Cardiovascular Institute of Southern Missouri
Poplar Bluff, USA

Pushpit Singh
Clinical Research Associate
Department of Clinical Research and Academics
Fortis Flt Lt Rajan Dhall Hospital
New Delhi, India

R Manivasagam
Interventional and Echo Cardiologist
Director, Heart Care and Cure Centre
Tiruchirappalli, Kerala, India

Raghav Khullar
Resident
Department of Nephrology
All India Institute of Medical Sciences
New Delhi, India

Rahul Mehrotra
Department of Cardiology
Artemis Hospitals
Gurugram, Haryana, India

Raj Singh Bhati
Resident in Medicine
Hind Institute of Medical Sciences
Barabanki, Uttar Pradesh, India

Raj Wasan
College of William and Mary
Williamsburg, VA, USA

Rajarshi Halder
Resident, RG Kar Medical College
Kolkata, West Bengal, India

Rajeev Garg
Senior Interventional Cardiologist
Gleneagles Hospitals
Hyderabad, Telangana, India

Rajeev Gupta
Department of Preventive Cardiology and Medicine
Eternal Heart Care Centre and Research Institute
Jaipur, Rajasthan, India

Rajeevalochana Parthasarathy
Senior Consultant and Nephrologist
Medway Hospitals
Chennai, Tamil Nadu, India

Rajesh Meena
Department of Medicine
Moolchand Medicity
New Delhi, India

Rajesh Mishra
Head, Department of Critical Care
Moolchand Medcity
New Delhi, India

Rajesh Natuva
Consultant Cardiologist
Star Hospitals
Hyderabad, Telangana, India

Rajesh Ranjan Behera
Consultant Physician
KIMS Hospital
Bhubaneswar, Odisha, India

Rakesh Varma
Former DG Health, Govt of India
Professor and Head
Department of Cardiology,
ESIC Medical College and Hospital
Faridabad, Haryana, India

Ramya Pechetty
Consultant and Cardiologist
Apollo Spectra Hospital
Hyderabad, Telangana, India

Ranjan Modi
Senior Consultant and Head of Unit
Interventional Cardiology and Structural Heart Disease
New Delhi, India

Ranjit K Nath
Director Professor and Head
Department of Cardiology
Atal Bihari Vajpayee Institute of Medical Sciences and and Dr Ram Manohar Lohia Hospital
New Delhi, India

Ranjit Mohan Anjana
Dr Mohan's Diabetes Specialities Centre
Madras Diabetes Research Foundation
Chennai, Tamil Nadu, India

Ranjit Unnikrishnan
Dr Mohan's Diabetes Specialties Centre and
Madras Diabetes Research Foundation
Chennai, Tamil Nadu, India

Ravi Komatireddy
C/o Dr Hanumanth K Reddy
Clinical Adjunct Professor
Department of Internal Medicine
St Louis University Medical School,
St Louis, MO
Medical Director, Cardiovascular Institute of Southern Missouri
Poplar Bluff, USA

Ravi R Kasliwal
Chairman (Clinical and Preventive Cardiology)
Medanta—The Medicity
Gurugram, Haryana, India

Reeta Varyani
Department of Cardiology
Sri Sathya Sai Institute of Higher Medical Sciences Whitefield
Bengaluru, Karnataka, India

Rekha Mishra
Senior Consultant
Department of Cardiology
Indraprastha Apollo Hospital
New Delhi, India

Rohan Patel
Senior Resident
Department of Cardiology
Dharma Vira Heart Center
Sir Ganga Ram Hospital
New Delhi, India

Rohit Tandon
Consultant Physician
Dayanand Medical College and Hospital
Hero DMC Heart Institute
Ludhiana, Punjab, India

Rohit Walia
Head
Department of Cardiology
Maharishi Markandeshwar Medical College
Ambala, Haryana, India

Roopali Khanna
Professor
Department of Cardiology
Sanjay Gandhi Postgraduate Institute
of Medical Sciences
Lucknow, Uttar Pradesh, India

Ruchi Sharma
ESIC Medical College
Faridabad, Haryana, India

Rupesh Salve
Medical Affairs and Clinical Research
Ipca Laboratories Limited
Mumbai, Maharashtra, India

S Shanmugasundaram
Former Professor of Cardiology
Stanley and Madras Medical Colleges
Cardiologist, Billroth Hospitals
Chennai, Tamil Nadu, India

Sahana Shetty
Professor and Head
Department of Endocrinology
Kasturba Medical College, Manipal
Manipal Academy of Higher Education
Manipal, Karnataka, India

Sameer Dani
Director (Cardiology Services)
Apollo CVHF Heart Institute, Ahmedabad
Apollo Hospital International
Gandhinagar, Gujarat, India

Sandeep Seth
Department of Cardiology
All India Institute of Medical Sciences
New Delhi, India

Sandeepan Saha
Assistant Professor
Department of Cardiology
Dr Ram Manohar Lohia Institute
of Medical Sciences
Lucknow, Uttar Pradesh, India

Sangeeta Dhir
Department of Cardiology
Max Superspeciality Hospital
New Delhi, India

Sanjay C Porwal
Head
Department of Cardiology
Jawaharlal Nehru Medical College
KLE Academy of Higher Education
and Research
Belagavi, Karnataka, India

Sanjay Mittal
Vice Chairman
Clinical Cardiology and Research
Medanta—The Medicity
Gurugram, Haryana, India

Saptadipa Das
Senior Resident
Department of Nephrology
Grant Government Medical College and
Sir JJ Group of Hospitals
Mumbai, Maharashtra, India

Sarika Verma
ENT Surgeon and Allergy Specialist
Director, AllergyDoc Clinics
Head
Department of Allergy
Moolchand Medicity
New Delhi, India

Sarita Bajaj
Senior Consultant and Endocrinologist
Former Director–Professor and Head
Department of Medicine
MLN Medical College
Prayagraj, Uttar Pradesh, India

Sarita Rao
Senior Interventional Cardiologist
and Director (Cathlab)
Department of Cardiology
Apollo Hospitals
Indore, Madhya Pradesh, India

Satyendra Tewari
Professor
Department of Cardiology
Sanjay Gandhi Postgraduate Institute
of Medical Sciences
Lucknow, Uttar Pradesh, India

Saumitra Ray
Consultant
Department of Cardiology
Manipal Hospitals
Kolkata, West Bengal, India

SB Gupta
Former Consultant, Physician,
and Cardiologist
Asian Heart Institute, Mumbai
Former Head, Department of Medicine
and Cardiology
Central Railway Headquarters Hospital
Mumbai, Maharashtra, India

Shaik Nafeez Javed
Cardiology Resident
Jawaharlal Nehru Medical College
KLE Academy of Higher Education and Research
Belagavi, Karnataka, India

Shaimaa Zakariya
C/o Hala Elmarsafawy
Professor
Department of Pediatrics and Pediatric Cardiology
Director, Cardiac Catheterization Laboratory
Children Hospital
Mansoura University, Egypt

Shakil Shaikh
Honorary Cardiologist
Fortis Hospital
Thane, Maharashtra, India

Shambo Samrat Samajdar
Department of Outpatient Clinic
Diabetes and Allergy-Asthma Therapeutics
Specialty Clinic
Kolkata, West Bengal, India

Sharad Chandra
Professor
Department of Cardiology
King George's Medical University
Lucknow, Uttar Pradesh, India

Sharvari Mahajan
University Hospitals Birmingham
NHS Foundation Trust

Sheeba George
Senior Interventional Cardiologist and Head
Department of Cardiology
Jubilee Memorial Hospital
Thiruvananthapuram, Kerala, India

Shekhar Kunal
Associate Professor
Department of Cardiology
ESIC Medical College and Hospital
Faridabad, Haryana, India

Shibba Takkar Chhabra
Professor
Department of Cardiology
Dayanand Medical College and Hospital
Hero DMC Heart Institute
Ludhiana, Punjab, India

Shipra Gupta
Associate Consultant (Medical Oncology)
Paras Hospital
Gurugram, Haryana, India

Shishu Shankar Mishra
Professor and Director
SOA University, Bhubaneswar
Professor and Director
DRIEMS University and Institute of Health Sciences
and Padmini Care Hospital, Cuttack
Director, Med-n-Heart Clinic
Cuttack, Odisha, India

Shitij Chaudhary
Assistant Professor
Department of Cardiology
Cardiothoracic Sciences Centre
All India Institute of Medical Sciences
New Delhi, India

Shivani Rao
Associate Professor
Department of Cardiology
Atal Bihari Vajpayee Institute of Medical Sciences and Dr Ram Manohar Lohia Hospital
New Delhi, India

Shraddha Ranjan
Senior Consultant
(Clinical and Preventive Cardiology)
Jay Prabha Medanta Super Specialty Hospital
Patna, Bihar, India

Shreyasee Borah
C/o Dr Sunil Prakash
Principal Director and Head
Department of Nephrology and Renal Transplant Service
BLK Max Super Specialty Hospital
New Delhi, India

Shubham Srivastava
Senior Resident
Department of Cardiology
Sanjay Gandhi Postgraduate Institute of Medical Sciences
Lucknow, Uttar Pradesh, India

Shweta Sharma
Medical Affairs and Clinical Research
Ipca Laboratories Limited
Mumbai, Maharashtra, India

Siddarth Varshney
Consultant and Interventional Cardiologist
Medanta—The Medicity
Gurugram, Haryana, India

Sidharth S Pattnaik
Assistant Professor
Department of Internal Medicine
Kalinga Institute of Medical Sciences
Bhubaneswar, Odisha, India

SN Pathak
Additional Director (Cardiology)
Fortis Hospital
New Delhi, India

SN Routray
Former Head
Department of Cardiology
Srirama Chandra Bhanja Medical College and Hospital
Cuttack, Odisha, India

Sneha Garg
Associate Consultant (Cardiology)
Max Superspecialty Hospital
New Delhi, India

Somnath Mukhopadhay
Consultant and Interventional Cardiologist
Nightingale Hospital
Kolkata, West Bengal, India

Soumit Sharma
Internal Medicine Resident
University of Alabama at Birmingham
Huntsville, Alabama, USA

Srichandran L
Senior Consultant and Cardiologist
Apollo Hospitals
Chennai, Tamil Nadu, India

Srikanta Sharma
Senior Consultant Physician
Kalinga Institute of Medical Sciences and Hospital
Bhubaneswar, Odisha, India

Srina Ray
Junior Clinical Fellow, ITU
Epsom and St Helier University Hospitals
NHS Trust, UK

SS Iyengar
Manipal Hospital
Bengaluru, Karnataka, India

Subhash Kumar Wangnoo
Apollo Centre for Obesity, Diabetes and Endocrinology
Apollo Hospitals
New Delhi, India

Sudhir Kumar Mathi
Resident
Department of Cardiology
Maharishi Markandeshwar Medical College
Ambala, Haryana, India

Sudhir Kumar Satpathy
Associate Professor
KIMS Pradyumna Bal Memorial Hospital
Bhubaneswar, Odisha, India

Suhas Erande
Professor
Pune, Maharashtra, India

Sujoy Majumdar
Senior Consultant
(Endocrinology and Diabetes)
Apollo Multi Specialty Hospital
Kolkata, West Bengal, India

Suman Kumar
Professor and Head
Department of Medicine
Armed Forces Medical College
Pune, Maharashtra, IndiaW

Sunil Modi
Senior Consultant and Cardiologist
Indraprastha Apollo Hospital
New Delhi, India

Sunil Prakash
Principal Director and Head
Department of Nephrology and Renal Transplant Service
BLK Max Super Specialty Hospital
New Delhi, India

Sunil Raheja
Senior Consultant
Department of Internal Medicine
Moolchand Hospital, New Delhi, India

Supraja Moorthy
Assistant Professor
Pondicherry Institute of Medical Sciences
Puducherry, India

Supratip Kundu
Consultant and Interventional Cardiologist
Manipal Hospitals
Kolkata, West Bengal, India

Sura Kishore Mishra
Department of Cardiology
Srirama Chandra Bhanja Medical College and Hospital, Cuttack, Odisha, India

Tapan Ghose
Senior Director and Head
Department of Cardiology
Head, Clinical Research and Academics
Fortis Flt Lt Rajan Dhall Hospital
New Delhi, India

Tarun Kumar
Associate Director and Head
Department of Cardiology
Medanta Moolchand Heart Center
New Delhi, India

Taruni Lalchandani
Assistant Professor
Department of ENT
Dr Ram Manohar Lohia Institute of Medical Sciences
Lucknow, Uttar Pradesh, India

Teena Jabir
Final Year General Medicine PG
Travancore Medical College Hospital
Kollam, Kerala, India

Thair Al Jumaily
Consultant and Cardiologist
Fujairah Hospital, EHS
Fujairah, UAE

Tiny Nair
Head, Department of Cardiology
PRS Hospital
Thiruvananthapuram, Kerala, India

Tripti Deb
Senior Consultant
Department of Cardiologist
Apollos Hospital Jubilee Hills
Hyderabad, Telangana, India

Umesh Chandra Tripathi
Assistant Professor
Department of Cardiology
King George's Medical College
Lucknow, Uttar Pradesh, India

Urvashi Gupta
Senior Consultant
Department of Gastroenterology
Moolchand Medcity
New Delhi, India

V Anand
Department of Medicine
Moolchand Medcity
New Delhi, India

V Mohan
Chairman
Madras Diabetes Research Foundation
ICMR-Collaborating Centre of Excellence
[ICMR-CCoE] and
Dr Mohan's Diabetes Specialties Centre
Chennai, Tamil Nadu, India

Vaibhav Deorari
Department of Neurosciences
Max Superspecialty Hospital
New Delhi, India

Vaidehi Mendpara
Internal Medicine Resident
Cleveland Clinic Foundation
Cleveland, USA

Varinder S Bedi
Institute of Vascular and Endovascular Sciences
Sir Ganga Ram Hospital
New Delhi, India

Veenaa Manjari S
Consultant Nephrologist
Medway Hospitals
Chennai, Tamil Nadu, India

Vidit Bhatia
Hamdard Institute of Medical Sciences
and Research
New Delhi, India

Vidyut Jain
Cardiologist
Choithram Hospital and Research Centre
Indore, Madhya Pradesh, India

Vijayadithyan Jaganathan
Internal Medicine Resident
University of Nevada
Reno, Nevada, USA

Vikash Kumar Maurya
Department of Cardiology
Institute of Medical Sciences
Banaras Hindu University
Varanasi, Uttar Pradesh, India

Vineet Behera
Consultant Nephrologist and
Professor (Medicine)
Armed Forces Medical College
Pune, Maharashtra, India

Vineet Bhatia
Director
Department of Cardiology
Medanta Hospital
Noida, Uttar Pradesh, India

Vinit Suri
Senior Consultant
Neurologist and Academic Coordinator
Indraprastha Apollo Hospital
New Delhi, India

Vinod Mittal
Senior Consultant Diabetologist
and Head
Centre for Diabetes and Metabolic Diseases
Delhi Heart and Lung Institute
New Delhi, India

Vinod Sharma
Senior Consultant Cardiologist
National Heart Institute
New Delhi, India

Vinus Taneja
Consultant
Department of Internal Medicine
Sir Ganga Ram Hospital
New Delhi, India

Vipin Kumar
Senior Consultant
Interventional Cardiologist
Ruban Memorial Hospital
Patna, Bihar, India

Vitull K Gupta
Health and Human Rights Activist
Consultant
Department of Medicine
Kishori Ram Hospital and
Diabetes Care Centre
Bathinda, Punjab, India
Chairman, API (Malwa Branch)
President, LAI (Punjab Chapter)
Chairman, CCDSI (Punjab)

Vivek Tandon
Director and In-charge
Noninvasive Cardiac Laboratory
Max Smart Super Specialty Hospital
New Delhi, India

Viveka Kumar
Principal Director and Chief of Cath Lab
Max Super Specialty Hospital
New Delhi, India

Vivudh Pratap Singh
Senior Consultant (Interventional Cardiology)
Fortis Escorts Heart Institute
New Delhi, India

VK Katyal
Medical Director
Positron Super Specialty and
Cancer Hospital
Rohtak, Haryana, India

Wael Al Mahmeed
Consultant Cardiologist
Heart Vascular and Thoracic Institute
Cleveland Clinic
Abu Dhabi, UAE

Wissam I Khalife
Department of Cardiovascular Medicine
University of Texas Medical Branch
Galveston, TX, USA

Yaser Ahmad
Internal Medicine Resident
University of Alabama Birmingham
Birmingham, Alabama, USA

Yashendu Sarda
Assistant Professor
Department of Nephrology
Sanjay Gandhi Postgraduate Institute
of Medical Sciences
Lucknow, Uttar Pradesh, India

Yugal K Mishra
Chief of Clinical Services
Chairman Manipal Institute
of Cardiac Sciences
Chief Cardiovascular Surgeon
Manipal Hospitals
New Delhi, India

Zakia A Khan
Senior Interventional Cardiologist
Fortis Hospital
Thane, Maharashtra, India

Foreword

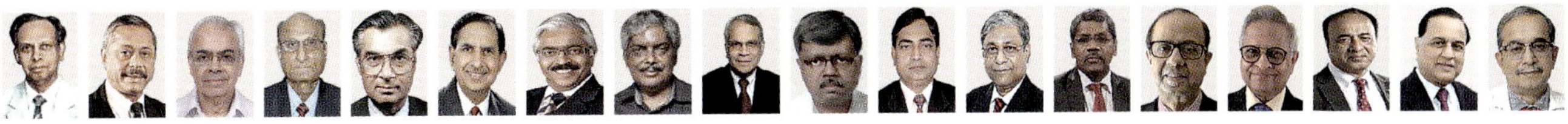

We are honored and have a great pleasure to write the Foreword for the state-of-art *Advances in Obesity and Lipid Management in CVD (Cutting Edge Strategies by Multispeciality Lens): A Textbook of Cardiology*. The textbook was long due considering the wealth of data, new strategies of management, and advances in diagnostic, prognostic, and therapeutic technology based in clinical practice.

It is one of the most needed, comprehensive, illustrative, well-structured books, published with enormous information about advances in clinical approach, imaging including advances in management of obesity-inflicted morbidity and mortality such as cardiovascular disease (CVD), chronic kidney disease (CKD), diabetes mellitus (DM), heart failure (HF) and cardiometabolic modulation by glucagon-like peptide-1 receptor agonist (GLP-1RA) such as semaglutide and tirzepatide and lipid management with statins, ezetimibe, bempedoic acid, PCSK9i, inclisiran apheresis, and gene therapy. The efficacy of drug therapy guided by biomarkers, echocardiography, and multimodality imaging is very well explained.

The book is an excellent and outstanding educational initiative by the joint efforts of 14 Editors-in-Chief, 60 National Principal Editors, 21 International Editors, 196 National Editors, and over 300 contributing authors. This book comprises 23 sections, including Clinical, Obesity and Diagnostic Markers, Obesity and Heart Failure, Obesity and Coronary Artery Disease, Obesity and Hypertension, Obesity with Diabetes, Obesity Cardiomyopathy with Heart Failure, Obesity with Arrhythmia, Obesity and Cardiolipidology, Obesity with Aortic Disease, Obesity with Stroke, Obesity and Kidney, Obesity and Sexual Dysfunction, Obesity and Women, Obesity, Heart Failure and Echocardiography, Obesity and Intensive Care Unit, Cardio-ophthalmology, Obesity, HFpEF, Cardio-ENT, and Cardiopulmonary Disease, Obesity, HFpEF and Pediatrics, Obesity, HFpEF and Cardio-oncology, Obesity and Therapeutics, Nonstatin Therapy and Dyslipidemia, and Future Directions and 172 chapters.

The chapters are well outlined, structured, well written, and referenced. The writing style of every chapter is vivid, concise, and practical. There are excellent graphics, tables, figures, and algorithms that present the relevant information. The printing and binding are of excellent quality. This book will represent a milestone for obesity and lipid management including advances in management of obesity-inflicted morbidity and mortality such as CVD, CKD, DM, HF, and cardiometabolic modulation by GLP-1RA such as Semaglutide and Tirzepatide and lipid management with statins, ezetimibe, bempedoic acid, PCSK9i, inclisiran apheresis, and gene therapy.

We congratulate the Chief Editors, Dr HK Chopra, Dr Navin C Nanda, Dr Jagat Narula, Dr GS Wander, Dr Sarita Bajaj, Dr Satyendra Tewari, Dr Praveen Chandra, Dr Viveka Kumar, Dr Tiny Nair, Dr CK Ponde, Dr Dinesh Khullar, Dr JPS Sawhney, Dr AK Pancholia, Dr S Shanmugasundaram, Principal Editors, International and National Editors, and all the contributors for accomplishing this prodigious achievement of great clinical relevance in cardiology practice of cardiometabolic approach today by meticulous obesity and lipid management.

M Khalilullah
Director and Senior Consultant Cardiologist
The Heart Centre
New Delhi, India
Past President, National CSI

Naresh Trehan
Chairman and Managing Director
Medanta—The Medicity
Gurugram, Haryana, India

SC Manchanda
Senior Consultant
Department of Cardiology
Dharma Vira Heart Center
Sir Ganga Ram Hospital
New Delhi, India

SK Parashar
Senior Consultant Cardiologist
The Heart Centre
New Delhi, India
Past President, CSI, IAE

DB Pahlajani
Head, Department of Interventional Cardiology
Breach Candy Hospital Research Centre
Mumbai, Maharashtra, India
Past President, CSI

Kamal K Sethi
Chairman and Managing Director
Director of Cardiology
Delhi Heart and Lung Institute
New Delhi, India
Past President, CSI

Ashok Seth
Chairman
Fortis Escorts Heart Institute
New Delhi, India
President, APSIC
Past President, National CSI

PK Deb
Former Chief, Cardiologist
ESI PG Institute of Medical Sciences
Kolkata, West Bengal, India
Past President, National CSI

C Venkata S Ram
Director, Apollo Institute for Blood Pressure Management
World Hypertension League/ South Asia Office, Apollo Hospitals
Hyderabad, Telangana, India
Texas Blood Pressure Institute
Dallas, Texas, USA

Santanu Guha
Professor and Head
Department of Cardiology
Medical College
Kolkata, West Bengal, India
Past President, National CSI

KC Goswami
Former Professor
Department of Cardiology
All India Institute of Medical Sciences
New Delhi, India
Past President, National CSI

MK Das
Senior Consultant and Interventional Cardiologist
CK Birla Hospital
Kolkata, West Bengal, India
Past President, National CSI

PP Mohanan
Director and Head
Department of Cardiology
Westfort Hi-Tech Hospital
Thrissur, Kerala, India
Past President, National CSI

Partha Sarathi Banerjee
Senior Consultant
Interventional Cardiologist
Columbia Asia Hospital
Kolkata, West Bengal, India
Past President, National CSI

Vijay Bang
Senior Interventional Cardiologist
Lilavati Hospital and Research Centre
Mumbai, Maharashtra, India
Past President, National CSI

PC Rath
Senior Consultant Cardiologist and Head
Department of Cardiology
Apollo Hospitals
Hyderabad, Telangana, India
Past President, National CSI

Sanjay Tyagi
Senior Consultant Cardiologist and Clinical Lead
Department of Cardiology
Apollo Hospitals Group
Northern Region
Immediate President
National CSI

Dhiman Kahali
Director, Interventional Cardiology
BM Birla Heart Hospital
Kolkata, West Bengal, India
President, CSI

Preface

A healthy Nation is the strongest foundation of progress. When science, policy, and clinical wisdom unite, they possess the power to reshape destinies, not only of individuals, but also of entire populations.

Aligned with the global vision of this textbook, "A healthy Heart is an expression of controlled Obesity and Controlled lipids", *Advances in Obesity and Lipid Management in CVD (Cutting Edge Strategies by Multispeciality Lens): A Textbook of Cardiology* represents a united commitment to address one of the most pressing health challenges of our time. Obesity and dyslipidemia are no longer isolated clinical entities; they are determinants of cardiovascular health, influencing disease onset, progression, and outcomes across the entire cardiometabolic spectrum.

Today, these conditions profoundly shape the landscape of cardiovascular medicine, spanning atherosclerosis, coronary artery disease, hypertension, arrhythmias, vascular disorders, and stroke, to heart failure, particularly HFpEF, and multiorgan complications, including renal, neurological, and metabolic diseases. As India advances toward a healthier and stronger future, it becomes imperative to understand these conditions not only scientifically but also contextually, addressing their impact across diverse populations and healthcare environments.

This textbook brings together an exceptional consortium of leading experts from India and across the globe to explore obesity and lipid disorders through a comprehensive, multidisciplinary, and clinically pragmatic lens. It examines the epidemiology, evolving definitions, global guidelines, and real-world practice frameworks from major cardiovascular and endocrine societies while thoughtfully contextualizing them for Indian and Asian populations, where unique genetic, metabolic, lifestyle, and healthcare factors shape disease expression and therapeutic outcomes through a multidisciplinary approach.

Moving from scientific insight to clinical application, the book delves deeply into mechanisms such as inflammation, neurohormonal dysregulation, endothelial dysfunction, adipose biology, metabolic remodeling, and their influence on cardiac structure and function. It addresses the broad clinical spectrum, highlighting obesity's intricate associations with cardiomyopathy, HFpEF, coronary artery disease, arrhythmias, vascular and cerebrovascular disorders, renal dysfunction, women's cardiovascular health, pediatric risks, critical care complexities, and neurocardiometabolic intersections.

One of the great strengths of this volume lies in its focus on diagnostic innovation and therapeutic advancement. It presents contemporary clinical evidence and real-world insights into transformative pharmacotherapies, including SGLT2 inhibitors such as Empagliflozin and Dapagliflozin, GLP-1 receptor agonists such as semaglutide encompassing trials including STEP 1–8, STEP HFpEF with and without diabetes mellitus, STEP TEEN, STEP-UP, SUSTAIN 6, SOUL, SELECT, SCORE and STEER, demonstrating mortality and morbidity benefits, in addition to weight reduction, diabetes control, and cardiovascular benefits, dual GIP–GLP-1 agonists such as tirzepatide with the SURPASS and SURMOUNT programs showing weight reduction, diabetes control and cardiometabolic benefits, with cardiovascular outcomes trial (CVOT) data awaited and new and emerging metabolic agents. Cardiorenometabolic benefits are evaluated using adipokines such as leptin and adiponectin; inflammatory markers such as C-reactive protein (CRP) and interleukin-6 (IL-6); echocardiography and multimodality imaging, including CT, MRI, and nuclear techniques; and artificial intelligence-based applications. Bariatric strategies, lifestyle interventions, cardionutrition, and cardiac rehabilitation are also addressed, thereby enhancing translational value and clinical applicability.

Equally important is the inclusivity reflected in this work. Women's health across the lifespan, elderly and pediatric populations, high-risk groups, oncology patients, individuals with multiple comorbidities, and vulnerable clinical subsets are all meaningfully addressed. Paradoxes, controversies, registries, real-world experiences, and future research directions enrich scientific discourse and stimulate continued inquiry.

As the burden of cardiometabolic disease continues to rise, one truth becomes increasingly evident: Effective prevention and management of obesity and lipid disorders lie at the heart of cardiovascular protection. This book reflects India's resolve to lead through knowledge, innovation, and compassionate care, not only for our nation, but also for the global medical community.

This textbook is the result of dedicated scholarly collaboration, clinical wisdom, and academic commitment. I extend my deepest gratitude to every contributing author, reviewer, section editor, and coordinator whose expertise and devotion have shaped this comprehensive resource. Their collective efforts have created a work that is scientifically rigorous, clinically relevant, and deeply aligned with patient-centric care.

The contributors to this book have brought together their expertise and experience to create a resource rich in knowledge and practical insights. Their dedication and efforts have made this textbook a repository of information, tailored to meet the needs of clinicians, researchers, and healthcare professionals striving to optimize patient care.

Our sincere gratitude extends to all the contributors and editors whose unwavering dedication and expertise have culminated in the realization of this edition. Their commitment to advancing the realm of cardiology is commendable, setting an exemplary standard for forthcoming endeavors.

We earnestly hope that *Advances in Obesity and Lipid Management in CVD (Cutting Edge Strategies in Multispeciality Lens): A Textbook of Cardiology*, the first of its kind from India to the world, will serve as a catalyst for the progression and development of effective and innovative methodologies in managing obesity and lipid disorders, thereby contributing to the betterment of the lives of innumerable individuals globally.

We have made every possible effort to maintain the quality and standards of this book. We are confident that this book will serve as an important reference guide for postgraduate students, fellows, internists, cardiologists, endocrinologists, nephrologists, neurologists, critical care specialists, pulmonologists, oncologists, ophthalmologists, ENT experts, dermatologists, pediatricians, pediatric surgeons, cardiovascular surgeons, imaging experts, and nutritionists. Bringing forth *Advances in Obesity and Lipid Management in CVD (Cutting Edge Strategies by Multispeciality Lens): A Textbook of Cardiology* was a phenomenal task and required well-structured team efforts with immense dedication, devotion, and coordination.

We express our gratitude to all the eminent cardiologists, including Professor M Khalilullah, Dr Naresh Trehan, Professor SC Manchanda, Dr SK Parashar, Dr DB Pahlajani, Dr KK Sethi, Dr Ashok Seth, Dr PK Deb, Dr C Venkata S Ram, Dr Santanu Guha, Dr KC Goswami, Dr MK Das, Dr PP Mohanan, Dr Partha Sarathi Banerjee, Dr Vijay Bang, Dr PC Rath, Dr Sanjay Tyagi, and Dr Dhiman Kahali, for writing the foreword for this book.

We also express our thanks to each and every member of the Cardiological Society of India (CSI); all physicians from India and abroad; manuscript contributors; Dr Anu Grover, Director, Scientific Communication Mangrove Creations for structuring the manuscript; industry partners; and our National Principal Editors, International Editors, and all the National Editors for their constant support.

We further extend our thanks to M/s Jaypee Brothers Medical Publishers (P) Ltd, New Delhi, India, for publishing this book so effectively. We also thank Shri Jitendar P Vij (Group Chairman), Mr Ankit Vij (Managing Director), Ms Pooja Bhandari [Director—Production (Books and Journals)], Ms Nikita Chauhan (Publishing Manager), Mr Ashwani Kumar Singh (Senior Manager), Ms Seema Dogra (Cover Visualizer), Mr Ashwani Kumar (Quality Controller), Mr Rajkumar (InDesign Operator), and Mr Gopal Singh Kirola (Graphic Designer) for their help, guidance, and timely active intervention in composing, designing, and editing this book.

Our sincere thanks also go to Soban Singh, who worked tirelessly to maintain records of every minor and detailed communication.

"Obesity affects every aspect of people's lives, from health to relationships.
The time to act is now by lifestyle optimization and timely intervention with GLP1RA"

HK Chopra (India), Navin C Nanda (USA), Jagat Narula (USA)
GS Wander, Sarita Bajaj, Satyendra Tewari, Praveen Chandra (India)
Viveka Kumar, Tiny Nair, CK Ponde, Dinesh Khullar (India)
JPS Sawhney, AK Pancholia, S Shanmugasundaram (India)

Preface

Obesity is now considered a disease, and its association with atherosclerotic cardiovascular disease and diabetes mellitus is well known. Taking into account the newer definitions of obesity, which assess not only the body mass index but also anthropometric indices such as the waist to hip ratio, the prevalence of obesity in the general population is very high, with over 70% being reported in a recent study from the United States. Obesity has been difficult and frustrating to treat because standard regimens such as recommended diets are difficult to follow for prolonged periods. However, as described in detail in this unique and comprehensive textbook primarily edited by none other than the eminent *Dr HK Chopra*, recently introduced medications together with lifestyle modifications show promise in revolutionizing the management of obesity, which has reached an epidemic proportion. These include glucagon-like peptide-1 (GLP-1) receptor agonists, dual receptor agonists (GLP-1 RAs), triple agonists as well as medications with non-GLP mechanisms. These medications result in profound and rapid weight loss by curbing appetite and increasing satiety in addition to other mechanisms and represent a most welcome game changer in the treatment of obesity.

The second component of the book deals with dyslipidemias, which are a major factor in the causation of atherosclerotic cardiovascular disease, especially in more vulnerable populations such as Asian Indians living in India as well as the Indian diaspora abroad. Some factors such as increased levels of highly atherogenic small, dense, low-density lipoprotein levels in Asian Indians living in the United States compared with the White ethnic group were demonstrated many years ago by the Kulkarni–Nanda group. The book also covers, among many other aspects, the more recently emphasized importance of assessing serum lipoprotein (a) and Apo lipoprotein B levels. Thus, this book provides an up-to-date knowledge of both these subjects.

This most impressive textbook consists of a vast number of 172 chapters written by a huge number of authors who are experts in their respective fields. The first part of the book deals with Advances in Obesity Management and includes a section on clinical perspectives with individual chapters on obesity definition, obesity association with cardiovascular disease, diabetes mellitus, dyslipidemia, autoimmunity, cardiometabolic risk, genetics, and guidelines and management strategies. The other sections deal with obesity and diagnostic markers, obesity and heart failure, obesity and coronary artery disease, obesity and hypertension, obesity with diabetes, obesity cardiomyopathy with heart failure, obesity with arrhythmias, obesity and cardiolipidology, obesity with stroke, obesity and kidney, obesity and sexual dysfunction, obesity and women, obesity, heart failure and echocardiography, obesity and intensive care unit, cardio-ophthalmology, obesity and cardiopulmonary disease, obesity and pediatrics, obesity and cardio-oncology, and last but not the least obesity and therapeutics which has the largest number of chapters.

The second part of the book deals with Advances in Lipid Management in Cardiovascular Disease. This consists of two sections titled Nonstatin Therapy and Dyslipidemia, and Future Directions.

Another unique feature of the book would be its impact on a huge number of medical as well as paramedical professionals because many of them deal with obesity and dyslipidemias in their day-to-day clinical practice.

Dr HK Chopra who is very well known in India for his vast experience and expertise in all aspects of clinical cardiology is also an author of several cardiology textbooks and is highly sought after as a speaker by many scientific institutions as well as public media and forums. He deserves all kudos for putting together this amazing and most useful textbook.

Navin C Nanda (USA)

Preface

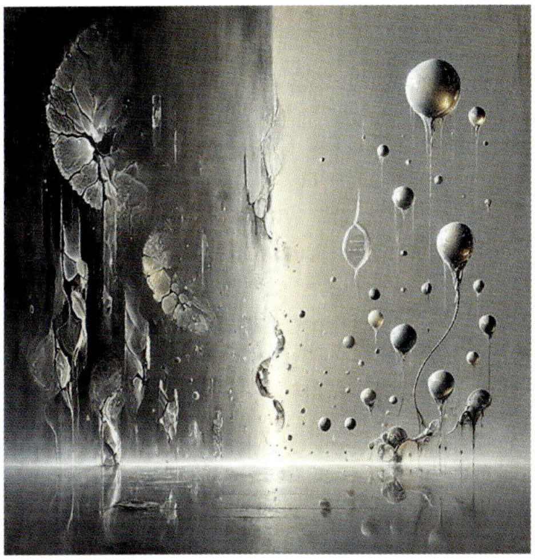

Management of Obesity and Lipid Disorders: Homeostasis Rising?

Historically and traditionally, but not inappropriately, we have trained at the targets after the pathology has set in. Some common examples include finding a way to restricting calories after the waist girth has increased uncontrollably or hepatocytes have been denuded of low-density lipoprotein (LDL) receptors. Similarities with other chronic diseases may include obvious hypertension, neurohumoral upregulation in heart failure, or revascularization in acute and chronic coronary syndromes. Modern medicine is likely to go more preemptive, respect physiology, and establish homeostasis. Could we prevent LDL receptor downregulation by nipping PCSK9 in the endoplasmic reticulum on a long-term basis? Could we reset the gut–brain axis to balance hunger, satiety, and energy expenditure? Could we contain neurohumoral modulation before overt heart failure or hypertension? An emerging and burgeoning field of ribonucleic acid (RNA) therapeutics is the most attractive and cost-effective step in this direction. Of course, gene editing would eventually become the destination for *raising homeostasis*!

Obesity: From Weight Loss to Adiposity Biology as a Treatable Disease

A middle-aged patient with lifelong *yo-yo dieting* frustratingly claims—"My body fights me, and it is not my willpower failure." It is *physiology*—when the hunger pangs rise, satiety sensation falls, and energy expenditure dwindles after dieting. Understanding it better, we have witnessed a conceptual shift that obesity is a *chronic, relapsing neuroendocrine disease* with *defended body-weight set point* (hypothalamic and brainstem circuits), *peripheral mediators* (GLP-1, GIP, glucagon, amylin, etc.), *adipose organ dysfunction* (inflammation, fibrosis, ectopic fat, altered adipokines), and *cardiometabolic complications* (MASLD-MASH, HFpEF, CKD, OSA, T2D). The concept justifies *long-term pharmacotherapy* and combination approaches, like we do for other chronic diseases such as hypertension. New therapeutic strategies work largely by *dialing down appetite and food noise* and changing what the brain perceives as *normal.*

The incretin era is evolving to be multihormonal. GLP-1 receptor agonists (such as semaglutide) are targeting cardiometabolic remodeling beyond glycemia quite like *medical bariatrics,* as one of our patients describes—"It's like someone turned off the constant background craving." And, it is indeed consistent with central appetite circuit modulation as a mesolimbic reward plus hypothalamic satiety integration, not just stomach slowing. Dual agonism, GLP-1 and GIP (such as tirzepatide) as a synergistic approach to satiety, has pushed weight loss even further. We still struggle to understand as to how GIP signaling in brain and adipose interacts with GLP-1 effects, especially since GIP alone could be obesogenic but might become favorable when co-activated. Could we consider GLP-1 as *reduce hunger drive plus slow intake* and GIP as *reshape nutrient handling and modulate reward to satiety circuits.* Together, they inflict a *behavioral rewrite.* Addition of glucagon as a triple agonist strategy could be a *metabolic amplifier,* the philosophy being *eat less* (i.e., a neuroendocrine effect) and *burn more or partition more efficiently* (i.e., hepatic and adipose thermogenesis effect).

And then, amylin is back to target satiety through a different mechanism. It is co-secreted with insulin and acts on the area postrema and hindbrain circuits to reduce meal size and slow gastric emptying, but for a patient the feel is totally different than for semaglutide.

So, if we added all drugs and created an approach quite like that of hypertension or heart failure management, the combination therapy would have different targets working in concert. The triple pathway would take care of food noise and appetite; amylin will influence meal termination or portion size. They all would add up in face of improved tolerability possibly as we might need lower doses of many medications. Imagine a patient claiming, "I stop halfway through and feel done—like never before." There is yet another group of thought leaders that believe in combination through *stepwise precision escalation*. The precision could be driven by *phenotype guidance*; for example, subjects reporting substantial hyperphagia or binge-like symptoms would receive central satiety agents with consideration of an amylin-pathway drug to restrict meal size. If a patient suffers from visceral adiposity and fatty liver, the agents best suited are those with effects on hepatic fat and insulin resistance. And patients presenting with obesity with heart failure with preserved ejection fraction (HFpEF) would deserve a focus not only on weight loss and cardiometabolic remodeling but also on volume status, renal function, and functional capacity. The newer drugs have radically shifted the fulcrum of management as the success of management would be increasingly judged by organ outcomes, not just loss of pounds from around the waist. The primary endpoints would be metabolic dysfunction-associated liver disease, obstructive sleep apnea, HFpEF, and chronic kidney disease. Hence, we must cater to liver fat and inflammation to fibrosis pathways (steatohepatitis biology including reduction in hepatic de novo lipogenesis and ectopic triglyceride with downstream inflammatory signaling and insulin resistance), sleep apnea severity (weight loss helps, but evaluate airway anatomy and neuromuscular tone), cardiac remodeling (diastolic function, LV mass, epicardial fat), and renal hemodynamics and albuminuria. There is one word of caution here. We must ensure muscle mass and quality weight loss as a first-class goal. We need to preserve lean mass and strength and avoid frailty, sarcopenia, or functional decline, especially in older adults, incorporate more protein targets (distributed across meals), and encourage progressive resistance-training prescriptions. An interest in anabolic-sparing adjuncts is being explored. If patients lose weight rather quickly and reports weakness, we must not stop treatment, but tweak rate of loss, increase resistance training, optimize protein, reassess micronutrients, and monitor function.

Does surgery have any role left? Beyond classic bariatric surgery, endoscopic bariatric therapies (e.g., sleeve gastroplasty) that reduce gastric volume without incisions and revisional and metabolic procedures tailored to reflux risk, diabetes severity, and anatomy will continue to have a limited role to play in patients' severe challenges. The surgical interventions would be more inclusive of bridging strategies, i.e., procedure and medication rather than procedure *or* medication, as a patient would use medication to lose 10–15% before surgery to reduce operative risk and then would continue medical therapy postoperation to defend the new set point. This "hybrid chronic care" model is going to become increasingly common, as we agree that the procedures alter way beyond restricting food or calories and may work through influencing bile acid, incretin, vagal tone, microbiome, and nutrient sensing to comprehensively reset appetite and glucose regulation.

Obesity management has shifted from calorie arithmetic to neuroendocrine set-point engineering, using multihormone pharmacology, procedure–drug combinations, and complication-focused endpoints while newly prioritizing lean mass, function, and organ health. It is moving toward mapping human appetite neurocircuitry with better imaging and neurobehavioral endpoints, understanding adipose organ as an immune-metabolic organ (comprising macrophage polarization and fibrosis), and equally importantly targeted gut microbiome interventions (unlike generic probiotics and based on signal molecules, bile acids, engineered strains). This is exactly where the obesity management field is likely to move, and this book is a primer for our readers who wait for our ADVANCES series year after year.

Dyslipidemias: Imagining Paradigmatic Shifts

Broadly, LDL and statin therapy remain the fulcrum of the management of lipid disorders. Drugs such as ezetimibe and bempedoic acid complement statin regimens (poststatin toolkit). However, manipulation of LDL has advanced to a stage that we are able to achieve the LDL levels that we were born with and must decide to take the same levels to grave with us. The magic number would fall between 25 and 30 mg/dL and would likely confront most chronic diseases like never before. These newer therapeutic interventions work through PCSK9 platform, be it antibodies, siRNA, and (emerging) oral approaches. PCSK9 regulates LDL receptor recycling, and inhibiting it increases hepatic LDL receptor density, accelerating clearance of apoB particles. The patients with premature ASCVD keep forgetting pills, and instead of labeling them noncompliant, we could now switch the model to infrequent dosing; LDL becomes predictable, and adherence becomes a *workflow* rather than a personality trait.

There is an increasing trend to focus beyond LDL cholesterol on apoB or non-HDL-C as the *best single summary* of atherogenic particle burden, especially when triglycerides are elevated or metabolic syndrome is present. It is so because atherosclerosis tracks better with the number of apoB-containing particles [LDL, VLDL remnants, Lp(a)] than with LDL cholesterol content per particle. Small cholesterol-poor particles can yield normal LDL-C but high apoB. Should we not be alarmed when we encounter a middle-aged man with central adiposity and prediabetes and LDL cholesterol of 82 who was reassured—until apoB returned at 118. Treating the particle burden, not just LDL cholesterol, and targeting remnant cholesterol and insulin resistance become even more attractive as elevated lipoprotein is going to be actionable. Lp(a) is an LDL with a tail of apo(a) with kringle repeats that are linked to pro-atherogenic effects (apoB particle), pro-inflammatory signaling, pro-thrombotic milieu, and pro-calcific biology. High Lp(a) may carry a hidden risk in genetically programmed particles—that LDL cholesterol would not reveal. It warrants earlier and more aggressive LDL lowering, tighter control of other risk factors, and consideration of therapies that lower Lp(a) modestly (such as nicotinic acid), while dedicated RNA-based therapeutics are in late stages of development.

The importance of triglycerides and remnants, even though less frequent, remains substantial as residual risk after LDL correction. Hypertriglyceridemia and the remnant cholesterol (cholesterol in triglyceride-rich lipoproteins) as causal in atherosclerosis are often a marker of insulin resistance and hepatic overproduction of VLDL, impaired lipolysis (LPL axis), alcohol, hypothyroidism, kidney disease, and genetic dyslipidemias. It is becoming important to focus on apoB and remnants, not just triglyceride number, and treat metabolic drivers (weight, glycemia, MASLD) because VLDL biology is upstream. It is important to recognize that TG 600 is not just TG 600, such as two patients may have TG 600 mg/dL, associated with either (patient A) uncontrolled diabetes and fatty liver (VLDL overproduction) or (patient B) genetic chylomicronemia physiology (LPL pathway failure). Same triglyceride value, different particle types, different pancreatitis risks, and very different therapeutic targets.

Emerging genetic and mechanistic exploration behooves us to deliberately step away from LDL cholesterol and TG numbers and treat dyslipidemia as a problem of particle flux, remodeling, and clearance across atherogenic and pancreatitis pathways. If we think of plasma lipoproteins as a circulating particle ecosystem, *what drives events may not necessarily be how much cholesterol is inside particles,* but *how many apoB particles are in circulation* (atherosclerotic particle burden), *what kind of apoB particles they are* (LDL vs. remnant-rich, cholesterol-poor vs. cholesterol-rich), *how long they circulate* (residence time, endothelial exposure), *how efficiently triglyceride-rich particles are lipolyzed and cleared* (LPL axis), *how particles are remodeled* (CETP axis, hepatic lipase, exchange of core lipids), and *which mediators gate these processes* (PCSK9, apoC-III, ANGPTLs, inflammation, insulin resistance). Therefore, the management construct could roughly become *particle number* × *residence time* × *atherogenicity,* modulated by *gates* (i.e., PCSK9, apoC-III, LPL, CETP).

Hypothetically, we could encapsulate the entire atherogenic dyslipidemia management paradigm as below in four steps:

Step 1: Replace lipid panels with particle-centric vital signs. The *core metrics* (the new ABCs) could include *ApoB* (*atherogenic particle count*: LDL + remnants + Lp(a)), *non–HDL particle surrogates* (non–HDL cholesterol still useful but secondary), *LDL-P/apoB discordance* (when LDL cholesterol lies), *remnant particle burden* (conceptually: VLDL/IDL remnants; clinically approximated by apoB + TG context and/or advanced lipoprotein testing if available), *ApoC-III level or apoC-III-rich lipoprotein signal* (where available), and *Lp(a) particle concentration* (separate genetic particle line). In addition, it would be important to define the *functional axes* (what is *wrong?*), such as the *clearance axis* (LDL receptor availability, i.e., PCSK9 gate), *lipolysis axis* (LPL pathway throughput, i.e., apoC-III/ANGPTL gates), *remodeling axis* (CETP-driven core lipid exchange and particle transformation), and *production axis* (hepatic VLDL-apoB secretion rate, i.e., insulin resistance, MDALD biology).

Step 2: Classification of four dyslipidemia phenotypes, instead of *hypercholesterolemia* versus *hypertriglyceridemia* segregation by *particle mechanics.*

Phenotype A: ApoB overload (high atherogenic particles)

- *Signature:* High apoB (could also be with discordantly acceptable LDL cholesterol)
- *Mechanism:* Increased apoB secretion and/or impaired LDLR clearance
- *Primary gate:* PCSK9–LDLR

Therapeutic construct should include:

- *First-line:* Maximize LDLR-mediated clearance, such as statin/ezetimibe that are *LDLR upregulators;* the paradigm here is not cholesterol—it is receptor density.
- Add PCSK9 inhibition, i.e., *residence time killer* for apoB particles.
- If persistent, newer therapies could be considered/developed that reduce apoB production flux, such as ApoB RNA therapeutics, especially in severe genetic phenotypes

Phenotype B: Remnant dominance (cholesterol-poor but highly atherogenic remnants)

- *Signature:* apoB elevated with high TG context, postprandial atherogenicity, metabolic syndrome
- *Mechanism:* Overproduction of VLDL-apoB plus delayed remnant clearance
- *Primary gates:* LPL throughput and apoC-III

Therapeutic construct could include:

- *Prioritize:* apoC-III suppression/LPL pathway derepression (conceptually, it is increasingly feasible as therapeutics mature)
- *Combine with:* LDLR clearance optimization (because remnants also clear via hepatic receptors)
- *Treat production drivers:* Insulin resistance, hepatic fat biology (which is the VLDL factory).

Phenotype C: Lipolysis failure/chylomicronemia spectrum (pancreatitis risk biology)

- *Signature:* Very high TG but the *event risk* is pancreatitis from chylomicrons
- *Mechanism:* Impaired LPL function or overinhibition (apoC-III high, ANGPTL up)
- *Primary gates:* LPL, apoC-III, ANGPTL3/4

Therapeutic construct could include:

- It is not about LDL; it is about restoring lipolytic throughput.
- *Target:* apoC-III and/or ANGPTL3 pathways, strict dietary fat control, and eliminate secondary inhibitors, such as alcohol and uncontrolled diabetes

Phenotype D: Remodeling pathology (CETP-driven particle reshaping)

- *Signature:* HDL cholesterol patterns, small dense LDL tendency, mixed dyslipidemia with insulin resistance
- *Mechanism:* CETP exchanges TG ↔ cholesteryl ester, reshaping particle composition and downstream catabolism
- *Primary gate:* CETP-mediated core lipid exchange

Therapeutic construct could include:

- CETP inhibition as *remodeling control* rather than *raising HDL cholesterol.*
- The goal is not pretty HDL; it is to *reduce atherogenic particle exposure* by altering particle kinetics and possibly apoB handling where the clinical benefit signal exists.

Step 3: The *Gates and Lever Model* and what to target. This could become the dominant basis of the new paradigm to treat dyslipidemia by manipulating *gates* or the mediators that control particle flow.

Gate 1: PCSK9, the LDLR gatekeeper, i.e., the clearance gate

- *Effect:* Determines LDLR density and controls apoB particle residence time.
- To be preferentially used when *apoB* is *high* or there exists premature ASCVD despite recommended LDL cholesterol levels or when adherence favors an infrequent dosing approach
- Think of it as a *turn-up hepatic particle vacuum power.*

Gate 2: ApoC-III, the LPL brake, and remnant clearance inhibitor, i.e., lipolysis or remnant gate

- *Effect:* Inhibits LPL-mediated TG hydrolysis and impairs hepatic uptake of remnants
- To be preferentially used when there is remnant dominance, hypertriglyceridemia spectrum, pancreatitis-prone physiology, i.e., metabolic remnant syndrome
- Think of it as a *release of the brake on lipolysis and remnant disposal.*

Gate 3: LPL, the throughput enzyme, i.e., the particle shredder for TG-rich lipoproteins

- *Effect:* Converts big TG-rich particles into remnants and facilitates clearance
- *Problem:* Increasing LPL without ensuring remnant clearance can theoretically shift risk from pancreatitis to atherogenesis if remnants accumulate. So *LPL must be paired with remnant clearance capacity.*
- Think of it as an *increase in processing capacity, but do not clog the exit.*

Gate 4: CETP, the remodeling engine, i.e., core lipid exchange

- *Effect:* Redistributes TG and cholesteryl ester between particles, influencing size, density, and clearance pathways
- The prospective value of CETP inhibition is not *HDL vanity*, but *changing particle kinetics and apoB behavior* that would reduce events.

Gate 5: Mediator layers of levers in lipid metabolism

- *ANGPTL3/4*: Physiologic inhibitors of LPL, i.e., a system-level throttle
- *Insulin resistance/hepatic fat*: Drives VLDL-apoB overproduction, i.e., production lever
- *Inflammation*: Modifies endothelial retention, oxidation susceptibility, and macrophage uptake, i.e., particle atherogenicity per unit apoB.

Step 4: A Practical Algorithm using the new construct

Step 4A—Identify and quantify the particle problem

- Measure *apoB* and Lp(a).
- Determine if it is primarily *ApoB overload* versus *remnant dominance* versus *lipolysis failure* versus *remodeling pathology*. It can be often inferred from apoB, clinical phenotype, and TG context by advanced lipoprotein testing.

Step 4B—Choose the dominant gate

- If *high apoB/ASCVD*, focus on *PCSK9–LDLR clearance gate* early.
- If *remnant dominance/metabolic syndrome*, focus on *apoC-III/LPL gate* and reduce production drivers.
- If *pancreatitis risk biology*, prioritize *LPL axis restoration*, i.e., apoC-III/ANGPTL strategies plus strict fat management.
- If *mixed small-dense patterns*, consider *remodeling axis (CETP)* where appropriate and fix production/clearance.

Step 4C—Treat particle targets, not lipid targets

- *Primary target: ApoB to a low-risk zone for the patient risk class*
- *Secondary targets: Remnant particle signal, apoC-III-mediated phenotype, Lp(a) independent risk*
- Exact numeric targets could vary by guideline recommendations, but in renewed paradigm, the *direction* is consistent, i.e., always maintaining lower apoB and shorter residence time.

How might the newer paradigm change therapeutic decisions?

- *LDL-C is fine, apoB is not:* A patient with family history and insulin resistance has LDL-C of 100 but apoB is high. An old approach would classify it as borderline. By particle-flux approach, this would be ApoB overload. We could directly target clearance, i.e., LDLR plus PCSK9 gate, because events track with particle number and exposure time.
- *TG fell, but remnants rose:* A patient's TG improves with lifestyle and better glycemia, but apoB stays high. Old approach would claim TG success. The particle-flux approach could have helped improve pancreatitis risk, but there is still an atherosclerotic particle burden. A shift to apoB and remnant clearance would need attention.
- *Pancreatitis phenotype:* In a patient with very high TG and recurrent pancreatitis, LDL cholesterol only focus is irrelevant in the acute frame. By particle-flux approach, this is lipolysis failure, and we must treat the LPL axis to remove brakes like apoC-III/ANGPTL signaling when feasible, with strict dietary fat strategy and prevent chylomicron accumulation.

Jagat Narula (USA)

The Editorial Board of

Advances in Obesity and Lipid Management in CVD

(Cutting Edge Strategies by Multispeciality Lens)

A Textbook of Cardiology

Express their gratitude and thanks to the following Academic Partners

Platinum Academic Partner

IPCA Laboratories Ltd.

Gold Academic Partners

Emcure Pharmaceutical Ltd.

JB Chemicals and Pharmaceuticals Ltd.

Silver Academic Partners

Merck Ltd.

Micro Labs Ltd.

Healthy Heart Society

Bronze Academic Partners

USV Pvt. Ltd.
Zydus Healthcare Ltd.
Three Dots Lifescience Pvt Ltd.
Lupin Ltd.
Cipla Ltd.
Eris Lifesciences Ltd.
KRBL Ltd.

Supporters

Zydus Lifesciences Ltd.
Intas Pharmaceuticals Ltd.
Nutrabuff Nutraceuticals
Mankind Pharma Ltd.
NATCO Pharma Ltd.
Bayer Pharmaceuticals Pvt. Ltd.
Apichem Healthcare
Optimal Pharmtech
United Drilling Tools Ltd.
Marico Ltd.

For rendering unrestricted education support which made this book possible in its current enhanced form as *"Global Education Initiative in Cardiology"*.

Contents

PART I

ADVANCES IN OBESITY MANAGEMENT

SECTION 1: CLINICAL

SECTION 2: OBESITY AND DIAGNOSTIC MARKERS

SECTION 3: OBESITY AND HEART FAILURE

SECTION 4: OBESITY AND CORONARY ARTERY DISEASE

SECTION 11: OBESITY WITH STROKE: CLINICAL INSIGHT AND MANAGEMENT

SECTION 12: OBESITY AND KIDNEY

SECTION 13: OBESITY AND SEXUAL DYSFUNCTION

SECTION 14: OBESITY AND WOMEN

SECTION 15: OBESITY, HEART FAILURE, AND ECHOCARDIOGRAPHY

SECTION 16: OBESITY AND INTENSIVE CARE UNIT

SECTION 17: CARDIO-OPHTHALMOLOGY

SECTION 18: OBESITY, HFpEF, CARDIO-ENT, AND CARDIOPULMONARY DISEASE

SECTION 19: OBESITY, HFpEF AND PEDIATRICS

SECTION 20: OBESITY, HFpEF AND CARDIO-ONCOLOGY

SECTION 21: OBESITY AND THERAPEUTICS

Obesity and Tirzepatide

Bempedoic Acid

Inclisiran and Dyslipidemia

PART I
Advances in Obesity Management

SECTION 1

Clinical

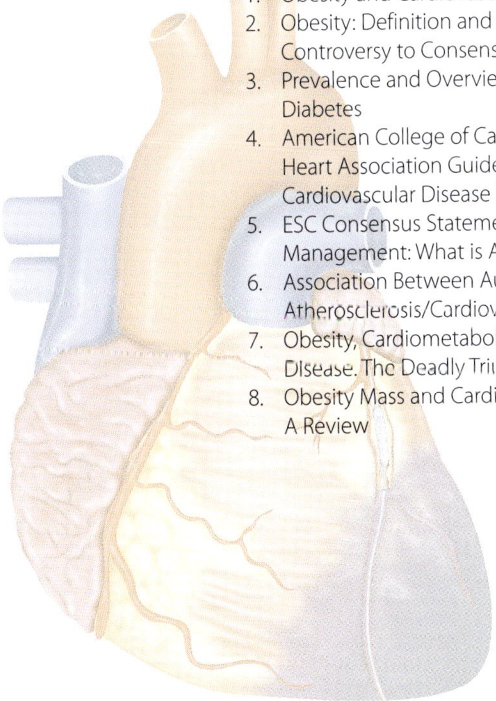

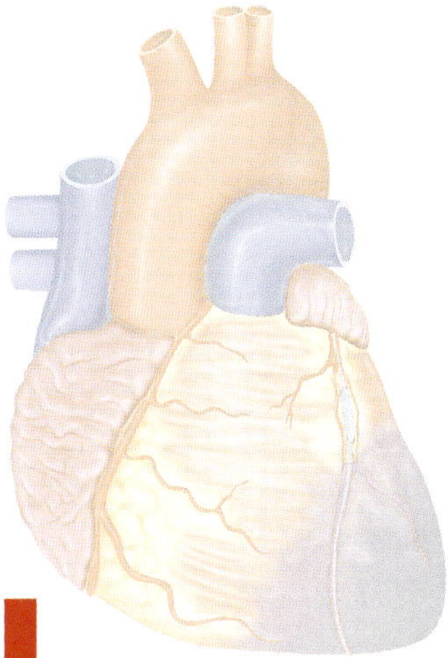

1

CHAPTER

Obesity and Cardiovascular Disease: An Overview

Abhishek Garg, Gurpreet Singh Wander

INTRODUCTION

Over the past two decades, obesity has emerged as a significant global public health concern, affecting both children and adults at an alarming rate. In India, findings from the ICMR-INDIAB study (phase I, 2015) indicated that obesity rates among adults varied widely across regions, ranging from 11.8 to 31.3%, and central obesity affected 16.9–36.3% of the population in different states.[1] More recent data from the National Family Health Survey-5 (2019–2021) demonstrated that approximately one in four women and one in five men aged 15 years and above were either overweight or obese [body mass index (BMI) ≥25 kg/m^2].[2] This rising trend has not only contributed to a reduction in overall life expectancy but has also been linked to increased rates of morbidity.[3]

The link between cardiovascular (CV) diseases and obesity has been widely documented and analyzed in numerous studies. Obesity is strongly implicated in the pathogenesis of a wide spectrum of CV conditions, including atherosclerosis, symptomatic coronary artery disease (CAD), heart failure (HF), and atrial fibrillation (AF). While obesity frequently leads to CV complications through the development of comorbid conditions such as hypertension, dyslipidemia, and type 2 diabetes mellitus (T2DM), it is now recognized that CV damage may also occur independently of these risk factors.[4]

Emerging evidence suggests that excessive adipose tissue can induce direct structural and functional changes in the myocardium, thereby contributing to CV pathology even in the absence of traditional risk factors.[5] However, paradoxically, obese individuals diagnosed with HF often demonstrate better survival outcomes compared to their nonobese counterparts—a phenomenon widely referred to as the "obesity paradox."[6-8] This paradoxical association has also been noted in post-percutaneous coronary interventions (PCI) outcome data.[9] In this chapter, we will review the effect of obesity on CV health.

MEASURES OF OBESITY

Obesity can be assessed using several anthropometric indices beyond just total body weight. The most widely used tool is the BMI, which calculates body weight in relation to height and serves as a general indicator of overweight and obesity. The Centers for Disease Control and Prevention (CDC) classifies weight categories based on specific BMI thresholds, as shown in **Table 1**.[10] In addition to BMI, waist circumference and waist-to-hip ratio (WHR) are also utilized to assess body fat distribution, especially central or abdominal obesity. Among these, waist circumference is considered a more accurate marker of visceral adiposity and demonstrates a stronger correlation with BMI compared to WHR.[11]

OBESITY AND CARDIOVASCULAR DISEASE RISK FACTORS

Hypertension

Excess body weight is a key contributor to elevated blood pressure and an increased risk of systemic hypertension, a significant factor in the development of CAD, HF, stroke, and AF.[12] According to the Framingham Heart Study,[13]

TABLE 1: Obesity threshold classification.

Category BMI (kg/m²)	*Europoid*	*Asian*
Healthy weight	18.5 to <25	18.5 to <23
Overweight	25 to <30	23 to <25
Obesity:	≥30	≥25
• Class 1	30 to <35	25 to <30
• Class 2	35 to <40	≥30
• Class 3 (Severe)	≥40	–
Additional anthropometric measures:		
Measure		*Threshold*
Waist circumference		*Women:* ≥35 in (Europoid), ≥31.5 in (South Asian, Chinese) *Men:* ≥40 in (Europoid), ≥35.5 in (South Asian, Chinese) *Japanese women:* ≥35.4 in *Japanese men:* ≥33.5 in
Waist-to-height ratio		≥0.50

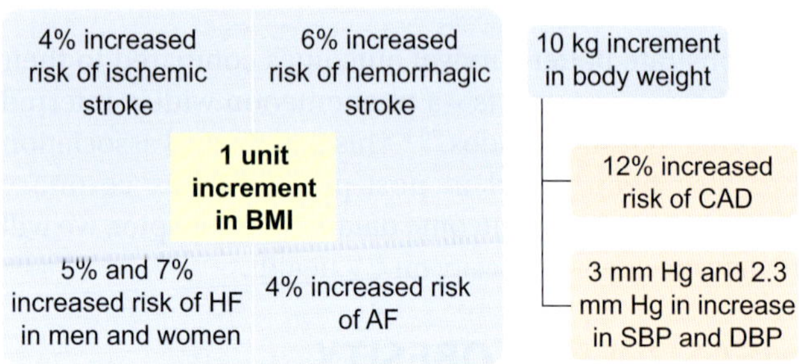

Fig. 1: Effect of weight gain on cardiovascular events.

over 30% of hypertension in men and >60% in women is linked to a BMI above 25 kg/m². Similarly, the Physician's Health Study reported an 8% increase in hypertension risk for each 1-unit rise in BMI.[14] Even a modest weight gain of over 5% in 8 years was strongly associated with an increased risk of hypertension in individuals with a normal BMI at baseline,[12] as shown in **Figure 1**.

Diabetes

Obesity is also closely tied to insulin resistance and metabolic syndrome, both of which elevate the risk for T2DM and cardiovascular disease (CVD).[12] A study from the Behavioral Risk Factor Surveillance System showed that every 1 kg increase in weight over 8 years raised the incidence of T2DM by 9%.[15] Metabolic syndrome, which includes abdominal obesity, atherogenic dyslipidemia (such as elevated triglycerides and low HDL cholesterol), hypertension, insulin resistance, and a pro-inflammatory state, more than doubles the risk of CAD, contributing to a 37% attributable risk in people over the age of 50.[15]

Dyslipidemia

The primary link between obesity and CAD risk is through metabolic syndrome and atherogenic dyslipidemia. Obese individuals may have normal low-density lipoprotein (LDL) cholesterol levels, but often possess smaller, denser LDL particles, which are more susceptible to oxidation and promote atherosclerosis.[12] Increased circulating free-fatty acids contribute to the formation of triglyceride-rich particles, especially very-low-density lipoproteins (VLDL), further elevating the levels of small, dense LDL particles. Beyond traditional risk factors, factors related to adiposity hormones and inflammatory cytokines (adipokines) also play a role in promoting a prothrombotic state and systemic inflammation in obesity.[12]

Elevated levels of IL-6, TNF-alpha, and C-reactive protein, along with low levels of adiponectin, heighten inflammation, fostering the development of atherosclerosis and increasing CV events.[12] Additionally, recent research has highlighted the role of lipotoxicity and fat infiltration into various organs in contributing to CVD, though these factors might also provide insights into the protective effects seen in the obesity paradox. Notably, epicardial adipose tissue and pericardial fat are now recognized as important risk factors for CV conditions, such as mortality, HF, and stroke, with regional fat distribution playing a critical role in these outcomes.[12]

OBESITY AND ATHEROSCLEROTIC DISEASE

Obesity and atherosclerosis share overlapping pathophysiological pathways, with lipid accumulation and chronic low-grade inflammation playing central roles.[16] The link between obesity and CAD can be explored in two clinical contexts: Its contribution to the development of atherosclerosis and chronic stable ischemic heart disease, and its impact on acute coronary syndromes (ACS) and outcomes after interventions. The Pathobiological Determinants of Atherosclerosis in Youth (PDAY) study[17] provided key insights by analyzing arterial changes in young individuals' postmortem, revealing that coronary atherosclerosis often begins early in life. A higher BMI is associated with more severe and complex atherosclerotic changes, such as fatty streak formation and plaque development. Other studies found that lesion complexity increased with subcutaneous fat thickness in individuals with a BMI over 30 kg/m^2.[17] Evidence from long-term cohort studies indicates that obesity must often be sustained for nearly two decades before it independently contributes to clinically significant CAD.[16] Furthermore, a weight increase of 10 kg has been linked to a 12% rise in CAD risk, along with concomitant increases in blood pressure.[18] Central obesity predicts poorer outcomes in patients with established CVD. Findings from the TRACE registry confirmed this association even after adjusting for common comorbidities such as diabetes and hypertension.[19] Furthermore, the INTERHEART study showed that waist-related measures—WHR, waist circumference, and waist-to-height ratio—were stronger predictors of myocardial infarction than BMI, emphasizing the dominant role of abdominal fat in CAD risk.[20]

Beyond its effects on the large coronary arteries, obesity also impacts the coronary microvasculature, which plays a vital role in regulating myocardial blood flow. Coronary microvascular dysfunction frequently occurs alongside obstructive or nonobstructive CAD, thereby worsening ischemia and adverse cardiac outcomes.[21] This dysfunction is closely related to endothelial impairment and may also involve structural changes in small vessels.[22] Higher BMI has been independently linked to microvascular disease, which itself serves as a predictor of increased CV risk in obese individuals. Importantly, prospective studies have shown that weight reduction, particularly through bariatric surgery, can lead to measurable improvements in coronary microvascular function.[21]

OBESITY AND ACUTE CARDIOVASCULAR SYNDROMES

Obesity significantly influences the risk and presentation of acute CV events, particularly in younger individuals. In a large cohort of over 100,000 patients with non-ST elevation myocardial infarction (NSTEMI), obesity emerged as the most prominent factor associated with NSTEMI in younger adults, followed by tobacco use. Notably, higher BMI was associated with a younger age of presentation, indicating an inverse relationship between BMI and age at onset of ACS.[22] This trend is similarly observed in patients with ST elevation myocardial infarction (STEMI),[23] and current evidence supports obesity as an independent risk factor for STEMI in the younger population. Beyond myocardial infarction, obesity is also associated with an elevated risk of acute cerebrovascular events. Each 1-unit rise in BMI increases the risk of ischemic stroke by 4% and hemorrhagic stroke by 6%.[16,18]

OBESITY AND PERCUTANEOUS CORONARY INTERVENTION OUTCOMES

Short-term Outcomes

Evidence from large registries highlights complex interactions between obesity and PCI outcomes. The Cath PCI Registry, which included more than 83,000 patients with severe obesity, demonstrated that obesity was independently linked to higher in-hospital mortality but paradoxically lower bleeding risk after adjustment for confounders.[24] Weight-based dosing protocols for anticoagulants such as unfractionated heparin pose challenges, as obese patients often require a prolonged time to achieve therapeutic anticoagulation.[21] Further registry analyses of over 227,000 patients showed that severe obesity was associated with increased risks of contrast-induced nephropathy, dialysis-requiring renal dysfunction, and vascular complications, particularly at femoral access sites, though gastrointestinal bleeding and major adverse cardiac events (MACE) were not significantly different.[25] Interestingly, data from the British Cardiovascular Intervention Society Registry indicated an "obesity paradox": Patients with BMI ≥25 kg/m^2 had lower 30-day mortality following PCI, and greater survival persisted up to 5 years, regardless of clinical presentation.[26] Similar findings from the APPROACH registry reinforced this paradox, as overweight and obese patients demonstrated lower 6-month mortality compared with normal-weight counterparts.[27]

Long-term Outcomes

In contrast, long-term follow-up reveals a more nuanced picture. Patients with lower BMI tend to experience more adverse events after PCI, while those with moderate obesity appear to have better outcomes. A pooled analysis of 23,000 patients from 11 prospective PCI trials found that individuals with very low BMI (<18.5 kg/m^2) had the highest risk of major CV events, whereas outcomes improved with higher BMI, particularly >30 kg/m^2.[28] A large meta-analysis involving >865,000 patients undergoing PCI or CABG confirmed a U-shaped association between BMI and all-cause mortality/MACE, with increased risk at both extremes of BMI.[29] However, this protective effect of obesity diminishes with severe obesity. Data from the APPROACH registry showed that patients with class 3 obesity and high-risk coronary anatomy had significantly worse long-term survival, with mortality rates higher at both 5 and 10 years compared to those with normal BMI.[27]

OBESITY AND HEART FAILURE

Despite advances in pharmacological and interventional therapies for HF, hospitalizations for acute decompensated HF continue to rise alongside the global obesity epidemic. In India, the prevalence of overweight and obesity has shown a rapid upward trend, with 23% of men and 24% of women aged 15 years and above as per NHFS-5. The link between obesity and HF is of growing clinical importance.[2] The association was first highlighted in 1956 through a case of morbid obesity-induced HF due to mechanical compression by excess adipose tissue.[16] Today, it is recognized that obesity contributes to HF through multiple mechanisms, including structural and functional myocardial changes. The concept of "obesity cardiomyopathy" was introduced in 1992, following a study of 519 patients, which demonstrated a higher prevalence of dilated cardiomyopathy among obese individuals based on right heart catheterization and myocardial biopsy findings.[16]

Evidence from large population studies has established obesity as an independent risk factor for HF. In a landmark analysis of 5,881 participants from the Framingham Heart Study, Kenchaiah et al.[30] found that each 1 kg/m^2 increase in BMI was associated with a 7% higher HF risk in women and 5% in men. Compared to individuals with normal BMI, the risk of developing HF was nearly twice as high in obese individuals, with hazard ratios of 2.17 for women and 1.90 for men.[30] This relationship remained significant even after adjusting for age, lifestyle factors, and comorbidities such as diabetes, hypertension, and prior myocardial infarction. Similarly, the Physician's Health Study, involving 21,094 men without known CAD, confirmed that both overweight and obesity were independently linked to increased HF incidence.[31]

Mechanism of Obesity-associated Heart Failure

Multiple mechanisms have been proposed to explain how obesity contributes to the development of HF, as shown in **Flowchart 1**. Obesity leads to hemodynamic alterations—including increased blood volume, cardiac output, and blood pressure—which over time can result

Flowchart 1: Interplay of various mechanisms of obesity that lead to heart failure.

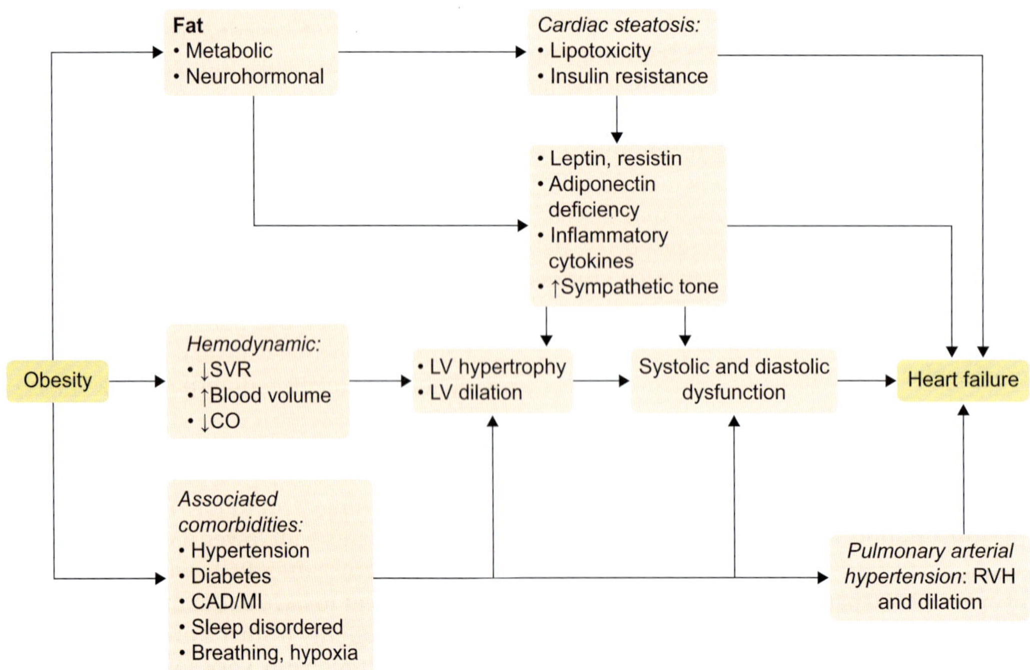

BOX 1: Obesity-induced hemodynamic effects and cardiovascular adaptations.

Hemodynamic and cardiac structural and functional adaptations associated with obesity:

- ↑ Intravascular blood volume
- ↑ Stroke volume
- ↑ Heart rate
- ↓ Heart rate variability
- ↑ Cardiac output
- ↑ Systemic vascular resistance
- ↑ Blood pressure
- ↑ Pulmonary artery systolic pressure
- ↑ Filling pressures in the left and right heart cavities
- LA enlargement
- LV dilatation
- LV hypertrophy (eccentric or concentric type)
- Abnormal LV diastolic filling

in left ventricular (LV) hypertrophy, systolic and diastolic dysfunction, and even right ventricular (RV) involvement, as shown in **Box 1**. Structural cardiac remodeling due to chronic volume and pressure overload is especially pronounced in individuals with severe obesity. This process, often referred to as "obesity cardiomyopathy," reflects the direct myocardial effects of adiposity.[16] While obesity-related HF with reduced ejection fraction is relatively uncommon and warrants evaluation for other causes, HF with preserved ejection fraction is significantly more prevalent in obese populations.

Moreover, the MESA study demonstrated that the obesity-HF relationship weakens after adjusting for inflammatory markers such as IL-6 and C-reactive protein, highlighting the central role of chronic inflammation in obesity-related HF pathogenesis.[32]

Obesity Paradox in Heart Failure

Although obesity is a well-established risk factor for developing HF, numerous studies have reported lower mortality among overweight and obese patients with established HF, a phenomenon termed the "obesity paradox."[6,7] One proposed explanation is that severe HF can lead to cardiac cachexia, a catabolic state causing weight loss.[7] However, newer data challenge this theory. A recent study showed that patients who were overweight or obese even before the onset of HF (premorbid obesity) had better long-term survival—up to 10 years—compared to normal-weight individuals, indicating that the obesity paradox extends beyond weight loss in advanced HF.[16]

An interesting aspect of the obesity paradox in HF is the observed inverse association between obesity and circulating levels of natriuretic peptides, particularly brain natriuretic peptide (BNP).[6,7] Multiple studies have confirmed that individuals with higher BMI, whether healthy or suffering from HF, tend to have lower BNP concentrations. A likely explanation is that increased adipose tissue leads to greater expression of natriuretic peptide clearance receptors (NPR-C), which enhances the peripheral removal of BNP. This mechanism, however, does not explain the simultaneous reduction of NT-proBNP, as this inactive fragment does not interact with NPR-C.[6,7]

OBESITY AND CORONARY CALCIUM SCORING

Coronary artery calcium (CAC) scoring is widely used as a marker to assess the burden of atherosclerosis.[33] Interestingly, the calcification seen in coronary arteries shares biological pathways with bone formation, involving similar cytokines, transcription factors, and cell types. While calcified plaques are often considered more stable, noncalcified plaques tend to be unstable and more likely to rupture.[33] Research has shown an inverse relationship between bone mineral density (BMD) and coronary calcification—individuals with higher BMD tend to have lower levels of CAC.[33] BMI plays a role here; increased body weight may exert mechanical stress that promotes higher bone density. In older adults (aged 60 and above), studies have found a linear association between BMI and BMD, with higher BMI linked to stronger bones.[33]

Supporting this, a large prospective study by Kovacic et al.[34] involving nearly 10,000 patients undergoing PCI revealed that higher BMI was independently associated with lower levels of coronary calcification. In contrast, older age, hypertension, diabetes, and peripheral vascular disease were linked to higher calcium levels. These findings raise the possibility that reduced CAC in obese individuals could partially explain the so-called obesity paradox,[33] where obese patients with CVD may sometimes experience better outcomes than leaner individuals.

OBESITY AND ATRIAL FIBRILLATION

Atrial fibrillation, one of the most prevalent arrhythmias globally, is significantly more common in obese individuals.[16] The Framingham Heart Study demonstrated that each 1-unit increase in BMI was associated with a 4% higher risk of developing AF, independent of other CV risk factors, myocardial infarction, or HF.[35] Compared to individuals with normal BMI, those with obesity had a 50% increased risk of AF. Similarly, findings from the Danish Diet, Cancer, and Health Cohort Study showed a positive association between AF risk and various anthropometric and body composition measures, including BMI, waist and hip circumference, total body fat, and even lean body mass.[16]

Mechanisms for Atrial Fibrillation with Obesity

The Framingham Heart Study identified left atrial (LA) enlargement as the primary mediator between obesity and increased AF risk. The greater the BMI, the larger the LA.[16] This dilation results from obesity-induced volume overload, elevated LV diastolic pressures, LV hypertrophy, and comorbidities such as hypertension, diabetes, and sleep apnea. In addition to structural changes, genetic factors may contribute. Variants such as the TaqIB polymorphism in the cholesteryl ester transfer protein gene and *CRP* gene polymorphisms have been linked to higher AF risk in obese men, as shown in **Figure 2.**[16]

Another important factor is epicardial adipose tissue (EAT). EAT thickness correlates with visceral adiposity and BMI and has been associated with higher AF burden. The Framingham study further demonstrated that pericardial fat volume independently predicts AF, beyond BMI or LA size,[36] suggesting EAT may play an active role in arrhythmogenesis.

Moreover, individuals with a lower BMI who experience a single episode of new-onset AF are less likely to transition to permanent AF compared to those with obesity. Evidence from the Australian LEGACY (Long-Term Effect of Goal-Directed Weight Management in an Atrial Fibrillation Cohort) trial further supports this, showing that sustained weight reduction markedly reduces AF recurrence.[36] In this trial, participants who achieved a weight loss of 10% or more had a six-fold higher likelihood of remaining free from AF over time.[37] Obese individuals are also at a markedly increased risk of developing comorbid conditions such as hypertension, T2DM, metabolic syndrome, CAD, and obstructive sleep apnea. These comorbidities, in turn, contribute to the increased incidence of AF seen in obese populations by promoting structural and electrophysiological remodeling of the atria.

OBESITY AND VENOUS THROMBOEMBOLISM

Numerous studies in recent years have consistently demonstrated a significant association between obesity and the development of venous thromboembolism (VTE). Observational data indicate that individuals with elevated BMI are two to three times more likely to experience VTE compared to those with normal weight profiles.[38] The risk is particularly amplified in those classified as morbidly obese (BMI >40 kg/m^2). A meta-analysis by Yang et al.,[39] which incorporated data from one cohort and eight case-control studies involving 8,125 VTE cases and 23,272 controls, revealed that individuals with obesity had over twice the odds of developing a first spontaneous VTE event compared to those with normal BMI (odds ratio: 2.33; 95% CI: 1.68–3.24). This analysis also highlighted the importance of fat distribution, especially visceral adiposity, as a key driver in the obesity-VTE link. Supporting this, Hanson et al.[33] followed 792 men for 26 years. They found that those with abdominal obesity (waist circumference >100 cm) had a significantly greater risk of VTE, even after accounting for other CV risk factors such as hypertension, diabetes, and stroke.[40] These findings support that individuals with higher levels of visceral fat are at substantially increased risk of developing thrombotic events.

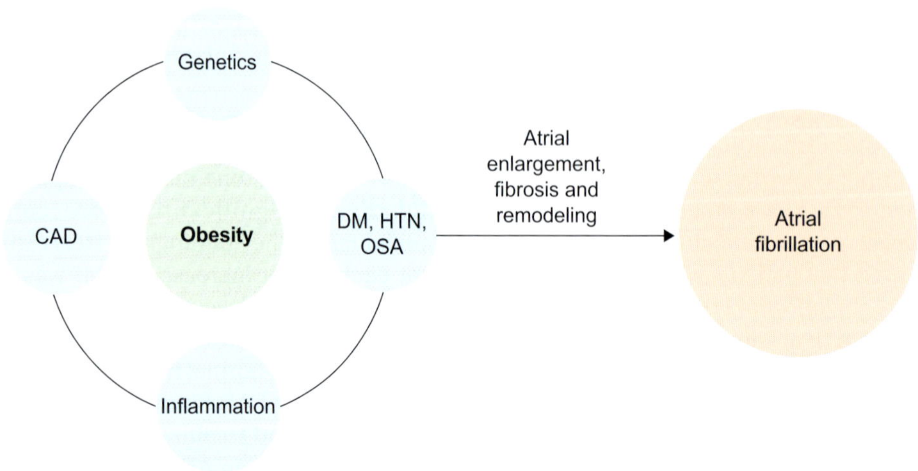

Fig. 2: Interplay mechanism of the development of AF in obesity.

MANAGEMENT

Management of obesity in CVD requires a multimodal approach. Lifestyle intervention remains foundational, but modern guidelines emphasize early integration of nutrient-stimulated hormone (NuSH) therapies such as GLP-1 and GIP/GLP-1 receptor agonists, which achieve substantial weight loss and reduce CV events. Bariatric surgery remains effective for select patients. Care is multidisciplinary, combining behavioral support, pharmacotherapy, and procedural strategies, with individualized goals.

CONCLUSION

Obesity is a well-established contributor to the pathogenesis of various CVDs. It serves not only as an independent risk factor but also as a risk marker for the onset and progression of CAD, HF, and AF. Excess adiposity promotes systemic inflammation, metabolic dysregulation, and structural cardiac changes that predispose individuals to both symptomatic and asymptomatic CV conditions. Emerging evidence also highlights the impact of weight loss in reducing CV risk, especially AF recurrence. Therefore, effective prevention and management of obesity are vital in reducing the growing burden of CVD worldwide.

REFERENCES

1. Pradeepa R, Anjana RM, Joshi SR, et al. Prevalence of generalized and abdominal obesity in urban and rural India: the ICMR-INDIAB study (phase I). Indian J Med Res. 2015;142(2):139-50.
2. International Institute for Population Sciences (IIPS), ICF. National Family Health Survey (NFHS-5), 2019-21: India Report. Mumbai: IIPS; 2021.
3. Fontaine KR, Redden DT, Wang C, et al. Years of life lost due to obesity. JAMA. 2003;289:187-93.
4. Poirier P, Giles TD, Bray GA, et al. Obesity and cardiovascular disease: pathophysiology, evaluation, and effect of weight loss. Circulation. 2006;113:898-918.
5. Poirier P, Martin J, Marceau P. Impact of bariatric surgery on cardiac structure, function and clinical manifestations in morbid obesity. Expert Rev Cardiovasc Ther. 2004;2:193-201.
6. Horwich TB, Fonarow GC, Hamilton MA, et al. The relationship between obesity and mortality in patients with heart failure. J Am Coll Cardiol. 2001;38:789-95.
7. Lavie CJ, Alpert MA, Arena R, et al. Impact of obesity and the obesity paradox on prevalence and prognosis in heart failure. JACC Heart Fail. 2013;1(2):93-102.
8. Shah RV, Gayat E, Januzzi JL Jr, et al. Body mass index and mortality in acutely decompensated heart failure across the world: a global obesity paradox. J Am Coll Cardiol. 2014;63:778-85.
9. Akin I, Nienaber CA. "Obesity paradox" in coronary artery disease. World J Cardiol. 2015;7(10):603-8.
10. Gilbert O, Gulati M, Gluckman TJ, et al. 2025 concise clinical guidance: an ACC expert consensus statement on medical weight management for optimization of cardiovascular health: a report of the American College of Cardiology Solution Set Oversight Committee. J Am Coll Cardiol. 2025;86(7):536-55.
11. Kurpad SS, Tandon H, Srinivasan K. Waist circumference correlates better with body mass index than waist-to-hip ratio in Asian Indians. Natl Med J India. 2003;16(4): 189-92.
12. Lavie CJ, Arena R, Alpert MA, et al. Management of cardiovascular diseases in patients with obesity. Nat Rev Cardiol. 2018;15(1):45-56.
13. Wilson PW, D'Agostino RB, Sullivan L, et al. Overweight and obesity as determinants of cardiovascular risk: the Framingham experience. Arch Intern Med. 2002;162(16):1867-72.
14. Gelber RP, Gaziano JM, Manson JE, et al. A prospective study of body mass index and the risk of developing hypertension in men. Am J Hypertens. 2007;20(4):370-7.
15. Mokdad AH, Ford ES, Bowman BA, et al. Diabetes trends in the US: 1990-1998. Diabetes Care. 2000;23:1278-83.
16. Mandviwala T, Khalid U, Deswal A. Obesity and cardiovascular disease: a risk factor or a risk marker? Curr Atheroscler Rep. 2016;18(5):21.
17. McGill HC Jr, McMahan CA, Herderick EE, et al. Obesity accelerates the progression of coronary atherosclerosis in young men. Circulation. 2002;105:2712-8.
18. Lau D, Dhillon B, Yan H, et al. Adipokines: molecular links between obesity and atherosclerosis. Am J Physiol Heart Circ Physiol. 2005;288:H2031-41.
19. Kragelund C, Hassager C, Hildebrandt P, et al. Impact of obesity on long-term prognosis following acute myocardial infarction. Int J Cardiol. 2005;98:123-31.
20. Yusuf S, Hawken S, Ounpuu S, et al. Effect of potentially modifiable risk factors associated with myocardial infarction in 52 countries (the INTERHEART study): case-control study. Lancet. 2004;364:937-52.
21. Powell-Wiley TM, Poirier P, Burke LE, et al. Obesity and cardiovascular disease: a scientific statement from the American Heart Association. Circulation. 2021;143(21):e984-1010.
22. Madala M, Franklin BA, Chen AY, et al. Obesity and age of first non-ST-segment elevation myocardial infarction. J Am Coll Cardiol. 2008;52:979-85.
23. Das SR, Alexander KP, Chen AY, et al. Impact of body weight and extreme obesity on the presentation, treatment, and in-hospital outcomes of 50,149 patients with ST-segment elevation myocardial infarction: results from the NCDR (National Cardiovascular Data). J Am Coll Cardiol. 2011;58(25):2642-50.
24. Payvar S, Kim S, Rao SV, et al. In-hospital outcomes of percutaneous coronary interventions in extremely obese and normal-weight patients: findings from the NCDR. J Am Coll Cardiol. 2013;62:692-6.

25. Buschur ME, Smith D, Share D, et al. The burgeoning epidemic of morbid obesity in patients undergoing percutaneous coronary intervention: insight from the Blue Cross Blue Shield of Michigan Cardiovascular Consortium. J Am Coll Cardiol. 2013;62:685-91.
26. Holroyd EW, Sirker A, Kwok CS, et al. The relationship of body mass index to percutaneous coronary intervention outcomes: does the obesity paradox exist in contemporary PCI cohorts? Insights from the British Cardiovascular Intervention Society Registry. JACC Cardiovasc Interv. 2017;10:1283-92.
27. Terada T, Forhan M, Norris CM, et al. Differences in short- and long-term mortality associated with BMI following coronary revascularization. J Am Heart Assoc. 2017;6:e005335.
28. Park DW, Kim YH, Yun SC, et al. Association of body mass index with major cardiovascular events and with mortality after percutaneous coronary intervention. Circ Cardiovasc Interv. 2013;6:146-53.
29. Ma WQ, Sun XJ, Wang Y, et al. Does body mass index truly affect mortality and cardiovascular outcomes in patients after coronary revascularization with PCI or CABG? A systematic review and network meta-analysis. Obes Rev. 2018;19:1236-47.
30. Kenchaiah S, Evans JC, Levy D, et al. Obesity and the risk of heart failure. N Engl J Med. 2002;347:305-13.
31. Kenchaiah S, Sesso HD, Gaziano JM. Body mass index and vigorous physical activity and the risk of heart failure among men. Circulation. 2009;119(1):44-52.
32. Bahrami H, Bluemke DA, Kronmal RA, et al. Novel metabolic risk factors for incident heart failure and their relationship with obesity: the MESA (Multi-Ethnic Study of Atherosclerosis) study. J Am Coll Cardiol. 2008;51(18):1775-83.
33. Ghoorah K, Campbell P, Kent A, et al. Obesity and cardiovascular outcomes: a review. Eur Heart J Acute Cardiovasc Care. 2016;5(1):77-85.
34. Kovacic JC, Lee P, Baber U, et al. Inverse relationship between body mass index and coronary artery calcification in patients with clinically significant coronary lesions. Atherosclerosis. 2012;221(1):176-82.
35. Wang TJ, Parise H, Levy D, et al. Obesity and the risk of new-onset atrial fibrillation. JAMA. 2004;292:2471-7.
36. Thanassoulis G, Massaro JM, O'Donnell CJ, et al. Pericardial fat is associated with prevalent atrial fibrillation: the Framingham Heart Study. Circ Arrhythm Electrophysiol. 2010;3(4):345-50.
37. Pathak RK, Middeldorp ME, Meredith M, et al. Long-term effect of goal-directed weight management in an atrial fibrillation cohort. J Am Coll Cardiol. 2015;65:2159-69.
38. Sanchez C, Miller K, Raj R, et al. The associations between obesity and deep vein thrombosis in patients with cardiovascular disease: a narrative review. Cureus. 2024;16(8):e66731.
39. Yang G, De Staercke C, Hooper WC. The effects of obesity on venous thromboembolism: a review. Open J Prev Med. 2012;2(4):499-506.
40. Hansson PO, Eriksson H, Welin L, et al. Smoking and abdominal obesity: risk factors for venous thromboembolism among middle-aged men: the study of men born in 1913. Arch Int Med. 1999;159(16):1886-90.

2

CHAPTER

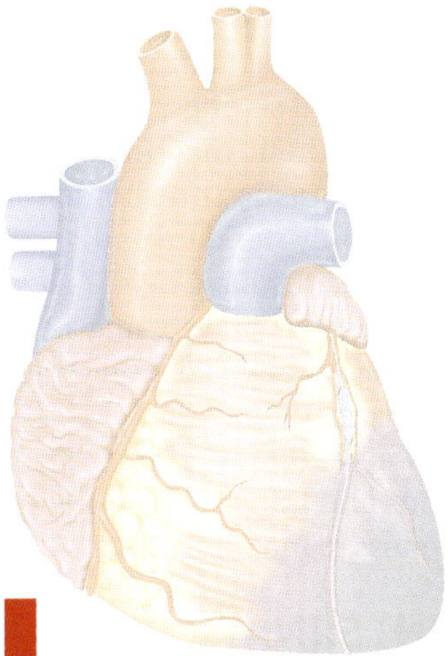

Obesity: Definition and Classification—From Controversy to Consensus

Saumitra Ray, Mainak Mukhopadhyay, Srina Ray

INTRODUCTION

Obesity is a global epidemic that has profound adverse impacts on cardiovascular and metabolic health, with more than one billion individuals affected worldwide. Its classification has long relied upon simplistic cutoffs such as BMI, but the ongoing obesity pandemic and the emergence of new therapeutics have exposed flaws in older definitions. Calls for change stem from controversies, including the inadequacy of BMI to differentiate between body fat and lean mass, its inability to capture metabolic health, and variability in risk by ethnicity and age. In 2025, major international panels—including the Lancet Commission—proposed an updated framework that emphasizes a comprehensive, patient-centered approach using modern diagnostic tools and functional assessment.[1,2]

HISTORICAL CONTEXT AND CONTROVERSIES

- Earlier definitions relied solely on the BMI threshold of ≥30 kg/m^2, despite long-standing awareness of its limitations, such as inability to distinguish between adiposity and muscle, and failure to account for fat distribution or metabolic health.
- Disproportionate risk among different populations (e.g., higher risk at lower BMI among Asian Indians) led to alternative criteria for some groups.[3]
- Increasing recognition that up to 20% of the population previously classified as overweight are at risk for obesity-related complications according to new tools, rendering them misclassified and untreated under older paradigms.[4]

2025 CONSENSUS ON DEFINITION[1,2]

- *Obesity is now defined as a condition characterized by excess adiposity, with or without abnormal distribution or function of adipose tissue, and causes, that are multifactorial and incompletely understood.*
- A distinction is made between "preclinical obesity" (excess adiposity with preserved organ/system function) and "clinical obesity" (excess adiposity causing functional impairment or comorbidities such as heart failure, diabetes, or limited mobility).
    - *Preclinical obesity:* A state of excess adiposity where tissues/organs function normally, but risk for future disease or organ dysfunction is increased.
    - *Clinical obesity:* Chronic and systemic illness characterized by measurable or observable impairment in organ/system function (e.g., cardiac dysfunction, diabetes, and sleep apnea) due to excess adiposity.
- *Diagnosis is now a two-step process:*
    1. *Confirmation of excess adiposity:* Best confirmed by direct body composition studies, or by anthropometric surrogates (waist circumference, waist-to-hip, or waist-to-height ratio) in addition to or instead of BMI, using cutoffs validated by age, gender, and ethnicity.

       For extreme BMI (>40 kg/m^2), further confirmation is generally unnecessary.
    2. *Assessment of functional impact or comorbidities:* Assessment for clinical manifestations or diagnostic

tests confirming organ/system dysfunction, or significant impairment in activities of daily life due to obesity.

- New frameworks (European, American, and Asian) now incorporate waist measures and comorbidity assessment into diagnosis, with several society guidelines aligning or adapting their thresholds as of 2025.[5]

CLASSIFICATION SYSTEMS[6-8]

- *Traditional BMI-based staging:* Retained for epidemiology, population risk screening, and research, but replaced by clinical criteria in diagnostic and therapeutic decision-making.
- *Functional staging:* Obesity is staged by impact on mobility, organ function, and associated diseases [e.g., Edmonton Obesity Staging System (EOSS), which considers metabolic, mechanical, and mental health domains].
- *Anthropometry plus assessment:* Combination of BMI, waist circumference/waist-to-height ratio, and clinical profile to determine risk and need for intervention.

DIAGNOSTIC CRITERIA (2025)[1,2,7]

Diagnostic criteria 2025 are given in **Table 1**.

LIMITATIONS[9,10]

- *Ethnic variation:* Cutoffs often need adjustment for specific populations, as risk at a given BMI is not the same worldwide (e.g., BMI ≥23 for South Asians).

TABLE 1: Diagnostic criteria.

Criterion	*Preclinical obesity*	*Clinical obesity*
Body fat confirmation	Required	Required
BMI alone	Not sufficient	Not sufficient
Waist/waist-to-height ratio	≥0.5 recommended	≥0.5 recommended
Organ/system dysfunction	Absent	Present (e.g., diabetes, CVD, reduced daily function, etc.)
Comorbidities	May be present (risk elevated)	Present (direct result of obesity)
Use of functional staging	Optional	Essential
Use in treatment decisions	Preventive strategies	Active therapeutic intervention

- *Measurement challenges:* Direct measures of body fat are not universally available or practical in routine care, especially in resource-limited settings.
- *Subjectivity:* Functional assessment may introduce inter-clinician variability; diagnostic thresholds for organ dysfunction may not be fully standardized.
- *Risk of stigma and access:* Concerns have been raised that patients labeled as "preclinical" obesity may have limited access to medical care or weight-loss therapies due to insurance or guideline restrictions.
- *Longitudinal data:* Need for validation of long-term outcomes of new definitions and impact on mortality, morbidity, and responsiveness to intervention.

GUIDELINES (2025 INTERNATIONAL RECOMMENDATIONS)[1,2]

- *BMI should be used primarily as a population-level risk marker, not as an individual-level diagnostic determinant.*
- *Diagnosis of obesity should involve confirmation of excess adiposity by best available direct or surrogate measures, not BMI alone.*
- *Classification into preclinical or clinical obesity should be based on the presence of objective organ/system dysfunction or significant impairment in function due to adiposity.*
- *Treatment and prevention should be tailored to the stage of obesity, functional impact, and comorbid profile, not merely BMI category.*

CONCLUSION

The definition and classification of obesity have evolved into a nuanced, patient-centered, and functionally driven framework. Reliance on BMI alone has been supplanted by multifactorial diagnostic processes that improve clinical decision-making, risk stratification, and access to therapy. Future research must focus on standardizing diagnostic instruments, refining functional criteria, and monitoring long-term clinical outcomes. The challenge for clinicians, policymakers, and researchers is now to implement and further validate these advances globally, ensuring equitable and effective management of obesity for all patient populations.

REFERENCES

1. Rubino F, Cummings DE, Eckel RH, et al. Definition and diagnostic criteria of clinical obesity. Lancet Diabetes Endocrinol. 2025;13(3):221-62.
2. World Health Organization. (2025). Obesity and overweight. [online] Available from https://www.who.int/

news-room/fact-sheets/detail/obesity-and-overweight [Last accessed January, 2026].

3. Medscape, Tucker ME. (2025). New Obesity Definition Raises the Number Who Have It. [online] Available from https://www.medscape.com/viewarticle/new-obesity-definition-raises-number-who-have-it-2025a1000i1u [Last accessed January, 2026].
4. Northwestern University Feinberg School of Medicine, News Center. (2025). Redefining Obesity With New Global Guidelines. [online] Available from https://news.feinberg.northwestern.edu/2025/01/15/redefining-obesity-with-new-global-guidelines/ [Last accessed January, 2026].
5. Iacobucci G. Define obesity as clinical or pre-clinical for more accurate diagnosis, says global commission. BMJ. 2025;388:r78.
6. Guglielmi G. New obesity definition sidelines BMI to focus on health. Nature. 2025;637(8047):773-4.
7. BBC. (2025). Global report calls for obesity to be redefined. [online] Available from https://www.bbc.com/news/articles/c79dz14d30ro [Last accessed January, 2026].
8. Misra A, Vikram NK, Ghosh A, et al. Revised definition of obesity in Asian Indians living in India. Diabetes Metab Syndr. 2025;19(1):102989.
9. Kalra S, Kapoor N, Verma M, et al. Defining and Diagnosing Obesity in India: A Call for Advocacy and Action. J Obes. 2023;2023:4178121. Erratum in: J Obes. 2025;2025:9806198.
10. ASMBS. Consensus Statement on Obesity as a Disease. [online] Available from https://asmbs.org/resources/consensus-statement-on-obesity-as-a-disease/ [Last accessed January, 2026].

3

CHAPTER

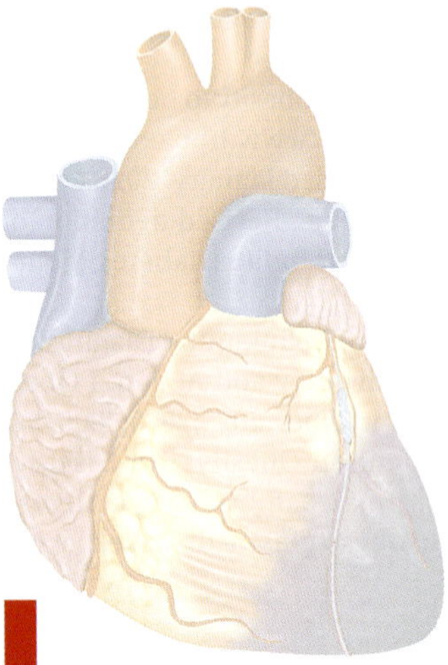

Prevalence and Overview of Obesity with Diabetes

Subhash Kumar Wangnoo, Asim Siddiqui

INTRODUCTION

Rapid urbanization and its benefits of socioeconomic growth have led to a problem of plenty! It has raised standards of living but has contributed to a more stressful and sedentary lifestyle coupled with unhealthy dietary habits. This phenomenon is being observed in all corners of the globe irrespective of the economic status; at the same time, the healthcare facilities are unable to keep up with the surge in the noncommunicable diseases. In the last 2–3 decades, obesity has become a silent global pandemic affecting all age groups and is now a severe public health problem as one of the most common noncommunicable diseases. One of the effects of this surge is an increase in the prevalence of metabolic diseases, especially type 2 diabetes, especially in the younger age group.

Overweight and obesity is now a big public health issue, with a doubling of the worldwide occurrence since 1975. Obesity is defined as excessive or abnormal storage of fat in the body and is operationally defined by body mass index (BMI), which has a lower cut-off for Asians—obese if the BMI is ≥25 kg/m^2. Studies have shown that the relative risk of developing type 2 DM is 4.6-fold higher for woman and 3.5-fold higher for men with a BMI >29.9 kg/m^2 compared to their same-sex peers with a BMI <24.9 kg/m^2, although the associations between central obesity and comorbidities vary among different races and ethnicities. Anatomically, body fat or adipose tissue is distributed unequally in varying proportion across the body. When the adipose tissue is excessively accumulated around the visceral organs in the abdomen, it is termed as central obesity or abdominal obesity (AO). In India, an estimated 30–65% of the population is affected by AO. Well-documented epidemiologic data from recent studies examining the prevalence of AO found that the age-standardized prevalence of AO was 46.6% among the urban population in Chennai, 26.6% in Tamil Nadu, 18.7% in Maharashtra, 16.9% in Jharkhand, and 36.1% in Chandigarh, respectively. The most extensive health and demographic survey in India, National Family and Health Survey, introduced a novel measure in its fifth iteration (NFHS-5) performed between 2019 and 2021, revealed that among women, overall or generalized obesity (GO) prevalence was recorded at 23%, whereas a significantly higher proportion, around 40%, exhibited AO. Among men, the prevalence of GO stood at 22%, while AO was prevalent at 12%. As per estimates, 77 million people were diabetic in India, which is expected to increase over 134 million by the end of 2045. The prevalence of diabetes in India has increased from 7.1 to 8.9% between 2009 and 2019, with several studies indicating a growing prevalence of obesity and diabetes across the country.

Although the association between the increasing prevalence of obesity leading to diabetes is not straightforward, empirical evidence linking the pathogeneses of these two common metabolic disorders has been demonstrated by the overlaps in their genetics/epigenetics revealed by the genome-wide association study, with researchers further providing evidence of associations at the molecular level. This is further evidenced by demonstration of shared etiological and pathophysiological features leading to amplification of genetic susceptibilities, the ectopic expansion of adipose tissue and excessive accumulation of certain nutrients and metabolites that lead to metabolic imbalance via insulin resistance, dysfunctional autophagy, and microbiome-gut-brain axis, further exacerbating the dysregulation of immunometabolism through chronic systemic inflammation, leading to an accelerated loss of β-cell function and gradual elevation of blood glucose.

INTERPLAY BETWEEN OBESITY AND DIABETES

The pathogenesis of diabetes is characterized by the inflammatory component inducing progressive loss of β-cell insulin secretion with coexisting insulin resistance, impacting early β-cell function, where coexisting overweight and obesity are deemed the most effective triggers. The expansion of adipose tissue in nonadipose sites—the ectopic fat—elevates the levels of certain metabolites, leading to overproduction of inflammatory cytokines that fuel systemic inflammation and cellular function disruption, contributing to impaired insulin signaling, locally induced loss of β-cell function, the onset of hyperglycemia, and the eventual occurrence of diabetes. Epidemiological studies have demonstrated that many patients with obesity have "prediabetes" before eventually developing hyperglycemia. This presents early intervention options directed toward mitigating diabetes onset.

Environmental factors and hyperglycemia contribute to epigenetic changes in DNA and histones, modulating gene expression in organs implicated in the pathogenesis and progression of diabetes and β-cell function. This is best demonstrated in studies documenting an association with higher maternal BMI before pregnancy, greater calorie intake, more significant gestational weight gain, and maternal hyperglycemia with childhood obesity and future risk of developing diabetes. Maternal hyperglycemia and gestational diabetes are associated with precursors of diabetogenic potential in offspring, further indicating a powerful effect of maternal hyperglycemia on pancreatic β-cell development and function.

ECTOPIC EXPANSION OF ADIPOSE TISSUE

Three types of adipocytes play an important role in the interplay between obesity and diabetes. The white adipocytes are the dominant subcutaneously stored and energy-producing adipocytes capable of secreting adipokines such as leptin and adiponectin. Brown adipocytes located within supraclavicular, paravertebral, mediastinal, and other adipose-tissue depots can be activated and produce heat during cold exposure, with their activity being negatively correlated with age, BMI, and fasting glycemia. Scattered within white adipose tissue (WAT) and characterized by their progenitor cellular origin, beige [thermogenic beige, or brown-and-white ("bright")] adipocytes, as their names imply, can turn into brown adipocytes in response to cold exposure, exercise, and endocrine signals. The distribution of adipose tissue is more critical in developing insulin resistance. Abdominal fat releases factors including nonesterified fatty acids and adipocytokines [including reduced adiponectin and tumor necrosis factor-α (TNF-α)] which increases the risk of diabetes. With the expansion of adipocytes, the cells become less responsive to insulin due to the reduced efficiency of glucose transport caused by stretched cell surface of enlarged adipocytes and oxidative stress caused by overnutrition. The overt accumulation and expansion of WAT is related to a remodeling of the microenvironment characterized by aberrant inflammation, fibrosis, hypoxia, dysregulated secretion of adipokines, and disrupted mitochondrial function, which impairs insulin signaling, triggers insulin resistance, reduces insulin-stimulated glucose-transport activity, and accelerates β-cell dysfunction, all of which play a role in the pathogenesis of diabetes. The WAT expansion in skeletal muscles and the liver increases the level of diacylglycerol (DAG), which activates the epsilon form of protein kinase C (PKCε), leading to decreased glucose uptake in muscles and disrupts insulin-induced activation of glycogen synthesis and suppression of glucose production in the liver, fueling hyperglycemia. Moreover, the expansion of adipose tissue in the liver leads to steatosis, exacerbating insulin resistance by causing lipotoxicity-induced cellular dysfunction and apoptosis.

INTERPLAY AT THE CELLULAR LEVEL

Hypoxia, fibrosis, and mitochondrial dysfunction associated with the microenvironment of obesity also contribute to the development of diabetes. Hypoxia activates the transcription factor hypoxia-inducible factor-1α (HIF-1α) that triggers fibrosis, enhances local inflammation, and lowers insulin sensitivity. Lipotoxicity induces mitochondrial dysfunction, mainly involving a reduction in mitochondrial mass and ATP production with overproduction of reactive oxygen species (ROS), which is detrimental to insulin sensitivity due to the critical role of mitochondria in regulating the adipogenesis, fatty acid synthesis, esterification, and lipolysis of adipocytes. Elevated levels of free fatty acids (FFAs) resulting from enhanced lipolysis may increase endoplasmic reticulum (ER) stress and impair β-cell function.

The obesity-induced low-grade inflammation affects many organs and involves activation of the innate immune system that impacts metabolic balance, resulting in tissue damage via increased fibrosis and necrosis at the same time. The elevation of circulating lipopolysaccharide (LPS), hypoxia, and fibrosis, and the consequent occurrence of systemic inflammation in obesity plays a causative role in insulin resistance, insulin deficiency, and dysregulation of energy homeostasis. Dysregulated secretion of proinflammatory cytokines, including TNF, interleukin (IL)-1β, IL-6, IL-8, leptin, resistin, and monocyte chemoattractant protein 1 (MCP1) by adipocytes and macrophages within adipose tissue, the low-grade systemic inflammation dampens insulin signaling.

MICROBIOME–GUT–BRAIN AXIS

The microbiome–gut–brain axis is one of the most critical mechanisms regulating whole-body metabolism, adiposity, energy balance, and central appetite and food reward signaling in humans. Microbiome dysfunction is the main culprit responsible for energy imbalance, fat deposition, inflammation, insulin resistance, glucolipotoxicity, and dysregulation of endocrine signaling pathways by either direct or indirect effect. The changes in gut microbial production have been suggested to induce a more considerable impact on the development of metabolic disorders compared to its direct influence on the metabolic process resulting from its altered composition. The composition of the microbiome is both endogenously and exogenously shaped by multiple factors, including maternal environment, age, ethnicity, diet, medication (especially antibiotics), and genetics, among which the diet is main determinant, and the composition of gut microbiome changes with the development of obesity and diabetes. Under normal conditions, the gut barrier only allows a minimal amount of LPS to enter the circulation, the elevated LPS in obesity and diabetes binds to TLR4 and activates NF-κB signaling pathways, promoting the secretion of inflammatory cytokines such as IL-1, IL-6, and TNF-α, which contributes toward metabolic dysfunction at cellular levels. The decrease in the diversity of the microbiome is related to the increase in BMI, fat mass, inflammatory markers, reduced insulin sensitivity, and dyslipidemia. The changes in the composition of the microbiome also affect fasting glucose, glycated hemoglobin levels, and diabetes development through inducing significant alterations such as changes in appetite, inflammation, insulin resistance, hepatic lipid metabolism, and hyperglycemia by converting dietary nutrients into metabolites thus regulating their central and peripheral effect.

CONCLUSION

A worldwide increase in the prevalence of obesity has led to the concomitant increase in the prevalence of diabetes. Obesity, particularly when associated with increased abdominal and intra-abdominal fat distribution and increased intrahepatic and intramuscular triglyceride content, is a major risk factor for developing prediabetes and diabetes due to its effects on insulin resistance and β-cell dysfunction. These alterations include adipose tissue fibrosis (increased rates of fibrogenesis and expression of genes involved in extracellular matrix formation), inflammation (increased proinflammatory macrophage and T-cell content and the production of PAI-1), and the production of exosomes that can induce insulin resistance. However, none of these factors can influence systemic metabolic function without a mechanism for adipose tissue communication with other organs. It is possible that several adipose tissue secretory products that are released into the bloodstream, including PAI-1, adiponectin, FFAs and exosomes, are involved in this signaling process, but additional research is needed to fully assess their clinical importance. In addition, it is also likely that crosstalk among adipose tissue, the liver, muscle, and pancreatic islets contribute to insulin resistance and hepatic steatosis. Decreasing body fat mass by inducing a negative energy balance, not by surgical removal, can ameliorate or normalize obesity-induced metabolic dysfunction and can even achieve diabetes remission if there is adequate restoration of β-cell function.

BIBLIOGRAPHY

1. Bhardwaj S, Misra A, Misra R, et al. High prevalence of abdominal, intra-abdominal and subcutaneous adiposity and clustering of risk factors among urban Asian Indians in North India. PloS One. 2011;6:e24362.
2. Cani PD, Amar J, Iglesias MA, et al. Metabolic endotoxemia initiates obesity and insulin resistance. Diabetes. 2007;56(7):1761-72.
3. Chait A, den Hartigh LJ. Adipose tissue distribution, inflammation and its metabolic consequences, including diabetes and cardiovascular disease. Front Cardiovasc Med. 2020;7:22.
4. Cryan JF, O'Riordan KJ, Cowan CSM, et al. The microbiota-Gut-Brain axis. Physiol Rev. 2019;99(4):1877-2013.
5. Deepa M, Farooq S, Deepa R, et al. Prevalence and significance of generalized and central body obesity in an urban Asian Indian population in Chennai, India (CURES:47). Eur J Clin Nutr. 2009;63:259-67.
6. Delisle HF. Poverty: The double burden of malnutrition in mothers and the intergenerational impact. Ann NY Acad Sci. 2008;1136:172-84.
7. De Vadder F, Kovatcheva-Datchary P, Goncalves D, et al. Microbiota-generated metabolites promote

metabolic benefits via gut-brain neural circuits. Cell. 2014;156(1-2):84-96.
8. Dhawan D, Sharma S. Abdominal obesity, adipokines and non-communicable diseases. J Steroid Biochem Mol Biol. 2020;203:105737.
9. Government of India, Ministry of Health and Family Welfare. National Family Health Survey (NFHS-5), 2019-21: Compendium of Fact Sheets—India and 14 States/UTs (Phase II). New Delhi: MoHFW; 2021. pP. 428-31.
10. Halberg N, Khan T, Trujillo ME, et al. Hypoxia-inducible factor-1 alpha induces fibrosis and insulin resistance in white adipose tissue. Mol Cell Biol. 2009;29(16):4467-83.
11. Keating ST, El-Osta A. Epigenetic changes in diabetes. Clin Genet. 2013;84(1):1-10.
12. Malone JI, Hansen BC. Does obesity cause type 2 diabetes mellitus (T2DM)? or is it the opposite? Pediatr Diabetes. 2019;20(1):5-9.
13. Misra A, Chowbey P, Makkar BM, et al. Consensus Group. Consensus statement for diagnosis of obesity, abdominal obesity and the metabolic syndrome for Asian Indians and recommendations for physical activity, medical and surgical management. J Assoc Physicians India. 2009;57:163-70.
14. Misra A, Khurana L. Obesity and the metabolic syndrome in developing countries. J Clin Endocrinol Metab. 2008;93(11 Suppl 1):S9-30.
15. Misra A. Ethnic-specific criteria for classification of body mass index: A perspective for Asian Indians and American diabetes association position statement. Diabetes Technol Ther. 2015;17:667-71.
16. Mohan V, Deepa R. Obesity and abdominal obesity in Asian Indians. Indian J Med Res. 2006;123:593-6.
17. Pradeepa R, Anjana RM, Joshi SR, et al. Prevalence of generalized and abdominal obesity in urban and rural India- the ICMR-INDIAB Study (Phase-I) [ICMR-INDIAB-3. Indian J Med Res. 2015;142:139-50.
18. Pradeepa R, Mohan V. Epidemiology of type 2 diabetes in India. Indian J Ophthalmol. 2021;69:2932-8.
19. Saltiel AR, Olefsky JM. Inflammatory mechanisms linking obesity and metabolic disease. J Clin Invest. 2017;127(1):1-4.
20. Shuster A, Patlas M, Pinthus JH, et al. The clinical importance of visceral adiposity: A critical review of methods for visceral adipose tissue analysis. Br J Radiol. 2012;85:1-10.
21. Sun K, Kusminski CM, Scherer PE. Adipose tissue remodeling and obesity. J Clin Invest. 2011;121(6):2094-101.
22. Yazıcı D, Sezer H. Insulin resistance, obesity and lipotoxicity. Adv In Exp Med Biol. 2017;960:277-304.

4

CHAPTER

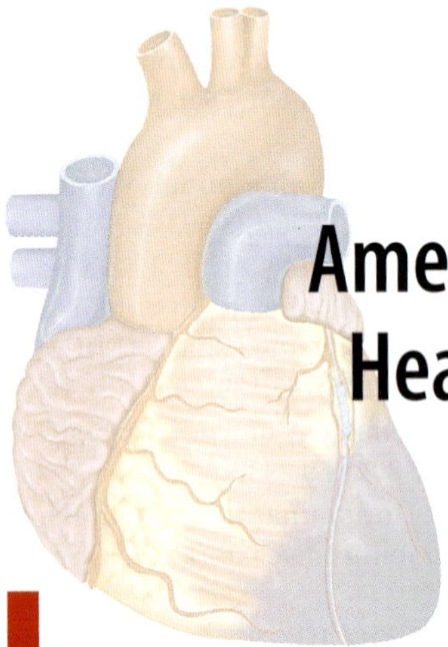

American College of Cardiology and American Heart Association Guidelines for Obesity and Cardiovascular Disease Management

Abhishek Garg, Akash Batta, Gurpreet Singh Wander

INTRODUCTION

Obesity is recognized as a chronic, relapsing disease that substantially increases cardiovascular (CV) risk, driving hypertension, type 2 diabetes mellitus (T2DM), dyslipidemia, atherosclerotic cardiovascular disease (ASCVD), heart failure (HF; especially HFpEF), atrial fibrillation, and sudden death. Early US guidance—the 2013 American College of Cardiology (ACC)/American Heart Association (AHA)/The Obesity Society (TOS)[1] guideline—organized care around body mass index (BMI) diagnosis, optional waist circumference (WC) when BMI was 25–35 kg/m^2, intensive lifestyle intervention, threshold-based pharmacotherapy (BMI ≥27 kg/m^2 with comorbidity or ≥30 kg/m^2), and bariatric surgery (BMI ≥40 or ≥35 kg/m^2 with comorbidity). This framework reflected limited therapy options, modest drug efficacy, and little recognition of obesity as a CV disease.

The 2024 European Society of Cardiology (ESC)[2] Clinical Consensus reframed obesity as a primary cardiometabolic disease, emphasizing central adiposity and WC (targets <94 cm for men, <80 cm for women). It promoted long-term, multidisciplinary programs, integrated obesity into CV care (including HF), and highlighted evidence for modern pharmacotherapy and surgery as CV-risk-reducing interventions. However, as a consensus rather than a full guideline, it lacked detailed treatment sequencing and predated major US pharmacotherapy recommendations.

The 2025 ACC Concise Clinical Guidance[3] reflects breakthroughs in incretin-based therapies (semaglutide, tirzepatide), stronger CV outcome data, and the need to abandon "lifestyle-failure-first" rules. It recommends glucagon-like peptide-1 (GLP-1) and glucose-dependent insulinotropic polypeptide (GIP)/GLP-1 agonists as first-line therapy, always alongside lifestyle measures, within team-based, equitable care **(Table 1)**.

DIAGNOSIS OF OBESITY

At the population level, BMI serves as a simple and effective tool for assessing excess body weight. However, its accuracy is limited at the individual level, as it does not distinguish between fat mass and lean muscle, nor does it account for variations in fat distribution, sex, ethnicity, or health risks. For example, South Asian and Chinese populations are at higher cardiometabolic risk at lower BMI values, leading to proposals for reduced cutoff points of ≥23 kg/m^2 for overweight and ≥25 kg/m^2 for obesity in these groups **(Table 2)**.[3]

Alternative anthropometric indicators such as WC, waist-to-hip ratio (WHR), and waist-to-height ratio (WHtR) provide additional information on central (abdominal) adiposity, which has a stronger association with CV events compared to overall BMI.[3] However, standardized cutoff values for these measures remain under discussion.

More precise assessments of body fat can be made using advanced imaging modalities such as dual-energy X-ray absorptiometry, CT, or MRI. However, these are not feasible for routine use in large populations.[3] Thus, in clinical and epidemiological practice, the diagnosis of obesity is generally made by combining BMI with anthropometric measures (WC, WHR, and WHtR) to better capture excess adiposity and its impact on organ function and overall health.[3]

TABLE 1: Comparison of various guidelines for obesity management.

Aspect	*2013 ACC/AHA/TOS1*	*2024 ESC/EASO2*	*2025 ACC3*
View of obesity	Overweight/obesity as a major risk factor for CVD; focus on weight reduction	Obesity as a chronic relapsing disease *and an* independent CVD risk factor	Obesity as a chronic disease is directly linked to CV risk; it integrates obesity therapy into CV prevention
Screening	Annual BMI; WC if BMI 25–35 kg/m^2	BMI, WC, and WHR; ethnicity-specific cutoffs (lower for Asians)	Same as prior, but focus on identifying patients for early pharmacotherapy
Lifestyle intervention	First-line: diet, exercise, behavioral therapy; intensive programs (≥14 sessions/ 6 months)	Structured, multidisciplinary, long-term support; target ≥5–10% weight loss	Still foundational, but always combined with pharmacotherapy in eligible patients
Weight-loss goal	5–10% over 6 months	5–10% reduction improves CV risk; more if comorbidities	Individualized; ≥10% often recommended; tied to CV outcomes
Pharmacotherapy	If BMI ≥27 (with comorbidity) or ≥30	Same thresholds; emphasizes GLP-1 receptor agonists (liraglutide, semaglutide) due to CV benefits	Paradigm shift: GLP-1 (semaglutide) and GLP-1/GIP (tirzepatide) recommended as first-line; no need to "fail" lifestyle first
Bariatric/ metabolic surgery	BMI ≥40, or ≥35 with comorbidities	Same; can consider BMI ≥30 with uncontrolled T2DM	Same, with continued support for surgery as an option in severe cases
CVD focus	Indirect—via control of comorbidities (DM, HTN, dyslipidemia)	Direct—obesity management embedded in CVD prevention and HF care	Strong CV focus—especially HFpEF patients; aligns weight management with CV event reduction
Long-term follow-up	At least 1 year of maintenance support	Lifelong multidisciplinary follow-up	Lifelong management emphasized addressing equity, stigma, and access barriers

(ACC/AHA/TOS: American College of Cardiology/American Heart Association/The Obesity Society; BMI: body mass index; CV: cardiovascular; CVD: cardiovascular disease; ESC: European Society of Cardiology; HF: heart failure; T2DM: type 2 diabetes mellitus; WC: waist circumference; WHR: waist–hip ratio)

TABLE 2: Diagnosis of obesity.

Category BMI (kg/m^2)	*Europoid*	*Asian*
Healthy weight	18.5–<25	18.5–<23
Overweight	25–<30	23–<25
Obesity	≥30	≥25
Class 1	30–<35	25–<30
Class 2	35–<40	≥30
Class 3 (severe)	≥40	–
Additional anthropometric measures		
Measure		Threshold
Waist circumference (inches)		• Women: ≥35 in Europoid, ≥31.5 in South Asian and Chinese • Men: ≥40 in Europoid, ≥35.5 in South Asian and Chinese • Japanese women: ≥35.4 • Japanese men: ≥33.5
Waist-to-height ratio		≥0.50

Source: Gilbert et al.[3]

BENEFITS OF WEIGHT LOSS IN CARDIOVASCULAR DISEASE

The primary objectives of weight management in individuals with obesity or overweight are to prevent further weight gain, promote weight reduction, and sustain long-term weight maintenance.[4] Regular monitoring of BMI and WC remains crucial for assessing progress and evaluating treatment effectiveness. Evidence suggests that dietary approaches, such as the Mediterranean diet, can reduce CV risk; however, the degree of adherence and personalization still require further investigation.[4] While the Look AHEAD trial[5] did not demonstrate overall reductions in major CV events, subgroup analyses suggested that losing at least 10% of body weight was associated with significant CV benefits. Physical activity, particularly aerobic exercise, further enhances insulin sensitivity, vascular health, and reduces inflammation, even beyond its effects on weight loss.[4] Pharmacological therapies like liraglutide have shown CV benefits in high-risk diabetic patients, whereas bariatric surgery has consistently been associated with reduced coronary and cerebrovascular events, highlighting its potential long-term CV advantage.[4]

WEIGHT LOSS IN OBESITY AND OVERWEIGHT

Both the ACC/AHA[1,3] and ESC guidelines[2] highlight weight reduction as an important strategy for individuals with overweight or obesity to lower CV risk. A modest but clinically relevant weight loss—defined as about 5% of baseline body weight—has been shown to improve blood pressure, lipid profile, glucose regulation, and even reduce premature all-cause mortality.[6] In contrast, the ESC[2] guidelines recommend caution in older adults, noting that weight loss may not always be advantageous because of the "obesity paradox," where carrying extra weight can sometimes appear to have a protective effect. In such patients, the focus should shift toward maintaining muscle mass and ensuring adequate nutrition, rather than aggressive weight reduction. Similarly, the ACC/AHA[1,3] guidelines recommend careful monitoring in elderly individuals to avoid loss of lean body mass and nutritional deficiencies when pursuing weight loss strategies.

MEASURES TO ADDRESS OBESITY AND OVERWEIGHT

Dietary Approaches

Both the 2019 ACC/AHA[7] and 2021 ESC[8] guidelines emphasize that weight reduction should begin with structured dietary interventions. A moderate calorie restriction, typically around 500 kcal/day, is recommended. In certain cases, very-low-calorie diets (<800 kcal/day) may be considered under strict medical supervision.[7] The ESC supports[8] several dietary patterns for weight loss, including plant-based or Mediterranean diets, low- or very-low-carbohydrate diets, low-fat diets, and high-protein diets. While these approaches show similar short-term effects, the Mediterranean diet has demonstrated better long-term CV and metabolic benefits. Carbohydrate-restricted or ketogenic diets may improve blood sugar control in people with diabetes but should ideally be plant-based and not followed for long durations.[6] High-protein diets may help preserve lean muscle mass and reduce hunger, while the overall focus should remain on reducing processed foods and prioritizing fruits, vegetables, whole grains, and healthy fats. Intermittent fasting and time-restricted eating are also acceptable, though their benefits appear similar to calorie-restricted diets.[6] Importantly, consistency and adherence to healthy eating patterns matter more than choosing a single "best" diet.[6]

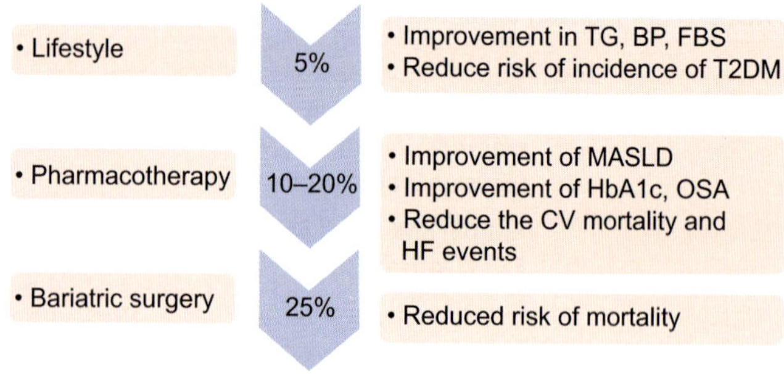

Fig. 1: Weight loss threshold associated with comorbidity improvement. (BP: blood pressure; CV: cardiovascular; CVD: cardiovascular disease; FBS: fasting blood sugar; HbA1c: hemoglobin A1c; HF: heart failure; MASLD: metabolic dysfunction-associated steatotic liver disease; TG: triglycerides)

Physical Activity

Exercise plays a crucial role alongside dietary changes to enhance and sustain weight loss. The ACC/AHA[7] recommends at least 150 minutes per week of moderate-intensity aerobic activity, such as brisk walking, for initial weight loss. To prevent weight regain and maintain results, 200–300 minutes per week may be required.[6] Combining aerobic and resistance training can improve muscle strength, CV fitness, and metabolic health.[6] For older adults, exercise programs should be individualized, with special attention to preventing muscle loss (sarcopenic obesity) and promoting safe, enjoyable activities.[6]

When diet and physical activity are combined into a structured lifestyle program, individuals typically achieve 5–10% weight loss, which leads to meaningful improvements in blood pressure, cholesterol, blood sugar, and overall CV risk[1] **(Fig. 1)**.

PHARMACOTHERAPY

Beyond lifestyle interventions, medications have been used for weight reduction for over a century. First-generation compounds such as thyroid hormone, dinitrophenol, and amphetamines were effective but carried serious CV or systemic risks, leading to regulatory bans or restrictions.[1] With evolving safety standards, second-generation agents such as fenfluramine, sibutramine, and lorcaserin were introduced but later withdrawn due to adverse effects.[1] Currently, approved therapies include orlistat, phentermine/topiramate, and naltrexone/bupropion.[1] These agents generally achieve 5–10% weight loss, though gastrointestinal or neuropsychiatric side effects and insufficient long-term CV outcome evidence limit their use.[1] The ESC guidelines[2] endorse orlistat, naltrexone/bupropion, whereas the ACC/AHA does not, reflecting regional regulatory differences clinicians must consider.

The 2025 ACC/AHA guidelines highlight obesity as a chronic, relapsing condition that necessitates sustained, multifaceted management approaches rather than short-term interventions.[1] A major advance in this update is that the third generation of antiobesity therapies, often referred to as nutrient-stimulated hormone (NuSH) agents, incretin-based therapies, has dramatically reshaped the treatment landscape. NuSH therapies are positioned as a pivotal component of obesity care for several reasons. First, they provide an intermediate treatment option between lifestyle intervention and bariatric surgery.[9] Second, these therapies directly target the underlying disease mechanisms of obesity, particularly the hormonal pathways involved in hunger, satiety, and food cravings.[1] By modifying appetite-regulating signals, NuSH agents address the physiological drivers of weight regain, something lifestyle approaches alone cannot reliably overcome.[1] Third, NuSH therapies offer flexibility through dose titration, allowing clinicians to balance effectiveness with tolerability.[1]

This enables personalized treatment planning, reduces adverse effects, and optimizes outcomes across diverse patient populations.[1] These agents originally developed for T2DM, liraglutide, semaglutide, and tirzepatide are now FDA-approved for obesity management as well.[1]

VARIOUS NUTRIENT-STIMULATED HORMONE AGENTS

In this section, we outline the currently available NuSH agents, presented in chronological order of their regulatory approval. For each therapy, details regarding the mechanism of action, recommended dosing, average weight reduction at 1 year, and common side effects are summarized.

Liraglutide

Liraglutide is a GLP-1 receptor agonist (RA) administered once daily via subcutaneous injection.[10] With 97% homology to native GLP-1, it enhances glucose-dependent insulin secretion, suppresses glucagon, delays gastric emptying, and promotes satiety through central appetite regulation.[10] Initially approved at 1.2–1.8 mg for T2DM, a higher 3.0 mg dose was later approved for chronic weight management in individuals with overweight or obesity.[10] The pivotal SCALE[11] obesity and prediabetes trial demonstrated that liraglutide 3.0 mg resulted in an average weight reduction of ~8% compared to ~2.6% with placebo, with 63% of patients achieving ≥5% weight loss **(Table 3)**. Additionally, liraglutide reduced progression to T2DM and improved cardiometabolic parameters. Common adverse effects include nausea, vomiting, diarrhea, and an increased risk of gallbladder disease.[10] A key precaution is that its use is contraindicated in patients with a personal or family history of medullary thyroid carcinoma or those with multiple endocrine neoplasia type 2.[10]

SEMAGLUTIDE

Semaglutide, like liraglutide, is a GLP-1 RA, but its long half-life of nearly 180 hours allows once-weekly subcutaneous dosing rather than daily administration.[10] It was initially developed for T2DM at lower doses and later evaluated for chronic weight management. To minimize gastrointestinal side effects, the full therapeutic dose is gradually achieved over a period of 16 weeks.

Its efficacy and safety were established through the STEP program, a series of large randomized controlled trials in individuals with overweight or obesity. In STEP 1, semaglutide plus lifestyle counseling resulted in an average weight reduction of 14.9% over 68 weeks, compared with 2.4% with placebo, with more than half of participants losing at least 15% of their baseline weight[13] **(Table 3)**. In STEP 2, participants with T2DM experienced somewhat smaller reductions (~9.6%), a trend also seen with other antiobesity medications.[13] STEP 3 showed that adding intensive behavioral therapy provided only modest additional benefit beyond semaglutide alone.[13] At the same time, STEP 4 demonstrated that ongoing therapy is necessary to sustain weight loss, as discontinuation led to substantial weight regain.[13] STEP 5 further confirmed durable weight reduction over 2 years with continued treatment.[13] Beyond weight loss, semaglutide improved blood pressure, glycemic control, triglycerides, inflammation markers, and functional capacity. Side effects are primarily gastrointestinal and are comparable to those of liraglutide.

Tirzepatide

Tirzepatide is a novel dual agonist that combines GIP and GLP-1 receptor agonism within a single molecule, administered as a once-weekly subcutaneous injection.[10] It was initially approved for T2DM management, with its weight reduction efficacy subsequently established through the SURMOUNT phase III trial program, paralleling the design of the semaglutide STEP studies. Each trial extended over 72 weeks, allowing gradual dose escalation to minimize gastrointestinal intolerance.[10]

Table 3: Dose, route, and side effects of various NuSH agents approved by FDA for obesity.

Medication	*FDA-approved indication for weight management*	*Dosage/titration/storage*	*Clinical efficacy for weight loss*	*Side effects*
Liraglutide	Adults with an initial BMI ≥30 kg/m^2 or ≥27 kg/m^2 with a weight-related comorbidity	• Start 0.6 mg subcutaneously daily • Increase weekly up to 3 mg for adults. Store 30 days at room temperature; longer with refrigeration	*SCALE*[11] obesity and prediabetes 56-week RCT (*n* = 3,731): • ↓ *Weight*: 8.0% liraglutide versus 2.6% placebo • ↓ *Weight* ≥5%: 63.2% liraglutide versus 27.1% placebo	Nausea, diarrhea, constipation, vomiting, injection-site reactions
Semaglutide	Adults with obesity or overweight with a weight-related comorbidity	• Start 0.25 mg subcutaneously weekly • Increase every 4 weeks up to 1.7 or 2.4 mg • Ozempic stable 56 days, Wegovy 28 days at room temperature; longer with refrigeration	*STEP-1*[12] 68-week RCT (*n* = 1,961): • ↓ *Weight*: 14.9% semaglutide versus 2.4% placebo • ↓ *Weight* ≥5%: 86.4% semaglutide versus 31.5% placebo	
Tirzepatide	Adults with obesity or overweight with a weight-related comorbidity	• Start 2.5 mg subcutaneously weekly • Increase every 4 weeks up to 5, 10, or 15 mg • Store 21 days at room temperature; longer with refrigeration	*SURMOUNT-1*[10] 72-week RCT (*n* = 2,539): • ↓ *Weight*: 15.0% with 5 mg, 19.5% with 10 mg, 20.9% with 15 mg, versus 3.1% placebo • ↓ *Weight* ≥5%: 85% with 5 mg, 89% with 10 mg, 91% with 15 mg, versus 35% with placebo	

In SURMOUNT-1, tirzepatide produced unprecedented weight reductions, with average losses of 19.5% at 10 mg and 20.9% at 15 mg, compared with just 3.1% with placebo. Remarkably, at the 15 mg dose, weight reductions of 10, 15, 20, and 25% or greater were achieved by 84, 71, 57, and 36% of participants, respectively[10] **(Table 3)**. SURMOUNT-2 mirrored STEP-2 findings, showing attenuated efficacy in patients with T2DM, with weight loss approximately one third lower than in nondiabetic participants.[14]

In contrast to semaglutide trials, SURMOUNT-3[15] demonstrated that a sequential approach—beginning with a 12-week intensive lifestyle intervention (mean 6.9% loss) followed by tirzepatide—led to cumulative reductions of 24.3% of baseline weight versus 4.5% with placebo. SURMOUNT-4[16] confirmed the importance of continued therapy: After an initial 20.9% reduction, patients maintained on tirzepatide lost an additional 5.5%, whereas those switched to placebo regained 14%.

Tirzepatide's side-effect profile largely resembles that of GLP-1 receptor agonists, predominantly gastrointestinal. Beyond weight loss, improvements in glycemia, lipids, blood pressure, and functional capacity have been observed.

Setmelanotide

Setmelanotide is a melanocortin 4 receptor (MC4R) agonist approved by the FDA in 2020 for patients ≥6 years with obesity due to proprotein convertase subtilisin/kexin type 1 (PCSK1), proopiomelanocortin (POMC), PCSK1, or leptin receptor (LEPR) deficiency.[17] It restores MC4R pathway activity, helping reduce appetite and increase energy expenditure. Phase III trials showed 25.6% weight loss in POMC deficiency and 12.5% in LEPR deficiency.[17] Adverse effects include hyperpigmentation, sexual arousal disturbances, and psychiatric symptoms. Its use is limited to rare, genetically defined obesity rather than general weight management.[17]

In summary, NuSH therapies—particularly semaglutide and tirzepatide—are transforming the treatment of obesity, offering potent weight loss, favorable cardiometabolic effects, and long-term efficacy. Yet, ensuring equitable access, sustained adherence, and careful patient selection remains critical for maximizing their impact in clinical practice.

TABLE 4: Cardiovascular outcomes of FDA-approved NuSH agents in various trials.

Trial	*Medication*	*Population*	*Size/duration (participants)/ years*	*Average baseline BMI and weight change in treatment group*	*Effect on primary outcome (composite of cardiovascular death, AMI, or CVA unless specified)*	*Effect on HF hospitalization*
LEADER[19]	Liraglutide 1.8 mg	T2DM and high cardiovascular risk or disease (81.3% with CVD)	9,340 participants/ 3.8 years	32.5 kg/m², –2.3 kg	Reduction HR: 0.87; 95% CI: 0.78–0.97	No difference HR: 0.87; 95% CI: 0.73–1.05
SUSTAIN-6[20]	Semaglutide 1.0 mg	T2DM and high cardiovascular risk (83.0% with CVD)	3,297 participants/ 2.1 years	33.0 kg/m², –4.3 kg	Reduction HR: 0.74; 95% CI: 0.58–0.95	No difference HR: 1.11; 95% CI: 0.77–1.61
SELECT[21]	Semaglutide 2.4 mg	CVD and BMI >27 kg/m²	17,604 participants/ 3.3 years	33.4 kg/m², –9.1 kg	Reduction HR: 0.80; 95% CI: 0.72–0.90	No difference HR: 0.79; 95% CI: 0.60–1.03
STEP-HFpEF[22]	Semaglutide 2.4 mg	HF with EF ≥45% and BMI ≥30 kg/m²	529 participants/ 12 months	37.0 kg/m², –13.9 kg	Improvement in KCCQ	No difference (exploratory endpoint)
SUMMIT[23]	Tirzepatide 15 mg	HF with EF ≥50% and BMI ≥30 kg/m²	731 participants/ 2.3 years	38.2 kg/m², weight change of –13.9%	Reduction in cardiovascular death, worsening HF HR: 0.62; 95% CI: 0.41–0.95	Reduction HR: 0.44; 95% CI: 0.22–0.87
SURMOUNT-MMO[24] (NCT05556512)	Tirzepatide 15 mg	CVD or risk, BMI ≥27 kg/m²	15,374 participants enrolled	Trial is fully recruited and ongoing	Estimated completion date 2027	Not available

IMPACT ON ASSOCIATED COMORBITIES BY NUTRIENT-STIMULATED HORMONE AGENTS

Nutrient-stimulated hormone therapies provide benefits that extend far beyond weight reduction, offering significant protection against CV complications. In patients with T2DM at high CV risk or with established CVD, these agents lower the incidence of CVD, myocardial infarction, and stroke[18] **(Table 4)**. Importantly, their value is not confined to individuals with diabetes. In patients with ASCVD and a BMI ≥27 kg/m², semaglutide has been shown not only to induce substantial weight loss but also to reduce major adverse cardiovascular events (MACE).[21] Ongoing trials are evaluating whether tirzepatide can deliver similar benefits, both in people with T2DM[24] and in those with lower BMI thresholds (≥25 kg/m²).[25]

HFpEF is another area where NuSH therapies demonstrate promise. Semaglutide therapy has been associated with improved symptoms, enhanced physical capacity, and better exercise performance.[26] While the degree of benefit appeared to be proportional to the amount of weight lost,[22] emerging evidence suggests that additional weight-independent mechanisms may also contribute.[27] Importantly, the SELECT trial[21] provided the first randomized evidence that an obesity drug can reduce major CV events, with a 20% risk reduction in patients with established CV disease **(Table 4)**. Similarly, tirzepatide has shown encouraging results in patients with obesity and HFpEF, reducing the combined outcome of CVD and worsening HF, potentially expanding the therapeutic role of these agents in this high-risk group. A large CV outcomes trial (SURMOUNT-MMO)[24] is ongoing to determine its impact on CV morbidity and mortality **(Table 4)**.

SURGICAL MANAGEMENT OF OBESITY

Bariatric surgery is recognized in the various guidelines as an effective treatment option for patients with obesity who remain at high CV risk despite comprehensive lifestyle-based strategies. In such cases, surgical intervention serves not only to facilitate weight reduction but also to improve long-term cardiometabolic outcomes. To help identify suitable candidates, the guidelines recommend applying the lifetime CV risk calculator, which provides an estimate of both near-term and lifetime risk. This approach enables clinicians to better stratify individuals who would gain the most benefit from surgery and to guide decision-making beyond immediate weight concerns. By incorporating CV risk prediction into the assessment process, bariatric surgery is framed as part of a broader strategy aimed at lowering the burden of obesity-related CV disease rather than being limited to weight management alone.

FUTURE DIRECTIONS IN OBESITY MANAGEMENT

The search for more effective and tolerable treatments for obesity has led to significant advancements, with a range of new antiobesity medications currently in development. Building on the success of incretin-based medications such as liraglutide, semaglutide, and tirzepatide, new therapies, collectively referred to as NuSH medications, are targeting multiple hormonal pathways involved in appetite regulation and energy expenditure. These include dual and triple receptor agonists that combine GLP-1 with other pathways such as GIP and glucagon, which could offer enhanced therapeutic benefits.[10]

Oral formulations of GLP-1 receptor agonists, such as oral semaglutide and orforglipron, are also in advanced stages of development.[10] While oral delivery improves convenience, gastrointestinal side effects remain a concern. Additionally, therapies targeting amylin receptors, cannabinoid receptors, and mitochondrial uncouplers are being explored for their potential in reducing weight and improving metabolic profiles.[10]

Emerging combination therapies, such as cagrilintide with semaglutide or retatrutide (a triple GIP, GLP-1, and glucagon receptor agonist), have demonstrated promising results in clinical trials, with significant reductions in body weight.[10] As research progresses, these new treatments will provide clinicians with more personalized, effective options for managing obesity, focusing on long-term weight loss, metabolic improvement, and CV risk reduction.[10]

CONCLUSION

The field of obesity care has entered a transformative stage, offering an expanding array of strategies for diagnosis, weight reduction, and CV risk management. Novel therapies, including newer generation NuSH agents, improve cardiometabolic health and reduce major CV events in obesity with ASCVD or HFpEF. Additional treatments are in development. With obesity's high prevalence and CV burden, cardiologists play a central role. Key challenges persist in initiating and sustaining long-term therapies to manage this chronic condition effectively.

REFERENCES

1. Jensen MD, Ryan DH, Apovian CM, et al. 2013 AHA/ACC/TOS guideline for the management of overweight and obesity in adults: a report of the American College of Cardiology/American Heart Association Task Force on Practice Guidelines and The Obesity Society. J Am Coll Cardiol. 2014;63(25 Part B):2985-3023.
2. Koskinas KC, Van Craenenbroeck EM, Antoniades C, et al. Obesity and cardiovascular disease: an ESC clinical consensus statement. Eur Heart J. 2024;45(38):4063-98.
3. Gilbert O, Gulati M, Gluckman TJ, et al. 2025 Concise Clinical Guidance: an ACC Expert Consensus Statement on medical weight management for optimization of cardiovascular health: a report of the American College of Cardiology Solution Set Oversight Committee. J Am Coll Cardiol. 2025;86(7):536-55.
4. Powell-Wiley TM, Poirier P, Burke LE, et al. Obesity and cardiovascular disease: a scientific statement from the American Heart Association. Circulation. 2021;143(21):e984-1010.
5. Wing R, Bolin P, Brancati FL, et al. Cardiovascular effects of intensive lifestyle intervention in type 2 diabetes. N Engl J Med. 2013;369:145-54.
6. Yurista SR, Eder RA, Feeley M, et al. A closer look at ACC/AHA and ESC guidelines for managing obesity and overweight in adults. JACC Adv. 2023;2(7):100570.
7. Arnett DK, Blumenthal RS, Albert MA, et al. 2019 ACC/AHA guideline on the primary prevention of cardiovascular disease: a report of the American College of Cardiology/American Heart Association Task Force on Clinical Practice Guidelines. J Am Coll Cardiol. 2019;74:e177-232.
8. Visseren FLJ, Mach F, Smulders YM, et al. 2021 ESC guidelines on cardiovascular disease prevention in clinical practice. Eur Heart J. 2021;42:3227-337.
9. Hall KD, Kahan S. Maintenance of lost weight and long-term management of obesity. Med Clin. 2018;102(1):183-97.
10. Chao AM, Taylor S, Moore M, et al. Evolving approaches for pharmacological therapy of obesity. Annu Rev Pharmacol Toxicol. 2025;65:169-89.
11. Pi-Sunyer X, Astrup A, Fujioka K, et al. A randomized, controlled trial of 3.0 mg of liraglutide in weight management. N Engl J Med. 2015;373(1):11-22.
12. Wilding JPH, Batterham RL, Calanna S, et al. Once-weekly semaglutide in adults with overweight or obesity. N Engl J Med. 2021;384:989-1002.
13. Kushner RF, Calanna S, Davies M, et al. Semaglutide 2.4 mg for the treatment of obesity: key elements of the STEP trials 1 to 5. Obesity. 2020;28:1050-61.
14. Garvey WT, Frias JP, Jastreboff AM, et al. Tirzepatide once weekly for the treatment of obesity in people with type 2 diabetes (SURMOUNT-2): a double-blind, randomised,

multicentre, placebo-controlled, phase 3 trial. Lancet. 2023;402:613-26.
15. Wadden TA, Chao AM, Machineni S, et al. Tirzepatide after intensive lifestyle intervention in adults with overweight or obesity: the SURMOUNT-3 phase 3 trial. Nat Med. 2023;29:2909-18.
16. Aronne LJ, Sattar N, Horn DB, et al. Continued treatment with tirzepatide for maintenance of weight reduction in adults with obesity: the SURMOUNT-4 randomized clinical trial. JAMA. 2024;331:38-48.
17. Clément K, van den Akker E, Argente J, et al. Efficacy and safety of setmelanotide, an MC4R agonist, in individuals with severe obesity due to LEPR or POMC deficiency: single-arm, open-label, multicentre, phase 3 trials. Lancet Diabetes Endocrinol. 2020;8:960-70.
18. Gerstein HC, Colhoun HM, Dagenais GR, et al. Dulaglutide and cardiovascular outcomes in type 2 diabetes (REWIND): a double-blind, randomised placebo-controlled trial. Lancet. 2019;394:121-30.
19. Marso SP, Daniels GH, Brown-Frandsen K, et al. Liraglutide and cardiovascular outcomes in type 2 diabetes. N Engl J Med. 2016;375:311-22.
20. Marso SP, Bain SC, Consoli A, et al. Semaglutide and cardiovascular outcomes in patients with type 2 diabetes. N Engl J Med. 2016;375:1834-44.
21. Lincoff AM, Brown-Frandsen K, Colhoun HM, et al. Semaglutide and cardiovascular outcomes in obesity without diabetes. N Engl J Med. 2023;389:2221-32.
22. Borlaug BA, Kitzman DW, Davies MJ, et al. Semaglutide in HFpEF across obesity class and by body weight reduction: a prespecified analysis of the STEP-HFpEF trial. Nat Med. 2023;29:2358-65.
23. Packer M, Zile MR, Kramer CM, et al. Tirzepatide for heart failure with preserved ejection fraction and obesity. N Engl J Med. 2025;392:427-37.
24. National Library of Medicine. (2024). A Study of Tirzepatide (LY3298176) on the Reduction on Morbidity and Mortality in Adults With Obesity (SURMOUNT-MMO). [online] Available from https://clinicaltrials.gov/study/NCT05556512. [Last accessed January, 2026].
25. Sattar N, García-Pérez LE, Rodríguez A, et al. Tirzepatide and cardiometabolic parameters in obesity: summary of current evidence. Diabetes Obes Metab. 2025;27(10):5386-92.
26. Kosiborod MN, Abildstrøm SZ, Borlaug BA, et al. Semaglutide in patients with heart failure with preserved ejection fraction and obesity. N Engl J Med. 2023;389:1069-84.
27. Petrie MC, Borlaug BA, Butler J, et al. Semaglutide and NT-proBNP in obesity-related HFpEF: insights from the STEP-HFpEF program. J Am Coll Cardiol. 2024;84:27-40.

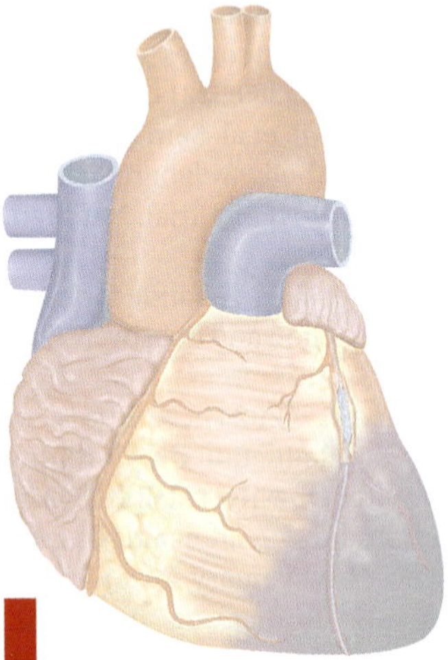

5

CHAPTER

ESC Consensus Statement for Obesity and CVD Management: What is Applicable for Indians?

Satyendra Tewari, Prashant Gautam

INTRODUCTION

Obesity is currently a global health epidemic and a disease in itself. The European Society of Cardiology (ESC) Clinical Consensus Statement on Obesity and Cardiovascular Disease (CVD) illustrates the complex interaction between obesity, various cardiovascular risk factors, and manifestations.[1] While these guidelines are derived largely from European data, the principles are very much applicable to Indian population, where obesity and CVD are increasing at alarming rates. Rapid urbanization, changes in dietary pattern, and physical inactivity have led to the increase in obesity and its related cardiovascular manifestations in India. This chapter discusses the applicability of the ESC guidelines in the Indian context, determining potential areas of prevention, early detection, and management of cardiovascular risk due to obesity.

DEFINITION OF OBESITY

Obesity is defined as excessive body fat accumulation that can impair health. The World Health Organization (WHO) classification of obesity is based on body mass index (BMI), which is calculated as BMI = weight (kg)/height (m^2) **(Table 1)**.

Asian Indians have higher body fat for a given BMI, and comorbidities such as type 2 diabetes occur at lower BMI levels than in other populations.[2,3] Therefore, obesity in Asian Indians is defined as BMI ≥25 kg/m^2 (overweight: 23–24.9 kg/m^2) and abdominal obesity as waist circumference ≥90 cm in men and ≥80 cm in women.[4]

TABLE 1: WHO classification for adults.

Category	*BMI (kg/m²)*
Underweight	<18.5
Normal weight	18.5–24.9
Overweight	25.0–29.9
Obesity (class I)	30.0–34.9
Obesity (class II)	35.0–39.9
Obesity (class III/severe/morbid)	≥40.0

EPIDEMIOLOGY AND INDIAN CONTEXT

According to WHO, in 2022, 1 in 8 people in the world were living with obesity and 2.5 billion adults (18 years and older) were overweight. Of these, 890 million were living with obesity.[5] In India, the National Family Health Survey (NFHS-5) reports that nearly one in four adults is overweight or obese.[6] According to recent Indian Council of Medical Research (ICMR-INDIAB) data, more than 250 million Indians live with generalized obesity and over 350 million with abdominal obesity.[7]

PATHOPHYSIOLOGY AND RISK FACTORS

Obesity results from an imbalance of energy intake and energy expenditure. Although genetics and biology affect personal risk of obesity, it is the prevailing environmental and societal factors that are mainly responsible for the global epidemic. Indians develop metabolic complications at lower BMI levels compared to Western populations. This is primarily due to a greater proportion of visceral fat, higher insulin resistance, and unique genetic predispositions. This highlights the relevance of waist circumference, waist-to-hip circumference ratio, and waist-to-height ratio over BMI as more reliable measures of CVD risk in India.

OBESITY AND CARDIOVASCULAR RISK FACTORS

The ESC statement emphasizes obesity as a complex, multifactorial disease, and a major cause of cardiovascular morbidity and mortality.

- *Type 2 diabetes mellitus (T2DM):* Nearly 80% of patients with T2DM are overweight or obese. Indians are predisposed to early diabetes due to their genetic makeup.
- *Hypertension:* Risk rises linearly with BMI, and obesity contributes to resistant hypertension.
- *Dyslipidemia:* Defined by the presence of high triglycerides, low HDL cholesterol, and small dense LDL particles, this pattern is very prevalent in South Asians.
- *Obstructive sleep apnea (OSA):* Extremely common in the obese population, OSA exacerbates hypertension, heart failure, and arrhythmias.

CLINICAL MANIFESTATIONS OF OBESITY-RELATED CARDIOVASCULAR DISEASE

According to the ESC consensus, obesity influences nearly every aspect of cardiovascular pathology **(Fig. 1)**:

- *Atherosclerotic cardiovascular disease (ASCVD):* Accelerated atherosclerosis leads to premature CAD, MI, and stroke. Recent studies have shown that obesity is associated with high ASCVD risk in Indians.[8-10]
- *Heart failure (HF):* Both HF with reduced EF (HFrEF) and HFpEF are linked to obesity. In India, the prevalence of heart failure with preserved ejection fraction (HFpEF) linked to obesity is rising rapidly.[11]
- *Arrhythmias:* Atrial fibrillation is particularly common, and obesity increases recurrence after ablation.
- *Thromboembolism:* Obese individuals are at greater risk of venous thromboembolism, DVT, and pulmonary embolism.
- *Valvular disease:* Obesity may accelerate calcific aortic stenosis progression.

Management Strategies

The ESC recommends organized approach to obesity management, starting with lifestyle modification as the foundation.

Early Screening

Use lower BMI thresholds for screening and intervention, measure waist circumference routinely, and initiate early screening for diabetes, hypertension, dyslipidemia, and obstructive sleep apnea in all overweight or obese adults.

Lifestyle Interventions

- *ESC recommendations:* Lifestyle modification is the cornerstone, including calorie restriction (500–750

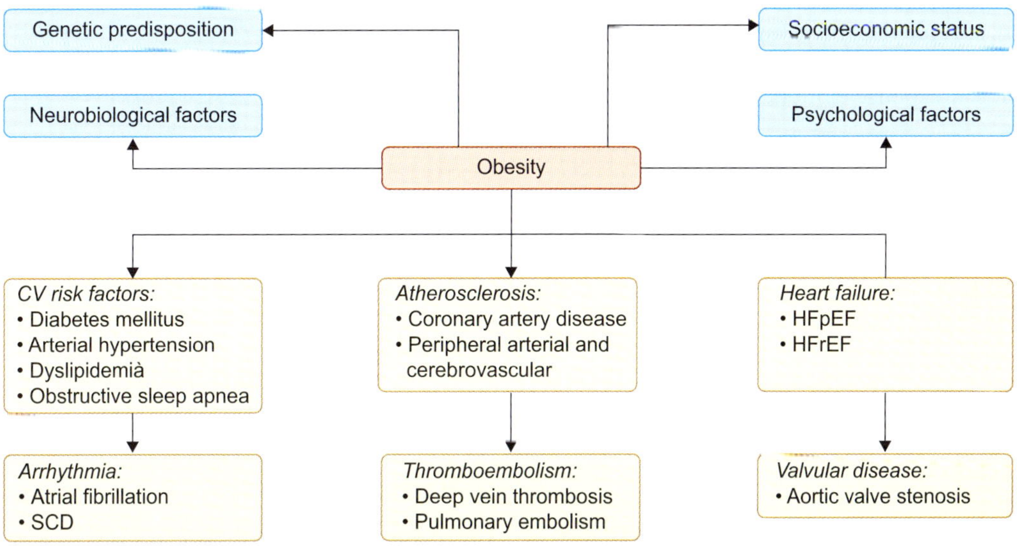

Fig. 1: Impact of obesity on cardiovascular system.

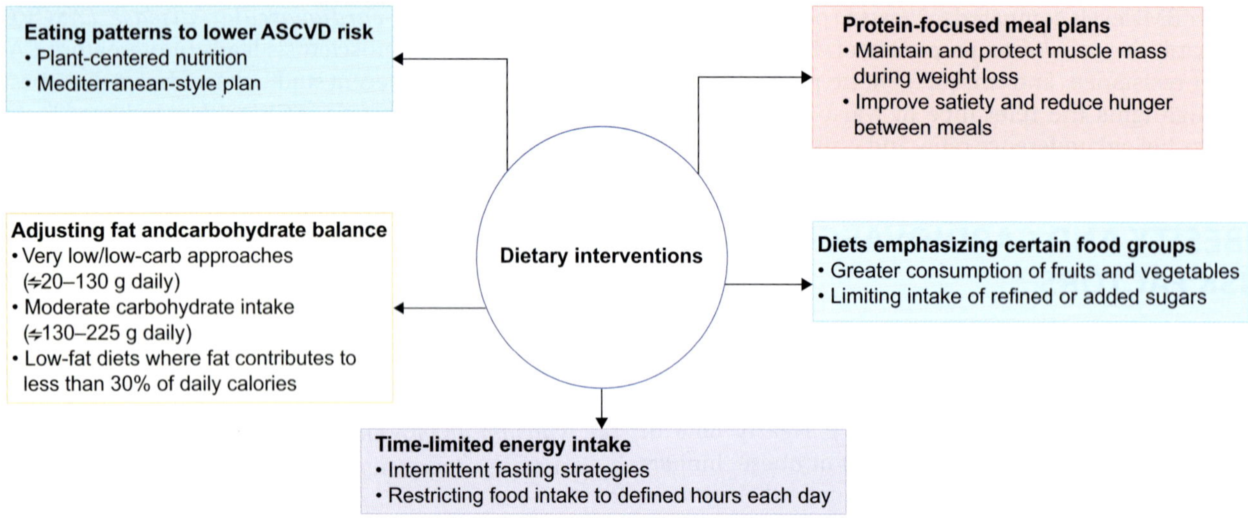

Fig. 2: Dietary interventions for obesity and CVD management.

kcal/day deficit), at least 150 minutes of moderate-intensity physical activity per week, and behavioral interventions.

- *Indian adaptation:* For Indian population, traditional diets rich in lentils, vegetables, and whole grains should be promoted while discouraging refined carbohydrates, deep-fried foods, and sugar-sweetened beverages **(Fig. 2)**. Physical activity interventions should leverage culturally acceptable options such as yoga, brisk walking, and cycling.

Pharmacological Approaches

- *Global perspective:* Approved agents include orlistat, liraglutide, semaglutide, tirzepatide, naltrexone-bupropion, and phentermine-topiramate.
- *Indian context:*
    - *Orlistat* is inexpensive but has gastrointestinal side effects.
    - *GLP-1 receptor agonists* (liraglutide and semaglutide) are highly effective but costly. Injectable semaglutide was recently approved in India.
    - *Tirzepatide***,** a dual GIP/GLP-1 agonist, shows >20% weight loss and significant cardiometabolic improvements.

Bariatric and Metabolic Surgery

Bariatric surgery (sleeve gastrectomy and Roux-en-Y gastric bypass) is recommended for patients with BMI ≥40 or ≥35 with comorbidities. While effective, barriers in India include cost, limited specialized centers, and lack of awareness.

PUBLIC HEALTH AND POLICY IMPLICATIONS

ESC Perspective

The ESC emphasizes systemic approaches, such as taxing sugar-sweetened beverages, restricting marketing of junk food, urban planning to encourage walking and cycling, and early childhood interventions.

Indian Adaptation

- *Government programs:* Initiatives such as the *Fit India Movement* and *Ayushman Bharat* offer platforms for obesity interventions.
- *Schools and workplaces:* Nutrition education, mandatory physical education, and corporate wellness programs can promote healthy behavior.

LIMITATIONS

ESC guidelines are broad but have limitations in their direct use in Indian populations. Socioeconomic inequalities restrict access to competent medical care, organized weight-reduction programs, and expensive pharmacologic agents. Cultural food habits, restricted public knowledge, and unavailability of open spaces for physical exercises further restrict use.

CONCLUSION

Obesity is major contributor of cardiovascular morbidity and mortality in India. The ESC consensus provides current evidence for obesity and CVD management but requires careful adaptation to Indian context. Comprehensive management strategies including early detection, culturally modified lifestyle interventions, cost-effective pharmacological strategies, and widespread public health policies are critical to CVD prevention and optimal management. Eliminating obesity will demand collaboration across healthcare providers, policymakers, and communities to reduce the burden of cardiovascular disease and improve population health.

REFERENCES

1. Koskinas KC, Van Craenenbroeck EM, Antoniades C, et al. Obesity and cardiovascular disease: an ESC clinical consensus statement. Eur Heart J. 2024;45:4063-98.
2. Dudeja V, Misra A, Pandey RM, et al. BMI does not accurately predict overweight in Asian Indians in northern India. Br J Nutr. 2001;86(1):105-12.
3. Vikram NK, Misra A, Pandey RM, et al. Anthropometry and body composition in northern Asian Indian patients with type 2 diabetes: receiver operating characteristics (ROC) curve analysis of body mass index with percentage body fat as standard. Diabetes Nutr Metab. 2003;16(1):32-40.
4. Misra A, Vikram NK, Ghosh A, et al.; India Obesity Commission Members. Revised definition of obesity in Asian Indians living in India. Diabetes Metab Syndr. 2025;19(1):102989.
5. World Health Organization. Obesity and overweight fact sheet. [online] Available from https://www.who.int/news-room/fact-sheets/detail/obesity-and-overweight [Last accessed January, 2026].
6. Ministry of Health and Family Welfare, Government of India. National Family Health Survey-5 (NFHS-5); 2021.
7. Indian Council of Medical Research. Indian Council of Medical Research (ICMR) Guidelines for Obesity Management; 2022.
8. Chaithra S, Sangeetha MD, Sreenath MPK. Cardiovascular Risk Assessment and its Components Using 10-year Atherosclerotic Cardiovascular Disease Risk Score Plus among Indian Population: A Hospital-based Cross-sectional Study. J Clin Preventive Cardiol. 2024;13(4):80-6.
9. Puri R, Bansal M, Mehta V, et al. Lipid Association of India 2023 update on cardiovascular risk assessment and lipid management in Indian patients: Consensus statement IV. J Clin Lipidol. 2024;18(3):e351-73.
10. Loitongbam L, Surin WR. The Rising Burden of Cardiovascular Disease and Thrombosis in India: An Epidemiological Review. Cureus. 2024;16(11): e73786.
11. Chandramouli C, Tay WT, Bamadhaj NS, et al. Association of obesity with heart failure outcomes in 11 Asian countries: A cohort study. PLOS Med. 2019;16(12):e1002916.

6

CHAPTER

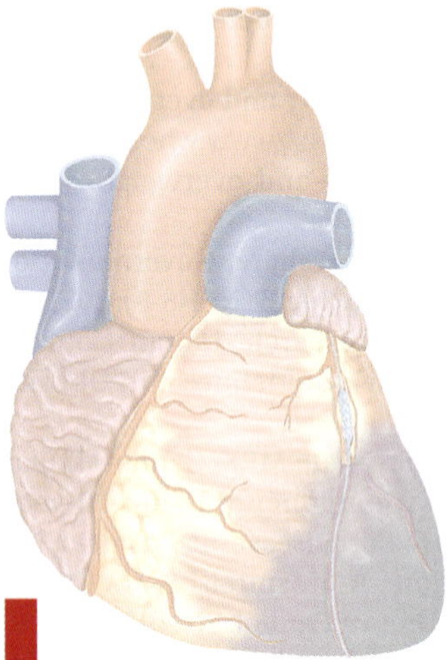

Association Between Autoimmunity, Obesity, and Atherosclerosis/ Cardiovascular Disease

Raj Wasan, Juliana Spanova, Nayna Nanda, Anita N Wasan, Anil Nanda, Navin C Nanda, HK Chopra

INTRODUCTION

Autoimmune disease, obesity and atherosclerosis/ cardiovascular disease are all significant health concerns each in their own right. It is important from a therapeutic standpoint to look into the possible associations between these three disease states. Autoimmune diseases consist of a group of conditions that result from an abnormal immune response that involves the formation of autoantibodies, overproliferation of B and T lymphocytes, and immune system dysregulation.[1] These diseases result in inflammation and organ dysfunction. Laboratory testing is the main diagnostic method to diagnose autoimmune disease; however, the association between the autoantibodies and specific pathological diseases is unclear. Autoimmune diseases affect patients of all ages, particularly women.[2] The pathogenesis of autoimmunity is multifactorial; this means that it can result from a combination of genetic disposition, lifestyle factors, as well as environmental exposures.[1] The purpose of this chapter is to discuss the association and relationship of autoimmunity with obesity and atherosclerosis/ cardiovascular disease and their therapeutic implications.

AUTOIMMUNITY AND OBESITY

There have been studies that have examined the link between obesity and the development of autoimmune disease.[1] Obesity is highly prevalent globally and is associated with increased mortality.[3] Obesity is also a risk factor for the development of atherosclerosis. It has been shown that there can be a link between obesity and the prevalence of most autoimmune diseases with the exception of systemic lupus erythematosus (SLE).[1] However, the causal link between obesity and autoimmune disease is not clear. There is an increased risk between an elevated basal metabolic index (BMI) and hypothyroidism, psoriasis, rheumatoid arthritis, and type 1 diabetes. Adipose tissue, specifically visceral and subepicardial, has been shown to secrete cytokines that are inflammatory.[3]

OBESITY AND ATHEROSCLEROSIS/ CARDIOVASCULAR DISEASE

Obesity causes chronic inflammation that results in atherosclerosis and cardiovascular disease. Patients with increased visceral and subepicardial adipose tissue are at an increased risk for atherosclerosis/cardiovascular disease, as well as diabetes, which is an independent risk factor for cardiovascular disease.[4] Adipose tissue is not only an energy store, as there is also an endocrine function playing a role in the release of cytokines that are involved in inflammation and immunity.[5] Obesity activates aldosterone and chemokines, which, in turn, cause oxidative stress, insulin resistance, and abnormalities in the metabolism of lipids. The chemokines include but are not limited to leptin, interleukin 6 (IL-6), and monocyte chemoattractant protein. Aldosterone contributes to the aggregation of platelets, thrombosis and fibrosis.[4]

Tumor necrosis factor (TNF) is a proinflammatory cytokine that has a broad range of biological activities, including playing a crucial role in driving the systemic effects of cancer: cachexia and "B symptoms" (fevers, chills, and night sweats). When released by adipocytes, it attracts immune cells to the tissue, which further promotes the inflammatory process by secreting more chemokines, leading to a positive feedback loop of chronic inflammation. Interleukin-1 beta (IL-1β) induces inflammation by promoting the expression of inflammatory genes in cells throughout the body, and Interleukin-18 (IL-18) works synergistically with other interleukins to upregulate the expression of other inflammatory cytokines. IL-1β, TNF and IL-18 are all secreted by adipose tissue, and together result in hyperpermeability of vascular endothelial junctions and endothelial cell dysfunction.[5]

Leptin is an example of a cytokine released from adipose tissue that is implicated in many immune pathways, including the production of Th1 cytokines, which include IFN-G and IL-2.[5] Th1 cells, also known as helper T-cells, are a subset of T-cells activated by macrophages that secrete IL-2, a key interleukin that upregulates cytotoxic T-cell activity as well as B-cell proliferation in the body. Increased leptin can increase the monocyte and macrophage secretion of TNF-α, MCP-1 and IL-6, which are inflammatory cytokines. Leptin can also increase the adhesion molecules such as VCAM-1, ICAM-1 and E-selectin, which increase vascular permeability, monocyte adhesion to vascular cell walls, and atheroma formation Leptin promotes the expression of PAI-1 which inhibits fibrinolysis. Increased concentrations of plasma leptin correspond to increased coronary artery calcifications and myocardial infarctions.[4]

The amount of IL-6, a proinflammatory cytokine, correlates with the amount of adipose tissue and increases the expression of TNF-α and MCP-1. It decreases lipoprotein lipase activity, which, in turn, then increases cellular uptake of lipids contributing to the formation of plaques. In overweight individuals, an IL-6 concentration >1 pg/mL is predictive of coronary artery disease. If the level of IL-6 can be reduced to <1.65 ng/mL, studies have shown a reduction in major cardiovascular events. MCP-1, also known as monocyte chemoattractant protein 1, is increased in patients with obesity. MCP-1 attracts monocytes that secrete IL-6 and TNF-α. Studies have shown that increased levels of MCP-1 are associated with cardiovascular disease.[4]

AUTOIMMUNITY AND ATHEROSCLEROSIS/ CARDIOVASCULAR DISEASE

There is more evidence that shows the association between autoimmune disease and cardiac disease. There is a risk of cardiovascular disease with autoimmune diseases such as SLE, connective tissue autoimmune diseases, and/or rheumatoid arthritis.[6] One comprehensive population-based study of 22 million individuals in the United Kingdom found that of the individuals who developed cardiovascular disease, those with a diagnosed autoimmune condition had nearly double the risk of developing cardiovascular disease before age of 65, years with the highest risk seen in systemic sclerosis, SLE, Addison's disease, and type 1 diabetes mellitus. The risk of having an autoimmune condition in the development of atherosclerosis was found to be akin to that of a 20 mm Hg increase in systolic blood pressure or a diagnosis of Type 2 diabetes. This is consistent with a >50% increased risk of atherosclerotic heart disease.[7] Abnormalities in leukocyte function and/or inflammatory cytokines can cause vascular issues. Endothelial dysfunction as well as abnormalities in B- and T-cell functions in autoimmune disease can contribute to atherosclerosis. Autoantibodies can also be involved in cardiovascular systemic inflammation, but it is unclear as to the functional mechanism. Anti-inflammatory therapies can help reduce the risk of atherosclerosis, especially in patients with autoimmune disease.[5] Autoimmunity is also associated with myocarditis.[8] It is important to control risk factors, including dyslipidemia and hypertension as well as lifestyle risks, in those patients with autoimmune disease.

THERAPEUTICS

Treatment of obesity involves a multifactorial approach. Lifestyle modifications, including diet and exercise, are traditional in reducing weight. One possible treatment to reduce the risk of cardiac disease is immunomodulatory therapy.[6] Some treatment goals can be the reduction of Th17 activity and promoting T-regulatory cell expansion.[5] These can reduce inflammation associated with obesity and possibly reduce the pathology associated with autoimmunity.

The ketogenic diet is a high fat, low carbohydrate diet that results in ketosis, which produces ketone bodies, such as beta-hydroxybutyrate.[7] Beta-hydroxybutyrate can help reduce inflammation associated with certain autoimmune diseases.[5] In addition, several antiobesity medications act on the central nervous system.[9] One of the oldest weight loss medications is phentermine. Phentermine is a sympathomimetic medication that increases norepinephrine in the hypothalamus. Phentermine is also combined with topiramate for weight loss, which both do by reducing appetite. Naltrexone-bupropion acts on the central nervous system to reduce appetite. In addition to central nervous system medications, intragastrointestinal medications are used to treat obesity. Orlistat is a medication that blocks the absorption and digestion of approximately 30% of ingested fat. Oral cellulose-citric acid hydrogel expands the stomach, creating a sense of satiety.[9]

Newer pharmacotherapies have revolutionized therapies for obesity. Glucagon-like peptide 1 (GLP-1) is used to treat diabetes by increasing insulin secretion. The GLP-1 reduces the release of glucagon and diminishes gastric emptying and motility, thus, decreasing appetite. GLP-1 also has anti-inflammatory activities.[10] Several GLP-1 medications are United States Food and Drug Administration (US FDA) approved including liraglutide and semiglutide.

Some pharmaceutical medications in development for obesity include small molecule GLP-1 medications, such as danuglipron. Amylin, a pancreatic islet cell hormone which delays gastric emptying, is also in development.[9] Glucagon, though it increases blood glucose, has been shown to be effective in increasing satiety. Glucagon, amylin, and GLP-1 combination medications are currently in development.

Promising data exist regarding immune therapies for cardiovascular disease.[11] Anti-IL-1 therapy, anakinra, has been associated with positive clinical benefit in Kawasaki disease.[12] Canakinumab, an IL-1B antagonist, has been associated with a reduced recurrence rate of cardiovascular events compared to placebo.[13] Ziltivekimab, an anti-IL-6 therapy, is currently being investigated for the treatment of cardiovascular disease due to improved inflammatory biomarkers, such as C-reactive protein, with therapy.[14] However, low dose methotrexate therapy did not have a significant beneficial effect on cardiovascular events compared to placebo.[15]

CONCLUSION

In conclusion, although there is not a clear link between autoimmunity and obesity, there are links between autoimmunity and atherosclerosis/cardiovascular disease as well as obesity and atherosclerosis/cardiac disease. Multiple current therapies for obesity, autoimmunity, and inflammation exist. However, additional research is needed with regards to anti-inflammatory and auto-immune modulatory therapies for cardiovascular disease.

REFERENCES

1. Spatocco I, Mele G, De Rosa G, et al. Obesity as a risk factor for autoimmune diseases: a systematic review and Meta-analysis. Obesity (Silver Spring). 2026;34(1): 36-50.
2. Pisetsky DS. Pathogenesis of autoimmune disease. Nat Rev Nephrol. 2023;19(8):509-24.
3. Xunliang Li, Jie Zhu, Wenman Zhao, et al. The Causal Effect of Obesity on the Risk of 15 Autoimmune Diseases: A Mendelian Randomization Study. Obes Facts. 2023;16(6):598-605.
4. Henning RJ. Obesity and obesity-induced inflammatory disease contribute to atherosclerosis: a review of the pathophysiology and treatment of obesity. Am J Cardiovasc Dis. 2021;11(4):504-29.
5. Colamatteo A, Fusco C, Matarese A, et al. Obesity and Autoimmunity Epidemic: The Role of Immunometabolism. Annu Rev Nutr. 2025;45(1):115-40.
6. Porsch, F., Binder, C.J. Autoimmune diseases and atherosclerotic cardiovascular disease. Nat Rev Cardiol. 2024;21:780-807.
7. Conrad N, Verbeke G, Molenberghs G, et al. Autoimmune diseases and cardiovascular risk: a population-based study on 19 autoimmune diseases and 12 cardiovascular diseases in 22 million individuals in the UK. Lancet. 2022;400(10354):733-43.
8. Won T, Song E, Kalinoski H, et al. Autoimmune myocarditis, old dogs and new tricks. Circ Research. 2024;134(12):1767-90.
9. Gudzune K, Kushner R. Medications for obesity. JAMA. 2024;332(7):571-84.
10. Jastreboff A, Kushner R. New frontiers in obesity treatment: GLP-1 and nascent nutrient-stimulated hormone-based therapeutics. Annu Rev Med. 2023;74:125-39.
11. Ridker P, Luscher T. Anti-inflammatory therapies for cardiovascular disease. Eur Heart J. 2014;35(27):1782-91.
12. Ferrera G, Giani T, Caparello M, et al. Anakinra for treatment-Resistant Kawasaki disease: Evidence from a literature review. Peds Drugs. 2020;22(6):645-52.
13. Ridker P, Everett BM, Thuren T, et al. Antiinflammatory therapy with canakinumab for atherosclerotic disease. N Engl J Med. 2017;377(12):1119-31.
14. Ridker P, Devalaraja M, Baeres FMM, et al. IL-6 inhibition with ziltivekimab in patients at high atherosclerotic risk (RESCUE): a double-blind, randomised, placebo-controlled, phase 2 trial. Lancet. 2021;397(10289):2060-9.
15. Ridker P, Everett BM, Pradhan A, et al. Low-dose methotrexate for the prevention of atherosclerotic events. N Engl J Med. 2019;380(8):752-62.

7

CHAPTER

Obesity, Cardiometabolic Risk, and Cardiovascular Disease: The Deadly Triumvirate

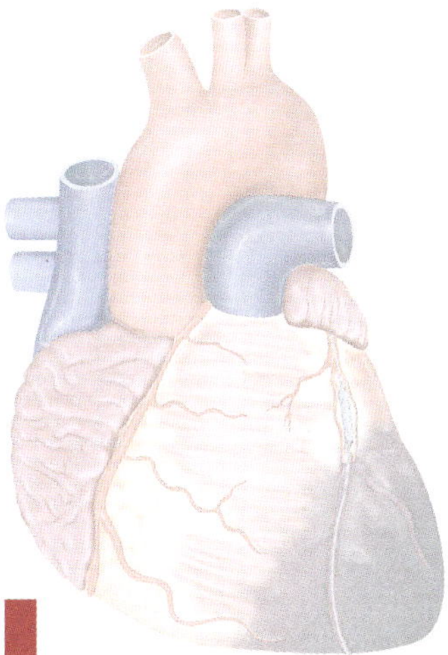

Rajeev Gupta

INTRODUCTION

The World Health Organization (WHO) defines obesity as a chronic complex disease with excessive fat deposits that can impair health.[1] Obesity also has a sociocultural definition that views body fatness as a symbol of health, beauty, status, or wealth, and in recent years as a symbol of ill-health, gluttony, and deprivation.[2] This condition is marked by excessive body fat accumulation, typically assessed using body mass index (BMI).[1] Adiposity refers to the amount and distribution of body fat, particularly visceral fat around organs, which is more metabolically active and more harmful than subcutaneous fat.[3] Both are influenced by genetics, diet, physical inactivity, and environmental factors.[4]

Excess adiposity, especially visceral fat, promotes insulin resistance, dyslipidemia [high triglycerides, low high-density lipoprotein (HDL) cholesterol], and hypertension.[4] Obesity often clusters with metabolic syndrome components: Abdominal obesity, raised blood pressure (BP), high blood glucose, and abnormal lipids, amplifying cardiovascular risk and contributing to atherosclerosis, arterial plaque buildup, and increased risk of acute coronary syndromes and stroke.[5] The adipose tissue also releases proinflammatory cytokines (e.g., IL-2a, IL-6, and TNF-α), which exacerbate vascular damage and endothelial dysfunction.[5] In this review, we shall present data on obesity and adiposity epidemiology with special focus on India, describe escalating cardiometabolic risk and cardiovascular conditions with increasing adiposity, and briefly dwell on the management of obesity for the prevention of cardiovascular disease (CVD) and associated multiple vascular morbidities.

OBESITY AND ADIPOSITY EPIDEMIOLOGY

Obesity has been defined as BMI ≥30 kg/m^2 by the WHO,[1] while the Asian consensus considers BMI ≥25 kg/m^2 as the marker of obesity and ≥23 kg/m^2 as overweight.[6,7] Adiposity encompasses total body fat and its distribution, with central (visceral) fat posing greater risks than peripheral (subcutaneous) fat due to metabolic effects.[5] Globally, in 2022, over 1 billion people lived with obesity, affecting one in eight individuals.[8] Adults overweight (BMI ≥25 kg/m^2) reached 2.5 billion (43%), with 890 million obese (16%). Among children under 5 years, 35 million were overweight in 2024; for ages 5–19 years, 390 million were overweight, including 160 million obese.[8] Trends show adult obesity doubling since 1990 and adolescent rates quadrupling. Projections indicate a 115% rise in adults with obesity to 1.13 billion by 2030.[8] Overweight and obesity prevalence may increase by 30.7% in 2050, nearing 60% globally.[8,9]

Regionally, overweight varies by 31% in Southeast Asia and Africa and up to 67% in the Americas.[8] Asia hosts nearly half of the overweight children under 5 years of age. Adiposity epidemiology highlights higher central fat in men and certain ethnic groups, linked to cardiometabolic risks; global body fat percentage averages vary, with BMI as a common proxy despite limitations in capturing distribution.[7] Socioeconomic development, urbanization, and unhealthy diet drive this epidemic, with low- and middle-income countries seeing rapid increases.[7,10] The global burden of obesity is shown in **Figure 1**.

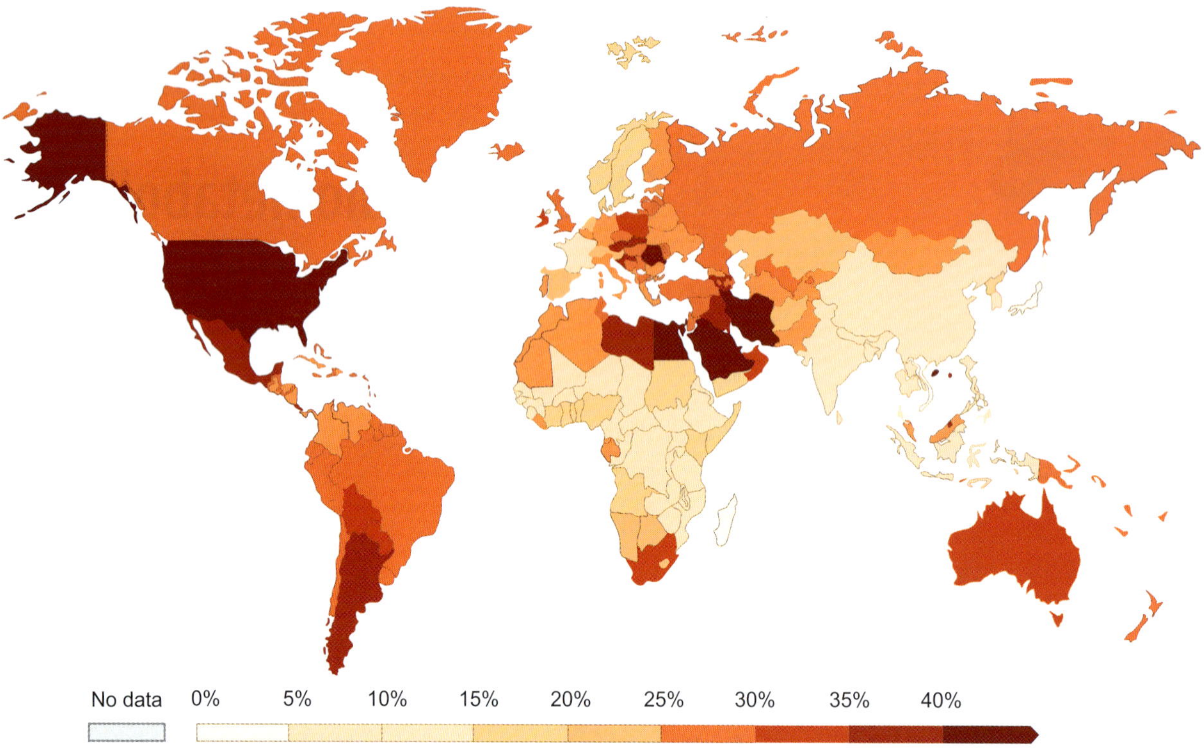

Fig. 1: Global burden of obesity in the year 2022. Estimated prevalence of obesity (BMI >30 kg/m^2) based on general population surveys and statistical modeling.
Source: Our World in Data. Available at Our World in Data. (2022). Data: Obesity in adults. [online] Available from https://ourworldindata.org/grapher/share-of-adults-defined-as-obese?time=latest&overlay=download-vis. [Last accessed January, 2025].

Obesity has emerged as an important problem in India, and Our World in Data site has reported increasing obesity from 1990 to 2021 from <2 to 7.2% presently, using the older WHO criteria of BMI ≥30 kg/m^2.[8] However, as the current guidelines have suggested a lower BMI for the classification of obesity in India,[7] either ≥25 kg/m^2 (or even ≥23 kg/m^2), the burden is significantly greater. In the nationwide ICMR-INDIAB study, obesity (BMI ≥25 kg/m^2) was observed in 28.6% of participants [95% confidence interval (CI), 26.9–30.3%].[11] This has been extrapolated to 254 million individuals (CI 239–269 million) with generalized obesity in India. There is significant regional variation of obesity, and state-level prevalence rates range from 11.6 to 53.3% with more individuals with obesity in northern and southern Indian states **(Figs. 2A and B)**. Obesity is widely prevalent in the urban regions of the whole country **(Figs. 2A and B)**.[11] In the Jaipur Heart Watch (JHW) study, we reported an exponential increase in the prevalence of obesity (BMI ≥25 kg/m^2) from 20% in the early 1990s to >40% by the mid-2010s.[12]

Abdominal obesity is considered a more important marker of cardiometabolic risk and is widely prevalent in India **(Figs. 2A and B)**.[7,11] It has been defined as high abdominal circumference with Asian-specific criteria of >90 cm in men and >85 cm in women. It has also been classified according to the raised waist–hip ratio (WHR) of >0.9 in men and >0.8 in women. According to the ICMR-INDIAB-17 study, it is more prevalent than generalized obesity in India, with a prevalence rate of 39.5% (CI 37.7–41.4%).[11] This has been extrapolated to 351 million individuals (CI 335–368 million) with abdominal obesity in the country. There is significant state-level variation ranging from 18.4 to 61.2% with higher prevalence in northern, central, and southern Indian states **(Figs. 2A and B)**. Similar to generalized obesity, abdominal obesity is highly prevalent in all the urban regions of the country **(Figs. 2A and B)**. There is a strong linear correlation between generalized obesity and abdominal obesity (Pearson's r >0.9), and many epidemiologists prefer BMI as a convenient measure of obesity instead of abdominal obesity due to greater interobserver variation in the measurement of the latter.[1]

OBESITY, ABDOMINAL OBESITY, AND CARDIOMETABOLIC RISK

Obesity and adiposity as the drivers of cardiovascular risk in India were reported in the JHW studies three decades

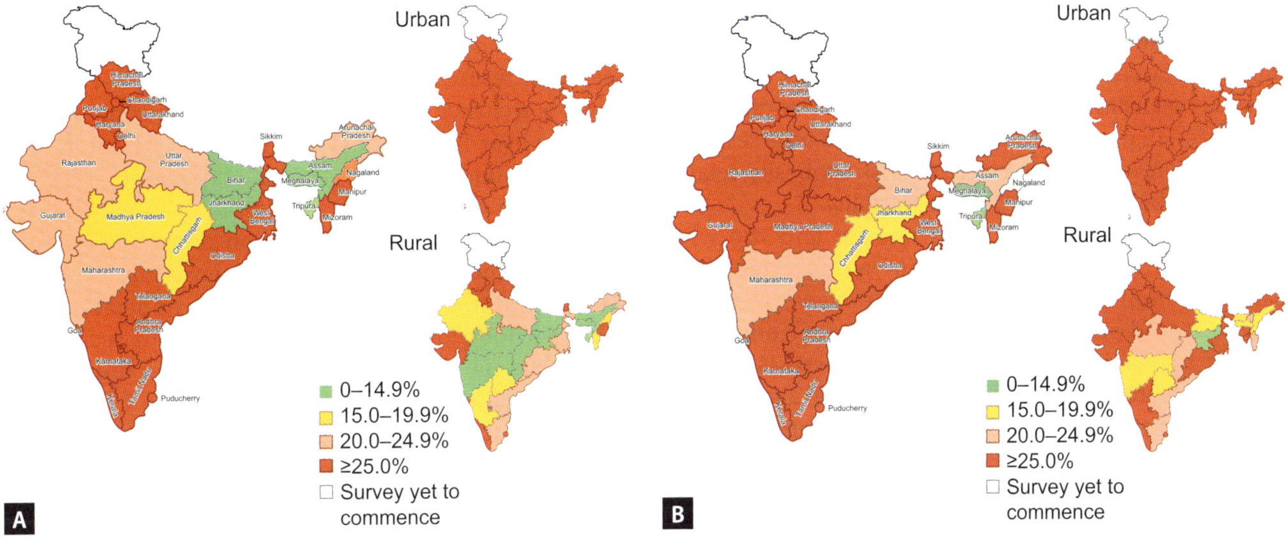

Figs. 2A and B: ICMR-INDIAB-17 study on prevalence of generalized obesity and abdominal obesity in different states of India. (A) Generalized obesity: BMI 25 kg/m^2; (B) Abdominal obesity: WHR ≥0.9 M/0.8 F.
Source: Modified from Anjana et al. (2023).

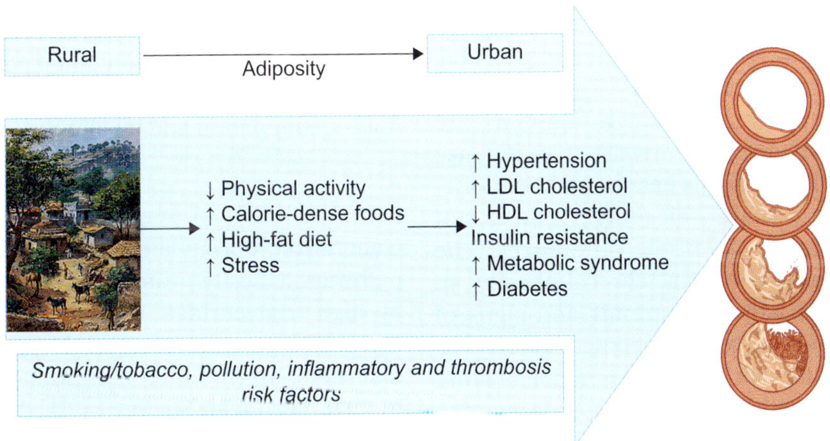

Fig. 3: Rural–urban difference in obesity (adiposity) as the central mechanism of cardiometabolic risk factors and increasing cardiovascular diseases in India: Jaipur Heart Watch study.

ago **(Fig. 3)**.[12,13] Rural-urban comparisons of risk factors in the first JHW studies demonstrated that urbanization was associated with increasing unhealthy lifestyles (sedentariness, unhealthy diet, and stress).[14-17] This transition was associated with an increase in generalized and abdominal obesity, which in turn led to increased hypertension, dyslipidemia (raised total and LDL cholesterol, triglycerides), insulin resistance, metabolic syndrome, and diabetes in urban populations. This, combined with the unhealthy urban milieu of tobacco use, indoor and ambient pollution, and thrombogenic factors, has sustained the CAD epidemic in India.[18] Increasing unplanned urbanization in India shall only fuel the CVD epidemic.[19]

Obesity and Adiposity

Although the excess adiposity is most commonly assessed using the BMI, its limitation is that it does not consider the body fat distribution or the amount of free fat mass, while several anthropometric (e.g., waist circumference, waist-height ratio, and WHR) and imaging measurements can be used to assess body fat distribution.[5,10] An analysis of pooled data from over 650,000 white adults in 2014 showed that waist circumference was positively associated with mortality at all BMI levels from 20 to 50 kg/m^2, leading to the conclusion that waist circumference should be assessed in combination with BMI to assess the risk of obesity-related cardiometabolic risks, CVDs, and mortality.[10]

Given the heterogeneity of obesity and the wide variability in health outcomes for any given BMI, a Lancet Commission proposed new frameworks for the diagnosis and staging of obesity that better align with current evidence.[10] European Atherosclerosis Society (EAS) and European Society of Obesity (ESO) also endorse this framework.[5] Both initiatives consider obesity as an adiposity-based chronic disease (ABCD) and emphasize its clinical consequences.[5] The basic defect in obesity is the dysfunctional subcutaneous adipose tissue (adiposopathy) that releases free fatty acids and many adipokines, leading to visceral obesity and fat deposition in other ectopic depots and associated adverse sequelae. The Lancet Commission also states that the diagnosis of obesity should be based on the recognition of abnormal and/or excessive fat accumulation (anthropometric component) and the analysis of its present and potential effects on health (clinical component).[10] The framework recommends using the waist-to-height ratio as the anthropometric component instead of waist circumference (in combination with BMI), as this has shown superiority as a cardiometabolic disease risk marker and is not dependent on sex-specific or ethnic differences. The Lancet Commission used the term "clinical obesity" to describe a situation in which symptoms and signs of excess adiposity are present, and "preclinical obesity" as a state of excess adiposity with preserved function of other tissues and organs but with increased risk of developing clinical obesity.[10] It concluded that the clinical assessment of obesity should include measures of adiposity in addition to BMI (such as other anthropometric measures) to determine whether an individual has excess adiposity. In JHW studies, we reported that increasing obesity (BMI) correlated significantly with increasing cardiovascular risk factors: Hypertension, hypercholesterolemia, hypertriglyceridemia, metabolic syndrome, and diabetes **(Figs. 4A to F)**.[13,20] Similar data are available for abdominal obesity.[20]

Obesity Associated Systemic Metabolic Disorder

The European Atherosclerosis Society consensus on clinical staging to guide management of metabolic disorders and their sequelae is focused on obesity leading to pathological processes affecting the heart, liver, and kidneys.[5] This adiposity-induced syndrome has been termed systemic metabolic disorder (SMD), which is a cluster of interrelated metabolic abnormalities affecting liver, heart, kidney, pancreas, etc. **(Table 1)**. The integrated model of SMD is based on pathophysiological stages characterized by (1) initiation from adiposity to insulin resistance, (2) propagation due to lipotoxicity and inflammation, and (3) decompensation leading to fibrosis and multiorgan failure.[5] There appears to be a feedback loop between adiposity, insulin resistance, and inflammation that is a consequence of lipotoxicity, inflammasome, and organ cross-talk.[5]

The pathophysiology-based SMD syndrome comprises three stages. Stage 1 is characterized by metabolic abnormalities such as dysfunctional adiposity and dyslipidemia without detectable organ damage.[5,21] Stage 2 is with early organ damage that is manifested as type 2 diabetes, asymptomatic left ventricular diastolic dysfunction, metabolic-associated steatohepatitis (MASH), and early-stage chronic kidney disease (CKD). Stage 3 is characterized by more advanced organ damage affecting multiple organs **(Table 1)**. Various forms of high-risk obesity, driven by maintained positive energy balance, are the most common cause of SMD, leading to ectopic lipid accumulation and insulin resistance.

Pathophysiology

Generalized obesity elevates CVD risk through multiple pathways. Obesity promotes dyslipidemia, characterized by high triglycerides, low HDL cholesterol, and small dense LDL particles, along with type 2 diabetes and sleep disorders, all of which compound CVD susceptibility. In 2025 European Society of Cardiology's (ESC) obesity consensus statement, obesity is highlighted as a key driver of these comorbidities, emphasizing its role in increasing type 2 diabetes and hypertension risks.[22] Furthermore, cumulative exposure to excess BMI over time, measured as BMI years, predicts CAD more robustly than snapshot measurements. Visceral adipose tissue (VAT) releases proinflammatory cytokines, fostering insulin resistance and endothelial dysfunction **(Fig. 5)**.[23-25] Ectopic fat deposits, such as epicardial and pericardial fat, correlate with arterial stiffness and CAD progression, even in nonobese populations.

Mechanistically, obesity induces systemic inflammation, oxidative stress, and hemodynamic alterations.[26-29] The lipotoxicity **(Fig. 5)** of adiposopathy involves excess uptake of free fatty acids, ceramides cause apoptosis and insulin resistance, diacylglycerols lead to protein kinase C activation, acylcarnitines lead

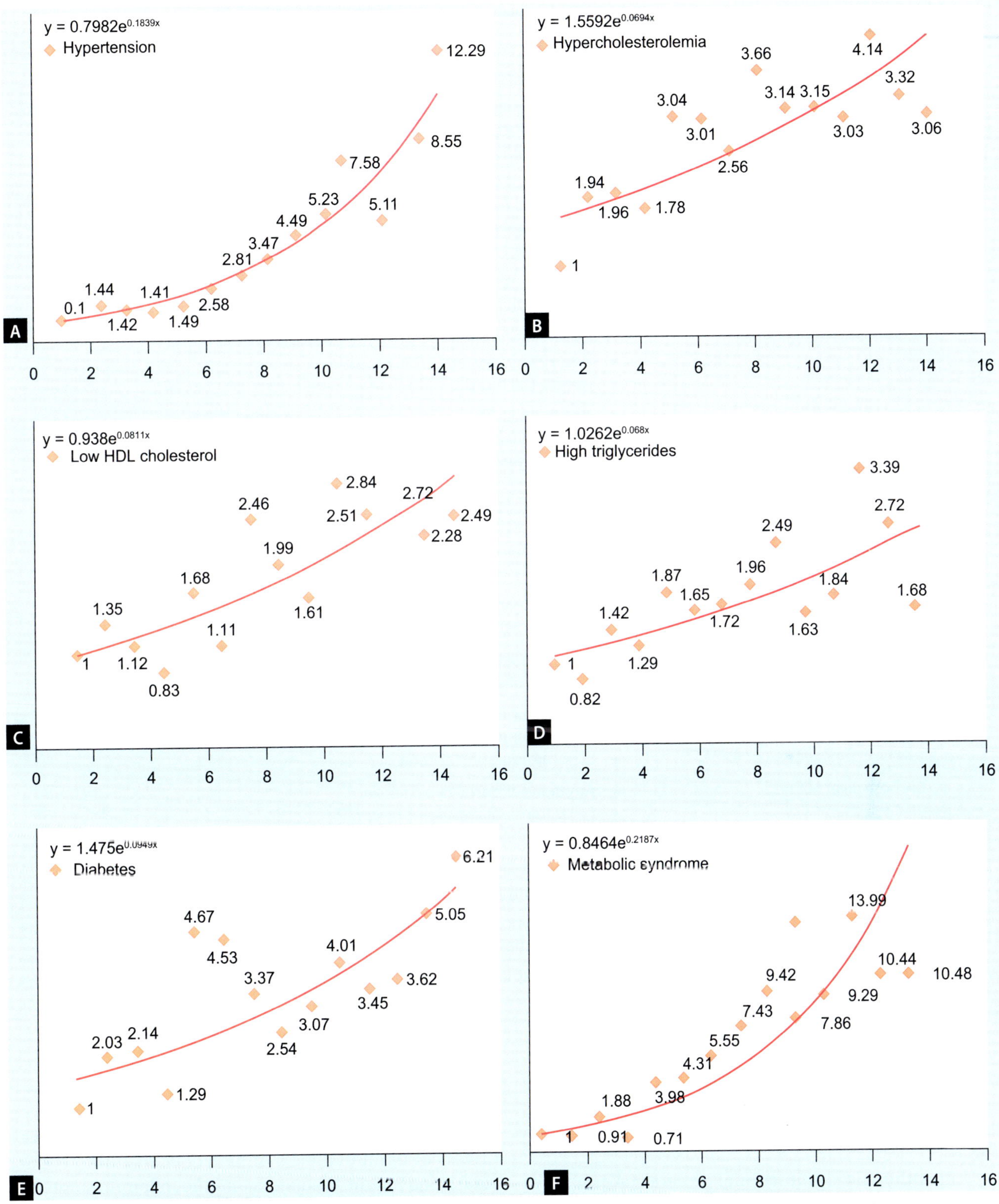

Figs. 4A to F: Obesity as driver of multiple cardiometabolic risk factors in India: Jaipur Heart Watch studies.
Source: Modified from Gupta et al. (2012).

TABLE 1: Stages of obesity associated systemic metabolic disorder.

Stages	Pathophysiology	Manifestations
Stage 1	Overweight/obesity	BMI >25 kg/m^2, waist >90M/85F cm (Asian)
	Insulin resistance/prediabetes	• HOMA insulin resistance >2.5 • Fasting glucose 100–124 mg/dL • OGTT glucose 141–199 mg/dL
	Isolated liver steatosis	• Increased liver triglycerides • FLI ≥60+ liver ultrasound • CAP score >275 dB/m by liver ultrasound • MRI >5.5%
	Hypertension	• BP ≥140/≥90 mm Hg • BP >120/70 in the presence of other comorbidities or risk factors
	Atherogenic dyslipidemia	• Fasting triglycerides ≥150 mg/dL (nonfasting ≥177 mg/dL) • Non-HDL cholesterol ≥130 mg/dL • ApoB ≥100 mg/dL
Stage 2	Type 2 diabetes	• HbA1c >6.5 • Fasting glucose ≥125 mg/dL • OGTT plasma glucose ≥200 mg/dL
	Asymptomatic diastolic dysfunction	Echocardiographic criteria
	MASH/fibrosis	• Elevated SGOT/SGPT • F2-F3 by transient elastography or MRI • F2-F3 by liver biopsy
	Albuminuria and CKD stages 1 and 2	• Estimated GFR >60 mL/min/1.72 m^2 • UACR 3–29 mg/mmol
	Subclinical atherosclerosis	• CAC score >100 • Evidence of atherosclerosis by imaging
Stage 3	Heart failure HFpEF	• Elevated BNP or NT-ProBNP • Dyspnea and congestion • Echocardiographic criteria
	Cirrhosis/liver failure	• Any signs of portal hypertension • F4 by transient elastography or MRI • F4 by liver biopsy
	Reduced kidney function/failure, CKD stages 3–5	• Estimated GFR <60 mL/min/1.73 m^2 • UACR at any level
	Clinical manifestations of ASCVD	History of myocardial infarction, ischemic stroke, peripheral artery disease, or any revascularization

(BMI: body mass index; BNP: B-type natriuretic peptide; BP: blood pressure; CAC: coronary artery calcium; CKD: chronic kidney disease; F: female; FLI: fatty liver index; GFR: glomerular filtration rate; HFpEF: heart failure with preserved ejection fraction; M: male; MASH: metabolism-associated steatohepatitis; MRI: magnetic resonance imaging; OGTT: oral glucose tolerance test; UACR: urine albumin creatinine ratio)

to mitochondrial dysfunction (reactive oxygen species activation and decreased β-oxidation), and oxidized lipids lead to inflammation and stressed endoplasmic reticulum **(Fig. 5)**.[29]

Unhealthy and dysfunctional visceral fat promotes renin–angiotensin–aldosterone system activation, leading to hypertension and left ventricular hypertrophy. Abdominal obesity exacerbates these harmful effects via paracrine effects on vessels, accelerating plaque formation and thrombosis. Recent reviews underscore that metabolically unhealthy obese phenotypes face amplified CVD events, necessitating screening. Key drivers of harmful effects of metabolic disturbances act via hemodynamic mediators and the inflammasome and involve both inflammatory factors (TNF-α, IL-1, IL-16, IL-18, SAA, MCP-1, MMP-9, ICAM-1, etc.) and fibrotic factors (TGF-β, fibronectin, collagen-1, PAI-1, CTGF, etc.) **(Fig. 6)**.[24]

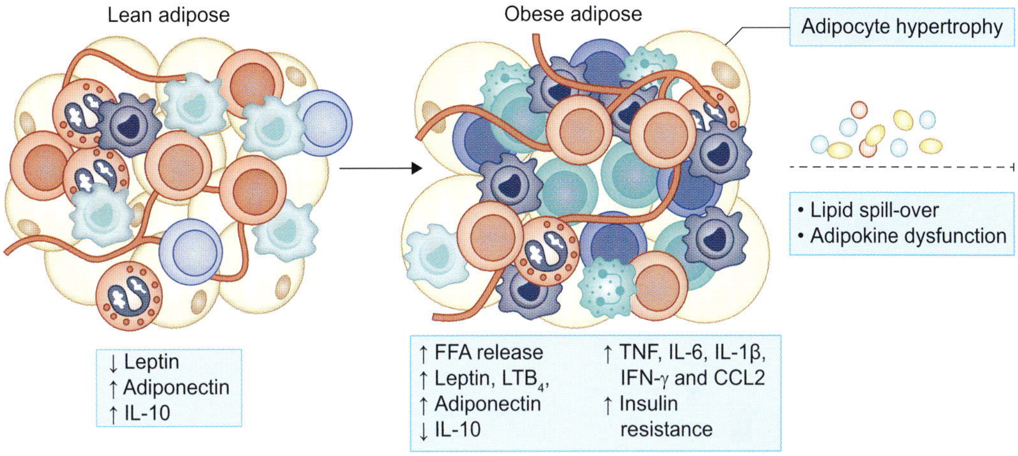

Fig. 5: Pathophysiology of obese adipose tissue and adipocyte hypertrophy with lipid spill-over and adipokine dysfunction. Multiple proinflammatory pathways are activated.
Source: Modified from Brennan et al. (2021).

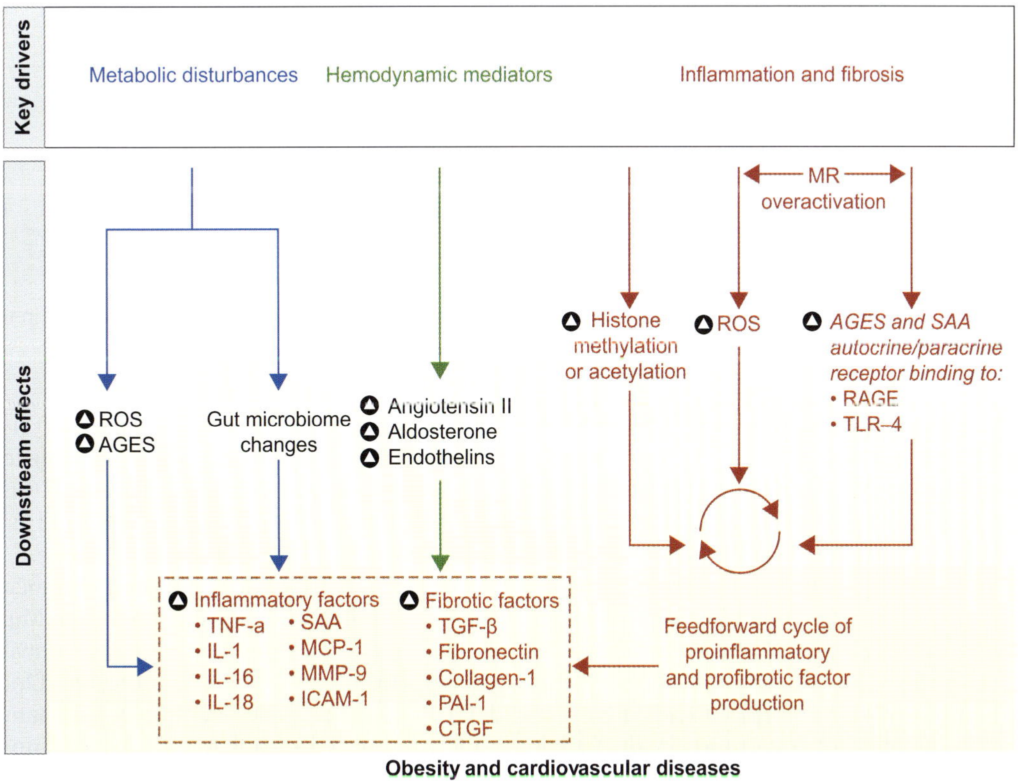

Fig. 6: Metabolic disturbances, hemodynamic mediators, and inflammation. Key drivers of the downstream effects of adiposity on the kidney.
Source: Modified from Tuttle et al. (2022).

OBESITY AND CARDIOVASCULAR DISEASES

There is considerable epidemiological evidence of a parabolic association of generalized and abdominal obesity with CVDs. Increasing BMI and waist circumference are parabolically associated with increasing CVD incidence and deaths. Prospective Studies Collaboration analyzed data on cause-specific mortality in 900,000 adults from 57 prospective studies and reported that BMI was a

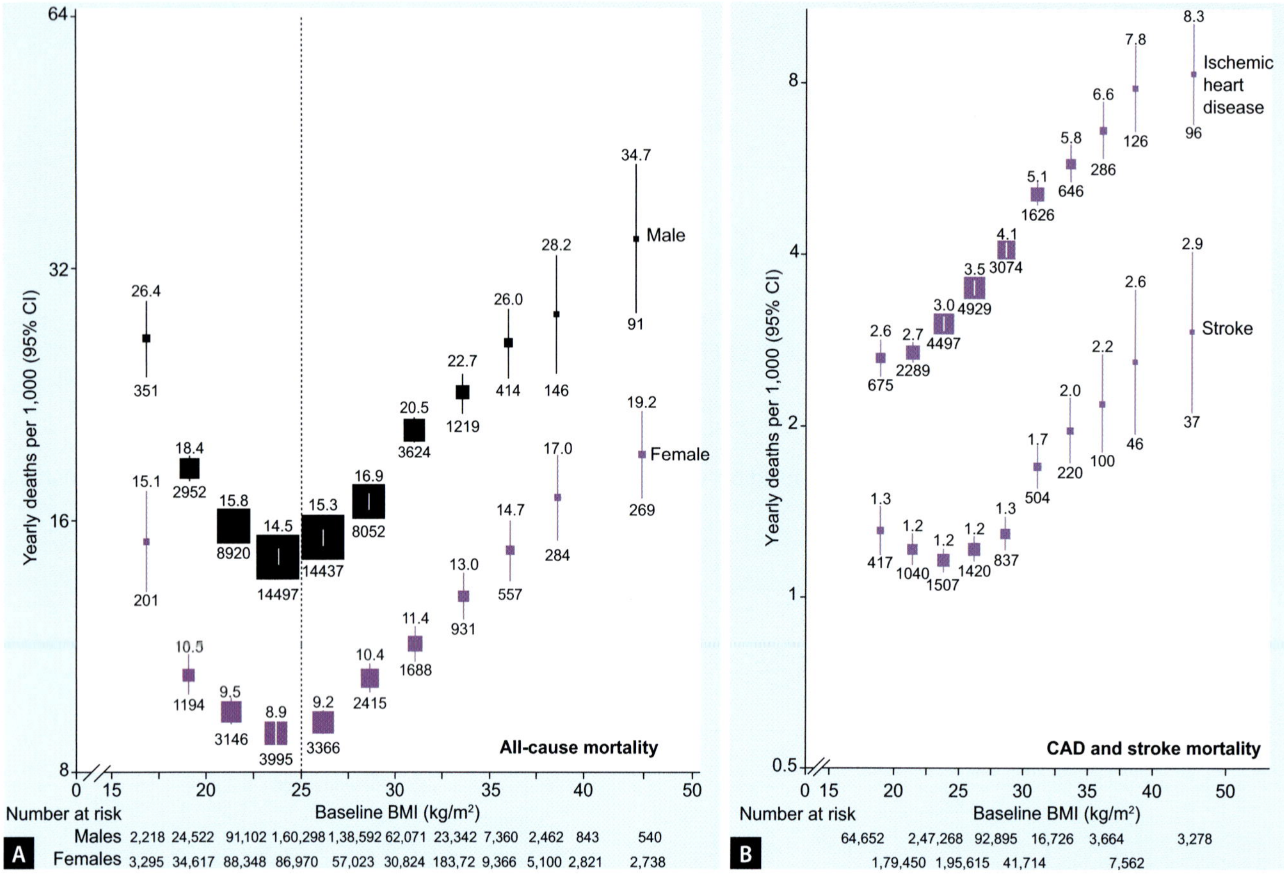

Figs. 7A and B: Association of BMI with overall mortality (A) and CAD and stroke mortality (B) in men and women in the Prospective Studies Collaboration study.
Source: Modified from Prospective Studies Collaboration et al. (2009).

strong predictor of overall mortality both above and below the apparent optimum of about 22.5-25 kg/m^2 **(Figs. 7A and B)**.[29] The excess mortality above this range is due mainly to CVD and is probably largely causal. At 30-35 kg/m^2, median survival is reduced by 2-4 years; at 40-45 kg/m^2, it is reduced by 8-10 years. The excess mortality below 22.5 kg/m^2 was due mainly to smoking-related diseases and is not fully explained. However, the association of BMI with CAD and stroke mortality was essentially linear within the range of BMI of 15-50 kg/m^2 **(Figs. 7A and B)**.

Association of abdominal obesity (waist circumference) with all-cause and CVD mortality is identical to the BMI-related adverse outcomes. The Emerging Risk Factors Collaboration conducted a collaborative analysis of 58 prospective studies and 221,934 people in 17 countries.[30] It was reported that in people with BMI of 20 kg/m^2 or higher, HRs for CVD were 1.23 (95% CI 1.17-1.29) with BMI, 1.27 (1.20-1.33) with waist circumference, and 1.25 (1.19-1.31) with WHR, after adjustment for age, sex, and smoking status **(Figs. 8A to F)**. It was also reported that the BMI, waist circumference, and WHR, whether assessed singly or in combination, did not improve CVD risk prediction when additional information was available for systolic BP, history of diabetes, and lipids. Based on this and similar studies, BMI and adiposity were relegated as risk markers rather than risk factors for CAD and stroke.

In India, prospective data on the association of BMI with CVD outcomes are available in the Mumbai Cohort Study, Kerala Cohort Study, and a nationwide study.[31-33] All reported a direct linear relationship of increasing BMI with CVD, although the strength of association was lower than in other countries in Asia and in most developed countries.[34,35] The case-control INTERHEART,[36,37] and prospective PURE studies,[38,39] provide more recent data on the association of obesity and abdominal obesity with cardiovascular outcomes in this region.

In the INTERHEART study, BMI showed a graded association with myocardial infarction (OR 1.44, CI 1.32-1.57 top quintile versus bottom quintile before adjustment), this substantially reduced after adjustment for WHR (OR 1.12, CI 1.03-1.22) and became nonsignificant after adjustment for other risk factors (0.98, 0.88-1.09).[36]

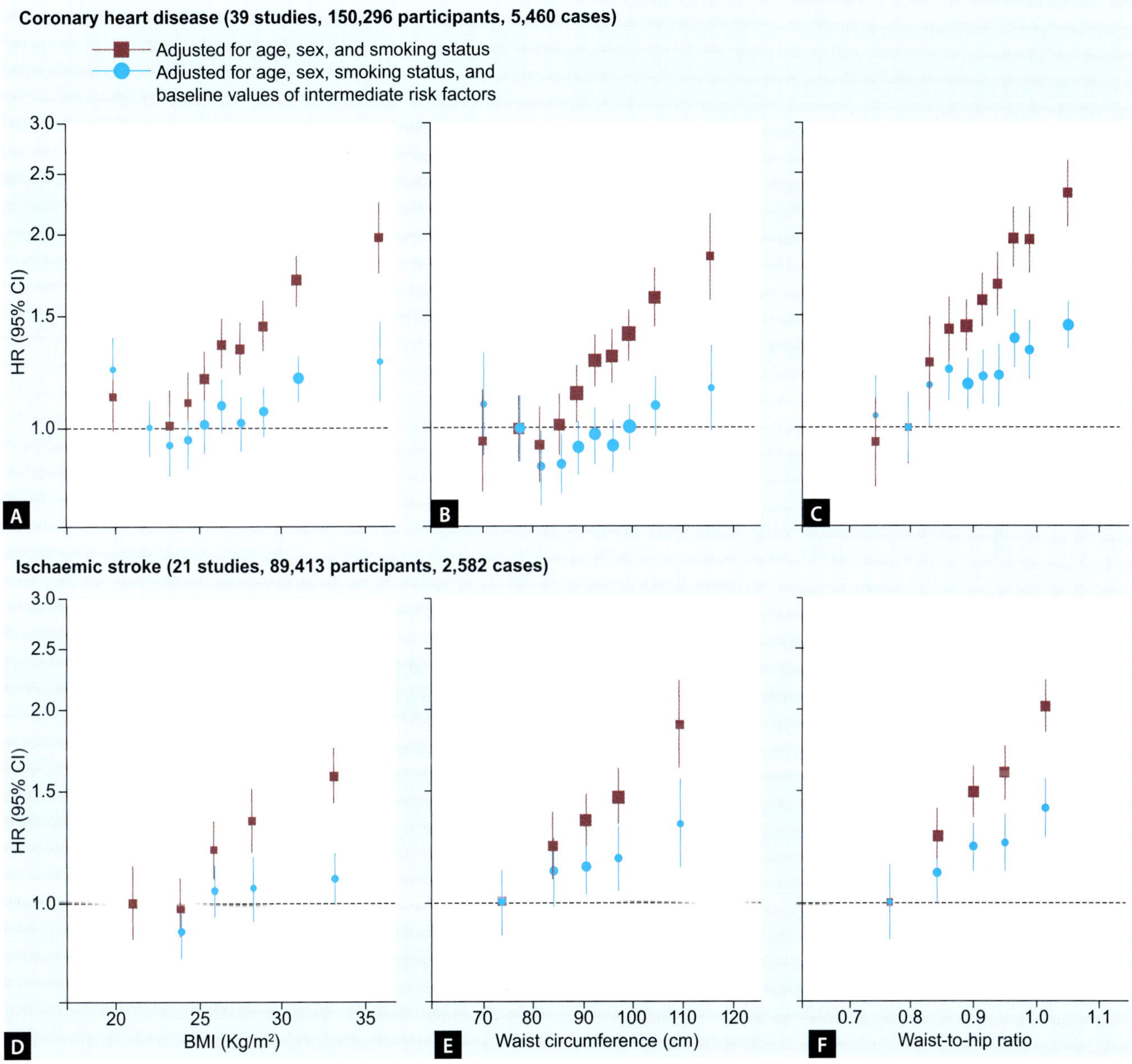

Figs. 8A to F: Association of BMI, waist circumference, and WHR with CAD (upper panel) and ischemic stroke events in the Emerging Risk Factors Collaboration study.
Source: Modified from Emerging Risk Factors Collaboration et al. (2011).

For WHR, the OR for every successive quintile was significantly greater than that of the previous one [second quintile: 1.15, 1.05–1.26; third quintile: 1.39; 1.28–1.52; fourth quintile: 1.90, 1.74 2.07; and fifth quintile: 2.52, 2.31–2.74 (adjusted for age, sex, region, and smoking)]. WHR and waist were closely ($p < 0.0001$) associated with risk of myocardial infarction even after adjustment for other risk factors (ORs for top quintile vs. lowest quintiles were 1.75, 1.33, and 0.76, respectively). This report concluded that WHR was a more robust indicator of acute myocardial infarction risk worldwide. Redefinition of obesity based on WHR instead of BMI increases the estimate of myocardial infarction attributable to obesity in most ethnic groups, including in South Asians.[37]

In the 12-year follow-up data from the PURE study, there was an insignificant association of BMI with CVD outcomes, and only WHR associations were reported.[38] In high versus low WHR groups, multivariate adjusted OR for incidence CVD was 1.26 (CI 1.18–1.34) while for CVD deaths, it was 1.13 (CI 1.05–1.20). The population attributable fraction [PAF (%)] for abdominal obesity was 5.7% (CI 1.7–9.8%) but was more for low-income countries (mainly from South Asia) (7.0%, CI 0.2–13.9) as compared to middle-income countries (5.2%, CI 1.8–8.6%) and high-income countries (6.8%, CI -6.5 to 20.1%). Long-term follow-up data in the South Asian countries reported similar outcomes.[39] In this report, only WHR was assessed as a marker of obesity, and the PAF was 6.9% (CI). This was lower than the PAFs for other risk factors: Hypertension 13.1%, high non-HDL cholesterol 11.1%, diabetes 8.9%, and low education 7.7%.[39]

OBESITY AND ATHEROSCLEROSIS PATHOPHYSIOLOGY

The ESC consensus statement[22] details how obesity accelerates atherosclerosis through multiple pathways. Most of the pathways have been reported above. Visceral adiposity is strongly associated with CVD, as excess free fatty acids overload the liver, increasing very low-density lipoprotein (VLDL) production and atherogenic dyslipidemia. This dyslipidemia, coupled with insulin resistance, elevates cardiovascular risk even in the absence of other metabolic abnormalities. The statement highlights that obesity-induced inflammation, driven by proinflammatory cytokines and hsCRP, promotes endothelial dysfunction by reducing nitric oxide bioavailability and increasing oxidative stress **(Fig. 5)**. This fosters a prothrombotic state, with elevated plasminogen activator inhibitor-1 (PAI-1) levels impairing fibrinolysis. Perivascular adipose tissue (PVAT) in obesity shifts from an anti-inflammatory to a proatherogenic state, secreting factors that enhance coronary inflammation **(Figs. 5 and 6)**.

Computed tomography (CT) imaging of pericoronary ectopic fat during routine CT coronary angiography can quantify coronary inflammation,[40] offering prognostic value for future cardiovascular events, though not yet routine in clinical practice.[41] Epicardial fat, correlated with subclinical atherosclerosis, further contributes to CAD risk. The key mechanisms are as follows:

- *Adipose tissue dysfunction:* Visceral fat and other ectopic fat deposits, such as epicardial fat, directly impair vascular function by promoting inflammation and oxidative stress. These tissues correlate with subclinical atherosclerosis and CAD, independent of BMI.
- *Inflammation and oxidative stress:* Obesity-induced low-grade inflammation, with elevated hsCRP and cytokines, drives endothelial dysfunction and plaque progression.
- *Dyslipidemia and insulin resistance:* Obesity exacerbates atherogenic dyslipidemia and insulin resistance, amplifying ASCVD risk. The statement notes that metrics like waist circumference (men >94 cm, women >88 cm) better reflect visceral fat and cardiovascular risk than BMI alone.
- *Environmental and societal factors:* While genetic factors contribute, the global obesity epidemic is largely driven by environmental influences, including poor diet and sedentary lifestyles, which exacerbate atherosclerotic risk.

Obesity is a critical, yet underaddressed, driver of atherosclerosis. Through visceral adiposity, systemic inflammation, dyslipidemia, and endothelial dysfunction, obesity accelerates plaque formation and cardiovascular risk. The ESC 2024 statement advocates for comprehensive weight loss strategies, including lifestyle interventions, antiobesity medications such as semaglutide, and bariatric procedures, to mitigate these effects.[22] By integrating metrics such as waist circumference and advanced imaging of adipose tissue, clinicians can better stratify risk and tailor interventions.

OBESITY AND OTHER CARDIOVASCULAR DISEASES

Important CVDs associated with obesity are (1) heart failure, especially heart failure with preserved ejection fraction (HFpEF), and (2) cardiac arrhythmia, especially atrial fibrillation (AF). Adiposopathy-related adipokines are important.

Heart Failure with Preserved Ejection Fraction

Obesity significantly increases the risk of HFpEF by promoting inflammation, hypertension, and insulin resistance, and it can also hinder diagnosis due to symptom overlap and altered biomarker levels. Obesity leads to HFpEF through multiple mechanisms including (1) metabolic dysfunction due to inflammation, hypertension, dyslipidemia, and insulin resistance; (2) mechanical effects as the excess body fat causes mechanical constraints on the heart and lungs, impairing cardiac and pulmonary function; (3) hormonal imbalance due to increased aldosterone levels which contributes to plasma volume expansion, and activation of various adipokines that lead to apoptosis and myocardial fibrosis **(Figs. 5 and 6)**; and (4) inflammation as the VAT is a source of inflammatory mediators that promote insulin resistance and mitochondrial dysfunction.[42] Diagnosis of HFpEF is challenging because of symptom overlap as breathlessness and exercise intolerance are common to both obesity and HFpEF; attenuated biomarkers as natriuretic peptide levels may not be increased in the obese; and imaging limitations.[42] Specific management strategies that have been found useful for obesity-associated HFpEF include focus on lifestyle changes and pharmacotherapies, including glucagon-like peptide-1 receptor agonists (GLP-1 RAs) and SGLT2 inhibitors, which have shown better outcomes in randomized controlled trials of HFpEF and are approved by various guidelines.[43]

Atrial Fibrillation

Obesity promotes AF by causing left atrial (LA) enlargement due to increased blood volume and filling pressures, leading to structural and electrical remodeling. Adipose tissue releases inflammatory and fibrotic factors, oxidative stress, and activates autonomic nerves, creating a substrate vulnerable to AF. The atrial remodeling occurs due to:

- Inflammation of adipose tissue releases proinflammatory cytokines and adipokines that promote atrial inflammation.
- Fibrosis due to elevated levels of signaling molecules and oxidative stress **(Fig. 6)** induces excessive collagen deposition in the atrium, leading to fibrosis and impaired conduction.
- Structural and functional changes leading to inflammatory and fibrotic changes that cause both structural remodeling (e.g., LA enlargement) and functional abnormalities, creating a "substrate" that promotes AF.
- Molecular pathways, including the renin–angiotensin–aldosterone system and endothelin-1, are activated, further contributing to fibrosis and remodeling.
- Metabolic changes due to associated conditions such as diabetes and insulin resistance, common in obesity, impair metabolic flexibility, and increase AF risk.
- Autonomic dysregulation due to obesity can lead to autonomic nervous system imbalances that are magnified by the presence of obstructive sleep apnea, a common accompaniment of obesity.
- Epicardial adipose tissue (EAT), the fat layer surrounding the heart, plays a direct role by releasing proinflammatory and profibrotic molecules and harboring ganglionated plexi that can trigger AF.

Obesity management including weight reduction early in the course of disease can prevent the occurrence of AF. Specific drugs that target obesity such as GLP-1 RAs are also useful.[22]

INTERVENTIONS

Both obesity and especially abdominal obesity are pivotal CVD risk modifiers, driving morbidity through metabolic and inflammatory pathways. Guidelines recommend WC monitoring alongside BMI for risk stratification, advocating lifestyle changes, pharmacotherapy, and weight management to mitigate threats. The Venice Declaration on Obesity by IFSO[42] has professed obesity as a disease condition and has appealed for a call to action for its early diagnosis and multimodal treatment. The Declaration also focuses on international and national policy changes, which are vital to mitigate the obesity burden worldwide.

A number of interventions are available for weight reduction and obesity management. These include the classic lifestyle interventions (dietary change, physical activity), which are not very successful, to older pharmacological agents (orlistat, phentermine, metformin, etc.), which were only partially successful. The modern era of obesity management began with surgical interventions listed in **Table 2** and GLP-1 RAs that have revolutionized obesity management.[22]

Obesity management requires a multifaceted approach, integrating lifestyle, pharmacological, and surgical interventions **(Table 2)**. The GLP-1 RAs have emerged as a cornerstone of pharmacological strategy. The ESC 2024 Consensus Statement and other guidelines highlight available GLP-1 RAs, such as liraglutide, semaglutide, and tirzepatide, for their efficacy in achieving significant weight loss (10–20%) and improving cardiovascular outcomes.[22,44] These agents mimic GLP-1, slowing gastric emptying, enhancing satiety, and reducing appetite via central and peripheral mechanisms. Semaglutide, administered weekly, and tirzepatide, a dual GLP-1/GIP agonist, demonstrate superior weight loss compared to earlier agents such as orlistat, with added benefits in managing diabetes and reducing atherosclerosis risk. Lifestyle interventions—calorie-restricted diets (500–750 kcal deficit) and 150–300 minutes/week of physical activity—remain foundational but are enhanced by GLP-1 RAs. Bariatric surgery, such as sleeve gastrectomy, offers durable weight loss for severe obesity (BMI ≥40 kg/m^2) but is invasive.

Glucagon-like peptide-1 receptor agonists are indicated for BMI ≥30 kg/m^2 or ≥27 kg/m^2 with comorbidities, with continuation dependent on achieving ≥5% weight loss at 3 months. Their integration with lifestyle changes optimizes obesity control and cardiovascular health.[44,45] The benefits of various weight loss interventions on multiple cardiovascular risk factors and overall cardiovascular risk are summarized in **Figure 9**.

TABLE 2: Interventions for obesity management.

Intervention	*Description*	*Indications*
Lifestyle		
Dietary modifications	• Calorie-restricted diet, aim for 500–750-calorie daily deficit • Healthy meal plans, such as Mediterranean, Indo-Mediterranean, or vegetarian diets	• Recommended as first-line for all BMI ≥25 kg/m^2 • Combined with other therapies for better outcomes
Physical activity	At least 150 minutes per week of moderate aerobic exercise for maintenance; 300 minutes per week for weight loss; include strength training	• Enhances weight loss and maintenance • Improves cardiovascular health and comorbidities such as hypertension and diabetes. Recommended as an adjunct to all other therapies
Behavioral modification	Intensive programs with counseling, motivational interviewing, goal setting, and self-monitoring; family-based programs for children	At least 26 contact hours over 3–12 months for children; addresses psychological aspects to prevent regain
Pharmacological		
Orlistat	Lipase inhibitor that reduces fat absorption	For BMI ≥30 kg/m^2 or ≥27 kg/m^2 with comorbidities, modest weight loss (3–5%)
Phentermine	Appetite suppressant for short-term use	For BMI ≥30 kg/m^2 or ≥27 kg/m^2 with comorbidities, monitor for cardiovascular risks
Liraglutide (GLP-1 RA)	Injectable that slows gastric emptying and reduces appetite	For BMI ≥30 kg/m^2 or ≥27 kg/m^2 with comorbidities; up to 8% weight loss, continue if ≥5% loss at 3 months
Semaglutide (GLP-1 RA)	Weekly injectable or oral; promotes satiety and weight loss	• Similar indications; average 15–20% weight loss • Beneficial for diabetes management
Tirzepatide (dual GLP-1/ GIP agonist)	Weekly injectable; dual action for enhanced efficacy	• For BMI ≥30 kg/m^2 or ≥27 kg/m^2 with comorbidities, up to 21% weight loss • Reduces diabetes and CV risks
Dual and triple incretin mimetics	Oral and injectable forms in clinical trials	Same as for other GLP-1 RAs
Others (e.g., metformin, SGLT-2 inhibitors)	Off-label use for weight management, especially in diabetes	Adjunct in type 2 diabetes; prioritize agents with weight-loss benefits
Surgical		
Roux-en-Y gastric bypass	Surgical rerouting of stomach and intestines to reduce absorption	For BMI ≥40 kg/m^2 or ≥35 kg/m^2 with comorbidities; 25–30% weight loss; durable, improves diabetes
Sleeve gastrectomy	Removal of a portion of the stomach to create a smaller sleeve	Similar indications: 25–30% weight loss; lower complication rate than bypass
Adjustable gastric banding	Placement of band around stomach to restrict intake	Less common now; for BMI ≥40 kg/m^2 or ≥35 kg/m^2 with comorbidities; adjustable but higher revision rates
Biliopancreatic diversion with duodenal switch	Complex procedure combining sleeve and bypass for malabsorption	For severe obesity (BMI ≥50 kg/m^2), the highest weight loss but higher nutritional risks
Endoscopic		
Intragastric balloon (IGB)	Temporary balloon placement in the stomach to promote fullness	For BMI ≥30–40 kg/m^2 where lifestyle failed, combined with lifestyle, temporary (6 months)
Endoscopic sleeve gastroplasty	Minimally invasive suturing to reduce stomach size	For BMI ≥30 kg/m^2 or ≥27 kg/m^2 with comorbidities; 13–16% weight loss; emerging long-term data
Policy interventions		
National- or state-level focused policies to mitigate obesogenic environment	• Focus on social determinants, urban infrastructure, and walkability • Food policies to reduce ultra-processed foods, sugar-sweetened beverages, transfats, simple sugars, and refined carbohydrates • Promote the availability of fruit, vegetables, and proteins	Population-level interventions are long-term solutions Primordial and primary prevention of obesity

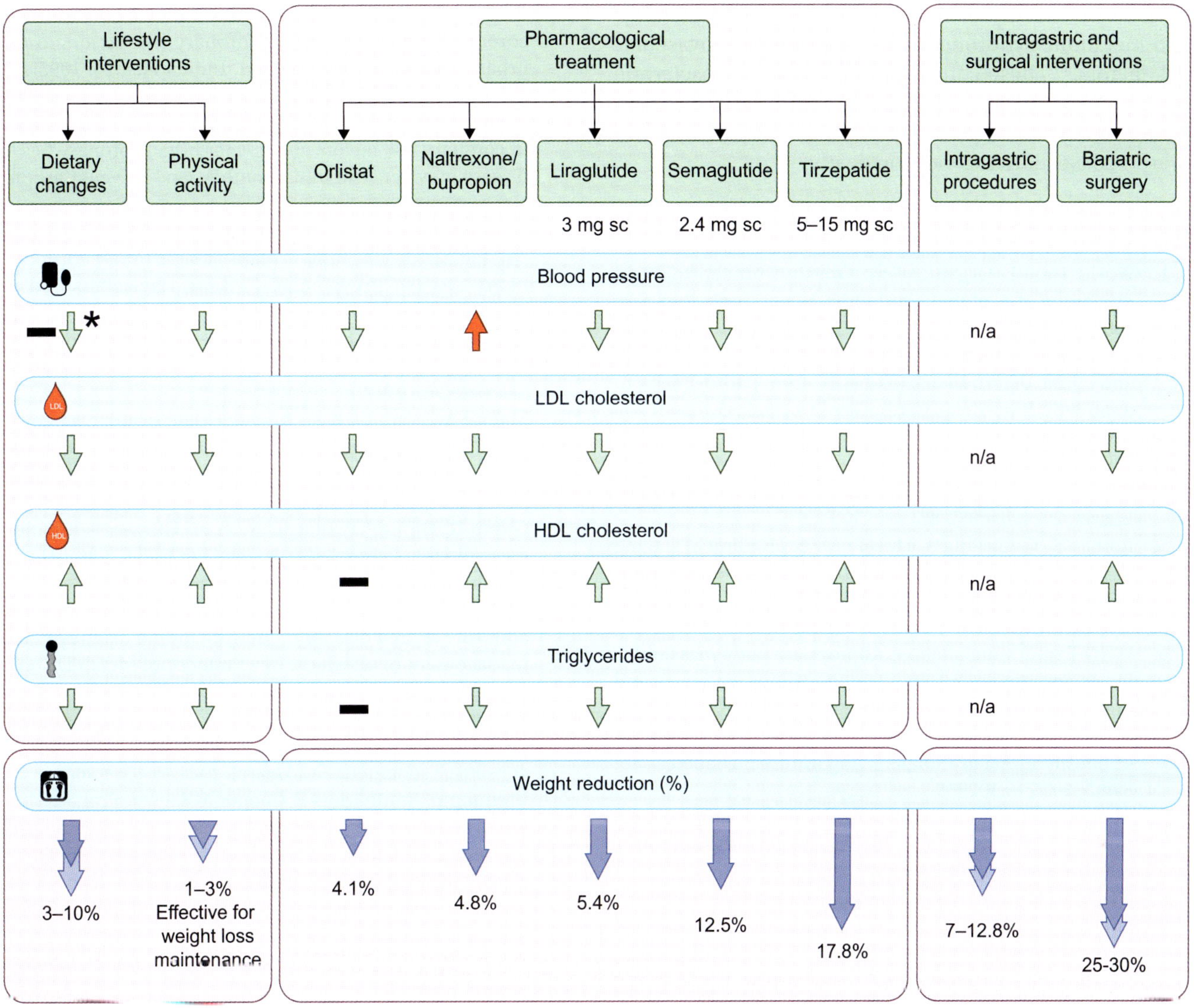

Fig. 9: Efficacy of various lifestyle, pharmacological, and surgical interventions for weight reduction.
Source: Modified from Koskinas et al. (2024).

The policy interventions are usually not mentioned in a cardiovascular textbook. However, I believe that if the obesity epidemic is to be curtailed, policy focus is crucial.[46,47] The focus should be on curtailing the obesogenic environment, so rampant in our communities.[44] This needs a major transformation in political vision with a health-in-all-policies approach, policy formulation, and its implementation.[46,47] Detailed discussion is beyond the scope of this chapter.

LOOKING AHEAD AND CONCLUSION

The obesity epidemic, currently sweeping the middle, lower middle, and low-income countries across the globe, is mainly driven by the increasing BMI of the rural populations.[48] CVDs, such as CAD, stroke, and peripheral arterial diseases, are not the only manifestations, and more than a hundred disease conditions have been attributed to them.[4,44] The list includes various serious illnesses, including heart disease, type 2 diabetes, fatty liver disease, certain cancers (such as colon, breast, and kidney cancer), and sleep apnea. Other associated health issues involve high BP, dyslipidemias, osteoarthritis, and various mental health conditions such as depression and anxiety. Future politicians, planners, health administrators, physicians, and the public should be aware of the myriad conditions and wholeheartedly implement obesity-reducing policies.[49] For a cardiologist, the adiposity epidemic presents as a deadly triumvirate of cardiovascular, kidney, and metabolic syndrome with increased cardiovascular risk factors.[50] These contribute to raised atherosclerotic coronary, cerebrovascular and peripheral arterial diseases, cardiac arrhythmias (AF), heart failure with reduced and preserved ejection fraction, and death.

REFERENCES

1. World Health Organization. Obesity: preventing and managing the global epidemic. WHO Tech Rep Ser. 2000;894:1-37.
2. Capoccia D, Milani I, Colangeli L, et al. Social, cultural and ethnic determinants of obesity: from pathogenesis to treatment. Nutr Metab Cardiovasc Dis. 2025;35:103901.
3. Haslam DW, James WPT. Obesity. Lancet. 2005;366: 1197-209.
4. Lingvay I, Cohen RV, le Roux CW, et al. Obesity in adults. Lancet. 2024;404:972-87.
5. Romeo S, Vidal-Puig A, Husain M, et al. Clinical staging to guide management of metabolic disorders and their sequelae: a European Atherosclerosis Society consensus statement. Eur Heart J. 2025;EPub:ehaf314.
6. WHO Expert Consultation. Appropriate body mass index for Asian populations and its implications for policy and intervention strategies. Lancet. 2004;363:157-63.
7. Misra A, Vikram NK, Ghosh A, et al. Revised definition of obesity in Asian Indians living in India. Diabetes Met Syndr. 2025;19:102989.
8. Ritchie H, Roser M. (2024). Obesity. Our World in Data. [online] Available from https://ourworldindata.org/obesity. [Last accessed January, 2025].
9. GBD 2021 Adult BMI Collaborators. Global, regional, and national prevalence of adult overweight and obesity, 1990-2021, with forecasts to 2025: a forecasting study for the Global Burden of Disease Study 2021. Lancet. 2025;405:813-38.
10. Rubino F, Cummings DE, Eckel RH, et al. Definition and diagnostic criteria of clinical obesity. Lancet Diabetes Endocrinol. 2025;13:221-62.
11. Anjana RM, Unnikrishnan R, Deepa M, et al. Metabolic non-communicable disease health report of India: the ICMR-INDIAB national cross-sectional study (ICMR-INDIAB 17). Lancet Diabetes Endocrinol. 2023;11: 474-89.
12. Gupta R, Guptha S, Gupta VP, et al. Twenty-year trends in cardiovascular risk factors in India and influence of educational status. Eur J Prev Cardiol. 2012;19: 1258-71.
13. Gupta R, Agrawal A, Misra A, et al. Metabolic cardiovascular risk factors worsen continuously across the spectrum of body mass index in Asian Indians. Indian Heart J. 2012;64:236-44.
14. Gupta R, Gupta VP, Ahluwalia NS. Educational status, coronary heart disease and coronary risk factor prevalence in a rural population of India. BMJ. 1994;309:1332-36
15. Gupta R, Prakash H, Majumdar S, et al. Prevalence of coronary heart disease and coronary risk factors in an urban population of Rajasthan. Indian Heart J. 1995;47: 331-8.
16. Gupta R, Prakash H, Gupta VP. Urban-rural differences in coronary risk factors and greater urban coronary heart disease prevalence in India. South Asian J Prevent Cardiol. 1997;1:27-33.
17. Gupta R, Gupta VP. Urban-rural differences in coronary risk factors do not fully explain greater urban coronary heart disease prevalence. J Assoc Physicians India. 1997;45:683-6.
18. Gupta R, Gupta VP. Lessons for prevention from a coronary heart disease epidemiology study in western India. Curr Sci. 1998;74:1074-7.
19. Mathur M, Wani VJ, Basu R, et al. Urban health resilience: strategies for strengthening public health systems in response to urbanisation challenges. Ind J Comm Med. 2024;49(Suppl2):S159-64.
20. Gupta R, Gupta VP, Bhagat N, et al. Obesity is a major determinant of coronary risk factors in India: Jaipur Heart Watch studies. Ind Heart J. 2008;60:26-33.
21. Perdomo CM, Aviles-Olmos I, Dicker D, et al. Towards an adiposity related disease framework for the diagnosis and management of obesities. Rev Endocrinol Metab Disord. 2023;24:795-807.
22. Koskinas KC, Van Craenenbroeck EM, Antoniades C, et al. Obesity and cardiovascular disease: an ESC clinical consensus statement. Eur Heart J. 2024;45:4063-98.
23. Brennan E, Kantharidis P, Cooper ME, et al. Proresolving lipid mediators: regulators of inflammation, metabolism and kidney function. Nat. Rev Nephrol. 2021;17:725-39.
24. Tuttle KR, Agarwal R, Alpers CE, et al. Molecular mechanisms and therapeutic targets for diabetic kidney disease. Kidney Int. 2022;102:248-60.
25. Fruhbeck G. The adipose tissue as a source of vasoactive factors. Curr Med Chem Cardiovasc Haematol Agents. 2004;2:197-208.
26. Fruhbeck G. The Sir David Cuthbertson Medal Lecture. Hunting for new pieces to the complex puzzle of obesity. Proc Nutr Soc. 2006;65:329-47.
27. Lim S, Meigs JB. Links between ectopic fat and vascular disease in humans. Arterioscl Thromb Vasc Biol. 2014;34:1820-6.
28. Cypess AM. Reassessing human adipose tissue. N Engl J Med. 2022;386:768-79.
29. Prospective Studies Collaboration; Whitlock G, Lewington S, et al. Body-mass index and cause-specific mortality in 900 000 adults: collaborative analyses of 57 prospective studies. Lancet. 2009;373:1083-96.
30. Emerging Risk Factors Collaboration; Wormser D, Kaptoge S, et al. Separate and combined associations of body-mass index and abdominal adiposity with cardiovascular disease: collaborative analysis of 58 prospective studies. Lancet. 2011;377:1085-95.
31. Pednekar MS, Hakama M, Heberts JR, et al. Association of body mass index with all-cause and cause-specific

mortality: findings from a prospective cohort study in Mumbai, India. Int J Epidemiol. 2008;37:525-34.
32. Sauvaget C, Ramadas K, Thomas G, et al. Body mass index, weight change and mortality risk in a prospective study in India. Int J Epidemiol. 2008;37:990-1004.
33. Gajalakshmi V, Lacey B, Kanimozhi V, et al. Body-mass index, blood pressure, and cause-specific mortality in India: a prospective cohort study of 500 810 adults. Lancet Glob Health. 2018;6:e787-94.
34. Zheng W, McLerran DF, Rolland B, et al. Association between body mass index and risk of death in more than 1 million Asians. N Engl J Med. 2011;364:719-29.
35. GBD 2015 Obesity Collaborators; Afshin A, Forouzanfar MH, et al. Health effects of overweight and obesity in 195 countries over 25 years. N Engl J Med. 2017;377:13-27.
36. Yusuf S, Hawken S, Ounpuu S, et al. Obesity and the risk of myocardial infarction in 27000 participants from 52 countries: a case-control study. Lancet. 2005;366: 1640-9.
37. Joshi P, Islam S, Pais P, et al. Risk factors for early myocardial infarction in South Asians compared with individuals in other countries. JAMA. 2007;297:286-94.
38. Yusuf S, Joseph P, Rangarajan S, et al. Modifiable risk factors, cardiovascular disease, and mortality in 155,722 individuals from 21 high-income, middle-income, and low-income countries (PURE): a prospective cohort study. Lancet. 2020;395:795-808.
39. Joseph P, Kutty VR, Mohan V, et al. Cardiovascular diseases, mortality and their associations with modifiable risk factors in a multinational South Asia cohort: a PURE substudy. Eur Heart J. 2022;43:2831-40.
40. Oikonomou EK, West HW, Antoniades C. Cardiac computed tomography: assessment of coronary inflammation and other plaque features. Arterioscl Thromb Vasc Biol. 2019;39:2207-19.
41. Tsiachristas A, Chan K, Wahome E, et al. Cost-effectiveness of a novel AI technology to quantify coronary inflammation and cardiovascular risk in patients undergoing coronary computed tomography angiography. Eur Heart J Qual Care Clin Outcomes. 2025;11:434-44.
42. De Luca M, Belluzzi A, Navarra G, et al. The Venice Declaration: obesity as a disease—a call to action for diagnosis, multimodal treatment, and policy change. Obes Surg. 2025;35:1999-2003.
43. Gupta R, Chaudhary M, Guptha S. Heart failure with preserved ejection fraction (HFpEF) in the Indian context. J Indian Coll Cardiol. 2025;15:42-54.
44. Ahmed SK, Mohammed RA. Obesity: prevalence, causes, consequences, management, preventive strategies and future research directions. Metabol Open. 2025;27:100375.
45. Gupta R. Relevance of polypill for primary prevention of cardiovascular diseases in the 21st century. RUHS J Health Sci. 2025;10:64-7.
46. Gupta R, Wood DA. Primary prevention of ischemic heart disease: populations, individuals, and healthcare professionals. Lancet. 2019;394:685-96.
47. Gupta R, Yusuf S. Challenges in management and prevention of ischemic heart disease in low socioeconomic status people in LLMICs. BMC Med. 2019;17:e209.
48. NCD Risk Factor Collaboration (NCD-RisC). Rising rural body-mass index is the main driver of the global obesity epidemic in adults. Nature. 2019;569:260-4.
49. Chusan YAC, Eneli I, Hennessy E, et al. Next steps in efforts to address the obesity epidemic. Annu Rev Public Health. 2025;46:171-91.
50. Ndumele CE, Neeland IJ, Tuttle KR, et al. A synopsis of the evidence for the scientific and clinical management of cardiovascular-kidney-metabolic (CKM) syndrome: a scientific statement from the American Heart Association. Circulation. 2023;148:1636-64.

8

CHAPTER

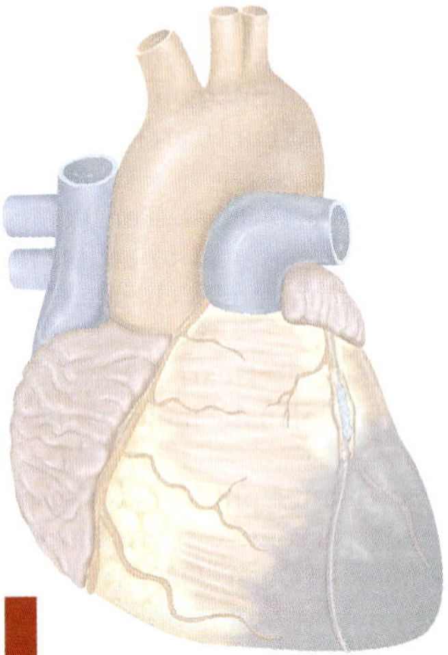

Obesity Mass and Cardiovascular Disease: A Review

Daran Amini, Deepika Misra

INTRODUCTION

Obesity is one of the most important public health problems facing the world today.[1] Between 1975 and 2022, the prevalence of obesity has more than tripled.[2] In 2024, the World Obesity Federation estimated that nearly 3 billion people are overweight or obese.[1] As a leading modifiable risk factor for death and disability, this chapter will explore six relevant clinical trials which examine the intersection between excess body mass and cardiovascular disease.[3-8]

Pharmacologic-based cardiovascular outcome trials where the intervention is the addition of a GLP-1 receptor agonist **(Table 1)**.

SEMAGLUTIDE EFFECTS ON CARDIOVASCULAR OUTCOMES IN PEOPLE WITH OVERWEIGHT OR OBESITY (SELECT)

Randomized study of semaglutide 2.4 mg weekly compared to placebo in subjects who are 45 years or older, had preexisting cardiovascular disease, and a BMI of ≥27, and no history of diabetes.[3] A total of 17,604 patients were enrolled, with a mean follow-up duration of 39.8 months.[3] The primary outcome was time to first cardiovascular death, nonfatal myocardial infarction, or nonfatal stroke.[3] This was significantly decreased in the treatment group (HR 0.80; 95% CI 0.72–0.90; $p < 0.001$).[3] Relevant secondary end points in the treatment group include a reduced heart failure composite end point, which was the first occurrence of death from CV causes or hospitalization or an urgent medical visit for heart failure (HR 0.82; 95% CI 0.71–0.93), and reduced coronary revascularization (HR 0.77; 95% CI 0.68–0.87).[3]

SEMAGLUTIDE TREATMENT EFFECT IN PEOPLE WITH OBESITY AND HEART FAILURE WITH PRESERVED EJECTION FRACTION (STEP-HFPEF)

In total, 529 patients with heart failure with preserved ejection fraction (HFpEF) and a BMI of ≥30 received either semaglutide 2.4 mg weekly, or placebo, for 52 weeks.[4] The dual primary end points were changes in the Kansas City Cardiomyopathy Questionnaire Clinical Summary Score (KCCQ-CSS) and percent weight change.[4] Secondary end points included a hierarchical composite of death, heart failure events, KCCQ-CSS difference, and 6-minute walk testing, in this order.[4] The treatment group scored 7.8 points higher (95% CI 4.8–10.9; $p < 0.001$) in the KCCQ-CSS, with higher scores indicating fewer symptoms and physical limitations, had –13.3% body weight change compared to –2.6% in the placebo group (–10.7%; 95% CI –11.9 to –9.4%; $p < 0.001$), produced more wins in a hierarchical composite end point (win ratio 1.72; 95% CI 1.37–2.15; $p < 0.001$), and had –43.5% change in C-reactive protein (CRP) compared to –7.3% with placebo (estimated treatment ratio 0.61; 95% CI 0.51–0.72; $p < 0.001$).[4]

TABLE 1: Pharmacologic-based cardiovascular outcome trials where the intervention is the addition of a GLP-1 receptor agonist.

	Select	*STEP-HFpEF*	*Leader*
Design	Multicenter, double-blind, randomized, placebo-controlled, event-driven superiority trial	Multicenter, double-blind, randomized, placebo-controlled trial	Multicenter, double-blind, randomized, placebo-controlled trial
Participants	17,604	529	9,340
Participant age	Mean age: 61.6 ± 8.9	Median age 69.0 (62–75)	Mean age 64.3 ± 7.2
Intervention and dosage (mg) versus control	Semaglutide 2.4 mg weekly (8,803) versus placebo (8,801)	Semaglutide 2.4 mg weekly (263) versus placebo (266)	Liraglutide 1.8 mg daily (4,668) versus placebo (4,672)
Baseline CVD/DM status	Participants had established CVD, defined as previous MI, stroke, or symptomatic PAD Participants were not diabetic	• Participants had EF of 45% or greater, NYHA class II, III, or IV, KCCQ-CSS < 90, 6MWD 100 m or greater, and one of the following: Elevated LV filling pressures, elevated natriuretic peptide levels plus echocardiographic abnormalities, or hospitalization for HF in the 12 months before screening plus ongoing diuretic therapy or echocardiographic abnormalities • Participants were not diabetic	• *2 cohorts for CVD status:* Age 50 or more with at least one cardiovascular condition (ASCVD, CKD3, or greater, NYHA II or III HF), or age 60 or more with at least one CV risk factor (microalbuminuria/ proteinuria, hypertension and LVH, LV systolic or diastolic dysfunction, or ABI of <0.9) • All participants had type 2 diabetes with HbA1c 7% or more
Baseline BMI	Mean BMI 33.4 ± 5.0	Median BMI 37.0 (33.7–41.4)	Mean BMI 32.5 ± 6.3
Follow-up (months)	39.8 ± 9.4	12	45.6
Primary outcomes	Composite of death from CV causes, nonfatal MI, nonfatal stroke (HR 0.80; 95% CI 0.72–0.90; $p < 0.001$)	• Change in KCCQ-CSS from baseline to week 52 (points): 7.8 (4.8–10.9; $p < 0.001$) • Percentage change in body weight from baseline to week 52: –10.7% (–11.9 to –9.4%; $p < 0.001$)	• Time-to-event analysis consisting of the first occurrence of death from CV causes (HR 0.78; 95% CI 0.66–0.93; $p = 0.007$), nonfatal MI (HR 0.88; 95% CI 0.85–1.03; $p = 0.11$), or nonfatal stroke (HR 0.89; 95% CI 0.72–1.11; $p = 0.30$) • The primary composite outcome was lower in the treatment group (HR 0.87; 95% CI 0.78–0.97; $p = 0.01$)
Secondary outcomes	• Death from CV causes (HR 0.85; 95% CI 0.71–1.01; $p = 0.07$) • First occurrence of death from CV causes or hospitalization or an urgent medical visit for heart failure: HF composite end point (HR 0.82; 95% CI 0.71–0.96) • Death from any cause (HR 0.81; 95% CI 0.71–0.93)	• Change from baseline to week 52 in 6MWD (m): 20.3 (8.6–32.1; $p < 0.001$) • Change from baseline to week 52 in CRP level: Estimated treatment ratio 0.61 (0.51–0.72; $p < 0.001$) • Hierarchical composite end point: Win ratio 1.72 (1.37–2.15; $p < 0.001$)	• Expanded composite outcome consisting of primary outcome, plus coronary revascularization (HR 0.91; 95% CI 0.80–1.04; $p = 0.18$), hospitalization from unstable angina (HR 0.98; 95% CI 0.76–1.26; $p = 0.87$) or hospitalization for heart failure (HR 0.87; 95% CI 0.73–1.05; $p = 0.14$) • Microvascular events: Retinopathy and nephropathy (HR 0.84; 95% CI 0.73–0.97; $p = 0.02$)
Adverse effects	Higher rate of GI disorders, metabolism and nutrition disorders, administration-site conditions, and gallbladder-related disorders	Higher rate of GI adverse events	Higher rate of GI adverse events

(6MWD: 6-minute walk distance; ABI: ankle–brachial index; ASCVD: atherosclerotic cardiovascular disease; CI: confidence interval; CKD: chronic kidney disease; CRP: C-reactive protein; CV: cardiovascular; DM: diabetes mellitus; EF: ejection fraction; HF: heart failure; HR: hazard ratio; KCCQ-CSS: Kansas City Cardiomyopathy Questionnaire Clinical Summary Score; LVH: left ventricular hypertrophy; MI: myocardial infarction; NYHA: New York Heart Association; PAD: peripheral artery disease)

LIRAGLUTIDE EFFECT AND ACTION IN DIABETES: EVALUATION OF CARDIOVASCULAR OUTCOME RESULTS (LEADER)

In total, 9,340 patients with type 2 diabetes who had a hemoglobin A1c of ≥7%, and either at least one cardiovascular condition or at least one cardiovascular risk factor were treated with either liraglutide 1.8 mg daily, or placebo in a time-to-event analysis, with median follow-up of 3.8 years.[5] The mean BMI of participants was 32.5 ± 6.3.[5] The treatment group experienced significantly fewer primary outcome events of CV death, nonfatal MI, or nonfatal stroke (HR 0.87; 95% CI 0.78–0.97; $p = 0.01$), with a significant reduction in CV death (HR 0.78; 95% CI 0.66–0.93; $p = 0.007$).[5] The rates of nonfatal MI, nonfatal stroke, and heart failure hospitalizations were nonsignificantly lower in the treatment group.[5]

Trials where the intervention involves bariatric surgery **(Table 2)**.

TABLE 2: Trials where the intervention involves bariatric surgery.

	SOS	*Stampede*
Design	Prospective, nonrandomized, matched, surgical intervention controlled trial	Prospective, randomized, surgical intervention controlled trial
Participants	4,047	134
Participant age	Mean age 46.1 ± 5.8	Mean age 48.7 ± 8.1
Intervention versus control	Bariatric surgery versus conventional treatment	Intensive medical therapy alone or intensive medical therapy plus Roux-en-Y gastric bypass or sleeve gastrectomy
Baseline BMI	41.3 ± 4.4	36.5 ± 3.5
Baseline CVD/DM status	Diabetes: 10.7% (treatment group) versus 11.4% (control). Previous MI: 31% (treatment group) versus 29% (control group)	• All patients had type 2 diabetes, with or without the use of insulin • Across all groups, 92.5% patients had metabolic syndrome, 84.3% had dyslipidemia, and 64.7% had hypertension
Primary outcomes	All-cause mortality reduced in the bariatric surgery group (HR 0.71; $p = 0.01$)	5.3% of participants on medical therapy alone achieved HbA1c of 6% or less, compared to 29% of gastric bypass participants ($p = 0.08$ in ITT analysis), and 23% of gastric sleeve ($p = 0.17$ in ITT analysis)
Secondary outcomes	• *Cardiovascular death:* HR 0.47 (95% CI 0.29–0.76; $p = 0.002$) • *First-time MACE:* HR 0.67 (95% CI 0.54–0.83; $p < 0.001$)	• Zero participants on medical therapy achieved an HbA1c of 6% or less without diabetes medication, compared to 22.4% with gastric bypass ($p = 0.006$) and 14.9% with sleeve gastrectomy ($p = 0.04$) • –2.1% change from baseline in A1c in both surgical groups compared to medical group ($p = 0.03$) • 58% ($p = 0.003$) reduction in fasting plasma glucose with gastric bypass and 35% ($p = 0.02$) reduction with gastric sleeve compared to medical group • 17.9 kg reduction in the gastric bypass group ($p = 0.03$) and 13.3 kg reduction in the gastric sleeve group ($p = 0.03$) compared to the medical therapy group • –24.9% change in serum LDL ($p = 0.012$) in the gastric bypass group • –22.6% change in serum LDL ($p = 0.016$) in the gastric sleeve group compared to medical therapy group • –31.5% change in serum triglycerides ($p = 0.03$) in the gastric bypass group and –21.1% change in serum LDL (0.04) in the gastric sleeve group compared to medical therapy group
Adverse effects	Reoperation rates (excluding operations due to postoperative complications): Banding, 31%; vertical banded gastroplasty, 21%; gastric bypass, 17%	• 49% occurrence of anemia in the gastric sleeve group compared to 16% in medical therapy ($p < 0.05$) • 64% of gastric bypass participants experienced an episode of hypoglycemia compared to 91% of medical therapy participants ($p < 0.05$)

(A1c: glycated hemoglobin; CI: confidence interval; CV: cardiovascular; DM: diabetes mellitus; HbA1c: hemoglobin A1c; ITT: intention-to-treat; LDL: low-density lipoprotein; MI: myocardial infarction)

EFFECTS OF BARIATRIC SURGERY ON MORTALITY IN SWEDISH OBESE SUBJECTS (SOS)

In this nonrandomized, prospective study, 2010 obese participants (BMI ≥ 34 in men and ≥38 in women) who received bariatric surgery were matched to 2,037 obese controls who received usual care, with a median follow-up of 14.7 years.[6] The primary end point was total mortality, but death from MI or stroke was predefined secondary end points.[6] In this study, bariatric surgery was associated with reduced CV death (HR 0.47; 95% CI 0.29–0.76; $p = 0.002$), and the surgery group had lower first-time CV events, fatal or nonfatal (HR 0.67; 95% CI 0.54–0.83; $p < 0.001$).[6]

SURGICAL THERAPY AND MEDICATIONS POTENTIALLY ERADICATE DIABETES EFFICIENTLY (STAMPEDE)

In total, 150 patients with type 2 diabetes and a BMI between 27 and 43 were randomly assigned to intensive medical therapy alone or intensive medical therapy plus Roux-en-Y gastric bypass or sleeve gastrectomy with 5-year follow-up.[7] The primary end point was the percentage of participants achieving glycated hemoglobin (HbA1c) of 6.0% or less with or without glucose-lowering medications in an intention-to-treat analysis.[7] In total, 5.3% of participants on medical therapy alone achieved this, compared to 29% of participants who underwent gastric bypass ($p = 0.08$), and 23% of participants who underwent sleeve gastrectomy ($p = 0.17$).[7] Patients who underwent surgical procedures had significant reductions in HbA1c, triglycerides, mean body weight, and increase in mean HDL compared to medical therapy alone (all $p < 0.05$).[7] At 5 years, the gastric bypass group experienced a significant reduction in cardiovascular medication burden.[7] This group had a higher percentage of participants on zero CV medications at 5 years (34.7 vs. 10.5%; $p < 0.05$), and a lower proportion on lipid-lowering therapy at 5 years versus medical therapy alone (38.8 vs. 71.1%; $p < 0.001$).[7] Overall, these results suggest that at 5 years, individuals with excess body mass who receive bariatric surgery plus intensive medical therapy (vs. medical therapy alone) experience reduced cardiovascular medication burden and improvements in cardiometabolic risk factors, such as weight, HbA1c, and triglyceride/HDL levels.[7]

Cardiovascular outcome trial where the intervention involves lifestyle modifications **(Table 3)**.

PRIMARY PREVENTION OF CARDIOVASCULAR DISEASE WITH A MEDITERRANEAN DIET SUPPLEMENTED WITH EXTRA-VIRGIN OLIVE OIL OR NUTS (PREDIMED)

In total, 7,447 participants who were at high cardiovascular risk and had no cardiovascular disease at baseline were

TABLE 3: Cardiovascular outcome trial where the intervention involves lifestyle modifications.

	Predimed
Design	Parallel group, multicenter, randomized controlled trial
Participants	7,447
Participant age	Mean age 67 ± 6.2 years
Intervention versus control	Mediterranean diet with EVOO or Mediterranean diet with mixed nuts versus control diet
Baseline BMI	Mean BMI 29.9 ± 3.8
Baseline CVD/DM status	48.9% of participants had a diagnosis of type 2 diabetes. 82.7% of participants had a diagnosis of hypertension. 72.3% of participants had a diagnosis of dyslipidemia, 22% of participants had a family history of premature CHD
Primary outcomes	Both Mediterranean diets had a significant decrease in 5 years absolute risk % (HR 0.7; 95% CI 0.55–0.89)
Secondary outcomes	Both Mediterranean diets had a significant decrease in stroke (HR 0.58; 95% CI 0.42–0.82), and neither diet had a significant decrease in MI, death from CV cause, or death from any cause
Adverse effects	No relevant adverse effects were reported

(CHD: coronary heart disease; CI: confidence interval; CV: cardiovascular; DM: diabetes mellitus; EVOO: extra-virgin olive oil; HR: hazard ratio; MI: myocardial infarction)

randomly assigned to one of three groups: Mediterranean diet supplemented with extra-virgin olive oil (EVOO), Mediterranean diet supplemented with mixed nuts, or a control diet based on advice to reduce dietary fat.[8] The trial was stopped at a median follow-up of 4.8 years on the basis of a prespecified interim analysis.[8] The primary outcome was the occurrence of a major adverse cardiovascular event (MACE): CV death, nonfatal MI, or nonfatal stroke.[8] MACE significantly decreased in the Mediterranean diet + EVOO arm (HR 0.69; 95% CI 0.53–0.91) and the Mediterranean diet + mixed nuts arm (HR 0.72; 95% CI 0.54–0.95), when compared to the control group.[8] MACE reduction was driven by significantly fewer strokes in both Mediterranean subgroups (HR 0.65; 95% CI 0.44–0.95 with EVOO; and HR 0.54; 95% CI 0.35–0.82 with mixed nuts), while changes in MI, death from CV causes, and death from any cause were not statistically significant.[8]

REFERENCES

1. World Obesity Federation. Prevalence of Obesity. [online] Available from https://www.worldobesity.org/about/about-obesity/prevalence-of-obesity. [Last accessed January, 2026].
2. GBD 2021 Adolescent BMI Collaborators. Global, regional, and national prevalence of child and adolescent overweight and obesity, 1990–2021, with forecasts to 2050: a forecasting study for the Global Burden of Disease Study 2021. Lancet. 2025;405:785-812.
3. Lincoff AM, Brown-Frandsen K, Colhoun HM, et al; SELECT Trial Investigators. Semaglutide and cardiovascular outcomes in obesity without diabetes. N Engl J Med. 2023;389(24):2221-32.
4. Kosiborod MN, Abildstrøm SZ, Borlaug BA, et al; STEP-HFpEF Trial Committees and Investigators. Semaglutide in patients with heart failure with preserved ejection fraction and obesity. N Engl J Med. 2023;389(12):1069-80.
5. Marso SP, Daniels GH, Brown-Frandsen K, et al; LEADER Trial Investigators. Liraglutide and cardiovascular outcomes in type 2 diabetes. N Engl J Med. 2016;375(4):311-22.
6. Sjöström L, Peltonen M, Jacobson P, et al. Bariatric surgery and long-term cardiovascular events. JAMA. 2012;307(1):56-65.
7. Schauer PR, Bhatt DL, Kirwan JP, et al; STAMPEDE Investigators. Bariatric surgery versus intensive medical therapy for diabetes—5-year outcomes. N Engl J Med. 2017;376(7):641-51.
8. Estruch R, Ros E, Salas-Salvadó J, et al; PREDIMED Study Investigators. Primary prevention of cardiovascular disease with a Mediterranean diet supplemented with extra-virgin olive oil or nuts (retraction and republication). N Engl J Med. 2018;378(25):e34.

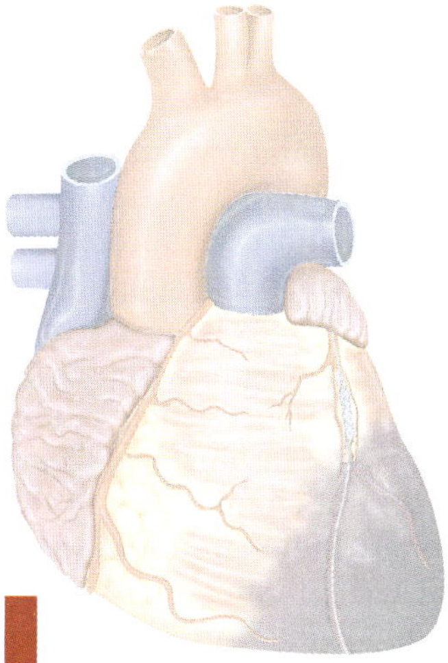

9

CHAPTER

Obesity and Cardiometabolic Risk Factor Relationship

Sarita Bajaj

INTRODUCTION

Obesity is a growing epidemic worldwide, with roughly 650 million adults and about 340 million young people affected. India has also seen a steady rise in the prevalence of obesity.[1] The Indian Council of Medical Research–India Diabetes (ICMR–INDIAB) study reported that about 254 million adults (28.6%) have generalized obesity and 351 million (39.5%) have abdominal obesity in India, as defined by the World Health Organization (WHO) Asia-Pacific criteria.[2]

Obesity is not only a key determinant of diabetes but is also directly associated with an increased risk of a spectrum of disorders, including metabolic dysfunction-associated steatotic liver disease (MASLD), dyslipidemia, hypertension, and atherosclerotic cardiovascular disease (CVD), thereby increasing overall cardiometabolic risk.

Studies have consistently shown a direct relationship between excess adiposity and increased risk of CVD. Understanding the link between the two and the underlying pathophysiology is key to the prevention and management of obesity and associated cardiometabolic risk.

OBESITY AND INCREASED CARDIOMETABOLIC RISK

Obesity has emerged as one of the strongest modifiable determinants of cardiovascular mortality worldwide. A recent analysis based on data from the Global Burden of Disease 2021 study reported that CVDs attributable to high body mass index (BMI) (>25 kg/m^2) accounted for approximately 1.9 million deaths and 45.43 million disability-adjusted life years (DALYs) across both urban and rural populations.[3] The global rise in obesity-attributable cardiovascular deaths is associated with the growing prevalence of type 2 diabetes, dyslipidemia, and hypertension, particularly in low- and middle-income countries, where urbanization and lifestyle transitions have intensified the cardiometabolic burden.

Large prospective cohorts have demonstrated a graded linear association between BMI and cardiovascular mortality. Each 5 kg/m^2 increment in BMI is associated with approximately a 30% higher coronary heart disease mortality and a 40% higher stroke mortality, independent of age and sex.[4] While a portion of this association is mediated by blood pressure, glucose, and lipid abnormalities, analyses from the Emerging Risk Factors Collaboration reveal a residual independent effect of adiposity on vascular death, potentially driven by systemic inflammation, endothelial dysfunction, oxidative stress, and prothrombotic pathways. Obesity is consistently associated with increased morbidity and early mortality, especially from CVD. In a pooled analysis of 10 large US cohorts including over 3.2 million person-years of follow-up, overweight and obesity were associated with significantly higher lifetime risks of CVD compared to normal BMI, with hazard ratios of 1.21–1.32 for overweight and 1.67–1.85 for obesity. Individuals with excess body weight developed CVD at younger ages and spent a greater proportion of their lifespan living with CVD morbidity, highlighting the long-term cardiovascular burden of obesity despite similar overall longevity.[5] Importantly, the duration of obesity exposure, referred to as *cumulative obesity*, has emerged as a major determinant of cardiometabolic risk, independent of current weight status. Long-term exposure to adiposity may promote irreversible vascular, metabolic, and structural changes that persist despite later weight reduction. Data from the Framingham Heart Study (FHS) demonstrated that the duration of obesity was independently associated with a higher risk of both all-cause mortality [adjusted heart rate (HR) 1.07, 95% CI 1.05–1.08] and cardiovascular mortality [adjusted HR: 1.06, 95% confidence interval (CI): 1.05–1.07].[6]

PATHOPHYSIOLOGY

Obesity is characterized by adipose tissue hypertrophy and hyperplasia, resulting in impaired vascularization and subsequent tissue hypoxia. This hypoxic state activates hypoxia-inducible factor-1α (HIF-1α), which in turn triggers an inflammatory cascade and upregulation of proinflammatory cytokines. Both adipocytes and infiltrating immune cells secrete tumor necrosis factor-α (TNF-α), interleukin-6 (IL-6), interleukin-1β (IL-1β), and resistin, while levels of the insulin-sensitizing adipokine adiponectin decline. These cytokines activate the nuclear factor-κB (NF-κB) and c-Jun N-terminal kinase (JNK) signaling pathways, leading to serine phosphorylation of insulin receptor substrate-1 (IRS-1) and the development of insulin resistance within adipose and peripheral tissues. These macrophage-derived cytokines again act on adipocytes to stimulate lipolysis, releasing free fatty acids (FFAs) that lead to macrophage activation, forming a vicious cycle of inflammatory and metabolic dysfunction. Elevated circulating FFAs and TNF-α levels impair insulin signaling in skeletal muscle and liver, promoting systemic insulin resistance.[7,8]

In addition, the anti-inflammatory adipokine adiponectin, secreted predominantly by white adipose tissue, exerts insulin-sensitizing and cardioprotective effects by enhancing fatty acid oxidation and suppressing cytokine production. In acute as well as chronic inflammation, as seen in obesity, circulating adiponectin levels decline, contributing to macrophage activation, endothelial dysfunction, and systemic insulin resistance.[7]

Adipocytes also secrete several components of the renin-angiotensin-aldosterone system (RAAS) system, including angiotensinogen (AGT), renin, angiotensin-converting enzyme (ACE), and angiotensin II receptors (AT1 and AT2). In obesity, adipose mass expansion increases secretion of angiotensinogen, leading to higher local and systemic levels of angiotensin II (Ang II) and aldosterone. Ang II, in turn, stimulates adipocyte hypertrophy, inflammation, and oxidative stress, leading to a vicious cycle of RAAS activation and adipose dysfunction. This RAAS activation leads to vasoconstriction, increased peripheral resistance, increased salt and water retention, sympathetic nervous system stimulation, and endothelial dysfunction. All these factors further contribute to the increased risk of hypertension and CVD in obesity. **Flowchart 1** illustrates the various mechanisms of obesity and excess adiposity leading to increased cardiometabolic risk.

Flowchart 1: Pathophysiology of cardiometabolic risk in obesity.

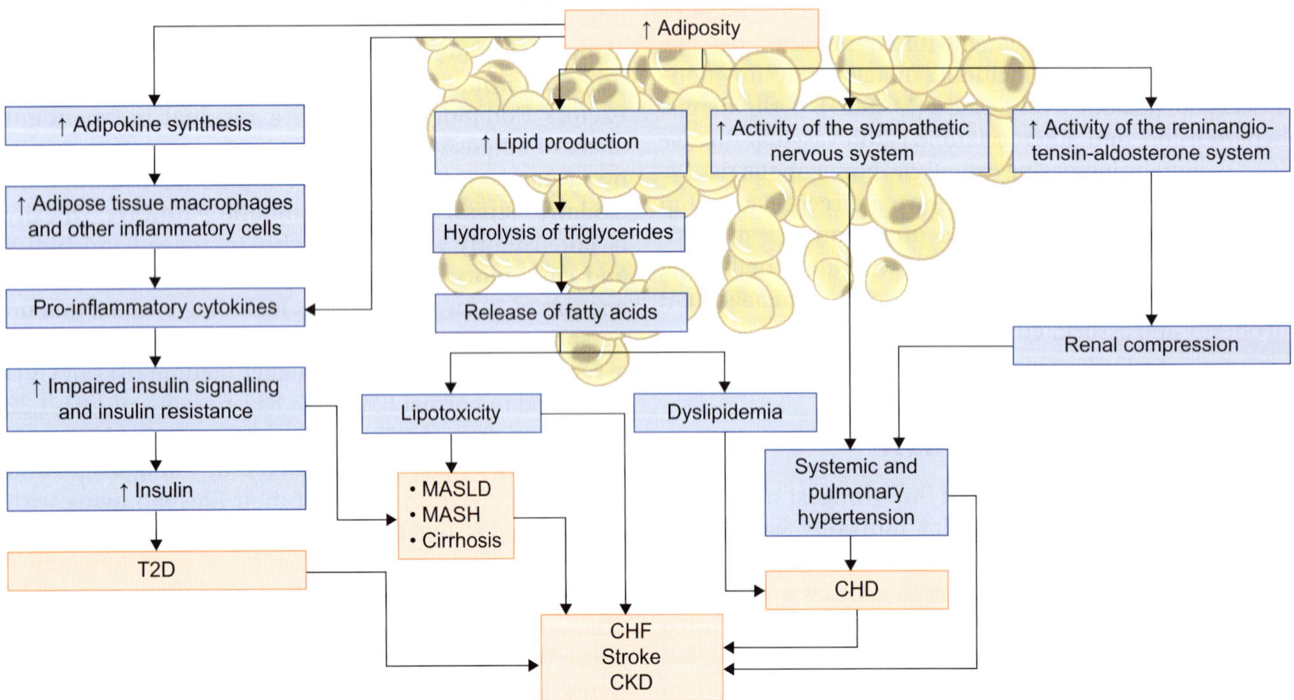

SUBCUTANEOUS ADIPOSE TISSUE VERSUS VISCERAL ADIPOSE TISSUE

Subcutaneous adipose tissue (SAT) expands primarily through adipocyte hypertrophy and, to a lesser extent, hyperplasia. In many individuals with obesity, the expandability of SAT is limited; once this threshold is exceeded, excess lipids are redirected to visceral adipose tissue (VAT) and ectopic sites, such as the liver, pancreas, and heart. This induces lipotoxicity, driving cellular apoptosis, inflammation, and insulin resistance. VAT exhibits distinct features that increase cardiometabolic risk. VAT expansion in obesity is typically not accompanied by a parallel increase in angiogenesis, which can lead to poor adipocyte oxygenation. Its expansion, hence, leads to inadequate vascular supply, creating hypoxia that provokes oxidative stress, fibrosis, and necrosis. Hypoxic VAT upregulates proinflammatory genes in tissue-resident macrophages, promoting adipocyte insulin resistance and recruitment of circulating leukocytes, forming crown-like structures around dying adipocytes. Activated adipocytes and infiltrating immune cells release the proinflammatory cytokines into the circulation, sustaining systemic low-grade inflammation. Also, VAT contains more macrophages as compared to SAT, leading to an enhanced inflammatory response. Both insulin resistance and low-grade inflammation are eventually responsible for increased cardiometabolic risk associated with obesity.[7]

NORMAL-WEIGHT OBESITY

South Asians are uniquely predisposed to develop obesity-related metabolic complications at lower BMI thresholds compared to Western populations. This was first described in the Yajnik Yudkin (YY) paradox, which highlighted the tendency of Indians to accumulate excess body fat despite having a normal BMI, a phenotype later termed "normal-weight obesity" (NWO) or the "thin–fat phenotype.[9]"

NWO is defined by an increased body fat percentage despite a normal BMI, with proposed Asian cut-offs of ≥20.6% for men and ≥33.4% for women. Individuals with this phenotype exhibit a higher prevalence of diabetes, hypertension, and dyslipidemia, comparable to those with overt obesity, and often show limited responsiveness to lifestyle interventions. This phenotype confers substantial cardiometabolic and vascular risk, being strongly associated with insulin resistance, metabolic syndrome, atherosclerosis, and cardiovascular events. Importantly, individuals with NWO have a higher all-cause and cardiovascular mortality than metabolically healthy normal-weight counterparts, with hazard ratios approaching those of obese individuals.[10]

These individuals with the thin–fat phenotype typically have lower skeletal muscle mass and greater visceral and hepatic fat accumulation, even at normal BMI. This pattern leads to insulin resistance, lipotoxicity, and chronic low-grade inflammation, predisposing to early-onset type 2 diabetes and CVD. The reduced oxidative capacity of skeletal muscle, along with adipocyte dysfunction and impaired adiponectin signaling, further aggravates metabolic abnormalities. Developmental factors, including intrauterine growth restriction and early-life undernutrition, followed by rapid postnatal weight gain, contribute to adipocyte hypertrophy and limited subcutaneous expandability, leading to ectopic fat deposition in metabolically active organs.

The high prevalence of NWO among South Asians, both in native and diaspora populations, underscores the need for ethnicity-specific definitions of adiposity and metabolic risk rather than reliance on BMI alone. Recognition of this metabolic obesity is critical for early identification and prevention of cardiometabolic disease in populations burdened simultaneously by undernutrition and noncommunicable diseases.

OBESITY INDICES AND CARDIOMETABOLIC RISK

Although BMI remains the most widely used measure of obesity, it poorly reflects fat distribution and therefore underestimates cardiometabolic risk in many individuals, especially Indians. In contrast, indices measuring central or visceral adiposity, such as waist circumference (WC), waist–hip ratio (WHR), and waist–height ratio (WHtR), better predict insulin resistance, dyslipidemia, hypertension, and CVD.[8,11] Large epidemiological studies, including INTERHEART (International Study of Risk Factors for Acute Myocardial Heart Attack) and PURE (Prospective Urban Rural Epidemiological Study), have shown that WHR and WC outperform BMI in predicting myocardial infarction and stroke, particularly in South Asian populations, where metabolic risk manifests at lower BMI levels. Imaging-based quantification of VAT and hepatic fat by CT or magnetic resonance imaging (MRI) remains the gold standard for defining cardiometabolic risk, as VAT expansion and ectopic lipid deposition are directly linked to insulin resistance, endothelial dysfunction, and atherogenesis.

RECENT GUIDELINES AND RECOMMENDATIONS

Recognizing the pitfalls of basing the diagnosis and staging of obesity on BMI alone, the latest guidelines on the definition and diagnostic criteria of obesity published in *The Lancet* have recommended the use of at least one additional anthropometric measurement, such as WC or percentage body fat, along with BMI for the diagnosis of obesity. Furthermore, the guidelines introduce a clinical criterion based on the presence of organ dysfunction (e.g., hepatic, musculoskeletal, reproductive, or respiratory impairment) or age-adjusted functional limitations in activities of daily living. This multidimensional framework indicates a shift from weight-centric assessment toward evaluating metabolic health and organ-specific consequences of adiposity, recognizing obesity as a chronic, multisystem disease rather than merely a risk factor.[12]

Similarly, the expert consensus published by Misra et al. has proposed a revised definition and staging of obesity for Asian Indians, acknowledging that conventional international cut-offs underestimate cardiometabolic risk in this population. The panel recommended lowering the BMI thresholds to ≥23 kg/m^2 for overweight and ≥25 kg/m^2 for obesity, reflecting the increased metabolic risk observed at lower BMI levels. Ethnicity-specific WC cut-offs of ≥90 cm for men and ≥80 cm for women, and a WHtR >0.5, have also been suggested as better indicators of central adiposity and cardiometabolic risk. Importantly, the consensus also proposed a staging system incorporating obesity-related comorbidities, including type 2 diabetes, hypertension, dyslipidemia, MASLD, and obstructive sleep apnea, to more accurately stratify severity and guide clinical management.[11]

CONCLUSION

Obesity is one of the most significant and modifiable risk factors for cardiometabolic disease worldwide. Beyond its well-established association with type 2 diabetes, obesity contributes directly to the development of dyslipidemia, hypertension, MASLD, and atherosclerotic CVD through mechanisms involving chronic inflammation, insulin resistance, oxidative stress, and ectopic fat deposition. The relationship between adiposity and cardiovascular morbidity is not only dose-dependent but also influenced by the duration and distribution of excess fat.

In the South Asian context, where individuals exhibit a higher propensity for visceral adiposity and metabolic complications at lower BMI thresholds, reliance on BMI alone underestimates true cardiometabolic risk. Incorporation of additional anthropometric measures such as WC, WHR, and body fat percentage, along with assessment of obesity-related comorbidities, allows for more precise risk stratification.

REFERENCES

1. Abad-Jiménez Z, Vezza T. Obesity: A Global Health Challenge Demanding Urgent Action. Biomedicines. 2025;13(2):502.
2. Anjana RM, Unnikrishnan R, Deepa M, , et al. Metabolic non-communicable disease health report of India: the ICMR-INDIAB national cross-sectional study (ICMR-INDIAB-17). Lancet Diabetes Endocrinol. 2023;11(7):474-89.
3. Li H, Liang L, Song Z, Li Y. Global, regional, and national burden of cardiovascular disease attributable to high body mass index from 1990 to 2021 and projection to 2045. Front Endocrinol (Lausanne). 2025;16:1546176.
4. Prospective Studies Collaboration. Body-mass index and cause-specific mortality in 900 000 adults: collaborative analyses of 57 prospective studies. Lancet. 2009;373(9669):1083-96.
5. Khan SS, Ning H, Wilkins JT, et al. Association of body mass index with lifetime risk of cardiovascular disease and compression of morbidity. JAMA Cardiol. 2018;3(4):280.
6. Sidhu SK, Aleman JO, Heffron SP. Obesity duration and cardiometabolic disease. Arterioscler Thromb Vasc Biol. 2023;43(10):1764-74.
7. Kawai T, Autieri MV, Scalia R. Adipose tissue inflammation and metabolic dysfunction in obesity. Am J Physiol Cell Physiol. 2021;320(3):C375-91.
8. Valenzuela PL, Carrera-Bastos P, Castillo-García A, et al. Obesity and the risk of cardiometabolic diseases. Nat Rev Cardiol. 2023;20(7):475-94.
9. Madhu SV, Kapoor N, Das S, et al. ESI Clinical Practice Guidelines for the Evaluation and Management of Obesity in India: an Update (2025). Indian J Endocrinol Metab. 2025;29(4):355-65.
10. Kapoor N. Thin Fat Obesity: The Tropical Phenotype of Obesity. In: Feingold KR, Ahmed SF, Anawalt B (Eds). South Dartmouth (MA): MDText.com, Inc; 2000.
11. Misra A, Vikram NK, Ghosh A, et al. Revised definition of obesity in Asian Indians living in India. Diabetes & Metabolic Syndrome: Clin Res Rev. 2025;19(1):102989.
12. Rubino F, Cummings DE, Eckel RH, et al. Definition and diagnostic criteria of clinical obesity. Lancet Diabetes Endocrinol. 2025;13(3):221-62.

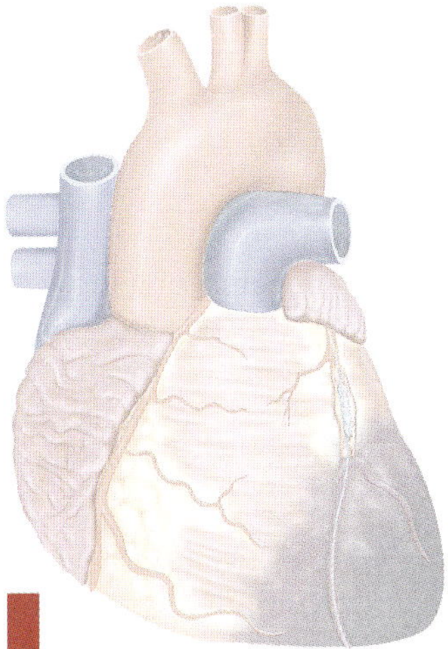

10

CHAPTER

Obesity, Cardiovascular Disease, and Salt: The Interlinked Relationship

Arvind Gupta, NK Singh

INTRODUCTION

Obesity, excessive salt intake, and cardiovascular disease (CVD) form a dangerous triad that drives a global health crisis. CVD, including heart attacks, strokes, and heart failures, remains the leading cause of death worldwide, claiming over 17 million lives annually.[1] Obesity affects nearly 40% of adults globally, while over 90% of people consume more salt than recommended, fueling high blood pressure (hypertension) and related heart complications.[2,3] This chapter explores how obesity and high salt intake interact to amplify CVD risk, the underlying mechanisms, clinical implications, and strategies for prevention and management. By understanding these conncctions, healthcare providers and policymakers can better address this preventable epidemic.[4,5]

INDEPENDENT EFFECTS OF OBESITY AND SALT ON CARDIOVASCULAR HEALTH

Obesity as a Cardiometabolic Risk Factor

Obesity, defined as a body mass index (BMI) of 30 kg/m^2 or higher, is a major driver of heart disease. Excess body fat, particularly visceral fat (fat around internal organs), disrupts normal body functions. It promotes insulin resistance, raising the risk of type 2 diabetes, and causes dyslipidemia, characterized by high levels of harmful fats in the blood.[6] Obesity also triggers inflammation by releasing proinflammatory molecules called cytokines, which damage blood vessels and increase blood pressure. Additionally, it activates the renin-angiotensin-aldosterone system (RAAS), a hormonal pathway that raises blood pressure and strains the heart.[7,8] These changes make the heart work harder, increasing the risk of heart failure, coronary artery disease, and stroke.[9] Obesity also affects the autonomic nervous system, which controls heart rate and blood pressure. Increased levels of leptin, a hormone produced by fat cells, overstimulate the sympathetic nervous system, leading to higher blood pressure and heart strain.[10] Over time, these effects cause structural changes in the heart, such as left ventricular hypertrophy (thickening of the heart muscle), further elevating CVD risk.[11]

Salt and Cardiovascular Risk

Dietary salt (sodium chloride) is essential for bodily functions, but excessive intake is harmful. The average global salt consumption is around 9–12 g/day, far exceeding the World Health Organization's (WHO) recommended limit of 5 g (about 2.3 g of sodium).[3] High salt intake raises blood pressure by causing the body to retain water, increasing the volume of blood in the arteries. This extra pressure damages blood vessel walls, leading to endothelial dysfunction (impaired blood vessel relaxation) and vascular stiffness (less flexible arteries).[12,13] Excess salt also disrupts the autonomic nervous system and promotes inflammation, further harming blood vessels and the heart.[14] Epidemiological studies, such as the International Study of Electrolyte Excretion and Blood Pressure (INTERSALT) and Prospective Urban Rural Epidemiology (PURE) studies, show a clear link between high salt intake and increased risks of hypertension, heart failure, stroke, and ischemic heart disease.[15,16] These effects are particularly pronounced in people who are salt-sensitive, meaning their blood pressure rises significantly with sodium intake.[17]

THE INTERPLAY OF OBESITY AND SALT IN CARDIOVASCULAR DISEASE

Additive and Synergistic Effects

Obesity and high salt intake do not act in isolation—they amplify each other's harmful effects. Obesity increases salt sensitivity, meaning that people with higher BMI are more likely to experience significant blood pressure spikes from salt consumption.[18] This synergy worsens hypertension and accelerates damage to the heart and blood vessels. For example, studies show that individuals with obesity have a stronger link between high salt intake and CVD events compared to those with normal BMI.[19] The combination of these risk factors creates a "perfect storm" for cardiovascular complications.

Shared and Synergistic Mechanisms

Several biological pathways explain how obesity and excess salt work together to harm the cardiovascular system **(Fig. 1)**.

Renin-angiotensin-aldosterone system activation: In obesity, fat cells produce angiotensinogen, a precursor to angiotensin II, which constricts blood vessels and raises blood pressure. High salt intake further activates RAAS, compounding these effects and promoting vascular remodeling (structural changes in blood vessels), which increases CVD risk.[7,20]

Leptin and sympathetic overdrive: Obesity elevates leptin levels, which overstimulate the sympathetic nervous system, increasing heart rate and blood pressure. High salt intake also raises leptin levels, intensifying this autonomic dysfunction and contributing to hypertension.[10,21]

Inflammation: Both obesity and excess salt trigger inflammation. Obesity causes fat cells to release proinflammatory cytokines, while high salt promotes immune cell infiltration into the kidneys and blood vessels.

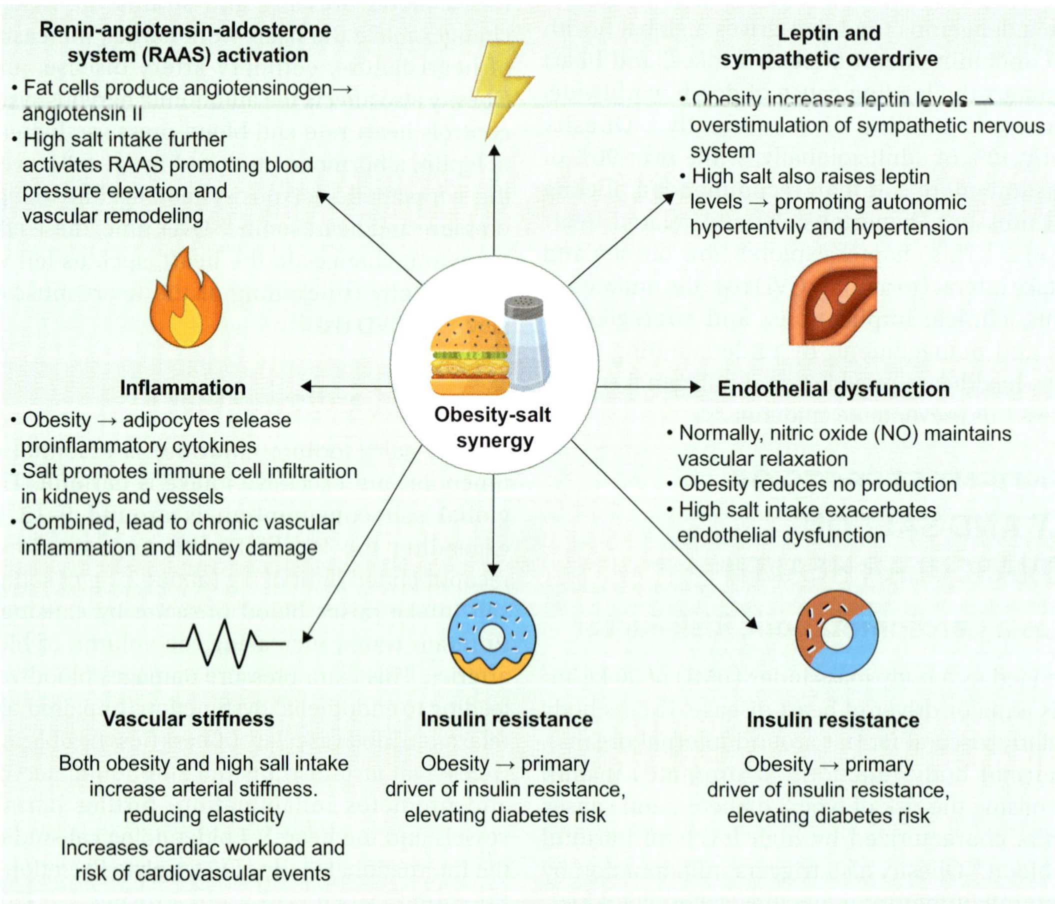

Fig. 1: Shared and synergistic mechanisms.

Together, these processes cause chronic inflammation, leading to vasoconstriction (narrowing of blood vessels) and kidney damage.[22,23]

Endothelial dysfunction: Healthy blood vessels rely on nitric oxide (NO) to relax and maintain proper blood flow. Obesity reduces NO production, and high salt intake worsens this dysfunction, leading to stiffer blood vessels and higher blood pressure.[13,24]

Vascular stiffness: Both obesity and high salt intake contribute to arterial stiffness, reducing the elasticity of arteries. This increases the workload on the heart and raises the risk of heart attack and stroke.[25]

Insulin resistance: Obesity is a primary cause of insulin resistance, which increases the risk of diabetes—a major CVD risk factor. High salt intake exacerbates insulin resistance by further activating RAAS, creating a vicious cycle.[20]

Role of Ultra-processed Foods

Ultra-processed foods, such as fast food, snacks, and sugary drinks, are a major source of both excess calories and sodium. These foods contribute to obesity by providing high amounts of sugar and unhealthy fats, while their high salt content drives hypertension.[26] For example, a single fast-food meal can contain more than the daily recommended sodium intake. The widespread availability and affordability of ultra-processed foods have fueled the global rise in obesity and salt-related CVD.[27]

EPIDEMIOLOGICAL EVIDENCE

Large scale studies provide strong evidence of the combined impact of obesity and high salt intake on CVD. The PURE study, involving over 150,000 participants across 17 countries, found that high sodium intake (above 6 g/day) was associated with a 20–30% higher risk of CVD events, particularly in individuals with obesity.[16] Similarly, the INTERSALT study, which examined sodium intake and blood pressure across 52 populations, showed that high salt consumption significantly increased blood pressure, with stronger effects in older adults and those with higher BMI.[15] The UK Biobank study further confirmed that frequent addition of salt to food (a proxy for high sodium intake) was linked to a higher risk of heart disease, especially in obese individuals.[28] These studies highlight that the combination of obesity and high salt intake disproportionately affects certain groups, including older adults and those with pre-existing hypertension.

CLINICAL IMPLICATIONS

Reducing Modifiable Risks

Addressing obesity and high salt intake is critical for preventing and managing CVD. Weight loss through diet and exercise can significantly lower blood pressure and improve heart health. Studies show that a 5–10% reduction in body weight can reduce systolic blood pressure by 5–10 mm Hg.[29] Similarly, reducing salt intake by 5 g/day can lower systolic blood pressure by 4–5 mm Hg and diastolic blood pressure by 1–3 mm Hg, with greater benefits in obese and hypertensive individuals.[13,30]

Guidelines and Recommendations

Major health organizations provide clear guidelines for managing these risk factors **(Fig. 2)**.

American Heart Association (AHA): It recommends a maximum of 2.3 g of sodium per day (about one teaspoon of salt), with an ideal limit of 1.5 g for people with hypertension or at high CVD risk.[31]

World Health Organization (WHO): It advocates for <5 g of salt per day and promotes policies to reduce sodium in processed foods.[3]

Dietary approaches to stop hypertension (DASH): This diet, rich in fruits, vegetables, whole grains, and low-fat dairy, is effective for lowering blood pressure and managing weight.[32]

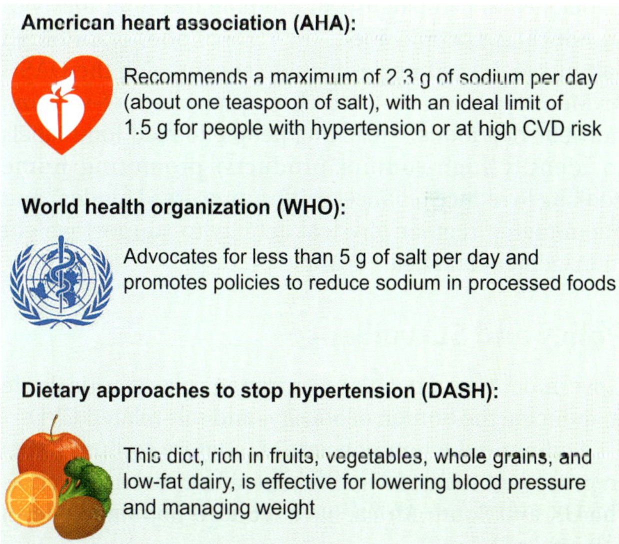

Fig. 2: Guidelines and recommendations.[3,31,32]

TABLE 1: Shared and synergistic mechanisms connecting obesity, high salt intake, and cardiovascular disease.

Mechanism	*Obesity*	*Excess salt*	*Synergistic effect*
RAAS activation	Increased angiotensinogen[7]	Further stimulates RAAS[20]	Worsens hypertension and vascular damage[7,20]
Endothelial dysfunction	Reduced NO[24]	Further impairs NO production[13]	Increases vascular stiffness and CVD risk[13,24]
Arterial stiffness	Increased stiffness[25]	Exacerbates stiffness[25]	Higher risk of heart attack and stroke[25]
Inflammation	Proinflammatory cytokines[22]	Immune cell infiltration[23]	Promotes vasoconstriction and kidney damage[22,23]
Sympathetic activity	Elevated leptin, autonomic dysfunction[10]	Salt-induced leptin increase[21]	Worsens blood pressure control[10,21]
Insulin resistance	Common in obesity[6]	Exacerbated via RAAS[20]	Increases diabetes and CVD risk[6,20]

Special Populations

Certain groups, such as individuals with obesity or African ancestry, are more salt-sensitive, meaning they experience larger blood pressure increases from salt intake.[18] These populations benefit most from targeted interventions, such as personalized dietary counseling and stricter sodium limits. Older adults also show increased salt sensitivity due to age-related declines in kidney function, making salt reduction particularly important.[33]

Mechanistic Overview

Table 1 summarizes the shared and synergistic mechanisms linking obesity, excess salt, and CVD.

PUBLIC HEALTH APPROACHES

Education and Behavioral Change

Public health campaigns can promote healthier lifestyles by educating people about the risks of obesity and high salt intake. Key strategies include encouraging the DASH or Mediterranean diet, which emphasizes low-sodium, nutrient-rich foods;[32] teaching people to read food labels to identify high-sodium products; promoting home cooking to reduce reliance on ultra-processed foods;[26] and encouraging regular physical activity to support weight management and heart health.[29]

Policy and Surveillance

Governments and health organizations play a critical role in reducing the burden of obesity- and salt-related CVD.

Sodium reduction policies: Mandatory sodium limits in processed foods, as implemented in countries such as the UK and South Africa, have reduced population-level salt intake.[34]

Food labeling: Clear, front-of-pack labels help consumers choose lower-sodium and healthier options.[3]

Obesity prevention: Policies such as taxes on sugary drinks and subsidies for healthy foods can curb obesity rates.[27]

Surveillance: Monitoring sodium intake and obesity trends through national health surveys allows for timely updates to guidelines.[3]

Community-based Interventions

Targeted programs in high-risk communities, such as those with high rates of obesity or limited access to healthy foods, can reduce CVD disparities. For example, community cooking classes and school-based nutrition programs have shown success in promoting healthier diets.[35]

CONCLUSION

Obesity and excessive salt intake are closely linked risk factors that amplify the global burden of cardiovascular disease. Their combined effects—through RAAS activation, inflammation, endothelial dysfunction, and vascular stiffness—create a synergistic threat to heart health. Addressing this triad requires a multifaceted approach, including individual lifestyle changes, clinical interventions, and robust public health policies. By prioritizing weight management, sodium reduction, and equitable access to healthy foods, we can significantly reduce CVD morbidity and mortality worldwide.

REFERENCES

1. World Health Organization. (2021). Cardiovascular diseases (CVDs). [online] Available from https://www.who.int/news-room/fact-sheets/detail/cardiovascular-diseases-(cvds) [Last accessed December, 2025].

2. Watso JC, Farquhar WB. The damaging duo: obesity and excess dietary salt contribute to hypertension and cardiovascular disease. Obesity Rev. 2023;24(8):e13589.
3. World Health Organization. (2025). Sodium reduction. [online] Available from https://www.who.int/news-room/fact-sheets/detail/sodium-reduction [Last accessed December, 2025].
4. Burnier M. Salt, blood pressure and cardiovascular risk. Int J Cardiol Hypertens. 2015;4:1-7.
5. Centers for Disease Control and Prevention. (2024). Heart disease risk factors. [online] Available from https://www.cdc.gov/heart-disease/risk-factors/index.html [Last accessed December, 2025].
6. Ahmed SK, Mohammed RA. Obesity: prevalence, causes, consequences, management, preventive strategies and future research directions. Metab Open. 2025;27:100375.
7. Lopez-Jimenez F, Almahmeed W, Bays HE, et al. Obesity and cardiovascular disease: mechanistic insights and management strategies. Eur J Prev Cardiol. 2022;29(17):2218-37.
8. Youssef GS. (2022). Salt and hypertension: current views. [online] Available from https://www.escardio.org/Journals/E-Journal-of-Cardiology-Practice/Volume-22/salt-and-hypertension-current-views [Last accessed December, 2025].
9. He FJ, Tan M, Ma Y, et al. Salt reduction to prevent hypertension and cardiovascular disease. J Am Coll Cardiol. 2020;75(6):632-47.
10. Han F, Li W, Duan N, et al. Relationship between salt intake and cardiovascular disease. J Clin Hypertens (Greenwich). 2025;27:e70078.
11. He J, Ogden LG, Vupputuri S, et al. Dietary sodium intake and subsequent risk of cardiovascular disease. JAMA. 1999;282(21):2027-34.
12. O'Donnell MJ, Mente A, Smyth A, et al. Salt intake and cardiovascular disease: why are the data inconsistent? Eur Heart J. 2013;34(14):1034-40.
13. He FJ, MacGregor GA. Role of salt in cardiovascular disease. Nat Rev Cardiol. 2009;6(11):678-85.
14. Vala DR, Azam MS. Salt and cardiovascular disease. Indian J Clin Cardiol. 2024;5(2):160-6.
15. INTERSALT Cooperative Research Group. INTERSALT: an international study of electrolyte excretion and blood pressure. BMJ. 1988;297(6644):319-28.
16. Mente A, O'Donnell M, Rangarajan S, et al. Associations of urinary sodium excretion with cardiovascular events in individuals with and without hypertension: a pooled analysis of data from four studies. Lancet. 2016;388(10043):465-75.
17. Weinberger MH. Salt sensitivity of blood pressure in humans. Hypertension. 1996;27(3):481-90.
18. Rocchini AP, Key J, Bondie D, et al. The effect of weight loss on the sensitivity of blood pressure to sodium in obese adolescents. N Engl J Med. 1989;321(9):580-5.
19. Strazzullo P, D'Elia L, Kandala N-B, et al. Salt intake, stroke, and cardiovascular disease: meta-analysis of prospective studies. BMJ. 2009;339:b4567.
20. Engeli S, Schling P, Gorzelniak K, et al. The adipose-tissue renin-angiotensin-aldosterone system: role in the metabolic syndrome? Int J Biochem Cell Biol. 2003; 35(6):807-25.
21. do Carmo JM, Hall JE, da Silva AA, et al. Leptin mediates the increase in blood pressure associated with obesity. Hypertension. 2014;64(6):1283-90.
22. Norlander AE, Madhur MS, Harrison DG, et al. The immunology of hypertension. J Exp Med. 2018;215(1):21-33.
23. Crowley SD. The cooperative roles of inflammation and oxidative stress in the pathogenesis of hypertension. Antioxid Redox Signal. 2014;20(1):102-20.
24. Frisbee JC. Obesity, insulin resistance, and microvascular dysfunction. Microcirculation. 2007;14(3):289-301.
25. Safar ME, Blacher J, Boutouyrie P, et al. Arterial stiffness and cardiovascular risk in hypertension. J Hypertens. 2018;36(4):689-96.
26. Thapsuwan S, Phulkerd S, Chamratrithirong A, et al. Relationship between consumption of high fat, sugar or sodium foods, obesity and non-communicable diseases. BMJ Nutr Prev Health. 2024;7:e000794.
27. Popkin BM, Adair LS, Ng SW, et al. Global nutrition transition and the pandemic of obesity in developing countries. Nutr Rev. 2012;70(1):3-21.
28. Ma H, Wang X, Li X, et al. Adding salt to food and risk of cardiovascular disease. J Am Coll Cardiol. 2022;80(22):2157-67.
29. Neter JE, Stam BE, Kok FJ, et al. Influence of weight reduction on blood pressure: a meta-analysis of randomized controlled trials. Hypertension. 2003;42(5):878-84.
30. Graudal NA, Galløe AM, Garred P, et al. Effects of sodium restriction on blood pressure, renin, aldosterone, catecholamines, cholesterols, and triglyceride: a meta-analysis. JAMA. 1998;279(17):1383-91.
31. American Heart Association. (2021). How much sodium should I eat per day? [online] Available from https://www.heart.org/en/healthy-living/healthy-eating/eat-smart/sodium/how-much-sodium-should-i-eat-per-day [Last accessed December, 2025].
32. Appel LJ, Moore TJ, Obarzanek E, et al. A clinical trial of the effects of dietary patterns on blood pressure. N Engl J Med. 1997;336(16):1117-24.
33. Luft FC, Weinberger MH, Grim CE, et al. Sodium sensitivity and resistance in normotensive humans. Am J Med. 1982;72(5):726-36.
34. He FJ, Brinsden HC, MacGregor GA, et al. Salt reduction in the United Kingdom: a successful experiment in public health. J Hum Hypertens. 2014;28(6):345-52.
35. Story M, Kaphingst KM, Robinson-O'Brien R, et al. Creating healthy food and eating environments: policy and environmental approaches. Annu Rev Public Health. 2008;29:253-72.

CHAPTER 11

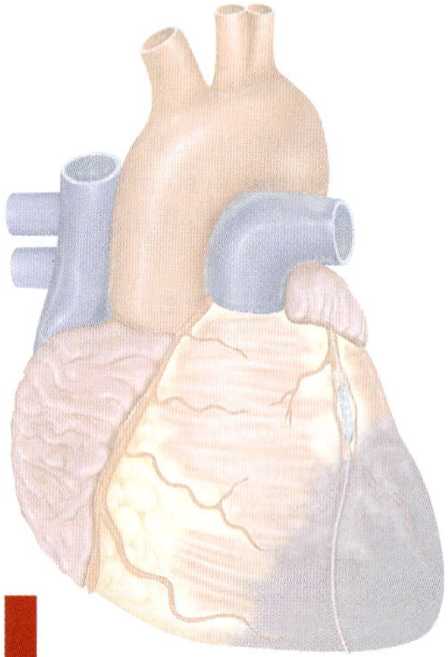

Obesity Paradox in Cardiovascular Disease

Shivani Rao, Nitish Naik, Ojas Jain

INTRODUCTION

Obesity has become a global health challenge, closely linked to numerous chronic conditions such as type 2 diabetes mellitus, cardiovascular diseases, and increased mortality. Despite the well-established risks of obesity, a paradoxical phenomenon has emerged in clinical literature, where overweight or mildly obese individuals with certain cardiovascular diseases may experience better survival outcomes than their normal-weight counterparts. This chapter explores this phenomenon, known as the "obesity paradox," by examining its epidemiology, clinical implications, pathophysiology, and evolving treatment perspectives.

EPIDEMIOLOGY AND GLOBAL IMPACT

According to data from the World Health Organization (WHO),[1] approximately 2.5 billion people worldwide are overweight, and nearly 890 million are living with obesity as of 2022. By 2030, nearly half of the adult population in the United States is projected to have obesity, with some states showing prevalence rates above 50%. This epidemic is not confined to developed countries; low- and middle-income countries in Asia, Latin America, and Africa are also experiencing rapid increases due to urbanization, sedentary lifestyles, and dietary changes.

In India, the obesity epidemic affects roughly 11.8–31.3% of the population, with abdominal obesity particularly common, ranging from 16.9% to 36.3%.

DEFINING OBESITY PARADOX

The term "obesity paradox" was coined nearly two decades ago by Gruberg[2] and colleagues to describe the observation that obesity might be associated with a better prognosis in patients with systolic heart failure or after percutaneous coronary intervention (PCI). Since then, this paradox has been reported in overweight patients with stable coronary heart disease (CHD), acute coronary syndromes, or coronary artery bypass grafting. However, the survival benefit does not generally extend to individuals with a body mass index (BMI) >30 kg/m^2.

This paradoxical association has also been observed in other cardiovascular conditions such as hypertension, atrial fibrillation (AF), pulmonary arterial hypertension, and congenital heart disease, sparking considerable debate in the cardiovascular community.

PARADOX IN HEART FAILURE

Obesity substantially increases the risk of developing heart failure. For each 1 kg/m^2 increase in BMI, the risk rises by 7% in women and 5% in men. Paradoxically, once heart failure develops, excess weight appears to have a protective effect. A meta-analysis[3] of nearly 22,000 patients with chronic heart failure followed over 3 years showed that underweight individuals had the highest mortality rates, whereas overweight and mildly obese individuals had the lowest mortality and readmission rates.

The DAPA-HF trial[4] demonstrated a U-shaped relationship, with optimal outcomes at a BMI near

30 kg/m^2. Proposed mechanisms include greater lean mass and metabolic reserves, reduced catabolism, favorable cytokine and inflammatory profiles, and lower natriuretic peptide levels, leading to earlier diagnosis and better treatment tolerance. The benefit is largely confined to overweight and class I–II obesity, while severe obesity (BMI ≥40 kg/m^2) is associated with adverse remodeling and poorer outcomes. Thus, preserving lean mass and improving fitness rather than aggressive weight loss is key in managing heart failure patients.

OBESITY PARADOX IN CORONARY ARTERY DISEASE

Obesity is a major independent risk factor for developing and progressing coronary artery disease (CAD). Each 5 kg/m^2 increase in BMI raises CAD risk by approximately 30%, even after adjusting for other factors like hypertension and dyslipidemia. Visceral adiposity, in particular, promotes oxidative stress, endothelial dysfunction, and systemic inflammation mediated by interleukins such as IL-1 and IL-18.

Despite these adverse effects, once CAD is established, overweight and mildly obese patients often exhibit improved survival—a phenomenon termed the obesity paradox. Meta-analyses[5] of over 1.3 million CAD patients demonstrate the lowest mortality rates in those with BMI between 25 and 35 kg/m^2, while mortality risk climbs sharply in severe obesity (BMI >35 kg/m^2), resulting in a U-shaped mortality curve.

Potential mechanisms behind this paradox include larger lean mass and metabolic reserves, lower natriuretic peptide levels enabling earlier therapy, and better drug tolerance. Patients who are underweight or sarcopenic tend to experience worse outcomes. Long-term physical activity over 5 years mitigates the paradox and its disappearance in cases of severe or central obesity highlights the critical role of fitness over mere calorie restriction in improving prognosis for obese CAD patients.

PARADOX IN ATRIAL FIBRILLATION

Obesity is a well-established independent risk factor for AF, second only to hypertension. The ARIC study found that nearly 18% of AF cases are attributed to overweight and obesity, with a 4% increase in risk per 1 kg/m^2 increase in BMI. Individuals with obesity may have up to a 50% higher incidence of AF.[6]

Structural remodeling in obese patients includes left atrial enlargement, interstitial fibrosis, and slowing of electrical conduction. Other contributing factors such as increased left ventricular filling pressures, diastolic dysfunction, hypertension, or heart failure exacerbate AF development. Moreover, sleep apnea quadruples AF risk, while diabetes worsens outcomes via glycosylation-induced myocardial fibrosis. Chronic low-grade inflammation and activation of the NLRP3 inflammasome (IL-1 and IL-18) further drive AF pathogenesis.

Despite the elevated risk, once AF develops, an obesity paradox emerges: Overweight and obese patients demonstrate lower all-cause and cardiovascular mortality compared to normal BMI individuals. Large cohorts such as AFFIRM and ARISTOTLE consistently confirm this protective association. Additionally, higher visceral adiposity measured by waist circumference is linked to decreased mortality in AF, contrasting with heart failure and CAD where central obesity diminishes the paradox.

Possible explanations include better metabolic and lean mass reserves, younger onset age, more frequent rhythm control therapy, and greater anticoagulant use. Importantly, higher cardiorespiratory fitness (CRF) independently improves outcomes and reduces AF recurrence, underscoring the importance of exercise-based management over weight loss alone in obese AF patients.

PATHOPHYSIOLOGICAL INSIGHTS

The pathophysiology underlying the obesity paradox **(Fig. 1)** is complex and multifactorial. One of the earliest and most accepted explanations is the metabolic reserve hypothesis, which proposes that excess adipose tissue in obese individuals serves as an energy and nutritional buffer, aiding survival during catabolic stress, acute illnesses, and chronic inflammation in diseases like heart failure and chronic kidney disease. This metabolic reserve provides a survival advantage compared to leaner individuals who lack such reserves.

Additionally, obesity alters the inflammatory and neurohormonal milieu. Increased circulating levels of leptin and soluble TNF-α receptors in obese patients may neutralize toxic proinflammatory cytokines, potentially creating a more balanced immune environment. Elevated concentrations of circulating lipoproteins in obese individuals bind and inactivate bacterial endotoxins, thereby reducing systemic inflammatory load and protecting against adverse cardiovascular remodeling.

Furthermore, increased mobilization of endothelial progenitor cells in severely obese patients enhances repair mechanisms for damaged myocardium and promotes new blood vessel growth, potentially mitigating atherogenic processes.[7]

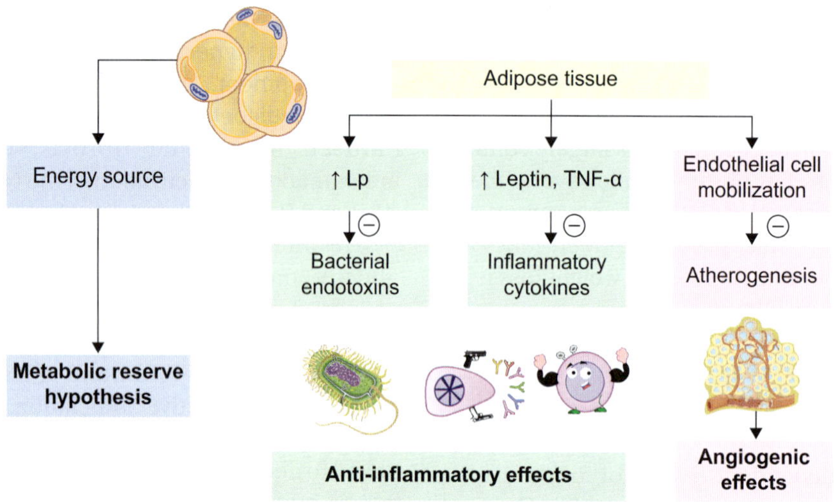

Fig. 1: Pathophysiology of obesity paradox.

TABLE 1: Clinical features of different obesity subsets.

Obesity phenotypes	*Normal weight*	*Athlete*	*Nonsarcopenic obese*	*Sarcopenic obese*
	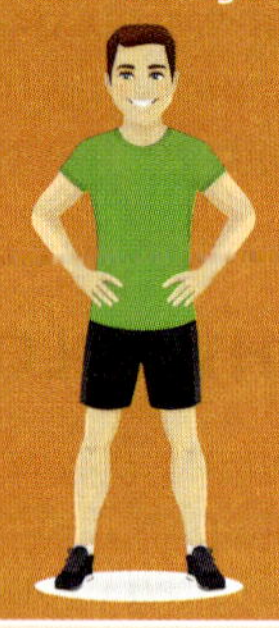	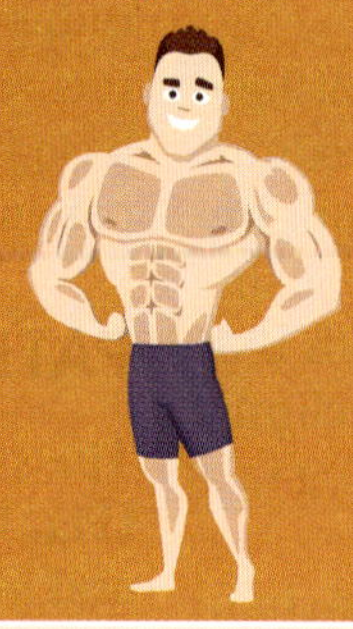	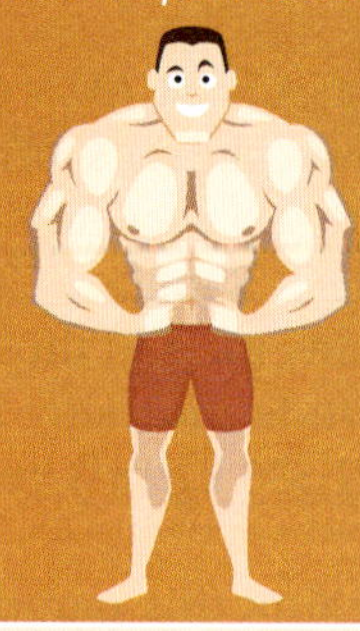	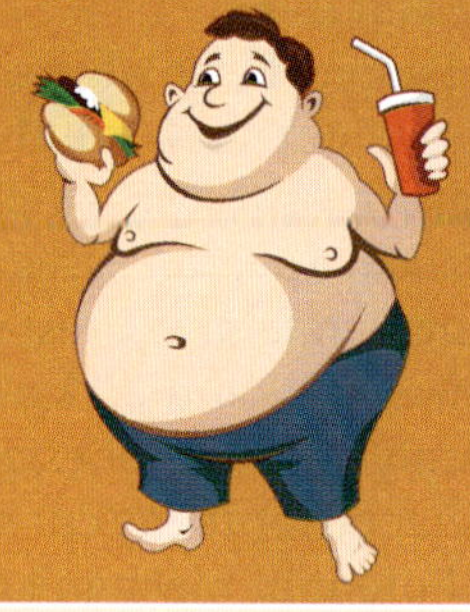
BMI (kg/m^2)	18.5–25	≥30	≥30	≥30
Fat mass	Normal	Decreased	Increased	Increased
Lean mass	Normal	Increased	Increased	Decreased
Cardiorespiratory fitness	Normal	Increased	Mildly impairment?	Severe impairment?

(BMI: body mass index)

METABOLICALLY HEALTHY OBESITY

Metabolically healthy obesity (MHO) describes a subset of individuals with obesity (BMI ≥30 kg/m^2) who do not exhibit typical metabolic syndrome features such as hypertension, dyslipidemia, insulin resistance, or hyperglycemia, and who often maintain preserved CRF. The clinical features of different obesity subsets are described in **Table 1**. Despite this seemingly favorable profile, emerging evidence indicates that MHO is a transient, intermediate state rather than a stable, benign phenotype.

Individuals with MHO tend to have higher amounts of subcutaneous fat relative to visceral fat, lower systemic inflammation, and better insulin sensitivity. Nonetheless, longitudinal studies reveal that up to 50% of MHO individuals eventually develop adverse metabolic profiles associated with obesity, especially with aging, physical inactivity, or weight gain.

Population-based analyses suggest that metabolically healthy obese individuals still face a 20–30% higher risk of major cardiovascular events, coronary diseases, and heart failure compared to their metabolically healthy lean counterparts.[8] The apparent protection observed in MHO may stem partly from confounding factors such as higher physical fitness and favorable fat distribution. Physically active "fat but fit" individuals often exhibit near-normal cardiometabolic risk, while low fitness levels sharply increase mortality risk.

Therefore, MHO should be recognized as a state posing increased cardiovascular risk, warranting lifestyle modifications focused on improving fitness, reducing abdominal fat, and preserving metabolic health.

REASSESSING PARADOX: BIASES AND CONFOUNDERS

The obesity paradox is increasingly interpreted as a methodological illusion rather than a genuine physiological benefit conferred by obesity. Several analytical and measurement biases distort the apparent relationship between adiposity and cardiovascular outcomes.

Confounding and Study Design Bias

Observational studies are susceptible to confounding. For instance, obese patients with heart failure often present earlier with more symptoms, prompting aggressive treatment. Higher blood pressure and preload in these patients may enhance neurohormonal therapy tolerance, while better nutritional reserves and less frequent cachexia improve survival statistics. Adjusting rigorously for age, comorbidities, treatment intensity, and follow-up often attenuates or nullifies the observed survival advantage in obesity within heart failure and CAD cohorts.[9]

Limitations of the Body Mass Index

Body mass index fails to distinguish lean mass from fat mass or evaluate fat distribution. While subcutaneous fat may be metabolically neutral, visceral fat promotes pathological remodeling and systemic inflammation. Alternative metrics such as waist-to-height ratio and weight-adjusted waist index more accurately reflect central adiposity and better predict outcomes. Studies using these measures often eliminate the apparent protective effect observed with BMI alone.

Reverse Causation and Frailty

Lower BMI in patients with chronic illnesses may reflect unintentional weight loss due to disease related cachexia, sarcopenia, or systemic illness rather than a healthy body composition. Such conditions increase mortality risk, creating a misleading appearance of survival benefit among heavier patients.[10]

Collider Stratification and Selection Bias

Statistical conditioning on disease presence may introduce collider bias, which can reverse the observed association between obesity and survival. Correcting for such biases often abolishes the obesity paradox.

Emerging Evidence (PCI and Heart Failure)

Recent analyses of patient-level data from randomized trials involving PCI reveal that a moderately elevated BMI correlates with better overall survival, primarily driven by reductions in noncardiac mortality rather than cardiovascular causes. Contemporary cohorts, however, do not show an independent protective effect of overweight or obesity after multivariate adjustment, with some studies reporting increased risks of repeat revascularization in overweight or obese nondiabetic individuals.

Similarly, refined adiposity measurements and improved confounder controls negate the previously reported survival advantage of obesity in patients with heart failure, highlighting the importance of accurate assessment and adjustment in evaluating obesity outcomes.

PHYSICAL FITNESS AND SURVIVAL

Cardiorespiratory fitness significantly modifies the relationship between obesity and cardiovascular outcomes. A landmark meta-analysis published in *JAMA* quantified that each 1-MET increase in CRF lowers all-cause and cardiovascular event risk by approximately 13–15%.[11] More recent analyses find even greater benefits, with reductions in heart failure risk nearing 18% per 1-MET increase in CRF.

In patients with heart failure, the obesity paradox largely appears in those with low fitness (e.g., peak VO_2 <14 mL/kg/min). Among high-fitness patients, BMI loses prognostic significance, and survival is superior regardless of weight. Similarly, in CAD populations, adherence to physical activity recommendations or higher CRF capacity eliminates the obesity paradox observed in more sedentary groups.

THERAPEUTIC ADVANCES AND THEIR IMPLICATIONS

Recent breakthroughs in glucagon-like peptide-1 (GLP-1) receptor agonists and dual GLP-1/glucose-dependent insulinotropic polypeptide (GIP) therapies have fundamentally challenged the concept of the obesity paradox. These therapies demonstrate that intentional weight loss improves cardiovascular outcomes across all levels of adiposity.

For instance, the SELECT trial[12] showed that semaglutide 2.4 mg reduces major adverse cardiovascular events by about 20%, with consistent benefits regardless of baseline BMI. The STEP-HFpEF trial[13] found that semaglutide improved exercise capacity, quality of life, and cardiac biomarkers in obese patients with heart failure with preserved ejection fraction (HFpEF), without compromising physiological reserve.

Similarly, tirzepatide, evaluated in the SURMOUNT-1[14] and SUMMIT[15] studies, induced approximately 20% weight loss, translating into enhanced heart failure outcomes and symptom relief. Meta-analyses confirm that GLP-1 agonists reduce major cardiovascular events across BMI categories, indicating that cardioprotection is independent of adiposity levels.

Collectively, these findings suggest that the obesity paradox largely results from measurement and analytical artifacts. When adiposity is safely and effectively reduced, cardiovascular risk declines, contradicting the idea that obesity confers a true survival advantage.

CONCLUSION

The obesity paradox remains one of the most intriguing and debated observations in cardiovascular medicine. Although overweight and mildly obese individuals with established cardiovascular disease often exhibit better short- and medium-term outcomes compared to their leaner peers, this phenomenon appears to result more from complex biases and limitations of measurement rather than a true protective effect of excess adipose tissue.

Obesity undoubtedly increases the risk of developing heart failure, CAD, and arrhythmias through inflammatory and neurohormonal pathways and adverse cardiac remodeling. However, within these disease states, factors such as lean body mass, metabolic reserves, and CRF may confer transient survival advantages.

Importantly, recent clinical trials with GLP-1 and dual GLP-1/GIP receptor agonists demonstrate that intentional weight loss improves cardiovascular function, symptoms, and clinical outcomes. These advances contradict the notion that obesity per se is protective in cardiovascular disease patients.

Future research should employ integrative phenotyping that transcends BMI to include assessments of visceral adiposity, sarcopenia, metabolic health, and CRF. While preventing obesity remains a public health priority, for patients with established cardiovascular diseases, strategies combining targeted weight loss, enhanced fitness, and preservation of lean mass are paramount to improve prognosis.

REFERENCES

1. World Health Organization. (2025). Obesity and overweight. [online] Available from https://www.who.int/news-room/fact-sheets/detail/obesity-and-overweight [Last accessed January, 2026].
2. Gruberg L, Weissman NJ, Waksman R, et al. The impact of obesity on the short- and long-term outcomes after percutaneous coronary intervention: the obesity paradox? J Am Coll Cardiol. 2002;39(4):578-84.
3. Nguyen HT, Vo TTT, Nguyen TMT, et al. Relationship between body mass index and prognosis of chronic heart failure: A meta-analysis. Front Cardiovasc Med. 2023;10:1145279.
4. McMurray JJV, Solomon SD, Inzucchi SE, et al. Dapagliflozin in patients with heart failure and reduced ejection fraction. N Engl J Med. 2019;381(21):1995-2008.
5. Lowenstern A, Ng N, Takagi H, et al. Influence of obesity on coronary artery disease and clinical outcomes in the ADVANCE registry. Circ Cardiovasc Imaging. 2023;16(5):373-85.
6. Huxley RR, Lopez F, Folsom AR, et al. Absolute and attributable risks of atrial fibrillation in relation to optimal and borderline risk factors: The Atherosclerosis Risk in Communities (ARIC) Study. Circulation. 2011; 123(14):1501-8.
7. Doehner W, Clark AL, van Veldhuisen DJ, et al. Heart failure and obesity: translational approaches and therapeutic implications. Eur J Heart Fail. 2024;26:5-17.
8. Čermáková E, Vaňhara P, Hubáček T. Metabolically healthy obesity and health risks: A meta-analysis of prospective cohort studies. Cent Eur J Public Health. 2024;32(1):11-20.
9. Butt JH, Petrie MC, Jhund PS, et al. Anthropometric measures and adverse outcomes in heart failure with reduced ejection fraction: Revisiting the obesity paradox. Eur Heart J. 2023;44(4):1136-53.
10. Prokopidis K, Fiorer A, Greco EA, et al. Prognostic and associative significance of malnutrition, unintentional weight loss, low BMI, and reduced lean mass in chronic illness. Clin Nutr ESPEN; 2025.
11. Kodama S, Saito K, Tanaka S, et al. Cardiorespiratory fitness as a quantitative predictor of all-cause mortality and cardiovascular events in healthy men and women: A meta-analysis. JAMA. 2009;301(19):2024-35.
12. Pfeffer MA, Sattar N, Foucault A, et al. Semaglutide and cardiovascular outcomes in obesity without diabetes. N Engl J Med. 2023;389(23):2096-108.
13. Butler J, Borlaug BA, Petrie MC, et al. Semaglutide in patients with heart failure with preserved ejection fraction and obesity. N Engl J Med. 2023;389(11):1069-84.
14. Frias JP, Palmer JP, Mehta A, et al. Tirzepatide once weekly for the treatment of obesity. N Engl J Med. 2022;387(3):205-16.
15. Packer M, Zile MR, Kramer CM, et al. Tirzepatide for heart failure with preserved ejection fraction and obesity. N Engl J Med. 2025;392(5):427-37.

12

CHAPTER

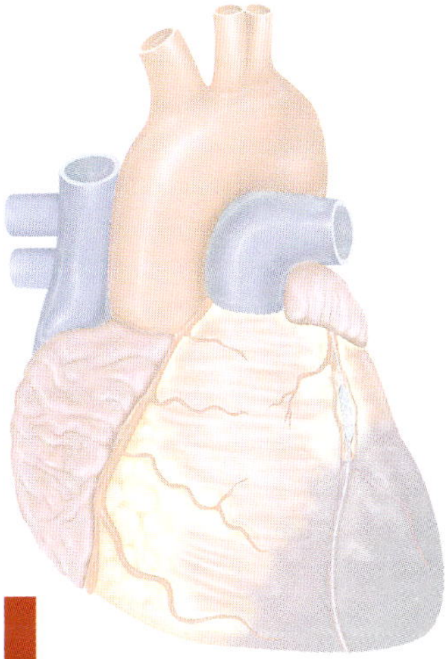

Obesity Paradox

AK Pancholia, HK Chopra

INTRODUCTION

The term "Obesity paradox," also sometimes called "reverse epidemiology," refers to the growing evidence that obesity in individuals with cardiovascular, pulmonary, or renal disease leads to better overall outcomes in terms of reduced mortality both in and out of the hospital, reduced morbidity, and improved survival rates.[1] The prevalence of obesity has increased dramatically over the last three decades and has reached global epidemic proportions in both adults and children in the United States.[2] It is associated with numerous comorbidities, including hypertension, type 2 diabetes mellitus, dyslipidemia, and cardiovascular disease.[2-4] Obesity is considered one of the five major risk factors for cardiovascular disease by the American Heart Association and has been shown to be associated with the development of heart failure, coronary heart disease, sudden cardiac death, atrial fibrillation, and reduced overall survival. Despite the associations between obesity and these health conditions, a number of recent studies have documented a puzzling phenomenon, termed the *"obesity paradox,"* in which overweight and obese individuals with established cardiovascular disease have a better prognosis compared with normal weight subjects.[5,6] Other recent studies have explored the role of fitness in the context of the obesity paradox and health outcomes. It has been demonstrated that irrespective of the presence of an obesity paradox or related risk markers, individuals who are relatively fit have significantly better survival and fewer cardiovascular events than unfit individuals.[7-9]

HOW THE CONCEPT EMERGED?

21 years ago, Gruberg and coworkers observed better outcomes in overweight and obese patients with coronary heart disease undergoing percutaneous coronary intervention compared with their normal-weight counterparts. This unexpected phenomenon was described as "an obesity paradox".[10] Normal-weight patients had higher incidence of major inhospital complications, including cardiac death. Moreover, at 1-year follow-up significantly higher mortality rates were observed in low- and normal-weight patients compared with obese and overweight. A systematic review of 40 cohort studies with 250, 152 patients found significantly lower risks for total mortality (RR 0.87) and cardiovascular mortality (RR 0.88) in overweight patients.[11] These mortality risks were not increased in obese patients [body mass index (BMI) 30–35 kg/m^2] compared with normal-weight subjects. However, severely obese patients (BMI 35 kg/m^2) exhibited the highest risk (RR 1.88) for cardiovascular mortality.[11]

Obesity paradox is seen in:

- Hypertension
- Heart failure
- Coronary artery disease
- Atrial fibrillation

OBESITY PARADOX IN HYPERTENSION

Obese patients have a higher prevalence of hypertension compared with lean subjects, and obesity adversely affects

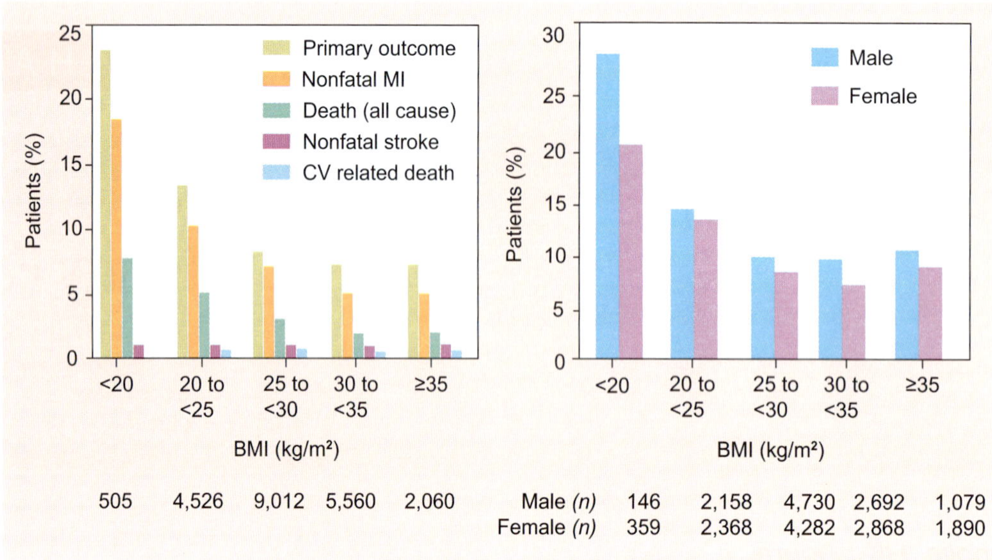

Fig. 1: Prognosis of obese hypertensive patients.
Source: Uretsky et al.[12]

CHD risk factors and leads to increased prevalence of LV hypertrophy, independent of arterial pressure. However, several studies demonstrate an obesity paradox in hypertensive subjects. The largest of such studies is from Uretsky et al.,[12] who investigated the effects of obesity on outcomes in 22,576 patients with treated hypertension and with known CHD. Despite an overall worse control of blood pressure during a 2-year follow-up, all-cause mortality was 30% lower in overweight and obese hypertensive patients compared with their lean counterparts **(Fig. 1)**. Other studies have either demonstrated the same finding or demonstrated a U-shaped relationship between BMI and all-cause, CV, and non-CV mortality, being that excess mortality was noted at both extremes of BMI.[2] Certainly, overweight and mildly obese hypertensive patients seem to have a better prognosis than their leaner counterparts. Possible mechanisms are low systemic vascular resistance and low plasma renin activity.

OBESITY PARADOX AND HEART FAILURE

Because obesity causes marked abnormalities in LV structure and function,[13] the increase in the prevalence of HF with obesity is not surprising. Another study of 5,881 Framingham Heart Study participants demonstrated a 5% increase in HF prevalence in men and a 7% increase in women for every 1 kg/m^2 increase in BMI.[14] However, in a study of 550 subjects without diabetes, increased BMI was not associated with increased risks of HF, whereas metabolic syndrome increased the risk of HF by 2.5-fold.[15] In this study, in contrast to normal weight patients with metabolic syndrome, metabolically healthy obese subjects had a decreased HF risk in a 6-year follow-up. However, a recent study from Norway demonstrated that in contrast to CHD, metabolically healthy obese patients still had an increased risk of HF.[16] Alpert et al.[17] demonstrated a very strong relationship between morbid obesity and HF prevalence. The obesity paradox in HF has recently been reviewed in detail.[6,18] In a meta-analysis of observational HF studies (N ¼ 28,209). Compared with patients with normal BMI, overweight, and obese HF patients had reductions in CV (–19% and –40%, respectively) and total mortality (–16% and –33%, respectively) during an average 2.7-year follow-up. The obesity paradox in HF has been demonstrated with BMI, % body fat (BF), and with waist circumference (WC) or central obesity[19-21] **(Fig. 2)**.

Recent evidence suggests that this does not typically apply to more morbid obesity, where prognosis is adversely affected in acute CHD,[22,23] CHD patients undergoing revascularization[24,25] including percutaneous intervention and coronary artery bypass grafting, as well as in patients with HF.[26,27]

OBESITY PARADOX AND CORONARY HEART DISEASE

Obesity is an important risk factor for CHD,[3] although some studies indicate that CHD may not be increased in "metabolically healthy" obesity.[16,28-30] Nevertheless, as

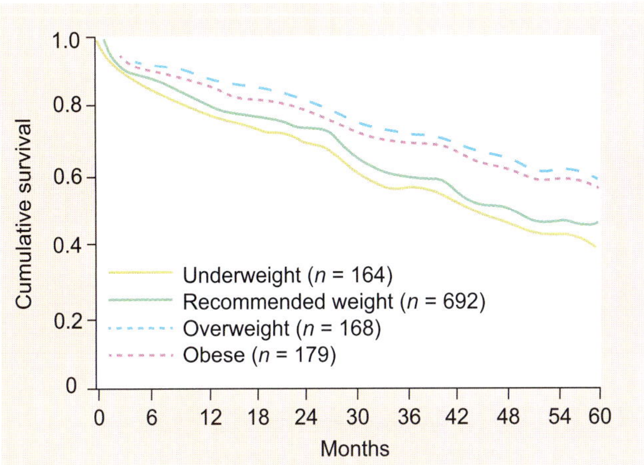

Fig. 2: Obesity and hear failure.
Source: Horwich TB, Fonarow GC, Hamilton MA, et al. The relationship between obesity and mortality in patients with heart failure. J Am Coll Cardiol. 2001;38:789-95.

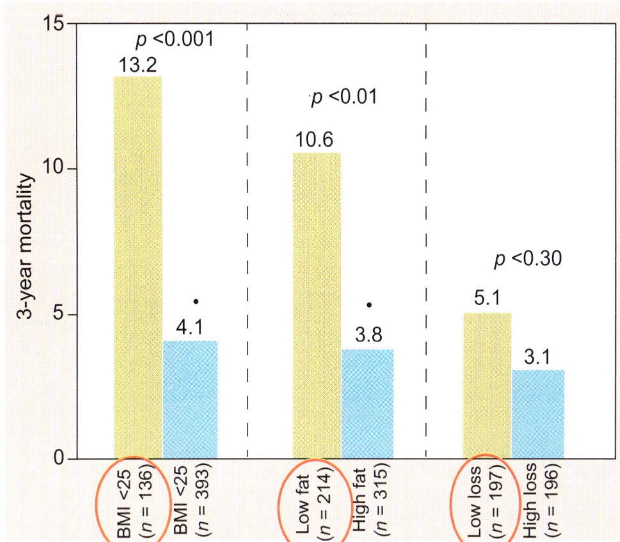

Fig. 3: Normal weight central obesity and mortality.
Source: Lavie CJ, et al.[38]

with hypertension, many studies using various measures of adiposity, including BMI,[11] % BF,[31-33] and some even with central obesity or WC,[31] have demonstrated an obesity paradox in CHD. A meta-analysis of 40 cohort studies in more than 250,000 patients with CHD found lower risk of total and CV mortality in underweight and normal-weight CHD patients.[11] However, those authors demonstrated that in patients with class II obesity (BMI 35–40 kg/m^2), there was an excess risk of CV mortality without any increase in total mortality. Recently, some studies have demonstrated an increased risk in CHD patients with "normal weight obesity" and "normal weight central obesity", in which % BF or WC, respectively, is high, although BMI is in the normal range,[34,35] whereas others have only demonstrated this finding in those with low fitness[32] **(Fig. 3)**.

Lower adiposity with the worst CV outcome may represent as a "lean paradox" instead of an obesity paradox.[31,33,36,37] It has been demonstrated that this obesity paradox with low BF (defined as <25% in men and <35% in women) and low BMI,[38] and both low BF and low BMI are independent predictors of worse outcomes. However, in a study of 581 patients with CHD, we demonstrated that only those with low BMI (<25 kg/m^2) and low BF had a high mortality rate compared with the other groups.[31] Most recently, we demonstrated that both low BF and low lean mass (or nonfat mass) are associated with the worst survival; patients with both high lean mass and BF had the best survival, whereas intermediate survival rates were noted in the other groups.[32] Other studies demonstrate that this may represent more of an "overweight paradox," where overweight CHD patients do particularly well compared with lean.[35,36] Therefore, in CHD, it appears that there is a strong obesity paradox, particularly with BMI, but also with BF and central obesity, with the best prognosis noted in overweight CHD patients, as opposed to those with more severe obesity.[39]

OBESITY PARADOX IN POST-CABG

There are several differences in opinions on the link between the BMI and post-CABG morbidity and mortality in the current literature. There is a school of thought maintaining that BMI is not a risk factor for mortality,[10,40] while some other investigators consider obesity as a protective factor in patients undergoing CABG.[41] Most experts agree on its relation with post CABG complications, however, is WC, which is deemed the best and most simple anthropometric measurement for central obesity **(Fig. 4)**.

OBESITY PARADOX AND ATRIAL FIBRILLATION

As with obesity, the prevalence of AF has been increasing and is expected to increase by 2.5-fold during the next 30 years.[2] A meta-analysis of 16 studies of more than 120,000 patients[42] demonstrates that obese patients had a 50% increased risk of developing AF. However, as in patients with hypertension, CHD, and HF, overweight and obese patients with AF have a considerably better prognosis than do those patients with normal BMI.

In a sub-analysis of the AFFIRM study[43,44] (Atrial Fibrillation Follow-up Investigation of Rhythm Management), an inverse relationship between obesity

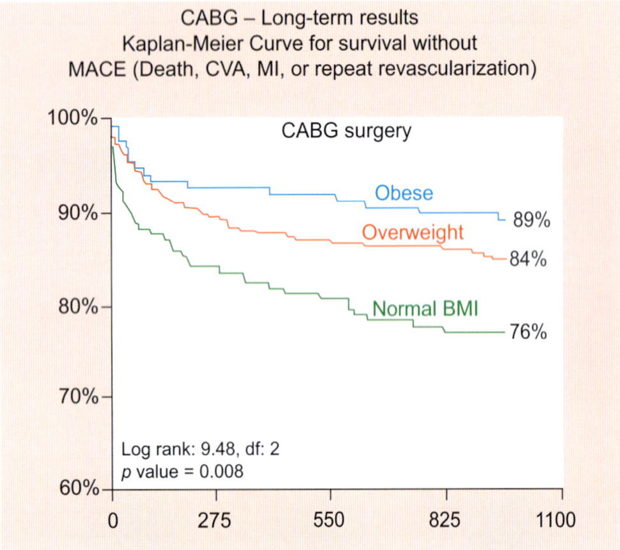

Fig. 4: ARTS Trial result.
Source: Gruberg L, Mercado N, Milo S, et al. Impact of body mass index on the outcome of patients with multivessel disease randomized to either coronary artery bypass grafting or stenting in the ARTS trial: the obesity paradox II? Am J Cardiol. 2005;95:439.

and prognosis was also described. Accordingly, rate of all-cause death was higher in the normal BMI group (5.8 per 100 patient-years) than in the overweight and obese groups (3.9 and 3.7, respectively).

OTHER MANIFESTATIONS OF OBESITY PARADOX

- *Peripheral arterial disease:* The overall mortality rates in patients with peripheral arterial disease decreased with increasing BMI, reaching 54% in underweight, 50% in normal weight, 40% in overweight, and 31% in obese subjects.[45]
- *Stroke:* Overweight and obese patients have significantly better survival rates after stroke than their normal-weight counterparts.[46] In another study, class I obesity was associated with decreased risk of postoperative stroke after carotid endarterectomy.[47]
- *Thromboembolism:* Obese patients with acute venous thromboembolism have less than one-half the mortality in normal-weight subjects.[48]
- *Complications during catheter ablation for atrial fibrillation:* Patients with less robust stature were more prone to complications during catheter ablation for atrial fibrillation with the use of intracardiac echocardiography. Low body weight was a significant risk factor (p = 0.013), with 0.8% increase of complication rate/10 kg body weight decrease.[49]
- *Mortality in patients undergoing nonbariatric general surgery:* Lower risk of death was observed in overweight and moderately obese patients undergoing nonbariatric general surgery than in those with normal weight.[50]
- *Amputation risk among nonelderly diabetic men:* Amputation risk decreased in diabetic men with increasing BMI.[51]
- *Hemodialysis patients:* Higher mortality rates were observed in hemodialysis patients who exhibited lower BMI and weight loss.[52]

POTENTIAL MECHANISMS FOR THE OBESITY PARADOX IN CARDIOVASCULAR DISEASES

- Nonpurposeful weight loss
- Younger age at presentation
- Lower prevalence of smoking
- Greater metabolic reserves
- Less cachexia
- Lower atrial natriuretic peptides
- Attenuated response to renin–angiotensin–aldosterone system
- High blood pressure, allowing for more cardiac medications
- Differing etiology, associated with a better prognosis
- Increased muscle mass and muscular strength
- Implications regarding cardiorespiratory fitness
- Unmeasured confounding factors

Other mechanisms are:

- *Cardiorespiratory fitness:* Increased cardiorespiratory fitness plays an important role in obesity paradox with lower all-cause mortality and lower risk of cardiovascular and metabolic diseases.[53] It also modifies the relation of adiposity to cardiovascular and all-cause mortality.[35]
- *Endothelial progenitor cells:* Explained through a greater mobilization of endothelial progenitor cells in obese.
- *Thromboxane production*: Explained through a decreased production of thromboxane in obese patients.[54]
- *Ghrelin sensitivity:* Ghrelin is a gastric peptide hormone with its CV benefits like improved left ventricular function, exercise capacity, and muscle wasting in patients with chronic heart failure and has been found more in obese patients and thus hypothesized to be cardioprotective in obese.
- *Soluble tumor necrosis factor receptor:* TNF-α increases the cardiometabolic risk.[55] Obese patients have lower

concentration of TNF-α, which may cause a better outcome in obese patients with heart failure.

CONCLUSION

Obesity is recognized as a major risk factor for cardiovascular diseases and diabetes, but it has been observed that a higher BMI may be associated with a lower mortality and a better outcome in several chronic diseases and health circumstances. This protective effect of obesity has been described as the "obesity paradox" or "reverse epidemiology." However, it should be emphasized that the BMI is a crude and flawed anthropometric biomarker that does not take into account fat mass/fat-free mass ratio, nutritional status, cardiorespiratory fitness, BF distribution, or other factors affecting health risks and the patient's mortality. Obese individuals may also demonstrate better outcome in response to certain therapeutic procedures. The obesity paradox was mostly reported in elderly. Therefore, the protective effect of nutritional status in overweight and obese elderly individuals and the health-deteriorating effect of undernutrition in non-overweight subjects probably contribute to this paradox. Besides the age and nutritional status, other factors such as less risky lower body obesity, favorable body composition, and cardiorespiratory fitness are potential contributors to the obesity paradox. Finally, the obesity paradox does not imply that obesity is healthy or that weight gain should be recommended. Obesity remains a critical risk factor for developing chronic diseases. However, in patients already suffering from certain serious chronic conditions, it highlights the importance of individual assessment, focusing on overall body composition (muscle mass vs. fat mass), nutritional status, and cardiorespiratory fitness rather than relying solely on BMI. Discussion over the existence of the obesity paradox cannot lead to an underestimation of obesity as a crucial risk factor for the development of cardiovascular and metabolic diseases that requires comprehensive prevention and management strategies.

REFERENCES

1. Motamed N, Sohrabi M, Poustchi H, et al. The six obesity indices, which one is more compatible with metabolic syndrome? A population based study. Diabetes Metab Syndr. 2017;11(3):173-7.
2. Poirier P, Giles TD, Bray GA, et al. Obesity and cardiovascular disease: pathophysiology, evaluation, and effect of weight loss. Arterioscler Thromb Vasc Biol. 2006;26:968-76.
3. Lavie CJ, Milani RV, Ventura HO. Obesity and cardiovascular disease: risk factor, paradox, and impact of weight loss. J Am Coll Cardiol. 2009;53:1925-32.
4. Klein S, Burke LE, Bray GA, et al. American Heart Association Council on Nutrition, Physical Activity, and Metabolism. Clinical implications of obesity with specific focus on cardiovascular disease: a statement for professionals from the American Heart Association Council on Nutrition, Physical Activity, and Metabolism. Circulation. 2004;110:2952-67.
5. Arena R, Lavie CJ. The obesity paradox and outcome in heart failure: is excess bodyweight truly protective? Future Cardiol. 2010;6:1-6.
6. Oreopoulos A, Padwal R, Kalantar-Zadeh K, et al. Body mass index and mortality in heart failure: a meta-analysis. Am Heart J. 2008;156:13-22.
7. McAuley P, Myers J, Abella J, et al. Body mass, fitness and survival in veteran patients: another obesity paradox? Am J Med. 2007;120:518-24.
8. McAuley PA, Kokkinos PF, Oliveira RB, et al. Obesity paradox and cardiorespiratory fitness in 12,417 male veterans aged 40 to 70 years. Mayo Clinic Proc. 2010;85:115-21.
9. McAuley P, Pittsley J, Myers J, et al. Fitness and fatness as mortality predictors in healthy older men: the Veterans Exercise Testing Study. J Gerontol A Biol Sci Med Sci. 2009;64:695-9.
10. Gruberg L, Weissman NJ, Waksman R, et al. The impact of obesity on the short-term and long-term outcomes after percutaneous coronary intervention: the obesity paradox? J Am Coll Cardiol. 2002;39:578-84.
11. Romero-Corral A, Montori VM, Somers VK, et al. Association of bodyweight with total mortality and with cardiovascular events in coronary artery disease: a systematic review of cohort studies. Lancet. 2006;368:666-78.
12. Uretsky S, Messerli FH, Bangalore S, et al. Obesity paradox in patients with hypertension and coronary artery disease. Am J Med. 2007;120:863-70.
13. Lavie CJ, Alpert MA, Arena R, et al. Impact of obesity and the obesity paradox on prevalence and prognosis in heart failure. J Am Coll Cardiol HF. 2013;1:93-102.
14. Kenchaiah S, Evans JC, Levy D, et al. Obesity and the risk of heart failure. N Engl J Med. 2002;347:305-13.
15. Voulgari C, Tentolouris N, Dilaveris P, et al. Increased heart failure risk in normal-weight people with metabolic syndrome compared with metabolically healthy obese individuals. J Am Coll Cardiol. 2011;58:1343-50.
16. Mørkedal B, Vatten LJ, Romundstad PR, et al. Risk of myocardial infarction and heart failure among metabolically healthy but obese individuals: a prospective population based study. J Am Coll Cardiol. 2014;63:1071-8.
17. Alpert MA, Terry BE, Mulekar M, et al. Cardiac morphology and left ventricular function in morbidly obese patients with and without congestive heart failure and effect of weight loss. Am J Cardiol. 1997;80:736-40.
18. Speakman JR, Selman C. Physical activity and resting metabolic rate. Proc Nutr Soc. 2003;62(3):621-34.
19. Lavie CJ, Osman AF, Milani RV, et al. Body composition and prognosis in chronic systolic heart failure: the obesity paradox. Am J Cardiol. 2003;91:891-4.

20. Clark AL, Chyu J, Horwich TB. The obesity paradox in men versus women with systolic heart failure. Am J Cardiol. 2012;110:77-82.
21. Clark AL, Fonarow GC, Horwich TB. Obesity and obesity paradox in heart failure. Prog Cardiovasc Dis. 2014;56:409-14.
22. Das SR, Alexander KP, Chen AY, et al. Impact of body weight and extreme obesity on the presentation, treatment, and in-hospital outcomes of 50,149 patients with ST-segment elevation myocardial infarction: results from the NCDR (National Cardiovascular Data Registry). J Am Coll Cardiol. 2011;58:2642-50.
23. Lavie CJ, Milani RV, Ventura HO. Impact of obesity on outcomes in myocardial infarction: combating the "obesity paradox". J Am Coll Cardiol. 2011;58:2651-3.
24. Payvar S, Kim S, Rao SV, et al. In-hospital outcomes of percutaneous coronary interventions in extremely obese and normal-weight patients: findings from the NCDR (National Cardiovascular Data Registry). J Am Coll Cardiol. 2013;62:692-6.
25. Buschur ME, Smith D, Share D, et al. The burgeoning epidemic of morbid obesity in patients undergoing percutaneous coronary intervention: insight from the Blue Cross Blue Shield of Michigan Cardiovascular Consortium. J Am Coll Cardiol. 2013;62:685-91.
26. Nagarajan V, Cauthen CA, Starling RC, et al. Prognosis of morbid obesity patients with advanced heart failure. Congest Heart Fail. 2013;19:160-4.
27. Lavie CJ, Ventura HO. Analyzing the weight of evidence on the obesity paradox and heart failure: is there a limit to the madness? Congest Heart Fail. 2013;19:158-9.
28. Ortega FB, Lee DC, Katzmarzyk PT, et al. The intriguing metabolically healthy but obese phenotype: cardiovascular prognosis and role of fitness. Eur Heart J. 2013;34:389-97.
29. Lavie CJ, Milani RV, Ventura HO. Disparate effects of metabolically healthy obesity in coronary heart disease and heart failure. J Am Coll Cardiol. 2014;63(11):1079-81.
30. Oliveros E, Somers VK, Sochor O, et al. The concept of normal weight obesity. Prog Cardiovasc Dis. 2014;56:426-33.
31. Lavie CJ, De Schutter A, Patel D, et al. Body composition and coronary heart disease mortality: an obesity or a lean paradox? Mayo Clin Proc. 2011;86:857-64.
32. McAuley PA, Artero EG, Sui X, et al. The obesity paradox, cardiorespiratory fitness, and coronary heart disease. Mayo Clin Proc. 2012;87:443-51.
33. Lavie CJ, De Schutter A, Patel DA, et al. Body composition and survival in stable coronary heart disease: impact of lean mass index and body fat in the "obesity paradox". J Am Coll Cardiol. 2012;60:1374-80.
34. Coutinho T, Goel K, Corrêa de Sá D, et al. Central obesity and survival in subjects with coronary artery disease: a systematic review of the literature and collaborative analysis with individual subject data. J Am Coll Cardiol. 2011;57:1877-86.
35. Coutinho T, Goel K, Corrêa de Sá D, et al. Combining body mass index with measures of central obesity in the assessment of mortality in subjects with coronary disease: role of "normal weight central obesity". J Am Coll Cardiol. 2013;61:553-60.
36. Azimi A, Charlot MG, Torp-Pedersen C, et al. Moderate overweight is beneficial and severe obesity detrimental for patients with documented atherosclerotic heart disease. Heart. 2013;99:655-60.
37. Lavie CJ, De Schutter A, Milani RV. Is there an obesity, overweight or lean paradox in coronary heart disease? Getting to the 'fat' of the matter. Heart. 2013;99:596-8.
38. Lavie CJ, Milani RV, Artham SM, et al. The obesity paradox, weight loss, and coronary disease. Am J Med. 2009;122:1106-14.
49. De Schutter A, Lavie CJ, Milani RV. The impact of obesity on risk factors and prevalence of coronary heart disease: the obesity paradox. Prog Cardiovasc Dis. 2014;56:401-8.
40. Engel AM, McDonough S, Smith JM. Does an obesity body mass index affect hospital outcomes after coronary artery bypass graft surgery? Ann Thorac Surg. 2009;88(6):1793-800.
41. Sung SH, Wu TC, Huang CH, et al. Prognostic impact of body mass index in patients undergoing coronary artery bypass surgery. Heart. 2011;97(8):648-54.
42. Wanahita N, Messerli FH, Bangalore S, et al. Atrial fibrillation and obesity results of a meta-analysis. Am Heart J. 2008;155:310-5.
43. Badheka AO, Rathod A, Kizilbash MA, et al. Influence of obesity on outcomes in atrial fibrillation: yet another obesity paradox. Am J Med. 2011;123:646-51.
44. Ardestani A, Hoffman HJ, Cooper HA. Obesity and outcomes among patients with established atrial fibrillation. Am J Cardiol. 2010;106:369-73.
45. Galal W, van Gestel YR, Hoeks SE, et al. The obesity paradox in patients with peripheral arterial disease. Chest. 2008;134:925-30.
46. Vemmos K, Ntaios G, Spengos K, et al. Association between obesity and mortality after acute first-ever stroke: the obesity stroke paradox. Stroke. 2011;42:30-6.
47. Jackson RS, Black JH 3rd, Lum YW, et al. Class I obesity is paradoxically associated with decreased risk of postoperative stroke after carotid endarterectomy. J Vasc Surg. 2012;55:1306-12.
48. Stein PD, Matta F, Goldman J. Obesity and pulmonary embolism: the mounting evidence of risk and the mortality paradox. Thromb Res. 2011;128:518-23.
49. Aldhoon B, Wichterle D, Peichl P, et al. Complications of catheter ablation for atrial fibrillation in a high-volume centre with the use of intracardiac echocardiography. Europace. 2013;15:24-32.
50. Mullen JT, Moorman DW, Davenport DL. The obesity paradox: body mass index and outcomes in patients

undergoing nonbariatric general surgery. Ann Surg. 2009;250:166-72.
51. Sohn M-W, Budiman-Mak E, Oh EH, et al. Obesity paradox in amputation risk among nonelderly diabetic men. Obesity (Silver Spring). 2012;20:460-2.
52. Kalantar-Zadeh K, Streja E, Molnar MZ, et al. Mortality prediction by surrogates of body composition: an examination of the obesity paradox in hemodialysis patients using composite ranking score analysis. Am J Epidemiol. 2012;175:793-803.
53. Hainer V, Toplak H, Stich V. Fat or fit: what is more important? Diabetes Care 2009;32(Suppl 2):S392-S397.
54. Graziani F, Biasucci LM, Cialdella P, et al. Thromboxane production in morbidly obese subjects. Am J Cardiol. 2011;107:1656-61.
55. Ledderose C, Kreth S, Beiras-Fernandez A. Ghrelin, a novel peptide hormone in the regulation of energy balance and cardiovascular function. Recent Pat Endocr Metab Immune Drug Discov. 2011;5:1-6.

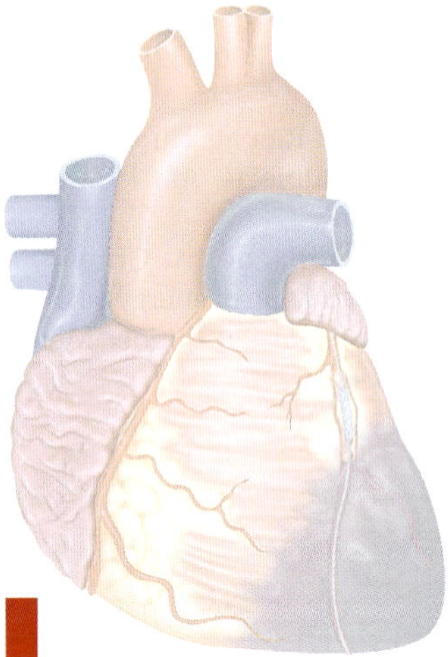

13

CHAPTER

Obesity and Smoking: A Complex, Paradoxical Relationship

Ankit Agarwal, Ranjit K Nath

INTRODUCTION

Obesity and tobacco use drive a large fraction of global cardiovascular and metabolic disease burden. While smoking prevalence has declined due to successful control efforts, obesity rates have risen ruthlessly, producing a shifting landscape of population risk. At an individual level, epidemiological data unexpectedly show that current smokers frequently have lower average body mass index (BMI) than never-smokers.[1,2] This has led to dangerous misinterpretations about smoking and weight. A mechanistic understanding clarifies that nicotine reduces appetite and increases resting energy expenditure—effects that commonly lower measured body weight—while smoking simultaneously promotes visceral and ectopic fat deposition, systemic inflammation, dyslipidemia, and insulin resistance. These latter changes drive cardiometabolic risk independently of BMI.[3-6] This chapter synthesizes current mechanistic, imaging, genetic, and clinical evidence, addresses apparent paradoxes, and presents practical recommendations for clinicians and policymakers.

This chapter comprises:

- Epidemiological patterns and paradoxes
- Review biological mechanisms linking nicotine with energy balance and fat distribution
- Formulate evidence from imaging, genetic (Mendelian randomization), and longitudinal clinical studies
- Recommend evidence-based clinical management strategies including cessation pharmacotherapy and weight-management approaches

MECHANISMS LINKING SMOKING AND BODY COMPOSITION

Nicotine's central effects include stimulation of nicotinic acetylcholine receptors that activate pro-opiomelanocortin (POMC) neurons in the arcuate nucleus, stimulating melanocortin pathways (MC4R) to suppress appetite and reduce caloric intake.[3] Peripherally, nicotine increases sympathetic outflow and catecholamine levels (epinephrine/norepinephrine), which modestly elevate resting metabolic rate and promote lipolysis.[4] Together these effects explain observed lower mean body weight among many smokers. On the other hand, chronic tobacco exposure is proinflammatory, increases oxidative stress, and enhances cortisol metabolism, biological changes that may promote visceral adiposity and ectopic lipid deposition (hepatic steatosis, pericardial fat), both strong drivers of cardiometabolic disease. Moreover, smoking is also associated with development of insulin resistance, which is another risk factor for cardiovascular diseases.[5,6] Behavioral and socioeconomic factors—dietary patterns, alcohol use, sedentary lifestyle, and social determinants of health—interact with these mechanisms to shape individual phenotypes.

EVIDENCE SYNTHESIS AND EPIDEMIOLOGY

Epidemiologic studies using direct imaging (CT/MRI) have acknowledged higher visceral adipose tissue (VAT) among current smokers versus never-smokers after controlling for BMI and other confounders. For instance, Kim et al.[7] reported significantly greater VAT measured by CT scans in smokers. Mendelian randomization analyses (e.g., Carrasquilla et al.[8]) support a causal effect of lifetime tobacco exposure on increased waist-to-hip ratio and central adiposity metrics, independent of BMI, strengthening reasoning beyond observational associations. Meta-analyses and pooled cohort studies examining weight trajectories after cessation demonstrate average gains of approximately 4–5 kg at 12 months, though with significant heterogeneity: Some quitters lose weight, most gain modestly, and a minority gain >10 kg.[9] Notably, pooled mortality analyses show that quitting smoking is associated with large reductions in all-cause and cardiovascular mortality compared with continued smoking; these benefits persist despite typical post-cessation weight gain.[10,11] Apparent clinical paradoxes—such as improved short-term outcomes among smokers with acute coronary syndromes—are attributable to confounding by younger age and fewer comorbidities; fully adjusted analyses remove the paradoxical effect. Similarly, reports of an "obesity paradox" in chronic disease frequently attenuate after controlling for smoking status and reverse causation.[11]

CLINICAL IMPLICATIONS AND MANAGEMENT

Clinical care should prioritize smoking cessation for all patients while emphasizing on weight and metabolic health. Crucial components include comprehensive assessment, evidence-based cessation, preventive weight-management strategies, and well-defined follow-up.

Assessment: Record tobacco use (status, intensity, and pack-years), motivation, and prior quit attempts; measure BMI, waist circumference, and baseline metabolic panel (fasting lipids, glucose/HbA1c). Consider early imaging (e.g., liver ultrasound, CT/MRI) when clinical suspicion for ectopic fat is high and results would alter management.[12]

Treatment: Combine behavioral support with pharmacotherapy. Nicotine replacement therapy (NRT), bupropion, and varenicline each increase quit rates; bupropion has demonstrated modest short-term weight-sparing effects, NRT blunts early gains, and varenicline—while weight neutral—offers the highest abstinence probabilities. Choice should be individualized.[13,14]

Concurrent weight management: Integrate dietary counseling with a focus on high-protein meals, low glycemic-index carbohydrates, portion control, and replacement of calorically dense snacks; prescribe

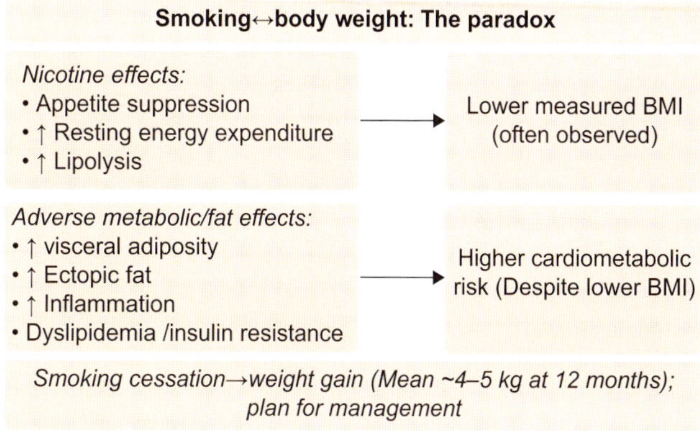

Fig. 1: Nicotine reduces appetite and increases metabolic rate while promoting visceral adiposity.

graduated exercise programs highlighting aerobic activity for visceral fat reduction plus resistance training to preserve lean mass.

For persistent, clinically meaningful weight gain, referral to obesity services and consideration of pharmacotherapy (e.g., GLP-1 receptor agonists) or bariatric assessment is appropriate **(Fig. 1)**.

Monitoring: Schedule follow-up at 1, 3, and 6 months post cessation to document weight, waist circumference, and metabolic markers; escalate interventions if weight gain exceeds 5–7% or metabolic parameters deteriorate.[15,16]

POLICY AND PUBLIC HEALTH IMPLICATIONS

At the population level, sustained tobacco control (taxation, advertising restriction, smoke-free laws, cessation services) delivers major cardiovascular mortality declines **(Flowchart 1)**.[17] The contrast of falling smoking and rising obesity requires parallel investments in obesity prevention and treatment, including improved access to behavioral programs and pharmacotherapy **(Fig. 2)**. Cohesive programs—quit lines offering weight-management modules, combined cessation and obesity trials, and training primary care teams—can magnify individual and public health benefits. Cost-effectiveness analyses favor combined approaches in high-risk groups.[1,2]

KEY MESSAGES

- Smoking lowers measured BMI in many individuals but increases visceral adiposity and cardiometabolic risk.
- Quitting smoking leads to considerable reductions in mortality; modest post-cessation weight gain should not discourage cessation efforts.

Flowchart 1: Obesity paradox.

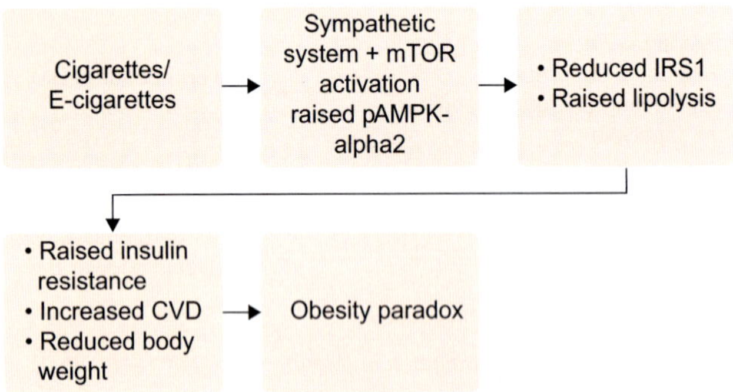

[AMPK-alpha2 (reactive oxygen species induction): 5′AMP activated protein kinase alpha-2; IRS-1: insulin receptor substrate 1; mTOR (skeletal muscle): mammalian target of rapamycin]

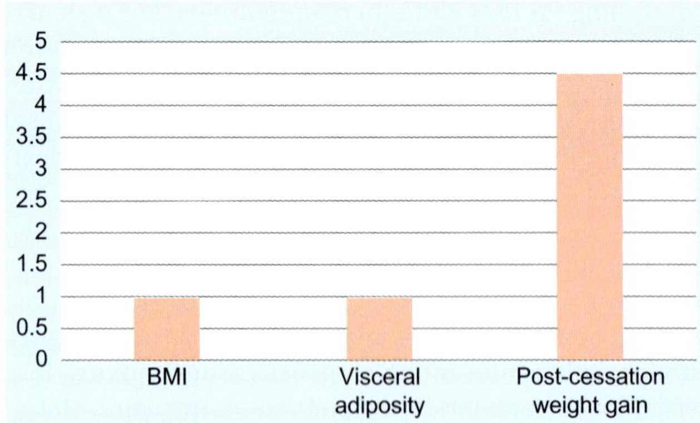

Fig. 2: Illustrative observations. Lower BMI in smokers; higher visceral adiposity on imaging; average post-cessation weight gain ≈ 4–5 kg at 12 months.

TABLE 1: Landmark studies on the association between smoking and body weight and mortality.

Study (year)	*Design*	*N/setting*	*Core finding*
Kim et al.[7] (2012)	Cross-sectional CT imaging	~3,000 (Korean cohort)	Higher VAT in smokers after BMI adjustment
Aubin et al.[9] (2012)	Meta-analysis	Pooled RCTs/cohorts	Mean post-cessation weight gain ≈4–5 kg at 12 months
Carrasquilla et al.[8] (2024)	Mendelian randomization	Genetic consortia	Genetic liability to smoking increases WHR independent of BMI
Freedman et al.[11] (2006)	Cohort mortality	Large US cohorts	Obese smokers have markedly higher mortality versus lean never-smokers
Yan et al.[10] (2022)	Prospective cohort	Large population sample	Cessation reduces mortality; post-cessation gain not linked to higher mortality

- Clinicians must measure waist circumference and monitor metabolic markers rather than relying merely on BMI.
- Comprehensive cessation pharmacotherapy with behavioral weight-management; consider specialist referral for persistent obesity.
- Public health policy should sustain tobacco control and multiply obesity-prevention and treatment resources.

LIMITATIONS AND RESEARCH PRIORITIES

Current knowledge relies heavily on observational data; residual confounding and reverse causation remain concerns. Measurement heterogeneity (self-reported smoking, differing adiposity metrics) complicates synthesis. Future directions include longitudinal imaging studies covering smoking initiation/cessation, randomized trials of integrated cessation-plus-weight interventions, mechanistic research on nicotine's adipocyte effects, and trials evaluating anti-obesity agents to mitigate post-cessation weight gain.

CONCLUSION

Smoking and obesity interact in complex and often counterintuitive ways. The net clinical imperative is clear: Promote and enable smoking cessation while implementing strategies to anticipate, manage, and prevent weight gain and metabolic risk. Multidisciplinary, patient-centered interventions that combine effective tobacco dependence treatment with attention to diet, activity, and, when appropriate, pharmacologic obesity therapies will yield the greatest improvements in cardiovascular and metabolic outcomes **(Table 1)**.

REFERENCES

1. World Health Organization. (2025). Obesity and overweight. [online] Available from https://www.who.int/news-room/fact-sheets/detail/obesity-and-overweight. [Last accessed January, 2026].
2. World Health Organization. (2025). Tobacco. [online] Available from https://www.who.int/news-room/fact-sheets/detail/tobacco. [Last accessed January, 2026].

3. Audrain-McGovern J, Benowitz NL. Cigarette smoking, nicotine, and body weight. Nicotine Tob Res. 2011;13(10):1095-106.
4. Walker JF, Collins LC, Rowell PP, et al. Smoking effects on energy expenditure and catecholamine levels. Nicotine Tob Res. 1999;1(4):365-70.
5. Koromilas E, Polyzos SA, Mantzoros C. Smoking cessation and weight: implications for metabolic disease. Int J Obes. 2021;45(4):861-71.
6. Khawaja T, Nied M, Wilgor A, et al. Impact of visceral and hepatic fat on cardiometabolic health. Curr Cardiol Rep. 2024;26(11):1297-307.
7. Kim JH, Hwang JH, Park SY, et al. Cigarette smoking increases abdominal and visceral obesity. PLoS One. 2012;7(5):e45815.
8. Carrasquilla GD, Holmes MV, Davey Smith G, et al. Mendelian randomization evidence linking smoking to abdominal adiposity. Addiction. 2024; 119(6):1024-34.
9. Aubin HJ, Farley A, Lycett D, et al. Weight gain in smokers after quitting: systematic review and meta-analysis. BMJ. 2012;345:e4439.
10. Yan J, Li X, Li Y, et al. Weight gain after smoking cessation and risk of chronic disease and mortality. JAMA Netw Open. 2022;5(8):e2235464.
11. Freedman DM, Mantzoros C, Falk RT, et al. The mortality risk of smoking and obesity combined. Am J Prev Med. 2006;31(5):355-62.
12. Jenkins DA, Bowden J, Robinson HA, et al. Adiposity-mortality relationships in type 2 diabetes and coronary disease. Diabetes Care. 2018;41(9):1878-86.
13. Jorenby D. Clinical efficacy of bupropion in the management of smoking cessation. Drugs. 2002;62 Suppl 2:25-35.
14. Bush T, Lovejoy J, Javitz H, et al. Randomized trial of combined treatments for smoking cessation and weight control. Contemp Clin Trials Commun. 2017;7:95-102.
15. Xavier D, Alves G, Oliveira IB, et al. GLP-1 receptor agonists and post-cessation weight: early evidence. 2025.
16. Pedersen SD, Manjoo P, Dash S, et al. Pharmacotherapy for obesity management in adults: 2025 clinical practice guideline update. CMAJ. 2025;197(27):E797-809.
17. World Health Organization. (2023). WHO Framework Convention on Tobacco Control (FCTC) implementation reports. [online] Available from https://www.who.int/teams/health-promotion/tobacco-control/who-framework-convention-on-tobacco-control. [Last accessed January, 2026].

14

CHAPTER

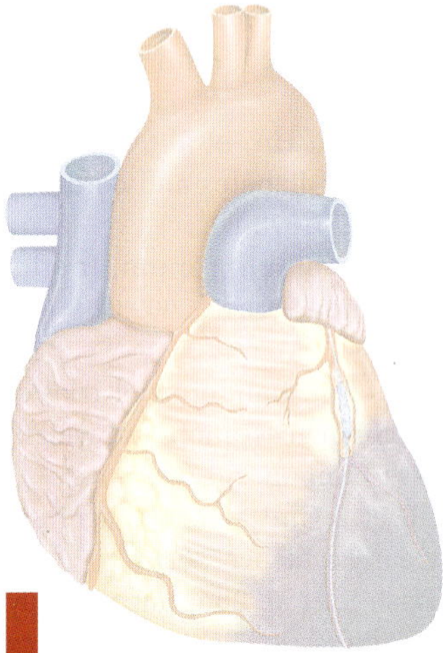

Obesity and Genetics: Understanding the Heritable Influence

Kamlesh Raut, Ankit Sahu, Aditya Kapoor

INTRODUCTION

Obesity is a major health problem worldwide. The World Health Organization (WHO) indeed describes the escalating global obesity crisis as *"21st century epidemic"* due to an alarming increase in the prevalence of obesity in the past two decades to pandemic levels, with >*1 billion* people worldwide living with obesity in 2022, affecting about one *in eight people*[1] globally. Worldwide adult obesity has *more than doubled* since 1990, while children and adolescent obesity has *quadrupled*. In 2022, 2.5 billion adults (18 years and older) were overweight, including 890 million who were living with obesity and over 390 million children and adolescents aged 5–19 years were overweight, including 160 million who were living with obesity.[2]

Obesity is *a complex multifactorial disorder* which results from the interaction of multiple genes with the environment. The increasing prevalence of obesity is due to a combination of individual factors, including genetics, epigenetics, metagenomics, as well as environmental, cultural, and behavioral factors. The modern environment often promotes overeating and inactivity—*an "obesogenic" environment* characterized by the easy availability of energy-dense foods and reduced opportunities for physical exercise. Research indicates that *genetic, endocrine, and metabolic factors modulate* one's propensity to gain weight.

GENETIC MODULATION OF OBESITY

Several studies on genetic obesity have found that genetic mutations, polymorphisms, and changes in gene expression all have a major role in predisposition for obesity. Initially, *candidate gene studies* identified certain genes to be pathogenic for severe early-onset obesity (monogenic obesity). Early studies for identification of causative genes in monogenic obesity had a case-focused design: Patients with severe early-onset obesity and their affected and unaffected family members were investigated for potential gene-disrupting causal mutations via Sanger sequencing.[3] Later, next-generation sequencing (NGS) and the development of *genome-wide association studies (GWAS)* have increased the discovery of genetic associations and awareness of monogenic and polygenic causes of obesity. Over the past two decades, the advances in *GWAS* accompanied by high-throughput genome-wide genotyping techniques have enabled the identification of genetic variants throughout the whole genome.[3]

There are three types of genetic obesity: *monogenic*, *polygenic*, and *syndromic*. Genes associated with obesity are shown in **Table 1**.

1. *Monogenic obesity:* It results from a mutation or deficiency of a *single gene* and is a *rare* but severe cause of obesity. It occurs when there is a mutation in one of the genes involved in the *leptin-melanocortin pathway*. The most common monogenic form of obesity is caused by mutations in the *melanocortin-4 receptor (MC4R) gene*.[4] Typical features of monogenic obesity are *hyperphagia* (insatiable hunger) and *early-onset obesity* (age 3–5 years). Patient with monogenic obesity gains body weight rapidly starting early in infancy, and the velocity of increasing body mass index (BMI) reaches to peak level during childhood.[5] The additional clinical manifestations of patients with monogenic obesity include short stature, red hair, susceptibility to

TABLE 1: Genes associated with genetic obesity.

Gene	*Encoding protein*	*Type of genetic obesity*
LEP	Leptin	Monogenic
LEPR	Leptin receptor	Monogenic
PCSK1	Proprotein convertase subtilisin/kexin enzyme 1	Monogenic
MC4R	Melanocortin-4 receptor	Monogenic, polygenic
POMC	Pro-opiomelanocortin neuropeptide	Monogenic
ASIP	Agouti signaling protein	Monogenic
BDNF	Brain-derived neurotrophic factor	Monogenic, polygenic
FTO	Fat-mass and obesity associated gene; Fe^{2+}α-ketoglutarate-dependent dioxygenase	Polygenic
SIM1	Single-minded 1 transcription factor	Monogenic
NTRK2/TRKB	Neurotrophic tyrosine receptor kinase 2 (receptor for BDNF)	Monogenic
KSR2	Kinase suppressor of Ras 2 protein	Monogenic
NPY	Neuropeptide Y	Monogenic
SH2B1	SH2B adaptor protein 1	Monogenic
ADCY3	Adenylyl cyclase 3	Monogenic
INSIG2	Insulin-induced gene 2 protein	Polygenic
MKRN3, MAGEL2, NDN, NPAP1, and SNURF-SNRPN (in Prader–Willi syndrome critical region)	Makorin ring finger protein 3, MAGE family member L2, necdin protein, nuclear pore-associated protein, SNRPN upstream reading frame–small nuclear ribonucleoprotein polypeptide N	Syndromic (Prader–Willi syndrome)
COH1/VPS13B	Vacuolar protein sorting 13 homolog B	Syndromic (Cohen's syndrome)
BBS 1–26	BBSome proteins	Syndromic (Bardet–Biedl syndrome)

infection, recurrent diarrhea, or endocrine defects, such as pituitary insufficiencies, diabetes insipidus, adrenal insufficiency, hypothyroidism, or hypogonadism.[5,6]

The Leptin–melanocortin Pathway

The leptin–melanocortin circuit in the hypothalamus has a key role in *appetite regulation*. Most studies on genetic obesity have revealed that genes expressed exclusively in this pathway have a pivotal role in obesity. Leptin is an appetite-regulating hormone secreted from adipose tissue and acts through leptin receptor located in the arcuate nucleus of the hypothalamus. It is mainly involved with *decrease in appetite*.[7] It stimulates the production of pro-opiomelanocortin (POMC) in the POMC neurons, located in the arcuate nucleus of the hypothalamus, which is converted to melanocyte-stimulating hormone (MSH) by proprotein convertase subtilisin/kexin type 1 (PCSK1). MSH interacts with the melanocortin receptors, including the MC4R, in the paraventricular nucleus of hypothalamus, and leads to activation of MC4R. The activation of MC4R results in *reduction of food intake* and concomitant *increase of energy consumption*.[8]

Most obese people do not lack leptin, but instead have *hyperleptinemia*, which leads to *leptin resistance*.[9] In obesity, an excess of leptin is secreted, which eventually leads to *leptin resistance* (similar to insulin resistance). When cells in the hypothalamus become resistant to leptin, the signal for satiety is not received and the person remains hungry.

In humans, >200 distinct genetic variants are associated with early-onset obesity and hyperphagia.[10] *MC4R*-associated obesity is the *most common monogenic form of obesity*, with a reported prevalence of up to 6%.

- *MC4R deficiency:* MC4R is a G protein-coupled receptor that is critical in the leptin–melanocortin pathway. MC4R deficiency is the *most common monogenic obesity disorder*.[4,5] Pathogenic variants in the MC4R gene cause approximately 2–5% of the cases of extreme early-onset obesity.[8,11] The variants in MC4R gene can be inherited either in an autosomal dominant or recessive pattern. Clinical manifestations of MC4R deficiency include *severe early-onset obesity, hyperphagia,* and hyperinsulinemia accompanied by lean body mass increase and rapid linear growth.

- *Leptin deficiency:* Leptin deficiency caused by the pathogenic variants in the *LEP* gene is *an extremely rare monogenic obesity disorder,* and <100 cases have been published to date.[3] The clinical manifestations include early-onset obesity and severe hyperphagia. The patients *can have additional manifestations, including frequent infections and endocrine defects,* such as hypogonadotropic hypogonadism and hypothyroidism, if they have biallelic variants in LEP.[12]
- *Leptin receptor deficiency:* Leptin receptor deficiency is a rare autosomal recessive disease caused by biallelic pathogenic variants in the LEPR gene. The phenotype is similar to leptin deficiency except *increase in serum leptin levels.* Individuals having leptin receptor deficiency show rapid weight gain, severe childhood obesity, hyperphagia, and insufficient satiety. The accompanied endocrine defects are comparable to the those of leptin deficiency, but *recurrent infections are nearly observed.*[13]
- *POMC deficiency:* POMC deficiency is an autosomal recessive monogenic obesity disorder. The clinical manifestations include hyperphagia, resulting in severe early-onset obesity, *pigmentary abnormalities* including red hair or pale skin color, and adrenal insufficiency.[14]
- *PCSK1 deficiency:* Patients with PCSK1 deficiency present with early-onset severe obesity accompanied by *diarrhea* in the infancy and *postprandial hypoglycemia.*[15] Additional clinical manifestations include neuroendocrine defects, such as diabetes insipidus, hypogonadotropic hypogonadism, adrenal insufficiency, and hypothyroidism.

Neuropeptide Y

Another gene of interest is the *Neuropeptide Y* (NPY) gene, which encodes *neuropeptide Y,* a potent hypothalamic orexigenic peptide. There is an association between the *NPY* gene and obesity. In fact, administration of neuropeptide NPY causes *increased food intake* and obesity. NPY neurons inhibit POMC neurons that decrease appetite, and they *activate orexin- and melanin-concentrating hormones,* which are *appetite-inducing peptides.*

1. *Polygenic obesity:* It results from the simultaneous presence of *multiple gene variants,* which have an accumulative effect. Polygenic obesity is certainly the *most common form of obesity,* which inevitably results from the interaction between obesogenic environmental factors and variants of different risk alleles. Unlike monogenic and syndromic obesity, *it is more difficult to study polygenic obesity* because, hypothetically, every individual has a different number of variants, which can contribute to the phenotype with a different "weight" and with complex allelic interactions that are difficult to evaluate. Over the past two decades, the advances in GWAS accompanied by high-throughput genome-wide genotyping techniques have enabled the identification of genetic variants throughout the whole genome.[3] In 2007, the GWAS for obesity phenotype demonstrated that several common variants in the intron of FTO (fat mass and obesity-associated gene) were *associated with BMI* in the large populations.[16] Numerous following GWAS identified >1,000 loci associated with the obesity trait to date.[17] The key features of monogenic and polygenic obesity are shown in **Table 2**.
2. *Syndromic obesity:* It is associated with other signs of a developmental disorder and may or may not be accompanied by a congenital malformation syndrome. The obesity associated with syndromic forms is *usually severe* and *has an early onset* with neurodevelopmental disorders and/or polymalformative syndrome. The typical signs are *dysmorphic features and organ abnormalities.* The syndromic forms of obesity are generally due to genomic segment *copy number variants (CNVs)* or consequence of chromosomal abnormalities.[18] It is estimated that there are at least 80 genetic syndromes in which obesity is considered a main feature. The examples of syndromes associated with obesity include the Prader–Willi syndrome, Cohen syndrome, and Bardet–Biedl syndrome. Prader–Willi syndrome occurs due to the *lack of expression* of the *paternal genes* of the *chromosome region 15*: 15q11.2–q13, and it is characterized by symptoms and signs such as developmental delay, intellectual disability,

TABLE 2: Key features of monogenic and polygenic obesity.

Monogenic	*Polygenic*
Early-onset, severe obesity	Common obesity
High genetic contribution	Modest genetic contribution
Single mutation in one gene	Hundreds of variants in or near many genes
Large genetic effect	Each variant has a small effect
Rare	Common
High penetrance	Low penetrance
No environmental influence	Environment is a key determinant

severe infant hypotonia, early-childhood onset obesity, and hyperphagia.

EPIGENETICS

Epigenetic changes are those that affect genetic expression without changing the sequence of DNA; these are acquired through interaction with the environment and, interestingly, are also heritable. Epigenetic changes can be influenced by environmental factors, such as diet, physical activity, and exposure to toxins. Studies have shown that maternal obesity and gestational diabetes can lead to epigenetic changes in offspring, which can increase the risk of obesity and metabolic disorders later in life.[19] Having a high-risk genetic profile makes a person more susceptible to an obesogenic environment. Studies concluded that the presence of these genes increases the risk of obesity but does not necessitate obesity. This risk can be ameliorated by healthy food choices, increased physical activity, and avoiding other causes of obesity.

CONCLUSION

Obesity is a complex health problem influenced by various factors, including genetics, environment, and behavior. The current obesity epidemic does not have a purely genetic basis, although *genetics do play a significant role in the susceptibility* to development of obesity. Changes to lifestyle over the past decades have created an "obesogenic environment" in which underlying individual genetic factors contributing to risk can be exposed. With the advent of GWAS, we have finally started to detect robust associations between common genetic variants and obesity. As GWAS have discovered more obesity-associated loci, *the majority of the loci identified in monogenic obesity involve the leptin–melanocortin pathway*. Although GWAs have been successful in identifying obesity loci, these only explain a small fraction of the interindividual variation, so additional genetic factors remain to be detected. Exploration of genetic factors and metabolic pathways is critical for the precise treatment and prevention of obesity.

REFERENCES

1. World Health Organization. (2024). One in eight people are now living with obesity. [online] Available from https://www.who.int/news/item/01-03-2024-one-in-eight-people-are-now-living-with-obesity. [Last accessed December, 2025].
2. World Health Organization. (2025). Obesity and overweight. [online] Available from https://www.who.int/news-room/fact-sheets/detail/obesity-and-overweight. [Last accessed December, 2025].
3. Loos RJ, Yeo GS. The genetics of obesity: from discovery to biology. Nat Rev Genet. 2022;23:120-33.
4. Farooqi IS. Monogenic human obesity syndromes. Handb Clin Neurol. 2021;181:301-10.
5. Hinney A, Korner A, Fischer-Posovszky P. The promise of new anti-obesity therapies arising from knowledge of genetic obesity traits. Nat Rev Endocrinol. 2022;18: 623-37.
6. Sohn YB. Genetic obesity: an update with emerging therapeutic approaches. Ann Pediatr Endocrinol Metab. 2022;27:169-75.
7. Spiegelman BM, Flier JS. Obesity and the regulation of energy balance. Cell. 2001;104:531-43.
8. Dayton K, Miller J. Finding treatable genetic obesity: strategies for success. Curr Opin Pediatr. 2018;30:526-31.
9. Myers MG Jr., Leibel RL, Seeley RJ, et al. Obesity and leptin resistance: distinguishing cause from effect. Trends Endocrinol Metab. 2010;21:643-51.
10. Botha R, Kumar SS, Grimsey NL, et al. A unique MC4R signaling profile for obesity-associated constitutively active variants. J Mol Endocrinol. 2023;71:e230008.
11. Lubrano-Berthelier C, Dubern B, Lacorte JM, et al. Melanocortin 4 receptor mutations in a large cohort of severely obese adults: prevalence, functional classification, genotype-phenotype relationship, and lack of association with binge eating. J Clin Endocrinol Metab. 2006;91:1811-8.
12. Wasim M, Awan FR, Najam SS, et al. Role of leptin deficiency, inefficiency, and leptin receptors in obesity. Biochem Genet. 2016;54:565-72.
13. Kleinendorst L, Abawi O, van der Kamp HJ, et al. Leptin receptor deficiency: a systematic literature review and prevalence estimation based on population genetics. Eur J Endocrinol. 2020;182:47-56.
14. Yeo GS, Chao DH, Siegert AM, et al. The melanocortin pathway and energy homeostasis: from discovery to obesity therapy. Mol Metab. 2021;48:101206.
15. Jackson RS, Creemers JW, Ohagi S, et al. Obesity and impaired prohormone processing associated with mutations in the human prohormone convertase 1 gene. Nat Genet. 1997;16:303-6.
16. Scuteri A, Sanna S, Chen WM, et al. Genome-wide association scan shows genetic variants in the FTO gene are associated with obesity-related traits. PLoS Genet. 2007;3:e115.
17. Buniello A, MacArthur JA, Cerezo M, et al. The NHGRI-EBI GWAS catalog of published genome-wide association studies, targeted arrays and summary statistics 2019. Nucleic Acids Res. 2019;47:D1005-12.
18. D'Angelo CS, Varela MC, de Castro CIE, et al. Chromosomal microarray analysis in the genetic evaluation of 279 patients with syndromic obesity. Mol Cytogenet. 2018;11:14.
19. Ling C, Ronn T. Epigenetics in human obesity and type 2 diabetes. Cell Metab. 2019;29:1028-44.

15

CHAPTER

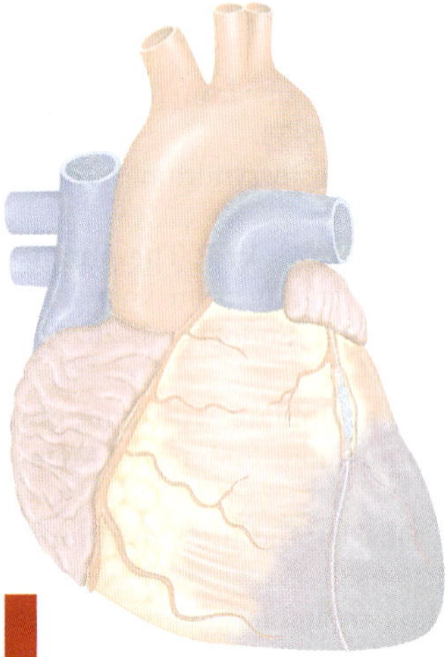

Guidelines for Obesity and Cardiovascular Disease Management

Anuj Maheshwari, Raj Singh Bhati

INTRODUCTION

Obesity is a long-term, recurring neurohormonal disease that speeds up atherosclerotic cardiovascular disease (ASCVD), heart failure with preserved ejection fraction (HFpEF), atrial fibrillation, high blood pressure, dyslipidemia, type 2 diabetes mellitus (T2DM), chronic kidney disease (CKD), and nonalcoholic fatty liver disease (NAFLD) in many ways, such as by causing visceral fat, systemic inflammation, ectopic fat deposition, and insulin resistance.[1,2] In South Asia, including India, rapid urbanization and changes in diet have led to a dual epidemic where cardiometabolic risk shows up at lower BMI levels (overweight ≥23 kg/m^2, obesity ≥25 kg/m^2) because of a higher percentage of visceral fat, a genetic tendency to insulin resistance, and atherogenic dyslipidemia.[3-5] The 2025 updates from the American College of Cardiology (ACC), Brazilian Society of Cardiology, and World Health Organization (WHO) bring together landmark cardiovascular outcomes trials (CVOTs), real-world evidence, and agreement from multiple societies to make weight loss a key strategy for preventing cardiovascular disease (CVD).[1,6,7] The goal is to lose 10–15% of your body weight to lower your risk of major adverse cardiovascular events (MACE) by 20–45%[1] **(Fig. 1)**.

DESCRIPTION

Epidemiology and Risk Stratification

In India, more than 30% of adults in cities are obese, and >40% of normal-weight people have central obesity, which leads to a two to three times higher rate of ASCVD than in Caucasians with the same body mass index (BMI). South Asians have 3–5% more body fat mass, smaller fat cells that promote hypertrophy and inflammation, and fat that accumulates in the wrong places too soon.[3,4] This is why the thresholds for overweight BMI are 23.0–24.9 kg/m^2, obesity is 25 kg/m^2, and abdominal obesity is a waist circumference ≥90 cm (men) or ≥80 cm (women).[3,5,8]

Risk stratification combines BMI/waist with other health issues.[1] Low risk means a BMI of 18.5–22.9 kg/m^2, a normal waist, and no other health issues. Moderate risk means being overweight and having 0–1 other health issues. High risk means being obese or having abdominal obesity and having 2 or more other health issues, such as hypertension (HTN), dyslipidemia, prediabetes/T2DM, CKD stage 3, OSA, or NAFLD. Very high-risk means having established ASCVD, HF, CKD stage 4, or T2DM for >10 years.[1,2]

Pathophysiological Links Between Obesity and Cardiovascular Disease

Excessive adiposity induces hypertrophic adipocytes to secrete proinflammatory cytokines [tumor necrosis factor-alpha (TNF-α), IL-6, and resistin], diminishes adiponectin levels, and promotes leptin resistance, thereby facilitating endothelial dysfunction, atherogenesis, and thrombosis.[2] Ectopic fat in the myocardium/pericardium disrupts diastolic function (HFpEF), whereas hepatic steatosis exacerbates insulin resistance and dyslipidemia [elevated triglycerides, diminished high-density lipoprotein cholesterol (HDL-C), and small dense low-density

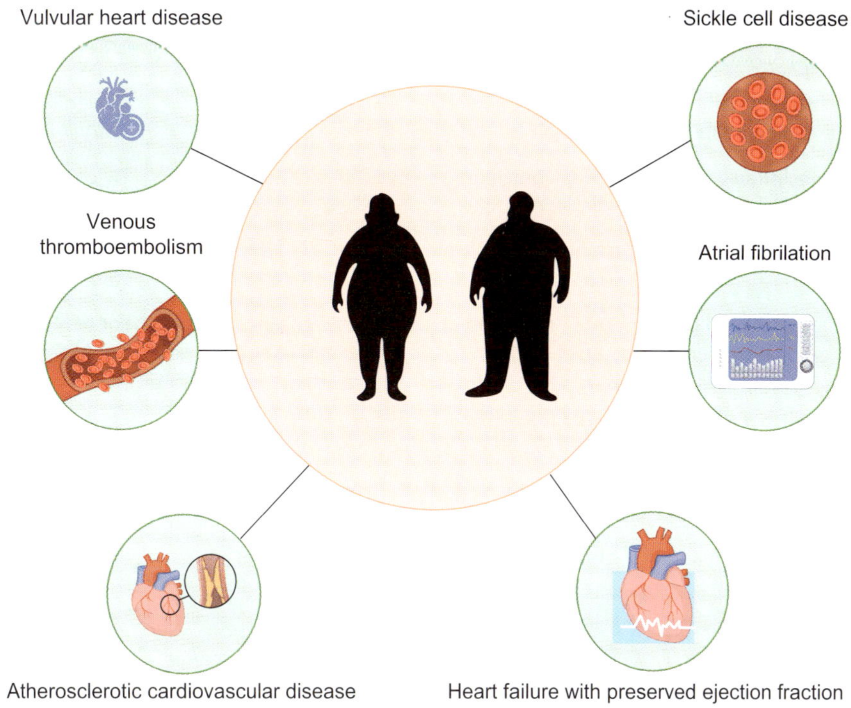

Fig. 1: Impact of obesity on cardiovascular disease (CVD).

lipoprotein (LDL)].[2,9] Neurohormonal activation [sympathetic overdrive, renin-angiotensin-aldosterone system (RAAS)] increases afterload, encourages left ventricular (LV) hypertrophy and sodium retention, and leads to concentric remodeling, arrhythmia, and pulmonary HTN.[2] Glucagon-like peptide-1 receptor agonists (GLP-1 Ras) counteract these pathophysiological mechanisms through a 10–20% reduction in weight, direct anti-inflammatory effects, and enhanced hemodynamics, demonstrating a more significant reduction in major adverse cardiac events (MACE) in individuals with a BMI exceeding 35 kg/m^2 [hazard ratio (HR) 0.72 compared to 0.92 in those with a lower BMI].[10]

Lifestyle and Behavioral Interventions

Intensive lifestyle therapy can help you lose 5–10% of your body weight in 6–12 months.[1] This leads to improvements in your heart and metabolism, such as a 0.5–1% drop in glycated hemoglobin (HbA1c), a 2–5 mm Hg drop in systolic blood pressure (SBP), a 10–20% drop in TG, and a 5–10% rise in HDL, regardless of how much fat you lose.[1,2] This is because the gut microbiome improves, and inflammation decreases.[1] Prescribe a Mediterranean or plant-based diet with a daily calorie deficit of 500–750 kcal (with an emphasis on vegetables, legumes, and nuts; limit refined carbs to <10% of calories and sodium to <2 g/day); moderate aerobic and resistance training for at least 150–300 minutes a week (two to three times a week), with cardiac rehabilitation for people with CVD to lower the risk of deconditioning. Self-monitoring, cognitive behavioral therapy (CBT), motivational interviewing, and digital tools are all behavioral components. Interventions at home and work can increase adherence by 20–30%.[1]

Pharmacological Management of Obesity in Cardiovascular Disease

Glucagon-like peptide-1 receptor agonists (semaglutide, liraglutide) and dual GLP-1/GIP RAs (tirzepatide) are first-line treatments that lower the risk of MACE [risk ratio (RR): 0.86, 95% confidence interval (CI): 0.79–0.94], CV death (RR: 0.86), and all-cause mortality (RR: 0.87).[1,9,10] They work even better for people with T2DM, HFpEF, and CKD.[1,10] According to the SURMOUNT-1/2 extensions, tirzepatide helps people lose 15–22% of their weight over three years.[9,11] It also helps lower their blood pressure (–7 mm Hg), triglycerides (–25%), and visceral fat –40%).[12] Indications include: BMI ≥27 kg/m^2 + comorbidity or ≥30 kg/m^2; South Asians ≥25 kg/m^2 + high CVD risk; titrate slowly while watching for GI intolerance and pancreatitis (rare, <0.5%).[1,6,13] For synergistic benefit, combine with

TABLE 1: Advances in lipid-lowering therapies.

Category	Agent	Mechanism	LDL/TG effect	Key clinical notes
PCSK9-Directed	Alirocumab/ evolocumab	PCSK9 monoclonal antibodies	↓ LDL-C ~60%	Proven MACE reduction; used in ASCVD, FH, statin intolerance[14]
	Inclisiran	siRNA blocking hepatic PCSK9	↓ LDL-C ~50%	Twice-yearly dosing; excellent adherence; guideline-endorsed[15]
ACL Inhibitor	Bempedoic acid	Inhibits ATP-citrate lyase	↓ LDL-C 20–25%	CLEAR Outcomes: reduced MACE in statin-intolerant patients[16]
TG/Residual Risk Therapies	ApoC-III inhibitors (volanesorsen and olezarsen)	ASO inhibition of ApoC-III	Large ↓ TG; ↓ remnant cholesterol	For severe HTG and chylomicronemia, the ASCVD benefit under study[17]
	ANGPTL3 inhibitors (evinacumab, RNA agents)	Inhibit ANGPTL3	↓ LDL-C, TG, non-HDL-C	Effective in refractory hypercholesterolemia, especially HoFH[18]
	Lp(a)-lowering (Pelacarsen and Olpasiran)	ASO/siRNA lowering Lp(a)	↓ Lp(a) >80%	Major outcome trials underway; will address residual risk[19]
	Saroglitazar	Dual PPAR-α/γ agonist	↓ TG 40–60%; ↓ non-HDL-C; modest glycemic improvement	Approved in India for diabetic dyslipidemia and NASH; improves TG-rich lipoproteins and insulin sensitivity[20]
RNA therapeutics	siRNA/ASO platforms	Gene-silencing (liver-targeted)	Deep, durable lipid lowering	Long-interval dosing (monthly–yearly) improves adherence[21]

(ANGPTL3: angiopoietin-like protein 3; ASO: antisense oligonucleotide; ATP: adenosine triphosphate; HoFH: homozygous familial hypercholesterolemia; MACE: major adverse cardiovascular events; PCSK9: proprotein convertase subtilisin/kexin type 9; PPAR-α/γ: peroxisome proliferator-activated receptor alpha/gamma; NASH: nonalcoholic steatohepatitis; non-HDL-C: nonhigh-density lipoprotein cholesterol; siRNA: small interfering ribonucleic acid; RNA: ribonucleic acid)

statins and sodium-glucose cotransporter 2 (SGLT2) inhibitors.[1] **Table 1** summarizes key lipid-lowering options.

METABOLIC/BARIATRIC SURGERY

Procedures like Roux-en-Y gastric bypass and sleeve gastrectomy lead to a sustained weight loss of 20–30%, a 30–45% decrease in MACE, a 0.47% decrease in HF hospitalizations, and a decrease in CV mortality, with a perioperative risk of 0.2–0.5% even in people who have had myocardial infarction (MI) or stenting before.[22-23] Benefits arise from glycemic remission (70% T2DM reversal), blood pressure normalization (50%), and resolution of inflammation; long-term data validate durability compared to medical therapy.[14] Indications include: BMI ≥40 kg/m^2 or ≥35 kg/m^2 with uncontrolled comorbidity; Asian-adjusted BMI ≥32.5–37.5 kg/m^2; all patients necessitate multidisciplinary optimization [echocardiogram, cardiopulmonary exercise testing (CPET) if heart failure].[1,5,23]

LIMITATIONS

Even though the 2025 guidelines have made great progress, there are still significant gaps in evidence and problems with implementing them into practice, especially in places like India, where the burden is high **(Table 2)**.[1,3,13]

GUIDELINES

2025 Integrated Algorithm for Obesity-Cardiovascular Disease Management

This algorithm adapts Brazilian PREVENT stratification with South Asian BMI/waist cut-offs and American College of Cardiology (ACC)/World Health Organization (WHO) priorities, aiming for a loss of ≥10–15% to reduce MACE/HF based on landmark trials (SELECT/SOS/STEP).[1,7]

Universal Screening and Risk Stratification (Annual for Adults ≥20 years)

- BMI (South Asian thresholds: Overweight 23–24.9, obesity ≥25 kg/m^2), waist ≥ 90/80 cm (M/F).[3,5]

TABLE 2: Evidence gaps and implementation challenges in 2025 obesity-CVD guidelines.

Domain	*Specific gap*	*Impact*	*2025 evidence status*
Elderly (>75 years)	Frailty/sarcopenia risks with GLP-1RA	Falls, muscle loss	Subgroup data only; no CVOTs
Advanced HF/CKD (eGFR<30)	Volume shifts, renal clearance	HF worsening	STEP-HFpEF signals; SURPASS-RENAL pending
Sarcopenic Obesity	BMI misses myosteatosis	Functional decline	40% relative muscle loss on tirzepatide
South Asian surgery	Limited CVOT representation	Uncertain MACE benefit	5% Asian cohorts; Indian registries are incomplete
Tirzepatide long-term	>10 years malignancy/bone/CV mortality	Unknown durability	SURMOUNT-4 (3 years); SURMOUNT-MACE 2028
LMIC access (India)	₹50K–1L/month; <10% rural reach	Inequity despite 80% mandates	Supply/cold-chain gaps
Infrastructure	<500 bariatric centers	Care deserts	70% districts lack MDT

(CKD: chronic kidney disease; CVD: cardiovascular disease; CVOT: cardiovascular outcome trials; GLP-1RA: glucagon-like peptide-1 receptor agonist; HF: heart failure; LMIC: low- and middle-income countries)

- Prevent 10-year ASCVD risk assessment (<5% low, 5–19.9% moderate, or 20% high) and heart failure risk (7.5% high); screen for T2DM, HTN, lipids, CKD, and obstructive sleep apnea (OSA).[1]

Lifestyle (All Patients)

- 500–750 kcal deficit (Mediterranean or plant-based diet, <10% refined carbs); ≥150 min/week aerobic + resistance training; CBT/self-monitoring.
- Aim for a weight loss of 5–10% every 3 months [1].

Pharmacotherapy Options for Obesity in CVD Patients (BMI ≥ 27 + Comorbidity or ≥30; Escalate if <5% Loss at 3 Months) are Detailed in Table 3[7,9]

Titrate slowly; monitor gastrointestinal (GI) side effects and heart rate q3 months.[1,13]

Surgery (Body Mass Index ≥35+ Failure or ≥40; Asians ≥32.5+)

- RYGB/sleeve (20–30% sustained weight loss; MACE ↓33%).[22-23]
- Preoperative cardiovascular optimization required.[1]

Monitor (q3-6 months Lifelong)

- Weight, blood pressure, A1c, lipids, and eGFR.
- Add statins and SGLT2 inhibitors for comprehensive cardioprotection.
- Adjust therapy to prevent relapse.[1]

Risk-target Matrix

The risk-target matrix **(Table 4)** outlines weight loss goals and treatment sequences based on ASCVD and HF risk levels.

TABLE 3: Pharmacological agents for obesity management.

Agent	*Weight loss*	*CV benefit*
Semaglutide 2.4 mg/week	15–20%	MACE ↓20% (SELECT)
Tirzepatide 10–15 mg/week	18–22%	TG ↓25–67% (SURMOUNT)

TABLE 4: Risk-target matrix for obesity-CVD management.

ASCVD risk	*HF risk*	*Target loss*	*Sequence*
Low (<5%)	Low	≥5%	Lifestyle only
Moderate (5–19.9%)	High	≥10%	Lifestyle + GLP-1RA
High (≥20%)	High	≥15%	GLP-1RA → Bariatric surgery

(ASCVD: atherosclerotic cardiovascular disease; CVD: cardiovascular disease; GLP-1RA: glucagon-like peptide-1 receptor agonist)

CONCLUSION

The 2025 guidelines establish obesity as a modifiable cardiovascular disease risk factor requiring integrated, evidence-based management. GLP-1 RAs and tirzepatide lower MACE by 14–35% and bariatric surgery by 45%, with even more pronounced effects in South Asians with elevated BMI. By 2030, India's projected 10 million cardiovascular disease events caused by obesity can be prevented through culturally appropriate, multidisciplinary implementation strategies.

REFERENCES

1. Valerio CM, Saraiva JFK, Valente F, et al. 2025 Brazilian evidence-based guideline on the management of obesity

and prevention of cardiovascular disease and obesity-associated complications: a position statement by five medical societies. Diabetol Metab Syndr. 2025;17(1):432.
2. Schiele F, Dievart F, Jacobi D, et al. Onboarding obesity management in cardiovascular care: A cardiologist's guide to the latest advances. Am J Prev Cardiol. 2025;22:100987.
3. Deshpande A, Shah NS, Kandula NR. Obesity and Cardiovascular Risk among South Asian Americans. Curr Cardiovasc Risk Rep. 2023;17(3):73-82.
4. Riaz M, Lodhi S. Beyond BMI: Exploring obesity trends in the South Asian region. Obes Pillars. 2024;13:100156.
5. Tham KW, Abdul Ghani R, Cua SC, et al. Obesity in South and Southeast Asia-A new consensus on care and management. Obes Rev. 2023;24(2):e13520.
6. World Health Organization. (2025). WHO issues global guideline on the use of GLP-1 medicines in treating obesity. [Online] Available from https://www.who.int/news/item/01-12-2025-who-issues-global-guideline-on-the-use-of-glp-1-medicines-in-treating-obesity [Last accessed January, 2026].
7. American College of Cardiology. (2025). New ACC Guidance Addresses Obesity Treatment Strategies Across the CV Spectrum. [Online] Available from https://www.acc.org/Latest-in-Cardiology/Articles/2025/07/07/17/05/New-ACC-Guidance-Addresses-Obesity-Treatment-Strategies-Across-the-CV-Spectrum [Last accessed January, 2026].
8. Prasad DS, Kabir Z, Dash AK, et al. Abdominal obesity, an independent cardiovascular risk factor in Indian subcontinent: A clinico epidemiological evidence summary. J Cardiovasc Dis Res. 2011;2(4):199-205.
9. Sattar N, García-Pérez LE, Rodríguez A, et al. Tirzepatide and cardiometabolic parameters in obesity: Summary of current evidence. Diabetes Obes Metab. 2025;27(10):5386-92.
10. Kalayci A, Januzzi JL, Mitsunami M, et al. Clinical features modifying the cardiovascular benefits of GLP-1 receptor agonists: a systematic review and meta-analysis. Eur Heart J Cardiovasc Pharmacother. 2025;11(6):552-61.
11. Guan H, Jiang H, Yuan H, et al. Long-term efficacy and safety of tirzepatide in participants with type 2 diabetes with inadequate glycaemic control on metformin and/or sulfonylurea: Post-hoc analysis of SURPASS-4. Diabetes Obes Metab. 2025;27(11):6480-90.
12. American College of Cardiology. (2025). Weight Loss Can Lead to Better CV Outcomes in Middle-Age, Patient-Provided WLM Treatment More Effective Than Professional Support Alone. [Online] Avaialble from https://www.acc.org/Latest-in-Cardiology/Journal-Scans/2025/06/03/16/38/Weight-Loss-Can-Lead-to-Better-CV-Outcomes [Last accessed January, 2025].
13. Alhowiti A, Mirghani H, Abdulrahman Qrmli A, et al. Barriers to glucagon-like peptide-1 agonists used for obesity management among the general population in Tabuk City, Saudi Arabia, and their relation to smoking cessation and antidepressants. Front Pharmacol. 2025;16:1510554.
14. Sabatine MS, De Ferrari GM, Giugliano RP, et al. Clinical Benefit of Evolocumab by Severity and Extent of Coronary Artery Disease: Analysis From FOURIER. Circulation. 2018;138(8):756-66.
15. Ray KK, Troquay RPT, Visseren FLJ, et al. Long-term efficacy and safety of inclisiran in patients with high cardiovascular risk and elevated LDL cholesterol (ORION-3): results from the 4-year open-label extension of the ORION-1 trial. Lancet Diabetes Endocrinol. 2023;11(2):109-19.
16. Nissen SE, Lincoff AM, Brennan D, et al. Bempedoic Acid and Cardiovascular Outcomes in Statin-Intolerant Patients. N Engl J Med. 2023;388(15):1353-64.
17. Gaudet D, Alexander VJ, Baker BF, et al. Antisense Inhibition of Apolipoprotein C-III in Patients with Hypertriglyceridemia. N Engl J Med. 2015;373(5):438-47.
18. Raal FJ, Rosenson RS, Reeskamp LF, et al. Evinacumab for Homozygous Familial Hypercholesterolemia. N Engl J Med. 2020;383(8):711-20.
19. Tsimikas S, Karwatowska-Prokopczuk E, Gouni-Berthold I, et al. Lipoprotein(a) Reduction in Persons with Cardiovascular Disease. N Engl J Med. 2020;382(3):244-55.
20. Sawhney JP, Ramakrishnan S, Madan K, et al. CSI clinical practice guidelines for dyslipidemia management: Executive summary. Indian Heart J. 2024;76 Suppl 1(Suppl 1):S6-19.
21. Miname MH, Rocha VZ, Santos RD. The Role of RNA-Targeted Therapeutics to Reduce ASCVD Risk: What Have We Learned Recently?. Curr Atheroscler Rep. 2021;23(8):40.
22. Schauer PR, Nissen SE. After 70 Years, Metabolic Surgery Has Earned a Cardiovascular Outcome Trial. Circulation. 2021;143(15):1481-3.
23. Liu Z, Wang H, Fan D, et al. Asia's Growing Contribution to Obesity Surgery Research: A 40-year Bibliometric Analysis. Obes Surg. 2024;34(6):2139-53.

CHAPTER 16

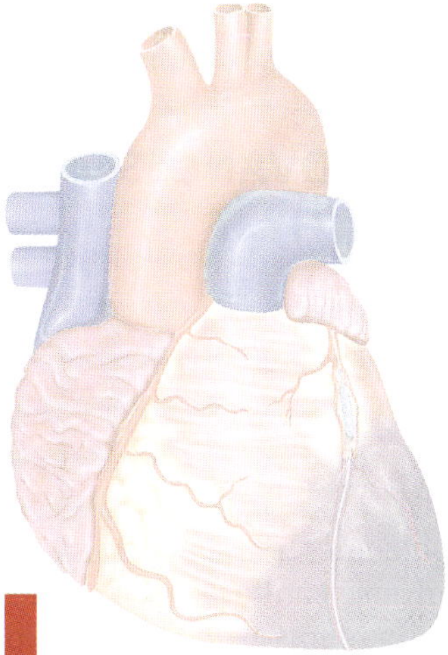

Advances in Obesity and Lipid Management in Cardiovascular Diseases: Cardiac Anesthetist Perspective

Poonam Malhotra Kapoor

INTRODUCTION

Obesity and dyslipidemia are tightly coupled drivers of atherosclerotic cardiovascular disease (ASCVD) and of perioperative risk in cardiac surgery. Over the last 5 years, the field has shifted from largely lifestyle-and-statin centric care to a multimodal pharmacologic and procedural armamentarium: High-potency statins remain foundational, but novel antiobesity agents [glucagon-like peptide-1 (GLP-1) receptor agonists and dual incretin agonists], second-line LDL-lowering therapies (PCSK9 monoclonal antibodies, siRNA agents such as inclisiran), and nonstatin small molecules (bempedoic acid)—plus agents targeted at triglyceride-related risk (icosapent ethyl)—have changed how we think about long-term risk reduction and short-term perioperative physiology. These advances have implications for preoperative optimization, intraoperative management, and early ICU care.[1]

PATHOPHYSIOLOGIC RATIONALE BACKGROUND THAT IS IMPORTANT

Adiposity as a multimodal stressor: Adipose tissue in obesity is not inert: visceral adiposity produces systemic inflammation, hypercoagulability, and adverse myocardial remodeling; it also predisposes to difficult airway, reduced functional residual capacity, obstructive sleep apnea (OSA), and altered pharmacokinetics of anesthetic agents. These mechanisms explain the increased incidence of postoperative atrial fibrillation, low cardiac output, and pulmonary complications in obese cardiac surgery patients.[2]

Targeting Obesity in Cardiovascular Disease Management: Cardiac Adipose Tissue Is a Real Biomarker!

There are different types of adipose tissue, including cardiac adipose tissue, which comprises epicardial and pericardial (or paracardiac) fractions. Epicardial adipose tissue (EAT) is unique due to its proximity to the heart and a distinct gene expression profile compared to other adipose depots, such as visceral and subcutaneous fat. EAT plays a crucial role in the development and progression of cardiovascular diseases (CVDs) with high morbidity and mortality, acting both as a metabolic and inflammatory mediator.

Cardiac adipose tissue, particularly EAT, is a key player in cardiometabolic disease. Understanding its pathophysiological role and incorporating imaging tools to evaluate EAT may enhance cardiovascular risk stratification and disease management.[3]

In a position statement by five medical societies, management of obesity and prevention of CVD and obesity-associated complications following cardiovascular risk assessment using the Predicting Risk of CVD Events risk score, individuals with obesity or overweight will be stratified according to their 10-year risk of developing atherosclerotic disease (low, moderate, or high) and heart failure (high-risk). Antiobesity treatment will then be guided by the best evidence-based recommendations designed to address excess adiposity and reduce associated complications, as shown in **Table 1**.

TABLE 1: Cardiovascular risk assessment in individuals with overweight or obesity.

High—20% at 10 years	• Established coronary artery disease, myocardial infarction (MI), ischemic stroke or transient ischemic attack (TIA), peripheral artery disease (PAD), arterial revascularization in any territory • Primary prevention with total CV risk by PREVENT score—20% at 10 years • Type 2 diabetes duration >10 years. • Chronic kidney disease stage 3b/4/5 • Coronary artery calcium (CAC) score >100 Agatston units (AU). (without diabetes) or >10 AU (with diabetes), Lp(a) >50 mg/dL or >125. nmol/L, familial hypercholesterolemia (FH), or LDL-C >190 mg/dL
High HF risk—20% at 10 years	• BMI >40 kg/m^2, even if asymptomatic • Individuals with obesity, plus diabetes and hypertension • Severe obstructive sleep apnea (OSA) • Atrial fibrillation • Chronic kidney disease stage 3b/4/5 • Elevated NT-proBNP or BNP • PREVENT HF risk score—20% at 10 years • Established ASCVD • Symptoms suggestive of HF

RESIDUAL LIPID RISK AND PLAQUES VULNERABLE TO PERIOPERATIVE STRESS

Low-density lipoprotein cholesterol (LDL-C) lowering reduces plaque progression and stabilizes lesions; inflammation and triglyceride-rich lipoproteins remain residual risk domains even when LDL is controlled. New agents lower these risks by complementary mechanisms (PCSK9 pathway, ACL-inhibition, and RNA interference) and—in trials—reduce events beyond statin monotherapy. Understanding the mechanism helps us anticipate effects (e.g., on inflammation, wound healing, and rare hepatic effects) that may be clinically relevant preoperatively.[4]

EPIDEMIOLOGY OF OBESITY IN HEART FAILURE

Avoidance of excess adiposity throughout the lifespan is key to the prevention of incident Heart Failure, particularly HFpEF. The "Heart failure obesity survival paradox" in part represents the negative implications of unintentional weight loss. Obesity treatments offer opportunities for improved heart failure symptom burden, functional capacity, quality of life, and fewer hospitalizations.[5]

MAJOR THERAPEUTIC ADVANCES–WHAT CHANGED AND WHY IT MATTERS?

Antiobesity Pharmacotherapy with Cardiovascular Benefit

Semaglutide (Weekly 2.4 mg)

The SELECT cardiovascular outcomes trial showed a ~20% relative reduction in major adverse cardiovascular events (MACE) in overweight/obese patients with established CVD (without diabetes), together with sustained weight loss and renal benefits. For the anesthetist, this class reduces body weight, improves hemodynamics and metabolic profile long-term, but has perioperative considerations.[1]

Tirzepatide (Dual Glucagon-like Peptide/Glucagon-like Peptide-1 Agonist)

Tirzepatide produces larger weight loss than first-generation GLP-1 RAs in obesity trials (SURMOUNT series) and favorable cardiometabolic improvements; cardiovascular outcome evidence is emerging (meta-analyses and real-world studies suggest safety and possible benefit), but large CVOTs are ongoing. From an anesthetic viewpoint, tirzepatide's potent weight loss and glycemic effects may change drug dosing, fluid distribution, and stress responses.[6]

Why are these clinically relevant? These drugs are shifting preoperative profiles (fewer BMI-related complications long term) but introduce short-term issues: Delayed gastric emptying, nausea, increased gallstone risk, and the need to manage hypoglycemia risk and changes in drug absorption and volume of distribution.

NEW AND REPURPOSED LIPID-LOWERING THERAPIES

Bempedoic Acid (Adenosine Triphosphate Citrate Lyase Inhibitor)

The CLEAR Outcomes trial in statin-intolerant patients demonstrated a statistically significant reduction in MACE versus placebo, with LDL lowering and favorable safety signals in the trial population. This provides an oral non-statin option for patients' intolerance of statins.[7]

Proprotein Convertase Subtilisin/Kexin Type 9 Inhibitors (Monoclonal Antibodies) and Ribonucleic Acid Therapeutics

Monoclonal PCSK9 inhibitors (evolocumab and alirocumab) remain in potent LDL-lowerers with proven cardiovascular event reduction in high-risk populations. Inclisiran (siRNA targeting PCSK9) offers twice-yearly dosing with meaningful LDL-C reductions; large outcomes trials (ORION/ORION-4/HPS-4) and recent data on broader populations have expanded clinical interest, though outcome-level evidence is still accruing.[8]

Icosapent Ethyl (High-dose Eicosapentaenoic Acid, Reduction of Cardiovascular Events with Icosapent Ethyl–Intervention Trial)

Reduces ischemic events in selected patients with elevated triglycerides despite statin therapy and remains a consideration for residual triglyceride-driven risk.[9]

Why is clinically relevant? For the cardiac anesthetist, these agents alter the patient's baseline risk and inflammatory milieu; they can influence perioperative LDL/inflammatory markers and, rarely, have hepatic or hematologic side effects to consider in perioperative laboratories/monitoring. Evidence for perioperative continuation is limited for the newer agents, but continuation of statins perioperatively is supported by guidelines and associated with improved short-term outcomes.

INTENSIVE CARE UNIT CONSIDERATIONS IN OBESITY AND DYSLIPIDEMIA

Metabolic Recalibration

If a patient is on GLP-1 RA or tirzepatide, document start date, dose, GI tolerance, and glycemic trends. For patients actively losing weight on these agents, reassess airway and pulmonary function (OSA screening), nutritional status, and liver function. GLP-1 agents commonly cause nausea and delay gastric emptying—treat as at-risk for aspirations.[1]

Lipid Therapy

Continue chronic statin therapy through the perioperative period (guideline supported); initiation of statin therapy at least 1–2 weeks of preoperative is reasonable for high-risk vascular patients. For PCSK9 or inclisiran recipients, evidence to guide perioperative continuation is limited—decisions should be multidisciplinary (cardiology, surgery, and anesthesia) and individualized; there is no class-wide recommendation to stop these agents before cardiac surgery at present.[10]

Nutritional and Adiposity Indices

Consider combining adiposity-nutritional indices (CANI) as predictors of MACCE after CABG (evidence from cardiac critical care literature); use such indices to inform risk discussion and ICU planning.[11]

Glycemia and Nutrition

Glucagon-like peptide-1-class drugs reduce gastric emptying and may increase nausea postoperatively—anticipate altered enteral feeding tolerance and avoid sudden discontinuation that could destabilize glycemic control. If the patient is nil per oral and requires intensive insulin therapy, follow institutional insulin protocols; coordinate with endocrinology for bridging.

Infectious Risk and Wound Healing

Weight loss and altered nutritional state (rapid or ongoing) can impact wound healing. Monitor for bile-related complications (increased gallstone risk with rapid weight loss) and pancreatitis if clinically suspected in patients on GLP-1 or dual agonists.

Continuation of Secondary Prevention

Restart statins early postoperatively unless contra-indicated; where PCSK9 monoclonal therapy or inclisiran has been used, coordinate timing of dosing with the cardiology team—no strong evidence yet to mandate routine perioperative withholding.

Airway and Ventilation

Expect decreased FRC, rapid desaturation and increased risk of difficult mask ventilation/intubation in higher BMI; have an OSA plan, use recruitment strategies, and protective ventilation (lower tidal volume, higher PEEP titrated to physiology).[2]

Hemodynamic Effects

Rapid weight loss or metabolic changes from antiobesity drugs may lead to altered vasomotor tone and myocardial energetics—be vigilant for exaggerated BP and HR responses during induction and rewarming. Adjust dosages carefully and monitor serum electrolytes and glucose intraoperatively.

Coagulation and Inflammation

Aggressive LDL-lowering and agents that modulate inflammation may blunt classic inflammatory surges, but data on immediate pro/anticoagulant effects peri-CABG are limited. Use standard point-of-care coagulation monitoring (ROTEM/TEG) as always.

DIAGNOSIS OF OBESITY

Although BMI is an inexpensive, easily acquired, and readily reproducible metric that is strongly embedded in research and clinical practice, significant limitations exist in the detection of excess adiposity, the location of adiposity, and applicability to diverse populations. To determine a diagnosis of clinical obesity in individuals with BMI <35 kg/m^2, direct assessment of excess adiposity with an anthropometric criterion [e.g., waist circumference (the most readily obtainable), waist-to-hip ratio, or waist-to-height ratio] or body composition assessment (e.g., dual X-ray absorptiometry, when available) may be used. Clinicians should be aware that obesity remains a stigmatized condition and that some individuals may experience discomfort with being weighed, abdominally measured, or talking about weight during a medical visit.

CHALLENGES OF THE DIAGNOSIS OF HEART FAILURE IN INDIVIDUALS WITH OBESITY

Because individuals with obesity have lower NP concentrations, lower thresholds are used in those who have obesity and exertional dyspnea to avoid underdiagnosis of HF in this population, although specific thresholds are not currently established. For individuals with HF and obesity, monitoring for T2DM, hypertension, atrial fibrillation, sleep disordered breathing, and objective evidence of exercise intolerance can identify the need for targeted interventions.

MANAGEMENT OF OBESITY IN HEART FAILURE

Behavioral changes aimed at intentional weight loss are appropriate to attempt for individuals with obesity because even modest changes in body weight can result in improvements in risk of cardiovascular events, although weight loss is often unsustainable. Exercise can improve functional status in individuals with HFpEF.

ROLE OF ANTIOBESITY MEDICATIONS IN HEART FAILURE WITH PRESERVED EJECTION FRACTION WITH OBESITY

The STEP-HFpEF program and SUMMIT trial show that, in people with BMI \$30 kg/m^2 and HF with EF \$45% (semaglutide) and EF \$50% (tirzepatide), weight loss is associated with improvements in symptoms and functional capacity. Insufficient evidence exists to date to confidently conclude that semaglutide and tirzepatide reduce HF events in individuals with HFpEF and obesity (with stronger evidence for tirzepatide), although exploratory analysis indicates favorable changes in biomarkers and imaging parameters, suggesting potential distinct mechanistic advantages outside of weight loss.

During early-phase gradual dose escalation of semaglutide or tirzepatide, which occurs every 4 weeks, monitor kidney function and electrolytes with adjustment of diuretics, antihypertensive agents, and antihyperglycemic agents as indicated, particularly if gastrointestinal adverse effects are prominent.

INVASIVE INTERVENTIONS

For individuals with HF and obesity, MBS appears effective for intentional weight loss and potentially to reduce the risk of HF events, including hospitalization for HF and death, although these possibilities are based only on data from observational studies. Individuals with HF who are undergoing MBS have an increased risk of postoperative cardiovascular morbidity and death, suggesting the need for preoperative optimization and perioperative care by clinicians with expertise in HF management.

EMERGING QUESTIONS AND AREAS FOR FUTURE STUDY (BRIEF)

- *Class effect vs agent specificity for CV protection:* SELECT (semaglutide) and SURMOUNT/SURPASS (tirzepatide) signal important cardio metabolic benefits, but head-to-head and mechanistic work to separate weight-mediated from pleiotropic effects is ongoing.[13]
- *Perioperative trials:* Trials that test perioperative continuation vs temporary suspension of novel lipid-lowering agents and GLP-1/dual agonists are sparse; cardiac surgery is an ideal setting to study whether rapid LDL/inflammatory modulation improves myocardial protection and short-term outcomes.
- *Implementation and equity:* Access, cost, and real-world adherence to twice-yearly inclisiran or expensive

GLP-1 therapy will shape outcomes; real-world comparative effectiveness studies are emerging.

CONCLUSION

Obesity confers increased risks of HF, coronary artery disease, and stroke[12] and weight loss can reduce CVD risk. Given emerging evidence of the benefits of semaglutide and tirzepatide in individuals with HFpEF and obesity in concert with healthy behavioral interventions, clinicians should be aware of optimal diagnosis, risk assessment, and management of obesity in individuals with HF. An essential future priority will be providing equitable access through policies and systems to ensure that individuals with adverse SDOH have access to evidence-based AOM, particularly so that we can avoid the unintended consequence of further exacerbating health inequities. With accurate evaluation of obesity as well as administration and monitoring of safe and effective interventions, clinicians may improve quality of life and functional capacity and potentially reduce HF events in individuals living with HF and obesity.

REFERENCES

1. Lincoff AM, Brown-Frandsen K, Colhoun HM, et al. Semaglutide and Cardiovascular Outcomes in Obesity without Diabetes. N Engl J Med. 2023;389(24):2221-32.
2. Seyni-Boureima R, Zhang Z, Antoine MMLK, et al. A review on the anesthetic management of obese patients undergoing surgery. BMC Anesthesiol. 2022;22(1):98.
3. D'Elia S, Luisi E, Solimene A, et al. Targeting Obesity in Cardiovascular Disease Management: Cardiac Adipose Tissue Is a Real Biomarker! Targets. 2025;3(2):17.
4. Priyanka FNU, Durga FNU, Affan M, Venjhraj FNU. The PCSK9 Inhibitors: A Lipid-lowering Therapy to Treat Atherosclerotic Cardiovascular Diseases. Nat Cell Science. 2025;3(2):92-9.
5. Breathett K, Lewsey S, Brownell NK, et al. Implementation science to achieve equity in heart failure care: a scientific statement from the American Heart Association. Circulation. 2024;149(19):e1143-63.
6. Jastreboff AM, Aronne LJ, Ahmad NN, et al. Tirzepatide Once Weekly for the Treatment of Obesity Ania M. N Engl J Med. 2022;387(3):205-16.
7. Nissen SE, Lincoff AM, Brennan D, et al; CLEAR Outcomes Investigators. Bempedoic Acid and Cardiovascular Outcomes in Statin-Intolerant Patients. N Engl J Med. 2023;388(15):1353-64.
8. Ray KK, Raal FJ, Kallend DG, et al. Inclisiran and cardiovascular events: a patient-level analysis of phase III trials. Eur Heart J. 2023;44(2):129-38.
9. Huston J, Schaffner H, Cox A, et al. A Critical Review of Icosapent Ethyl in Cardiovascular Risk Reduction. Am J Cardiovasc Drugs. 2023;23(4):393-406.
10. Halvorsen S, Mehilli J, Cassese S, et al. ESC Scientific Document Group. 2022 ESC Guidelines on cardiovascular assessment and management of patients undergoing non-cardiac surgery. Eur Heart J. 2022;43(39):3826-924.
11. Bansal N, Magoon R, Dey S, et al. Preoperative Combined Adiposity-Nutritional Index predicts MACCE following OPCABG (PANDORA). J Card Criti Care TSS. 2022;5(3);214-21.
12. Huston J, Schaffner H, Cox A, et al. A critical review of icosapent ethyl (IPE) for cardiovascular risk reduction: clinical outcomes and evidence from REDUCE-IT and related studies. Am J Cardiovasc Drugs. 2023;23(5): 393-406.
13. Jastreboff AM, Aronne LJ, Ahmad NN, et al. Tirzepatide once weekly for treatment of obesity (SURMOUNT-1). N Engl J Med. 2022;387(3):205-16.

SECTION 2

Obesity and Diagnostic Markers

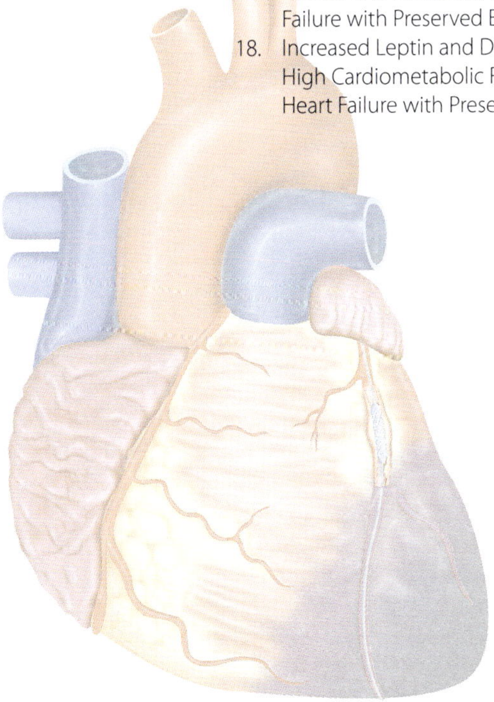

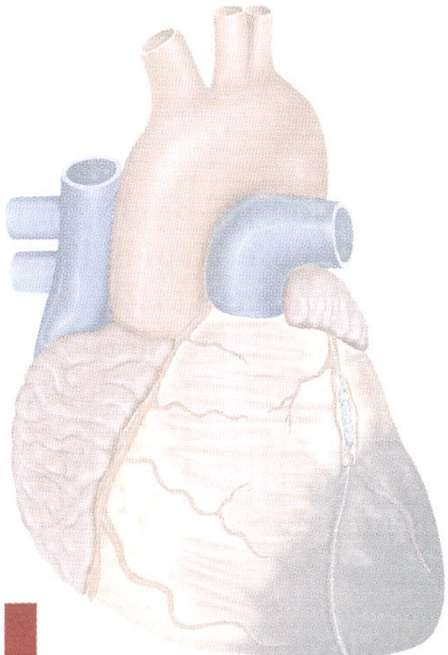

17

CHAPTER

Clinical and Molecular Tools in Obese Heart Failure with Preserved Ejection Fraction

Srikanta Sharma, Sidharth S Pattnaik, Soumit Sharma, HK Chopra

INTRODUCTION

Heart failure with preserved ejection fraction (HFpEF) represents more than half of all heart failure cases today and is increasingly recognized as a systemic, heterogeneous, and comorbidity-driven syndrome. Among its several phenotypes, obesity-related HFpEF has emerged as one of the most prevalent and clinically distinct variants. Obesity modifies cardiac structure, mechanics, and metabolism—contributing to concentric remodeling, diastolic dysfunction, and exercise intolerance through hemodynamic, metabolic, and inflammatory mechanisms.[1] New evidence now makes it clear that obesity is not just a background factor or a mechanical cause of breathlessness, but a direct driver of HFpEF. It damages the heart and other organs including the lungs, muscles, kidneys, and liver collectively mediated by systemic inflammation, neurohormonal activation, autonomic dysregulation, and altered hemodynamic load.[2]

Importantly, the prevalence of obesity has paralleled the rise in HFpEF, creating an urgent need for accurate diagnostic and molecular tools tailored to this subgroup. Traditional markers (e.g., natriuretic peptides) may be blunted in obese individuals, while novel omics-based biomarkers and advanced imaging have begun to refine our understanding of pathophysiology and guide therapy.[3]

CONTENTS AND DESCRIPTION

Clinical Characterization and Bedside Tools

Clinical History and Phenotyping

Patients typically present with exertional dyspnea, reduced exercise tolerance, and peripheral congestion. However, in obesity-HFpEF, classic symptoms such as orthopnea or paroxysmal nocturnal dyspnea are less prominent, because elevated filling pressures are often masked by high intrathoracic pressure and chest wall mass.[4]

A detailed history should assess comorbidities—hypertension, type 2 diabetes, sleep apnea, metabolic syndrome, and deconditioning.

Physical Examination

Look for jugular venous distention, peripheral edema, S4 gallop, and evidence of metabolic dysregulation (acanthosis nigricans and central adiposity). However, obesity may obscure some findings such as displaced apical impulse or muffled heart sounds.[5]

Cardiopulmonary Exercise Testing

Cardiopulmonary exercise testing (CPET) differentiates cardiac from noncardiac limitations. Obese HFpEF patients demonstrate reduced peak VO_2 (oxygen consumption), steep VE (minute ventilation)/VCO_2 (carbon dioxide production) slope (ventilatory efficiency), and impaired oxygen pulse, reflecting combined cardiac and peripheral inefficiency.[6]

Diagnostic algorithms: H2FPEF and HFA-PEFF in obesity:

Two structured pathways are commonly used to quantify the probability of HFpEF in patient presenting with unexplained exertional dyspnea:

1. *H2FPEF (Heavy meaning BMI >30 kg/m², Hypertensive, Atrial fibrillation, Pulmonary hypertension, Elder, Filling pressure)*: A clinical echo score that explicitly awards two points for obesity, reflecting the high pretest probability of HFpEF in obese patients with dyspnea.[7]
2. *HFA-PEFF (ESC algorithm):* Integrates functional testing and biomarkers with echocardiography. Its strengths include modularity and the option for diastolic stress testing; however, the biomarker arm can misclassify obese patients if standard NP cutoffs are used.[8]

Echocardiography

Echocardiography remains the cornerstone:

- *Structural changes:* Concentric LV hypertrophy, left atrial (LA) enlargement, and increased relative wall thickness
- *Functional parameters:* Elevated E/e′, reduced tissue Doppler velocities, and impaired longitudinal strain despite preserved EF.[9] LA strain may be impaired even when conventional LA size/volume looks normal.
- Strain imaging improves sensitivity for early myocardial dysfunction.
- Right heart assessment is essential due to frequent pulmonary hypertension and right ventricular dysfunction.
- Obesity-hypoventilation, OSA, and increased blood volume predispose to pulmonary hypertension and RV dysfunction in HFpEF.

Cardiac MRI

When echocardiographic windows are poor, cardiac magnetic resonance (CMR) imaging provides detailed assessment of:

- Ventricular mass and volumes
- Diffuse fibrosis (via T1 mapping)
- Epicardial adipose tissue (EAT) quantification. High EAT volume and low T1 times are independently associated with adverse outcomes in obese HFpEF.[10]

Laboratory and Circulating Biomarkers—Molecular Tools

Natriuretic Peptides

Brain natriuretic peptide (BNP) and NT-proBNP are often disproportionately low in obese HFpEF, likely due to reduced peptide synthesis, increased clearance, and sequestration in adipose tissue.[11] In obese HFpEF, proposed NT-proBNP to rule-out thresholds as low as <50 pg/mL improves sensitivity.

Clinicians should interpret results using BMI-adjusted thresholds or rely more on imaging when suspicion remains high.

Inflammatory Markers and Adipokines

Obesity triggers chronic low-grade inflammation. Elevated CRP, IL-6, TNF-α, and altered adipokines (↑leptin, ↓adiponectin) correlate with symptom burden and reduced exercise capacity.[12]

Leptin reflects EAT activity and myocardial inflammation, whereas adiponectin reduction signals metabolic stress.

Oxidative and Metabolic Biomarkers

Markers like uric acid, free fatty acids, and insulin resistance indices (HOMA-IR) track metabolic overload. Elevated high-sensitivity troponin (hs-TnT) suggests ongoing subclinical myocardial injury in HFpEF.[13]

Proteomic and Metabolomic Signatures

High-throughput proteomics identify circulating protein patterns linked to extracellular matrix remodeling and inflammation. A "proteomic signature" of obese HFpEF includes upregulated leptin, IL-1 receptor antagonist, and matrix metalloproteinases.[14]

Metabolomics reveal impaired nitric oxide bioavailability and branched-chain amino acid metabolism—potential therapeutic targets.

Imaging Biomarkers and Molecular Imaging

Epicardial Adipose Tissue

Epicardial adipose tissue is both a biomarker and an active participant in disease. Quantified by computer tomography (CT) or CMR, it secretes proinflammatory cytokines and correlates with LV stiffness and exercise intolerance.[15]

Positron Emission Tomography and Magnetic Resonance Molecular Imaging

Positron emission tomography (PET) using 18F-FDG or 11C-acetate assesses myocardial inflammation and metabolism, while MRI T1 mapping measures diffuse fibrosis. These modalities help distinguish inflammatory versus fibrotic HFpEF phenotypes.[16]

Functional and Hemodynamic Evaluation

Invasive Hemodynamics

Right heart catheterization during supine or upright exercise remains the gold standard for diagnosis.

Hallmarks of obese HFpEF include:

- Elevated LV end-diastolic pressure (>15 mm Hg at rest or >25 mm Hg with exercise)
- Steep LV pressure-volume relationship. The end-diastolic pressure-volume relationship (EDPVR) reflects LV diastolic stiffness. Steeper slope is in the stiffer ventricle. Chronic volume overload leads to ventricular remodeling initially, and over time fibrosis and myocyte hypertrophy occur, which reduces compliance. This test is especially valuable when noninvasive parameters are discordant.[17]

Genomic and Epigenetic Tools

While no monogenic cause is identified, genome-wide studies reveal polymorphisms in genes regulating inflammation, extracellular matrix turnover, and adipose metabolism that predispose to obese HFpEF.[18]

Epigenetic markers (e.g., microRNAs miR-21 and miR-29) correlate with fibrosis and hypertrophy and may emerge as early diagnostic or therapeutic targets

LIMITATIONS OF CURRENT TOOLS

- *Reduced biomarker reliability:* Natriuretic peptide suppression leads to false negatives.[11]
- *Heterogeneity:* HFpEF overlaps with COPD, anemia, and deconditioning.
- *Accessibility:* Advanced imaging and omics profiling remain expensive and not universally available.
- *Lack of standardization:* No validated cut-off values for novel biomarkers (leptin, resistin, and proteomic panels).
- *Limited prognostic data:* Most molecular findings are associative; prospective validation is pending.[14]

GUIDELINES

Current guidelines from the AHA/ACC/HFSA (2022) and ESC (2023) provide the following recommendations:[3,19]

- *Diagnosis:* Combine symptoms, signs, elevated filling pressures, and preserved LVEF ≥50%.
- *Use of natriuretic peptides:* Interpret cautiously in obesity; low values do not exclude HFpEF.
- *Imaging:* Echocardiography with diastolic assessment is mandatory; consider strain and CMR when feasible.
- *Therapy:*
    - *SGLT2 inhibitors (empagliflozin and dapagliflozin):* Class I recommendation to reduce hospitalization.
    - Mineralocorticoid receptor antagonists may benefit selected patients with elevated filling pressures.
    - *Lifestyle and weight reduction:* Foundational for obese HFpEF.
- *Weight-loss interventions:*
    - GLP-1 receptor agonists (semaglutide) and dual GLP-1/GIP agonists (tirzepatide) improve functional status and quality of life in HFpEF with obesity.[20]
    - Bariatric surgery can reverse concentric remodeling and improve diastolic function in severe cases.

ALGORITHMS

Diagnostic Algorithm

Symptoms → ECG + TTE + BNP/NT-proBNP (consider BMI)

↓

If diagnostic uncertainty → CPET ± strain imaging

↓

If still inconclusive → CMR (fibrosis + EAT quantification)

↓

Persistent ambiguity → Invasive hemodynamic exercise testing

↓

Confirmed Obese HFpEF → Risk stratification and therapy

Management Algorithm

- *Volume control:* Loop diuretics titrated to euvolemia.
- *Disease-modifying therapy:* SGLT2 inhibitor for all eligible patients.
- *Comorbidity optimization:* Hypertension, diabetes, OSA, AF, and coronary disease.
- *Lifestyle and pharmacologic weight loss:*
    - Calorie restriction, exercise programs
    - GLP-1/GIP agonists for BMI ≥30 kg/m^2 or ≥27 kg/m^2 + comorbidities.[20]
    - Bariatric referral in severe obesity.
- *Follow-up:* Functional capacity, natriuretic peptide trend, and imaging at 6–12 months.

SUMMARY ILLUSTRATION (CONCEPTUAL)

Mechanistic Pathway

Obesity → Adipose dysfunction (↑EAT, ↑visceral fat) → Systemic inflammation (↑IL-6, ↑leptin, ↓adiponectin) → Microvascular endothelial dysfunction → Myocardial stiffening + fibrosis → Diastolic dysfunction → HFpEF symptoms

Diagnostic Toolbox

Clinical assessment + BMI-aware biomarkers + imaging (echo + strain + CMR) + CPET + molecular panels

Therapeutic Toolbox

Symptom control (diuretics), disease-modifying therapy (SGLT2i), comorbidity control, and weight reduction through lifestyle, pharmacologic, or surgical interventions.

KEY CLINICAL CLUES OF OBESE HEART FAILURE WITH PRESERVED EJECTION FRACTION

- Obese patient (BMI >30 kg/m²) with exertional dyspnea and preserved EF
- Low/normal BNP or NT-proBNP despite HF symptoms
- Concentric LV remodeling and LA enlargement
- Elevated EAT volume on imaging
- Severe exercise intolerance disproportionate to resting findings.[4,9,15]

PRACTICAL MOLECULAR MARKERS

Practical molecular markers are given in **Table 1**.

TABLE 1: Practical molecular markers in obese heart failure with preserved ejection fraction (HFpEF) and their clinical interpretation.

Category	*Key marker*	*Interpretation in obese HFpEF*
Natriuretic peptides	BNP, NT-proBNP	Lowered levels; adjust thresholds
Inflammatory	CRP, IL-6, and TNF-α	Elevated; reflect systemic inflammation
Adipokines	Leptin ↑, Adiponectin ↓	Correlate with EAT activity
Fibrosis	Galectin-3, ST2	Mark myocardial fibrosis/ remodeling
Metabolic	hs-TnT, insulin resistance	Reflect subclinical injury, metabolic stress

CONCLUSION

The obese HFpEF phenotype embodies a multisystem disorder integrating cardiovascular, metabolic, and inflammatory dysfunctions. Accurate identification demands the combined use of clinical assessment, functional testing, advanced imaging, and molecular biomarkers.

KEY MESSAGES

- Interpret natriuretic peptides with BMI context.
- Use imaging (strain, MRI, and EAT quantification) for diagnostic confidence.
- Recognize the molecular network—adipokines, inflammatory cytokines, and proteomic markers—as emerging precision medicine tools.
- *Target upstream drivers*: Weight loss and metabolic optimization remain the most disease-modifying interventions.
- *Future direction*: Multi-omic integration and artificial intelligence models may enable earlier detection and individualized therapy.

Through systematic use of these clinical and molecular tools, clinicians can better phenotype, stratify, and manage obese HFpEF—transforming a challenging syndrome into one of the most promising frontiers of precision cardiology.[1,14,20]

REFERENCES

1. Borlaug BA. Heart Failure With Preserved Ejection Fraction. J Am Coll Cardiol. 2023;81(7):623-39.
2. Borlaug BA, Jensen MD, Kitzman DW. Obesity and heart failure with preserved ejection fraction: new insights and pathophysiological targets. Cardiovasc Res. 2022;118(18):3434-50.
3. Heidenreich PA, Bozkurt B, Aguilar D, et al. 2022 AHA/ ACC/HFSA Guideline for the Management of Heart Failure: A Report of the American College of Cardiology/ American Heart Association Joint Committee on Clinical Practice Guidelines. Circulation. 2022;145:e895-e1032.
4. Obokata M, Reddy YNV, Pislaru SV, et al. Mechanisms of Dyspnea in Obese HFpEF. Circulation. 2017;136:1889-901.
5. Packer M. Obesity-Related Heart Failure Phenotypes. Eur Heart J. 2022;43:4316-26.
6. Kitzman DW, et al. Exercise Intolerance in Obese HFpEF. J Appl Physiol. 2023;135(1):12-22.
7. Basha M, Stavropoulou E, Nikolaidou A. Diagnosing Heart Failure with Preserved Ejection Fraction in Obese Patients. J Clin Med. 2025;14(6):1980.
8. van Dalen BM, Chin JF, Motiram PA. Challenges in the diagnosis of heart failure with preserved ejection fraction in individuals with obesity. Cardiovasc Diabetol. 2025;24(1):71.

9. Shah SJ, et al. Echocardiographic and Hemodynamic Characteristics of HFpEF Subgroups. JAMA Cardiol. 2023;8(2):120-30.
10. Packer M, et al. Epicardial Fat and Cardiac Function in HFpEF. Eur J Heart Fail. 2023;25:1032-44.
11. Clerico A, et al. Impact of Obesity on Natriuretic Peptides. Clin Chem Lab Med. 2022;60:1579-87.
12. Lam CS, et al. Inflammation and Adipokines in HFpEF. Circulation. 2023;147:415-29.
13. Matsue Y, et al. High-Sensitivity Troponin in HFpEF Prognosis. Eur Heart J. 2022;43:2010-21.
14. Tromp J, et al. Proteomic Signatures in HFpEF and Obesity. Circulation. 2024;150:1212-30.
15. Kapa S, et al. Epicardial Adipose Tissue and Diastolic Dysfunction. J Cardiovasc Magn Reson. 2023;25:34.
16. Taqueti VR, et al. PET and MRI in HFpEF Phenotyping. JACC Imaging. 2023;16(9):1021-34.
17. Reddy YNV, et al. Invasive Hemodynamic Assessment in HFpEF. Circulation. 2023;148:1802-1816.
18. Lindman BR, et al. Genetic and Epigenetic Insights into HFpEF. Nat Rev Cardiol. 2023;20:490-507.
19. McDonagh TA, Metra M, Adamo M, et al. 2023 Focused Update of the 2021 ESC Guidelines for the diagnosis and treatment of acute and chronic heart failure. Eur Heart J. 2023;44:3620-726.
20. Nassif ME, et al. Semaglutide in Obesity-Related HFpEF (STEP-HFpEF Trial). N Engl J Med. 2023;389:105-18.

18

CHAPTER

Increased Leptin and Decreased Adiponectin: High Cardiometabolic Risk Markers in Obese Heart Failure with Preserved Ejection Fraction

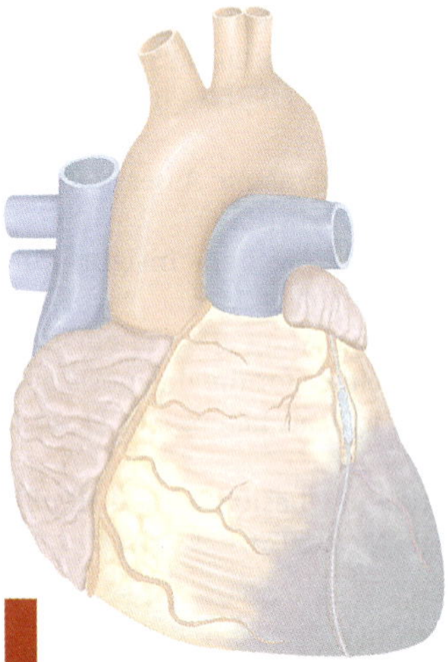

Kavita Tyagi, D Santosh

INTRODUCTION

Heart failure with preserved ejection fraction (HFpEF) now accounts for nearly 65% of all heart failure cases. Its rising prevalence parallels global increases in obesity and metabolic syndrome.[1,5] Cardiometabolic HFpEF is increasingly understood as an adipose tissue-driven disease.[1,4]

Adipose tissue functions as a dynamic endocrine organ that secretes adipokines, notably leptin and adiponectin, which directly influence systemic inflammation, myocardial remodeling, and vascular stiffness.[2,3] In obesity, elevated leptin and reduced or dysfunctional adiponectin represent potent markers of cardiometabolic risk and are central to HFpEF disease biology.[1,3]

CONTENTS AND DESCRIPTION

Adipose Tissue Dysfunction in Cardiometabolic Heart Failure with Preserved Ejection Fraction

Visceral adipose tissue (VAT) is metabolically active and highly pro-inflammatory. Expansion of VAT promotes immune cell infiltration, oxidative stress, and dysregulated adipokine secretion **(Table 1)**, creating a chronic low-grade inflammatory milieu that contributes to cardiometabolic HFpEF.[4,5]

Increased Leptin: Proinflammatory and Profibrotic

- Leptin correlates directly with fat mass; chronic elevation leads to central/peripheral leptin resistance.[2]
- Hyperleptinemia contributes to:
  - Myocardial hypertrophy and fibrosis.
  - Endothelial dysfunction.
  - Sympathetic activation and systemic inflammation.[1,2]
- High leptin is also linked with platelet activation, oxidative stress, and microvascular dysfunction—all characteristic of HFpEF.[1,4]

Decreased Adiponectin: Loss of Cardiometabolic Protection

- Adiponectin enhances insulin sensitivity, promotes lipid homeostasis, and reduces inflammation.[3]
- Obese HFpEF patients exhibit low or dysfunctional adiponectin.[1,3]

Adiponectin Paradox

Advanced HFpEF may show elevated adiponectin due to:

- Maladaptive compensation from cardiac stress (high BNP states).
- Adiponectin resistance, wherein the myocardium/endothelium no longer responds to the hormone.[6]

Leptin/Adiponectin Ratio

- A superior biomarker reflecting the net inflammatory and metabolic burden.[1,3]
- Elevated L/A ratio = high cardiometabolic risk, increased myocardial fibrosis, and adverse HFpEF prognosis.[1,6]

TABLE 1: Key adipokines and their pathophysiological roles in obese HFpEF.

Adipokine	*Change in obese HFpEF*	*Primary cardiovascular effect*	*Underlying mechanism*
Leptin	↑ Hyperleptinemia	Hypertrophy, fibrosis, endothelial dysfunction, ↑ cardiometabolic risk	Pro-inflammatory, profibrotic, leptin resistance
Adiponectin	↓ or paradoxically ↑	Loss of protection; may signal disease severity	Loss of anti-inflammatory/insulin-sensitizing effects; adiponectin resistance
L/A Ratio	↑	Integrated biomarker of high cardiometabolic risk	Reflects net inflammatory and fibrotic burden

Note: Left atrial (L/A) ratio is "currently an investigational risk marker; not yet recommended for routine decision-making."

Flowchart 1: VAT dysfunction.

VAT dysfunction pathway leading to HFpEF development

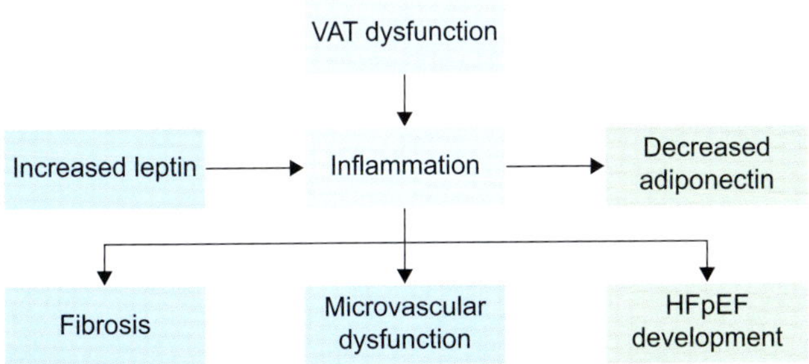

Source:

1. Borlaug BA, Jensen MD, Kitzman DW, et al. Obesity and heart failure with preserved ejection fraction: new insights and pathophysiological targets. Cardiovasc Res. 2023;118(18):3434-50.
2. Radakrishnan et al. PMC. 2025.
3. Rao et al. PMC. 2020.

IMAGES/CHARTS

Conceptual diagram showing VAT dysfunction **(Flowchart 1)** leading to increased leptin and decreased adiponectin, promoting inflammation, fibrosis, microvascular dysfunction, and HFpEF development.

LIMITATIONS

- Adiponectin paradox complicates biomarker interpretation.[6]
- Leptin resistance limits the therapeutic use of leptin analogues.[2]
- HFpEF is heterogeneous, influenced by sex, ethnicity, and metabolic phenotype.
- No validated thresholds for clinical decision-making using the L/A ratio yet.[1,5]

PROPOSED MANAGEMENT ALGORITHM

Step 1: Identify Cardiometabolic Heart Failure with Preserved Ejection Fraction

- HFpEF diagnosis + obesity/metabolic syndrome.
- Elevated L/A ratio as supportive evidence.[1]

Step 2: Initiate Foundational Heart Failure with Preserved Ejection Fraction Therapy

- BP, glycemic, and lipid control.
- Diuretics, sodium-glucose cotransporter 2 (SGLT2) inhibitors, mineralocorticoid receptor antagonists.[1]

Step 3: Target Adipose Tissue Dysfunction

- SGLT2 inhibitors (improve visceral adiposity + metabolic health).
- GLP-1 receptor agonists (substantial weight/VAT reduction).
- Structured exercise + caloric restriction.[1,5]

STEP 4: FUTURE THERAPIES

- Agents reducing leptin resistance.
- Adiponectin pathway enhancers.
- Anti-inflammatory adipokine modulators.[2,3]

Left atrial ratio is "currently an investigational risk marker; not yet recommended for routine decision-making."

CONCLUSION

The imbalance of increased leptin and decreased/dysfunctional adiponectin is a hallmark of cardiometabolic derangement in obese HFpEF. This adipokine dysregulation drives inflammation, vascular stiffness, and myocardial fibrosis. Understanding and targeting these pathways represent promising directions for 2025 and beyond, with the L/A ratio emerging as a clinically meaningful biomarker of cardiometabolic risk.[1,3,6]

REFERENCES

1. Theodorakis N, Kreouzi M, Hitas C, et al. Adipokines and Cardiometabolic Heart Failure with Preserved Ejection Fraction: A State-of-the-Art Review. Diagnostics. 2024;14(23):2677.
2. Flier JS, Ahima RS. Leptin physiology and pathophysiology: knowns and unknowns 30 years after its discovery. J Clin Invest. 2024;134(1):e174595.
3. Clemente-Suárez VJ, Redondo-Flórez L, Beltrán-Velasco AI, et al. The role of adipokines in health and disease. Biomedicines. 2023;11(5):1290.
4. Zhang P, Konja D, Wang Y. Adipose tissue secretory profile and cardiometabolic risk in obesity. Endocrine Metabolic Science. 2020;1(3-4):100061.
5. Shetty S, Suvarna R, Bhattacharya S et al. Visceral adiposity and cardiometabolic risk: Clinical insights and assessment. Cardiol Rev. 2025.
6. Theodorakis N, Kreouzi M, Anagnostou D, et al. Adiponectin as a biomarker of disease severity in HFpEF. Diagnostics. 2024;14:2677.

19
CHAPTER

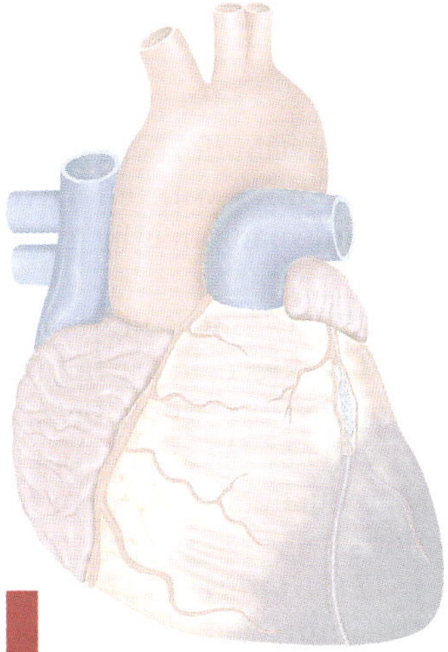

NT-proBNP in Obese Heart Failure with Preserved Ejection Fraction: Diagnostic, Prognostic, and Therapeutic Implications

Srikanta Sharma, Soumit Sharma, HK Chopra

INTRODUCTION

Heart failure with preserved ejection fraction (HFpEF) now represents more than half of all heart failure cases globally, and obesity is one of its most prominent drivers. The coexistence of obesity and HFpEF creates unique diagnostic and therapeutic challenges, particularly in the interpretation of natriuretic peptides such as N-terminal pro-B-type natriuretic peptide (NT-proBNP). Pro-BNP breaks down to form NT-proBNP and BNP. The natriuretic peptide (NP) system impacts salt and water (natriuresis and diuretics) handling and pressure (hypotension) regulation, and may influence myocardial structure and function. It also inhibits renin–angiotensin–aldosterone system and sympathetic activity. Unlike heart failure with reduced ejection fraction (HFrEF), where NT-proBNP is usually elevated and correlates strongly with disease severity, in obese HFpEF patients the biomarker is often deceptively low. This phenomenon complicates the diagnosis, risk stratification, and management of these patients.

The "natriuretic peptide paradox" in obesity is well recognized: Higher adiposity correlates with lower circulating NT-proBNP despite the presence of clinical congestion and hemodynamic derangements. Mechanisms include increased clearance through natriuretic peptide clearance receptors (NPRs) in adipose tissue, hormonal and metabolic modulation (hyperinsulinemia and leptin resistance), and plasma volume expansion leading to hemodilution. This attenuation of biomarker response has led to underdiagnosis of HFpEF in obese patients and misclassification of cardiovascular risk.

As obesity rates rise worldwide, and with HFpEF now the dominant form of heart failure in women and the elderly, the accurate interpretation of NT-proBNP has become a cornerstone of clinical cardiology. This chapter reviews the diagnostic, therapeutic, and prognostic implications of NT-proBNP in obese HFpEF, supported by recent guideline recommendations and clinical trial data up to 2025.

DIAGNOSTIC INTERPRETATION OF NT-proBNP IN OBESE HFPEF

Pathophysiological Considerations

N-terminal pro-B-type natriuretic peptide is secreted in response to myocardial wall stretch and neurohormonal activation. In HFpEF, diastolic dysfunction, increased left atrial pressure, and impaired relaxation trigger secretion. However, in obese patients, multiple mechanisms blunt NT-proBNP release or increase its clearance.

- *Adipose tissue clearance:* Adipocytes express NPR-C, which binds and internalizes circulating BNP, reducing its measurable concentration. Emerging evidence in 2025 highlights adipose tissue-derived hormonal modulation as a key regulator of NT-proBNP suppression in obesity.[1]
- *Hyperinsulinemia and leptin effects:* Insulin resistance reduces NP gene expression, while leptin signaling enhances NPR-C expression.
- *Plasma dilution:* Higher plasma volume in obesity leads to relative hemodilution.

- *Reduced myocardial wall stress transmission:* In obese individuals, pericardial restraint and altered ventricular geometry reduce the stimulus for NP release despite increased filling pressures. Recent mechanistic studies underscore that the blunted natriuretic peptide response in obese HFpEF is a reflection of altered pathobiology.[2]

Impact on Diagnostic Cut-offs

Obese patients often have NT-proBNP values below standard diagnostic thresholds, even in clinically overt HFpEF. Large cohort studies demonstrate that up to 20–30% of obese HFpEF patients present with NT-proBNP below guideline-recommended thresholds for ruling in heart failure.

- ESC 2023 guidelines recommend natriuretic peptide testing as the initial step for suspected HFpEF, with NT-proBNP cut-offs of >125 pg/mL in nonacute and >300 pg/mL in acute settings.[3] The negative predictive value of NT-pro-BNP is very high (0.94–0.98), while the positive predictive value is low (0.64–0.67), making them a good tool to rule out HF. However, in obesity, up to 50% of patients with HFpEF may fall below these thresholds.
- Proposed BMI-adjusted thresholds: For patients with BMI ≥35 kg/m^2, lowering NT-proBNP thresholds by approximately 50% has been suggested.[4] Recent registry data (2024) confirm that a BMI-adjusted algorithm improves sensitivity for HFpEF without sacrificing specificity.

Integration with Scoring Systems

Given NT-proBNP limitations, scoring systems such as HFA-PEFF (Heart Failure Association of European Society of Cardiology for evaluating HFpEF) and H_2FPEF (Clinical scoring-Heavy BMI >30 kg/m^2, Hypertensive, atrial Fibrillation, Pulmonary hypertension, Elderly, Filling pressure E/e >9) incorporate additional parameters: Echocardiographic diastolic indices, left atrial size, pulmonary pressures, and comorbidities. For obese patients, reliance on multiparametric approaches is essential.

THERAPEUTIC INTERPRETATION OF NT-proBNP IN OBESE HFPEF

Monitoring Treatment Response

N-terminal pro-B-type natriuretic peptide remains useful for monitoring therapy, but interpretation should focus on relative change rather than absolute value. A >30% reduction from baseline is considered clinically meaningful, even if values remain "low" in obese patients.

- *Diuretics:* Loop diuretics remain first line for congestion relief. NT-proBNP typically declines with effective decongestion, though the absolute nadir may be lower in obese patients.
- *SGLT2 inhibitors:* Trials such as EMPEROR-Preserved and DELIVER demonstrated reduced heart failure hospitalization irrespective of baseline NT-proBNP.[5,6] Subgroup analyses confirm efficacy in obese HFpEF patients, although biomarker reduction was attenuated compared to nonobese cohorts.
- *GLP-1 receptor agonists (STEP-HFpEF, 2023–2024):* Semaglutide significantly improved symptoms, exercise capacity, and reduced NT-proBNP modestly.[7] Importantly, weight loss itself contributed to reduced wall stress.
- *ARNI (sacubitril/valsartan):* In PARAGON-HF, sacubitril/valsartan lowered NT-proBNP compared with valsartan, but obese subgroups showed smaller absolute changes.[8]
- In *chronic* HF therapy, 20–25% reduction in mortality with NP-guided therapy[9] was observed.

Case Vignette

A 58-year-old woman, BMI 38 kg/m^2, presents with exertional dyspnea. NT-proBNP is 180 pg/mL. Echocardiography shows preserved EF, left atrial enlargement, and diastolic dysfunction. Despite a "borderline" NT-proBNP, diagnosis of HFpEF is supported. After initiation of dapagliflozin and semaglutide, she reports symptom improvement, NT-proBNP falls to 120 pg/mL, and 8 kg weight reduction occurs. This illustrates that trend monitoring and multiparametric assessment outweigh absolute NP levels in obese HFpEF.

PROGNOSTIC INTERPRETATION OF NT-proBNP IN OBESE HFPEF

Retained Prognostic Value

Despite lower absolute values, NT-proBNP retains its prognostic significance in obese HFpEF when assessed serially. Multiple cohort studies confirm that each doubling of NT-proBNP predicts a twofold increase in mortality and hospitalization risk, independent of BMI.

The Obesity Paradox

Paradoxically, obese HFpEF patients often exhibit better survival than lean counterparts, despite more symptoms, lower NT-proBNP and higher comorbidity burden.[10] This "obesity paradox" may relate to metabolic reserves, altered cytokine signaling, or limitations of current biomarkers. However, recent evidence suggests that adipose tissue-derived hormonal modulation also contributes, blunting NT-proBNP release and complicating prognostic interpretation.[1]

Prognostic Algorithms

In the acute setting, both elevations of the initial value at the time of presentation[11] and changes with therapy (value at hospital discharge) are strong predictors of short[12] and long-term outcomes.[13] Persistence of higher than 5,000 pg/mL NT-proBNP levels long after decongestion portends poor outcomes, as per PROTECT (ProBNP Outpatient Tailored Chronic HF trial).[14] For chronic cases, data from Val-HeFT, where both baseline values and changes over 3 months in NT Pro BNP have been shown to be among the most powerful predictors of future outcomes.[15]

Serial NT-proBNP measurements combined with clinical risk models [MAGGIC (Meta Analysis Global Group In Chronic heart failure) score, HFA-PEFF] improve prognostication. BMI-specific thresholds remain under investigation, but the trajectory of NT-proBNP is consistently more predictive than absolute value.

ALGORITHMS

Practical clinical use requires integrating NT-proBNP into structured algorithms.

- *Diagnosis*: Begin with NT-proBNP, apply BMI-adjusted cut-offs (e.g., >250 pg/mL in obese for acute HF), proceed to echocardiography and multiparametric scoring.
- *Prognosis:* Repeat NT-proBNP at follow-up; a >30% fall indicates favorable prognosis.
- *Therapy monitoring:* Use NT-proBNP trend with symptom score and weight/BMI trajectory **(Table 1)**.

CLINICAL CASE-BASED LEARNING

Case: A 62-year-old man with BMI 37 kg/m^2, hypertension, and type 2 diabetes presents with exertional dyspnea (NYHA II–III) and lower limb edema.

Examination: Elevated JVP, mild pedal edema, and BMI-adjusted BP 138/78 mm Hg

Laboratories: NT-proBNP 210 pg/mL

Echocardiography: LVEF 60%, left atrial enlargement, E/e′ ratio 16, and mild pulmonary hypertension

1. *Step 1: Diagnostic dilemma:*
    i. NT-proBNP = 210 pg/mL → below standard HFpEF diagnostic threshold (>300 pg/mL in acute, >125 pg/mL in nonacute)
    ii. However, the patient has BMI 37 kg/m^2 → apply BMI-adjusted threshold (~50% lower).
    iii. Corrected threshold ≈ >150 pg/mL → patient exceeds cut-off
    iv. Echo supports HFpEF (raised filling pressures).
    v. Diagnosis: Obese HFpEF
2. *Step 2: Therapeutic strategy:*
    i. Initiate SGLT2 inhibitor (dapagliflozin) for outcome benefit.
    ii. Add loop diuretic for congestion relief.
    iii. Consider GLP-1 RA (semaglutide) for weight reduction and symptom improvement (STEP-HFpEF evidence).
    iv. Lifestyle modification: Sodium restriction and exercise rehabilitation.
3. *Step 3: Prognostic consideration:*
    i. NT-proBNP relatively low, but serial monitoring is important.
    ii. *Goal:* >30% reduction from baseline at follow-up (e.g., from 210 → ~150 pg/mL).
    iii. Recognize obesity paradox: Despite more symptoms, prognosis may be more favorable compared to lean HFpEF.

TABLE 1: Clinical implications of NT-proBNP in obese HFpEF.

Domain	*Implication*	*Key notes*
Diagnostic	NT-proBNP often falsely low due to obesity-related mechanisms	Adjust thresholds ↓ ~50% for BMI ≥35 kg/m^2; integrate with echo and HFA-PEFF/H_2FPEF scores
Therapeutic	Guides monitoring of congestion and therapy response	Focus on trend (>30% reduction), not absolute value; response attenuated with obesity
Prognostic	Retains predictive value despite lower baseline levels	Serial changes predict outcomes better; obesity paradox complicates interpretation
Guideline use	ESC 2023 and AHA 2022 recommend NP testing, but caution in obesity	2025 consensus supports BMI-adjusted cut-offs and recognition of GLP-1 RAs as therapeutic tools

LIMITATIONS

- *Assay variability:* Different NT-proBNP assays have variable sensitivity at low ranges.
- *Comorbidities:* Chronic kidney disease, sleep apnea, and pulmonary hypertension confound interpretation.
- *Under-representation in trials:* Severe obesity (BMI >40 kg/m^2) remains under-studied.
- *Threshold ambiguity:* No universally accepted BMI-adjusted cut-offs; current practice relies on expert consensus.
- Additionally, comorbidities, such as atrial fibrillation, renal dysfunction, and aging, can all modify natriuretic peptide levels.[16]

GUIDELINES

- *ESC 2023:* NT-proBNP testing recommended as initial diagnostic step; cut-offs of 125 pg/mL (nonacute) and 300 pg/mL (acute) remain standard, but caution advised in obesity.[3]
- *AHA/ACC/HFSA 2022:* Multiparametric evaluation emphasized; NT-proBNP integrated with echo and risk scoring.[17]
- 2025 updates (emerging): Preliminary consensus statements endorse BMI-adjusted thresholds, particularly lowering NT-proBNP cut-offs by ~50% in patients with BMI ≥ 35 kg/m^2. This emphasizes trend monitoring, and supports the role of GLP-1 RAs for obese HFpEF.

CONCLUSION

N-terminal pro-B-type natriuretic peptide remains a cornerstone biomarker in HFpEF but requires careful interpretation in obese patients. Diagnostic thresholds must be adjusted, and emphasis placed on serial changes rather than absolute values. Therapeutically, NT-proBNP guides monitoring of congestion and response to modern therapies, though attenuation of biomarker decline in obesity must be recognized. Prognostically, NT-proBNP retains predictive power, but its paradoxical relationship with obesity necessitates integration with clinical scoring systems and imaging.

KEY LEARNING POINTS

- N-terminal pro-B-type natriuretic peptide is often deceptively low in obese HFpEF due to increased clearance, hormonal modulation, and plasma dilution.
- BMI-adjusted cut-offs improve diagnostic accuracy, with values lowered by ~50% for BMI ≥ 35 kg/m^2.
- Serial NT-proBNP changes (>30% fall from baseline) are more reliable than absolute values for monitoring therapy.
- SGLT2 inhibitors and GLP-1 receptor agonists improve outcomes in obese HFpEF; NT-proBNP decline may be modest but still prognostically meaningful.
- The obesity paradox complicates prognostic interpretation: Obese HFpEF patients may have better survival despite lower NT-proBNP.
- Guidelines (2023–2025) endorse multiparametric assessment: NT-proBNP should always be interpreted alongside echocardiography and clinical scoring systems.

REFERENCES

1. Nagueh SF, et al. Hemodynamic correlates of natriuretic peptide attenuation in obese HFpEF. J Am Coll Cardiol. 2025;85:215-29.
2. Obokata M, et al. Pathophysiology of obese HFpEF: Hemodynamic and metabolic mechanisms. Circulation. 2024;149:1450-65.
3. McDonagh TA, et al. 2023 ESC Guidelines for the diagnosis and treatment of acute and chronic heart failure. Eur Heart J. 2023;44(31):2659-758.
4. Obokata M, et al. Clinical impact of obesity on natriuretic peptide levels and diagnostic accuracy in HFpEF. J Am Coll Cardiol. 2023;81(5):453-66.
5. Anker SD, Butler J, Filippatos G, et al. Empagliflozin in heart failure with a preserved ejection fraction. N Engl J Med. 2021;385(16):1451-61.
6. Solomon SD, McMurray JJV, Claggett B, et al. Dapagliflozin in heart failure with mildly reduced or preserved ejection fraction. N Engl J Med. 2022;387(12):1089-98.
7. Kosiborod MN, Abildstrøm SZ, Borlaug BA, et al. Semaglutide in Patients with Heart Failure with Preserved Ejection Fraction and Obesity. N Engl J Med. 2023;389(12):1069-84.
8. Solomon SD, McMurray JJV, Anand IS, et al. Angiotensin-Neprilysin Inhibition in Heart Failure with Preserved Ejection Fraction. N Engl J Med. 2019;381(17):1609-20.
9. Troughton R, Felker GM, Januzzi JL, Jr. Natriuretic peptide-guided heart failure management. Eur Heart J. 2014;35(1):16-24.
10. Packer M. The obesity paradox in heart failure: reappraisal in the era of SGLT2 inhibitors. Eur J Heart Fail. 2024;26:893-902.
11. Fonarow GC, Peacock WF, Phillips CO, et al. the ADHERE Scientific Advisory Committee and Investigators Admission B-type natriuretic peptide levels and in-hospital mortality in acute decompensated heart failure. J Am Coll Cardiol. 2007;49:1943-50.
12. Bettencourt P, Azevedo A, Pimenta J, et al. N-terminal-pro-brain natriuretic peptide predicts outcome after

hospital discharge in heart failure patients. Circulation. 2004;110:2168-74.
13. Kociol RD, Horton JR, Fonarow GC, et al. Admission, discharge, or change in B-type natriuretic peptide and long-term outcomes: data from Organized Program to Initiate Lifesaving Treatment in Hospitalized Patients with Heart Failure (OPTIMIZE-HF) linked to Medicare claims. Circ Heart Fail. 2011;4:628-36.
14. Gaggin HK, Truong QA, Rehman SU, et al. Characterization and prediction of natriuretic peptide "nonresponse" during heart failure management: results from the ProBNP Outpatient Tailored Chronic Heart Failure (PROTECT) and the NT-proBNP-Assisted Treatment to Lessen Serial Cardiac Readmissions and Death (BATTLESCARRED) study. Congest Heart Fail. 2013;19:135-42.
15. Masson S, Latini R, Anand IS, et al. the Val-HeFT Investigators Prognostic value of changes in N-terminal pro-brain natriuretic peptide in Val-HeFT (Valsartan Heart Failure Trial). J Am Coll Cardiol. 2008;52:997-1003.
16. Hildebrandt P, Collinson PO, Doughty RN, et al. Age-dependent values of N-terminal pro-B-type natriuretic peptide are superior to a single cut-point for ruling out suspected systolic dysfunction in primary care. Eur Heart J. 2010;31:1881-9.
17. Heidenreich PA, Bozkurt B, Aguilar D, et al. 2022 AHA/ACC/HFSA Guideline for the management of heart failure: A Report of the American College of Cardiology/American Heart Association Joint Committee on Clinical Practice Guidelines. J Am Coll Cardiol. 2022;79(17):e263-e421.

SECTION 3

Obesity and Heart Failure

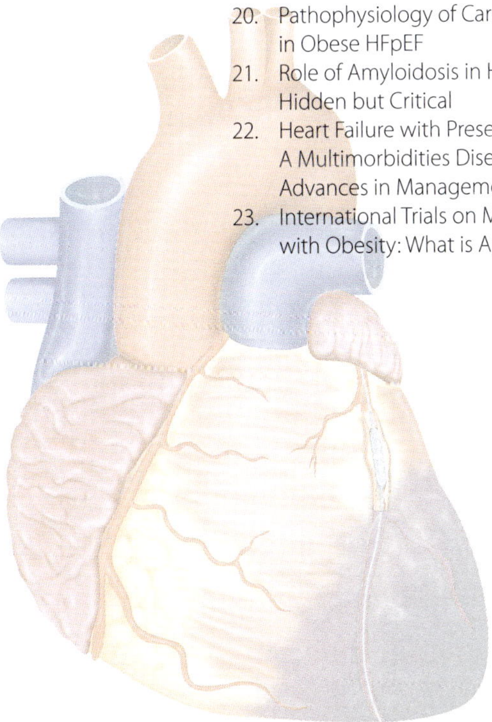

20

CHAPTER

Pathophysiology of Cardiometabolic Syndrome in Obese HFpEF

Hanumanth K Reddy, Ravi Komatireddy, Priyanka Gurram Reddy, Moaz Ahmad, Khizer Anees

INTRODUCTION

Several centuries ago, during the hunter-gatherer era, humans were busy with intense physical activity, just to procure their food. Now, there is an abundant availability of food and a marked decline in physical activity. With insatiable amount of food consumption, there has been a global pandemic of obesity/inactivity and the prevalence of heart failure with preserved ejection fraction (HFpEF). Although some patients with HFpEF have genetic/hereditary basis, a majority of cases are due to cardiometabolic syndrome. It is interesting to muse that this condition was unheard of 50 years ago and now it is a daily talk of medical community. The rise of HFpEF has run parallel with an alarming increase in obesity and so is atrial fibrillation as an integral part of HFpEF.

With rising affluence and concomitant decrease in physical activity, there has been a global epidemic of cardiometabolic syndrome and HFpEF in several developing countries.[1] The Centers for Disease Control and Prevention (CDC) of US reported that there was a prevalence of 40% obesity among adults from 2021 to 2023. The highest prevalence of obesity (39%) was during the prime age of 45–54 years. Furthermore, severe obesity affected 9% of the individuals. Obviously, these trends are nonsustainable for US and for that matter, for all of humanity. Serious societal reforms are of highest order to preserve longevity of human race on this planet.

CARDIOMETABOLIC HFpEF AS AN END-STAGE ENTITY OF CARDIOMETABOLIC SYNDROME

All patients with cardiometabolic syndrome are not affected by HFpEF, however, the HFpEF in patients with cardiometabolic syndrome represents the end stage sequela of the syndrome. Excess adiposity associated with reduced bioavailability of nitric oxide (NO) leads to diffuse microvascular dysfunction. This process and a cluster of other factors including inflammation, hypertension, insulin resistance, microvascular dysfunction, and hyperlipidemia **(Fig. 1)** set up ominous pathophysiological processes leading pathological LVH, interstitial fibrosis, reduction in the size of LV cavity, impaired relaxation, diastolic dysfunction, decreased cardiac output, fluid congestion with volume overload and full-blown HFpEF. There is evidence to suggest that HFpEF is a multiorgan disease involving liver, heart, liver, and kidney. Obesity, hypertension, hyperglycemia, hyperlipidemia, and sedentary lifestyle leading to systemic inflammation, enhanced oxidative stress, cardiac steatosis, immune modulation, insulin resistance, and adipokine dysregulation. The complex interplay of these morbid factors mediate structural, functional, and electrical remodeling of the cardiovascular system leading to LVH, myocardial fibrosis, left ventricular diastolic dysfunction, decreased LV end-diastolic volume, and cardiac output and congestive heart failure.

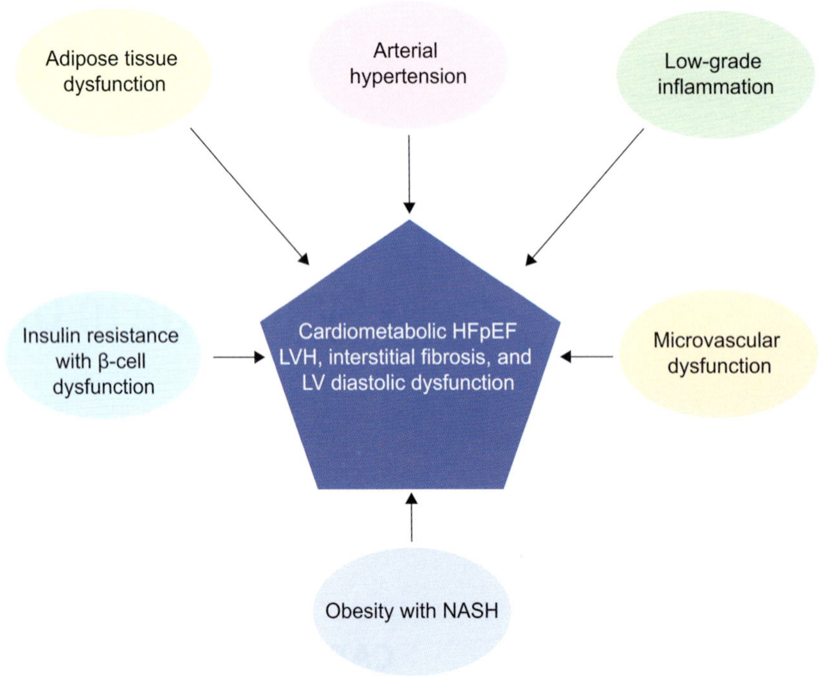

Fig. 1: Multiple metabolic processes in cardiometabolic HFpEF.

Inflammation

Obesity and visceral adiposity cause increased free fatty acids, adipokines, leptin, and decreased adiponectin. Type 2 diabetes mellitus and insulin resistance lead to hyperglycemia and hyperinsulinemia. Hypertension and dyslipidemia which add to oxidative stress with release of proinflammatory cytokines, IL-6, TNF-α, CRP, and MCP-1 into the circulation.[2]

Endothelial Dysfunction of Coronary Microvasculature

Coronary microvascular endothelial dysfunction and spasm occur with decreased bioavailability of NO caused by circulating cytokines. Reduced NO also causes impaired cGMP and PKG signaling in cardiomyocytes. Decreased PKG leads to titin (cardiomyocyte spring protein) hypophosphorylation making it stiffer.

Advanced glycation end-products (AGEs) of hyperglycemic state promote cross-linking of extracellular matrix. This together with excess collagen deposition, cardiomyocyte hypertrophy, and titin cause LV diastolic dysfunction.

Other Pathophysiological Mechanisms

Excess epicardial adipose tissue causes myocardial inflammation. Hyperaldosteronism with obesity results in sodium retention and expansion of plasma volume. Because of skeletal muscle myopathy, there is reduced VO_2, increased CO_2, and lactate production, rise in ventilation and dyspnea during exercise. As the disease progresses in patients with HFpEF, pulmonary hypertension, RV dysfunction, and atrial fibrillation will lead to their downhill course.

GENETIC BASIS OF CARDIOMETABOLIC HFpEF

Cardiometabolic HFpEF is mostly the end result of a heterogeneous cluster of risk factors. Because of this heterogeneity, there is a limited amount of genetic information. Available data indicates that there is a host of underlying genetic predispositions uncovered by environmental factors such as diet and physical activity. It is the end result of complex interplay of genetic substrate with acquired lifestyle changes. Similar to hepatic steatosis, lipids accumulate in the heart. Adipokine such as leptin dysregulation and immune cell activation lead to chronic low-grade systemic inflammatory state associated with elevated levels of proinflammatory cytokines and increased oxidative stress. Recurrent inflammation and repair result in fibrosis, impaired LV diastolic relaxation, elevated filling pressures and HFpEF.

Epigenetics denotes structural changes with environmental influences on the expression of the underlying

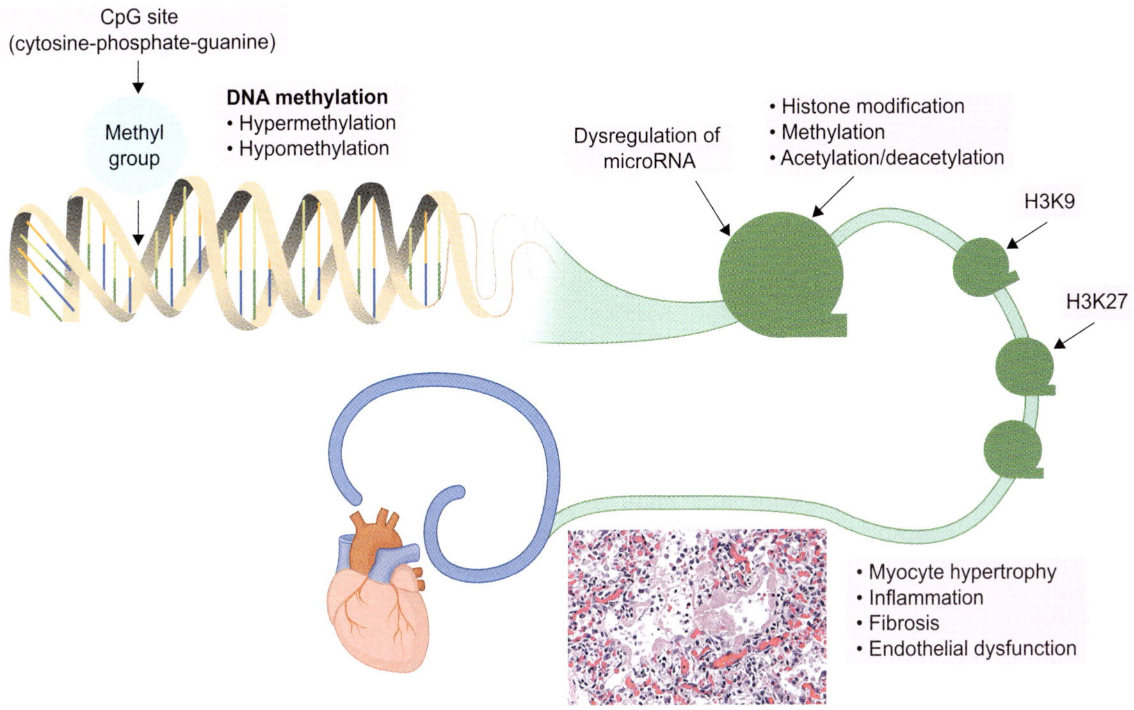

Fig. 2: Epigenetic dysregulation in cardiometabolic HFpEF.
Source: Gorica E, Geiger MA, Di Venanzio L, et al. Cardiometabolic heart failure with preserved ejection fraction: from molecular signatures to personalized treatment. Cardiovasc Diabetol. 2025;24(1):265.

genes. Gene expression such as changes in DNA methylation patterns and post-translation histone modification were shown to mediate myocyte hypertrophy, inflammation and fibrosis, and microvascular dysfunction **(Fig. 2)**.

Hypermethylation of DNA: Addition of methyl group to cytosine bases located in gene promoters turn off the fibrosis deactivating genes thus leading to excessive cardiac interstitial fibrosis.[3] This process occurs through transformation of fibroblasts into collagen producing myofibroblasts.

Fibrosis is an essential part of healing process, tissue repair, and organ preservation in response to acute injury and chronic inflammation. However, excessive accumulation of extracellular matrix (collagen and fibronectin) leads to organ disorder such as LV diastolic dysfunction in cardiometabolic HFpEF.

Cardiac fibroblasts are the primary regulators of cardiac structure by producing and maintaining extracellular matrix and myofibroblast in various disease processes. TGF-β is a seminal profibrotic factor acting through different pathways. During the cardiac remodeling process, TGF-β, interleukin 10, matricellular proteins, and fibroblasts are activated by macrophages, mast cells, and lymphocytes. Activated TGF-β stimulates Smad2 and Smad3 phosphorylation. These bind with Smad4 forming a trimeric complex which then enters the nucleus and binds to certain DNA sequences known as Smad binding elements which transcribe collagen producing profibrotic genes.

Fibroblasts get transformed into myofibroblasts with biochemical (TGF-β, TNF-α, and chemokines), physical, and mechanical stimuli (stiffness, tension, hypoxia, and mechanical damage).

Normally after adequate wound healing, the myofibroblasts undergo apoptosis and disappear. However, in disease states with persistent activation, myofibroblasts cause excessive fibrosis and organ dysfunction in various organs such as heart, lungs, liver, and kidneys.

MicroRNAs (miRNAs) are noncoding RNAs (19–25 nucleotides) located in the nucleus and cytoplasm and are released into the circulation and their expression is dependent on tissue-specific epigenetic changes. They play an important role in cardiac fibrosis.[4] In fact, at least 60 miRNAs have been identified in relation to cardiac remodeling. MiRNAs bind to messenger RNAs, modulate TGF-β/Smad pathway, influence proliferation of fibroblasts, and their transformation into myofibroblasts in producing extracellular matrix. There are several anti- and

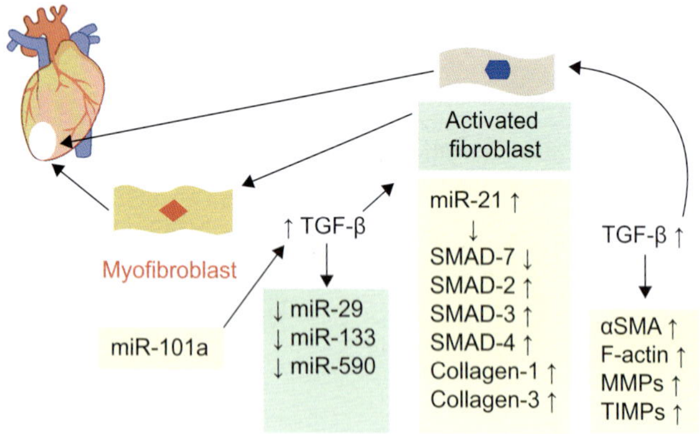

Fig. 3: Regulation of microRNAs in myocardial myofibrosis.

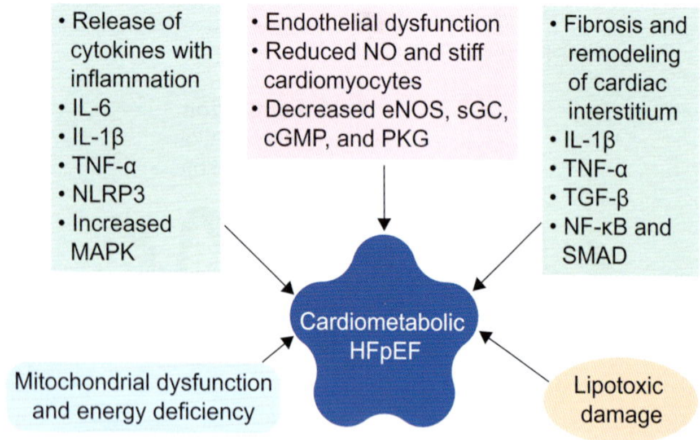

Fig. 4: Molecular basis of HFpEF.

profibrotic miRNAs, some examples depicted in **Figure 3**. More information about miRNAs is still evolving.

The delicate portion of extracellular matrix in a normal heart is maintained by finely regulated actions of matrix metalloproteinases (MMPs) and tissue inhibitors of metalloproteinases (TIMPs). An imbalance of MMPs and TIMPs leads to different types of cardiomyopathies. For example, high levels of MMP-9 are associated with fibrosis and enlarged LV chamber. MMP-2 degrades titin and troponin causing increased LV stiffness and impaired relaxation.

Thus, myocyte hypertrophy and cardiac extracellular matrix formation play an important role in LV diastolic dysfunction.

CONCLUSION

Hypertrophy and stiffness of cardiomyocytes from endomyocardial biopsies were showed to be responsible for diastolic dysfunction in patients with HFpEF. Animal models of cardiometabolic HFpEF have confirmed cardiomyocyte hypertrophy and stiffness. Comorbidity-mediated endothelial inflammation and dysregulation of the eNOS—cyclic guanosine monophosphate—PKG axis were noted to decrease PKG activity and hypophosphorylation of N2B of titin. Interestingly, in genetically normal mice, a combination of high-fat diet and suppression of NO synthases showed a strong HFpEF phenotype.[5]

Hypophosphorylation of N2Bus and PEVK were noted to cause myocardial stiffness in ZSF1 rats. In HFpEF patients, sodium-glucose cotransporter 2 inhibitor empagliflozin improved phosphorylation of troponin I, myosin-binding protein C, and titin thereby promoting myocardial chamber compliance and diastolic function **(Fig. 4)**.

REFERENCES

1. Borlaug BA, Sharma K, Shah SJ, et al. Heart Failure With Preserved Ejection Fraction: JACC Scientific Statement. J Am Coll Cardiol. 2023;81(18):1810-34.
2. Sabbah MS, Fayyaz AU, de Denus S, et al. Obese-inflammatory phenotypes in heart failure with preserved ejection fraction. Circ Heart Fail. 2020;13:e006414.
3. Gorica E, Paneni F. Cardiometabolic HFpEF with focus on type 2 diabetes mellitus. Cardiovasc Diabetol. 2025;24(1):390.
4. Rech M, Barandiarán Aizpurua A, van Empel V, et al. Pathophysiological understanding of HFpEF: microRNAs as part of the puzzle. Cardiovasc Res. 2018;114(6):782-93.
5. Porrello ER, Delbridge LMD. HFpEF-Time to Explore the Role of Genetic Heterogeneity in Phenotypic Variability: New Mechanistic Insights Offer Promise for Personalized Therapies. Circulation. 2019;140(20):1607-19.

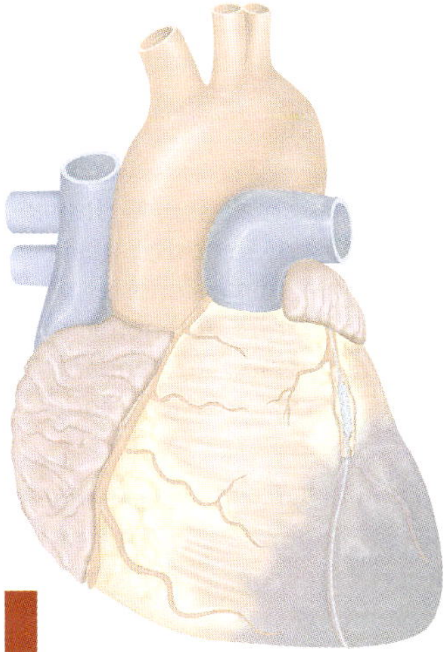

21

CHAPTER

Role of Amyloidosis in HFpEF and Obesity: Hidden but Critical

Somnath Mukhopadhay, Srina Ray, Saumitra Ray

INTRODUCTION

Heart failure with preserved ejection fraction (HFpEF) is now the dominant form of heart failure among older adults. It accounts for approximately 50% of all heart failure cases and its prevalence is rising due to aging populations and increasing rates of obesity. It is defined by typical heart failure symptoms and signs, a left ventricular ejection fraction (LVEF) ≥50%, and objective evidence of elevated filling pressures.[1] HFpEF is heterogeneous; it is more a syndrome than a single disease entity, with multiple phenotypes driven by aging, hypertension, obesity, diabetes, chronic kidney disease, and infiltrative processes **(Fig. 1)**.[2]

Among the latter, cardiac amyloidosis—especially transthyretin-related (ATTR)—has emerged as a "hidden but critical" cause of HFpEF.[3] The rising prevalence of obesity further complicates detection, phenotype expression, and management.[4] This chapter reviews the interplay between amyloidosis and HFpEF in the setting of obesity, highlighting diagnostic clues and therapeutic implications for cardiologists.

CARDIAC AMYLOIDOSIS: TYPES AND PATHOPHYSIOLOGY

Two main types affect the heart:

1. Transthyretin amyloidosis (ATTR):
    - *Wild type (ATTRwt):* Age-related misfolding of normal transthyretin protein is the main cause. It primarily affects the myocardium in older adults.[5]
    - *Variant/hereditary (ATTRv):* Mutant transthyretin leads to systemic deposition with cardiac involvement in this type.[5]
2. *Immunoglobulin light-chain (AL) amyloidosis:* Plasma cell dyscrasia can produce misfolded light chains which deposit rapidly in multiple organs, including the heart. Cardiac involvement is most common. More than 75% of patients exhibit symptoms of cardiac amyloid infiltration at the time of diagnosis. Prognosis is also very poor, median survival is around 4 months for advanced disease.[6]

Amyloid fibril deposition increases ventricular stiffness, reduces chamber compliance, causes thickened walls with small cavities, diastolic dysfunction, and restrictive physiology. Atrial infiltration usually contributes to higher chance of developing atrial fibrillation (AF). Electromechanical dissociation may also result from atrial infiltration. There may be higher risk of thrombus formation even in sinus rhythm. Microvascular infiltration and direct cardiomyocyte toxicity add to impaired relaxation and conduction abnormalities.[7]

PREVALENCE OF AMYLOIDOSIS IN HEART FAILURE WITH PRESERVED EJECTION FRACTION

- Recent studies demonstrate that a significant minority of HFpEF patients harbor amyloidosis, especially ATTRwt.
- Autopsy and biopsy studies show 10–25% of elderly HFpEF patients have myocardial amyloid deposits.[8]

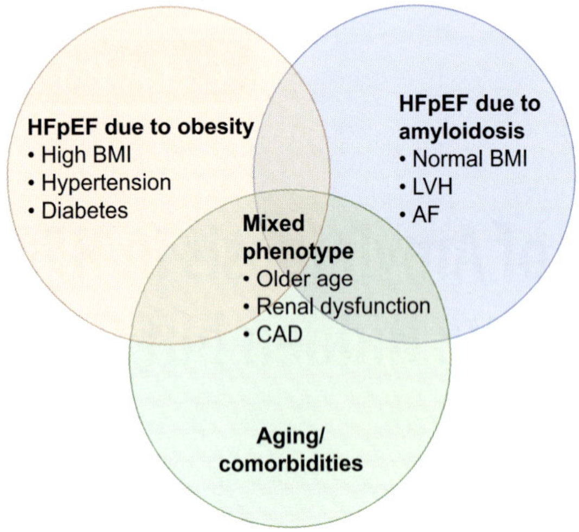

Fig. 1: Overlap of HFpEF phenotypes.

- Prospective screening of older HFpEF patients with LV wall thickness ≥12 mm finds ATTR cardiac amyloidosis (ATTR-CM) in 5–14%.[3,9]
- In the ATTR-ACT trial placebo arm, the mean age was 74 years and ~30% met HFpEF criteria at baseline.[10]

Thus, amyloidosis is underdiagnosed and often masquerades as "hypertensive" or "obesity-related" HFpEF.

OBESITY AND HEART FAILURE WITH PRESERVED EJECTION FRACTION

Obesity is a major driver of HFpEF: Over 80% of HFpEF patients are overweight or obese in many cohorts.[11] Pathophysiological mechanisms include:
- Increased plasma volume and preload
- Pericardial restraint from increased epicardial fat
- Myocardial stiffening and concentric remodeling
- Neurohormonal activation and systemic inflammation

Obesity leads to a distinct HFpEF phenotype with more volume overload, right heart dysfunction, and exercise intolerance.

INTERSECTION OF AMYLOIDOSIS AND OBESITY

When obesity coexists with amyloidosis, several challenges arise:
- *Masking of classic features:* Obesity attenuates ECG voltages and increases LV wall thickness, obscuring the "red flag" of low voltage despite hypertrophy.
- *Diagnostic confusion:* Concentric LV thickening may be ascribed to obesity or hypertension, delaying amyloidosis diagnosis.

TABLE 1: Clinical, imaging, and biomarker clues suggestive of cardiac amyloidosis in patients presenting with heart failure with preserved ejection fraction (HFpEF).

Domain	*Clues suggestive of amyloidosis in HFpEF*
Clinical	Age ≥65–70 years; male sex (ATTRwt); family history of amyloidosis; carpal tunnel syndrome, spinal stenosis, biceps tendon rupture; autonomic neuropathy; intolerance to standard HF therapies; unexplained low blood pressure
Anthropometry	Lower BMI than expected for severity of HFpEF; disproportionate dyspnea vs. obesity; lack of response to weight-loss interventions
Echocardiography	LV wall thickness >14 mm; "granular sparkling" myocardium; restrictive filling; biatrial enlargement; apical-sparing strain pattern ("cherry on top"), reduced S' velocity on the mitral annulus, reduced Global Longitudinal Strain with apical sparing, paradoxically low stroke volume relative to LV function
Electrocardiography	Low limb-lead voltages despite thick LV walls; pseudoinfarct Q waves; conduction disease or AV block; atrial fibrillation
Advanced imaging	Diffuse subendocardial/transmural late gadolinium enhancement and elevated extracellular volume on cardiac MRI; positive ^{99m}Tc-PYP or DPD scan with grade 2–3 myocardial uptake for ATTR
Biomarkers	NT-proBNP or troponin elevated out of proportion to blood pressure or obesity; abnormal serum free light chains or monoclonal protein (AL)

- *Opposite BMI trends:* In some cohorts, ATTR-CM patients had lower BMI than nonamyloid HFpEF despite similar wall thickness.[12]
- *Imaging limitations:* Obesity impairs echocardiographic (poor window) and nuclear scan image quality, hindering detection.

  Red flags: When to suspect amyloidosis in HFpEF (especially with obesity) **(Table 1)**.[13]
- Scores such as the AMY score [wall thickness >14 mm (1 point), absence of obesity (2 points), E/e' >14 (3 points)] improve discrimination of ATTR-CM from typical HFpEF. Total score over 3 suggests ATTR-CM and indicates the need for further specific testing.[14]

PATHOPHYSIOLOGICAL LINKS

- *Mechanical load:* Obesity increases preload and afterload, which may exacerbate the diastolic dysfunction from amyloid infiltration.
- *Inflammatory milieu:* Adipose tissue secretes cytokines and alters proteostasis, potentially accelerating amyloid deposition (hypothesis under investigation).
- *Diagnostic delay:* Misclassification as "obesity cardiomyopathy" leads to missed opportunities for disease-specific therapy.

CATHETER ABLATION IN CONTEMPORARY HEART FAILURE WITH PRESERVED EJECTION FRACTION TRIALS

Although most trials of HFpEF excluded diagnosed cases of infiltrative cardiomyopathy including CA, undiagnosed cases of CA have always been suspected to have been included inadvertently. Applying the echocardiographic and clinical criteria discussed above, an enriched subset from the TOPCAT trial showed the prevalence of CA to be close to 23%. It used simple echocardiographic measures like a reduced S′ velocity <6 cm/second of the mitral annulus and interventricular septum (IVS) thickness >1.2 cm to identify patients with suspected CA. This subgroup had a worse outcome compared to the rest of the patients.[15]

Similarly, in the PARAGON trial, male sex and high LVEF—the two subsets where the efficacy of valsartan sacubitril was conspicuously diminished—are typically seen in patients with wild-type ATTR CA. Differences in geographic responses of ARNI to CA in western Europe and America compared to rest of Asia are possibly due to more stringent and effective exclusion of CA in the former due to robust screening facilities.[3]

In most randomized clinical trials of sodium-glucose cotransporter 2 inhibitors (SGLT2i), transthyretin cardiomyopathy (ATTR-CM) was an exclusion criterion. Thus, it is difficult to evaluate the role of SGLT2i in ATTR-CM. A recently published study assessed the efficacy and tolerability of SGLT2i in patients with ATTR-CM. A total number of 2,356 consecutive ATTR-CM patients between 2014 and 2022 were analyzed of whom 260 (11%) were found to get SGLT2i. After a thorough comparison done between the groups according to the treatment, 14 variables were found to be significantly different including age and NT-proBNP. A propensity score reflecting the likelihood of being treated with SGLT2i for each patient was determined using 16 variables. The study concluded that SGLT2i was well tolerated by ATTR-CM patients and was beneficial for HF symptoms, renal function, and need for diuretics. More importantly, SGLT2i treatment reduced the risk of HF hospitalization and cardiovascular and all-cause mortality, regardless of the ejection fraction, despite the effect size being likely overestimated. In the absence of randomized trials, these data may encourage clinicians to use SGLT2i in patients with ATTR-CM.[16]

THERAPEUTIC IMPLICATIONS

Disease-specific Therapy for Amyloidosis

- *ATTR amyloidosis:* Tafamidis, a transthyretin stabilizer, reduced all-cause mortality and cardiovascular hospitalizations in ATTR-ACT.[10] Gene silencers (patisiran, inotersen, eplontersen, and vutrisiran) and investigational antiamyloid antibodies offer additional options.[17]
- *AL amyloidosis:* Urgent plasma cell-directed therapy (e.g., bortezomib-based chemotherapy) ± autologous stem cell transplant is critical.[6]

Heart Failure with Preserved Ejection Fraction Management

Standard measures (diuretics for congestion, blood pressure, and rhythm control) remain, but care is needed: amyloidosis patients are often preload-dependent and hypotensive. SGLT2 inhibitors, recently recommended for HFpEF, have not yet been tested extensively in amyloidosis but are being used cautiously.[18]

Obesity Management

Intentional weight loss via calorie restriction, supervised exercise, or bariatric surgery can improve functional capacity in obese HFpEF. GLP-1 receptor agonists may help both weight loss and metabolic control. However, in amyloidosis patients who are already prone to frailty or cachexia, aggressive weight loss may be harmful; individualized plans are essential.

Multidisciplinary Care

Early recognition through systematic screening of high-risk HFpEF patients, combined with amyloidosis specialist referral, optimizes outcomes.

PROGNOSIS

Heart failure with preserved ejection fraction patients with unrecognized amyloidosis deteriorate faster and have higher mortality and hospitalization rates than nonamyloid HFpEF.[3,9] Disease-specific therapy (e.g., tafamidis) slows progression and improves survival, especially if initiated early.[10] Obesity independently worsens symptoms and quality of life; its prognostic effect in amyloidosis remains complex ("obesity paradox").[12]

PROPOSED DIAGNOSTIC WORKFLOW

- Confirm HFpEF (LVEF ≥50%, elevated natriuretic peptides, structural heart disease, or diastolic dysfunction).
- Screen for red flags (clinical, ECG, and echo).
- Measure NT-proBNP/troponin and screen for monoclonal proteins (serum and urine immunofixation, and free light chains).
- Advanced imaging if suspicion high: cardiac MRI and ^{99m}Tc-PYP/DPD/HMDP scintigraphy.
- Endomyocardial biopsy if noninvasive tests equivocal or AL suspected. Initiate disease-specific therapy and optimize HFpEF and obesity management.

CONCLUSION

Amyloidosis, particularly ATTR, is an underrecognized yet critical cause of HFpEF. Its prevalence in older HFpEF cohorts approaches 5–15%. Obesity, a dominant HFpEF driver, both overlap with and obscure amyloidosis. Cardiologists should maintain a high index of suspicion, apply structured diagnostic pathways, and combine disease-specific amyloidosis therapy with tailored HFpEF and obesity management. Early recognition can meaningfully alter prognosis.

REFERENCES

1. McDonagh TA, Metra M, Adamo M, et al. 2021 ESC Guidelines for the diagnosis and treatment of acute and chronic heart failure. Eur Heart J. 2021;42(36):3599-726. Erratum in: Eur Heart J. 2021;42(48):4901.
2. Nagueh SF. Heart failure with preserved ejection fraction: insights into diagnosis and pathophysiology. Cardiovasc Res. 2021;117(4):999-1014.
3. González-López E, Gallego-Delgado M, Guzzo-Merello G, et al. Wild-type transthyretin amyloidosis as a cause of heart failure with preserved ejection fraction. Eur Heart J. 2015;36(38):2585-94.
4. Harada T, Obokata M. Obesity-Related Heart Failure with Preserved Ejection Fraction: Pathophysiology, Diagnosis, and Potential Therapies. Heart Fail Clin. 2020;16(3): 357-68.
5. Maurer MS, Bokhari S, Damy T, et al. Expert Consensus Recommendations for the Suspicion and Diagnosis of Transthyretin Cardiac Amyloidosis. Circ Heart Fail. 2019;12(9):e006075.
6. Wechalekar AD, Fontana M, Quarta CC, et al. AL Amyloidosis for Cardiologists: Awareness, Diagnosis, and Future Prospects: JACC: CardioOncology State-of-the-Art Review. JACC CardioOncol. 2022;4(4):427-41.
7. Siddiqi OK, Ruberg FL. Cardiac amyloidosis: An update on pathophysiology, diagnosis, and treatment. Trends Cardiovasc Med. 2018;28(1):10-21.
8. Tanskanen M, Peuralinna T, Polvikoski T, et al. Senile systemic amyloidosis affects 25% of the very aged and associates with genetic variation in alpha2-macroglobulin and tau: a population-based autopsy study. Ann Med. 2008;40(3):232-9.
9. Healy L, Giblin G, Gray A, et al. Prevalence of transthyretin cardiac amyloidosis in undifferentiated heart failure with preserved ejection fraction. ESC Heart Fail. 2025;12(2):1176-82.
10. Maurer MS, Schwartz JH, Gundapaneni B, et al. Tafamidis Treatment for Patients with Transthyretin Amyloid Cardiomyopathy. N Engl J Med. 2018 Sep 13;379(11):1007-16.
11. Obokata M, Reddy YNV, Pislaru SV, et al. Evidence Supporting the Existence of a Distinct Obese Phenotype of Heart Failure With Preserved Ejection Fraction. Circulation. 2017;136(1):6-19.
12. Timothy J Poterucha, et al. Abstract 13438: Obesity is Uncommon in Patients With Transthyretin Cardiac Amyloidosis. Circulation. 2021;144(Suppl_1).
13. Ray S, Kar A. Role of Amyloidosis in HFpEF Trials. Advances in HFpEF Management (AHM): A Textbook of Cardiology, 1st edition. New Delhi: Jaypee Brothers Medical Publishers (P) Ltd.; 2025. pp. 115-7.
14. Gioia G, Schrutka L, Jozwiak-Nozdrzykowska J, et al. Transthyretin amyloid cardiomyopathy among patients with heart failure and preserved ejection fraction: the AMY score. ESC Heart Fail. 2024;11(4):2172-81.
15. Sperry BW, Hanna M, Shah SJ, et al. Spironolactone in patients with an echocardiographic HFpEF phenotype suggestive of cardiac amyloidosis: results from TOPCAT. Heart Failure. 2021;9(11):795-802.
16. Porcari A, Cappelli F, Nitsche C, et al. SGLT2 Inhibitor Therapy in Patients With Transthyretin Amyloid Cardiomyopathy. J Am Coll Cardiol. 2024;83:2411-22.
17. Dave P, Anand P, Kothawala A, et al. RNA Interference Therapeutics for Hereditary Amyloidosis: A Narrative Review of Clinical Trial Outcomes and Future Directions. Cureus. 2024;16(6):e62981.
18. Garcia-Pavia P, Gonzalez-Lopez E, Anderson LJ, et al. Non-amyloid specific treatment for transthyretin cardiac amyloidosis: a clinical consensus statement of the ESC Heart Failure Association. Eur Heart J. 2025:ehaf710.

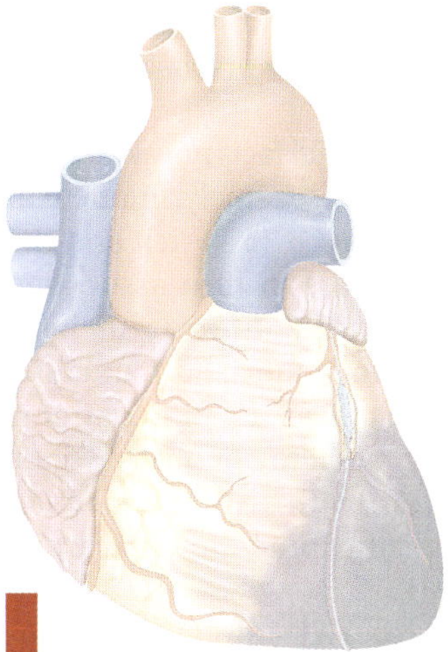

22

CHAPTER

Heart Failure with Preserved Ejection Fraction: A Multimorbidities Disease in Obesity—Advances in Management

Jostol Pinto, A George Koshy

DEFINITIONS AND PREVALENCE

Heart failure with preserved ejection fraction (HFpEF) is a complex clinical syndrome with impaired ventricular structure or function despite a left ventricular (LV) ejection fraction (EF) of ≥50%, causing impaired ejection of blood or elevated LV filling pressures, characterized biochemically by raised natriuretic peptides. While obesity is traditionally defined as having a body mass index (BMI) of over 30 kg/m^2, cardiovascular (CV) risk is often conferred with increasing central obesity and visceral adipose tissue (VAT).[1] Worldwide prevalence of HFpEF is over 32 million, while that of obesity far exceeds it at nearly 900 million (2.5 billion considering overweight/obese).[2] In the Western world, nearly 80% of patients with HFpEF are overweight/obese.[3,4]

CHALLENGES IN DIAGNOSIS

The diagnosis of HFpEF is limited by the fact that one of the essential parameters is that of healthy individuals—an EF of ≥50%. The onus of diagnosis now relies on clinical signs and symptoms, blood pressure, atrial fibrillation, structural features on echocardiography, and an elevated N-terminal probrain natriuretic peptide (NT-proBNP) in blood. It is even more challenging if the patient is already on heart failure (HF) drugs but are prescribed for other indications; for example, beta-blockers for hypertension, which have reverted atrial fibrillation; anti-hypertensive therapy, which normalizes blood pressure recordings; and diuretics, which relieve dyspnea and resolve edema. While an elevated NT-proBNP remains the cornerstone in the diagnostic armamentarium, it is typically depressed in the obese.[1] Although the reason is not clear, its validity is seen when NT-proBNP rises paradoxically with healthy weight loss.[5] It could be due to enhanced natriuretic peptide degradation in adipose tissue or due to less LV wall stress due to mild constraint on the heart. For the same reason, the E/e′ ratio during echocardiography underestimates the degree of HFpEF in the obese.[6] While dyspnea is a fundamental symptom in the clinical diagnosis of HFpEF, it is often considered to be caused by the obese abdomen per se, which limits diaphragmatic excursion. Jugular venous pulsations may be masked under an obese neck. All these factors can confound the diagnosis of HFpEF in the obese. Further, the obese patients have often been excluded from clinical trials, citing likely symptom-overlap of obesity and HF or the lack of an NT-proBNP cut-off for the obese.

PATHOPHYSIOLOGICAL LINKS IN "OBESE HFpEF"

Unlike the direct relationship between atherosclerosis and coronary artery disease, the link between obesity and the development of HFpEF needs better understanding; this "causation" is supported by epidemiological studies.[7] There is no obvious mechanism to the unread mind why adipose tissue causes HFpEF (not the case for hypertension causing HFpEF). For long, it was reckoned that obese patients with HFpEF were merely obese and HF was a confounding diagnosis. It was in 2013 that Paulus and Tschöpe proposed a novel paradigm for HFpEF in a state-of-the-art commentary in the Journal of the American College of Cardiology, shifting emphasis from LV afterload excess to coronary microvascular and systemic inflammation (Paulus hypothesis of HFpEF). Similarly, obesity is now no longer considered just a mechanical impediment to diaphragmatic excursion or a comorbid bystander in HFpEF—it is, in fact, now designated "from Pariah to Central Player" and rightly so.[8] Hypertension has been postulated to be the commonest cause of HFpEF for several years, but most antihypertensive drug trials for HFpEF have been negative despite blood pressure reduction. Upper body obesity (both visceral/omental and subcutaneous) is more deleterious to CV health than lower body obesity (gluteofemoral); this is in part due to the fact that it is upper body obesity [especially visceral adipose tissue (VAT)], which results in a greater release of free fatty acids (FFAs) and adipokines into circulation.[9] These excess FFAs cause insulin resistance in the liver and skeletal muscle and increase oxidation of FFAs (Randle cycle). Further, hypertrophic adipocytes are more insulin resistant, have greater lipolysis, and are more often seen in VAT as compared to hyperplastic adipocytes.[1] Although counterintuitive, abdominal fat (visceral and subcutaneous) with a greater proportion of hypertrophic adipocytes are less efficient in storing fat because they release proportionally more FFAs. Those with smaller abdominal fat deposits have greater efficiency in storing fat as they are associated with less hypertrophic adipocytes and thus lesser proportional lipolysis.[10]

Further, VAT is more strongly associated with HFpEF than abdominal subcutaneous fat.[4,9] It is proinflammatory, metabolically active, and oxidative; it increases insulin sensitivity and mediates the metabolic syndrome due to which "obese HFpEF" is also sometimes called "metabolic HFpEF."[4] While excess caloric intake contributes to obesity and VAT alike, cortisol preferentially enhances VAT while causing muscle catabolism.

Increased adiposity demands higher cardiac output and blood volume, and resultant LV dilation followed by hypertrophy. Obese HFpEF tend to have greater LV dilation and hypertrophy, and even more epicardial fat than nonobese HFpEF.[11] For any given LV transmural distending pressure, obesity results in a greater pulmonary capillary wedge pressure (PCWP) due to the external pressure on the heart.[1] Diastolic chamber stiffness is increased in obesity, and although systolic function is only subtly reduced, systolic reserve during exercise is grossly impaired.[12,13] This creates a vicious cycle where impaired systolic reserve begets impaired diastolic reserve (converse of Starling's law).[1]

Like the ventricle, the left atrium (LA) also undergoes remodeling in HFpEF and in obesity (LA myopathy).[14] However, atrial remodeling and atrial fibrillation is more often seen in nonobese HFpEF than in obese HFpEF; the confounder here is age: The latter are often a decade younger than the former. In other words, while LA myopathy does worsen obese HFpEF, it worsens nonobese HFpEF more.

Once thought to be inert, epicardial fat is now known to produce similar cytokines as VAT does, namely, interleukin (IL)-1β, IL-6, tumor necrosis factor α (TNF-α), and the adipofibrokine activin A. These are in turn associated with remodeling, dysfunction, and fibrosis of both cardiac and skeletal muscle, mitochondrial dysfunction, and capillary rarefaction.[8,15] Obese HFpEF patients have greater epicardial fat [compared to nonobese HFpEF and compared to heart failure with reduced ejection fraction (HFrEF)], and this contributes to pericardial restraint.[8,11]

Macrophage infiltration of VAT upregulates proinflammatory leptin, IL-6, TNF-α, and resistin and downregulates anti-inflammatory adiponectin and omentin-1, leading to metaboinflammation. CV effects of such adipokines include capillary rarefaction, endothelial and mitochondrial dysfunction. VAT also secretes profibrotic osteopontin, which promotes myocardial senescence.[16]

The normal heart derives 70–80% of its energy from free fatty acids (FFAs) and 20–30% from glucose during fasting. During exercise or ischemia, the heart preferentially shifts to glucose uptake as it is more energy efficient and generates less reactive oxygen species and lipid species. In obesity, the surplus circulating FFAs enhance myocardial FFA uptake initially, but this soon leads to cardiac lipotoxicity (cardiomyocyte steatosis), which is seen to correlate with diastolic impairment.[17] Here, during exercise, impaired glucose uptake could contribute to cardiac dysfunction. Indeed, myocardial injury is more often seen in HFpEF even in the absence of coronary artery disease.[18]

The heart needs continued substrate delivery during both systole and diastole, the latter being more energy-demanding. Phosphocreatinine/adenosine-triphosphate (PCr/ATP) ratio, which reflects myocardial energetics, has been observed to be lower in obesity; this affects diastole more as cytosolic calcium during diastole decreases. This is compensated by increased creatine kinase activity in obesity to maintain ATP delivery at rest (but not compensating enough during exercise).[19] Weight loss reduces creatine kinase activity and increases PCr/ATP ratio.[20]

ADIPOKINE LEPTIN: A CENTRAL OR PERIPHERAL ROLE IN OBESE HFpEF? OR BOTH?

Increased metabolic demand in the obese results in systemic vasodilation. Then ensues the well-studied cascade of arterial underfilling, activation of the sympathetic nervous system (SNS) and renin angiotensin aldosterone system (RAAS), sodium retention, and cardiomyocyte hypertrophy and fibrosis. Now, the initial step (vasodilation) is also brought about directly by leptin from perivascular fat. Incidentally, the final step (cardiomyocyte hypertrophy and fibrosis) is also brought about directly via cardiac leptin receptors (apart from indirect action via angiotensin II, aldosterone, and endothelin-1 receptors). Further, leptin is a direct activator of the RAAS and SNS; again, both can also be activated in morbid obesity by physical compression of the kidneys.[21] Rarely, obesity-related high-output HFpEF can occur.[22] Obesity-mediated glomerulopathy via hyperfiltration and inflammation also contributes to increased total blood volume.[23]

REGIONAL AND SEX DISTRIBUTION OF OBESE HFpEF

Visceral obesity harms women more than men and Asian women more than those in the West.[1,4,24] Although VAT is seen more in men, and gluteofemoral obesity is seen more in women, post-menopausal women tend to have increased VAT accompanied by a greater prevalence of HFpEF. Women gain an average of 2.5 kg after menopause, and most of it is VAT.[4] Further, women with HFpEF are found to have more visceral fat compared to women without HFpEF after matching for age and even BMI. This difference is not seen among men.[25] Excess VAT can contribute to developing HFpEF even in the absence of obesity, more so in Asians. This increased VAT also accounts for the greater prevalence of diabetes even in the nonobese.[4]

MANAGEMENT AND ITS EVIDENCE

Evidently, one of the arms of the management of "obese HFpEF" would be achieving weight loss. Weight loss in obesity has shown to reduce blood pressure and total body oxygen consumption, and most relevantly, up to 25% reduction in pulmonary wedge pressure (PCWP) and pulmonary arterial pressure.[26] However, this meta-analysis data was from the obese but not from HFpEF cohorts. Apart from dietary optimization, exercise and lifestyle modification, which form the foundation of healthy (but sometimes limited) weight loss in morbid obesity, pharmacotherapy and bariatric surgery are beneficial therapies here. Bariatric surgery is the most dramatic modality to bring about sustained weight loss and reduce the incidence of HF.[27]

Semaglutide (glucagon-like peptide-1 receptor agonist, GLP-1 RA) has shown positive results for weight loss and symptomatic clinical benefit in obese HFpEF in the trials STEP-HFpEF DM and STEP-HFpEF (Kosiborod MN et al., NEJM, 2024 and 2023, respectively) (median BMI: 37 kg/m^2). Through the SUMMIT trial (Packer M et al., NEJM, 2024) (731 patients followed up for 2 years; median BMI: 38.3kg/m^2), tirzepatide [dual agonist of glucose-dependent insulinotropic polypeptide (GIP) and GLP-1] (GIP/GLP-1 RA) has shown promise by reducing the composite of CV death and worsening HF [hazard ratio (HR) 0.62, $p = 0.026$] despite gastrointestinal adverse events. The SURMOUNT MMO (Study of Tirzepatide (LY3298176) on the Reduction of Morbidity and Mortality in Adults With Obesity) trial is yet to start recruiting, but it aims to find out CV outcomes and mortality benefit in obese patients who receive tirzepatide.

The pharmacotherapeutic options of HFpEF are limited, at least those options prolonging longevity. While diuretics relieve symptoms, congestion, and LV filling pressures (and thus HFpEF), obese HFpEF patients have poorer prerenal tolerance of diuresis as compared to their nonobese counterparts.[28] Spironolactone/eplerenone may have some benefit in obese HFpEF,[29] and ongoing trials such as SPIRRIT (recruiting in Sweden and the US) and SPIRIT-HF (based from Germany) may shed more evidence in the days to come. The recently published SOGALDI-PEF trial (Ferreira JP et al., JACC, July 2025) (median BMI: 28.3kg/m^2) showed that adding spironolactone to background dapagliflozin therapy for 3 months showed greater reduction in NT-proBNP (11% relative reduction), systolic blood pressure (by 5.2 mm Hg) and albuminuria but at the cost of hyperkalemia and worsening renal function.

The recently published FINEARTS-HF trial enrolled around 6,000 patients (EF >40%) and followed them up for a median of 32 months (Solomon SD et al., NEJM, 2024); it showed reduction in the composite of HF events and CV death (HR: 0.87, 95% CI, 0.74–0.94, $p = 0.007$) by finerenone; with a HF event HR of 0.82 (842 vs. 1024, $p = 0.006$) and a CV death HR of 0.93 (8.1% vs. 8.7%). Another finerenone study of hospitalized acute decompensated HF patients (EF >40%) called REDEFINE-HF is still recruiting. CONFIRMATION-HF is recruiting patients hospitalized for HF (any EF) to analyze the combination of finerenone with empagliflozin. EASi-HF, in its recruiting phase, is studying the potential benefit of oral vicadrostat (an aldosterone synthase inhibitor) in HF with EF >40%.

Sacubitril valsartan did show a trend towards reducing the composite of HF hospitalization and CV death but without statistical significance (HR: 0.87, $p = 0.06$) in the PARAGON-HF trial which enrolled around 4,800 patients

(Solomon SD et al., NEJM, 2019) [notably, the same author, same journal, same date (September 1st), 5 years apart, and same composite HR of 0.87 as FINEARTS-HF!].

Statins benefit patients with obese HFpEF in non-lipid-lowering mechanisms, namely, systemic anti-inflammatory activity and epicardial fat regression (which in turn reduces its adipokine release and cascading effects as described above). Similarly, sodium-glucose cotransporter 2 inhibitors (SGLT2i) reduce epicardial fat and VAT and their secretion of adipokines and TNF-α, and increase adipocyte glucose uptake. SGLT2i reduced HF hospitalization and CV death (HR: 0.79, 95% CI, 0.69–0.90, p <0.001) in the EMPEROR-Preserved trial (Anker SD et al., NEJM, 2021) which enrolled around 6,000 patients followed up for a median of 26 months and the DELIVER trial (Solomon SD, NEJM, 2022) (HR: 0.82, 95% CI, 0.73–0.92, p <0.001) which enrolled around 6,200 patients followed up for a median of 30 months. Although, around 1–2 kg weight loss is typically observed after SGLT2i therapy, it is unlikely to account for the clinical benefit in both obese and nonobese HFpEF.[1]

Suggested novel therapies for obese HFpEF include splanchnic nerve ablation,[30] percutaneous pericardial resection,[31] adipokine modification, targeted therapy for senescent cells and increasing satiety.[1] Yet another approach could be to increase catabolism or uncouple oxidative phosphorylation from the electron transport chain of the inner mitochondrial membrane. This was incidentally tried 85 years ago using a protonophore called 2,4-dintrophenol as a weight loss medication, but had to be withdrawn due to malignant hyperthermia. Its prodrug HU6 (metabolic accelerator for obese HFpEF) has undergone a phase 2a trial (HuMAIN-HFpEF) (Pandey A et al., JAMA, June 2025) displaying a reduction in weight, fat mass, and percentage visceral fat without significant muscle mass over 19 weeks. Other drugs being studied include ziltivekimab (IL-6 inhibitor), perhexiline (carnitine palmitoyltransferase-1 inhibitor), and mitochondrial antioxidants.[32] Paulus (mentioned earlier) proposed that treating HFpEF lies in combating the underlying vascular and oxidative mechanisms and thus could include nitrates, sildenafil, isosorbide-dinitrate/hydralazine, statins, and resveratrol. Despite their vasculoprotective effects, RAAS inhibitors have not shown any benefit in HFpEF.[33] Estrogen replacement therapy has been suggested to reduce VAT in postmenopausal women.[4,34] CV benefits are likely to be looked for in various incretin-based antiobesity drugs like dual GLP-1 and glucagon RAs (survodutide (SYNCHRONIZE trial), permvidutide), a triple GIP/GLP-1/glucagon RA (retatrutide) (TRIUMPH-3 trial), an oral GLP-1 RA (orforglipron), and an amylin/calcitonin RA with GLP-1 RA (cagrilintide/semaglutide) combination (RESPIRE HFpEF trial).[35]

CONCLUSION

The approach to finding therapies for HFpEF lies in targeting the systemic inflammation/VAT hypothesis and not cardiac mechanisms. This is why many trials of HFpEF to date have been negative, as the same beneficial drugs in HFrEF were tried in HFpEF with the hope of extended benefit. Notably, HFpEF seldom transitions to HFrEF, suggesting that the mechanism and thus therapeutic approach should be different.[36,37] Exercise and dietary caloric restriction reduce VAT and HFpEF.[4,7,34] Although not pharmacological, they suggest that mitigating the former resolves the latter. Further, weight regains on stopping GLP-1 RA therapy. Today, finerenone, sodium-glucose cotransporter-2 inhibitors (SGLT2i), GLP-1 RAs, and tirzepatide have trial evidence for the therapy of obese HFpEF.[1,35] The antiobesity drugs, more specifically anti-VAT drugs and incretin-based therapies, are likely to manifest as anti-HFpEF therapy in the days to come.

REFERENCES

1. Borlaug BA, Jensen MD, Kitzman DW, et al. Obesity and heart failure with preserved ejection fraction: new insights and pathophysiological targets. Cardiovasc Res. 2022;118(18):3434-50.
2. NCD Risk Factor Collaboration (NCD-RisC). Worldwide trends in underweight and obesity from 1990 to 2022: a pooled analysis of 3663 population-representative studies with 222 million children, adolescents, and adults. Lancet. 2024;403(10431):1027-50.
3. Kittleson MM, Panjrath GS, Amancherla K, et al. 2023 ACC Expert Consensus Decision Pathway on management of heart failure with preserved ejection fraction: a report of the American College of Cardiology Solution Set Oversight Committee. J Am Coll Cardiol. 2023;81(18):1835-78.
4. Kitzman DW, Nicklas BL. Pivotal Role of Excess Intra-abdominal Adipose in the Pathogenesis of Metabolic/Obese HFpEF. JACC Heart Fail. 2018;6(12):1008-10.
5. Kitzman DW, Shah SJ. The HFpEF Obesity Phenotype: The Elephant in the Room. J Am Coll Cardiol. 2016;68(2):200-3.
6. Obokata M, Reddy YNV, Melenovsky V, et al. Uncoupling between intravascular and distending pressures leads to underestimation of circulatory congestion in obesity. Eur J Heart Fail. 2022;24(2):353-61.
7. Rao VN, Zhao D, Allison MA, et al. Adiposity and Incident Heart Failure and its Subtypes: MESA (Multi-Ethnic Study of Atherosclerosis). JACC Heart Fail. 2018;6(12):999-1007.
8. Kitzman DW, Lam CSP. Obese heart failure with preserved ejection fraction phenotype: from Pariah to Central Player. Circulation. 2017;136(1):20-3.

9. Jensen MD, Haymond MW, Rizza RA, et al. Influence of body fat distribution on free fatty acid metabolism in obesity. J Clin Invest. 1989;83(4):1168-73.
10. Ali AH, Koutsari C, Mundi M, et al. Free fatty acid storage in human visceral and subcutaneous adipose tissue: role of adipocyte proteins. Diabetes. 2011;60(9):2300-7.
11. Obokata M, Reddy YN, Pislaru SV, et al. Evidence supporting the existence of a distinct obese phenotype of heart failure with preserved ejection fraction. Circulation. 2017;136(1):6-19.
12. Russo C, Jin Z, Homma S, et al. Effect of obesity and overweight on left ventricular diastolic function: a community-based study in an elderly cohort. J Am Coll Cardiol. 2011;57(12):1368-74.
13. Borlaug BA, Lam CS, Roger VL, et al. Contractility and ventricular systolic stiffening in hypertensive heart disease insights into the pathogenesis of heart failure with preserved ejection fraction. J Am Coll Cardiol, 2009;54(5):410-8.
14. Wang TJ, Parise H, Levy D, et al. Obesity and the risk of new-onset atrial fibrillation. JAMA. 2004;292(20):2471-7.
15. Mazurek T, Zhang L, Zalewski A, et al. Human epicardial adipose tissue is a source of inflammatory mediators. Circulation. 2003;108(20):2460-6.
16. Sawaki D, Czibik G, Pini M, et al. Visceral adipose tissue drives cardiac aging through modulation of fibroblast senescence by osteopontin production. Circulation. 2018;138(8):809-22.
17. Wu C-K, Lee J-K, Hsu J-C, et al. Myocardial adipose deposition and the development of heart failure with preserved ejection fraction. Eur J Heart Fail. 2020;22(3):445-54.
18. Obokata M, Reddy YNV, Melenovsky V, et al. Myocardial injury and cardiac reserve in patients with heart failure and preserved ejection fraction. J Am Coll Cardiol. 2018;72(1):29-40.
19. Rider OJ, Francis JM, Ali MK, et al. Effects of catecholamine stress on diastolic function and myocardial energetics in obesity. Circulation. 2012;125(12):1511-9.
20. Rider OJ, Francis JM, Tyler D, et al. Effects of weight loss on myocardial energetics and diastolic function in obesity. Int J Cardiovasc Imaging. 2013;29(5):1043-50.
21. Hall JE, do Carmo JM, da Silva AA, et al. Obesity-induced hypertension: interaction of neurohumoral and renal mechanisms. Circ Res. 2015;116(6):991-1006.
22. Reddy YN, Melenovsky V, Redfeld MM, et al. High-output heart failure: a 15-year experience. J Am Coll Cardiol. 2016;68(5):473-82.
23. Camara NO, Iseki K, Kramer H, et al. Kidney disease and obesity: epidemiology, mechanisms and treatment. Nat Rev Nephrol. 2017;13(3):181-90.
24. Lai YH, Liu ME, Su CH, et al. Obesity-related changes in cardiac structure and function among Asian men and women. J Am Coll Cardiol. 2017;69(23):2876-8.
25. Sorimachi H, Obokata M, Takahashi N, et al. Pathophysiologic importance of visceral adipose tissue in women with heart failure and preserved ejection fraction. Eur Heart J. 2021;42(16):1595-605.
26. Reddy YNV, Anantha-Narayanan M, Obokata M, et al. Hemodynamic effects of weight loss in obesity: a systematic review and meta-analysis. JACC Heart Fail. 2019;7(8):678-87.
27. van Veldhuisen SL, Gorter TM, van Woerden G, et al. Bariatric surgery and cardiovascular disease: a systematic review and meta-analysis. Eur Heart J. 2022;43(20):1955-69.
28. Reddy YNV, Obokata M, Testani JM, et al. Adverse renal response to decongestion in the obese phenotype of heart failure with preserved ejection fraction. J Card Fail. 2020;26(2):101-7.
29. Packer M. Obesity-associated heart failure as a theoretical target for treatment with mineralocorticoid receptor antagonists. JAMA Cardiol. 2018;3(9):883-7.
30. Fudim M, Kaye DM, Borlaug BA, et al. Venous tone and stressed blood volume in heart failure: JACC review topic of the week. J Am Coll Cardiol. 2022;79(18):1858-69.
31. Borlaug BA, Carter RE, Melenovsky V, et al. Percutaneous pericardial resection: a novel potential treatment for heart failure with preserved ejection fraction. Circ Heart Fail. 2017;10(4):e003612.
32. Noordali H, Loudon BL, Frenneaux MP, et al. Cardiac metabolism: a promising therapeutic target for heart failure. Pharmacol Ther. 2018;182:95-114.
33. Paulus WJ, van Ballegoij JJM. Treatment of heart failure with normal ejection fraction: An inconvenient truth! J Am Coll Cardiol. 2010;55(6):526-37.
34. Kitzman DW, Brubaker P, Morgan T, et al. Effect of caloric restriction or aerobic exercise training on peak oxygen consumption and quality of life in obese older patients with heart failure with preserved ejection fraction: a randomized clinical trial. JAMA. 2016;315(1):36-46.
35. Kim S, Yoo B. Obesity and heart failure with preserved ejection fraction: focus on new drugs and future direction in medical treatment. Korean J Intern Med. 2025;40(3):357-70.
36. Borlaug BA, Redfeld MM. Diastolic and systolic heart failure are distinct phenotypes within the heart failure spectrum. Circulation. 2011;123(18):2006-14; discussion 2014.
37. Zheng W, Qi Q, Li J, He C, et al. Heart failure with preserved ejection fraction and obesity: emerging metabolic therapeutic strategies. Diabetol Metab Syndr. 2025;17(1):336.

23

CHAPTER

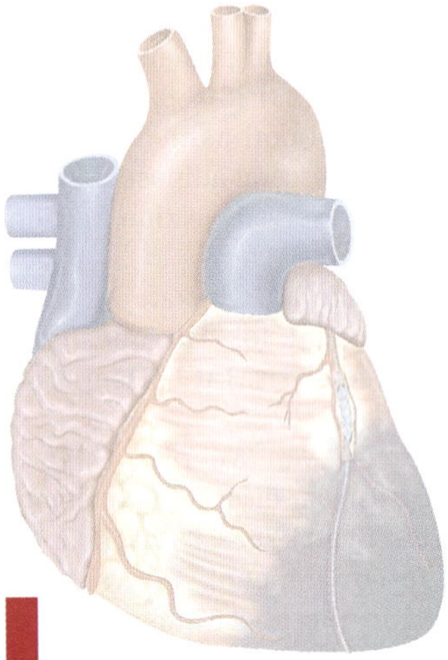

International Trials on Management of HFpEF with Obesity: What is Applicable for Indians?

Naveen Grag, KK Kapur

INTRODUCTION

Heart failure with preserved ejection fraction (HFpEF) amounts about 50% of all heart failure cases. The attributable causes are multifactorial including hypertension, diabetes, obesity, etc. Obesity related HFpEF (O-HFpEF) is recently emerge as cardiometabolically distinct entity as it independently contributes in systemic inflammation and alters cardiac hemodynamic and stiffness.[1-4]

Epicardial adiposity, i.e., fat deposition between myocardial and epicardial layer of heart is thought to be one of the main culprit of HFpEF. This deposit fat releases inflammatory molecules that induces changes in microvasculature of coronary arteries as well as to atrium. This insult leads to stiffness and fibrosis in left atrial (LA) wall as well as in left ventricular musculature. This enhanced deposition of collagen and fibrosis due to microvascular inflammation results into HFpEF. Furthermore, enhanced renin-aldosterone-angiotensin-system (RAAS) due to increased body mass, also contributes to cardiac remodeling. These changes in cardiac musculature affects mitral inflow velocities (E-velocity and A-velocity) as well as annular velocities (e'-velocity). The ratio of these velocities, i.e., E/A ratio depicts LV diastolic dysfunction (LVDD) and E/e' ratio indicates LV filling pressures. The increased ratio of these indices depicts the progression of LVDD or HFpEF. The altered ratios of these indices are often observed in obesity; and so obesity as a disease considered to be one of the prime factor for causation of O-HFpEF. Although, the magnitude of E/e' ratio has varied over time and also in relation to different publications; in general E/e' ratio of <8 for mean of medial and lateral annuli; indicates normal LV filling pressures, whereas E/e' >10 is considered indicator of elevated LV filling pressures. In those patients where tissue Doppler was not available, other indices such as elevated E/A ratio, LA volume index (LAVI) and LV hypertrophy was considered as indicators of LVDD.[5-9]

India is presently facing a unique challenge; with increasing diagnostic facilities, the HFpEF cases are rising. India may become a global hub for HFpEF patients; not because of increasing phenotypical obesity, but due to increased prevalence of visceral obesity. Even at low body mass index (BMI) levels in contrast to western population, Indians are more prone for microvascular damage caused by epicardial adiposity. In addition to it, the western cut-off for diagnosing HFpEF often underdiagnose Indian population due to their small cardiac chamber sizes. These differences also pose therapeutic outcomes while treating "thin" Indian patients with signs/symptoms of O-HFpEF.[10-16]

PATHOPHYSIOLOGY OF OBESITY RELATED HFpEF

The effects of obesity on heart can be summarized in **Figure 1**.

Hemodynamic Stress

Increased body mass causes heart to pump more blood. This results in high cardiac output among obese patients. Plasma volume expansion occurs due to retention of sodium and water in response to activation of RAAS, sympathetic nervous system, and arginine-vasopressin

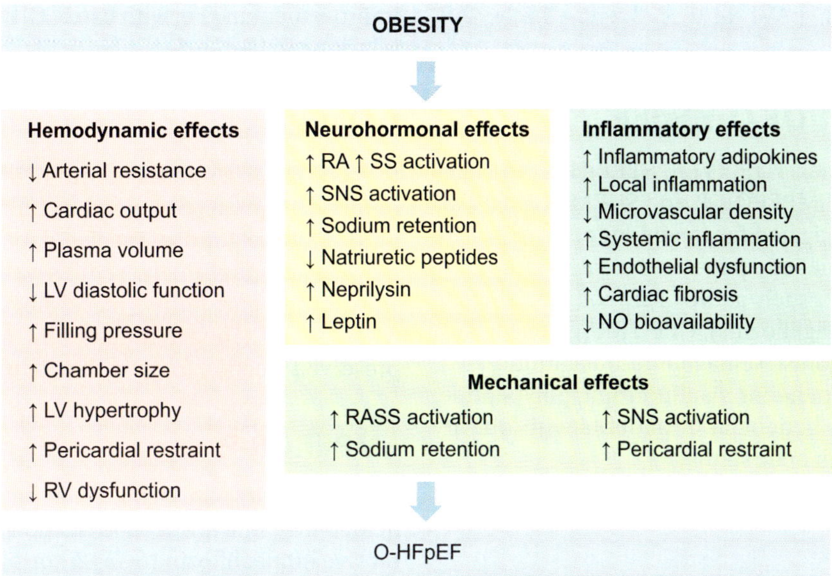

Fig. 1: Pathophysiological mechanisms leading to obesity related HFpEF.

axis. This neurohormonal activation increases systemic hypertension and so cardiac stress with high afterload, resulting in elevated LV pressures and LA dilatation.

Epicardial Adiposity

The epicardial fat around the coronary arteries and atrium is thought to be the main culprit of inducing inflammation. Many substances (such as leptin, omentin, visfatin, resistin, TNF, etc.) are found to be released by epicardial fat, that induces fibrotic changes in coronaries as well as in left atrium. Growing evidence also suggests that increased epicardial fat directly linked to atrial fibrillation (AF), heart failure, microvascular dysfunction, sudden cardiac death, and cardiomyopathies as well as predicting major adverse cardiovascular events (MACEs).[17-22]

ECHOCARDIOGRAPHY

The noninvasive diagnosis of HFpEF is often made by echocardiography. The ratio of mitral inflow and mitral annular velocities, i.e., E/e′ is often considered as a marker of HFpEF. The increased ratio of E/e′ indicates progression toward HFpEF.[23-25] *Jeannine von-der Bor et al.* studied E/e′ in children; grouped according to BMIz (WHO) in one group with a BMIz<1.04 and in other as overweight/obese with a BMIz ≥1.04 (**Fig. 2**).[26]

Giovanni Di Salvo et al. investigated 150 obese children and adolescents and showed a significant higher E/e′ ratio in obese children in comparison to a control group.[27]

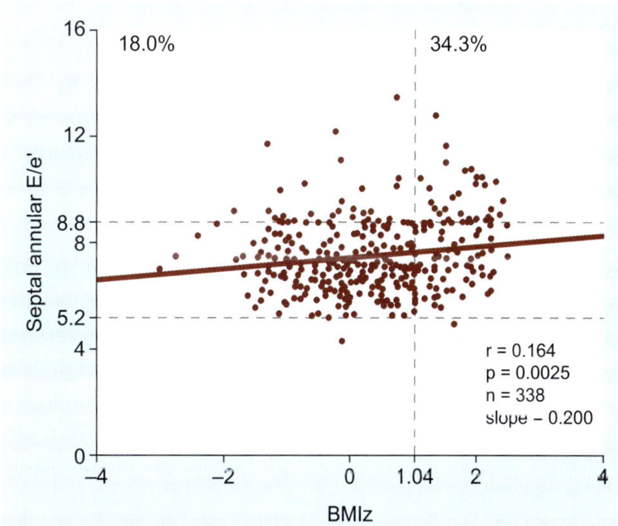

Fig. 2: Increase in BMI results in increase in E/e′.

Nowrin Kashem, et al. had also analyzed that tissue Doppler assessment showed lower e′ velocity (9.10 ± 3.76 cm/s vs. 10.50 ± 2.87 cm/s; p = 0.039) and higher E/e′ ratio (7.83 ± 2.79 vs. 6.25 ± 1.67; p = 0.001) among obese participants, consistent with impaired myocardial relaxation and elevated LV filling pressure.[28]

Joanna Bartkowia, et al. had also concluded in analysis of 457 school children that the mean mitral E/E′ ratio and LAVI were significantly higher in obese than those in nonobese individuals (E/E′: 5.2 ± 1.1 vs. 4.9 ± 0.8,

p adjusted = 0.043; LAVI 11.0 ± 3.2 vs. 9.6 ± 2.9, p adjusted = 0.001).[29]

MANAGEMENT OF O-HFpEF

Many randomized trials (DELIVER, STEP-HFpEF, STEP-HFpEF-DM, SUMIT, EMPEROR-P, and SURMOUNT-Trial) that were initially instigated for treatment of heart failure in diabetic and nondiabetic patients; revealed that many of antidiabetic drugs such as SGLT2i (sodium-glucose co-transporter 2, dapagliflozins), GLP-1RA (glucagon-like peptide-1 receptor agonist; semaglutide, dulaglutide, etc.), and GIP (glucose-dependent insulinotropic polypeptide; tirzepatide) are also beneficial in patients with obesity irrespective of their diabetic status.[30-36]

STEP-HFpEF

This trial conducted on 529 obese persons with HFpEF to evaluate the efficacy of semaglutide. The study was observed for 52 weeks and concluded that semaglutide (*GLP-1RA*) was effective in improving the life quality of life, physical limitations, hospital readmissions as well as weight reduction and reductions in symptoms. In addition to it, echocardiographic substudy of this trail also concluded that treatment with semaglutide significantly decreases E/A ratio, as well as E/e' ratio (improvement in diastolic dysfunction), in comparison to placebo group.[37]

STEP-HFpEF-DM

Similar to STEP-HFpEF trial, it was conducted on 616 obese diabetic patients with HFpEF. The end points resulted in larger reductions in heart failure-related symptoms and physical limitations and greater weight loss than placebo at 1 year. *Paolo Basile et al.* in their small pilot study concluded that treatment with *GLP-1RA* in diabetic patients largely improves LV global longitudinal strain (LV-GLS);[38] *Jong Shin Woo et al.* assessed the effectiveness of GLP-1RAs in patients with ST-segment-elevation MI and primary percutaneous coronary intervention. In this study, Exenatide *(GLP-1RA)* therapy was associated with lower cardiac enzyme values, lower E/e' values, better global longitudinal strain and global circumferential strain than of control group.[39]

SUMMIT and SURMOUNT

In these international, double-blind, randomized, placebo-controlled trials, obese patients with HFpEF received tirzepatide (*GIP*) for 1 year. Treatment with tirzepatide led to lower MACEs and improved health status in patients with O-HFpEF. The echocardiographic evidence by improvement in E/e' with use of GIP in O-HFpEF however is lacking in literature.

DELIVER

In this trial, 6,263 patients with heart failure and a mildly reduced or preserved ejection fraction (EF >40%) were randomly assigned to receive dapagliflozin (*SGLT2i*) or placebo. Dapagliflozin reduced the combined risk of worsening heart failure or cardiovascular death among patients with heart failure and a mildly reduced or preserved ejection fraction than of placebo group.

EMPEROR-P

In this double-blind trial, 5,988 patients with class II–IV heart failure and an ejection fraction of >40% to assigned to receive empagliflozin (*SGLT2i*) or placebo. Empagliflozin reduced the combined risk of cardiovascular death or hospitalization for heart failure in patients with heart failure and a preserved ejection fraction, regardless of the presence or absence of diabetes.

Tanaka et al. analyzed in prospective multicenter study the effect of dapagliflozin on LV diastolic function in patients with T2DM and stable heart failure. This study concluded that dapagliflozin promoted improvement in LV longitudinal myocardial function and improvement in LV diastolic function. There was a significant decrease in E/e' after 6 months of therapy.[40]

Prochaska et al. in their randomized, double-masked, controlled clinical trial, evaluated the effectiveness of empagliflozin compared to the placebo group on left ventricular diastolic function in patients with type 2 diabetes mellitus and elevated left ventricular end-diastolic pressure covered by the *EmDia clinical trial.* After 12 weeks of intervention, empagliflozin resulted in a significantly greater decrease in the E/e' ratio compared to placebo.[41]

Many of such landmark studies had shown long-term therapy with SGLT2i had resulted in markable decrease in E/e' in patients having elevated E/e'. The use of SGLT2i has been strongly recommended in many guidelines for treatment of HFpEF.

These trials led to a newer concept that antidiabetic drugs are useful in patients with O-HFpEF irrespective of their diabetic status. The efficacy of GIP/GLP-1RA and SGLT2i in treating patients with O-HFpEF is well established in many of earlier sited studies. These group of drugs not only help in weight reduction but also reduce the LV filling pressures and improves cardiac remodeling. Though recognized initially as "antidiabetic drugs"; these drugs now has extended role in patients with O-HFpEF irrespective of their diabetic status. Such conclusions had led to new era of treatment in patients with HFpEF.[42]

THE INDIAN PERSPECTIVE

As per the WHO, the obesity is defined as having BMI >30 kg/m^2. Most of the international trails also defines obesity as per earlier-mentioned guidelines only, but in case of Indians these guidelines underdiagnose the problem. The obesity-related heart failure for Indians is more common even at BMI >25 kg/m^2 (newer guidelines for Indians).[43-50] Many studies had shown that LVDD is common in Indians with BMI >25. *Manish Chandey et al.* described in their study that all patients who were having BMI >25 were shown to have LVDD. *C Mamatha Shree et al.* had shown that LVDD and LV filling pressures (E/e') was more prevalent in obese hypertensive patients than of nonobese hypertensives. Similarly, Shubhda *Gade et al.* also confirmed that the indices of contractility such as ejection fraction and mitral inflow velocities (E/A ratio as well as E/e') were significantly altered in obese subjects as compared to nonobese subjects. *Shobitha Muthukrishnan et al.* described lower heart rate variability in obese patients indicating altered autonomous nervous system among obese Indian subjects at BMI >25 kg/m^2.[7,12,51,52]

All these studies indicates, as compared to obese western population, Indians develop clinical signs of heart failure early. The obesity in India is growing fast, the latest national survey (National Family Health Survey-5, NFHS-5) concluded that obesity is more prevalent in Indian women than men (40% vs. 12%). Thus, the prevalence and burden of HFpEF among Indians is also increasing. The increasing obesity and early onset of metabolic dysfunctions challenges the treatment strategies.

The study, *ICMR-INDIAB 23,* is one of the detailed study of Indian population which revealed that metabolic disarray was present in both group of patients with BMI >25 kg/m^2 and in some patients with BMI < 25 kg/m^2. This study further unmask the iceberg problem of cardiometabolic problem among Indian population who are nonobese ("thin-fat" phenotype—characterized by a normal body weight but a high body fat percentage). Phenotypical obesity though increasing in India, but lean Indians also suffer with cardiac issues that leads to HFpEF. This is hypothesized due to epicardial adiposity. Diagnosing epicardial adiposity is another challenge in India due to lack of diagnostic facilities. This postulates that Indians (South Asians) are more prone for metabolic syndromes including cardiovascular and type 2 diabetes.[53-58]

This Indian phenotype and modified obesity grading of WHO (BMI >25 kg/m^2) for Indians had posed a unique challenge in treatment. Most of studies had advocated the use of antidiabetics and GIP/GLP-1 agonists for O-HFpEF with BMI >30 kg/m^2 (international criteria); whereas the Indian perspective obesity is at BMI >25 kg/m^2.

IS Kochar et al. had concluded the usefulness of GLP-1 agonists in weight reduction among Indian adolescents with BMI >27 kg/m^2. *EV Stryukova et al.* had shown that obese patients with BMI>25, have low levels of GIP/GLP hormones, which are inversely associated with the risk of having vulnerable atherosclerotic plaque.[59,60]

Liraglutide (*GLP-1RA*) Effect and Action in Diabetes (LEAD) program had also predicted cardiovascular benefits along with weight loss and improves β-cell function with use of liraglutide in type 2 diabetic patients.

However, since the phenotypical obesity as well as visceral adiposity being much more prevalent in India; many of such studies indicate the potential utility of GIP/GLP agonist medications for patients with obesity in India irrespective of their diabetic status with BMI >25 kg/m^2. Authors do recommend the use of GIP/GLP agonists for weight reduction in Indian patients. Owing to improvement in diagnostic facilities in India as well as change in lifestyle; the incidence of O-HFpEF is also increasing. Use of GIP/GLP agonist drugs not only help in reducing weight but also reduce epicardial/visceral fat and so symptoms/signs of HFpEF. The use of SGLT2i in patients with obesity is also important, but the weight loss is lower than of GIP/GLP drugs; however, the cardiovascular protection effect is thought to be better with SGLT2i than of GIP/GLP agonists. Thus, the choice is often goal oriented; for mild to moderate weight loss and for strong cardiovascular protection; SGLT2i is preferred, whereas for weight loss as primary goal GIP/GLP agonists are preferred. Authors recommend primarily use of GIP/GLP agonist among Indian patients with BMI >23 kg/m^2 with HFpEF or BMI >25 kg/m^2 with/without HFpEF with primary goal of visceral fat reduction. The use of SGLT2i may be recommended in addition to conventional antidiabetic drugs in diabetic patients, who are at more risk of HFpEF.

The impact of E/e' ratio >10 or the impact of E/e' ratio <10; in such patients being categorized as "obesity paradox"; is yet to be fully documented or appreciated.[61-64]

CONCLUSION

- Indians are more prone for obesity-induced diseases such as diabetes, HFpEF, hypertension, and atherosclerosis. Theses obesity-related diseases appear early in Indians than of western population. Thus, the obesity is considered at BMI >25 kg/m^2 in Indian continent whereas in western BMI >30 kg/m^2.
- Epicardial/visceral adiposity is considered as the main causes of cardiovascular events occurring

early in Indian patients as compared to western population. The "thin-fat" phenotype recognized in Indian population is more vulnerable population for cardiovascular diseases.

- The newer "antidiabetic drugs", viz., GIP/GLP-1RA/SGLT2i are now recommended for use of weight reduction and to improve LV filling pressures in obese patients irrespective of their diabetic status.
- As the signs/symptoms of O-HFpEF in Indian patients sets early at BMI >25 kg/m^2; these drugs are recommended for weight reductions and improvement in signs/symptoms of HFpEF.

REFERENCES

1. Binu AJ, Srinath SC, Cherian KE, et al. A Pilot Study of Electrocardiographic Features in Patients with Obesity from a Tertiary Care Centre in Southern India (Electron). Med Sci (Basel). 2022;10:56.
2. Kossaify A, Nicolas N. Impact of Overweight and Obesity on Left Ventricular Diastolic Function and Value of Tissue Doppler echocardiography. Cardiology. 2013;7:43-50.
3. Banerjee S, Kumar P, Srivastava S, et al. Association of anthropometric measures of obesity and physical activity with cardio-vascular diseases among older adults: Evidence from across-sectional survey, 2017–18. PLoS One. 2021;16(12):e0260148.
4. Seo JS, Jin HY, Jang JS, et al. The Relationships between Body Mass index and Left Ventricular Diastolic Function in a Structurally Normal Heart with Normal Ejection Fraction. J Cardiovasc Ultrasound. 2017;25(1):5-11.
5. Gupta RD, Tamanna N, Siddika N, et al. Obesity and Abdominal Obesity in Indian Population: Findings from a Nationally Representative Study of 698,286 Participants. Epidemiologia (Basel) 2023;4:163-72.
6. Saito Y, Obokata M. Diagnostic and therapeutic implications of obesity in heart failure with preserved ejection fraction. Eur J Heart Fail. 2024;26:190-2.
7. Gade S, Sahasrabuddhe AV, Mohite KA, et al. Effect of Obesity on Left Ventricular Systolic and Diastolic Functions Based on Echocardiographic Indices. Cureus. 2023;15(4):e37232.
8. Sharma AK, Kumar H, Razi MM, et al. To determine the correlation between echocardiographic diastolic parameters and invasively measured left ventricular end diastolic pressure in patients with heart failure with preserved ejection fraction- an observational, descriptive study. (CEAL-HFpEF study). Indian Heart J.2021;73:470-5.
9. Liyun L, Songbiao L, Chengshan W, et al. Left Ventricular Diastolic Dysfunction and Obesity: A Systematic Review and Meta-analysis of Echocardiographic Studies. Int J Cardiovasc Cerebrovasc Dis. 2016;4:27-34.
10. Sundaresan M, Velmurugan G, Dhivakar M, et al. Differential Prevalence of Overweight and Obesity, Hypertension and Diabetes in South India: A Population Based Cross-Sectional Study. Global Heart. 2024;19(1):72.
11. Singh G, Agrawal R, Tripathi N, et al. Overweight and obesity, the clock ticking in India? A secondary analysis of trends of prevalence, patterns, and predictors from 2005 to 2020 using the National Family Health Survey. Int J Noncommun Dis. 2023;8:31-45.
12. Muthukrishnan S, Vashishta S, Bhat S. The impact of overweight–obesity on heart rate variability among Indian adults—A cross-sectional study. J Family Med Prim Care. 2025;14:1952-7.
13. Lumori BAE, Nuwagira E, Abeya FC, et al. Association of body mass index with left ventricular diastolic dysfunction among ambulatory individuals with diabetes mellitus in rural Uganda: a cross-sectional study. BMC Cardiovasc Disord. 2022;22(1):279.
14. Ahirwar R, Mondal PR. Prevalence of obesity in India: A systematic review. Diabetes Metab Syndr. 2019;13:318-21.
15. Chaudhary M, Sharma P. Abdominal obesity in India: analysis of the National Family Health Survey-5 (2019–2021) data. Lancet Reg Health Southeast Asia. 2023;14:100208.
16. Mishra S, Murry B, Devi NK, et al. Obesity in dyslipidemia and hypertension: A study among young adults of Delhi/NCR. Clin Epidemiol Glob Health. 2023;22:101335.
17. Shen Q, Hiebert JB, Rahman FK, et al. Understanding Obesity-Related High Output Heart Failure and Its implications. Int J Heart Fail. 2021;3(3):160-71.
18. Rodrigues MM, Falcão LM. Pathophysiology of heart failure with preserved ejection fraction in overweight and obesity - Clinical and treatment implications. Int J Cardiol. 2025;430:133182.
19. Zhou Y, Yan H, Zhu Y, et al. Multifactorial mechanisms of obesity-related HFpEF: the central role of epicardial adipose tissue and therapeutic perspectives. Front Cardiovasc Med. 2025;12:1701459.
20. Dronkers J, van Veldhuisen DJ, van der Meer P, et al. Heart Failure and Obesity: Unraveling Molecular Mechanisms of Excess Adipose Tissue. J Am Coll Cardiol. 2024;84(17):1666-77.
21. Aurigemma GP, de Simone G, Fitzgibbons TP. Cardiac Remodeling in Obesity. Circ Cardiovasc Imaging. 2013;6(1):142-52.
22. Heidenreich P. Weight Loss and Cardiac Reverse Remodeling. J Am Coll Cardiol. 2022;80(16):1513-5.
23. Singh M, Sethi A, Mishra AK, et al. Echocardiographic Imaging Challenges in Obesity: Guideline Recommendations and Limitations of Adjusting to Body Size. J Am Heart Assoc. 2020;9:e014609.
24. Mei J, Li Y, Dong J, et al. Impacts of obesity on global subclinical left cardiac function represented by CMR-derived myocardial strain, TyG index may be a predictor. Sci Rep. 2023;13(1):16031.
25. Russo C, Jin Z, Homma S, et al. Effect of Obesity and Overweight on Left Ventricular Diastolic Function A Community-Based Study in an Elderly Cohort. J Am Coll Cardiol. 2011;57:1368-74.
26. von-der Born J, Baberowski S, Memaran N, et al. Impact of Sex and Obesity on Echocardiographic

Parameters in Children and Adolescents. Pediatr Cardiol. 2022;43(7):1502-16.

27. Di Salvo G, Pacileo G, Del Giudice EM, et al. Abnormal myocardial deformation properties in obese, non-hypertensive children: an ambulatory blood pressure monitoring, standard echocardiographic, and strain rate imaging study. Eur Heart J. 2006;27(22):2689-95.
28. Kashem N, Ahmed F, Tanu S, et al. Effects of body mass index on left ventricular function: An echocardiographic comparison between obese and nonobese individuals. Physiol Rep. 2025;13(24):e70705.
29. Bartkowiak J, Spitzer E, Kurmann R, et al. The impact of obesity on left ventricular hypertrophy and diastolic dysfunction in children and adolescents. Sci Rep. 2021;11:13022.
30. Kosiborod MN, Abildstrøm SZ, Borlaug BA, et al. Semaglutide in Patients with Heart Failure with Preserved Ejection Fraction and Obesity. N Engl J Med. 2023;389:1069-84.
31. Kumbhani DJ, Eagle KA. Semaglutide Treatment Effect in People With Obesity and Heart Failure With Preserved Ejection Fraction and Diabetes Mellitus - STEP-HFpEF DM. N Engl J Med. 2024;390:1394-407.
32. Milton Packer, Zile MR, Kramer CM, et al. Tirzepatide for Heart Failure with Preserved Ejection Fraction and Obesity. N Engl J Med. 2025;392:427-37.
33. Le Roux C, Zhang S, Aronne LJ, et al. Tirzepatide for the Treatment of Obesity: Rationale and Design of the SURMOUNT Clinical Development Program. Obesity. Obesity (Silver Spring). 2023;31(1):96-110.
34. Jastreboff AM, Aronne LJ, Ahmad NN, et al. Tirzepatide Once Weekly for the Treatment of Obesity. N Engl J Med. 2022;387:205-16.
35. Solomon SD, McMurray JJV, Claggett B, et al. Dapagliflozin in Heart Failure with Mildly Reduced or Preserved Ejection Fraction. N Engl J Med. 2022;387:1089-98.
36. Anker SD, Butler J, Filippatos G, et al. Empagliflozin in Heart Failure with a Preserved Ejection Fraction. N Engl J Med. 2021;385:1451-61.
37. Solomon SD, Ostrominski JW, Wang X, et al. Effect of Semaglutide on Cardiac Structure and Function in Patients With Obesity-Related Heart Failure. J Am Coll Cardiol. 2024;84(17):1587-602.
38. Basile P, Guaricci AI, Piazzolla G, et al. Improvement of Left Ventricular Global Longitudinal Strain after 6-Month Therapy with GLP-1RAs Semaglutide and Dulaglutide in Type 2 Diabetes Mellitus: A Pilot Study. J Clin Med. 2023;12(4):1586.
39. Woo JS, Kim W, Ha SJ, et al. Cardioprotective effects of exenatide in patients with ST-segment-elevation myocardial infarction undergoing primary percutaneous coronary intervention: results of exenatide myocardial protection in revascularization study. Arterioscler Thromb Vasc Biol. 2013;33(9):2252-60.
40. Tanaka H, Soga F, Tatsumi K, et al. Positive effect of dapagliflozin on left ventricular longitudinal function for type 2 diabetic mellitus patients with chronic heart failure. Cardiovasc Diabetol. 2020;19:6.
41. Prochaska JH, Jünger C, Schulz A, et al. Effects of empagliflozin on left ventricular diastolic function in addition to usual care in individuals with type 2 diabetes mellitus-results from the randomized, double-blind, placebo-controlled EmDia trial. Clin Res Cardiol. 2023;112(7):911-22.
42. Garg N. Effects of SGLT2i and GLP-1RA on Epicardial Fat, New Delhi: Jaypee Brothers Medical Publishers (P) Ltd.; 2025.
43. Ibrahim R, William P. Managing Obesity in Heart Failure: Latest Evidence and Knowledge Gaps. Curr Treat Options Cardiovasc Med. 2024;26:355-67.
44. Powell-Wiley TM, Poirier P, Burke LE, et al. Obesity and Cardiovascular Disease a Scientific Statement from the American Heart Association. Circulation. 2021;143:e984-1010.
45. Deshpande A, Shah NS, Kandula NR. Obesity and Cardiovascular Risk among South Asian Americans. Curr Cardiovasc Risk Rep. 2023;17(3):73-82.
46. Albakri A. Obesity cardiomyopathy: a review of literature on clinical status and meta-analysis of diagnostic and clinical management. Med Clin Arch. 2018;2:39.
47. Martinez-Amezcua P, Haque W, Khera R, et al. The Upcoming Epidemic of Heart Failure in South Asia. Circ Heart Fail. 2020;13:e007218.
48. Bays HE, Shrestha A, Niranjan V, et al. Obesity Pillars Roundtable: Obesity and South Asians. Obes Pillars. 2022;1:100006.
49. Misra A, Vikram NK, Ghosh A, et al. Revised definition of obesity in Asian Indians living in India. Diabetes Metab Syndr. 2025;19(1):102989.
50. Aziz N, Kallur SD, Nirmalan PK, et al. Implications of the Revised Consensus Body Mass Indices for Asian Indians on Clinical Obstetric Practice. J Clin Diagn Res. 2014;8(5):OC01-3.
51. Chandey M, Kamboj R, Vaid A, et al. A Study of the Impact of Body Mass Index on Diastolic Function in Patients with Normal Left Ventricular Ejection Fraction. AMEI's Curr Trends Diagn Treat. 2020;4(1):17-20.
52. Mamatha SC, Ks P, B G. Effect of obesity and hypertension on left ventricular geometry and function among asymptomatic Indian adults. Bioinformation. 2024;20(8):862-7.
53. Mohan D, Pradeepa R, Venkatesan U, et al. High prevalence of metabolic obesity in India: The ICMR-INDIAB national study (ICMR-INDIAB-23). Indian J Med Res. 2025;161:461-72.
54. Kittleson MM, Benjamin EJ, Blumer V, et al. 2025 ACC Scientific Statement on the management of Obesity in Adults With Heart Failure: A Report of the American College of Cardiology. J Am Coll Cardiol. 2025;86(20):1953-75.
55. Kapoor N. Thin Fat Obesity: The Tropical Phenotype of Obesity. South Dartmouth (MA): MDText.com, Inc.; 2021.

56. Balaji K, Chahil V, Shakoor A, et al. Inflammation and cardiometabolic disease in South Asians: The fire and fire tenders. J Clin Lipidol. 2025.
57. Savarese G, Schiattarella GG, Lindberg F, et al. Heart failure and obesity: Translational approaches and therapeutic perspectives. A scientific statement of the Heart Failure Association of the ESC. Eur J Heart Fail. 2025;27(7):1273-93.
58. Harrington J, Felker GM, Lingvay I, et al. Managing Obesity in Heart Failure A Chance to Tip the Scales? JACC Heart Fail. 2024;12:28-34.
59. Kochar IS, Sethi A. Efficacy and safety of liraglutide in Indian adolescents with obesity. Obes Sci Pract. 2019;5(3):251-7.
60. Garbuzova Striukova EV, Shramko VS, Kashtanova EV, et al. Adipokine-Cytokine Profile in Patients with Unstable Atherosclerotic Plaques and Abdominal Obesity. Int J Mol Sci. 2023;24(10):8937.
61. Marso SP, Daniels GH, Brown-Frandsen K, et al. Liraglutide and Cardiovascular Outcomes in Type 2 Diabetes. N Engl J Med. 2016;375:311-22.
62. Nagarajan V, Kohan L, Holland E, et al. Obesity paradox in heart failure: a heavy matter. ESC Heart Fail. 2016;3:227-34.
63. Reinhardt M, Schupp T, Abumayyaleh M, et al. Obesity Paradox in Heart Failure with Mildly Reduced Ejection Fraction. Pragmat Obs Res. 2024;15:31-43.
64. Packer M, Butler J, Lam CSP, et al. Central Adiposity or Hypertension: Which Drives Heart Failure With a Preserved Ejection Fraction? J Am Coll Cardiol. 2025;86(20): 1935-49.

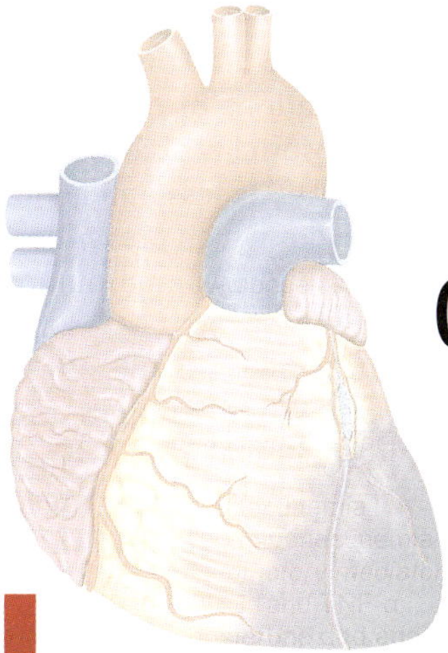

24

CHAPTER

Obesity and Left Ventricular Hypertrophy: The Link Unraveled

S Shanmugasundaram

INTRODUCTION

Obesity is widely prevalent across all countries contributing to a wide variety of health hazards that include metabolic syndrome, type 2 diabetes mellitus, systemic hypertension (SHT), atherosclerotic cardiovascular disease (ASCVD) which includes coronary artery disease (CAD), peripheral arterial disease (PAD) and stroke, heart failure, particularly the phenotype with preserved ejection fraction (HFpEF), cancers, neurological disorders, chronic lung diseases, and digestive disorders. The prevalence of overweight and obesity has almost doubled in the last three decades with one out of eight suffering from obesity. Nearly 43% of adults are overweight and 16% are obese. What was once a problem of developed countries some years ago is becoming common in low- and middle-income countries, because of globalization and industrialization. Low- and middle-income countries have to face both the extremes of nutrition, malnutrition among the underprivileged and obesity among the privileged people. Left ventricular hypertrophy (LVH) occurs commonly among the obese and contributes to heart diseases, mainly heart failure and arrhythmias. The mechanisms of LVH in obesity are multifactorial and it is recognized as a strong surrogate marker for increased cardiovascular risk in them.

OBESITY AS A CARDIOVASCULAR RISK FACTOR

Nearly one third in the population is either overweight or obese and obesity-related conditions are some of the leading causes of death. Obesity is one of the modifiable conventional risk factors for ASCVD. The causes for increased prevalence of ASCVD, atrial fibrillation, sudden death, and heart failure among obese include higher prevalence of other ASCVD risk factors such as diabetes, hypertension, physical inactivity, dietary indiscretion, as well as the proinflammatory milieu of obesity. Metabolic syndrome and type 2 diabetes are the consequences of increased visceral fat, both of which may lead to insulin resistance and increase the CV risk. Obese individuals are three times more likely to develop diabetes than normal-weight individuals (20~7.3%). About 80–85% of diabetics are overweight or obese. The relative risk of developing hypertension among obese is 78% in men and 65% in women. The increased blood volume, cardiac output, and higher arterial stiffness contribute to development of hypertension. Retroperitoneal fat excess may compress renal vasculature and nerves and may increase the plasma renin activity, angiotensinogen, angiotensin-converting enzyme activity, angiotensin II, and aldosterone, all of which lead to hypertension. Obstructive sleep apnea (OSA) which may increase sympathetic activity, insulin resistance, and hyperleptinemia is an additional source for increased arterial pressure in obese. LDL cholesterol level generally does not show linear relationship with BMI but atherogenic dyslipidemia (increased triglyceride, VLDL, and small dense LDL particles with lower HDL levels) is common among obese. The incidence rate ratios for CAD in obese subjects are 1.81 (M) and 2.69 (F); stroke 1.51 (M) and 1.49 (F); heart failure 1.79 (M) and 1.78 (F); and pulmonary embolism 3.51 (M) and 3.51 (F).[1]

MEASURES OF OBESITY

The severity of obesity is indirectly assessed by anthropometric measurements, among which body mass index (BMI) or Quetelet index is popular. BMI is the ratio of body weight in kilograms divided by height in meters squared. In the Western population, BMI of 18.5–24.9 is considered normal weight, 25–29.9 as overweight, and ≥30 as obesity. In the Asian population, BMI of 18.5–22.9 is considered as normal, 23–24.9 as overweight, ≥25 as obesity, and ≥27.5 as high-risk obesity. However, BMI does not take into account the height or body frame; hence, a tall, muscular person with a larger body frame may have a high BMI but with no increased adiposity. Moreover, there are subjects with overall obesity with predominant accumulation in subcutaneous tissue in the hip, buttocks, thighs, and arms in whom BMI is a poor indicator of harmful visceral adiposity. On the contrary, there are some with normal weight or lean but with increased visceral fat in whom BMI may be misleadingly normal or low. The extent of abdominal (visceral) obesity is better assessed by waist circumference (WC) and waist/hip ratio (WHR). In Western population, WC ≥94 cm in men and ≥80 cm is considered abnormal. Much higher risk is encountered when WC exceeds 102 cm in men and 88 cm in women. Lower thresholds are used for Asians; ≥90 cm in men and >80 cm in women. Much lower thresholds are proposed for Indians; ≥78 cm in men and ≥72 cm in women. The other measure of abdominal obesity is WHR—the ratio of WC (measured midway between lower margin of rib cage and iliac crest) to the hip circumference (measured at the level of maximum size of buttocks). WHR of ≥0.90 in men and ≥0.85 in women is considered abnormal. In recent times, waist-height ratio (WHtR) has been given importance because of its simplicity of measurement and applicability in all races, both in children and adults and in both sexes. A value of ≥0.5 is considered abnormal. BMI seems to be a marker of general obesity while WC, WHR, and WHtR are markers of abdominal obesity.

PREVALENCE AND IMPORTANCE OF LEFT VENTRICULAR HYPERTROPHY IN OBESITY

It is important to recognize the presence, extent, and pattern of LVH in obese because of prognostic implications. In obese subjects, LVH is induced by various hemodynamic and metabolic factors. LVH is accompanied by varying degrees of diastolic dysfunction which eventually promotes the development of HFpEF. Prevalence of HFpEF is increasing and is becoming more common than the other phenotype, namely heart failure with reduced ejection fraction (HFrEF). Adverse outcomes like worsening of heart failure leading to unplanned visits to emergency rooms and hospitalizations or cardiovascular deaths are common in HFpEF. Mortality exceeds 50% at 5 years of diagnosis. Because HFpEF is less amenable to treatment, prevention is a priority for which prevention and management of LVH and diastolic dysfunction are essential.

In a meta-analysis of 22 studies with 5,486 obese subjects, LVH was present in 56%. When compared to nonobese individuals, obese individuals had a relative risk of 4.19 for manifesting LVH. LV mass (LVM) index ranged from 91 to 194 g/m^2 and from 43 to 73 g/h$^{2.7}$ in various studies that were included. In the studies that indexed LVM to BMI, LVH prevalence ranged from 22 to 67%. When LVM was indexed to height$^{2.7}$, LVH was reported in 20–85%. There appeared to be a positive correlation between LVM and BMI. In that study, the presence of SHT failed to show an increased prevalence of LVH.[2]

In populations with a high prevalence of obesity, the population risk attributable to LV hypertrophy when LVM was normalized to height$^{2.7}$ is much greater than with normalization for body surface area (BSA) or height as a linear measure or using other allometric signals. Using LV mass/height$^{2.7}$, the prevalence of LV hypertrophy ranges between 13% in obese, normotensive individuals, and over 75% in individuals with morbid obesity, in the presence of hypertension.[3]

Left Ventricular Hypertrophy as a Risk Predictor

In general, LVH predicts increased risk for clinical events such as CAD, heart failure, and atrial fibrillation irrespective of the presence of CAD or SHT. In the meta-analysis of 20 studies with 48,545 subjects, the presence of LVH diagnosed by ECG or ECHO predicted increased risk of cardiovascular morbidity (OR 1.5–3.5 with a weighted mean risk rate ratio of 2.3) and increased risk of all-cause mortality (OR 1.5–8.0 with weighted mean risk ratio of 2.5).[4] Risk prediction appears to be independent of race, the presence of hypertension, or CAD, or between clinical and epidemiologic studies. There is a trend toward a worse outlook among women.

In those with obesity, the occurrence of LVH is one of the reasons for increased mortality and higher rate of cardiovascular events. LVH tends to manifest commonly in metabolically unhealthy obese but less often in metabolically healthy obese. The cross-sectional study of 10,804 adults in China revealed an odds ratio (OR) for LVH of 2.675 among the metabolically unhealthy nonobese persons, OR of 9.067 among metabolically unhealthy obese, and an OR of 1.968 for metabolically healthy obese. Among the five components of metabolic abnormalities, hypertension and WC were significantly associated with LVH.[5] While detection of the presence of LVH is used for risk prediction, the pattern of LV remodeling or alteration of geometry provides additional prognostic information. In a network meta-analysis of 22 echocardiographic studies (76,142 subjects of diverse cardiovascular diseases), concentric LVH (cLVH) was associated with the highest risk for all-cause mortality (OR 1.97) followed by eccentric hypertrophy (OR 1.71) and concentric remodeling (OR 1.56).[6]

Detection of Left Ventricular Hypertrophy

ECG and ECHO are the conventional methods used for diagnosis of LVH. Though ECG is less sensitive for detection of LVH when compared to ECHO, the widespread availability and simplicity of ECG allow it to be a commonly used tool for the diagnosis of LVH. At present, 37 different ECG criteria have been endorsed by the American Heart Association, a figure that suggests wide variability of sensitivity and specificity of each criterion that leads to uncertainty and lack of consensus among clinicians.[7] Commonly used ECG criteria for LVH include Sokolow-Lyon voltage criteria (R in V5 or V6 + S in V1 >3.5 mV); Cornell criteria (R in aVL + S in V3 >2.8 mV for men and >2.0 for women); R in aVL >1.1 mV; R in lead I >1.4 mV; and Romhilt-Estes criteria which uses voltage criteria with left axis deviation, ST-T changes, left atrial abnormality, QRS duration, and R peak time. The specificity of the Cornell voltage criteria, the method considered to be the most accurate, is approximately 90%, but the sensitivity is poor ranging from 20 to 40%. In Peguero and Lo Presti criteria, deepest S in any lead is added to S in V4. A value of >28 mm for men and >23 mm in women is considered to indicate LVH. The sensitivity of this sign is 70% and the specificity is 89%.[8]

Echocardiography is superior in the detection of LVH with a sensitivity of 80% and specificity of 90%. LVH is diagnosed in ECHO by measuring LVM. The formula of Devereux used for estimation of LVM from LV linear dimensions in M-mode is based on modeling the LV as a prolate ellipse and assumes that the major/minor axis ratio is 2:1. $LVM = 0.8 \{1.04[(LVIDd + PW + IVSd)^3 (LVIDd)^3]\} + 0.6$ g. LVM is standardized to either BSA or height. LVM of >95 g/m^2 (>44 g/ht$^{2.7}$) in females and >110 g/m^2 (48 g/ht$^{2.7}$) in males is considered to indicate LVH. This method is inaccurate in a distorted LV. LVM indexed to lean body mass is the best way to compare between subjects of different habitus, but difficult to do in routine practice. Though commonly indexed to BSA, this method often underestimates LVH in obese and overweight patients. Due to these shortcomings, indexing LVM to height raised to allometric powers such as 1.7 or 2.7 is adopted as it approximates lean body mass. Raising to allometric power is done to obtain linear relationship between body size and LVM. A value of LVM/height$^{2.7}$ >48 in men and 44 in women is considered abnormal.[9] In young adults, indexing LVM to height$^{2.7}$ may not account for gender differences and may lead to misclassification of subjects with respect to the presence of LVH. Hence, it may be appropriate to index LVM to height$^{1.7}$.[10]

2D and 3D ECHO-based LVM calculations are more reliable in remodeled/deformed ventricles. For 2D-based LVM calculation, one needs to measure LV muscle area from short axis view at the level of papillary muscle and the LV cavity long axis and short axis measurements from apical four-chamber view. These values are incorporated in complex equation for area length or truncated ellipsoid methods for obtaining LVM. The upper limit of LVM calculated by 2D ECHO is 88 g/m^2 for women and 102 g/m^2 for men. 3D LVM calculations are mostly done by automated algorithms. The upper limit of LVM by 3D ECHO is 90 g/m^2 for women and 97 g/m^2 for men.

In addition to estimating LVM, the type of LV remodeling in response to increased body mass can also be identified in ECHO, akin to what has been described in states of increased afterload such as SHT or aortic stenosis. cLVH is characterized by normal cavity size, uniformly increased LV wall thickness, increased LVM, and relative wall thickness (RWT - LV posterior wall thickness × 2/LV dimension in end-diastole) of >0.42. In concentric LV remodeling (CR), LV wall thickness is increased, LVM is normal, LV cavity size is normal or reduced, and RWT is >0.42. In eccentric hypertrophy (eLVH), LV is dilated, wall thickness is normal, LVM is increased, and RWT is <0.42. Traditionally, obesity is considered to induce eccentric hypertrophy pattern because of obesity related volume overload.[3] In the meta-analysis of Cuspidi, eccentric hypertrophy was more prevalent, being present in 66% while cLVH was seen in 34%.[2] However, there is a wide variation of structural adaptations to obesity with all the three patterns of LV remodeling being described in different cohorts. In a study of 11,972 obese subjects, abnormal LV geometry was found in 49% in whom CR was the most prevalent (34%) with eLVH and cLVH detected in 7 and 8%, respectively.[11] Gender specific differences have also been observed in the type of LV remodeling in response to increased BMI. In a cardiac MRI study of 741 subjects with no cardiovascular risk factors, increased LVM was found to positively correlate with BMI. Men showed greater hypertrophic response, with LVM being +2.3 g/BMI point increase. In women, LVM increase was

+1.6 g/BMI point. Moreover, cLVH was the most common pattern in men while eLVH was common among women. Since cLVH is known to be associated with higher CV mortality, this gender difference is a probable explanation for higher risk of CV death in obese men than obese women.[12] It is also believed that in those with subcutaneous obesity, eccentric hypertrophy is common [increased cardiac output and decreased peripheral vascular resistance (PVR)] and in those with visceral obesity, cLVH (increased cardiac output with elevated arterial stiffness) is the predominant pattern of LV remodeling.

Mechanisms of Left Ventricular Hypertrophy in Obesity

In obesity, LVH is caused by hemodynamic and a variety of nonhemodynamic factors.[13] In obesity, there is disproportionate growth of adipose tissue and lean body mass with a substantial increase in their ratio. Subcutaneous fat is metabolically inert and does not require increased blood supply, while visceral fat including abdominal, mediastinal, and epicardial adipose tissue (EAT) is metabolically active performing autocrine, paracrine, and endocrine activities, thereby requiring increased blood flow, thereby imposing additional hemodynamic load on the cardiovascular system. Blood volume is increased in obesity and the cardiac output tends to be higher in them in order to meet the increased energy demands. Increased salt intake adds to the increased blood volume. Blood viscosity is higher and there is an impaired adaptation of PVR all of which increase the stroke work of left ventricle and induce hypertrophy. OSA and central apnea often coexist with obesity. Sleep disordered breathing increases sympathetic activity which increases the heart rate and PVR adding to the hemodynamic load.

In addition to the direct hemodynamic effects of obesity, hypertension which often coexists may impose an additional load to LV thereby contributing to LVH. SHT occurs in two thirds of overweight/obese individuals. Prevalence of hypertension increases with body weight. SHT has been reported to occur in 56% of overweight individuals with a 2.5-fold increase in classes I and II obesity and up to 4.5-fold increase in morbidly obese.[14] Obesity increases the risk for SHT by 65–75% which is a major contributor for cardiovascular and kidney disease. Obese people have a 3.5-fold increased likelihood of having hypertension, and for every 5% increment in weight gain, the risk of developing hypertension increases by 20–30%. The increased prevalence of SHT in obese subjects is due to various factors. Increased adipose tissue leads to higher levels of leptin which increases renal sympathetic nervous activity by stimulating pro-opiomelanocortin–melanocortin 4 receptor pathway in the central nervous system. Accumulation of excessive amounts of visceral, perirenal, and renal sinus fat exert a compressive effect on kidneys which result in activation of renin–angiotensin–aldosterone system (RAAS). Obesity may lead to relative deficiency of natriuretic hormones. In addition, adipose tissue may produce inflammatory cytokines/chemokines that lead to vascular and target organ injury which in turn exacerbate hypertension.[15]

Obesity per se may induce LVH and coexisting hypertension increases the occurrence and severity of LVH. In a cross-sectional study conducted in China, the OR for developing LVH was 3.94 for hypertension and 1.90 for global obesity and 1.45–1.69 for abdominal obesity. The OR for LVH was much higher when obesity and hypertension occurred together (nearly 10–14).[16] In a cohort of hypertensive patients, LVH was prevalent in 12% in normal weight patients, 25% of overweight patients, and 48% of obese patients.[13] It is important to recognize that even the upper limit of normal blood pressure could contribute to the occurrence of LVH. In addition, normal office blood pressure value does not rule out the contribution of blood pressure in causation of LVH, as masked hypertension is prevalent in obese. It is not exactly known how the altered hemodynamics due to obesity ± hypertension lead to altered LV geometry. In obesity, there is volume overload as a result of expanding circulating blood volume attributed to increased salt intake associated with increased food intake. Additional pressure overload often coexists and is due to increased arterial stiffness and coexisting hypertension. In addition, increased salt intake is directly linked to increased LVM irrespective of the presence of hypertension. The normal phenomenon of suppression of RAAS after salt loading is blunted in insulin-resistant obese individuals.

There are multiple nonhemodynamic or metabolic pathways by which obesity may increase LVM. These pathways are particularly active in central obesity. Visceral adipose tissue produces leptin, resistin, and adipsin and may be a source of inflammatory cytokines such as TNF and IL-6. Inflammation may lead to edema and fibrosis which may increase the wall thickness. Adipocytes may also produce mineralocorticoid-releasing factors which may lead to myocardial hypertrophy and fibrotic changes. Insulin resistance and the resultant hyperinsulinemia may also result in growth promotion in myocardium. Epicardial fat correlates with visceral obesity and apart from its infiltration into myocardium, it may also create a proinflammatory milieu in the adjacent myocardium. Release of excessive free fatty acids may exert lipotoxicity. Increased LVM in obesity may be because of hypertrophy of myocardial cells, addition of myocardial cells in series or parallel, and increase in the interstitium.[13] These hemodynamic and nonhemodynamic stimuli increase protein synthesis, induce reexpression of fetal genes, and change the expression and function of several proteins, leading to progressive alterations in the size, geometry, composition, and function of heart. At the cellular level, there is altered growth, contraction, Ca^{2+} handling, ionic flux, energy metabolism, extracellular matrix arrangement, cytoskeletal structure, collagen deposition, etc.

Increase in EAT is currently viewed as an important contributor to atrial fibrillation and CAD because of the proximity to heart. EAT may be beneficial if present in small amounts in terms of cushioning effect as well as a source of fuel for the myocardium. When present in large amounts and when metabolically active, it may prove detrimental by creating an atherogenic and proinflammatory milieu to the myocardium in proximity. Infiltration of fat into myocardium, called myocardial steatosis, may also be responsible for the apparent increase in LVM.[17] In the Multi-Ethnic Study of Atherosclerosis, both visceral obesity and subcutaneous obesity were found to correlate with LVM. But only in visceral obesity, higher LV volumes and height-indexed LVM and higher LVM to volume ratio were encountered. This association of visceral obesity with LV concentricity may be precursor to development of heart failure.[18]

THERAPEUTIC IMPLICATIONS

There is evidence that weight reduction may lead to regression of LVM, though it may be incomplete if interstitial component is the dominant cause of increased LVM. BP control may also help in reducing LVM which is again incomplete if concomitant weight loss is not achieved. Regression of LVM may be a surrogate marker for improved cardiovascular outcome. Moreover, higher levels of fitness were found to improve the global longitudinal strain of LV among the obese. However, the improved fitness did not impact the prevalence of hypertension or LVH among the obese.[19] Thus, exercise may improve cardiovascular health in obese even if weight loss is incomplete or not achievable.

CONCLUSION

There is ample evidence that LVH occurs commonly in obese for which hemodynamic, metabolic, and inflammatory factors contribute. The increased cardiovascular risk in obese is at least partly mediated by increased LVM. Apart from recognizing the increase in LVM, delineating the pattern of LV remodeling is important in prognostication. The presence of LVH, particularly the cLVH or eLVH geometry, should prompt the physician to intensify efforts to reduce body weight and aggressively control hypertension, thereby improving the cardiovascular outlook of obese subjects.

REFERENCES

1. Guh DP, Zhang W, Bansback N, et al. The incidence of co-morbidities related obesity and overweight: a systematic review and meta-analysis. BMC Public Health. 2009;9:88.
2. Cuspidi C, Rescaldani M, Sala C, et al. Left-ventricular hypertrophy and obesity: a systematic review and meta-analysis of echocardiographic studies. J Hypertens. 2014;32(1):16-25.
3. Aurigemma GP, de Simone G, Fitzgibbons TP. Cardiac remodeling in obesity. Circulation. 2013;6(1):142-52.
4. Vakili BA, Okin PM, Devereux RB. Prognostic implications of left ventricular hypertrophy. Am Heart J. 2001; 141:334-41.
5. Zhang N, Chen Y, Guo X, et al. Metabolic abnormalities, but not metabolically healthy obesity, are associated with left ventricular hypertrophy. Heart Lung Circ. 2017;26:251-7.
6. Zheng Q, Loo G, Le TT, et al. Prognosis associated with geometric patterns of left ventricular remodeling: systematic review and network meta-analysis. F1000Research. 2019;8:1130.
7. Hancock EW, Deal BJ, Mirvis DM, et al. AHA/ACCF/HRS recommendations for the standardization and interpretation of the electrocardiogram: part V: electrocardiogram changes associated with cardiac chamber hypertrophy: a scientific statement from the American Heart Association Electrocardiography and Arrhythmias Committee, Council on Clinical Cardiology; the American College of Cardiology Foundation; and the Heart Rhythm Society. Endorsed by the International Society for Computerized Electrocardiology. J Am Coll Cardiol. 2009;53:992-1002.
8. Peguero JG, Lo Presti S, Perez J, et al. Electrocardiographic criteria for left ventricular hypertrophy. J Am Coll Cardiol. 2017;69:1694-1703.
9. Marwick TH, Gillebert TC, Aurigemma G, et al. Recommendations on the use of echocardiography in adult hypertension: a report from the European Association of Cardiovascular Imaging (EACVI) and the American Society of Echocardiography (ASE). J Am Soc Echocardiogr. 2015;28:727-54.
10. Taylor HCM, Chaturvedi N, Smith GD, et al. Is height$^{2.7}$ appropriate for indexation of left ventricular mass in healthy adolescents? The importance of sex differences. Hypertension. 2023;80:2033-42.
11. Lavie CJ, Milani RV, Ventura HO, et al. Disparate effects of left ventricular geometry and obesity on mortality in patients with preserved left ventricular ejection fraction. Am J Cardiol. 2007,100(9):1460-4.
12. Rider OJ, Lewandowski A, Nethononda R, et al. Gender-specific differences in left ventricular remodelling in obesity: insights from cardiovascular magnetic resonance imaging. Eur Heart J. 2013;34(4):292-9.

13. de Simone G, Izzo R, De Luca N, et al. Left ventricular geometry in obesity: Is it what we expect? Nutr Metab Cardiovasc Dis. 2013;23:905-12.
14. Sampson UK, Edwards TL, Jahangir E, et al. Factors associated with the prevalence of hypertension in the southeastern United States: insights from 69,211 blacks and whites in the Southern Community Cohort Study. Circ Cardiovasc Qual Outcomes. 2014;7:33-54.
15. Hall JE, Mouton AJ, da Silva AA, et al. Obesity, kidney dysfunction and inflammation: interactions in hypertension. Cardiovasc Res. 2021;117:1859-76.
16. Zhang X, Li G, Zhang D, et al. Influence of hypertension and global or abdominal obesity on left ventricular hypertrophy: a cross-sectional study. J Clin Hypertens (Greenwich). 2024;26(12):1342-50.
17. Murdolo G, Angeli F, Reboldi G, et al. Left ventricular hypertrophy and obesity: only a matter of fat? High Blood Press Cardiovasc Prev. 2015;22:29-41.
18. Abbasi SA, Bluemke DA, Jerosch-Herold M, et al. Visceral obesity and left ventricular remodeling: the multi-ethnic study of atherosclerosis. Nutr Metab Cardiovasc Dis. 2015;25:667-76.
19. Halland H, Matre K, Einarsen E, et al. Effect of fitness on cardiac structure and function in overweight and obesity (the FATCOR study). Nutr Metab Cardiovasc Dis. 2019;29:710-17.

25

CHAPTER

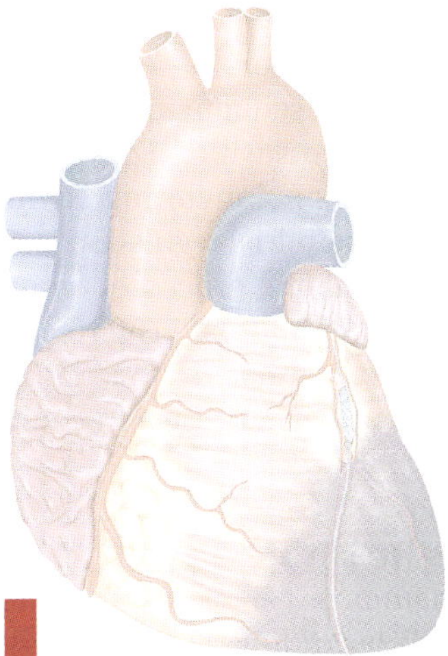

Epicardial Fat in Obesity with CVD and HFpEF: Diagnostic, Prognostic, and Therapeutic Implications

Vidyut Jain, Avani Jain

INTRODUCTION

Noninvasive imaging biomarkers can now be utilized to identify high-risk phenotypes in patients with coronary artery disease, allowing for the individualization of treatment, targeted prevention, and enhanced prognosis. Epicardial adipose tissue (EAT) serves as a visceral active fat depot, situated within the visceral layer of the pericardium and in direct contact with the myocardium and coronary arteries. This tissue and the myocardium share the same microcirculation and interact through paracrine and vasocrine pathways.[1,2]

Increasing evidence indicates that an increase in the volume of EAT leads to the release of adipokines, proinflammatory cytokines, and free fatty acids, which may influence the myocardium and contribute to the progression of coronary artery disease.[3,4] The volume of EAT is linked to various cardiovascular risk factors associated with the development and progression of not only coronary artery disease but also other cardiovascular conditions, including atrial fibrillation (AF) and heart failure.[5,6]

According to recent studies, EAT has higher rates of proinflammatory cytokine release and fatty acid degradation than subcutaneous and omental adipose tissue.[4] Although EAT contains only 1% of the overall fat mass, studies have shown that its quantity is strongly related to different cardiac and metabolic risk factors, independent of intra-abdominal visceral adiposity.[6] The majority of EAT is located in atrioventricular and interventricular grooves of the heart asymmetrically, and the association of EAT with atherosclerosis is region-specific.[7]

Macrophages in the EAT become active and contribute to the growth of atherosclerotic plaques. These macrophages can be classified into two main types: M1 and M2. M2 macrophages, which express CD206, have anti-inflammatory effects mediated by the PPARγ and IL-4-STAT6 pathways.[8,9] On the other hand, M1 macrophages, identified by their CD11c markers, use the TLR and NF-κB pathways to produce inflammatory substances such as TNF-α and IL-1β. The transformation of M1 macrophages into M2 macrophages can help to reduce inflammation and promote the healing of atherosclerotic plaques, thereby preventing the progression of atherosclerosis.[10]

Atherosclerotic plaque formation can be predicted by looking at the ratio of CD11c to CD206-positive cells, which relates to how macrophages are polarized. Research shows that vascular issues, inflammation, insulin resistance, and connections between metabolic processes play key roles in the development of coronary atherosclerosis. In cases of epicardial disease and heart attacks, this is also linked to the production of both proinflammatory and anti-inflammatory fat-related hormones, which in turn trigger macrophage activity. Higher levels of resistin in the blood and in EAT are connected to coronary artery disease and heart attacks.

The ratio of CD11c/CD206-positive cells after macrophage polarization may be used to predict the development of atherosclerotic plaque. The development of coronary atherosclerosis has been shown to be significantly influenced by vascular dysfunction, inflammation, insulin resistance, and connecting metabolic pathways. It is also linked to the development of pro- and anti-inflammatory adipocytokines and the subsequent activation of macrophages in myocardial infarction and epicardial disease. Myocardial infarction and CAD have been linked to elevated blood and EAT resistin levels.[11]

On the other hand, apelin is involved in energy metabolism and cardiovascular regulation; it is reduced in CAD patients, suggesting that it may have anti-ischemic qualities. The conflicting roles of resistin and apelin emphasize their significance in CAD pathogenesis and may lead to the discovery of novel treatment targets.[12]

Epicardial adipose tissue is located around the coronary arteries, interventricular and atrioventricular grooves, atria, right ventricle, and apex. EAT is anatomically contiguous with the underlying myocardium and shares a blood supply, allowing for paracrine signaling.[13] Primarily consisting of adipocytes, EAT also includes macrophages, lymphocytes, stromovascular cells, and nerve ganglia.[14] Physiologically, it serves as a buffer between the myocardium and excess peripheral fatty acids, reduces mechanical stress on the heart, functions as a storage of macromolecules such as free fatty acids and adiponectin (ADPN), and additionally plays a role in thermogenesis.[15]

Many explanations have been proposed to explain how elevated EAT affects heart failure with preserved ejection fraction (HFpEF) myocardial dysfunction. One is the "infiltrative lipotoxicity" paradigm, which emphasizes the paracrine activity and heart infiltration of EAT. The second is the "pericardial restraint" paradigm, which describes how cardiac function is mechanistically compromised by EAT enlargement inside a fixed pericardial space. A third possible explanation is EAT-induced alterations in left atrial function, which result in atrial arrhythmias that worsen cardiac function in HFpEF.[5]

The pathophysiologic disorders in HFpEF may be mediated by a number of mechanisms, even though this study presents each model separately. EAT typically functions as a direct modulator for paracrine signaling by secreting and releasing anti-inflammatory cytokines like ADPN. More proinflammatory and profibrotic cytokines, including interleukin-6 (IL-6), tumor necrosis factor-α (TNF-α), and monocyte chemotactic protein-1 (MCP-1), are released with EAT expansion, which alters its secretome profile.[15]

Parameters such as high EAT density, calcium score, macrophage polarization, and cytokine expression levels also contribute to the worsening of HFpEF.[16] In addition, cardiac fibrosis is ultimately caused by increased oxidative stress, mitochondrial dysfunction, and altered lipid and collagen metabolism. In addition to its paracrine and vasocrine-mediated effects, EAT may directly enter the heart and change the triglyceride content of cardiomyocytes. Age, body mass index (total adiposity), and other comorbidities are not related to these alterations, which result in diastolic dysfunction.[17]

Finally, ribonucleic acid (RNA) sequencing investigations of EAT obtained from patients with HFpEF have revealed differential expression of noncoding RNAs associated in inflammation, mitochondrial regulation, cell death, fibrosis, and primary metabolic processes when compared to individual controls without HF. The role of noncoding RNAs in EAT-mediated cardiac dysfunction is relatively poorly understood, and further research could yield new therapeutic options.[18]

PERICARDIAL RESTRICTION

Excessive EAT buildup compresses the myocardium and reduces ventricular strain and systolic function, impacting both the ventricle and atria. EAT takes up space between the visceral pericardium and myocardium. Exercise causes these changes to become more noticeable, and the patient starts to experience symptoms.[19]

Higher EAT thickness by echocardiography, along with the "square root sign" on invasive hemodynamic study, correlates well with pericardial restriction, and it also suggests increased ventricular interaction.[20] Due to poor ventricular filling and cardiac output, all of these alterations eventually result in increased sympathetic tone, volume redistribution, and venous return during exercise, aggravating pericardial limitation in HFpEF.[21] The result may explain the abnormal changes seen in HFpEF patients, such as elevated filling pressures, deteriorating peak oxygen demand, and peripheral oxygen extraction, all of which lead to exercise intolerance.[22] AF coexists with or develops in many HFpEF patients. One theory is that the atrial contractile reserve is compromised by high EAT.[23]

Therefore, in patients with concurrent HFpEF and AF, lower left atrial compliance is associated with increased pulmonary congestion and impaired exercise capacity.[24]

Additionally, AF may be linked to noncoaptation of the tricuspid and mitral valves, which can worsen pulmonary congestion and reduce cardiac output.[25]

Because of anomalies in atrial conduction caused by paracrine signaling, NLRP3 inflammasome activity, and adipose infiltration into the atrial myocardium, higher EAT in HFpEF may therefore enhance the burden of AF. By comprehending this pathophysiologic pathway, new treatment targets for atrial function in HFpEF may be investigated.[26]

DIAGNOSTIC IMAGING

It is possible to quantify EAT using a range of imaging techniques used in clinical practice, i.e., computed tomography (CT), cardiac magnetic resonance imaging (CMR), and transthoracic echocardiography (TTE). All these techniques are noninvasive. Each of these clinical imaging techniques has unique advantages and some limitations when it comes to measuring EAT.

Transthoracic echocardiography is a commonly utilized, repeatable, and readily accessible method that can be performed even at the patient's bedside. The most popular modality for evaluating EAT is TTE. EAT can occasionally exhibit greater echogenicity at higher levels or in the presence of inflammation, but it usually manifests as an anechoic region between the visceral pericardium anteriorly and the myocardium posteriorly.[27]

The two-dimensional EAT thickness can be measured at end-systole using the right ventricular free wall. There is a high association between three-dimensional volumetric measures of EAT and EAT thickness as measured by TTE. It is a readily accepted method for measuring EAT even though it is less reliable than CT and MRI, especially when it comes to interobserver and intraobserver reliability.[28]

Computed tomography and CMR are more reliable for the three-dimensional evaluation of EAT, although these procedures are time-consuming, and their cost and accessibility may prevent routine quantification of EAT. As an alternative, single-slice methods have been used, but similar to TTE, they are unable to take into consideration the different myocardial distribution of EAT, which may restrict minute variations in the overall volume of EAT.[29]

With encouraging first findings, a number of researchers have investigated how artificial intelligence and machine-based learning might be used to speed up image capture and segmentation and EAT volumetric quantification.[30,31]

The fat attenuation index, which is measured in CT Hounsfield units (HU), is another method of evaluating the features of EAT, fat density, inflammatory state, and fibrosis potential. The relative lipid content and adipocyte size within EAT volumes are described by FAI. In patients with established HFpEF, FAI may be a better predictor of cardiovascular risk than EAT volume. Increased adipocyte hypertrophy, proliferation, fibrosis, inflammation, and an increase in the amount of white adipose tissue (WAT) are hypothesized to be linked to this low-density EAT.[32]

The brown-to-white fat ratio within EAT can be distinguished using a new method that makes use of proton magnetic resonance spectroscopy. It is possible to investigate the connection between cardiac function and brown adipose tissue.[33]

Differences in heart shape may cause variations in EAT levels, and regional variations in distribution may have an impact on the accurate estimation. Additionally, it has been demonstrated that the position of EAT along the myocardium affects its protein expression, indicating the potential for activation and inhibition of several cytokine and metabolic pathways under pathological stress.[34]

Greater left ventricular mass and volume, as well as worse diastolic dysfunction when EAT directly covers the left ventricle, are linked to quantified larger regional variation in EAT among individuals with established HFpEF. Similarly, there is a strong correlation between increased EAT covering the right ventricle and deficiencies in right ventricular longitudinal strain with exercise.[35]

PROGNOSTIC IMPLICATION

Through the release of inflammatory mediators, EAT—which is regarded as a metabolically active organ—plays a crucial part in cardiovascular diseases and is connected with both vascular remodeling and oxidative stress. Adverse events are more common in patients with HFpEF due to the dysfunctional nature of EAT.[36]

The average volume of EAT is about 94 ± 40 mL, and the average volume indexed to BSA was 47 ± 18 mL/m^2. The volume of epicardial fat rose with the 10-year cardiovascular risk score, age, and male sex ($p < 0.001$ for all). EAT volume was larger in patients with obstructive coronary artery disease and increased across the coronary artery calcium score groups. Recent studies also emphasize that increased EAT harms cardiac biology, myocardial redox state, and intracellular calcium cycling.[37]

EPICARDIAL ADIPOSE TISSUE ATTENUATION

The mean EAT attenuation is -73.0 ± 5.6 HU, and it increases in elderly people ($p < 0.001$). Higher EAT attenuation is found to have a moderate link to CAD in patients with pericoronary adipose tissue attenuation and those with atherosclerotic coronary artery disease (rho = 0.51, $p < 0.001$). It was discovered that (1) the correlation between EAT volume and the composite outcome remained robust in patients with HFmrEF and HFpEF after adjusting for BMI;[2] (2) In patients with HFmrEF and HFpEF, EAT volume by CMR provides incremental prognostic value for the composite outcome; (3) Patients with high EAT are more symptomatic and regardless of obesity incidence; (4) Patients with increased EAT have lower LV GLS and higher ECV. These data support the concept that the accumulation of EAT is important in the pathophysiology and risk stratification of HFmrEF and HFpEF. Therefore, assessing EAT may be considered in the evaluation of these patients with HF.[38]

A meta-analysis of 1,939 HF patients revealed that those with AEs had a greater EAT than those without (SMD: 3.33, CI: 0.96–5.69, $p = 0.006$, I2 = 98%). The composite outcome of HF hospitalization and all-cause death (HR: 1.28, CI: 1.42–1.85, $p = 0.0002$, I2 = 93%) and HF readmission ($p < 0.001$, I2 = 10%) was also associated with increased EAT per unit.[39]

THERAPEUTIC IMPLICATION

Numerous studies have shown that the development of obesity-related cardiomyopathy is significantly influenced by the EAT. An increased risk of HFpEF and atrial arrhythmias results from EAT's direct crosstalk with the nearby myocardium, which affects both its structural integrity and electrophysiological function. There are several cardiovascular advantages of lowering EAT, particularly in people with aberrant glucolipid metabolism.[40]

NONPHARMACOLOGICAL

The mainstay of managing and preventing CVD is still changing one's lifestyle. It has been demonstrated that EAT thickness is decreased by weight loss attained through calorie restriction and increased physical activity. In overweight and somewhat obese people, a 12-week aerobic exercise program dramatically lowers EAT.[41]

Patients with AF who follow heart-healthy diets, like the Mediterranean diet, which is high in anti-inflammatory elements, have much lower levels of EAT, hence recommended.[42]

Bariatric surgery provides an additional nonpharmacological method of lowering adipose tissue depots. Bariatric surgery considerably lowers total body weight and visceral adipose tissue (VAT), but the decrease in EAT is very small and less noticeable than the loss of VAT. Additionally, myocardial triglyceride content did not change after surgery, indicating that bariatric surgery had a limited impact on cardiac ectopic fat depots.[43]

PHARMACOLOGICAL

Many studies have highlighted that the EAT plays a critical role in the development of obesity-related cardiomyopathy. EAT is involved in direct crosstalk with the adjacent myocardium, influencing both its structural integrity and electrophysiological function, leading to a higher chance of HFpEF and atrial arrhythmias. Reducing EAT has multiple cardiovascular benefits, especially in those with abnormal glucolipid metabolism. Regardless of diabetes status, selective sodium-glucose cotransporter 2 (SGLT2) inhibitors—which were first developed as oral antidiabetic medications—have shown promise as therapies for HFpEF apart from in HFrEF. Their effectiveness in lowering heart failure, cardiovascular death, and significant adverse cardiovascular events has been shown in clinical trials. Notably, regardless of weight reduction, SGLT2 inhibitors, such as dapagliflozin and empagliflozin, dramatically decrease EAT thickness or volume.[44,45]

Sodium-glucose cotransporter 2 inhibitor medication enhances cardiac glucose metabolism and increases fatty acid oxidation, lipolysis, and ketogenesis through changes in substrate use brought on by glycosuria.[46]

According to a recent study, human preadipocytes within EAT are the primary source of SGLT2 expression, which dramatically decreases as preadipocytes go through terminal differentiation. Human epicardial preadipocyte development and maturation are successfully inhibited by the SGLT2 inhibitor empagliflozin, which also improves the paracrine secretory profile of EAT by controlling IL-6 production.[47] Dapagliflozin is also able to increase the absorption of glucose in EAT, decrease the release of proinflammatory chemokines, and enhance EAT cell differentiation.[48]

A recent study demonstrated that SGLT2 inhibitors may provide benefits beyond EAT reduction, by retarding interstitial myocardial fibrosis and inflammation markers irrespective of diabetic status. The SGLT2 inhibitors have the potential to decrease EAT, improve metabolic pathways, and have a positive impact on both systolic and diastolic functions.[44]

Role of GLP-1R: In a study utilizing another oral hypoglycemic drug, it was revealed that GLP-1R expression in EAT directly correlates with genes promoting β-oxidation and white-to-brown adipocyte differentiation and is inversely correlated with proadipogenic genes. Genes involved in adipogenesis and lipid synthesis showed a positive correlation with GLP-2R expression, while genes that promote β-oxidation showed a negative correlation. Circulating levels of glucagon-like peptide-1 (GLP-1) and GLP-2 are elevated in CAD patients, particularly those with increased EAT thickness, indicating potential cardiovascular implications of these hormones.[49]

Glucagon-like peptide-1 analogs may reduce local adipogenesis and promote brown fat differentiation by targeting GLP-1R in EAT. Beyond controlling blood sugar, the GLP-1R agonists used to treat type 2 diabetes and obesity also improve cardiovascular health by reducing EAT thickness and altering metabolic pathways. GLP-1/GLP-1R in EAT can lead to improved fat utilization and the induction of brown fat differentiation, potentially contributing to overall cardiovascular benefits. Importantly, the presence of GLP-1R in human cardiomyocytes adds an intriguing dimension to the potential cardiovascular impact of these medications.[50]

Lipid-lowering drug therapy, statins, may also reduce EAT by modulating peroxisome proliferator-activated receptors (PPARs), via activation of PPARα and PPARγ, which improves insulin sensitivity and glucose uptake in EAT.[51]

Newer lipid-lowering drug, proprotein convertase subtilisin/kexin 9 (PCSK9) inhibitors, have also shown a significant reduction in EAT after a 6-month consumption (~20%), independent of low-density lipoprotein cholesterol (LDL-C) levels. These results demonstrate that effective lipid-lowering medications can reduce EAT and inflammation.[52]

FUTURE DIRECTION

Transcriptional analysis revealed that EAT displays elevated expression of the beige adipocyte-specific marker CD137, as well as the thermogenic genes *UCP-1, PRDM16, PGC-1α,* and *PPARγ* in patients who have increased EAT volume.[15]

However, the thermogenesis ability of EAT may decrease with age, obesity, and CAD.[53] Notably, there may be cardiovascular advantages to browning or beiging EAT. Adipose-derived EVs, a new type of interorgan and intercellular communication between EAT and the circulatory system, aid in the browning of WAT. A study found that macrophages get exosomes from adipose tissue-derived stem cells (ADSCs) in a one-way fashion, which polarizes them toward the anti-inflammatory M2 subtype and reduces the inflammatory component to impact EAT.[54]

Exosomes are potent cell-to-cell communication mediators that affect a number of biological processes, such as immunological regulation, inflammation, and tissue repair. Proteins, lipids, and RNAs (microRNAs) are examples of bioactive substances found in these vesicles that can affect the behavior of nearby or even distant cells. Cardiac EVs, which have proinflammatory qualities and worsen heart injury, are released more often during myocardial ischemia-reperfusion (IR), but IR injury was lessened by employing GW4869 to limit EV release.[55]

In comparison to non-AF patients, Shaihov-Teper et al. showed that EVs from EAT (EAT EVs) from AF patients had a unique proinflammatory, profibrotic, and proarrhythmic profile. These EAT EVs triggered arrhythmic re-entry in cardiomyocytes and increased fibrosis and inflammation in the atrial myocardium, indicating a unique mechanism by which EAT contributes to the pathophysiology of AF.[53] Upcoming work on PKR1 agonist, ADPN, and prohibitin 1 (PHB1), which are specific to *EAT* genes, will explore the effectiveness of a novel approach. Agents like ALY688 (an ADPN peptide analog) aim to restore the protective anti-inflammatory and antiatherogenic properties of EAT, though off-target effects are a current challenge.

RNA activation technology (saRNA): This novel technology is being investigated to specifically overexpress beneficial genes such as *ADIPOQ* and *PHB1* directly within adipose tissue, potentially minimizing systemic side effects.[56]

CONCLUSION

Recent interest in EAT and its impact on CVD and HFpEF is not only because of its close anatomical proximity and vascular supply to the myocardium, but also due to proinflammatory substances, which possibly deteriorate cardiovascular function as EAT exhibited elevated levels of interleukin-18 (IL-18) and IL-6.

Increased EAT is a strong predictor for new-onset HFpEF, myocardial dysfunction, enhanced pericardial restraint, and atrial arrhythmias, which may lead to myocardial fibrosis, impaired energy utilization, elevated filling pressures, and reduced exercise tolerance in HFpEF. The activation of macrophages in the EAT further promotes the development of atherosclerotic plaque. In addition, a shift in macrophage polarization from M2 to M1, as indicated by decreased CD206 and increased CD11c levels, also contributes to the elevated risk of developing coronary artery disease. Novel drugs, like SGLT2 inhibitor and GLP-1R, which are recommended in HFpEF, have shown the capability of reducing EAT, thus translating into therapeutic benefit. As the use of clinical imaging in suspected and established cases of HFpEF patients increases for proper and early identification of EAT load, therapeutic intervention across HFpEF populations will change the prognosis.

REFERENCES

1. Lacobellis G, Corradi D, Sharma AM. Epicardial adipose tissue: anatomic, biomolecular, and clinical relationships with the heart. Nat Clin Pract Cardiovasc Med. 2005;2: 536-43.
2. Gaborit B, Sengenes C, Ancel P, et al. Role of epicardial adipose tissue in health and disease: a matter of fat? Compr Physiol. 2017;7:1051-82.
3. Sacks HS, Fain JN. Human epicardial adipose tissue: a review. Am Heart J. 2007;153:907-17.
4. Mazurek T, Zhang LF, Zalewski A, et al. Human epicardial adipose tissue is a source of inflammatory mediators. Circulation. 2003;108:2460-66.
5. Rosito GA, Massaro JM, Hoffmann U, et al. Pericardial fat, visceral abdominal fat, cardiovascular disease risk factors, and vascular calcification in a community-based sample: the Framingham Heart Study. Circulation. 2008; 117:605-13.

6. Ansaldo AM, Montecucco F, Sahebkar A, et al. Epicardial adipose tissue and cardiovascular diseases. Int J Cardiol. 2019;278:254-60.
7. Abbara S, Desai JC, Cury RC, et al. Mapping epicardial fat with multi-detector computed tomography to facilitate percutaneous transepicardial arrhythmia ablation. Eur J Radiol. 2006;57(3):417-22.
8. Kang K, Reilly SM, Karabacak V, et al. Adipocyte-derived Th2 cytokines and myeloid PPARdelta regulate macrophage polarization and insulin sensitivity. Cell Metab. 2008;7(6):485-95.
9. Bouhlel MA, Derudas B, Rigamonti E, et al. PPARgamma activation primes human monocytes into alternative M2 macrophages with anti-inflammatory properties. Cell Metab. 2007;6(2):137-43.
10. Peled M, Fisher EA. Dynamic Aspects of Macrophage Polarization during Atherosclerosis Progression and Regression. Front Immunol. 2014;5:579.
11. Christou GA, Andriopoulou CE, Liakopoulou A, et al. Unraveling the role of resistin, retinol-binding protein 4 and adiponectin produced by epicardial adipose tissue in cardiac structure and function: evidence of a paracrine effect. Hormones (Athens). 2023;22(2):321-30.
12. Fraga-Silva RA, Seeman H, Montecucco F, et al. Apelin-13 treatment enhances the stability of atherosclerotic plaques. Eur J Clin Invest. 2018;48(3).
13. Iacobellis G. Epicardial adipose tissue in contemporary cardiology. Nat Rev Cardiol. 2022;19(9):593-606.
14. Iacobellis G, Bianco AC. Epicardial adipose tissue: emerging physiological, pathophysiological and clinical features. Trends Endocrinol Metab. 2011;22(11):450-7.
15. Doukbi E, Soghomonian A, Sengenès C, et al. Browning epicardial adipose tissue: Friend or foe? Cells. 2022;11(6):991.
16. Jolfayi AG, Beheshti AT, Hosseini SM, et al. Epicardial adipose tissue features as a biomarker and therapeutic target in coronary artery disease. Sci Rep. 2025;15(1):14786.
17. Wu CK, Tsai HY, Su MM, et al. Evolutional change in epicardial fat and its correlation with myocardial diffuse fibrosis in heart failure patients. J Clin Lipidol. 2017;11(6):1421-31.
18. He S, Zhu H, Zhang J, et al. Genome-wide screening for circRNAs in epicardial adipose tissue of heart failure patients with preserved ejection fraction. Am J Transl Res. 2023;15(7):4610-9.
19. Pugliese NR, Paneni F, Mazzola M, et al. Impact of epicardial adipose tissue on cardiovascular haemodynamics, metabolic profile, and prognosis in heart failure. Eur J Heart Fail. 2021;23(11):1858-71.
20. Crum Y, Hoendermis ES, van Veldhuisen DJ, et al. Epicardial adipose tissue and pericardial constraint in heart failure with preserved ejection fraction. ESC Heart Fail. 2024;11(3):1698-706.
21. Rao VN, Fudim M, Mentz RJ, et al. Regional adiposity and heart failure with preserved ejection fraction. Eur J Heart Fail. 2020;22(9):1540-50.
22. Koepp KE, Obokata M, Reddy YNV, et al. Hemodynamic and Functional Impact of Epicardial Adipose Tissue in Heart Failure With Preserved Ejection Fraction. JACC Heart Fail. 2020;8(8):657-66.
23. Wu A, Yang Z, Zhang X, et al. Association between epicardial adipose tissue and left atrial and ventricular function in patients with heart failure: A systematic review and meta-analysis. Curr Probl Cardiol. 2023;48(12):101979.
24. Reddy YNV, Borlaug BA, Gersh BJ. Management of atrial fibrillation across the spectrum of heart failure with preserved and reduced ejection fraction. Circulation. 2022;146:339-57.
25. Zoghbi WA, Levine RA, Flachskampf F, et al. Atrial Functional Mitral Regurgitation: A JACC: Cardiovascular Imaging Expert Panel Viewpoint. JACC Cardiovasc Imaging. 2022;15(11):1870-82.
26. Yao C, Veleva T, Scott L Jr, et al. Enhanced cardiomyocyte NLRP3 inflammasome signaling promotes atrial fibrillation. Circulation. 2018;138(20):222742.
27. Iacobellis G, Willens HJ. Echocardiographic epicardial fat: A review of research and clinical applications. J Am Soc Echocardiography. 2009;22:1311-9.
28. Flüchter S, Haghi D, Dinter D, et al. Volumetric assessment of epicardial adipose tissue with cardiovascular magnetic resonance imaging. Obesity (Silver Spring). 2007;15(4):870-8.
29. Requena-Ibáñez JA, Santos-Gallego CG, Rodriguez Cordero AJ, et al. Not only how much, but also how to, when measuring epicardial adipose tissue. Magn Reson Imaging. 2022;86:149-51.
30. Rodrigues ÉO, Rodrigues LO, Oliveira LSN, et al. Automated recognition of the pericardium contour on processed CT images using genetic algorithms. Comput Biol Med. 2017;87:38-45.
31. Commandeur F, Goeller M, Betancur J, et al. Deep Learning for Quantification of Epicardial and Thoracic Adipose Tissue From Non-Contrast CT. IEEE Trans Med Imaging. 2018;37(8):1835-46.
32. Liu J, Yu Q, Li Z, et al. Epicardial adipose tissue density is a better predictor of cardiometabolic risk in HFpEF patients: a prospective cohort study. Cardiovasc Diabetol. 2023;22(1):45.
33. Ouwerkerk R, Hamimi A, Matta J, et al. Proton MR Spectroscopy Measurements of White and Brown Adipose Tissue in Healthy Humans: Relaxation Parameters and Unsaturated Fatty Acids. Radiology. 2021;299(2):396-406.
34. Gaborit B, Venteclef N, Ancel P, et al. Human epicardial adipose tissue has a specific transcriptomic signature depending on its anatomical peri-atrial, peri-ventricular, or peri-coronary location. Cardiovasc Res. 2015;108(1):62-73.
35. Schulz A, Backhaus SJ, Lange T, et al. Impact of epicardial adipose tissue on cardiac function and morphology in patients with diastolic dysfunction. ESC Heart Fail. 2024;11(4):2013-22.
36. Antoniades C, Kotanidis CP, Berman DS. State-of-the-art review article. Atherosclerosis affecting fat: What can we

learn by imaging perivascular adipose tissue? J Cardiovasc Comput Tomogr. 2019;13(5):288-96.

37. Braescu L, Gaspar M, Buriman D, et al. The role and implications of epicardial fat in coronary atherosclerotic disease. J Clin Med. 2022;11(16):4718.
38. Wang W, Gao Y, Wang J, et al. Prognostic Value of Epicardial Adipose Tissue in Heart Failure With Mid-Range and Preserved Ejection Fraction: A Multicenter Study. J Am Heart Assoc. 2024;13(24):e036789.
39. Wu Q, Guo J, Liu F, et al. Prognostic value of epicardial adipose tissue in heart failure: a systematic review and meta-analysis. Front Cardiovasc Med. 2025;12:1618614.
40. Bao Y, Hu Y, Shi M, et al. SGLT2 inhibitors reduce epicardial adipose tissue more than GLP-1 agonists or exercise interventions in patients with type 2 diabetes mellitus and/or obesity: A systematic review and network meta-analysis. Diabetes Obes Metab. 2025;27(3):1096-112.
41. Bairapareddy KC, Maiya AG, Kumar P, et al. Effect of aerobic exercise on echocardiographic epicardial adipose tissue thickness in overweight individuals. Diabetes Metab Syndr Obes. 2018;11:303-12.
42. Barrio-Lopez MT, Ruiz-Canela M, Goni L, et al. Mediterranean diet and epicardial adipose tissue in patients with atrial fibrillation treated with ablation: a substudy of the 'PREDIMAR' trial. Eur J Prev Cardiol. 2024;31(3):348-55.
43. Gaborit B, Jacquier A, Kober F, et al. Effects of bariatric surgery on cardiac ectopic fat: lesser decrease in epicardial fat compared to visceral fat loss and no change in myocardial triglyceride content. J Am Coll Cardiol. 2012;60(15):1381-9.
44. Requena-Ibáñez JA, Santos-Gallego CG, Rodriguez-Cordero A, et al. Mechanistic Insights of Empagliflozin in Nondiabetic Patients With HFrEF: From the EMPA-TROPISM Study. JACC Heart Fail. 2021;9(8):578-89.
45. Iacobellis G, Gra-Menendez S. Effects of Dapagliflozin on Epicardial Fat Thickness in Patients with Type 2 Diabetes and Obesity. Obesity. 2020;28:1068-74.
46. Lopaschuk GD, Ussher JR, Folmes CD, et al. Myocardial fatty acid metabolism in health and disease. Physiol Rev. 2010;90(1):207-58.
47. Takano M, Kondo H, Harada T, et al. Empagliflozin Suppresses the Differentiation/Maturation of Human Epicardial Preadipocytes and Improves Paracrine Secretome Profile. JACC Basic Transl Sci. 2023;8(9):1081-97.
48. Díaz-Rodríguez E, Agra RM, Fernández ÁL, et al. Effects of dapagliflozin on human epicardial adipose tissue: modulation of insulin resistance, inflammatory chemokine production, and differentiation ability. Cardiovasc Res. 2018;114(2):336-46.
49. Dozio E, Vianello E, Malavazos AE, et al. Epicardial adipose tissue GLP-1 receptor is associated with genes involved in fatty acid oxidation and white-to-brown fat differentiation: A target to modulate cardiovascular risk? Int J Cardiol. 2019;292:218-24.
50. Gerstein HC, Colhoun HM, Dagenais GR, et al. Dulaglutide and cardiovascular outcomes in type 2 diabetes (REWIND): a double-blind, randomised placebo-controlled trial. Lancet. 2019;394:121-30.
51. Grosso AF, de Oliveira SF, Higuchi Mde L, et al. Synergistic anti-inflammatory effect: simvastatin and pioglitazone reduce inflammatory markers of plasma and epicardial adipose tissue of coronary patients with metabolic syndrome. Diabetol Metab Syndr. 2014;6(1):47.
52. Rivas Galvez RE, Morales Portano JD, Trujillo Cortes R, et al. Reduction of epicardial adipose tissue thickness with PCSK9 inhibitors. Eur Heart J. 2020;41:3008.
53. Shaihov-Teper O, Ram E, Ballan N, et al. Extracellular Vesicles From Epicardial Fat Facilitate Atrial Fibrillation. Circulation. 2021;143:2475-93.
54. Zhao H, Shang Q, Pan Z, et al. Exosomes From Adipose-Derived Stem Cells Attenuate Adipose Inflammation and Obesity Through Polarizing M2 Macrophages and Beiging in White Adipose Tissue. Diabetes. 2018;67(2):235-47.
55. Ge X, Meng Q, Wei L, et al. Myocardial ischemia-reperfusion induced cardiac extracellular vesicles harbour proinflammatory features and aggravate heart injury. J Extracell Vesicles. 2021;10(4):e12072.
56. Liu D, Chen W, Guo Z, et al. Advances and challenges of targeting epicardial adipose tissue (EAT) and perivascular adipose tissue (PVAT). Cardiovasc Diabetol. 2025;24(1):319.

26

CHAPTER

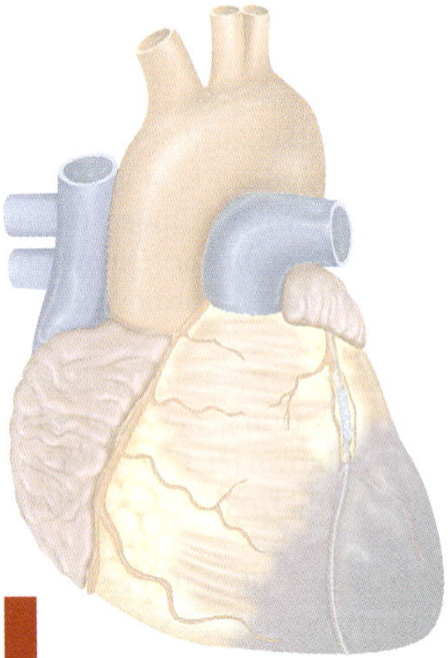

Advances in Obesity and Lipid Management in Cardiovascular Disease

Sheeba George

INTRODUCTION

Cardiovascular disease (CVD) is a leading cause of death worldwide, and a growing epidemic of obesity substantially contributes to its burden and adverse outcomes.[1,2] The Obesity Medicine Association has defined obesity as a "serious, chronic, progressive, relapsing, and treatable multi-factorial, neurobehavioral disease, wherein an increase in adiposity promotes adipose tissue dysfunction and abnormal fat mass physical forces, resulting in adverse metabolic, biomechanical, and psychosocial health consequences".[3] Since 1975, the rate of obesity has tripled and is projected to reach 1.9 billion adults (approximately 25% of the world population) by 2035.[4] Obesity directly contributes to the incidence of cardiovascular (CV) risk factors such as dyslipidemia, type 2 diabetes, hypertension, and sleep disorders, which together act as independent risk factors derived from multiple pathways and may ultimately lead to CVD.[5] The majority of deaths related to high body mass index (BMI) are due to CVD.[6]

Adipose tissue is richly supplied by a capillary network, with adipocytes located close to highly permeable vessels, which facilitates efficient exchange of molecules. Despite its larger mass, adipose tissue has relatively low perfusion per unit weight, which further decreases with increased obesity. Regulation via β-adrenergic receptors limits fluid mobilization from the interstitial space of adipose tissue, influencing volume status in obese patients with heart failure (HF). Hence, the increase in cardiac output in obesity is closely related to lean body mass rather than fat mass.[7] Additionally, adipokines, free fatty acids, and pro-inflammatory cytokines derived from excess adiposity promote endothelial dysfunction, dyslipidemia, and plaque instability, thereby accelerating atherogenesis.[7,8] Interventions for weight reduction with improved CVD outcomes are generally associated with the reduction of blood triglycerides (TG) levels and increased blood high-density lipoprotein cholesterol (HDL-C) levels among obese patients.[3] The current book chapter highlights the recent advances in obesity and lipid management, and their clinical implications in CVD prevention.

PATHOPHYSIOLOGICAL LINK BETWEEN OBESITY, DYSLIPIDEMIA, AND CARDIOVASCULAR DISEASE

Obesity and CVD are the worldwide public health challenges, associated with increased morbidity and mortality, with dyslipidemia being a major modifiable risk factor. Low-density lipoprotein (LDL), as the predominant apolipoprotein B (ApoB)-containing lipoprotein, plays a central role in cholesterol delivery to the arterial wall and is strongly associated with an increased risk of atherosclerotic cardiovascular disease (ASCVD).[9]

Obesity causes adipose tissue hypertrophy, dysfunction, and inflammation, which leads to structural and functional CV changes, mainly including left ventricular (LV) remolding with increased LV mass, left atrial enlargement, higher stroke volume, expanded total and central blood volume, reduced systemic vascular resistance, elevated cardiac output, LV filling pressure, and pulmonary atrial pressure.[10] Dyslipidemia contributes to atherosclerosis and CV events through plaque formation and oxidative stress. Elevated LDL-C penetrates the arterial endothelium, undergoes oxidation, and triggers inflammation, which leads to foam cell formation and atherosclerotic plaques. Oxidative stress promotes endothelial and smooth muscle damage, accelerates plaque proregression and increases plaque instability, ultimately raising the risk of rupture and thrombosis, myocardial infarction (MI), and stroke.[11]

Cardiac adipose tissue, particularly epicardial adipose tissue, is a distinct fat depot with unique gene expression, which, due to its close anatomical and functional relationship with the heart, acts as an important metabolic and inflammatory mediator in the development and progression of CVD.[12]

ADVANCEMENT IN OBESITY ASSESSMENT AND RISK STRATIFICATION

Weight loss in obesity is consistently associated with improvement in CV risk factors, including blood pressure (BP), lipid parameters, and glycemic control, with greater weight reduction yielding larger benefits in individuals.[13] The World Health Organization (WHO) defined overweight as a BMI between 25 and 29.9 kg/m^2 and obesity as a BMI ≥30 kg/m^2.[14] While BMI is useful for population-level screening, it is an indirect and imprecise measure of adiposity and should not be used in isolation to diagnose overweight or obesity. The BMI may overestimate fat mass in muscular individuals or individuals with edema, and underestimate adiposity in patients with sarcopenia who have reduced lean mass.[15] Although obesity is commonly defined using BMI, BMI does not predict cardiometabolic risk in individuals. The measure of central obesity, particularly the waist-to-hip ratio (WHR), is a superior predictor of metabolic diseases and MI.[16] Other challenges in individuals with CVD and obesity are listed in **Flowchart 1**.

Lifestyle Interventions

Lifestyle interventions, such as diet, physical activity, and behavioral therapy, often complemented by pharmacotherapy or bariatric procedures, show beneficial outcomes among individuals. However, long-term commitment and nutritional restriction should be avoided or closely monitored in individuals with advanced HF.[17] Mediterranean diet, rich in plant-based food and monounsaturated fat, low in saturated fat, meats, and dairy products, is considered one of the ideal nutritional models for CV health, especially for reducing the rates of coronary heart diseases, and ischemic stroke.[18] Whereas the dietary approaches to stop hypertension combination diet (DASH-CD) lowers BP levels, it also reduces oxidative stress induced by acute hyperlipidemia and raises

Flowchart 1: Challenges in individuals with CVD and obesity.

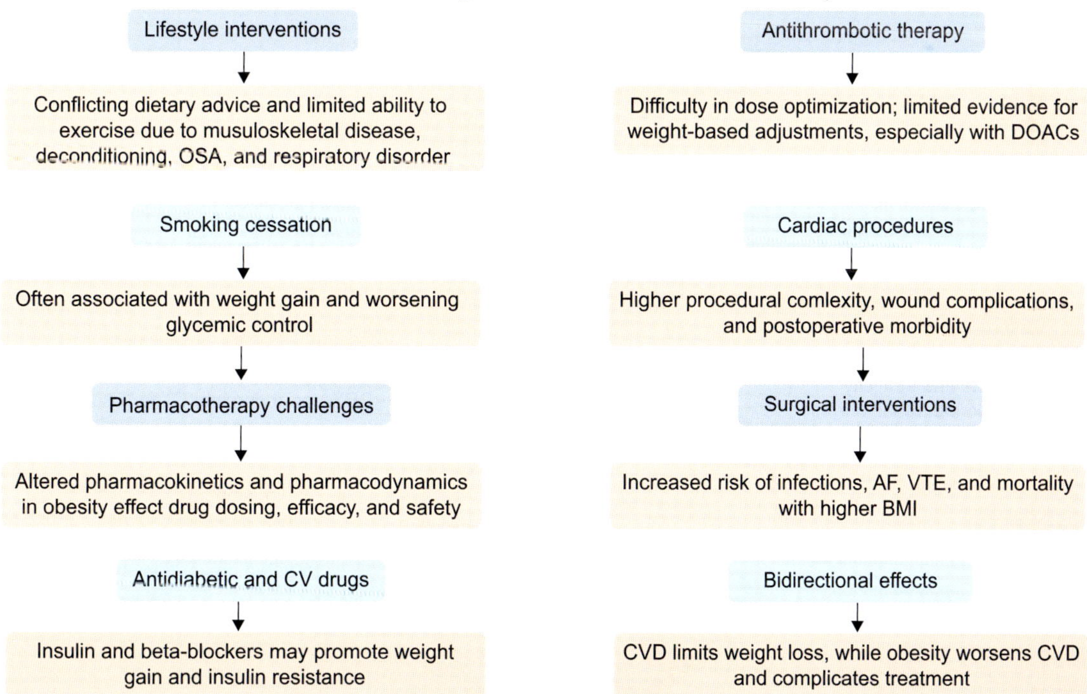

(AF: atrial fibrillation; CV: cardiovascular; CVD: cardiovascular disease; DOACs: direct oral anticoagulants; OSA: obstructive sleep apnea; VTE: venous thromboembolism)

antioxidant capacity.[19] The latest American College of Cardiology (ACC) guidelines strongly recommended weight reduction through dietary modification and regular physical activity, due to their substantial beneficial effects on lipid parameters and CV risk.[20] Additionally, Korean society recommended that a moderately low and low-carbohydrate diet can contribute to weight reduction in adults with overweight or obesity.[21] Intermittent fasting should be implemented cautiously in CV care, as its short-term metabolic benefits appear largely driven by caloric restriction, while long-term CV effects are uncertain.[22]

Cardiac rehabilitation in patients with obesity demonstrated significant benefits, including positive effects on weight reduction, CV risk factors, mental health, functional capacity, and adherence to lifestyle and pharmacological therapies.[3] Integration interventions, including physical activity with dietary modifications and smoking cessation, were the most effective strategies for improving CV risk factors.[23]

Pharmacotherapeutic Interventions

The glucagon-like peptide-1 receptor agonists (GLP-1 RA) are the first anti-obesity pharmacotherapies that have demonstrated CV benefits. The reduction in ASCVD risk and improvement in the lipid profiles with GLP-1RA therapy contribute to favorable CV outcomes.[24] Incretin-based therapies have shown a reduction of ≥5% body weight. Currently, FDA-approved incretin-based therapies include liraglutide, semaglutide, and tirzepatide, while retatrutide, the cagrilintide/semaglutide 2.4 mg combination, high-dose oral semaglutide, and oral orforglipron are in advanced stages of development.[25]

Metabolic and Bariatric Surgery

Among therapeutic options, bariatric surgery achieves the most substantial and sustained weight reduction and associated with greater reduction in CV events. Metabolic and bariatric surgery appears effective for intentional weight loss, reducing the risk of HF and death in obese HF individuals.[20] Laparoscopic vertical sleeve gastrectomy is the most common bariatric procedure used globally. Metabolic and bariatric surgery results in early cardiac remodeling, with reduced LV mass, improved diastolic function, and decreased left atrial size.[26] Metabolic surgery is associated with a significant reduction in all-cause and CV events, including MI and HF, particularly in individuals with obesity and established CVD.[27] A study by Wang L, et al. demonstrated that bariatric surgery significantly reduces estimated CV risk, especially reducing the risk of HF by 47–56% within 1–2 years after surgery.[28]

ADVANCEMENT IN LIPID ASSESSMENT AND RISK STRATIFICATION

The comprehensive CV risk assessment in individuals is depicted in **Figure 1**. Advances in lipid assessment

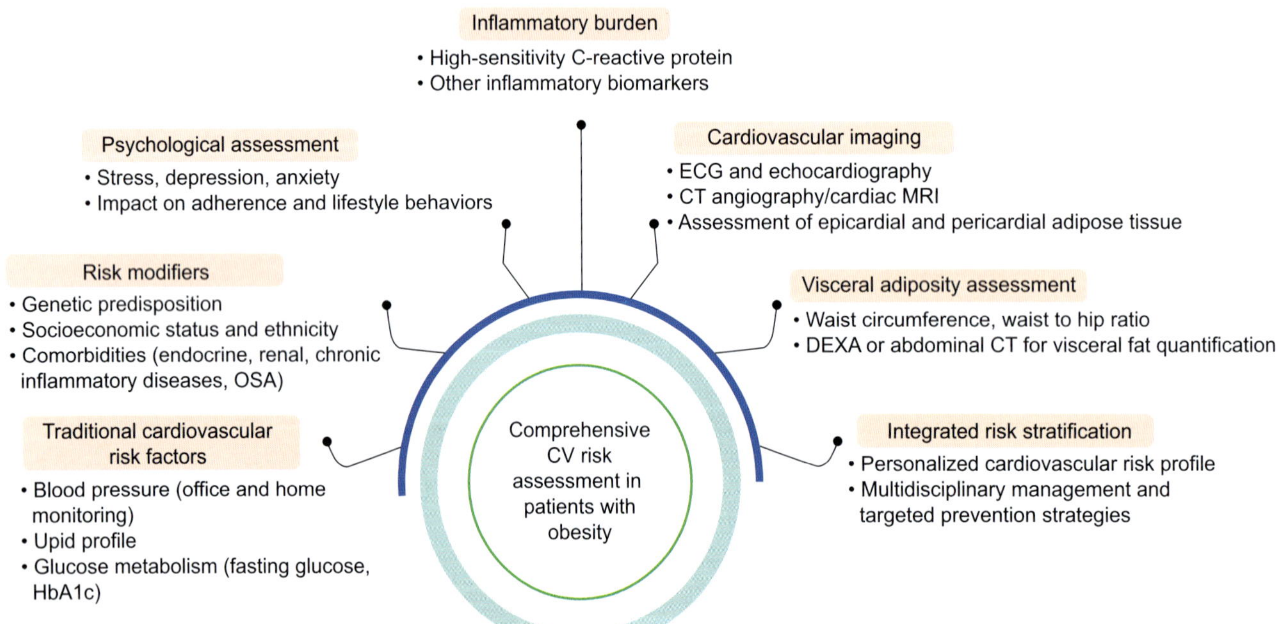

Fig. 1: Comprehensive CV risk assessment in patients with obesity. (CV: cardiovascular; CT: computed tomography; DEXA: dual-energy X-ray; ECG: electrocardiograph; OSA: obstructive sleep apnea)

extend far beyond traditional LDL-C evaluation, enabling more efficient discrimination of CV risk. Non-HDL-C captures the total cholesterol carried by all atherogenic particles and can be calculated from a routine lipid panel. It works in the non-fasting state and outperforms LDL-C in risk prediction, especially when triglycerides are elevated.[3] Guidelines recommend ApoB as a primary biomarker with a risk-adjusted target. Lipoprotein levels are genetically determined and confer a lifetime ASCVD risk comparable to heterozygous familial hypercholesterolemia (FH), adding incremental predictive value even after adjustment for traditional factors. High levels [lipoprotein(a) [LP(a)] >30 mg/dL] markedly raised premature CAD risk in young Indians.[29] TG-rich lipoproteins, including very LDL remnants, are ApoB containing particle that contribute substantially to residual CV risk. Non-HDL-C demonstrates the total atherogenic burden more comprehensively, thereby reducing the need for separate TG targets in routine risk assessment.[30]

Image-based assessment, particularly coronary artery calcium scoring, provides a direct measure of subclinical atherosclerotic burden and effectively reclassifies individuals at intermediate risk.[30] Precision medicine approaches, such as the lipidomic-enhanced risk score, further improve CV risk prediction by integrating hundreds of lipid species with the Framingham risk score, resulting in a significant improvement in CV risk assessment.[31]

NOVEL PHARMACOLOGICAL ADVANCES IN LIPID MANAGEMENT

Statins are the first-line agents for reducing the risk of ASCVD. Among patients with high CV risk, initiation of high-intensity statin therapy is strongly recommended to achieve an LDL-C reduction of >50%.[32] High intensity therapy remains the foundation of treatment, particularly in high and very high-risk individuals, where combination strategies are more suitable.[3] The addition of ezetimibe to high-intensity statin can yield an approximately 65% reduction in LDL-C.[32] However, statin intolerance represents a major barrier to optimal lipid control. In such cases, dose adjustment, alternate dosing schedules, and adjunctive non-statin agents such as ezetimibe or bempedoic acid are recommended.[3]

Ezetimibe is recommended after optimization in high- and very high-risk patients and has demonstrated benefits in primary prevention among older adults. The proprotein convertase subtilisin/kexin type 9 (PCSK9) monoclonal antibodies, including alirocumab and evolocumab, reduce LDL-C. Inclisiran, a PCSK9-targeted small interfering RNA, provides durable LDL-C lowering with twice-yearly dosing, potentially improving long-term adherence and population-level cholesterol control.[32] Bempedoic acid, an oral adenosine triphosphate (ATP) citrate lyase inhibitor, lowers LDL-C without skeletal muscle exposure and has shown CV benefit in statin-intolerant patients, positioning it as a valuable option in combination therapies, reduces hepatic cholesterol synthesis, and upregulates LDL receptor activity.[11] A study by Yamashita S et al. demonstrated that bempedoic acid produced dose-dependent and clinically significant LDL-C reductions, with minimal muscle and liver-related adverse events, supporting 180 mg as the optimal dose.[33] Despite optimal LDL-C lowering, residual CV risk persists, particularly in patients with hypertriglyceridemia or elevated LP(a). Elevated TG is recognized as a risk modifier, and optimal interventional strategies continue to evolve.[30]

INTEGRATED OBESITY AND LIPID MANAGEMENT IN CARDIOVASCULAR DISEASE PREVENTION

Therapeutic strategies that concurrently target adiposity and lipid pathways, such as a combination of GLP-1 receptor agonists (e.g., semaglutide, liraglutide) with statins, achieve an additive reduction in LDL-C and visceral adiposity, along with modest but clinically relevant lowering of systolic blood pressure.[34]

An individualized management algorithm typically begins with lifestyle modification, incorporates pharmacotherapy when ≥5% weight loss is not achieved or maintained, and escalates to bariatric surgery in patients with BMI ≥35 kg/m^2 or refractory cardiometabolic disease.[11] Effective implementation of these approaches requires a multidisciplinary care team, including cardiologists, gastrologists, dietitians, surgeons, and psychologists, to ensure coordination in treatment, patient education, adherence, and long-term follow-ups and monitoring.

FUTURE DIRECTIONS AND EMERGING THERAPIES

Emerging gene editing and RNA interference strategies, including CRISPR-Case9-based approaches targeting PCSK9, ApoB, or ANGPTL3, hold promise for achieving durable LDL-C lowering beyond what is currently possible with monoclonal antibodies.[35] Concurrent advances in omics-driven phenotyping and artificial intelligence are enabling more precise, personalized selection of obesity therapies by integrating genetic, metabolic, and microbiome data, thereby further guiding dietary, pharmacological, and procedural interventions.[36]

Modulation of the gut microbiome through targeted pre- or probiotics or fecal microbiota transplantation is also emerging as a potential strategy to improve lipid metabolism and insulin sensitivity.[37]

CONCLUSION

Obesity and dyslipidemia are closely interconnected risk factors for CVD. Effective prevention of these conditions requires sustained weight reduction, optimized lipid-lowering, and individualized risk stratification to address inflammatory metabolic pathways, which may help reduce CV risk and improve long-term outcomes.

REFERENCES

1. Lopez-Jimenez F, Di Cesare M, Powis J, et al. The Weight of Cardiovascular Diseases: Addressing the Global Cardiovascular Crisis Associated with Obesity. Global Heart. 2025;20(1):68.
2. Hao J, Lu M, Sun R, et al. Contribution of high BMI to the global burden of cardiovascular disease among young adults aged 20-39 from 1990 to 2021: A systematic analysis for the Global Burden of Disease Study 2021. Am J Prevent Cardiol. 2025:101283.
3. Bays HE, Kirkpatrick CF, Maki KC, et al. Obesity, dyslipidemia, and cardiovascular disease: A joint expert review from the Obesity Medicine Association and the National Lipid Association 2024. J Clin Lipidol. 2024;18(3):e320-50.
4. Ahmed SK, Mohammed RA. Obesity: Prevalence, causes, consequences, management, preventive strategies and future research directions. Metabolism Open. 2025:100375.
5. Powell-Wiley TM, Poirier P, Burke LE, et al. Obesity and cardiovascular disease: a scientific statement from the American Heart Association. Circulation. 2021; 143(21):e984-1010.
6. Feingold KR. Obesity and Dyslipidemia. In: Feingold KR, Ahmed SF, Anawalt B, et al. (Eds). Endotext. South Dartmouth (MA): MDText.com, Inc.; 2000.
7. Poirier P, Giles TD, Bray GA, et al. Obesity and cardiovascular disease: pathophysiology, evaluation, and effect of weight loss: an update of the 1997 American Heart Association Scientific Statement on Obesity and Heart Disease from the Obesity Committee of the Council on Nutrition, Physical Activity, and Metabolism. Circulation. 2006;113(6):898-918.
8. Luo J, He Z, Li Q, et al. Adipokines in atherosclerosis: unraveling complex roles. Front Cardiovasc Med. 2023;10:1235953.
9. Du Z, Qin Y. Dyslipidemia and cardiovascular disease: current knowledge, existing challenges, and new opportunities for management strategies. J Clin Med. 2023;12(1):363.
10. Jin X, Qiu T, Li L, et al. Pathophysiology of obesity and its associated diseases. Acta Pharm Sin B. 2023;13(6):2403-24.
11. Okoh P, Olusanya DA, Erinne OC, et al. An Integrated Pathophysiological and Clinical Perspective of the Synergistic Effects of Obesity, Hypertension, and Hyperlipidemia on Cardiovascular Health: A Systematic Review. Cureus. 2024;16(10):e72443.
12. D'Elia S, Luisi E, Solimene A, et al. Targeting Obesity in Cardiovascular Disease Management: Cardiac Adipose Tissue Is a Real Biomarker!. Targets. 2025;3(2):17.
13. Iwamoto SJ, Abushamat LA, Zaman A, et al. Obesity management in cardiometabolic disease: state of the art. Current atherosclerosis reports. 2021;23(10):59.
14. Purnell JQ. Definitions, Classification, and Epidemiology of Obesity. In: Feingold KR, Ahmed SF, Anawalt B, et al., editors. Endotext. South Dartmouth (MA): MDText.com, Inc.; 2000.
15. Sweatt K, Garvey WT, Martins C. Strengths and Limitations of BMI in the Diagnosis of Obesity: What is the Path Forward?. Current Obes Rep. 2024;13(3):584-95.
16. Yusuf S, Hawken S, Ounpuu S, et al. INTERHEART Study Investigators. Obesity and the risk of myocardial infarction in 27,000 participants from 52 countries: a case-control study. Lancet. 2005;366(9497):1640-9.
17. Escardio.org. (2024). Council for Cardiology Practice. [online] Available from https://www.escardio.org/Councils/Council-for-Cardiology-Practice-(CCP)/Cardiopractice/part-i-highlights-from-the-clinical-consensus-statement-by-the-European-society [Last accessed January 2026].
18. Martínez-González MA, Gea A, Ruiz-Canela M. The Mediterranean Diet and Cardiovascular Health. Circ Res. 2019;124(5):779-98.
19. Lopes HF, Martin KL, Nashar K, et al. DASH diet lowers blood pressure and lipid-induced oxidative stress in obesity. Hypertension. 2003;41(3):422-30.
20. Kittleson MM, Benjamin EJ, Blumer V, et al. 2025 ACC Scientific Statement on the Management of Obesity in Adults with Heart Failure: A Report of the American College of Cardiology. J Am Coll Cardiol. 2025;86(20): 1953-75.
21. Choi JH, Cho YJ, Kim HJ, et al. Effect of carbohydrate-restricted diets and intermittent fasting on obesity, type 2 diabetes mellitus, and hypertension management: consensus statement of the Korean Society for the Study of Obesity, Korean Diabetes Association, and Korean Society of Hypertension. Clin Hypertens. 2022;28(1):26.
22. Eliopoulos AG, Gkouskou KK, Tsioufis K, et al. A perspective on intermittent fasting and cardiovascular risk in the era of obesity pharmacotherapy. Front Nutr. 2025;12:1524125.
23. Tegegne TK, Shifti DM, Rawstorn JC, J et al. Digital lifestyle interventions for cardiovascular risk reduction: a systematic review and network meta-analysis. Health Policy Technol. 2024;13(3):100879.
24. Suter B, Rhodes A, Bigeh A, et al. The Role of GLP-1RA Medications in Medical Weight Loss and the Positive

Impacts on Lipid Management. Curr Cardiovasc Risk Rep. 2025;19(1):1-1.

25. Caruso I, Cignarelli A, Sorice GP, et al. Incretin-based therapies for the treatment of obesity-related diseases. NPJ Metabol Health Dis. 2024;2(1):31.
26. English WJ, Spann MD, Aher CV, et al. Cardiovascular risk reduction following metabolic and bariatric surgery. Ann Transl Med. 2020;8(Suppl 1):S12.
27. Piché ME, Poirier P, Wong JA. Impact of Metabolic Surgery on Cardiovascular Disease Outcomes. Can J Cardiol. 2025;41(9):1794-1808.
28. Wang L, Zhang X, Chen Y, et al. Reduced Risk of Cardiovascular Diseases After Bariatric Surgery Based on the New Predicting Risk of Cardiovascular Disease EVENTs Equations. J Am Heart Assoc. 2025;14(6): e038191.
29. Kumar Jinger DM. Advanced Lipid Markers as Predictors of Premature Coronary Artery Disease in Young Indians: Insights from A Case-Control Study. Int J Acad Med Pharm. 2025;7(2):1071-6.
30. Puri R, Bansal M, Mehta V, et al. Lipid Association of India 2023 update on cardiovascular risk assessment and lipid management in Indian patients: Consensus statement IV. J Clin Lipidol. 2024;18(3):e351-73.
31. Wu J, Giles C, Dakic A, et al. Lipidomic Risk Score to Enhance Cardiovascular Risk Stratification for Primary Prevention. J Am Coll Cardiol. 2024;84(5):434-46.
32. Komnianou A, Kyriakoulis KG, Menti A, et al. Cardiovascular Risk Assessment and Lipid-Lowering Therapy Recommendations in Primary Prevention. J Clin Med. 2025;14(7):2220.
33. Yamashita S, Fujita H, Yokota D, et al. Efficacy and Safety of Bempedoic Acid for Hypercholesterolemia in Japan: A Phase 2 Multicenter, Randomized, Double-Blind, Placebo-Controlled, Parallel-Group, Dose-Finding Trial. J Atheroscler Thromb. 2025;32(8):1053-70.
34. Schiele F, Dievart F, Jacobi D, et al. Onboarding obesity management in cardiovascular care: A cardiologist's guide to latest advances. Am J Prevent Cardiol. 2025:100987.
35. Safarova M, Bimal T, Soffer DE, et al. Advances in targeting LDL cholesterol: PCSK9 inhibitors and beyond. Am J Prevent Cardiol. 2024;19:100701.
36. Molla G, Bitew M. Revolutionizing Personalized Medicine: Synergy with Multi-Omics Data Generation, Main Hurdles, and Future Perspectives. Biomedicines. 2025;12(12):2750.
37. Mubarak G, Devasena I, Lavanya D, et al. The Impact of Gut Microbiota Modulation on Cardiovascular Risk: A Systematic Review. Eur J Cardiovasc Med. 2025;15(4).

SECTION 4

Obesity and Coronary Artery Disease

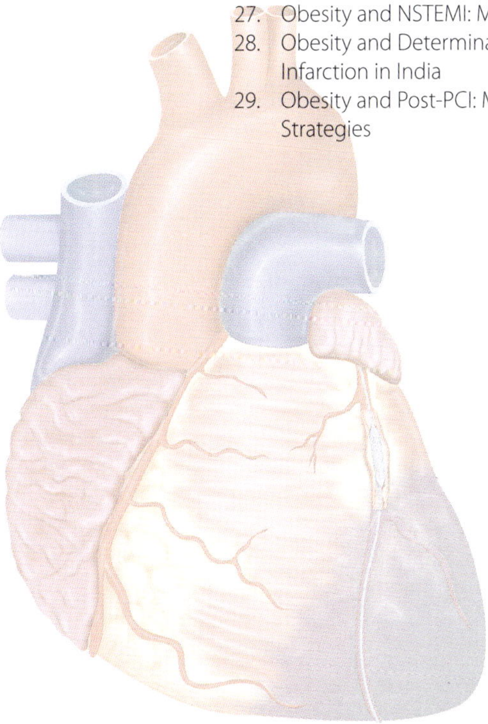

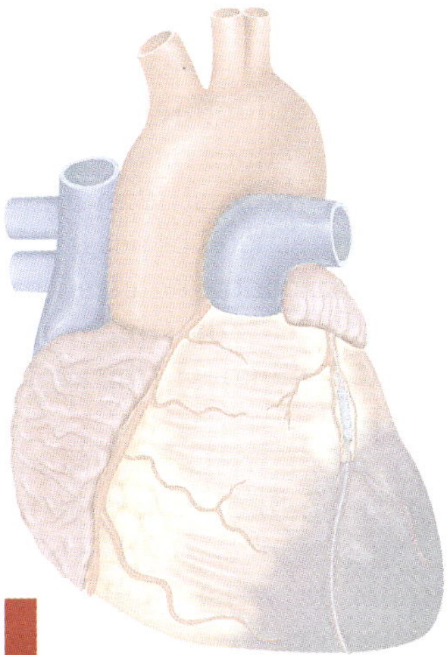

27 CHAPTER

Obesity and NSTEMI: Management Strategies

Debasish Das, Kaushik Manna, Debabrata Roy

INTRODUCTION

Obesity is the new pandemic that has emerged in the last few decades and is a major contributing factor behind the cardiovascular diseases. People with obesity face 50–100% higher all-cause mortality risk than normal weight individuals. About two-thirds of deaths in the obese patients are contributed to cardiovascular causes.[1] One large ACS registry found that roughly 71% of patients were suffering from obesity. And this high prevalence of obesity further increases our interest to investigate how much it influences development of NSTEMI in patients close.

Another important phenomenon called "obesity paradox" comes into play in this respect.[2] Studies have shown that 1-year mortality was higher in underweight patients in comparison to overweight or obese patients. This highlights that while obesity sharply increases cardiovascular risk, overweight individuals with ACS often paradoxically have a better short- and long-term survival than the linear patients. However, this paradox is likely explained by confounding factors, such as younger age, larger metabolic reserve, and more aggressive treatment rather than a true protective effect.

Obesity intertwins with traditional risk factors such as hypertension, type 2 diabetes mellitus, dyslipidemia and sleep apnea, as well as an independent risk factor for MACE. Excess visceral fat is proinflammatory as well as prothrombotic. Adipose tissues secret cytokines such as TNF-a, IL-6, leptin, and resist that promote endothelial dysfunction and atherosclerotic plaque formation. Obesity acts as an independent risk factor causing adverse cardiac remodeling, LV hypertrophy, diastolic dysfunction, and coronary artery disease. Obesity not only contributes to well-established cardiovascular risk factors like type 2 diabetes mellitus, dyslipidemia, hypertension, but also has direct adverse effects on cardiac structure and function.

Obese NSTEMI patients tend to be younger with higher prevalence of metabolic syndrome. The Framingham study and other subsequent studies showed that overweight individuals suffer from ACS about a decade earlier than normal weight patients. Obesity patients tend to have higher prevalence of multivessel disease and more diffuse atherosclerosis at angiography. However, in some patients, obesity seems to be protective: Some overweight ACS patients often have greater collateral flow, allowing more aggressive management. This may be a contributing factor for lower short-term mortality, as seen in some studies. Nonetheless, obese NSTEMI patients carry greater comorbidity burden and requires tailored care.

PATHOPHYSIOLOGY

Obesity induces a proatherogenic state. Adipose tissue is essentially an endocrine organ and releases adipocytes when inflammatory cytokines and thus, alters lipid metabolism. These chemicals released in response to obesity causes insulin resistance and chronic inflammation, accelerating the process of plaque development. In obesity, atheroma tends to be lipid rich and unstable. Obesity also increases platelet reactivity and coagulation factors. Obesity and type 2 diabetes mellitus runs hand in hand and thus accelerating the process of metabolic injury.[3] NSTEMI patients with obesity frequently have the metabolic ACS phenotype, that is, hyperglycemia, hypertriglyceridemia, and proinflammatory state.

Obese NSTEMI patients often have hypertension and LV hypertrophy at base. Often, they have coexisting metabolic syndrome, sleep apnea, and nonalcoholic fatty liver disease. Sleep apnea further predisposes to atrial fibrillation and worsens nocturnal hypoxia following myocardial infraction.

Obesity shifts the spectrum of ACS in younger expanding the pool of NSTEMI survivors who subsequently suffered the chronic sequel. Since most of the obese patients have coexisting type 2 diabetes mellitus, hypertension, and dyslipidemia, an aggregated cardiometabolic burden is triggered in the NSTEMI patients, causing a cascade of complications such as acute heart failure, arrhythmias, and CDK progression, unless aggressive aggressively managed.

Paradoxically, many observational studies show overweight and obese NSTEMI patients have lower in-hospital and 1-year mortality in comparison to normal weight patients. In one large registry, underweight patients had about 25% 1-year mortality, while only 7–8% mortality in the overweight/obese group. This obesity paradox may be a result of bias where lean patients may have other illnesses, causing body wasting and differences in treatment intensity. Patients with central obesity have a higher cardiac risk than those with peripheral fat. In practice, measuring waist circumference in addition to BMI helps risk stratification of obese NSTEMI patients.

To summarize, obesity in NSTEMI patients comprises complex interplay of inflammatory metabolic and hemodynamic factors that both raise baseline risk and influence acute presentation.

Understanding those mechanisms influences our management approaches, even though acute care protocols remained largely the same, as for nonobese patients.

MANAGEMENT STRATEGIES

Acute Management

Although all NSTEMI patients, regardless of BMI, should undergo rapid risk stratification and management according to standard ACS algorithms, obesity poses practical considerations that should be addressed while treatment planning. For risk assessment, validated scores like GRACE are applied uniformly. Obesity itself, however, is not a separate score variable. ESC and ACC recommend an early invasive coronary angiography within 24 hours of presentation, for high-risk NSTEMI patients, with GRACE score ≥140, dynamic changes, and recurrent angina.[4]

Large trials and meta-analyses demonstrate the benefit of invasive management across all BMI spectrum, and Class I recommendation for early angiography applies equally to all obese patients, wherever feasible. All obese NSTEMI patients should receive guideline-directed antithrombotic therapy. Current guidelines recommend dual antiplatelet therapy (DAPT) for at least 12 months with a potent P2Y12 inhibitors like prasugrel or ticagrelor in preference to clopidogrel, unless contraindicated by bleeding risk. There is no BMI-based adjustment for standard doses of aspirin or P2Y12 inhibitors in the acute setting.

Anticoagulation dosing should be weight adjusted. Low-molecular-weight heparins, like enoxaparin, should be given as 1–1.5 mg/kg once daily, while unfractionated heparin is titrated by weight and aPTT values. In morbid obesity, some experts recommend anti-Xa level monitoring or capping the dose to avoid overdose, though evidence is limited. Recent year ESC guidelines state that there is no clear ischemic advantage to bivalirudin over heparin when redial access is used and modern stents are applied.

Radial artery should be preferred for vascular access. RIVAL[5] and MATRIX[6] trials showed that transradial access significantly reduces bleeding and vascular complications in ACS, without compromising reperfusion. As a result, radial axis is recommended as the preferred approach in instrument patients undergoing invasive assessment whether without PCI. In obese patients, a large waist can make femoral puncture technically challenging and prone to bleeding and hematoma formation further supporting the use of radial access.

Obesity itself does not preclude CABG. But extreme obesity with BMI > 40 kg/m^2 BSA increases risks of wound infection and ventilation problems. Revascularization decisions (PCI vs. CABG) should be made on clinical grounds. The catheterization laboratory equipment size must be considered. Longer catheters and guidewires may be needed depending on large body habitus. Radiation scatter and X-ray dose are higher in obese patients, so operator should use image collimation and protective shielding diligently.

All eligible patients, irrespective of obesity, should receive high-intensity statin, beta blockers, ACE inhibitors/ARBs, and DAPT, as tolerated. Obesity often coexists with insulin resistance and hypertension that demand aggressive secondary prevention.[4]

Secondary Prevention

Secondary prevention in obese NSTEMI patients targets all modifiable risk factors, with added emphasis on weight reduction. Lifestyle modification remains the first line of therapy: Dietary counseling increases physical activity and gradual weight loss should be initiated inhospital or at discharge. Even a modest weight loss of 5–10% of body weight has shown to improve blood pressure, glycemic control, and lipid profile.[7] ESC and AHA/ACC guidelines recommend to set realistic weight loss goals and follow up lifestyle changes.

Recent guidelines and consensus documents recognize obesity as a chronic disease that merits direct intervention. ESC clinical consensus 2024 on obesity emphasizes that cardiologist should be actively involved in obesity management as part of holistic cardiovascular disease care. Routine BMI screening, referral to nutritionist, structured weight-loss programs, and early discussion of medical therapy for weight control are increasingly advocated.

In the recent years, pharmacotherapy has been available for obesity management. GLP-1 receptor agonists (liraglutide and semaglutide) have robust data for cardiovascular risk reduction in obese patients. In the landmark SELECT trial, overweight/obese nondiabetic patients with established CVD treated with subcutaneous semaglutide 2.4 mg weekly experience 26% relative reduction in MACE versus placebo. This antiobesity drug is one of its kind which has proven cardiovascular benefit.

Bariatric surgery is recommended for suitable patients. Current indications for bariatric surgery are BMI ≥40 kg/m^2 and BMI ≥35 kg/m^2 with significant comorbidities like diabetes and OSA. Observational studies and metanalysis have shown that bariatric surgeries like sleeve gastrectomy or gastric bypass markedly lowers long-term cardiovascular events, lowers all costs of cardiovascular mortality, and reduce rates of myocardial infarction and heart failure.

Aggressive LDL lowering, often to ≤55 mg/dL in very high-risk patients, is mandatory. High-dose statins are recommended, which can be complemented by ezetimibe and PCSK9 inhibitors.

Hypertension and diabetes should be managed appropriately. Apolipoprotein b is to be measured for risk stratification.[3] Cardiac rehabilitation is especially beneficial for obese patients; structured exercise and nutritional support can improve fitness and help sustain weight loss. Complete cessation of smoking is crucial; combination of smoking and obesity is particularly deleterious for black progression and thrombosis.

LIMITATIONS

Despite growing awareness, evidence, specifically addressing NSTEMI management in obesity, has limitations. Most of the trials did not stratify patients according to BMI, and morbidly obese patients were often under-represented. Thus, many recommendations for obese patients are extrapolated, rather than evidence base. Observational studies suggesting and obesity paradox suffer from confounding: Differences in age, fitness, and treatment between BMI groups can skew results. The true impact of obesity on post-MI prognosis remains complex and registry data may not capture unmeasured confounders like frailty and sarcopenia. Bariatric surgery, although promising, has not been evaluated in randomized CVD trials does recommendations rely on observational meta-analyses.

There is no clear consensus on how to adjust antithrombotic or heart failure drugs doses in extreme obesity. Many cardiology programs lack structured obesity clinics or protocols. Access to bariatric surgery or GLP-1 agonist drugs varies by region and financial conditions of the patients.

Finally, obesity is heterogeneous. Body composition (muscle vs. fat), fat distribution, fitness level, and metabolic health vary widely among patients with the same BMI. Current guidelines rely on BMI cutoffs. However, two patients with the same BMI may have very different risks. New imaging techniques, like body fat scans, and biomarkers, like adiponectin levels, might better characterize risk, although they are not in routine use as of now.

CONCLUSION

Obesity is common among ACS patients and raises all-cause and cardiovascular mortality; about two-thirds of deaths in obese patients are cardiovascular. Obese patients tend to develop ACS a decade earlier, have more metabolic syndrome, and have multivessel and diffuse atherosclerosis disease. Obesity contributes to accelerated adverse remodeling of the heart. Timely pharmacological as well as nonpharmacological interventions are the cornerstone in the management protocol of enzyme in obese patients.

REFERENCES

1. Koskinas KC, Van Craenenbroeck EM, Antoniades C, et al. Obesity and cardiovascular disease: an ESC clinical consensus statement. Eur Heart J. 2024;45(38):4063-98.
2. Gurevitz C, Assali A, Mohsan J, et al. The obesity paradox in patients with acute coronary syndromes over 2 decades – the ACSIS registry 2000–2018. Int J Cardiol. 2023;380:48-55.
3. Jackson EA. ESC Consensus Statement on Obesity and CVD: Key Points. Am Coll Cardiol. 2024. [Epub ahead of print].
4. Collet JP, Thiele H, Barbato E, et al. 2020 ESC Guidelines for the management of acute coronary syndromes in patients presenting without persistent ST-segment elevation. Eur Heart J. 2021;42(14):1289-367.

5. Jolly SS, Yusuf S, Cairns J, et al. Radial versus femoral access for coronary angiography and intervention in patients with acute coronary syndromes (RIVAL): a randomised, parallel-group, multicentre trial. Lancet. 2011;377(9775):1409-20.
6. Shah R, Khan B. The MATRIX trial. Lancet. 2019; 393(10183):1803.
7. Christodorescu R. (2024). Part II. Highlights from the ESC clinical consensus statement on obesity and cardiovascular disease: pharmacological and bariatric treatment strategies. [online] Available from https://www.escardio.org/communities/councils/cardiology-practice/education/cardiopractice/part-II-highlights-from-the-clinical-consensus-statement-by-the-european-society/ [Last accessed January, 2026].

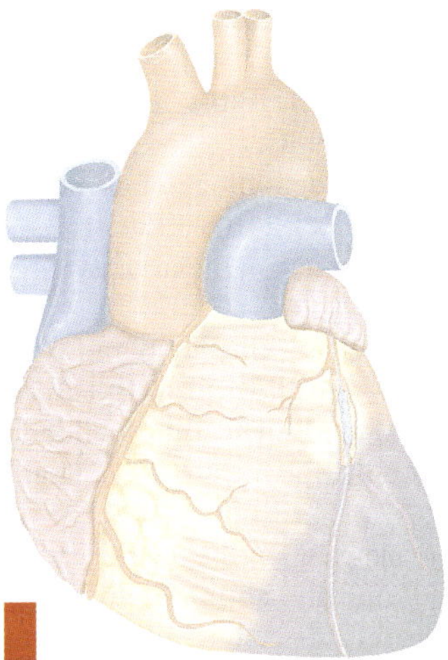

28 CHAPTER

Obesity and Determinants of Myocardial Infarction in India

Dhiman Kahali

INTRODUCTION

India has undergone a major epidemiological transition over the past few decades. While infectious diseases and undernutrition were predominant in earlier eras, contemporary India faces a growing burden of obesity and metabolic disease. This shift has contributed directly to the rising incidence of premature myocardial infarction (MI), often occurring in individuals without overt obesity by Western definitions.

OBESITY IN THE INDIAN POPULATION

Asian Indians exhibit a unique body composition marked by higher visceral adiposity and insulin resistance at lower body mass index (BMI) levels. This so-called thin-fat phenotype predisposes individuals to early atherosclerosis and coronary events, prompting lower BMI cut-offs in Indian clinical guidelines.

PATHOPHYSIOLOGICAL MECHANISMS LINKING OBESITY AND MYOCARDIAL INFARCTION

Obesity promotes MI through insulin resistance, atherogenic dyslipidemia, chronic inflammation, endothelial dysfunction, and a pro-thrombotic state. These mechanisms interact synergistically to accelerate coronary plaque formation and destabilization.

EPIDEMIOLOGICAL EVIDENCE

Large international studies and Indian registries consistently demonstrate that central obesity is a stronger predictor of MI than BMI. Indian patients tend to present younger and with more diffuse coronary artery disease compared to Western cohorts.

CENTRAL OBESITY AND RISK STRATIFICATION

Measures of abdominal adiposity, such as waist circumference and waist-hip ratio, outperform BMI in predicting MI risk among Indians. Visceral fat burden correlates closely with plaque instability and clinical events.

OBESITY AND PREMATURE MYOCARDIAL INFARCTION

An increasing proportion of MIs in India occur before the age of 40 years. Obesity often clusters with diabetes and smoking, resulting in aggressive and multivessel coronary disease.

THE OBESITY PARADOX

Although some studies describe lower short-term mortality among overweight MI patients, this so-called obesity paradox diminishes after adjustment for fat distribution and cardiorespiratory fitness.

IMPACT OF WEIGHT REDUCTION

Weight loss through lifestyle intervention, metabolic surgery, or pharmacotherapy improves cardiometabolic risk factors and reduces coronary events. Glucagon-like peptide-1 (GLP-1) receptor agonists have demonstrated cardiovascular benefit in obese diabetic individuals.

CLINICAL IMPLICATIONS

Body mass index alone is insufficient for cardiovascular risk assessment in Indians. Routine waist measurement, early metabolic screening, and integration of weight management into cardiac care are essential.

CONCLUSION

In the Indian context, obesity—particularly central obesity—is a powerful and early determinant of MI. Addressing obesity is fundamental to reducing the national burden of premature cardiovascular disease.

BIBLIOGRAPHY

1. Anjana RM, Deepa M, Pradeepa R, et al. Prevalence of diabetes and prediabetes in 15 states of India: results from the ICMR-INDIAB population-based cross-sectional study. Lancet Diabetes Endocrinol. 2017;5(8):585-96.
2. Enas EA, Dharmarajan TS, Varkey B. Dyslipidemia in Asian Indians. Indian Heart J. 2018;70:829-35.
3. Gupta R, Mohan I, Narula J. Epidemiology of coronary heart disease in India. Indian Heart J. 2016;68:130-42.
4. Lakdawala M, Vaze S. Bariatric surgery in India. Obes Surg. 2013;23:373-81.
5. Lavie CJ, De Schutter A, Milani RV. Obesity paradox in coronary heart disease. J Am Coll Cardiol. 2014;63:1345-54.
6. Marso SP, Daniels GH, Brown-Frandsen K, et al. Liraglutide and cardiovascular outcomes in type 2 diabetes. N Engl J Med. 2016;375(4):311-22.
7. Misra A, Chowbey P, Makkar BM, et al. Consensus statement for diagnosis of obesity, abdominal obesity and the metabolic syndrome for Asian Indians and recommendations for physical activity, medical and surgical management. J Assoc Physicians India. 2009;57:163-170.
8. Ridker PM, Cushman M, Stampfer MJ, et al. Inflammation, aspirin, and the risk of cardiovascular disease. Circulation. 2004;109:2818-25.
9. Xavier D, Pais P, Devereaux PJ, et al. Treatment and outcomes of acute coronary syndromes in India (CREATE): a prospective analysis of registry data. J Am Coll Cardiol. 2008;51:1422-9.
10. Yusuf S, Hawken S, Ounpuu S, et al. Effect of potentially modifiable risk factors associated with myocardial infarction in 52 countries (the INTERHEART study): case-control study. Lancet. 2004;364(9438):937-52.

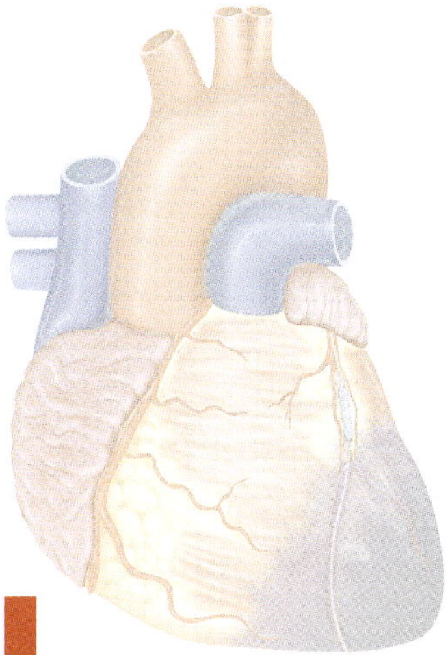

CHAPTER 29

Obesity and Post-PCI: Management Strategies

Deepti Yadav, Siddarth Varshney, Nagendra Chauhan, Praveen Chandra

INTRODUCTION

Obesity is no longer just a cosmetic concern—it is a major, modifiable driver of cardiovascular risk. For patients who have undergone percutaneous coronary intervention (PCI), excess adiposity influences short- and long-term outcomes: Restenosis, stent thrombosis risk via proinflammatory and prothrombotic states, recurrence of ischemia from progressive atherosclerosis, heart failure (HF) progression, and worsening of cardiometabolic comorbidities (diabetes, hypertension, dyslipidemia). Managing obesity after PCI, therefore, must be treated as an integral, multidisciplinary component of secondary prevention—not an optional add-on. Contemporary cardiology guidance (including recent ESC and AHA scientific statements) emphasizes structured weight management integrated into cardiac care, with lifestyle, pharmacologic, and procedural options now demonstrating cardiovascular benefit.[1]

This chapter outlines a practical, evidence-based, and patient-centered approach for clinicians in 2025—with attention to Indian/South Asian phenotypes and health-system realities—covering assessment, in-hospital and outpatient strategies, pharmacotherapies (notably GLP-1/GIP agents), bariatric options, cardiac rehabilitation (CR), monitoring, algorithms, and communication tips for a humanized delivery of care.

EPIDEMIOLOGY AND THE SOUTH ASIAN CONTEXT

Globally, obesity prevalence has been rising rapidly and is a major contributor to the surge in cardiovascular disease. South Asians present a particular challenge: For a given BMI, they tend to have higher visceral adiposity, greater insulin resistance, and earlier cardiometabolic disease compared with Europeans. Consequently, BMI thresholds and risk interpretation need local calibration—many Indian experts and consensus documents recommend lower BMI cutoffs and greater use of waist circumference and body-fat measures to assess risk in South Asian populations.[2]

Practical point: For Indian patients, use a low threshold for intensive risk management when BMI ≥23 kg/m^2 (overweight per Asian cutoffs) or waist circumference ≥90 cm (men)/≥80 cm (women)—and evaluate body composition where possible.

WHY OBESITY MATTERS AFTER PERCUTANEOUS CORONARY INTERVENTION—PATHOPHYSIOLOGY IN BRIEF

Key mechanisms by which obesity worsens post-PCI prognosis:

- Chronic systemic inflammation (elevated CRP, IL-6) that accelerates atherogenesis and neointimal hyperplasia
- Prothrombotic milieu (platelet hyperreactivity, altered fibrinolysis) that may increase early and late thrombotic risk
- Metabolic comorbidities (poorly controlled diabetes, dyslipidemia, hypertension) that raise recurrent ischemic events
- *Hemodynamic effects:* Increased blood volume, higher left ventricular workload, predisposition to HF

- *Procedural challenges:* Vascular access and imaging may be more difficult; accurate stent sizing and apposition can be affected by vessel size and technical considerations.

All these mechanisms make weight-focused secondary prevention both biologically plausible and clinically important.

ASSESSMENT AFTER PERCUTANEOUS CORONARY INTERVENTION—WHAT TO MEASURE AND WHEN

A structured post-PCI obesity assessment improves triage and personalized planning.

Immediate (In-hospital or Before Discharge)

- Height, weight, BMI (document baseline)
- Waist circumference and hip circumference (calculate waist-to-hip)
- Brief dietary, physical-activity, and psychosocial screen (food access, stress, sleep, tobacco/alcohol)
- Screen for diabetes (HbA1c or fasting glucose), lipid profile, liver enzymes, renal function, thyroid function, where indicated.
- Medication review (statins, antiplatelet, antihypertensive, diabetes drugs)
- *Brief motivational conversation:* Link weight to heart recovery and stent longevity—set realistic first goals (e.g., 5–10% weight reduction over 6 months).

Early Outpatient (2–6 Weeks)

- *Detailed cardiometabolic risk reassessment:* HbA1c, fasting lipids, BP, uric acid (if gout risk), sleep apnea screening (STOP-BANG)
- Functional capacity assessment; referral to CR
- Consider body composition (bioimpedance/DEXA) if available for nuanced counseling.

Follow-up Schedule

- At 1, 3, 6, 12 months—weight, BP, lipids, and medication adherence; more frequent visits if starting antiobesity pharmacotherapy or after bariatric surgery

MANAGEMENT STRATEGIES—A LAYERED APPROACH

Management should be stepped and personalized: Start broad (lifestyle + risk factor control), then add medications or procedures for patients who meet criteria or who fail initial measures. Shared decision-making is essential **(Flowchart 1)**.

Flowchart 1: Post-PCI obesity management pathway (2025).

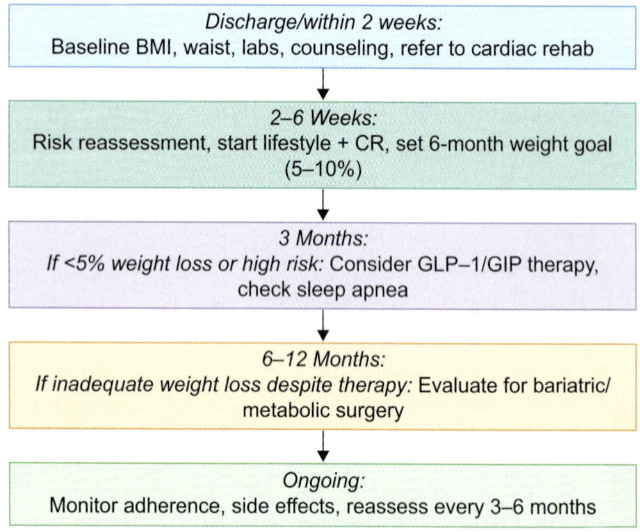

Optimize Secondary Prevention (Nonweight Specific but Essential)

- *Antiplatelet therapy and stent care:* Adhere to guideline-based DAPT duration per stent type and bleeding risk. Obesity alone does not usually change DAPT choice, but ensures adherence, counseling, and drug access.
- *Intensive lipid lowering:* High-intensity statin ± ezetimibe/PCSK9 as indicated—lipid control reduces progression and recurrent events.
- BP control and glycemic optimization (team with diabetology/endocrinology)
- Smoking cessation, vaccination, and control of other comorbidities

These measures form the foundation on which weight management adds incremental benefit.

Lifestyle Interventions—The Universal First Step

- *Dietary strategy:* Individualized calorie-reduction plan (generally 500–750 kcal/day deficit aiming for 0.5–1 kg/week), emphasizing whole grains, legumes, vegetables, modest carbohydrates (important in India), healthy fats, and portion control. Consider culturally sensitive meal plans (e.g., revised traditional Indian plates, timing of meals).
- *Physical activity:* Aim for at least 150 minutes/week moderate aerobic activity + 2 sessions/week resistance training; start with low-impact options after PCI and tailor to functional status. CR is ideal.

- *Behavioral support:* Structured counseling, goal setting, self-monitoring (apps or diaries), motivational interviewing, and problem-solving for barriers. Group or family involvement helps in India's collectivist households.
- *Sleep and stress:* Treat sleep apnea (common with obesity), promote sleep hygiene, and address psychosocial stressors that drive emotional eating.
- *Effectiveness:* Even modest weight loss (5–10%) improves blood pressure, lipids, and glycemic indices and reduces inflammatory markers; in the post-PCI patient, these improvements translate into lower recurrent risk when combined with other therapies.[3]

Cardiac Rehabilitation—Central, Underused, and Powerful

- Enroll every eligible post-PCI patient in an exercise-based CR program. In India, where CR access varies, hybrid or home-based CR with periodic center visits is a practical model. CR improves exercise tolerance, promotes weight loss, enhances medication adherence, and reduces rehospitalization. Integrate nutritional counseling and psychosocial therapy within CR.

Antiobesity Pharmacotherapy—New Era, Proven Cardiovascular Signals

The last 3–4 years have transformed pharmacologic options for obesity. GLP-1 receptor agonists (e.g., semaglutide) and the GIP/GLP-1 dual agonist tirzepatide produce marked, sustained weight loss and favorable cardiometabolic effects. Importantly, semaglutide (in the SELECT trial) demonstrated reductions in major adverse cardiovascular events in people with overweight/obesity and established cardiovascular disease; tirzepatide has shown benefit in HF and cardiometabolic endpoints in recent trials. These agents are now recognized as valid options for patients with cardiovascular disease who meet eligibility criteria.[4]

Practical Considerations (Post-PCI)

- *When to consider:* BMI ≥30 kg/m^2 (or ≥27 kg/m^2 with obesity-related comorbidity such as T2DM, or lower Asian cutoffs) who do not achieve adequate weight loss with lifestyle + CR; or patients who need rapid, clinically meaningful weight reduction and for whom benefits outweigh risks
- *Benefits:* Meaningful weight loss (often >10–15% over months), improved BP, lipids, glycemic control, and emerging CV outcome data. Semaglutide/other GLP-1s may lower MACE in selected populations.[5]
- *Safety and monitoring:* Gastrointestinal (GI) side effects are common; monitor for gallstones, pancreatitis (rare), and for interactions with oral medications (altered gastric emptying may affect absorption of some drugs). In post-PCI patients, monitor for symptoms and ensure continuity of antiplatelet therapy; there is no routine contraindication to combining GLP-1 agents with DAPT. Coordinate with endocrinology.
- *Access and cost:* In India, cost and availability limit broad use; discuss affordability, duration, and realistic goals with patients.

Semaglutide (GLP-1 Receptor Agonist)

- *Dose:* 2.4 mg weekly SC (obesity indication)
- *Efficacy:*
  - *Weight loss:* 12–15%
  - *HbA1c:* Reduction ~1–1.5%
  - *SELECT trial:* Reduces MACE by ~20% in overweight/obese patients *without diabetes* + established ASCVD
- *Post-PCI advantages:*
  - Lowers recurrent MI/stroke risk.
  - Improves BP, LDL, and HbA1c.
  - Well tolerated with DAPT
- *Cautions:* GI intolerance, gallstones, and rare pancreatitis
- *Best suited for:* Broad post-PCI population, especially nondiabetics with obesity + CAD

Tirzepatide (Dual GIP/GLP-1 Agonist)

- *Dose:* Weekly SC, titrated 10–15 mg
- *Efficacy:*
  - *Weight loss:* 18–22% (largest to date)
  - *HbA1c:* reduction by ~2–2.5%
  - *SUMMIT/SURPASS-CVOT:* Reduces HF hospitalization; emerging evidence for reduced MACE
- *Post-PCI advantages:*
  - Potent weight/metabolic control
  - Stronger benefit in obese diabetics with HF
- *Cautions:* More GI side effects, pancreatitis risk, high cost
- *Best suited for:* Obese post-PCI patients with *T2DM + HF/metabolic syndrome* needing aggressive weight control **(Table 1)**

Bariatric/Metabolic Surgery—For Selected High-risk Patients

Indications generally follow international standards (BMI ≥40 kg/m^2, or BMI ≥35 kg/m^2 with significant comorbidity; Asian cutoffs may be lower). Bariatric surgery produces the greatest sustained weight loss and dramatic improvement in cardiometabolic risk factors; observational data

TABLE 1: Comparison of semaglutide and tirzepatide.

Feature	*Semaglutide*	*Tirzepatide*
Drug class	GLP-1 agonist	Dual GIP/GLP-1 agonist
Average weight loss	12–15%	18–22%
CV outcome trial	SELECT (↓ MACE by 20%)	SUMMIT/SURPASS (↓ HF hospitalization; MACE benefit emerging)
Diabetes control	HbA1c ↓ ~1–1.5%	HbA1c ↓ ~2–2.5%
Heart failure benefit	Moderate (data emerging)	Stronger evidence for ↓ HF hospitalization
Adverse effects	GI upset, gallstones, and rare pancreatitis	GI upset (slightly more), rare pancreatitis
Formulation	Weekly injection (2.4 mg), oral 14 mg (less potent)	Weekly injection (10–15 mg)
Cost/accessibility	Moderate-high (oral + injection available)	High (injectable only, limited access in India)
Best use case post-PCI	Broad use: Overweight/obese with/without diabetes, proven CV benefit	Obese post-PCI with diabetes, metabolic syndrome, or HF where rapid/greater weight loss is desirable

suggest lower cardiovascular events in eligible patients. For post-PCI patients, timing and perioperative planning are critical: Optimize antiplatelet management, assess ischemic risk, and involve the cardiac team and anesthesia for perioperative hemodynamic management. In Indian practice, careful selection, counseling, and long-term follow-up for nutritional sequelae are essential.

Novel and Procedural Adjuncts

- Endoscopic bariatric therapies (e.g., intragastric balloons, endoscopic sleeve gastroplasty) are evolving options for certain patients who are not surgical candidates. Evidence in cardiovascular outcomes is still emerging; consider these therapies in tertiary centers with appropriate expertise.
- Device-drug interactions: No current evidence requires alteration of cardiac device therapy purely for weight-management devices, but multidisciplinary review is advised.

MONITORING, SAFETY, AND DRUG INTERACTIONS

- *Antiplatelet and anticoagulants:* Continue per cardiology guidance; weight-loss interventions generally do not mandate changes in antiplatelet regimens, but discuss perioperative DAPT strategy before surgery.
- *GLP-1 agents:* Monitor GI tolerance, gallbladder symptoms, and blood glucose (if diabetic). Watch for dehydration in elderly patients with vomiting. Coordinate with endocrinology.[6]
- *Drug absorption:* Slowed gastric emptying with GLP-1s can alter absorption of some oral agents— review critical drug dosing if needed.
- *Nutritional deficits after bariatric surgery:* Schedule long-term nutrition follow-up (iron, B_{12}, vitamin D, calcium).

LIMITATIONS, EVIDENCE GAPS, AND EQUITY ISSUES (2025)

- While SELECT (semaglutide) and SUMMIT (tirzepatide data) provide encouraging cardiovascular and HF signals, long-term data in diverse post-PCI Indian populations remain limited. Generalizability to lower-income settings and to patients with different comorbidity profiles needs more research.[4]
- Cost and access to GLP-1/GIP therapies and bariatric surgery remain major barriers in India; equitable delivery requires policy innovation and possible tiered reimbursement.
- Cultural patterns (dietary preferences, urban vs. rural activity levels) require locally adapted interventions and implementation research.
- Safety in specific subgroups (advanced CKD, frail elderly) calls for cautious personalized approaches.

CONCLUSION

Managing obesity after PCI in 2025 is a multidisciplinary blend of classic secondary prevention and modern metabolic therapeutics **(Flowchart 2)**. The evidence base has evolved: Lifestyle and CR remain core, while GLP-1/GIP agents and metabolic surgery offer powerful new tools. In India, the imperative is to tailor interventions to South Asian risk profiles, to overcome cost and access barriers, and to deliver care with empathy and realistic goals. Framing weight management as an integral part of stent-care and recovery—with clear algorithms,

Flowchart 2: Key practical takeaways—obesity and post-PCI management pathway (2025).

Treat obesity as a cardiac risk target after PCI—not optional

↓

Use asian-specific thresholds and waist measures for Indian patients

↓

Start with lifestyle + cardiac rehabilitation for everyone

↓

GLP–1/GIP pharmacotherapy—semaglutide, tirzepatide (CV benefit)

↓

Reserve bariatric surgery for selected patients

↓

Humanized, culturally sensitive, family-inclusive approach

team-based delivery, and measurable short-term goals—will improve both patient well-being and cardiovascular outcomes.

REFERENCES

1. Koskinas KC, Van Craenenbroeck EM, Antoniades C, et al. Obesity and cardiovascular disease: an ESC clinical consensus statement. Eur Heart J. 2024;45(38):4063-98.
2. Riaz M, Lodhi S. Beyond BMI: exploring obesity trends in the South Asian region. Obes Pillars. 2024;13:100156.
3. Laddu D, Neeland IJ, Carnethon M, et al. Implementation of obesity science into clinical practice: a scientific statement from the American Heart Association. Circulation. 2024;150(1):e7-19.
4. Deanfield J, Verma S, Scirica BM, et al. Semaglutide and cardiovascular outcomes in patients with obesity and prevalent heart failure: a prespecified analysis of the SELECT trial. Lancet. 2024;404(10454):773-86.
5. Ryan DH, Lingvay I, Deanfield J, et al. Long-term weight loss effects of semaglutide in obesity without diabetes in the SELECT trial. Nat Med. 2024;30:2049-57.
6. Binu AJ, Kapoor N. Cardiovascular implications of semaglutide in obesity management: redefining cardiovascular health strategies. Heart Int. 2024;18(1):3-4.

30

CHAPTER

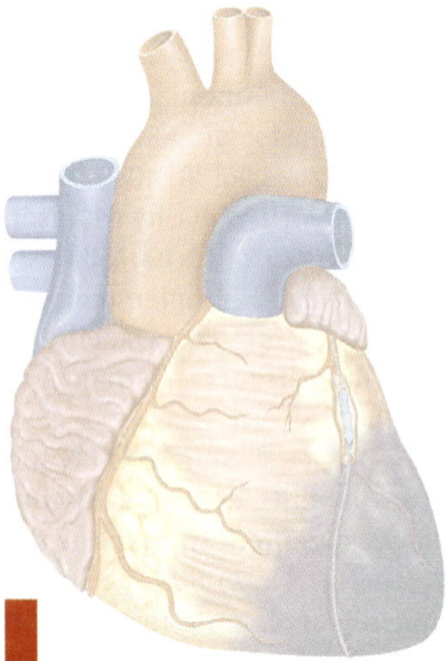

Obesity and Postcoronary Artery Bypass Graft Outcomes: Is it Different?

Yugal K Mishra, Manasmukul Dutta

INTRODUCTION

Obesity has emerged as a global health crisis, with over 650 million adults worldwide categorized as obese and nearly 1.9 billion overweight (WHO, 2024).[1] The condition is a major risk factor for coronary artery disease (CAD), which remains the leading cause of death globally. Surgical revascularization in the form of coronary artery bypass grafting (CABG) continues to be a cornerstone of management for advanced CAD.

India, too, is experiencing this rising burden. The ICMR-INDIAB study (2021) reported nearly 135 million Indians as overweight or obese, with prevalence rates reaching 30–35% in urban areas and 15–20% in rural areas.[2] South Asians also develop diabetes, hypertension, and CAD at younger ages, making obesity a particularly important determinant of CABG outcomes in this population.[3]

Understanding how obesity alters short- and long-term CABG outcomes is vital, since it not only increases perioperative risks but also shapes long-term survival and quality of life.[4]

EPIDEMIOLOGY AND PREVALENCE

Global burden: In developed countries such as the US and Europe, 40–50% of CABG patients are obese. This mirrors general obesity trends in the population and highlights how obesity has become a defining feature of surgical cohorts.

Indian context: Rising urbanization and lifestyle transitions have driven obesity rates upward in India. Patients often present with obesity in combination with diabetes, hypertension, and dyslipidemia. These comorbidities appear a decade earlier compared to Western populations, resulting in younger but higher-risk surgical candidates.

Thus, epidemiologically, obesity is no longer incidental but is central to the CABG population worldwide.

OBESITY PARADOX

Some studies have described an "obesity paradox," where overweight or mildly obese patients undergoing CABG do not fare worse, and occasionally show slightly better short-term outcomes than their normal-weight counterparts.[5,6]

Protective adipokines: Molecules like adiponectin improve endothelial function, while leptin supports angiogenesis and repair. In the early perioperative setting, these may buffer stress.

Nutritional reserves: Obese patients may better withstand catabolic stress due to greater metabolic stores.

Confounding and bias: Younger age, reverse causation (illness-related weight loss in "normal" groups), and closer follow-up also contribute.

Importantly, these effects are short-lived. In the long run, obesity consistently predisposes complications and higher mortality.

SHORT-TERM OUTCOMES AFTER CORONARY ARTERY BYPASS GRAFTING IN OBESE PATIENTS

Wound Infection and Delayed Healing

Obese patients face higher rates of superficial and deep wound infections, especially mediastinitis. Poorly vascularized adipose tissue impairs oxygen delivery and healing, while coexistent diabetes worsens the risk. Saphenous vein harvest sites also heal slowly.

Respiratory Complications and Prolonged Ventilation

Obesity reduces lung compliance and functional residual capacity. Postoperatively, this translates to prolonged mechanical ventilation, frequent atelectasis, and pneumonia. Each of these increases ICU stay and costs.

Sternal Instability

The heavy chest wall exerts mechanical strain on the sternum, raising the risk of instability or dehiscence. This risk is amplified in diabetics and COPD patients and leads to longer recovery and infection risk.

Metabolic Derangements

Surgical stress causes hyperglycemia, which is exaggerated by insulin resistance in obese patients. Elevated blood sugars promote infection and impair healing. Persisting dyslipidemia also destabilizes vascular physiology, impacting graft outcomes.

Renal and Hemodynamic Stress

Obesity increases circulating blood volume and cardiac output. These changes can complicate perioperative fluid balance and predispose to acute kidney injury (AKI), further prolonging hospitalization.

Summary: While mortality in the short term is not dramatically higher, obese patients experience disproportionately more morbidity, making their recovery more complex and resource intensive **(Table 1)**.

LONG-TERM COMPLICATIONS AFTER CORONARY ARTERY BYPASS GRAFTING

Recurrent CAD and graft failure: Persistent systemic inflammation and dyslipidemia accelerate atherosclerosis and intimal hyperplasia, especially in saphenous vein grafts, leading to occlusion within 5–10 years. Patients develop recurrent angina or MI and often require PCI or redo CABG, both riskier in obesity due to wound and respiratory vulnerabilities. Even arterial grafts, while more durable, are not immune to the hostile metabolic milieu.

Heart failure progression: Chronic volume load increases cardiac output demands, driving LV hypertrophy, and reduced compliance. Despite revascularization, diastolic dysfunction progresses and many patients evolve to HFpEF, with recurrent decompensation episodes, heightened filling pressures, and exercise intolerance compounded by deconditioning and OSA.

Arrhythmias: Obesity promotes atrial enlargement and fibrosis, alters autonomic tone, and, with OSA-related hypoxia, creates an arrhythmogenic substrate. Atrial fibrillation and ventricular ectopy become more frequent over time, increasing stroke risk, precipitating HF exacerbations, and contributing to rehospitalizations and mortality.

Metabolic deterioration: Insulin resistance typically worsens postoperatively, fueling poor glycemic control and persistent atherogenic dyslipidemia. This combination undermines graft patency, accelerates native-vessel disease, and amplifies microvascular injury in the heart, kidney, and brain, shortening long-term survival.

Renal dysfunction: Obesity-related glomerular hyperfiltration, intensified by diabetes and hypertension,

TABLE 1: BMI categories and post-CABG outcomes.

BMI category (kg/m^2)	*Short-term mortality*	*Long-term mortality*	*Common complications*	*Prognosis*
Underweight (<18.5)	↑ High	↑ High	Malnutrition, poor healing	Worst
Normal (18.5–24.9)	Reference	Reference	Balanced risk	Baseline
Overweight (25–29.9)	Neutral/↓	Neutral	Respiratory, metabolic complications	Acceptable
Obese I (30–34.9)	Neutral/↑ slight	↑	Wound infections, AF	Mixed
Obese II (35–39.9)	↑	↑ Higher	Renal dysfunction, respiratory failure	Poor
Obese III (≥40)	↑↑	↑↑↑	Severe wound infections, graft failure	Poorest

TABLE 2: Long-term complications in obese CABG patients.

Complication	Mechanism	Clinical impact
Graft failure	Inflammation, dyslipidemia	Angina, reintervention
Heart failure	LV hypertrophy, diastolic dysfunction	Rehospitalization
Arrhythmias	Sleep apnea, atrial fibrosis	Stroke, mortality
Diabetes progression	Insulin resistance	Vascular complications
Renal dysfunction	Hyperfiltration injury	CKD, dialysis
Stroke	AF, prothrombotic state	Disability, mortality
Poor recovery	Mobility limitations	Low quality of life
OSA/cancers	Hypoxia, tumor promotion	Competing mortality

advances to CKD. Declining eGFR complicates medication choices (e.g., antithrombotics and RAAS inhibitors), increases fluid-management complexity, and independently predicts adverse cardiovascular outcomes.

Stroke and thromboembolism: A prothrombotic state (elevated fibrinogen and PAI-1) combined with higher AF burden raises cerebrovascular event risk. Strokes often leave lasting disability, negating surgical gains; long-term anticoagulation mitigates risk but adds bleeding considerations.

Reduced functional recovery: Musculoskeletal pain, sarcopenic obesity, and breathlessness limit participation in rehab. Lower adherence to exercise and diet perpetuates deconditioning, reduces peak VO_2, and compromises return-to-work and quality-of-life metrics compared with nonobese counterparts.

OSA and obesity-associated cancers: Persistent sleep-disordered breathing sustains sympathetic overdrive and intermittent hypoxemia, aggravating hypertension, arrhythmias, and HF. Over years, obesity-associated malignancies (colon, breast, and pancreatic) contribute to competing, noncardiac mortality, reducing net survival gains **(Table 2)**.

MECHANISMS LINKING OBESITY TO OUTCOMES

Chronic inflammation: Adipose tissue secretes IL-6 and TNF-α, sustaining low-grade systemic inflammation that impairs leukocyte function, weakens wound healing, and accelerates atherosclerosis in native vessels and grafts—raising infection risk and hastening graft failure.

Adipokine dysregulation: Protective adiponectin levels fall with increasing adiposity, reducing endothelial nitric oxide signaling and anti-inflammatory effects; simultaneous leptin resistance and elevations in resistin/visfatin foster vascular injury and insulin resistance, worsening outcomes.

Hemodynamic burden: Increased blood volume and cardiac output remodel the left ventricle toward eccentric hypertrophy and reduced compliance; even after ischemia is corrected, diastolic dysfunction persists and predisposes to HFpEF and exercise intolerance.

Endothelial dysfunction: Oxidative stress reduces nitric oxide bioavailability and increases vascular stiffness; this impairs vasodilation, compromises microcirculatory perfusion, and promotes graft intimal hyperplasia and early occlusion.

Metabolic derangements: Persistent hyperglycemia and atherogenic dyslipidemia damage endothelium and smooth muscle integrity, diminish graft patency, and fuel systemic vascular complications involving brain, kidney, and myocardium.

SURGICAL AND PERIOPERATIVE PRINCIPLES

Preoperative planning: Careful preoperative evaluation is critical in obese patients, who often have coexisting diabetes, hypertension, and sleep apnea. Weight optimization and strict glycemic control, when feasible, reduce perioperative risks. Preoperative pulmonary assessment and OSA management with CPAP can also significantly improve postoperative outcomes.

Conduit choice: Internal mammary artery (IMA) remains the gold standard graft, but harvesting is technically more difficult in obese patients. Skeletonization reduces wound complications by preserving blood supply. Radial artery grafts are often preferred over saphenous vein grafts to avoid slow healing at leg sites, while bilateral IMA use must be cautiously weighed against infection risks.

Endoscopic/minimally invasive conduit harvesting: Endoscopic vein harvesting (EVH) or radial artery harvesting using minimally invasive techniques significantly reduces leg wound infections, hematoma formation, and delayed healing—all common in obese patients. This approach shortens recovery, lowers pain scores, and minimizes cosmetic concerns, making it especially beneficial in this high-risk group.

Sternal protection: Obese patients are particularly prone to sternal instability due to mechanical stress from the heavy chest wall. Techniques such as reinforced wiring, rigid fixation with plates, and prophylactic NPWT are essential to prevent dehiscence and mediastinitis, which carry high morbidity and mortality.

Minimally invasive and robotic CABG (sternum-sparing surgery): Sternotomy carries major wound-related risks in obese patients. Minimally invasive direct CABG (MIDCAB), totally endoscopic CABG (TECAB), and robotic-assisted CABG avoid full sternotomy, reducing infection risk and promoting faster recovery. These approaches preserve chest wall stability, improve pulmonary mechanics, and are increasingly recognized as superior long-term strategies for obese patients, especially when limited grafting is required.

On-pump versus off-pump CABG: Cardiopulmonary bypass may exacerbate systemic inflammation and fluid retention in obese patients. Off-pump CABG can help mitigate these risks and shorten ventilation time, but it requires surgical expertise and is best reserved for suitable anatomies.

Anesthetic and intraoperative management: Airway difficulty, altered drug pharmacokinetics, and respiratory compromise are frequent challenges. Strategies like careful preoxygenation, PEEP application, and appropriate drug dosing are required. Meticulous positioning reduces pressure injuries, while protective ventilation strategies prevent atelectasis.

Respiratory management: Early extubation, incentive spirometry, and chest physiotherapy are critical to reduce pulmonary complications. Obese patients are particularly vulnerable to hypoventilation and atelectasis, making aggressive respiratory care a cornerstone of postoperative management.

ICU and postoperative care: Intensive monitoring for respiratory compromise, arrhythmias, and metabolic instability is essential. Aggressive mobilization and physiotherapy aid recovery, while prophylactic anticoagulation and compression devices reduce thromboembolic events. Continuous glucose monitoring ensures metabolic stability.

Multidisciplinary approach: Optimal care requires coordinated input from surgeons, anesthesiologists, endocrinologists, physiotherapists, and nutritionists. This team-based strategy ensures holistic management, addressing both surgical risks and long-term rehabilitation needs.

OTHER MANAGEMENT STRATEGIES

Lifestyle interventions: Caloric restriction, Mediterranean or DASH diets, structured exercise programs, smoking cessation, and sleep hygiene form the foundation of long-term care. Weight loss improves graft patency and reduces comorbidities.

Pharmacological therapy: Statins reduce cholesterol and systemic inflammation, improving graft survival. Glycemic control with insulin remains perioperatively essential, while newer therapies like GLP-1 receptor agonists and SGLT2 inhibitors provide dual metabolic and cardiovascular benefits. Antiplatelet therapy and, when needed, anticoagulation remain crucial for preventing thrombosis.

Rehabilitation: Tailored cardiac rehabilitation is essential for obese patients, who often face orthopedic and mobility challenges. Supervised exercise, nutritional counseling, and psychological support improve adherence, reduce anxiety, and enhance functional recovery.

GUIDELINES

International guidelines (AHA/ACC, ESC/EACTS, and STS) consistently highlight obesity as a risk modifier in CABG.[7-9] They caution against using BMI alone as a risk tool, recommending assessment of metabolic health and fat distribution. Preoperative optimization of diabetes, hypertension, and OSA is strongly advised. Enhanced wound care, perioperative glucose control, and structured rehabilitation are recommended. Importantly, obesity is not a contraindication to CABG but mandates a tailored, multidisciplinary approach to maximize benefit.

CONCLUSION

Obesity significantly alters outcomes following CABG. In the short term, obese patients face higher risks of wound infections, respiratory complications, sternal instability, and metabolic derangements. In the long term, the burden of graft failure, arrhythmias, heart failure, renal dysfunction, stroke, and impaired rehabilitation is disproportionately greater than in normal-weight patients.

Awareness of these challenges is vital for both clinicians and patients. Prevention strategies aimed at reducing obesity through lifestyle measures and public health interventions remain the most effective long-term solution. For those who undergo CABG, perioperative optimization, careful surgical planning, and long-term rehabilitation tailored to obesity are critical.

Equally important is the role of patient education, since adherence to rehabilitation, diet, and medication can significantly alter outcomes. By recognizing obesity as a major modifier of CABG results and acting proactively, healthcare teams can improve both survival and quality of life.

Ultimately, the significance of obesity lies not only in its role as a risk factor for CAD, but also in its ability to reshape the recovery and long-term trajectory of patients after surgery. Tackling this challenge requires a combination of preventive strategies, clinical vigilance, and coordinated multidisciplinary care.

REFERENCES

1. WHO. (2025). Obesity and overweight: Factsheet. [online] Available from https://www.who.int/news-room/fact-sheets/detail/obesity-and-overweight [Last accessed January, 2026].
2. ICMR-INDIAB Study. Prevalence of Obesity in India. 2021.
3. Niskanen L, et al. Impact of Obesity on Mortality and Morbidity After CABG: A Meta-Analysis. J Thorac Cardiovasc Surg. 2016.
4. Reeves BC, et al. Obesity and Survival After Coronary Artery Bypass Surgery. Circulation. 2011.
5. Stamou SC, et al. The Obesity Paradox in Cardiac Surgery. J Thorac Cardiovasc Surg. 2014.
6. Lavie CJ, et al. The Obesity Paradox and Cardiovascular Disease. Prog Cardiovasc Dis. 2016.
7. AHA/ACC. Guidelines on CABG. 2021.
8. Neumann FJ, Sousa-Uva M, Ahlsson A, et al. 2018 ESC/EACTS Guidelines on myocardial revascularization. Eur Heart J. 2019;40(2):87-165.
9. Society of Thoracic Surgeons (STS). Adult Cardiac Surgery Database Risk Models. 2020.

31

CHAPTER

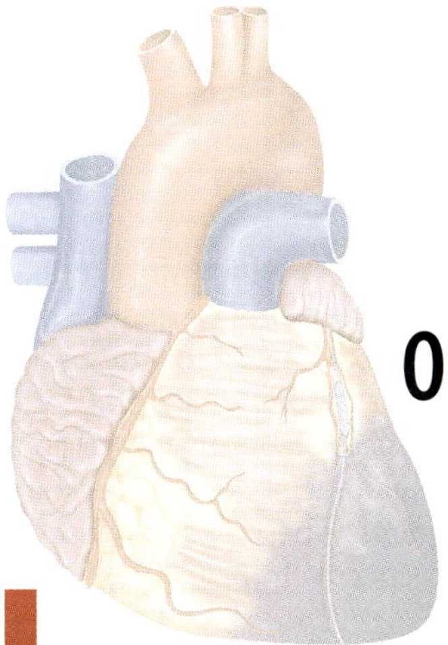

Obesity and Coronary Artery Calcium Score

Priya Jagia, Alamelu Alagappan

INTRODUCTION

Obesity is a multifactorial disease characterized by a complex pathogenesis and variability in the pathways and mechanisms that result in detrimental health outcomes. Numerous cardiovascular diseases such as atherosclerotic disease, heart failure, thromboembolic disease, arrhythmias, and sudden cardiac death, are associated with obesity. In the development of coronary artery disease (CAD) associated with obesity, the pathogenic role of atherogenic dyslipidemia is well established.

Obesity, particularly central obesity, is linked to abnormalities in bone regulatory proteins, dysregulated adipokines (lower adiponectin, increased free leptin), and chronic low-grade inflammation (elevated high sensitive C-reactive protein). By encouraging inflammation and vascular smooth muscle cell change, these factors contribute to arterial wall calcification.[1]

CORONARY ARTERY CALCIUM SCORE

One of the best markers of CAD is coronary artery calcium (CAC) score. The CAC score has become a widely available, dependable, and effective method of determining the risk of major cardiac events, particularly in asymptomatic individuals targeted for primary prevention interventions like aspirin and statins.

The CAC score is computed using 3-mm CT slices that are taken prospectively in synchrony with the ECG at a specific point in the R-R interval, typically in the mid/late diastole, are restricted to the cardiac region, have no overlap or gaps, and are obtained without the use of intravenous contrast material. Areas exhibiting at least 1 mm of hyperattenuation and >130 Hounsfield units (HU) or less than three consecutive pixels are referred to be calcified.

The Agatston methodology, which is recognized in the majority of population databases and studies, is the most commonly used method in clinical practice among the different approaches for assessing CAC scores. **Table 1** shows CAC scores with risk analysis and clinical correlation.[2]

TABLE 1: CAC scores with risk analysis and clinical correlation.[2]

CAC score (Agatston method)	*Risk analysis*	*Clinical correlation*
0	Absent/No risk	Low risk of future cardiovascular events
1–10	Minimal	Minimal atherosclerosis may be present with a low risk of future cardiovascular events
11–100	Mild	There is likely mild to minimum coronary artery stenosis. A mild risk of coronary artery disease exists
101–400	Moderate	Reasonable amount of plaque can be confirmed. Has a moderately increased risk of future cardiovascular events
>400	High	A high coronary calcium score correlated with a significant risk of having a cardiovascular event (such as myocardial ischemia) in near future

OBESITY AND CORONARY ARTERY CALCIUM SCORE

Obesity and CAC have a complicated association with neurobiological, epidemiological, and clinical ramifications that influence risk assessment and management techniques. CAC evaluation is a vital tool for risk stratification in this population since elevated CAC scores in obese people are strong predictors of future cardiac events and reflect an increased burden of coronary atherosclerosis. Numerous extensive research have shown that obesity, especially central obesity, is positively correlated with higher CAC prevalence and severity scores.

In a multicenter retrospective study, of the 36,509 people, 10.5% had CAC ≥400, 46.6% had zero CAC, and the median BMI was 26.6 kg/m^2 (interquartile range: 24.1–30.1). Overweight [risks ratio: 1.13 (95% CI: 1.1–1.2)] and obese [odds ratio: 1.5 (95% CI: 1.4–1.6)] people had higher multivariable adjusted odds of CAC >0 than people with normal BMI. Obese people had increased risk of coronary heart disease, and all-cause death than those with a normal BMI. In a sex-stratified analysis, obese men had higher risk of CAD, cardiovascular disease, and all-cause mortality.[3]

In research, obesity population is classified into metabolically healthy obese (MHO), metabolically unhealthy obese (MUO), and sarcopenic obese. Compared to people of normal weight, coronary calcification was more common in MHO individuals. When comparing MHO with normal-weight patients in multivariable-adjusted models, the CAC score ratio was 2.26 (95% CI: 1.48–3.43).

Metabolically healthy obese people may be more susceptible to cardiovascular disease events and death than those of normal weight who are metabolically healthy, according to new longitudinal studies. The MHO phenotype may be unstable and develop into overt metabolic conditions.[4]

In a study by Rhee et al., five CAC categories were used as the dependent variables in a multinomial logistic regression analysis; the MHO and MUO groups showed significantly higher odds ratios for increasing CAC categories compared with no calcification status (5.221 for CAC >400 in MUO group with 95% CI: 2.856~5.032) after controlling for age, sex, and smoking status.[5]

The worst-case scenario is sarcopenic obesity, which is defined by high-fat content and low muscle mass. Regardless of other risk factors, the risks of having a high CAC score are twice as high as those of sarcopenia or obesity alone. In addition to fat toxicity, it also includes increased inflammatory signals, poor glucose handling, and the loss of protective muscle-derived proteins.[6] **Figures 1 and 2** show CAC score in nonobese and obese patients.

CORONARY AGE

Coronary age estimates the age at which an average healthy individual would have the same estimated risk of coronary heart disease. It is calculated for the index patient, using clinical risk factors and CAC scoring data. CAC score has a significant impact on coronary age. In a study by Lemanowicz et al., difference between coronary age and metrical age was higher in obese patients than in controls (+5.6 vs. –4.8 years, respectively, $p < 0.005$).[7]

OTHER CT PARAMETERS

Pericoronary adipose tissue (PCAT) surrounds the coronary arteries and can be measured through CT-based fat attenuation index (FAI) measurements. Normally, the fat attenuation ranges around –95 to –70 Hounsfield units (HU). In obesity, due to increased inflammation and lipid infiltration, PCAT attenuation becomes less negative. Studies show that individuals with BMI ≥25 kg/m^2 and metabolic risk factors such as hypertension or dyslipidemia have higher PCAT attenuation values compared to normal-weight subjects, even when no Frank CAD is present.[8]

Epicardial adipose tissue (EAT) is a visceral fat depot located between the myocardium and the visceral pericardium. Obesity triggers adipocyte proliferation within EAT, expanding epicardial fat depots and promoting local inflammation and oxidative stress that predispose to CAD. Bakkum et al. in his study reported that EAT volume rise in obese individuals is an independent predictor of left ventricular mass and myocardial remodeling.[9]

Jagia et al. in their study of 799 Indian patients done in AIIMS, New Delhi, India, concluded that epicardial fat volume **(Figs. 3A to D)** was the standalone significant prognostic factor for both the existence of obstructive CAD and major adverse cardiovascular events (MACE) in patients with atypical chest pain and no known history of CAD. Apart from obstructive CAD and high-risk plaque features, CAC was a significant independent predictor of MACE.[10]

LIMITATIONS

- Image noise and beam hardening artifacts due to large body habitus
- Reduced spatial resolution due to larger chest circumference
- Vendor-dependent variability of CAC

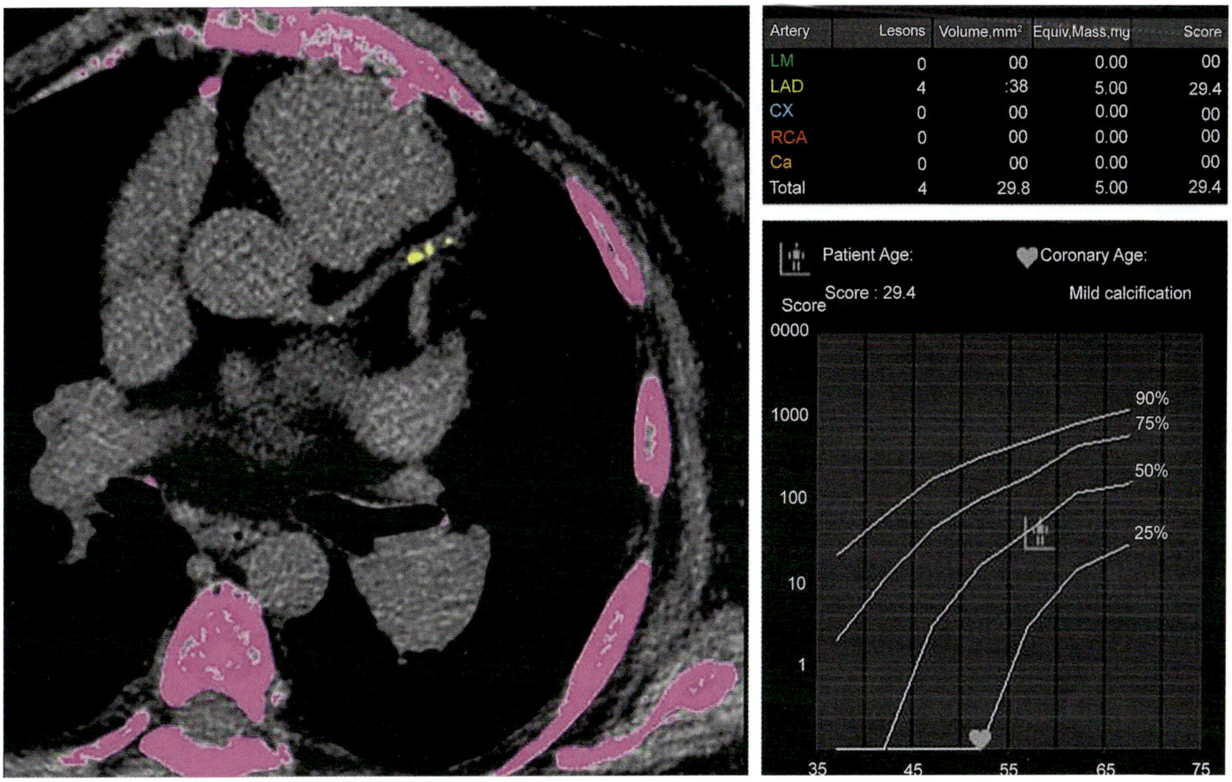

Fig. 1: CAC score in nonobese patient.

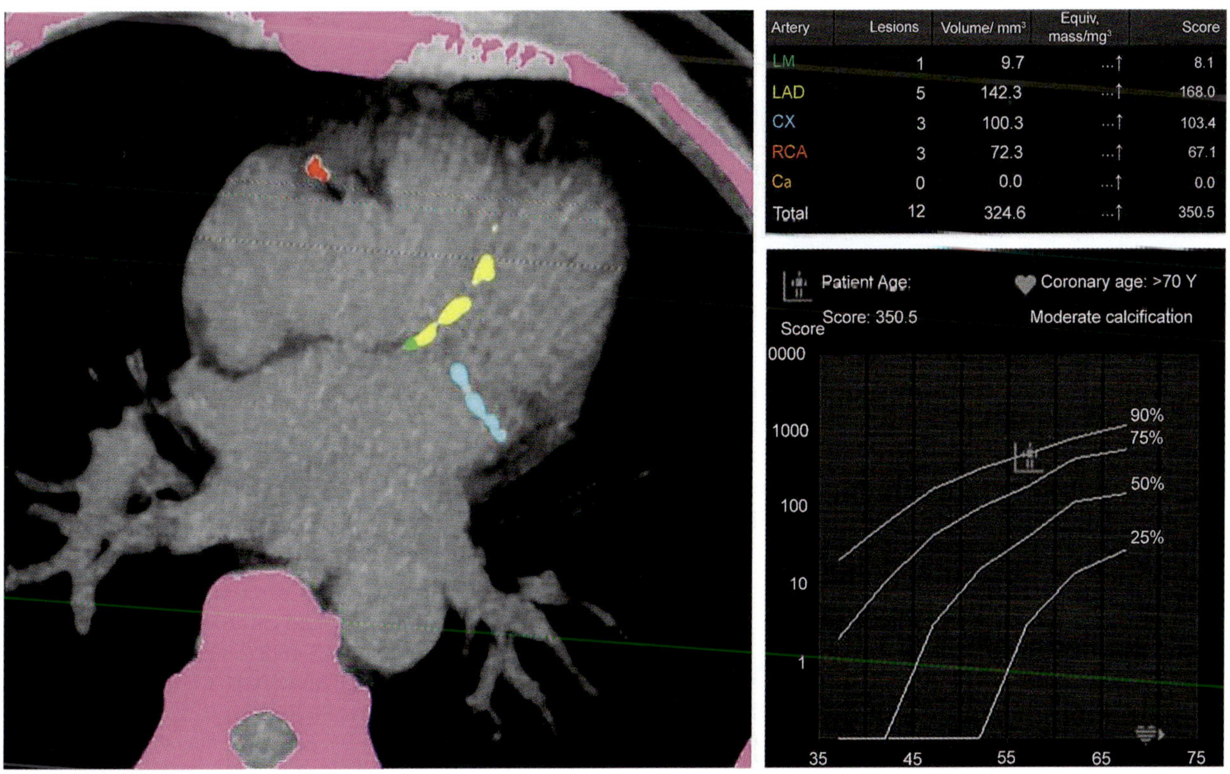

Fig. 2: CAC score in obese patient.

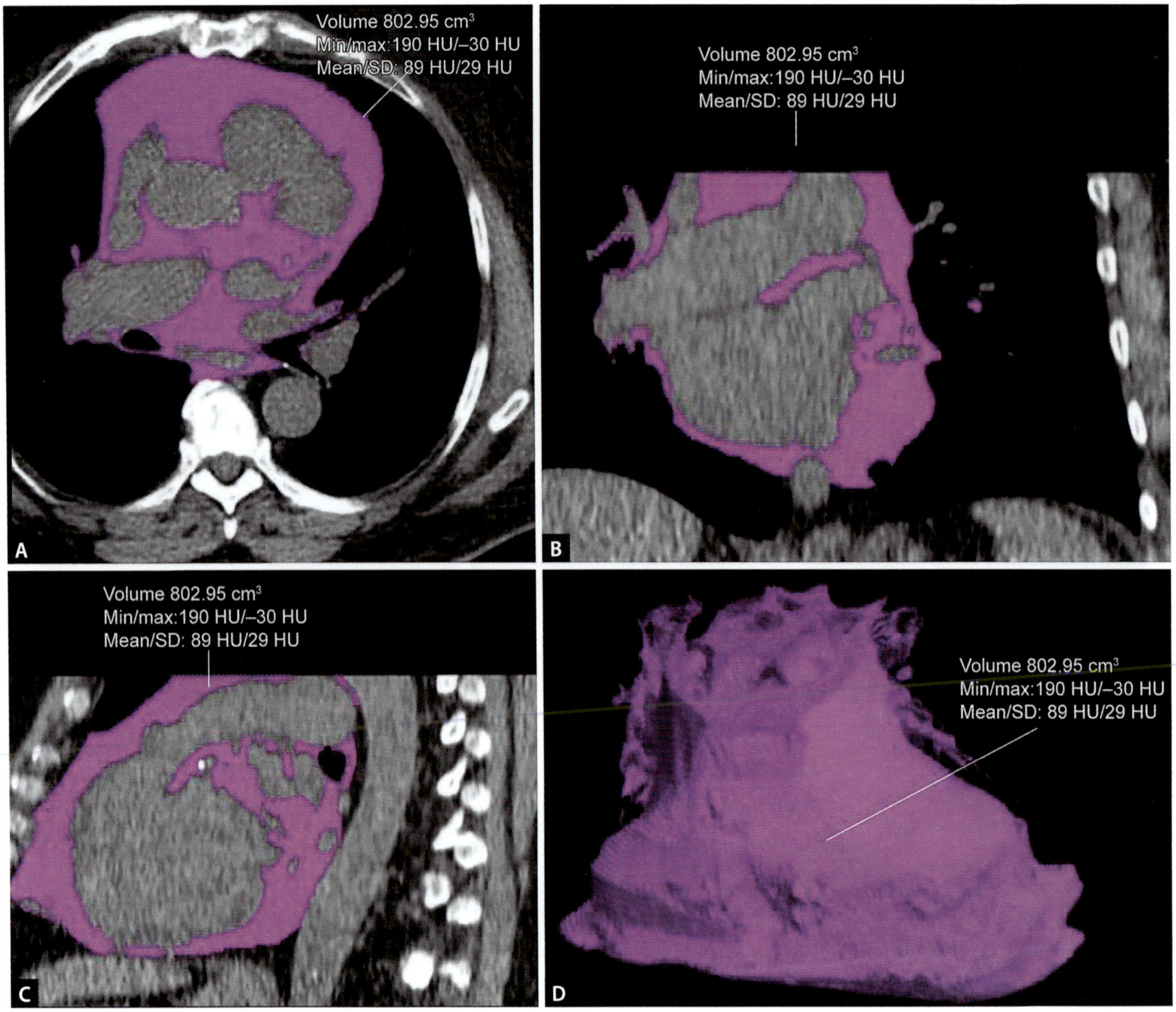

Figs. 3A to D: Elevated epicardial fat volume (505 cc) with the epicardial fat attenuation of –85 HU in a 70-year-old male with atypical chest pain.

- *Obesity paradox*: Although obese patients often show higher CAC prevalence, the prognostic link between CAC and mortality is less consistent, because some obese individuals—particularly those metabolically healthy—exhibit relatively lower cardiovascular mortality despite elevated calcium scores.[10]

CONCLUSION

Obesity independently increases the likelihood and extent of coronary calcification, reinforcing that CAC scoring remains a valuable risk stratification tool in obese patients. However, interpretation should account for the obesity paradox and possible confounding from metabolic health status when predicting outcomes.

REFERENCES

1. Koskinas KC, Van Craenenbroeck EM, Prescott EB. European Society of Cardiology clinical consensus statement on obesity and cardiovascular disease: 10 key points. Eur Heart J. 2025;46(37):3611-12.
2. Neves PO, Andrade J, Monção H. Coronary artery calcium score: current status. Radiol Bras. 2017;50(3):182-9.
3. Jensen JC, Dardari ZA, Blaha MJ, et al. Association of body mass index with coronary artery calcium and subsequent

cardiovascular mortality: the coronary artery calcium consortium. Circ Cardiovasc Imaging. 2020;13(7):e009495.

4. Chang Y, Kim BK, Yun KE, et al. Metabolically-healthy obesity and coronary artery calcification. J Am Coll Cardiol. 2014;63(24):2679-86.
5. Rhee EJ, Seo MH, Kim JD, et al. Metabolic health is more closely associated with coronary artery calcification than obesity. PLoS One. 2013;8(9):e74564.
6. Chung GE, Park HE, Lee H, et al. Sarcopenic obesity is significantly associated with coronary artery calcification. Front Med (Lausanne). 2021;8:651961.
7. Lemanowicz A, Białecki M, Leszczyński W, et al. Coronary age, based on coronary calcium measurement, is increased in patients with morbid obesity. Pol J Radiol. 2018;83:e415-e420.
8. Wang G, Jing M, Xi H, et al. Association of mean pericoronary adipose tissue attenuation with different demographic factors in a subgroup of patients without coronary artery disease stratified by sex, body mass index, and age. Quant Imaging Med Surg. 2024;14(1): 503-13.
9. Bakkum MJ, Danad I, Romijn MA, et al. The impact of obesity on the relationship between epicardial adipose tissue, left ventricular mass and coronary microvascular function. Eur J Nucl Med Mol Imaging. 2015;42(10): 1562-73.
10. Jagia P, Vidiyala P. Correlation of intrathoracic fat parameters and extra coronary calcium with severity of coronary artery disease. J Cardiovasc Comput Tomogr. 2024;18(4):81.

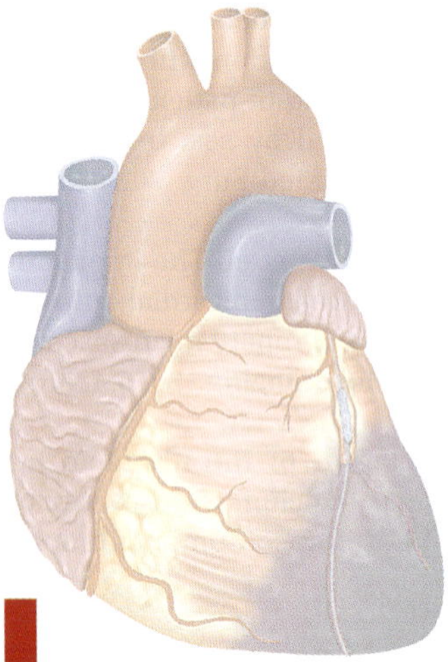

32 CHAPTER

Obesity and Vulnerable Plaque: Pathophysiology and Clinical Insights

Sandeepan Saha, Aditya Kapoor

INTRODUCTION

Cardiovascular disease (CVD) remains the leading cause of death worldwide, and within its spectrum, acute coronary syndromes (ACSs) are among the most devastating manifestations. The underlying substrate of most ACS events is the rupture or erosion of atherosclerotic plaques within coronary arteries, leading to thrombus formation and vessel occlusion. Importantly, not all atherosclerotic plaques are equal—while some remain stable and clinically silent, others demonstrate biological features that predispose them to rupture. These rupture-prone lesions are referred to as "*vulnerable plaques*."

Obesity, a global epidemic with rapidly rising prevalence, is strongly associated with cardiovascular morbidity and mortality. Traditionally, obesity has been linked to increased ASCVD risk through its contribution to hypertension, diabetes mellitus, and dyslipidemia. However, evidence now suggests that obesity has direct effects on plaque biology, modulating the inflammatory and metabolic environment that drives plaque vulnerability. This chapter explores the interface between obesity and vulnerable plaque: How excess adiposity contributes to plaque instability, how imaging modalities allow us to identify these high-risk features in vivo, and how therapies targeting obesity and inflammation may influence clinical outcomes.

VULNERABLE PLAQUE: DEFINITIONS AND FEATURES

Pathological Basis

Autopsy studies by Virmani et al. established the concept of plaque vulnerability, identifying *thin-cap fibroatheroma (TCFA)* as the most common precursor lesion to plaque rupture.[1] The vulnerable plaque is characterized by:

- A thin fibrous cap (<65 μm in histopathology)
- A large lipid necrotic core
- Abundant macrophage infiltration
- Neovascularization and intraplaque hemorrhage
- Microcalcifications, which contribute to mechanical instability

The major and minor criteria for defining vulnerable plaque are summarized in **Table 1**.

Plaque erosion, another important mechanism of ACS, is less dependent on lipid burden but still influenced by endothelial dysfunction and local inflammation.

Pathophysiological Mechanisms Linking Obesity to Plaque Vulnerability

Obesity is not merely a condition of excess weight but a *state of chronic metabolic inflammation* (metainflammation). Multiple mechanisms connect obesity to plaque vulnerability.

TABLE 1: Criteria for defining vulnerable plaques on the basis of the study of "Culprit" plaques.[2]

Major	• *Active inflammation:* Monocyte and macrophage and sometimes T-cell infiltration • Thin cap with large lipid-necrotic core • Endothelial denudation with superficial platelet aggregation • Fissured plaque • Stenosis >90%
Minor	• Superficial calcified nodule • Glistening yellow plaque seen at angioscopy • Intraplaque hemorrhage • Endothelial dysfunction • Outward (positive) remodeling

Epicardial and Perivascular Adipose Tissue

Epicardial adipose tissue (EAT) and perivascular adipose tissue (PVAT) are visceral fat depots in close proximity to coronary arteries. Unlike subcutaneous fat, these tissues lack fascial boundaries and exert paracrine and vasocrine effects on the coronary wall. Cytokines and adipokines secreted by EAT/PVAT directly diffuse into the vessel wall, promoting endothelial dysfunction, oxidative stress, and local inflammation.[3] This "outside-to-inside" signaling mechanism further amplifies local vascular inflammation and destabilization. Imaging biomarkers, such as pericoronary fat attenuation index (FAI), provide in vivo evidence of this link. A higher FAI values reflect inflamed PVAT and correlate with high-risk plaques (HRPs).[4]

Adipose Tissue as an Endocrine Organ

Adipose tissue is no longer considered a passive energy store but an active endocrine organ that secretes a variety of adipokines and cytokines. In obesity, hypertrophied adipocytes and infiltrating macrophages release proinflammatory mediators such as tumor necrosis factor-α (TNF-α), interleukin-6 (IL-6), and monocyte chemoattractant protein-1 (MCP-1). These factors enhance systemic and vascular inflammation, key drivers of plaque vulnerability.

Conversely, the secretion of protective adipokines like adiponectin is markedly reduced in obesity. Adiponectin exerts anti-inflammatory, antiatherogenic, and endothelial-protective effects. Thus, the imbalance between pro- and anti-atherogenic adipokines fosters an environment conducive to plaque destabilization.

Key mediators include:

- *Leptin:* In obese individuals, adipose tissue secretes excess leptin, leading to *hyperleptinemia*. Despite leptin's normal role in suppressing appetite and regulating metabolism, most obese patients develop *leptin resistance*, where tissues become less responsive to leptin's signals. This state contributes to persistent obesity and dyslipidemia. High leptin levels and leptin resistance promote atherosclerosis (AS) through multiple mechanisms:
  - *Endothelial dysfunction and inflammation:* Leptin stimulates monocytes and macrophages to produce proinflammatory cytokines (IL-6, TNF-α), promotes foam cell formation, and induces vascular inflammation.
  - *Lipid metabolism disturbance:* Hyperleptinemia disrupts cholesterol and triglyceride regulation, worsening dyslipidemia.
  - *Insulin resistance and diabetes link:* Excess leptin aggravates insulin resistance, further accelerating AS risk.
  - *Hypertension:* Leptin activates the sympathetic nervous system and increases aldosterone, raising blood pressure.

  Thus, in obesity, abnormal leptin signaling not only reflects excessive adiposity but also directly accelerates AS through vascular inflammation, metabolic dysregulation, and hemodynamic changes.[5]
- *Adiponectin*: Adiponectin is an adipokine with anti-inflammatory, insulin-sensitizing, and antiatherogenic effects. It protects vascular endothelium, enhances nitric oxide (NO) production, inhibits macrophage foam cell formation, and stabilizes plaques. Paradoxically, its circulating levels are reduced in obesity and metabolic syndrome, contributing to endothelial dysfunction, insulin resistance, and accelerated AS.[6]
- *Proinflammatory cytokines:* Resistin, TNF-α, IL-6, and MCP-1 are secreted by dysfunctional adipocytes and infiltrating macrophages, fueling vascular inflammation.

The paracrine secretion of these factors creates a local proinflammatory microenvironment that accelerates atherogenesis and destabilization.

Endothelial Dysfunction and Oxidative Stress

Obesity reduces NO bioavailability, impairs vasodilation, and promotes leukocyte adhesion. Oxidative stress damages endothelial integrity, setting the stage for plaque erosion and thrombosis.

Prothrombotic State

Obesity is associated with increased platelet activation, elevated plasminogen activator inhibitor-1 (PAI-1), and elevated fibrinogen levels.[7] Thus, plaque rupture in obese patients is more likely to be followed by occlusive thrombus, linking vulnerable plaque with a vulnerable patient.

Insulin Resistance and Metabolic Dysregulation

Obesity is strongly associated with insulin resistance, leading to compensatory hyperinsulinemia, glucose intolerance, and type 2 diabetes mellitus. Hyperglycemia induces endothelial dysfunction via increased advanced glycation end-products (AGEs), oxidative stress, and activation of prothrombotic pathways. Dyslipidemia, characterized by elevated triglycerides, small dense LDL particles, and reduced HDL cholesterol, further accelerates lipid deposition within plaques.

Small dense LDL particles are particularly atherogenic due to their greater arterial wall penetration, susceptibility to oxidation, and prolonged plasma half-life. Oxidized LDL promotes foam cell formation and necrotic core enlargement—hallmarks of vulnerable plaque.

Systemic and Vascular Inflammation

Obesity induces a chronic low-grade inflammatory state. Circulating C-reactive protein (CRP), IL-6, and TNF-α are elevated and correlate with adverse cardiovascular outcomes. Within the vascular wall, these mediators upregulate adhesion molecules, facilitate monocyte recruitment, and promote macrophage activation.[8] Activated macrophages secrete MMPs, which degrade extracellular matrix and thin fibrous cap. A schematic diagram of the mechanistic link between obesity and AS is illustrated in **Figure 1**.

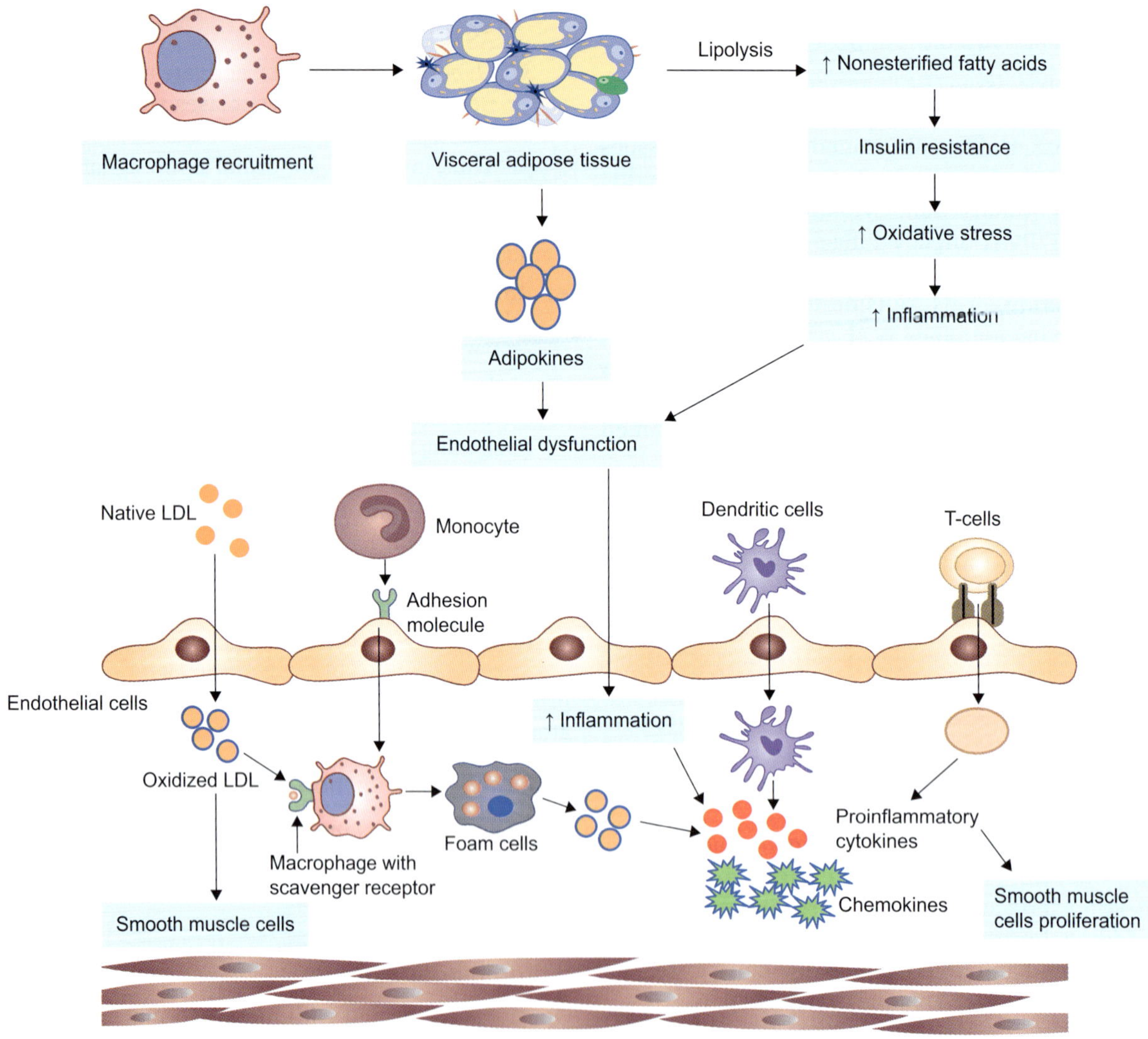

Fig. 1: Pathophysiological pathways linking obesity and atherosclerosis. Atherosclerosis begins with LDL retention and oxidation in the vessel wall, leading to foam cell formation, inflammation, and smooth muscle cell proliferation. Immune cells, including dendritic and T-cells, are recruited into the plaque, driving progression. In obesity, macrophage infiltration of adipose tissue promotes adipokine release, lipolysis, and elevated nonesterified fatty acids, fostering insulin resistance. This proinflammatory, pro-oxidative milieu aggravates endothelial dysfunction, smooth muscle growth, and accelerates plaque development.

TABLE 2: Endothelial function in healthy versus obese states.

Factor	*Healthy endothelium*	*Obese endothelium*
Vasoconstrictors	↓ (Reduced)	↑ (Increased)
Vasodilators	↑ (Increased)	↓ (Reduced)
Anticoagulant factors	↑ (Enhanced)	↓ (Reduced)
Procoagulant factors	↓ (Suppressed)	↑ (Enhanced)
Inflammatory mediators	↓ (Low)	↑ (Elevated)
Growth factors	↓ (Controlled)	↑ (Excessive)
Reactive oxygen species	↓ (Low oxidative stress)	↑ (High oxidative stress)

The key differences in endothelial function between healthy and obese states are summarized in **Table 2**.

Imaging Correlates

Noninvasive and invasive imaging modalities have enabled in vivo identification of vulnerable plaques.

Coronary CT angiography (CCTA): Beyond quantifying luminal stenosis, CCTA can characterize *HRP* features associated with ACS.[9] Hallmarks of HRP include:

- Low-attenuation plaque (LAP) (<30 HU)
- Napkin-ring sign
- Spotty calcification
- Positive remodeling index

Studies show these features are more prevalent in obese and metabolically unhealthy individuals. LAP burden, in particular, is a powerful predictor of events, outperforming luminal stenosis severity. Furthermore, pericoronary FAI correlates with local vascular inflammation, providing a direct link between adiposity and plaque biology.[10] CCTA also quantifies EAT volume and density. Increased EAT correlates with HRP features, reinforcing its pathogenic role.

Advances such as computational fluid dynamics (FFRCT, wall shear stress, axial plaque stress) and pericoronary adipose tissue (PCAT) attenuation analysis allow integration of hemodynamic forces and vascular inflammation into plaque evaluation, improving prediction of rupture-prone lesions. CCTA has demonstrated independent prognostic value in identifying patients at increased risk of ACS, even when stenosis is nonobstructive. Emerging tools combining anatomical, functional, and perivascular assessments further enhance risk stratification.[9] The SCOT-HEART trial highlighted that LAP burden on CCTA independently predicted myocardial infarction, underscoring the prognostic relevance of vulnerable plaque features.[11]

Cardiac Magnetic Resonance and Positron Emission Tomography

Emerging imaging modalities explore adipose inflammation. Positron emission tomography (PET) tracers such as 18F-FDG and novel inflammation-targeted tracers can assess PVAT activity, offering potential tools for obesity-related plaque research.

Intravascular Imaging Studies

- *Intravascular ultrasound (IVUS):* VH-IVUS reveals larger necrotic cores and higher remodeling indices in obese patients. Importantly, progression studies demonstrate accelerated transformation of fibroatheroma into TCFA among individuals with metabolic syndrome. Amano et al. showed using integrated backscatter IVUS (IB-IVUS) that patients with metabolic syndrome had plaques with a higher lipid volume and lower fibrous content, identifying MetS as an independent predictor of lipid-rich, vulnerable plaques.[12]
- *Optical coherence tomography (OCT):* OCT provides high-resolution imaging of fibrous caps. Obesity has been linked with thinner caps, greater lipid arc, and higher frequency of macrophage accumulations. In a study by Kataoka et al. involving 308 patients with coronary artery disease who underwent frequency-domain (FD)-OCT, obese patients were found to have more vulnerable atherosclerotic plaques than nonobese patients, characterized by thinner fibrous caps and a higher prevalence of TCFAs.[13]
- *Near-infrared spectroscopy (NIRS):* Obese individuals show higher lipid core burden index (LCBI), supporting a link between adiposity and lipid-rich plaques. Park et al. demonstrated that patients with thicker EAT had a significantly higher maximum LCBI on NIRS-IVUS, identifying epicardial fat as an independent predictor of lipid-rich vulnerable plaques in coronary artery disease.[14]

Autopsy Studies

Autopsy analyses of obese individuals reveal larger necrotic cores, greater macrophage infiltration, and thinner fibrous caps compared to lean individuals with CAD. Obesity correlates with increased prevalence of plaque rupture as the mechanism of sudden cardiac death. *Burke et al.* conducted an autopsy study of sudden coronary death and demonstrated that plaque rupture, compared with erosion, was significantly associated with higher body mass index, implicating obesity as a determinant of the rupture phenotype.[15]

TABLE 3: Summary of key studies linking obesity and vulnerable plaque.

Study/author	*Method/population*	*Key findings in obese patients*	*Implication for plaque rupture*
Kataoka et al.[13] (FD-OCT, 308 patients with CAD)	Frequency-domain optical coherence tomography	Thinner fibrous caps, higher prevalence of thin-cap fibroatheroma	Obesity promotes plaque vulnerability and rupture risk
Stone et al.[18] (ADAPT-DES Study)	Intravascular ultrasound in patients post-PCI	Highest BMI tertile had more plaque rupture and larger necrotic core	Obesity independently associated with higher prevalence of plaque rupture
Nishihira et al.[19] (Histology, 390 carotid plaques)	Carotid endarterectomy specimens	Obese males (<70 years) had ~6-fold higher odds of unstable plaques	Obesity predisposes to plaque destabilization and rupture
Amano et al.[12] (IB-IVUS, mild–moderate CAD)	Integrated backscatter intravascular ultrasound	Metabolic syndrome (often obesity-related) → larger lipid pool and necrotic core	Obesity contributes to vulnerable plaque phenotype
Schreuder et al.[20] (coronary CT in diabetics)	Coronary CTA in type 2 diabetes patients	BMI strongly correlated with larger, softer plaque volume	Obesity linked to higher burden of rupture-prone plaque
Burke et al.[15]	Autopsy study of sudden coronary death victims	Higher BMI observed in individuals with plaque rupture compared to those with plaque erosion	Obesity predisposes to rupture-prone plaque morphology
Holmström et al.[16]	600 autopsies of sudden coronary death due to CAD	Majority of decedents were overweight or obese	Supports obesity as a background factor in rupture-related sudden death
Michaud et al.[17]	Autopsy cases with acute coronary thrombosis (22 ruptures, 6 erosions)	BMI data indicated increased adiposity among rupture cases	Adiposity may enhance susceptibility to fatal plaque rupture
Hogea et al.[21]	Autopsy study of sudden cardiac death with epicardial adipose tissue measurement	Epicardial fat thickness correlated with BMI and silent MI	Obesity-related epicardial fat may contribute to plaque vulnerability and rupture

Holmström et al. analyzed 600 autopsies of sudden coronary death due to coronary artery disease and reported that plaque rupture represented the dominant substrate, with the majority of decedents categorized as overweight or obese.[16]

Michaud et al. investigated autopsy cases of acute coronary thrombosis and identified plaque rupture in 22 and erosion in six individuals, with body weight and BMI records supporting a contributory role of adiposity in rupture-related mortality.[17]

Table 3 summarizes key studies, their methodologies, and findings in obese patients, highlighting the implications for plaque rupture.

THERAPEUTIC STRATEGIES TARGETING OBESITY AND PLAQUE VULNERABILITY

Lifestyle Interventions

Weight loss through caloric restriction and exercise reduces systemic inflammation and regresses EAT.[22] Importantly, even modest weight loss (5–10%) improves endothelial function and lowers CRP.[23]

Pharmacological Interventions

- *Statins*: Statins stabilize plaques by reducing lipid core, promoting calcification, and reducing inflammation. Imaging trials demonstrate statin-induced regression of HRP.
- *PCSK9 inhibitors*: Potently lower LDL-C and promote regression of necrotic core volume on IVUS.
- *GLP-1 receptor agonists (GLP-1RAs)*: Reduce EAT volume and improve endothelial function.
- *SGLT2 inhibitors*: Show reductions in visceral fat and improvements in vascular inflammation, though direct plaque imaging evidence is emerging.
- *Anti-inflammatory therapies*: The CANTOS trial demonstrated that IL-1β inhibition reduces recurrent cardiovascular events independent of lipid lowering.[24]

Bariatric Surgery

Bariatric surgery induces substantial and sustained weight loss. MRI and CCTA studies reveal reductions in EAT and pericardial fat postsurgery.[25] Long-term observational studies confirm reductions in cardiovascular events, likely mediated by both risk factor improvement and direct changes in plaque biology.

Flowchart 1: The mechanistic links between obesity and the formation of vulnerable plaques—through pathways involving inflammation, endothelial dysfunction, and adipokine imbalance—are illustrated in the flowchart.

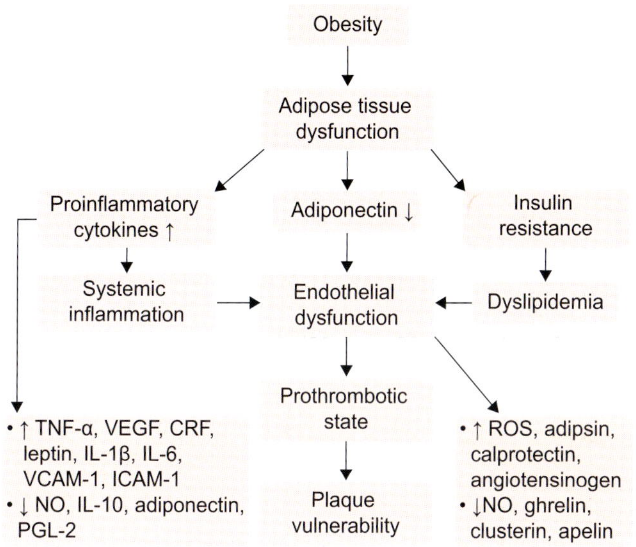

FUTURE DIRECTIONS

Despite accumulating evidence, many mechanistic links between obesity and plaque vulnerability remain incompletely understood. Future research priorities include:

- *Integration of adiposity measures into risk models*: Combining BMI with EAT volume, PVAT inflammation (FAI), and imaging-based plaque characteristics could refine ASCVD risk prediction.
- *Novel therapies targeting adipokines*: Restoring the leptin/adiponectin balance or modulating adipose tissue inflammation may provide new avenues for stabilizing plaques.
- *Synergy of therapies*: Future studies should explore combinations of GLP-1RAs, SGLT2 inhibitors, and anti-inflammatory agents in obese CAD patients.
- *Longitudinal imaging trials*: Needed to confirm that regression of EAT and LAP translates into fewer plaque rupture events.
- Integrating *artificial intelligence* in imaging to predict plaque vulnerability in obese individuals.

The mechanistic links between obesity and the formation of vulnerable plaques—through pathways involving inflammation, endothelial dysfunction, and adipokine imbalance—are illustrated in **Flowchart 1**.

CONCLUSION

Obesity plays a central role in the pathobiology of vulnerable plaque. Through complex interactions involving epicardial fat, adipokines, endothelial dysfunction, and systemic inflammation, obesity fosters the development of plaques with features prone to rupture and thrombosis. Modern imaging provides unprecedented insights into these relationships, enabling identification of high-risk individuals. Therapeutic strategies including lifestyle modification, pharmacological therapies, and bariatric surgery demonstrate potential for reversing plaque vulnerability. Targeting obesity thus represents a dual opportunity: Reducing global cardiovascular risk factors and directly stabilizing the atherosclerotic plaque.

REFERENCES

1. Virmani R, Kolodgie FD, Burke AP, et al. Lessons from sudden coronary death: a comprehensive morphological classification scheme for atherosclerotic lesions. Arterioscler Thromb Vasc Biol. 2000;20(5):1262-75.
2. Saam T, Hatsukami TS, Takaya N, et al. The vulnerable, or high-risk, atherosclerotic plaque: noninvasive MR imaging for characterization and assessment. Radiology. 2007;244(1):64-77.
3. Iacobellis G. Local and systemic effects of the multifaceted epicardial adipose tissue depot. Nat Rev Endocrinol. 2015;11(6):363-71.
4. Antoniades C, Antonopoulos AS, Deanfield J. Imaging residual inflammatory risk by perivascular fat attenuation index. J Am Coll Cardiol. 2018;72(4):323-6.
5. Wang C, Chang L, Wang J, et al. Leptin and risk factors for atherosclerosis: a review. Medicine. 2023;102(46):e36076.
6. Choi HM, Doss HM, Kim KS. Multifaceted physiological roles of adiponectin in inflammation and diseases. Int J Mol Sci. 2020;21(4):1219.
7. Samad F, Ruf W. Inflammation, obesity, and thrombosis. Blood. 2013;122(20):3415-22.
8. Hajjar DP, Gotto Jr AM. Biological relevance of inflammation and oxidative stress in the pathogenesis of arterial diseases. Am J Pathol. 2013;182(5):1474-81.
9. Lu G, Ye W, Ou J, et al. Coronary computed tomography angiography assessment of high-risk plaques in predicting acute coronary syndrome. Front Cardiovasc Med. 2021;8:743538.
10. Antonopoulos AS, Sanna F, Sabharwal N, et al. Detecting human coronary inflammation by imaging perivascular fat. Sci Transl Med. 2017;9(398):eaal2658.
11. Williams MC, Kwiecinski J, Doris M, et al. Low-attenuation noncalcified plaque on coronary computed tomography angiography predicts myocardial infarction: results

from the multicenter SCOT-HEART trial (Scottish Computed Tomography of the HEART). Circulation. 2020;141(18):1452-62.
12. Amano T, Matsubara T, Uetani T, et al. Impact of metabolic syndrome on tissue characteristics of angiographically mild to moderate coronary lesions: integrated backscatter intravascular ultrasound study. J Am Coll Cardiol. 2007;49(11):1149-56.
13. Kataoka Y, Puri R, Hammadah M, et al. Plaque vulnerability at non-culprit lesions in obese patients with coronary artery disease: frequency-domain optical coherence tomography analysis. Eur J Prev Cardiol. 2015;22(10):1331-9.
14. Park SS, Jung J, Mintz GS, et al. Epicardial adipose tissue thickness is related to plaque composition in coronary artery disease. Diagnostics. 2022;12(11):2836.
15. Burke AP, Farb A, Malcom GT, et al. Coronary risk factors and plaque morphology in men and women with coronary disease-causing sudden death. Circulation. 1998;97(3):213-6.
16. Holmström L, Agewall S, Yan C, et al. Culprit plaque morphology in sudden coronary death due to coronary artery disease: an autopsy study. Eur Heart J. 2022;43(20):1926-36.
17. Michaud K, Fellmann F, Giroud C, et al. Coronary artery calcifications and acute coronary thrombosis at autopsy: correlation with sudden cardiac death. Front Cardiovasc Med. 2021;8:692176.
18. Stone GW, Maehara A, Lansky AJ, et al.; PROSPECT Investigators. A prospective natural-history study of coronary atherosclerosis. N Engl J Med. 2011;364(3):226-35.
19. Nishihira K, Ishizaka N, Sumi M, et al. Obesity is associated with destabilized carotid plaques: a histological study. J Atheroscler Thromb. 2018;25(5):415-23.
20. Schreuder MM, van der Graaf Y, van der Velde AE, et al. SMART Study Group. Relation between body mass index and morphological features of coronary atherosclerotic plaques as assessed by multislice computed tomography in patients with type 2 diabetes mellitus. Cardiovasc Diabetol. 2014;13:91.
21. Hogea B, Popescu C, Dican L, et al. Epicardial adipose tissue, obesity, and silent myocardial infarction in sudden cardiac death victims: an autopsy study. Diagnostics (Basel). 2023;13(7):1345.
22. Liu Y, Hong F, Lebaka VR, et al. Calorie restriction with exercise intervention improves inflammatory response in overweight and obese adults: a systematic review and meta-analysis. Front Physiol. 2021;12:754731.
23. Tiezzi M, Vieceli Dalla Sega F, Gentileschi P, et al. Effects of weight loss on endothelium and vascular homeostasis: impact on cardiovascular risk. Biomedicines. 2025;13(2):381.
24. Ridker PM, Everett BM, Thuren T, et al. Anti-inflammatory therapy with canakinumab for atherosclerotic disease. N Engl J Med. 2017;377(12):1119-31.
25. Gaborit B, Jacquier A, Kober F, et al. Effects of bariatric surgery on cardiac ectopic fat: lesser decrease in epicardial fat compared to visceral fat loss and no change in myocardial triglyceride content. J Am Coll Cardiol. 2012;60(15):1381-9.

SECTION 5

Obesity and Hypertension

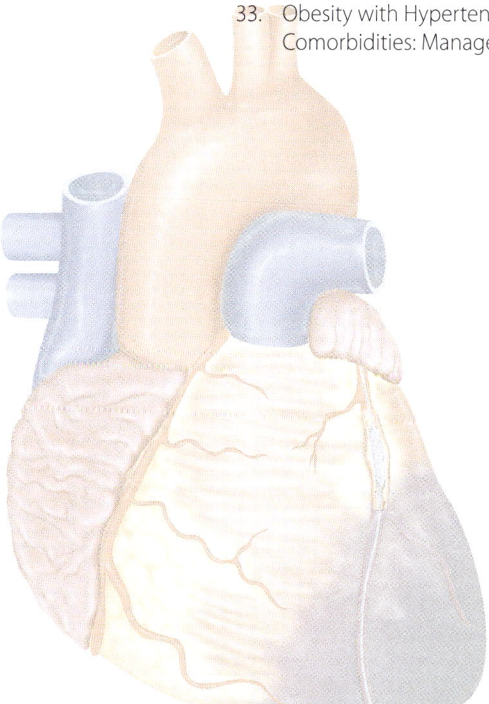

33

CHAPTER

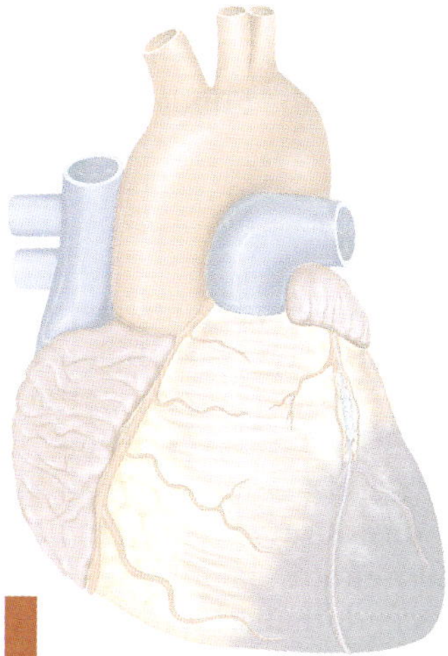

Obesity with Hypertension with Multiple Comorbidities: Management Strategies

Jabir Abdullakutty, Teena Jabir

INTRODUCTION

Obesity-related hypertension[1,2] has become a major cardiovascular problem in clinical practice. As people gain weight around the world, blood pressure is also rising, which together accelerates heart and kidney[3] disease. This form of hypertension[1] is unique because of its complex causes. Extra body fat disrupts normal blood flow by overstimulating nerve and hormone systems and putting stress on several organs.

This condition involves an overactive sympathetic nervous system[2] and increased activity of the renin-angiotensin-aldosterone[4,5] system. Insulin resistance, mild inflammation, and fat pressing on the kidneys[3] also contribute. Many patients have salt-sensitive, volume-related hypertension[1] that may not respond well to standard medications. Over time, high blood pressure harms the heart and kidneys[3] and makes metabolic syndrome worse. Managing these patients requires a plan that lowers blood pressure and addresses the underlying metabolic issues.

PATHOPHYSIOLOGY

Excess weight causes long-term high blood pressure through several connected factors. These include increased nerve activity,[1] hormone imbalances, pressure on the kidneys,[3] blood vessel problems, and inflammation that weakens normal blood vessel function **(Flowchart 1)**.

Flowchart 1: Pathophysiology of obesity-related hypertension.

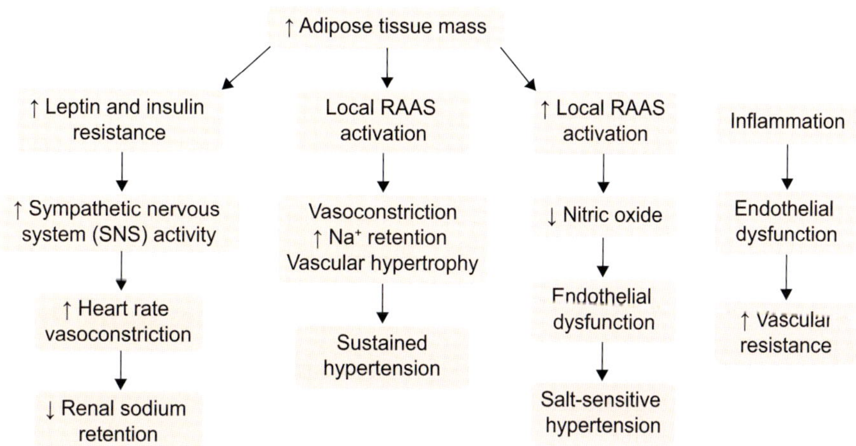

Sympathetic Stimulation

More body fat raises leptin[2] levels and changes how the brain responds to insulin. These changes activate the hypothalamus, which increases nerve activity to the heart, blood vessels, and kidneys.[3] This makes the heart pump harder, blood vessels tighten, and the kidneys[3] hold onto more sodium. As a result, blood pressure remains high, especially in people with insulin resistance or sleep apnea.[1]

Hormonal Activation (RAAS)[4,5]

Adipose tissue produces its own renin-angiotensin-aldosterone[4,5] hormones. Locally made angiotensin II and aldosterone cause blood vessels to narrow, increase sodium retention,[3] and promote tissue scarring. Ongoing exposure leads to stiff arteries and changes in the heart's left ventricle. Along with increased nerve activity,[1] these hormones are central to the development of obesity-related hypertension.

Mechanical Influence on the Kidneys

Large amounts of fat around and near the kidneys[3] increase pressure inside the kidney.[3] This pressure makes it harder for the kidneys[3] to filter blood and affects how they handle sodium. The body then needs higher blood pressure to remove the same amount of sodium. Over time, this leads to salt-sensitive hypertension,[1] small amounts of protein in the urine, and gradual loss of kidney[3] units.

Endothelial and Metabolic Changes

Inflamed fat tissue releases chemicals that use up nitric oxide,[6] which is important for relaxing blood vessels. Without enough nitric oxide,[6] arteries become stiff and more reactive, which increases resistance in the blood vessels. At the same time, insulin resistance[2] and abnormal blood fats speed up artery hardening, making blood pressure stay high.

Obstructive Sleep Apnea

Repeated low-oxygen episodes during sleep trigger bursts of nerve activity. Each episode briefly raises blood pressure, and over the years, this leads to lasting hypertension and worsened insulin resistance.[2] Treating sleep apnea[1] often improves both night and day blood pressure and helps with overall metabolic control.

MANAGEMENT

Successful control demands a strategy that addresses body weight, neurohormonal imbalance, and vascular damage together. No single measure suffices; lifestyle reform, pharmacologic therapy, and sometimes surgical intervention must be combined under ongoing supervision.

Lifestyle and Nutrition

Structured lifestyle change is the most effective and sustainable therapy. Calorie reduction using balanced diets such as DASH[7] or the Mediterranean pattern consistently lowers both weight and pressure. The goal is to restrict salt to <2 g daily and to emphasize fruits, vegetables, legumes, and unsaturated fats. Regular aerobic exercise—about 150 minutes each week—plus resistance training enhances endothelial[6] function and insulin action. Even modest weight loss of 5–10% can reduce systolic pressure by several millimeters of mercury. Attention to sleep quality, stress reduction, and correction of sleep apnea[1] further strengthens results.

Pharmacologic Therapy

- Drug treatment complements lifestyle measures.
- ACE inhibitors[8] or angiotensin-receptor blockers counter hormonal activation and protect renal function.
- Calcium-channel blockers relax arterial smooth muscle.
- Thiazide-like diuretics such as chlorthalidone relieve volume excess.
- Mineralocorticoid antagonists (spironolactone[8] or eplerenone) are valuable in resistant cases.
- Vasodilating β-blockers such as nebivolol[8] suit patients with coronary or heart failure overlap.
- Therapy should be individualized, often requiring combinations to reach target pressures.

Weight-targeted Drugs

Modern pharmacotherapy now allows weight reduction alongside pressure control. Agents that mimic or enhance incretin hormones—semaglutide[9] or tirzepatide—achieve double-digit percentage weight loss and improve metabolic flexibility. Sodium-glucose cotransporter-2 inhibitors aid natriuresis and protect both heart and kidney.[3] Using these drugs with diet and exercise[7] bridges the gap between medical and surgical approaches.

Surgical and Metabolic Procedures

When obesity is severe, with a body mass index over 40 kg/m^2 or over 35 kg/m^2 with complications, metabolic surgery is a practical option. Procedures like sleeve gastrectomy[10] and Roux-en-Y gastric bypass change gut hormones, improve insulin sensitivity, and lower aldosterone[4,5] levels. Many patients see their hypertension[1] partly or fully go away, and their heart size return to normal within months. Over the long term, these surgeries can help people live longer and need fewer medications.

Continuing Multidisciplinary Care

Long-term stability depends on regular follow-up[11,12] with a team that includes heart, kidney,[3] hormone, and nutrition specialists. Checking blood pressure, kidney[3] function, and waist size regularly helps catch problems early. Using mobile health apps or structured programs can keep patients motivated and help them stick to their treatment, turning short-term gains into lasting control.[13,14]

LIMITATION

This discussion summarizes current knowledge but is not based on a systematic review. How patients respond can vary by genetics, ethnicity, environment, and available resources. Differences in access to medicines and surgery also affect results. More long-term studies are needed to find out which treatment order works best over time.

ALGORITHMIC OUTLINE

The clinical evaluation starts by measuring body mass index, waist size, fasting blood sugar, cholesterol, and kidney[3] function. It is also essential to check for sleep apnea[1] and other possible causes.

Initial management focuses on improving diet, limiting salt, and increasing physical activity. Managing stress and getting enough sleep also help support these changes. Begin pharmacologic therapy with ACE inhibitors[8] or ARBs, followed by calcium-channel blockers and thiazide-type diuretics. In resistant hypertension,[1] add mineralocorticoid antagonists. If metabolic problems continue, use incretin-based drugs or SGLT2 inhibitors.[9]

If conservative treatments do not work or obesity is very severe, metabolic surgery[10] can provide lasting benefits. Ongoing monitoring of weight, kidney[3] function, and cardiovascular risk ensures that gains are maintained and complications prevented **(Flowchart 2)**.

Flowchart 2: Algorithm for the evaluation and management of obesity-associated hypertension.

Patient with obesity + hypertension ± multiple comorbidities

↓

Confirm phenotype:
- Waist circumference/BMI/OSA screen (stop-bang)
- 24-h ABPM or HBPM; check dipping pattern
- *Labs:* eGFR, K^+, UACR, fasting lipids, HbA1c; PRA/aldosterone if resistant

↓

Foundation therapy (ALL):
- Sodium <2 g/day: Weight-loss program
- Physical activity ≥150 min/week + resistance
- Treat OSA (CPAP) when present

↓

Antihypertensive backbone:
- ACE inhibitor or ARB
- + Dihydropyridine calcium-channel blocker
- + Thiazide-like diuretic (chlorthalidone/indapamide) if volume expanded

↓

Resistant or aaldosterone phenotype:
- Add mineralocorticoid receptor antagonist
- Consider loop diuretic if reduced eGFR
- Evaluate for primary aldosteronism

↓

Weight-centric pharmacotherapy:
- GLP-1 receptor agonist/dual incretin
- SGLT2 inhibitor (renal–cardio benefit)
- Consider metabolic surgery if BMI ≥40 or ≥35 with comorbidities

CONCLUSION

Obesity-related hypertension[1,2] shows how too much metabolic stress can change how the heart and blood vessels work. The goal of treatment is not just to reach certain blood pressure numbers, but to restore the body's natural balance. Lifestyle changes are the mainstay, with medications to address both blood flow and metabolic problems, and surgery for some patients.

New treatments that affect incretin[9] or kidney[3] pathways are bringing metabolic and heart care closer together, giving doctors more ways to treat several problems at once. When used by a team and supported by patient involvement, these methods can lower blood pressure and help heal affected organs. The main goal is to restore balance between metabolism, blood flow, and organ health, which is central to modern precision medicine.

REFERENCES

1. Canadian Journal of Cardiology Editorial Team. (2025). The obesity epidemic and its impact on hypertension. Can J Cardiol. [online]. Available from https://www.onlinecjc.ca/ [Last accessed December, 2025].
2. Shariq OA, McKenzie TJ. Obesity-related hypertension: a review of pathophysiology, management, and the role of metabolic surgery. Gland Surg. 2020;9(1):80-93.

3. National Center for Biotechnology Information (NCBI). (2025). Hypertension related to obesity: pathogenesis, characteristics and clinical implications. Clin Exp Hypertens. [online] Available from https://www.ncbi.nlm.nih.Gov/pmc/articles/.
4. Parvanova A, Reseghetti E, Abbate M, et al. Mechanisms and treatment of obesity-related hypertension—part 1: mechanisms. Clin Kidney J. 2023;17(1):sfad282.
5. Parvanova A, Abbate M, Reseghetti E, et al. Mechanisms and treatment of obesity-related hypertension—part 2: treatments. Clin Kidney J. 2025;18(3):sfaf035.
6. American Heart Association Journal Editors. (2025). Obesity in hypertension: the expanding waistline over time. Hypertension. [online] Available from https://www.ahajournals.org/journal/hyp [Last accessed December, 2025].
7. Lim Y, Haq N, Boster J. Obesity and comorbid conditions. StatPearls [Internet]. Treasure Island: StatPearls Publishing; 2025.
8. Jiang SZ, Lu W, Zong XF, et al. Obesity and hypertension. Exp Ther Med. 2016;12(4):2395-9.
9. Elsevier Health Sciences Editorial Team. Pathophysiology of obesity and its associated diseases. Elsevier Rev Metab Disord. 2023.
10. Nature Reviews Cardiology Editorial Team. (2025). The relationship between obesity and hypertension. Nat Rev Hypertens. [online] Available from https://www.nature.com/articles/.
11. Hall ME, Cohen JB, Ard JD, et al. Weight-loss strategies for prevention and treatment of hypertension. Hypertension. 2021;78(5):e38-50.
12. Obesity Medicine Association. (2025). OMA clinical practice statement: obesity and hypertension. Obes Med. [online] Available from https://www.sciencedirect.com/journal/obesity-medicine [Last accessed December, 2025].
13. American Diabetes Association. Obesity and weight management for prevention and treatment of type 2 diabetes. Diabetes Care. 2025;48(Suppl. 1):S167-79.
14. AHA/ACC Joint Committee Members. 2025 AHA/ACC hypertension guideline (living document). Hypertension. 2025;85(2):e1-65.

SECTION 6

Obesity with Diabetes

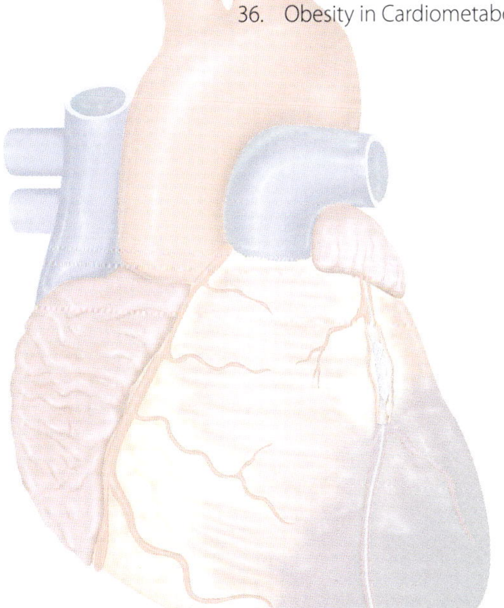

CHAPTER 34

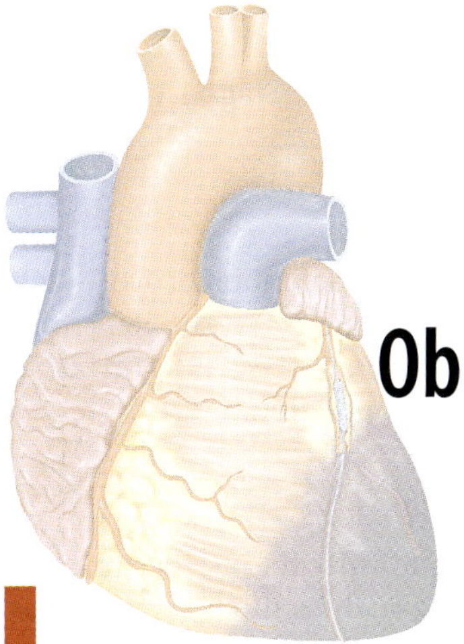

Obesity, Cardiorenal–Metabolic Continuum

I Sathyamurthy, KN Srinivasan

INTRODUCTION

Cardiovascular-renal-metabolic disease has been found to play an interlinked pathophysiological mechanism, which led to the definition of cardiovascular-kidney-metabolic (CKM) syndrome by the American Heart Association (AHA) in 2023. This group of diseases often begins with dysfunction or excessive accumulation of adipose tissue.[1]

DEFINITION AND PREVALENCE OF CARDIOVASCULAR-KIDNEY-METABOLIC SYNDROME

Cardiovascular-kidney-metabolic syndrome is defined as a systemic disorder characterized by pathophysiological interactions among metabolic risk factors, cardiovascular disease (CVD), and chronic kidney disease (CKD), leading to multiorgan dysfunction resulting in a high incidence of adverse cardiovascular outcomes.[1] Older age, male sex, racial or ethnic background, and socioeconomic status are associated with a higher comorbidity burden.[2] The greater burden observed in males has been attributed to increased visceral and hepatic fat accumulation.[3]

RISK FACTORS FOR CARDIOVASCULAR-KIDNEY-METABOLIC SYNDROME

The major risk factors contributing to CKM syndrome include diabetes mellitus (DM), hypertension, overweight or obesity, CKD, and hypertriglyceridemia. Inflammatory diseases such as systemic lupus erythematosus (SLE), rheumatoid arthritis, psoriasis, and HIV/AIDS, as well as family history of DM or kidney disease, sleep disorders, and elevated high-sensitivity C-reactive protein (hs-CRP) levels (>2.0 mg/L), have also been found to play a role in CKM syndrome.[1,4]

Gender-specific factors, including premature menopause, pregnancy complications, polycystic ovary syndrome (PCOS), and erectile dysfunction, may further influence disease progression and outcomes.[4]

PATHOPHYSIOLOGICAL MECHANISMS OF CARDIOVASCULAR-KIDNEY-METABOLIC CONNECTION

Obesity occurs when caloric intake exceeds energy expenditure, resulting in fat accumulation. The build-up and dysfunction of adipose tissue lead to increased production of cytokines, which in turn decrease insulin receptor function and elevate blood glucose levels.[5] Elevated free fatty acids (FFAs) contribute to increased triglyceride and very low-density lipoprotein (VLDL) levels, as well as higher concentrations of lipoprotein(a) [Lp(a)], all of which promote atherogenesis.[6]

Activation of the sympathetic nervous system (SNS) and the renin–angiotensin–aldosterone system (RAAS) further contributes to endothelial dysfunction and reduced nitric oxide availability. This results in increased peripheral vascular resistance, elevated heart rate, and enhanced aldosterone secretion. Consequently, sodium retention occurs, leading to hypertension.[7]

In CKD, the accumulation of uremic toxins also induces endothelial dysfunction and nitric oxide depletion, contributing to cardiac remodeling and dysfunction. Sex hormones influence fat distribution and metabolism, thereby contributing to gender-specific differences in the prevalence of obesity.[8]

EPIDEMIOLOGICAL EVIDENCE OF CARDIOVASCULAR-KIDNEY-METABOLIC NEXUS

Obesity

Obesity is defined by the World Health Organization (WHO) expert group as a body mass index (BMI) > 25 kg/m^2 for the Asian population. However, cases of *lean obesity* may be overlooked if BMI is used as the sole criterion.[9] In the Indian population, a waist circumference (WC) of ≥90 cm for men and ≥80 cm for women is considered central obesity, which is associated with a high metabolic risk. The National Family Health Survey (NFHS)-5 (2019–2021) reported that nearly one-quarter of Indian adults are overweight or obese.[10,11] Overall, type I diabetes accounts for only 9–10% of cases, while the remainder are type II DM.[12] Individuals with type II DM have a twofold increased risk of coronary artery disease (CAD), major stroke subtypes, and death due to other vascular causes (meta-analysis).[13] The CAPTURE study established that CVD is present in approximately 25% of individuals with type II DM.[14] Diabetic kidney disease (DKD) is the fourth leading cause of death worldwide and affects one-third of patients with type I DM and half of those with type II DM.[15]

Heart Failure

Heart failure is a clinical syndrome that increases the risk of a decline in glomerular filtration rate (GFR). Nearly 50% of patients with heart failure (HF) suffer from CKD.[16]

STAGING OF CARDIOVASCULAR-KIDNEY-METABOLIC SYNDROME

Cardiovascular-kidney-metabolic syndrome is classified into four stages (Stage 0–Stage 4).

Stage 0

In this stage, there are no cardiovascular risk factors. The BMI, WC, blood glucose, blood pressure (BP), and lipid profile are normal. There is no evidence of CKD, and the prevalence of Stage 0 CKM syndrome is 15% in women and 8.5% in men.[16]

Stage 1

Stage 1 is divided into two substages: Stage 1A and Stage 1B.

Stage 1A: Excess Adiposity

There are ethnic differences in the definition of overweight and obesity. The WHO recommends a WC of ≥80 cm for women and ≥90 cm for men, and a BMI ≥ 27.5 kg/m^2 as the cutoff for obesity in the Asian population.[17]

Stage 1B: Dysfunctional Adiposity

Dysfunctional adiposity manifests as ectopic fat deposition in visceral organs such as the liver, pancreas, kidneys, skeletal muscles, and heart. It is a marker of higher cardiovascular risk independent of BMI[17] and contributes to systemic inflammation, oxidative stress, and prediabetes.[18]

The visceral fat index is calculated based on BMI, WC, triglycerides, and HDL cholesterol (HDL-C) and is independently associated with an increased risk of HF and diastolic dysfunction.[19] The prevalence of Stage 1 CKM syndrome is 27.1% in women and 24.3% in men.[1]

Stage 2

Cardiovascular-kidney-metabolic syndrome is characterized by the presence of metabolic risk factors such as hypertension, hypertriglyceridemia, metabolic syndrome (MS), or DM and/or low to moderate risk of CKD, according to the Kidney Disease: Improving Global Outcomes (KDIGO) classification.[1]

Metabolic syndrome is defined by the presence of three or more of the following criteria:

- WC ≥80 cm for women and ≥90 cm for men (Asian origin)
- HDL-C ≤40 mg/dL for men and ≤50 mg/dL for women
- Triglycerides ≥150 mg/dL
- Elevated BP [systolic blood pressure (SBP) ≥130 mm Hg or diastolic blood pressure (DBP) ≥80 mm Hg] or current use of antihypertensive medications
- Fasting glucose ≥100 mg/dL.[20]

Metabolic syndrome is a known risk factor for type II DM and atherosclerotic cardiovascular disease (ASCVD).[20] DM should be suspected when symptoms such as polyuria, polydipsia, weight loss, delayed wound healing, or recurrent infections are present. It remains asymptomatic in >40% of adults worldwide.[12]

Chronic kidney disease is defined as an eGFR <60 mL/min/1.73 m^2 or a urinary albumin-to-creatinine ratio (UACR) ≥30 mg/g (≥3 mg/mmol) (KDIGO).[21]

Stage 3: Subclinical Cardiovascular Disease

Stage 3 CKM syndrome includes patients with subclinical HF or subclinical ASCVD in individuals with excess or dysfunctional adiposity and metabolic risk factors or CKD.[1]

Subclinical heart disease is defined as asymptomatic cardiac dysfunction, where biomarkers such as BNP (≥35 pg/mL), NT-pro BNP (≥125 pg/mL), and/or high-sensitivity Troponin-I (≥12 ng/L for men, ≥10 ng/L for women) or troponin-T (≥22 ng/L for men, ≥14 ng/L for women) are elevated. Echocardiography may reveal ventricular dysfunction or elevated filling pressures.[22] The prevalence of Stage 3 CKM syndrome is 14.3% in women and 22.4% in men.[3]

Stage 4

Stage 4 CKM syndrome is characterized by the presence of overt CVDs such as CAD, HF, stroke, peripheral arterial disease (PAD), or atrial fibrillation (AF) in individuals with excess/dysfunctional adiposity and risk factors such as CKD.[1] It is further divided into Stage 4A and Stage 4B, depending on the presence or absence of end-stage kidney disease (ESKD).[23] The prevalence of Stage 4 CKM syndrome is 7.2% in men and 6.0% in women, with higher cardiovascular mortality observed in women.[3]

SCREENING FOR CARDIOVASCULAR-KIDNEY-METABOLIC SYNDROME

Screening for CKM syndrome should begin early in life. Individuals under 21 years of age need to be assessed for overweight/obesity, BP, social determinants of health (SODH), fasting lipid profile, plasma glucose, and other metabolic biomarkers. In addition, components of MS, including screening for liver fibrosis, coronary calcium score, subclinical HF, and renal impairment, should be assessed in individuals over 21 years of age.[24]

Obesity screening is conducted by assessing BMI, WC, direct measurement of body fat, and blood leptin levels.[25] Cardiovascular evaluation includes measuring BP (both home and ambulatory) and cardiac biomarkers, such as high-sensitivity troponin-T (hs-trop-T) and NT-pro BNP.[26]

Prediabetes and diabetes are assessed by measuring fasting plasma glucose (FPG), glycosylated hemoglobin (HbA1c), oral glucose tolerance test (OGTT), and the Homeostatic Model Assessment of Insulin Resistance (HOMA-IR).[27] Insulin resistance is assessed using the triglyceride-glucose (TyG) index, which is based on fasting glucose and triglyceride levels.[28]

The modified TyG index is calculated using fasting glucose, BMI, WC, and the weight-to-height ratio, and has been found to detect CKM syndrome early and predict response to intervention.[29]

Lipid profiling helps in the early detection and management of MS. The atherogenic index of plasma (AIP) is calculated as the ratio of triglycerides to HDL-C levels and has been found to correlate directly with an increased incidence of CVD in individuals with CKM syndrome stages 1–3.[30] Lipoprotein(a) levels predict cardiovascular risk, and reducing them helps lower the risk of ASCVD.[31]

Other biomarkers, such as uric acid, soluble neprilysin, lipocalin-type prostaglandin D synthase, and endocan, have been found to potentially play a role in CKM syndrome staging.[24]

Inflammatory indices, such as the systemic immune-inflammation index (SII), have been found to be significantly associated with various components of CKM syndrome. SII is calculated from platelet, neutrophil, and lymphocyte counts. The systemic inflammation response index (SIRI) is calculated using neutrophil, lymphocyte, and monocyte counts. Patients with advanced CKM syndrome and a SIRI >0.81 have the highest mortality risk, especially those under 60 years of age.[32]

Renal function is assessed by calculating eGFR and UACR. It should be performed annually in patients with type I DM starting 5 years after diagnosis and in patients with type II DM from the first visit.[33]

The presence of fatty liver (hepatic steatosis) should be assessed by abdominal ultrasound and FibroScan, in addition to measuring serum transaminase levels. When fatty liver is associated with any one of the following criteria—overweight/obesity, type II DM, or other types of metabolic disturbances—it is classified as NAFLD or MASLD. It can be a precursor to fibrosis, cirrhosis, and hepatocellular carcinoma.[34]

Newer cardiac biomarkers, such as ST2, galectin-3, GDF-15, IL-6, and procalcitonin, have been found to be associated with an increased risk of HF. An ST2 level >35 ng/mL is associated with adverse outcomes and increased mortality.[35]

Subclinical atherosclerosis can be assessed using the coronary artery calcium (CAC) score, coronary angiography (CAG), and carotid intima-media thickness (CIMT). The CAC score can be repeated every 5 years in patients with mild-to-moderate, calculated 10-year CVD risk.[1]

MANAGEMENT OF CARDIOVASCULAR-KIDNEY-METABOLIC SYNDROME

Stage 0

The management of patients with Stage 0 involves education regarding maintaining a healthy lifestyle.[36]

Stage 1

The management of patients with Stage 1 focuses on addressing excessive or dysfunctional adiposity. It emphasizes behavioral changes, dietary measures, and physical activity. Anti-obesity medications (AOMs) are most effective when combined with lifestyle modifications. Currently recommended AOMs include Orlistat, glucagon-like peptide-1 receptor agonists (GLP-1 RAs) such as liraglutide and semaglutide, and the dual glucose-dependent insulinotropic polypeptide (GIP)/GLP-1 RA tirzepatide.[37] The ACC/AHA recommends a weight loss of 5–10% within 6 months. Intragastric interventions are used to reduce gastric capacity and motility, thereby increasing satiety.[38]

These procedures are considered for patients with a BMI ≥30 and <40 kg/m², or for those with a BMI >27 kg/m² who have one or more obesity-related comorbidities. Bariatric surgery is considered for patients with a BMI ≥40 kg/m², or with a BMI ≥35 kg/m² in the presence of DM. Orlistat has only a modest effect on weight and should be used cautiously in patients with CVD due to potential long-term cardiovascular risks.[37]

Tirzepatide, a dual GIP/GLP-1 RA administered as a once-weekly subcutaneous injection, results in significant weight loss (mean weight reduction of 20.9%), improvement in WC, BP, and lipid profile, in addition to a reduction in HbA1c (up to 1.94%).[39]

Similarly, semaglutide has been shown to produce significant weight loss and improvement in cardiometabolic risk factors. These agents tend to reduce appetite, delay gastric emptying, and increase satiety. Side effects such as nausea, vomiting, and diarrhea are very common with higher therapeutic doses.[40]

Stage 2

Therapy involves controlling cardiometabolic risk factors such as diabetes, hypertension, and dyslipidemia, in addition to lifestyle modifications, with the aim of preventing ASCVD and its progression.

Hypertension

Patients with hypertension should begin antihypertensive therapy in addition to lifestyle modifications and a low-salt diet, with the goal of achieving a target SBP of 120–129 mm Hg and DBP of 70–99 mm Hg.[41] Sodium-glucose cotransporter-2 (SGLT2) inhibitors lower BP through osmotic diuresis and natriuresis in the short term, and by improving arterial compliance and reducing sympathetic activity in the long term. Similarly, GLP-1 RAs have also been shown to reduce BP through weight reduction.[12]

Diabetes

Patients with diabetes should be started on antidiabetic medications in addition to lifestyle modifications and a low-carbohydrate diabetic diet, with the aim of achieving a target HbA1c of <7%. The target HbA1c may be relaxed to <8% in older, frail patients or those with a short life expectancy. For patients with high cardiovascular risk, established ASCVD (as per ESC 2023), HF, or CKD.[12]

Dyslipidemia

Risk scoring helps in assessing cardiovascular risk. Statin therapy should be considered, along with diet and lifestyle modification, to achieve the target LDL-C level. Coronary calcium scoring also aids in risk assessment and in the decision to initiate statin therapy. In primary prevention, LDL-C should be reduced by 30–49%, whereas in secondary prevention, LDL-C should be reduced by at least 50% from baseline. According to the Lipid Association of India, the LDL-C goals for extremely high-risk, very high-risk, and high-risk patients are <30, <55, and <70 mg/dL, respectively.[42]

When the target LDL-C level is not achieved with statins alone, combination therapy with other agents such as ezetimibe, bempedoic acid, PCSK9 inhibitors, or inclisiran should be considered.[12]

Hypertriglyceridemia with triglyceride levels >500 mg/dL should be treated with fibrates in combination with statins. When triglyceride levels are between 135 and 499 mg/dL, saroglitazar or icosapent ethyl can be added to statin therapy to reduce ASCVD risk.[1]

CKD

Drugs such as renin-angiotensin-aldosterone system inhibitors (RAASi) and SGLT2 inhibitors should be initiated in all patients with CKD. An initial transient decline in eGFR and a rise in serum creatinine may occur after starting these drugs, up to ≤30% with RAASi and 3–10% with SGLT2 inhibitors. However, therapy should be continued after confirming the absence of extracellular volume depletion.[21]

All patients with HF, regardless of their left ventricular ejection fraction, diabetic status, or urinary albumin excretion level, should be treated with SGLT2 inhibitors, similar to patients with CKD and an eGFR ≥20 mL/min/1.73 m^2.[43]

Finerenone should be considered in addition to SGLT2 inhibitors to reduce HF hospitalization, cardiovascular mortality and morbidity, as well as to slow the progression of renal failure and DKD in patients with type II diabetes.[43]

Stage 3

The goal of management in Stage 3 focuses on preventing subclinical HF and high-risk CKD from progressing to overt HF and advanced CKD, respectively. Comorbidities such as DM, hypertension, and obesity should be aggressively managed to prevent the progression of asymptomatic left ventricular dysfunction to overt HF.[1]

Stage 4

In patients with HF with reduced ejection fraction (HFrEF), the four pillars of HF management—ARNIs, SGLT2 inhibitors, MRAs, and beta-blockers—should be considered based on the patient's BP, renal function, electrolyte status, and degree of congestion. Regardless of ejection fraction and diabetic status, SGLT2 inhibitors are recommended for all patients with HF, as they improve ASCVD outcomes by reducing HF hospitalizations and cardiovascular mortality.[44]

Finerenone has become one of the key pillars in the management of HFmrEF and HFpEF, as its use has shown a significant effect in reducing cardiovascular events and preventing worsening HF.[45]

Similarly, incretin-based anti-obesity drugs have shown efficacy in patients with HFpEF. The use of semaglutide has been associated with a 31% reduction in the combined end point of cardiovascular death or HF events in HFpEF trials such as the STEP Heart Failure trials (STEP-HFpEF and STEP-HFpEF DM), SELECT (in patients with prior ASCVD or PAD), and FLOW (in patients with type II diabetes and CKD). Likewise, tirzepatide has demonstrated significant improvement in the composite outcomes of cardiovascular death or worsening HF in patients with HFpEF and obesity.[46]

CONCLUSION

Cardiovascular-kidney-metabolic syndrome is a well-recognized, distinct entity that needs to be addressed through an integrated approach involving cardiologists, nephrologists, and endocrinologists. This approach facilitates patient adherence to treatment and helps to avoid polypharmacy and contradictory therapies.

REFERENCES

1. Ndumele CE, Rangaswami J, Chow, SL, et al. Cardiovascular-kidney-metabolic health: a presidential advisory from the American Heart Association. Circulation 2023;148(20):1606-35.
2. Ostrominski JW, Arnold SV, Butler J, et al. Prevalence and overlap of cardiac, renal, and metabolic conditions in US adults, 1999-2020. JAMA Cardiol. 2023;8(11):1050-60.
3. Ji H, Sabanayagam C, Matsushita K, et al. Sex differences in cardiovascular-kidney-metabolic syndrome: 30-year US trends and mortality risks—brief report. Arterioscler Thromb Vasc Biol. 2025;45(1):157-61.
4. Massy ZA, Drueke TB. Combination of cardiovascular, kidney, and metabolic diseases in a syndrome named cardiovascular-kidney-metabolic, with new risk prediction equations. Kidney Int Rep. 2024;9(9):2608-18.
5. Larque E, Labayen I, Flodmark CE, et al. From conception to infancy: early risk factors for childhood obesity. Nat Rev Endocrinol. 2019;15(8):456-78.
6. Klop B, Elte JWF, Cabezas MC. Dyslipidemia in obesity: mechanisms and potential targets. Nutrients. 2013;5(4):1218-40.
7. El Meouchy P, Wahoud M, Allam S, et al. Hypertension related to obesity: pathogenesis, characteristics and factors for control. Int J Mol Sci. 2022;23(20):12305.
8. Guldan M, Unlu S, Abdel-Rahman SM, et al. Understanding the role of sex hormones in cardiovascular kidney metabolic syndrome: toward personalized therapeutic approaches. J Clin Med. 2024;13(15):4354.
9. Rubino F, Cummings DE, Eckel RH, et al. Definition and diagnostic criteria of clinical obesity. Lancet Diabetes Endocrinol. 2025;13(3):221-62.
10. GBD 2021 Diabetes Collaborators. Global, regional, and national burden of diabetes from 1990 to 2021, with projections of prevalence to 2050: a systematic analysis for the Global Burden of Disease Study 2021. Lancet. 2023;402(10397):203-34.
11. Sun H, Saeedi P, Karuranga S, et al. IDF Diabetes Atlas: global, regional and country-level diabetes prevalence estimates for 2021 and projections for 2045. Diabetes Res Clin Pract. 2023;204:110945.
12. Marx N, Federici M, Schutt K, et al. ESC Guidelines for the management of cardiovascular disease in patients with diabetes. Eur Heart J. 2023;44(39):4043-40.
13. Emerging Risk Factors Collaboration. Diabetes mellitus, fasting blood glucose concentration, and risk of vascular disease: a collaborative meta-analysis of 102 prospective studies. Lancet. 2010;375(9):2215-22.
14. Mosenzon O, Alguwaihes A, Leon JLA, et al. CAPTURE: a multinational, cross-sectional study of cardiovascular disease prevalence in adults with type 2 diabetes across 13 countries. Cardiovasc Diabetol. 2021;20(1):154.
15. Thomas MC, Brownlee M, Susztak K, et al. Diabetic kidney disease. Nat Rev Dis Primers. 2015;1:15018.
16. Szlagor M, Dybiec J, Młynarska E, et al. Chronic kidney disease as a comorbidity in heart failure. Int J Mol Sci. 2023;24(3):2988.

17. Palaniappan LP, Wong EC, Shin JJ, et al. Asian Americans have greater prevalence of metabolic syndrome despite lower body mass index. Int J Obes. 2011;35(3):393-400.
18. Longo M, Zatterale F, Naderi J, et al. Adipose tissue dysfunction as determinant of obesity-associated metabolic complications. Int J Mol Sci. 2019;20(9):2358.
19. Massy ZA, Drueke TB. Combination of cardiovascular, kidney, and metabolic diseases in a syndrome named cardiovascular-kidney-metabolic, with new risk prediction equations. Kidney Int Rep. 2024;9(9):2608-18.
20. Alemany M. The metabolic syndrome, a human disease. Int J Mol Sci. 2024;25(4):2251.
21. Kidney Disease: Improving Global Outcomes CKD Work Group. KDIGO 2024 clinical practice guideline for the evaluation and management of chronic kidney disease. Kidney Int. 2024;105(4S):S117-314.
22. Heidenreich PA, Bozkurt B, Aguilar D, et al. AHA/ACC/HFSA guideline for the management of heart failure: a report of the American College of Cardiology/American Heart Association Joint Committee on Clinical Practice Guidelines. Circulation. 2022;145(18):e895-1032.
23. McDonagh TA, Metra M, Adamo M, et al. 2021 ESC guidelines for the diagnosis and treatment of acute and chronic heart failure: developed by the Task Force for the Diagnosis and Treatment of Acute and Chronic Heart Failure of the European Society of Cardiology (ESC) with the special contribution of the Heart Failure Association (HFA) of the ESC. Eur Heart J. 2021;42(36):3599-726.
24. Kittelson KS, Gasparotto Junior A, Fillmore N, et al. Cardiovascular-kidney-metabolic syndrome—an integrative review. Prog Cardiovasc Dis. 2024;87:26-36.
25. Rubino F, Cummings DE, Eckel RH, et al. Definition and diagnostic criteria of clinical obesity. Lancet Diabetes Endocrinol. 2025;13(3):221-62.
26. Claudel SE, Schmidt IM, Gopal DM, et al. Elevated cardiac biomarkers in relatively healthy U.S. adults. Eur J Intern Med. 2024;121:152-4.
27. Claudel SE, Ashish V. Cardiovascular-kidney-metabolic syndrome: a step toward multidisciplinary and inclusive care. Cell Metab. 2023;35(12):2104-06.
28. Lanlan W, Zheng H. Elevated triglyceride glucose index is associated with advanced cardiovascular kidney metabolic syndrome. Sci Rep. 2024;14(1):31352.
29. Hong J, Zhang R, Tang H, et al. Comparison of triglyceride glucose index and modified triglyceride glucose indices in predicting cardiovascular diseases incidence among populations with cardiovascular-kidney-metabolic syndrome stages 0–3: a nationwide prospective cohort study. Cardiovasc Diabetol. 2025;24(1):98.
30. Zhang Y, Song Y, Lu Y, et al. Atherogenic index of plasma and cardiovascular disease risk in cardiovascular-kidney-metabolic syndrome stage 1 to 3: a longitudinal study. Front Endocrinol. 2025;16:1517658.
31. Kronenberg F, Mora S, Stroes ESG, et al. Lipoprotein(a) in atherosclerotic cardiovascular disease and aortic stenosis: a consensus statement of the European Atherosclerosis Society. Eur Heart J. 2022;43(39):3925-46.
32. Cao Y, Wang W, Xie S, et al. Joint association of the inflammatory marker and cardiovascular-kidney-metabolic syndrome stages with all-cause and cardiovascular disease mortality: a national prospective study. BMC Public Health. 2025;25(1):10.
33. Sindhu D, Sharma GSM, Kumbala DM. Management of diabetic kidney disease: where do we stand?: A narrative review. Medicine. 2023;102(14):e33366.
34. Chalasani N, Younossi Z, Lavine JE, et al. The diagnosis and management of nonalcoholic fatty liver disease: practice guidance from the American Association for the Study of Liver Diseases. Hepatology. 2018;67(1):328-57.
35. Gaggin HK, Januzzi JL Jr. (2023). Cardiac biomarkers and heart failure. expert analysis. [online] Available from https://www.acc.org/Latest-in-ardiology/Articles/2015/02/09/13/00/Cardiac-Biomarkers-and-Heart-Failure [Last accessed January, 2026].
36. Lloyd-Jones DM, Allen NB, Anderson CAM, et al. Life's essential 8: updating and enhancing the American Heart Association's construct of cardiovascular health: a presidential advisory from the American Heart Association. Circulation. 2022;146(5):e18-43.
37. Koskinas KC, Van Craenenbroeck EM, Antoniades C, et al. Obesity and cardiovascular disease: an ESC clinical consensus statement. Eur Heart J. 2024;45(41):4063-98.
38. Garvey WT, Mechanick JI, Brett EM, et al.; Reviewers of the AACE/ACE Obesity Clinical Practice Guidelines. American Association of Clinical Endocrinologists and American College of Endocrinology comprehensive clinical practice guidelines for medical care of patients with obesity. Endocr Pract. 2016;22(Suppl S3):1-203.
39. Jastreboff AM, Aronne LJ, Ahmad NN, et al. Tirzepatide once weekly for the treatment of obesity. N Engl J Med. 2022;387(3):205-16.
40. Sharaiha RZ, Shikora S, White KP, et al. Summarizing consensus guidelines on obesity management. J Clin Gastroenterol. 2023;57(10):967-76.
41. McEvoy JW, McCarthy CP, Bruno RM, et al. ESC guidelines for the management of elevated blood pressure and hypertension. Eur Heart J. 2024;45(39):3912-4018.
42. Visseren FLJ, Mach F, Smulders YM, et al. 2021 ESC guidelines on cardiovascular disease prevention in clinical practice. Eur Heart J. 2021;42(34):3227-337.
43. Herrington WG, Staplin N, Wanner C, et al.; The EMPA-KIDNEY Collaborative Group. Empagliflozin in patients with chronic kidney disease. N Engl J Med. 2023;388(2):117-27.
44. Bhatt DL, Szarek M, Steg PG, et al. Sotagliflozin in patients with diabetes and recent worsening heart failure. N Engl J Med. 2021;384(2):117-28.
45. Solomon SD, McMurray JJV, Vaduganathan M, et al.; FINEARTS-HF Committees and Investigators. Finerenone in heart failure with mildly reduced or preserved ejection fraction. N Engl J Med. 2024;39(16):1475-85.
46. Stefanska K, Sattar N. Incretin-based weight loss therapies and heart failure with preserved ejection fraction: guideline impactful results, but mechanisms unclear. Cardiovasc Res. 2025;121(1):1-3.

35

CHAPTER

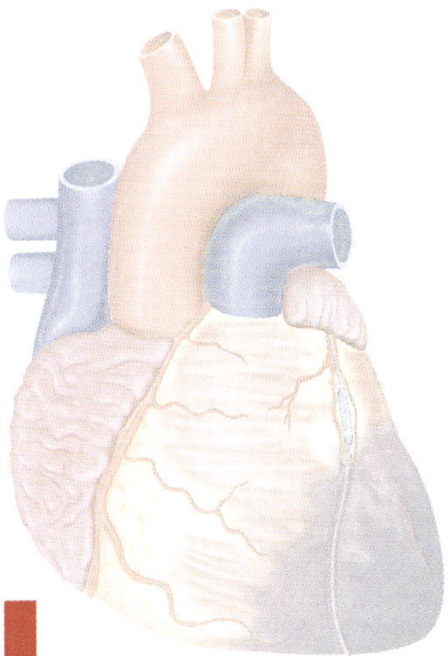

Obesity in Middle-aged Diabetes: Clinical Impact

Mohan Deepa, Ranjit Mohan Anjana, Ranjit Unnikrishnan, V Mohan

INTRODUCTION

The global rise in obesity has become a major medical and public health concern. According to the World Health Organization (WHO),[1] about 16% of adults worldwide are classified as obese, which translates to 890 million people living with obesity. As per the WHO estimates,[1] the global prevalence of adult obesity has more than doubled since 1990, with one in eight people living with obesity currently. Obesity, defined as "abnormal or excessive fat accumulation that may impair health," increases the risk of numerous disorders, both metabolic and weight-related, including cardiovascular disease, type 2 diabetes (T2D), dyslipidemia, fatty liver, gallstones, and atherosclerosis.[2,3] The strong link between obesity and T2D is well established.[4] Studies show that obesity is the most significant risk factor for developing T2D, increasing the risk multiple-fold due to mechanisms such as insulin resistance and pancreatic β-cell dysfunction. Individuals with obesity face a significantly higher risk of developing T2D compared to those with normal weight, although not all obese individuals develop the disease. This increased risk is driven by complex genetic, metabolic, and inflammatory mechanisms that impair insulin sensitivity and pancreatic β-cell function, contributing to the onset and progression of diabetes. These pathways highlight obesity as a potent accelerator of T2D development. The term "diabesity" describes the close interdependence between obesity and diabetes. It refers to the progressive process where an increase in body fat leads to impaired insulin secretion and a continual rise in insulin resistance, facilitating the transition from obesity to T2D.

OBESITY IN MIDDLE AGE

Obesity has become increasingly prevalent among the middle-aged productive population, posing significant challenges for individual health and economic productivity. This age group faces a high risk of developing obesity-related conditions that can impair work capacity and quality of life. T2D, often driven by obesity, accelerates this problem by causing further metabolic impairments and complications, which can reduce functional ability and increase healthcare costs during the prime working years. The dual burden of obesity and diabetes in middle-aged adults threatens not only their health but also has broader societal and economic implications, emphasizing the urgent need for preventive and management strategies targeted at this critical population group. With declining deaths from infectious diseases, many developed nations now face an epidemic of obesity-related conditions, which are rapidly spreading to low- and middle-income countries. This global upsurge is driven by urbanization, sedentary lifestyles, increased consumption of high-calorie foods, and reduced physical activity. Technological advances have lowered daily energy expenditure, and even small, sustained energy surpluses can lead to obesity over time.

OBESITY AND METABOLIC CHANGES IN MENOPAUSE

The menopausal transition represents a critical period of increased susceptibility to metabolic disturbances, particularly obesity and T2D. Declining estrogen levels

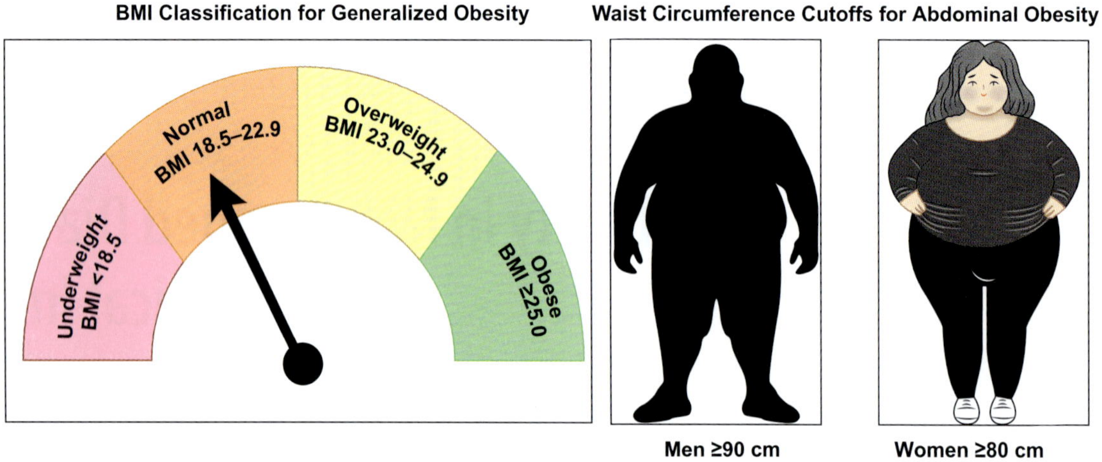

Fig. 1: Classification for obesity by BMI and waist circumference for Asian Indians.
Source: WHO Expert Consultation[8]

during menopause lead to a redistribution of body fat from peripheral to central depots, promoting visceral adiposity, insulin resistance, and dyslipidemia.[5] A systematic review has reported that postmenopausal women have a higher prevalence of metabolic syndrome and impaired glucose metabolism compared with premenopausal counterparts, independent of chronological aging.[6] Lifestyle factors, including reduced physical activity and dietary transitions during midlife, further exacerbate central obesity and insulin resistance, compounding diabetes risk.[7] These metabolic changes highlight the relevance of integrating early metabolic screening, lifestyle management, and preventive approaches into the routine care of menopausal women, providing a framework for reducing long-term risk of obesity-related comorbidities such as T2D.

OBESITY MEASURES

The most widely used for measurement of overweight and obesity is the body mass index (BMI), which is derived from height and weight measures of an individual. The interpretations of this measurement vary in different ethnic groups. For adults, WHO defines overweight as BMI ≥25 kg/m^2 and obesity as BMI ≥30 kg/m^2.[1] For Asian Indians, the recommended BMI cutoffs are lower than the standard WHO global criteria. Specifically, a BMI of 23.0–24.9 kg/m^2 is considered overweight, and a BMI ≥25.0 kg/m^2 is classified as obesity for this population.[8] These lower cutoffs reflect the increased risk of T2D, cardiovascular diseases, and other comorbidities observed at lower BMI values in Asian Indians.[9-11] Waist circumference (WC) is also used as an obesity measure, providing a more sensitive approach to classification. The WC cut point values differ for males and females, the standard WHO cut points being ≥102 cm for males and ≥88 cm for females. There are also ethnic specific cutoffs; for instance, in the Asian population, the cut points for abdominal obesity are ≥90 cm for males and ≥80 cm for females **(Fig. 1)**.

Defining obesity by either BMI or WC is inherently arbitrary, and risk estimates can vary significantly depending on the cutoff values applied. An epidemiological study on Asian Indians[12] reported obesity prevalence as 4.0% when using the international BMI cutoff of ≥30 kg/m^2, 9.9% with BMI ≥27.5 kg/m^2, 26.5% with the Asia Pacific definition of BMI ≥25 kg/m^2, and 45.9% using the BMI ≥23 kg/m^2. Thus, the reported prevalence of generalized obesity in the same population ranged widely from 4 to 45.9%, depending solely on the BMI threshold chosen. Similarly, using different cut points for WC would also lead to varying prevalences of abdominal obesity. Therefore, comparing obesity prevalence across different ethnic groups using varying cut points requires cautious interpretation.

REVISIONS TO OBESITY MEASURES

Misra et al.[13] presented a revised definition of obesity tailored specifically for Asian Indians. Recognizing the limitations of relying solely on BMI, the new framework incorporates both generalized and abdominal adiposity measures, such as WC and waist-to-height ratio, alongside clinical symptoms and obesity-related comorbidities. The definition classifies obesity into two stages: (1) Preclinical obesity with BMI >23 kg/m^2 without evidence of excess body fat, significant organ dysfunction, or daily activity impairment; (2) Clinical obesity with higher adiposity, accompanying functional limitations, and comorbid conditions. This approach addresses the greater metabolic risk seen in Asian Indians at lower BMI levels compared to Western populations and aligns with global efforts to refine obesity diagnosis based on health impact rather than weight alone.

Metabolic dysfunction, including diabetes, is commonly associated with obesity, yet some individuals with excess body fat do not show cardiometabolic risk factors. The recent Lancet Commission[14] on Clinical Obesity differentiates between individuals with excess adiposity who exhibit obesity-related illness, termed "clinical obesity," and those who do not, referred to as "preclinical obesity." The Commission recommends using BMI primarily as a surrogate measure for population-level health risk, epidemiological research, and screening rather than for assessing individual health. For accurate identification of excess adiposity, direct body fat measurement is preferred, or alternatively, at least one validated anthropometric measure (such as WC, waist-to-hip ratio, or waist-to-height ratio) tailored for age, sex, and ethnicity should be combined with BMI.

EPIDEMIOLOGICAL OVERVIEW OF OBESITY

The NCD Risk Factor Collaboration (NCD-RisC) data indicate a steep global rise in overweight and obesity from 1990 to 2040.[15] Prevalence of overweight (BMI 25.0–29.9 kg/m^2) increased from 17.5% in 1990 to 28.0% in 2022 and is projected to reach 43.97% by 2040. Prevalence of obesity (BMI ≥30.0 kg/m^2) rose from 6.44 to 16.06% during the same period and is expected to reach 38.96% by 2040. The prevalence of overweight and obesity by region is provided in **Figure 2**. The study reports that regional disparities in obesity prevalence will persist and intensify through 2040. The projections underscore widening global inequalities, with obesity increasing fastest in countries undergoing socioeconomic and nutrition transitions.

Growing evidence indicates that the Indian subcontinent is witnessing a rapid increase in overweight and obesity. Asian Indians are known to have a higher tendency for abdominal obesity and visceral fat accumulation; a pattern often referred to as the "Asian Indian phenotype."[16] Several population-based studies have reported varying obesity prevalence across India. In the late 1990s, an epidemiological survey in six districts of Kashmir Valley (5,083 adults) found an overall prevalence of 15.0%, higher in women (23.7%) than men (7.0%).[17] Among 532 rural-urban migrants in northern India's urban slums, obesity affected 15.6% of women and 13.3% of men.[18] In the New Delhi Birth Cohort, prevalence was 20% in men and 35% in women (BMI >30 kg/m^2), rising

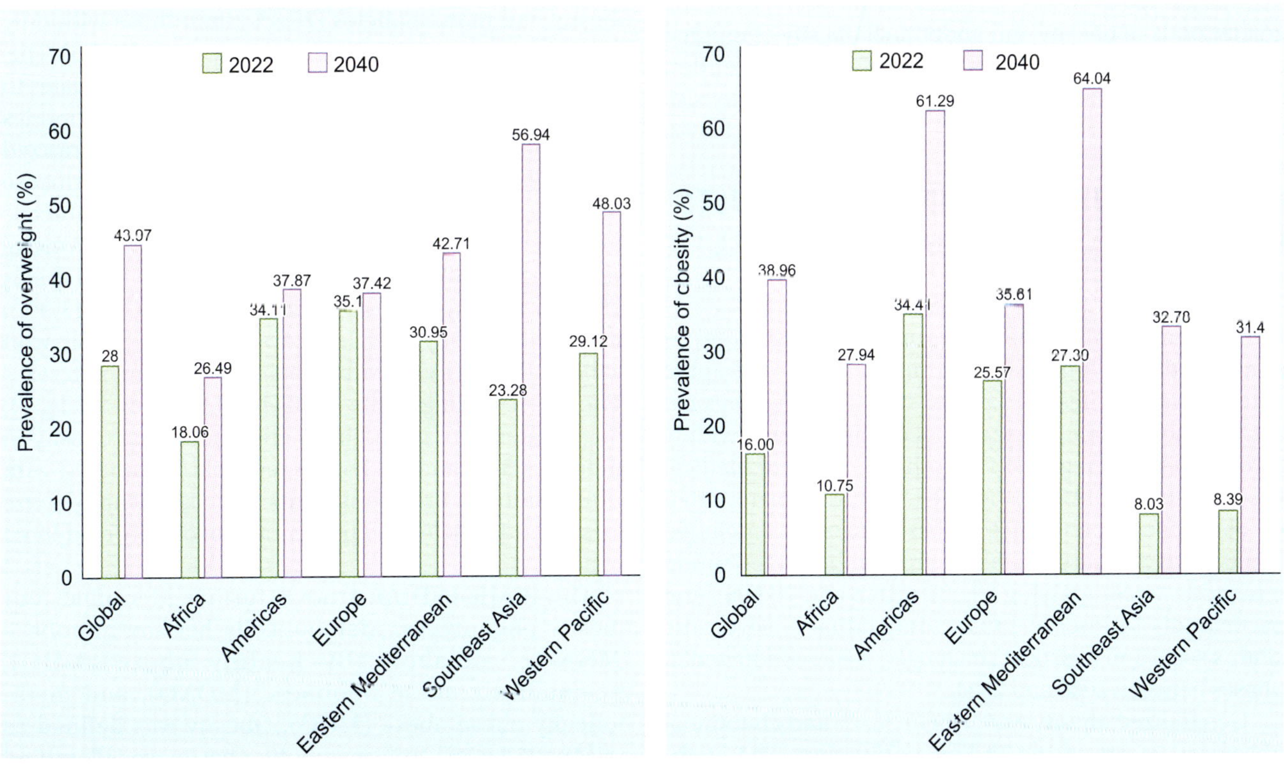

Overweight: BMI 25.0–29.9 kg/m^2 and *Obesity:* BMI ≥30.0 kg/m^2

Fig. 2: Global and region-wise prevalence of overweight and obesity in 2022 and projections for 2040.
Source: Liu et al.[15]

to 54 and 66%, respectively, when using BMI >25 kg/m^2.[19] The Chennai Urban Rural Epidemiology Study (CURES) conducted in Chennai city in Tamil Nadu, South India reported the age standardized prevalence of generalized obesity to be 45.9% (women: 47.4%; men: 43.2%), while that of abdominal obesity was 46.6% (women: 56.2%; men: 35.1%).[12] A representative survey of 99,598 adults in Mumbai reported that 19.0% of men and 30.0% of women had a BMI >25 kg/m^2.[20] A few studies have assessed obesity across multiple Indian regions. National Family Health Survey (NFHS) data show rising overweight/obesity prevalence, increasing from 18.9 to 22.9% in men and from 20.5 to 24.0% in women between NFHS-4 (2015–2016) and NFHS-5 (2019–2021).[21] A study published in 2023 highlights that the prevalence of abdominal obesity increased from 49.3% among women aged 30–39 years to 56.7% among those aged 40–49 years.[22] A study on spatial clustering of overweight and obesity among Indian women found 24% of women of reproductive age were affected, with the highest prevalence in Punjab (41%) and lowest in Meghalaya (11%), highlighting regional disparities.[23] Urban areas show higher obesity rates than rural ones, with significant increases in states such as Odisha, Sikkim, and Manipur.[21] Obesity prevalence is higher among women, urban residents, and those with higher education, with older age groups, especially 45–54 years, showing greater odds of obesity and abdominal obesity compared to younger groups.[24] This pattern reflects gender, socioeconomic, and regional differences in obesity risk across India.

OBESITY BURDEN IN INDIA—RESULTS FROM THE ICMR–INDIAB NATIONAL STUDY

India is a highly diverse nation with substantial regional, ethnic, linguistic, cultural, and demographic heterogeneity. Lifestyle factors such as diet, physical activity, social practices, and occupation vary widely across states and regions. The Indian Council of Medical Research–India DIABetes (ICMR-INDIAB) study reported on state-specific prevalence of obesity in India. It included adults aged 20 years and above from all 31 states/union territories, encompassing 33,537 urban and 79,506 rural participants (a total of 113,043 individuals). Given the study's scale and logistical challenges, it was conducted in phases between 2008 and 2020.

Generalized obesity was seen in 28.6% and abdominal obesity in 39.5% of the Indian population. The state-wise prevalence of generalized and abdominal obesity is presented in **Figures 3 and 4**. The prevalence of generalized obesity ranged from 11.6% in Jharkhand to 53.3% in Puducherry. The prevalence of abdominal obesity ranged from 21.0% in Assam to 61.2% in Puducherry. The prevalence of both was significantly higher in urban than in rural areas, and generalized obesity was markedly higher among females. The projections for the entire country are that an alarming 254 million had generalized obesity, and 351 million had abdominal obesity as of 2021. The INDIAB study highlighted that the widespread prevalence of obesity across India, even in areas with relatively low diabetes rates, is likely to be a precursor to the intensification of the diabetes epidemic, as Asian Indians are known to develop diabetes at lower levels of obesity than white Caucasians.[25,26]

METABOLICALLY HEALTHY AND UNHEALTHY OBESITY

Abdominal obesity (characterized by an elevated WC and accumulation of central or visceral fat) is associated with worse metabolic health than generalized obesity (characterized predominantly by elevated BMI). The CURES[12] reported that men with abdominal obesity had a higher diabetes rate (32.7%) than those with combined obesity (24.9%). In contrast, women with combined obesity had more diabetes (20.4%) than those with only abdominal (12.0%) or general obesity (11.8%) **(Fig. 5)**. This gender-specific variation in diabetes prevalence relates to differences in fat distribution and metabolic risk profiles between men and women. Among men, generalized obesity was most common in those with impaired glucose tolerance (IGT) (62.8%) compared to normal glucose tolerance (NGT) (39.8%) or diabetes (61.4%). Among women, generalized obesity was highest with diabetes (72.6%), followed by IGT (66.2%) and NGT (43.9%). Abdominal obesity prevalence was higher in people with diabetes than in those with impaired or NGT in both sexes **(Fig. 6)**. According to the ICMR-INDIAB study[27] **(Fig. 7)**, the prevalence of generalized and abdominal obesity in India was 51.4 and 68.3%, respectively. Compared with rural residents, urban residents had significantly more obesity, and females had higher rates of obesity compared to males.

The ICMR-INDIAB study[28] further identified four obesity phenotypes: Metabolically healthy nonobese (MHNO), metabolically healthy obese (MHO), metabolically obese nonobese (MONO), and metabolically obese obese (MOO). Obesity was defined as a BMI ≥25 kg/m^2, and metabolic obesity was identified when any two of the following risk factors were present: High WC, elevated blood pressure, high blood glucose,

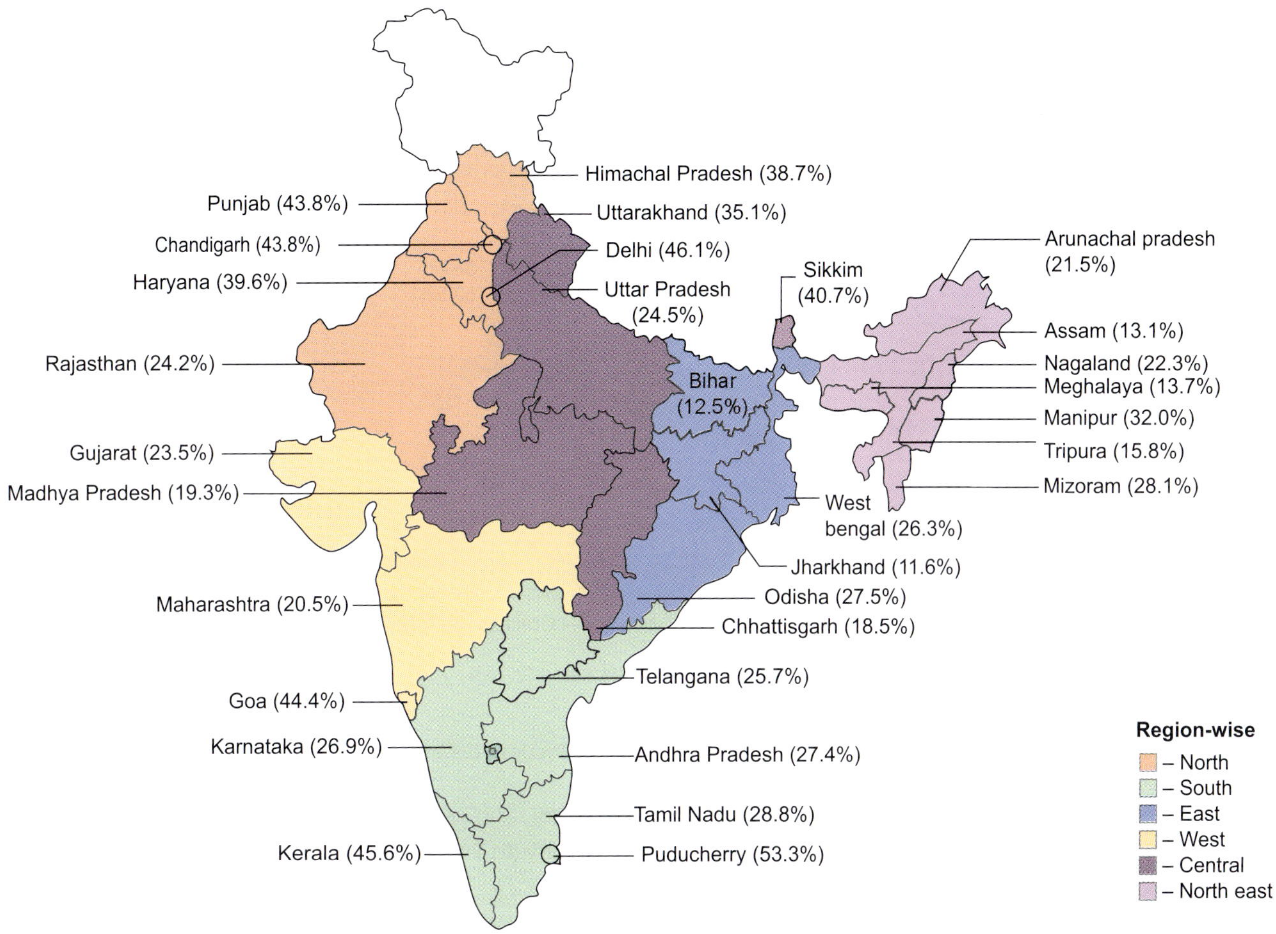

Fig. 3: Prevalence of generalized obesity by states/union territories within the different regions of India (ICMR-INDIAB study).
Source: Anjana et al.[30]

raised serum triglycerides, or low HDL cholesterol. MONO was present in 43.3% of the population, followed by MOO (28.3%), MHNO (26.6%), and MHO (1.8%). Both MOO and MONO showed strong association with T2D, coronary artery disease (CAD), and chronic kidney disease (CKD). While MOO showed highest risk for T2D and CAD, MONO showed the highest risk of CKD, especially among females. This study highlighted the fact that adults with MONO have a unique phenotype with adverse metabolic consequences. They pose a major public health challenge in India, accounting for a significant proportion of adults (43%), with a higher risk of T2D, CAD, and CKD. As they lack easily recognizable phenotypic markers of obesity, they can be identified only through targeted screening tests and may be missed if the diagnosis of obesity is based only on anthropometric parameters such as BMI.

DIABETES EPIDEMIC PARALLELS THE OBESITY EPIDEMIC

The WHO[1] describes diabetes as a global epidemic driven by lifestyle and economic transitions. It is among the most common chronic diseases, affecting people worldwide regardless of ethnicity. The International Diabetes Federation (IDF) Diabetes Atlas 2025[29] estimates that 589 million adults had diabetes in 2024 (11.1% of adults), a number expected to rise to 853 million by 2050. The substantial burden of diabetes in India was confirmed by a recent publication from the ICMR-INDIAB study,[30] which documented that there are an alarming 101 million adults with diabetes in India. T2D accounts for about 90% of all cases and, once prevalent mainly in high-income countries, now poses a major global health threat, especially in low- and middle-income nations where nearly three-quarters of

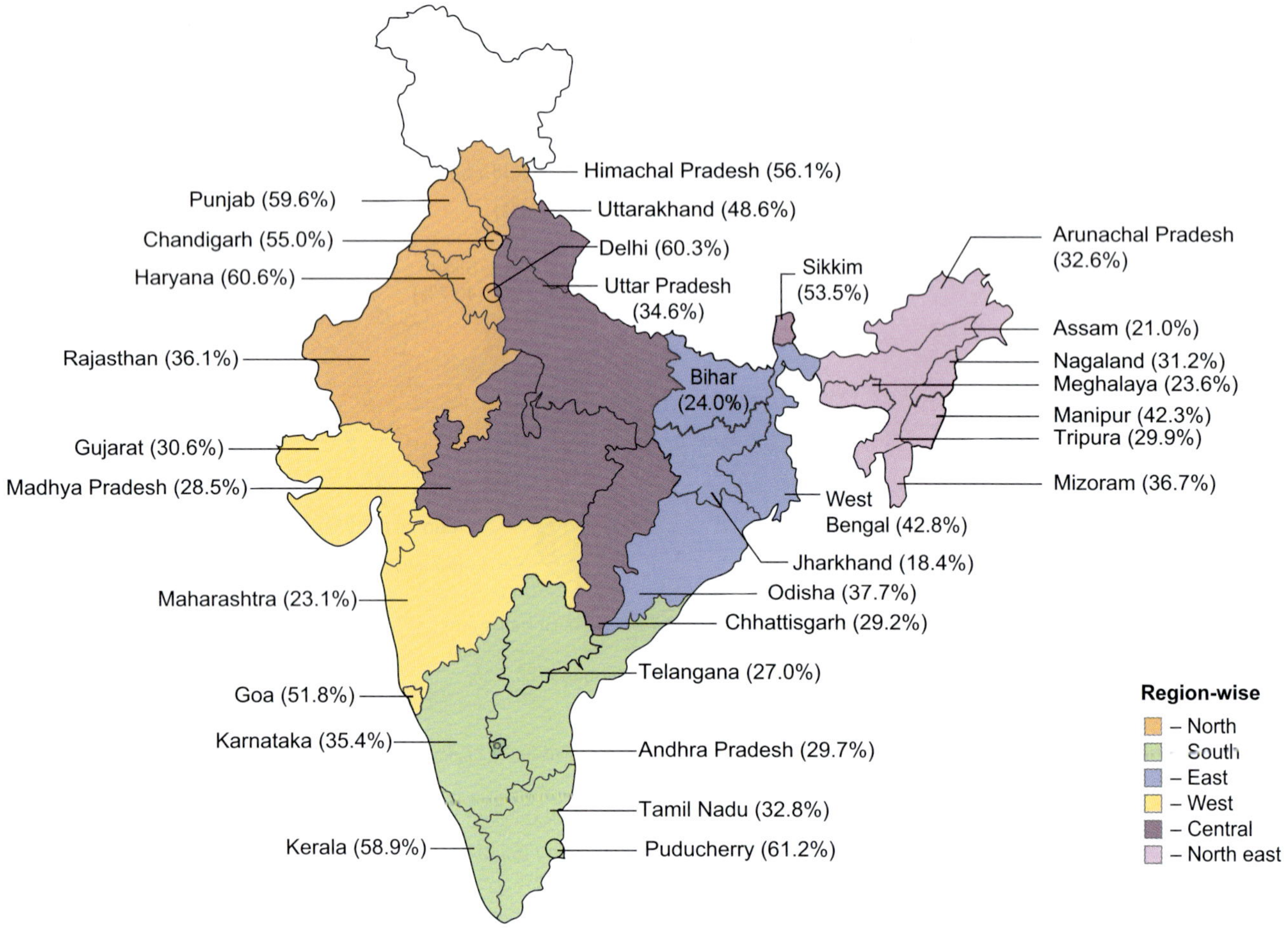

Fig. 4: Prevalence of abdominal obesity by states/union territories within the different regions of India (ICMR-INDIAB study).
Source: Anjana et al.[30]

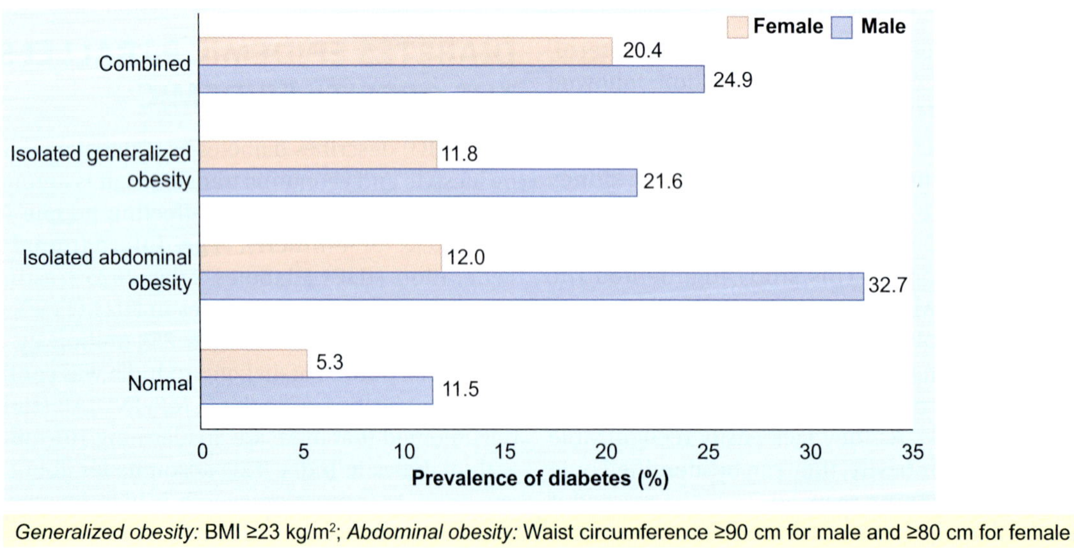

Fig. 5: Prevalence of diabetes by BMI and waist circumference categories.
Source: Deepa et al.[12]

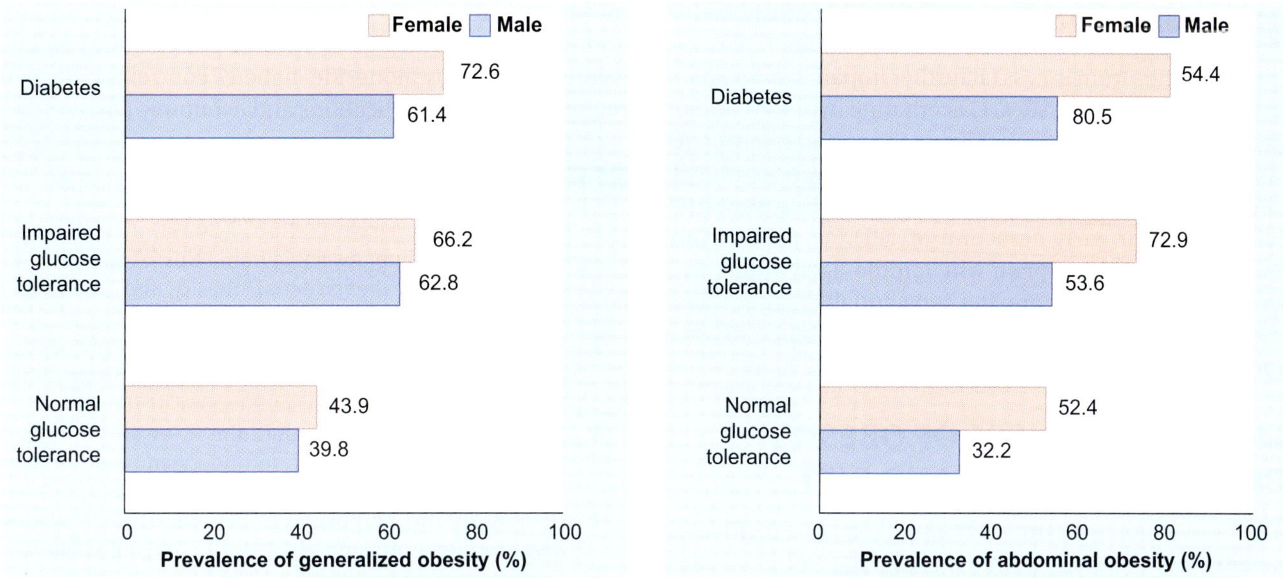

Generalized obesity: BMI ≥23 kg/m^2; *Abdominal obesity:* Waist circumference ≥90 cm for male and ≥80 cm for female

Fig. 6: Prevalence of generalized and abdominal obesity by glycemic status.
Source: Deepa et al.[12]

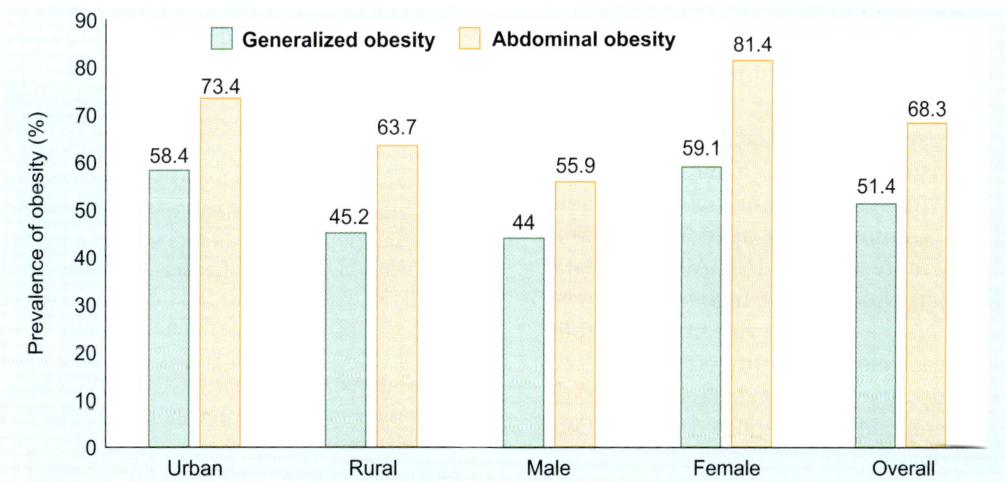

Generalized obesity: BMI ≥23 kg/m^2; *Abdominal obesity:* Waist circumference ≥90 cm for male and ≥80 cm for female

Fig. 7: Prevalence of generalized and abdominal obesity among those with self-reported diabetes in India.
Source: Anjana et al.[27]

affected individuals reside. Rapid urbanization, unhealthy diets, and physical inactivity are key drivers. As a progressive disease, T2D leads to serious complications affecting the eyes, kidneys, nerves, feet, and heart, imposing heavy costs on individuals and health systems.

PATHOPHYSIOLOGY OF OBESITY AND DIABETES

With the global prevalence of obesity increasing, mitigating the growing burden of T2D among middle-aged and adult populations is both crucial and challenging. Diabesity has reached critical proportions, imposing serious public health and economic burdens.[31] Excess adipose tissue, especially visceral fat, not only increases BMI but also disrupts normal glucose metabolism.[32] Adipose tissue secretes signaling molecules called adipokines, such as leptin and adiponectin, which influence insulin sensitivity; in obesity, leptin levels are elevated while adiponectin levels decrease, promoting insulin resistance.[33,34] Additionally, obesity triggers chronic low-grade inflammation, with increased proinflammatory cytokines such as interleukin-6 (IL-6) and tumor necrosis factor-alpha (TNF-α) interfering with insulin signaling.[35] Elevated free fatty acids from excess fat further impair insulin action in liver and muscle tissues, exacerbating hyperglycemia.[36] Emerging evidence also highlights the role of microRNAs, such as miR-34a, whose altered expression in obesity contributes to insulin resistance, providing potential biomarkers for early detection of T2D.[35,37] Collectively, these mechanisms explain why middle-aged adults with overweight or obesity are at a substantially higher risk of developing T2D, underscoring the importance of early prevention and targeted interventions.

LIFESTYLE DRIVERS OF OBESITY—PHYSICAL ACTIVITY AND DIET

The ICMR-INDIAB study (Phase-1) assessed physical activity and inactivity patterns using the Global Physical Activity Questionnaire (GPAQ) and reported that 54.4% of individuals were inactive, with inactivity higher in urban (65%) compared to rural areas (50%).[38] Females were significantly less active than males. Most physical activity occurred during work, with very low recreational physical activity reported. Over 88–94% of participants in each region reported no recreational activity. The proportion of individuals reporting no recreational activity steadily increased with increasing age from 86.7 to 95.9%. The proportion of middle-aged adults with no recreational activity was 93% among those aged 40–49 years and 94.7% among those aged 50–59 years. Analysis of nationally representative INDIAB study data showed that Indian diets typically have high levels of low-quality carbohydrates (such as white rice, milled whole grains, and added sugar), elevated saturated fat, and low protein intake.[39] Participants with the highest carbohydrate consumption had greater odds of generalized obesity (OR: 1.22) and abdominal obesity (OR: 1.15) compared to those with the lowest intake. The study emphasized that public health measures aimed at lowering total carbohydrate and saturated fat consumption while increasing plant and dairy protein intake could help reduce the risk of metabolic diseases in India.

CONCLUSION

Middle-aged individuals with concurrent obesity and diabetes face substantially increased risk of cardiometabolic diseases. The clinical management of diabetes is made more challenging by obesity due to increased insulin resistance, greater medication requirements, and slower response to standard therapies. The intertwined epidemics of obesity and diabetes in middle age demand integrated screening, prevention, and treatment strategies in clinical practice and policy. Addressing obesity alongside diabetes control is critical to reducing future complications and economic costs.

REFERENCES

1. World Health Organization. (2025). Obesity and overweight. [online] Available from https://www.who.int/news-room/fact-sheets/detail/obesity-and-overweight [Last accessed January, 2026].
2. Wyatt SB, Winters KP, Dubbert PM. Overweight and obesity: prevalence, consequences, and causes of a growing public health problem. Am J Med Sci. 2006;331(4):166-74.
3. Bischoff SC, Boirie Y, Cederholm T, et al. Towards a multidisciplinary approach to understand and manage obesity and related diseases. Clin Nutr. 2017;36(4):917-38.
4. Golay A, Ybarra J. Link between obesity and type 2 diabetes. Best Pract Res Clin Endocrinol Metab. 2005;19(4):649-63.
5. Gumpeny N, Lakshmi G, Gumpeny SR. Metabolic syndrome in menopause. Explor Endocr Metab Dis. 2025; 2:101440.
6. Hallajzadeh J, Khoramdad M, Izadi N, et al. Metabolic syndrome and its components in premenopausal and postmenopausal women: a comprehensive systematic review and meta-analysis on observational studies. Menopause. 2018;25(10):1155-64.
7. Ahuja M, Sharma JB, Perumal V, et al. A survey on relation of menopause to metabolic syndrome-SAFOMS study (South Asian Federation of Menopause Societies)-Interim Analysis. J Midlife Health. 2023;14(4):291-8.
8. WHO Expert Consultation. Appropriate body-mass index for Asian populations and its implications for policy and intervention strategies. Lancet. 2004;363:157-63.
9. Unnikrishnan R, Anjana RM, Mohan V. Diabetes in South Asians: is the phenotype different? Diabetes. 2014;63:53-5.
10. Gujral UP, Pradeepa R, Weber MB, et al. Type 2 diabetes in South Asians: similarities and differences with white Caucasian and other populations. Ann N Y Acad Sci. 2013; 1281:51-63.
11. Mohan V, Ramachandran A, Snehalatha C, et al. High prevalence of maturity-onset diabetes of the young (MODY) among Indians. Diabetes Care. 1985;8(4):371-4.
12. Deepa M, Farooq S, Deepa R, et al. Prevalence and significance of generalized and central body obesity in an urban Asian Indian population in Chennai, India (CURES: 47). Eur J Clin Nutr. 2009;63(2):259-67.
13. Misra A, Vikram NK, Ghosh A, et al. Revised definition of obesity in Asian Indians living in India. Diabetes Metab Syndr. 2025;19(1):102989.
14. Rubino F, Cummings DE, Eckel RH, et al. Definition and diagnostic criteria of clinical obesity. Lancet Diabetes Endocrinol. 2025;13(3):221-62.
15. Liu J, Fang Z, Lu Q, et al. Projecting global trends and inequalities in adult overweight and obesity, 2023-2040: findings from the NCD-RisC database. Obesity (Silver Spring). 2025;33(10):1955-67.

16. Deepa R, Sandeep S, Mohan V. Abdominal obesity, visceral fat and type 2 diabetes- Asian Indian phenotype. In: Mohan V, Rao GHR (Eds). Type 2 Diabetes in South Asians: Epidemiology, Risk Factors and Prevention. New Delhi: Jaypee Brothers Medical Publishers; 2006. pp.138-52.
17. Zargar AH, Masoodi SR, Laway BA, et al. Prevalence of obesity in adults—an epidemiological study from Kashmir Valley of Indian Subcontinent. J Assoc Physicians India. 2000;48(12):1170-4.
18. Misra A, Pandey RM, Devi JR, et al. High prevalence of diabetes, obesity and dyslipidaemia in urban slum population in northern India. Int J Obes Relat Metab Disord. 2001;25(11):1722-9.
19. Huffman MD, Prabhakaran D, Osmond C, et al.; New Delhi Birth Cohort. Incidence of cardiovascular risk factors in an Indian urban cohort results from the New Delhi birth cohort. J Am Coll Cardiol. 2011;57(17):1765-74.
20. Shukla HC, Gupta PC, Mehta HC, et al. Descriptive epidemiology of body mass index of an urban adult population in western India. J Epidemiol Community Health. 2002;56(11):876-80.
21. Singh G, Agrawal R, Tripathi N, et al. Overweight and obesity, the clock ticking in India? A secondary analysis of trends of prevalence, patterns, and predictors from 2005 to 2020 using the National Family Health Survey. Int J Non-Commun Dis. 2023;8:31-45.
22. Chaudhary M, Sharma P. Abdominal obesity in India: analysis of the National Family Health Survey-5 (2019-2021) data. Lancet Reg Health Southeast Asia. 2023;14:100208.
23. Chakrabarty M, Let S. Spatial clustering of overweight/obesity among women in India: insights from the latest National Family Health Survey. PLoS One. 2024; 19(7):e0305205.
24. Gupta RD, Tamanna N, Siddika N, et al. Obesity and abdominal obesity in Indian population: findings from a nationally representative study of 698,286 participants. Epidemiologia (Basel). 2023;4(2):163-72.
25. Anjana RM, Shanthi Rani CS, Deepa M, et al. Incidence of diabetes and prediabetes and predictors of progression among Asian Indians: 10-year follow-up of the Chennai Urban Rural Epidemiology Study (CURES). Diabetes Care. 2015;38:1441-8.
26. Narayan KMV, Kanaya AM. Why are South Asians prone to type 2 diabetes? A hypothesis based on underexplored pathways. Diabetologia. 2020;63:1103-9.
27. Anjana RM, Unnikrishnan R, Deepa M, et al.; ICMR-INDIAB collaborators. Achievement of guideline recommended diabetes treatment targets and health habits in people with self-reported diabetes in India (ICMR-INDIAB-13): a national cross-sectional study. Lancet Diabetes Endocrinol. 2022;10(6):430-41.
28. Mohan D, Pradeepa R, Venkatesan U, et al; ICMR-INDIAB Collaborative Study Group. High prevalence of metabolic obesity in India: the ICMR-INDIAB national study (ICMR-INDIAB-23). Indian J Med Res. 2025;161(5):461-72.
29. International Diabetes Federation (IDF). (2024). Diabetes Atlas. [online] Available from https://diabetesatlas.org/data-by-location/global/ [Last accessed January, 2026].
30. Anjana RM, Unnikrishnan R, Deepa M, et al.; ICMR-INDIAB Collaborative Study Group. Metabolic non-communicable disease health report of India: the ICMR-INDIAB national cross-sectional study (ICMR-INDIAB-17). Lancet Diabetes Endocrinol. 2023;11:474-89.
31. GBD 2021 Diabetes Collaborators. Global, regional, and national burden of diabetes from 1990 to 2021, with projections of prevalence to 2050: a systematic analysis for the Global Burden of Disease Study 2021. Lancet. 2023;402(10397):203-34.
32. Dhokte S, Czaja K. Visceral adipose tissue: the hidden culprit for type 2 diabetes. Nutrients. 2024;16(7):1015.
33. Yadav U, Kumar N, Sarvottam K. Role of obesity related inflammation in pathogenesis of peripheral artery disease in patients of type 2 diabetes mellitus. J Diabetes Metab Disord. 2023;22(1):175-88.
34. Clemente-Suárez VJ, Redondo-Flórez L, Beltrán-Velasco AI, et al. The role of adipokines in health and disease. Biomedicines. 2023;11(5):1290.
35. Kern L, Mittenbühler MJ, Vesting AJ, et al. Obesity-induced TNF-α and IL-6 signaling: the missing link between obesity and inflammation-driven liver and colorectal cancers. Cancers (Basel). 2018;11(1):24.
36. Naito H, Kaga H, Someya Y, et al. Fat accumulation and elevated free fatty acid are associated with age-related glucose intolerance: Bunkyo Health Study. J Endocr Soc. 2023;8(2):bvad164.
37. Benavides-Aguilar JA, Torres-Copado A, Isidoro-Sánchez J, et al. The regulatory role of microRNAs in obesity and obesity-derived ailments. Genes (Basel). 2023;14(11):2070.
38. Anjana RM, Pradeepa R, Das AK, et al.; ICMR– INDIAB Collaborative Study Group. Physical activity and inactivity patterns in India-results from the ICMR-INDIAB study (Phase-1) [ICMR-INDIAB-5]. Int J Behav Nutr Phys Act. 2014;11(1):26.
39. Anjana RM, Sudha V, Abirami K, et al. Dietary profiles and associated metabolic risk factors in India from the ICMR-INDIAB survey-21. Nat Med. 2025;31(11):3813-24.

CHAPTER 36

Obesity in Cardiometabolic Syndrome

Alok Modi, Vinod Mittal

INTRODUCTION

Obesity is recognized as the central driver of cardiometabolic syndrome (CMS), a cluster of abnormalities encompassing insulin resistance, abdominal adiposity, dyslipidemia, and hypertension. Together, these factors magnify the risk of type 2 diabetes mellitus (T2DM), cardiovascular disease (CVD), and premature mortality.[1,2] By 2025, projections estimate that over half of the global adult population will be overweight or obese, with South Asia, Latin America, and urbanized regions facing disproportionate burdens.[3,4] Importantly, CMS is no longer confined to adults; childhood and adolescent obesity has surged, with early-life exposures such as maternal obesity, tobacco use during pregnancy, and adolescent lifestyle behaviors shaping long-term cardiometabolic risk.[5]

The recognition of obesity as a chronic, progressive, and relapsing disease has reframed management strategies. No longer viewed as a cosmetic or lifestyle issue, obesity in CMS represents a systemic disorder with neurohormonal, inflammatory, and genetic underpinnings.[6,7] Advances in polygenic risk profiling and adipocentric mechanisms underscore the heterogeneity of CMS while highlighting potential pathways for targeted therapy.[1,3]

At the clinical front, 2025 marks the advent of pharmacotherapies that rival bariatric surgery in efficacy, most notably incretin-based dual and triple agonists, alongside established GLP-1 receptor agonists.[8-10] However, despite therapeutic optimism, the global prevalence continues to climb, calling for integrated strategies spanning prevention, risk stratification, and lifelong treatment **(Fig. 1)**.[11-13] This chapter provides a consolidated 2025 insight into obesity in CMS, synthesizing epidemiology, pathophysiology, clinical manifestations, diagnostic approaches, and therapeutic frontiers.[14]

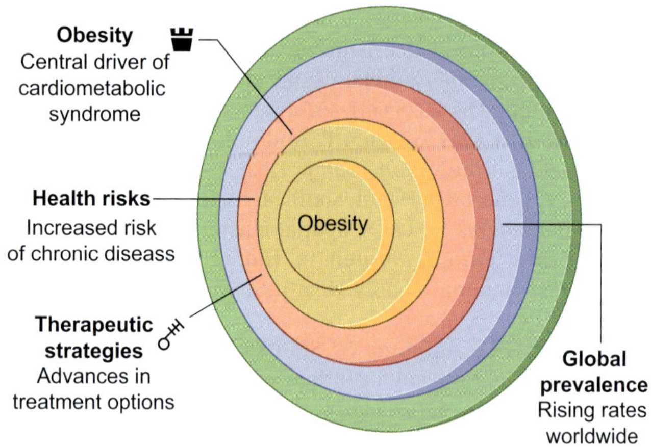

Fig. 1: Concentric 3D framework of obesity and cardiometabolic syndrome. *Obesity forms the central driver, surrounded by layers of cardiometabolic abnormalities, health risks, global prevalence, and therapeutic strategies.*

EPIDEMIOLOGY AND TRENDS

The prevalence of obesity has accelerated globally, with projections suggesting that by 2035, over 1.5 billion adults will meet criteria for obesity, accounting for more than half of the world's adult population **(Table 1)**.[3,4] This epidemiological shift is accompanied by a parallel increase in CMS, creating a synergistic burden on health systems and economies worldwide.[2] While historically concentrated in high-income nations, the epidemic has

TABLE 1: Global epidemiology and early-life determinants of obesity in cardiometabolic syndrome.

Domain	*Key findings*	*Source(s)*
Global prevalence (2025)	>1.5 billion adults projected to be obese by 2035; >50% of adult population affected	3,4,7
Regional susceptibility	South Asia, Latin America: Higher CMS risk at lower BMI due to visceral adiposity	1,3
Research trends	2014–2024: Surge in studies on VAT, oxidative stress, and NAFLD	5
Childhood onset	30% overweight/obese at 4 years; 46% at 9 years; ~29% by adolescence	15
Prenatal risk factors	Maternal obesity, smoking in pregnancy, and gestational diabetes linked to adolescent CMS risk	15
Protective factors	Adolescent physical activity inversely related to central adiposity and cardiometabolic risk	15

Note: This table summarizes epidemiological trends and developmental determinants linking obesity to cardiometabolic syndrome across the lifespan.

now penetrated low- and middle-income countries, driven by rapid urbanization, dietary transition, and sedentary behaviors.[4,7]

Regional heterogeneity is evident: South Asian and Latin American populations exhibit disproportionately high susceptibility to metabolic complications at lower body mass indices, reflecting a stronger contribution of visceral adiposity and genetic predispositions.[1,3] Bibliometric analyses of research trends between 2014 and 2024 reveal a steep rise in publications linking obesity to CVD, with visceral adipose tissue, oxidative stress, and nonalcoholic fatty liver disease emerging as major research hotspots.[5]

Another concerning trend is the early onset of obesity. Longitudinal cohort studies highlight that nearly one-third of children exhibit overweight or obesity by age four, rising to almost half by age nine, before declining slightly in adolescence.[15] Importantly, prenatal exposures such as maternal obesity and tobacco consumption during pregnancy have been directly associated with elevated adolescent cardiometabolic risk scores, including higher BMI, central adiposity, and blood pressure.[15]

These epidemiological observations reinforce obesity as a chronic, progressive disease with early origins and lifelong consequences. They underscore the urgency of early prevention, targeted screening, and culturally adapted interventions to address the expanding global cardiometabolic burden.[7,11]

PATHOPHYSIOLOGY AND MECHANISTIC INSIGHTS

The pathophysiology of CMS reflects a convergence of adipose, vascular, hepatic, and neurohormonal dysfunctions. Central to this process is visceral adiposity, which acts as an endocrine organ, releasing free fatty acids, adipokines, and proinflammatory mediators that drive insulin resistance, endothelial dysfunction, and atherogenesis.[1,3] Adipocentric models highlight how excess ectopic fat in the liver, muscle, and pancreas perturbs glucose and lipid metabolism, ultimately amplifying cardiometabolic risk.[2]

Genetic studies reveal that obesity is highly heritable, influenced by polygenic variants regulating appetite, satiety, and energy expenditure. Genome-wide association analyses have identified loci in neural and metabolic pathways that predispose to obesity-related diabetes and CVD, though ancestral representation remains limited.[1] These findings emphasize heterogeneity, underscoring the need for precision-based approaches in CMS.

At the molecular level, insulin resistance emerges as the keystone abnormality. Impaired insulin signaling elevates hepatic gluconeogenesis, reduces peripheral glucose uptake, and promotes hyperglycemia, thereby fostering progression to T2DM.[6] Dyslipidemia characterized by elevated triglycerides and low HDL cholesterol, along with hypertension, accelerates vascular remodeling and arterial stiffness.[4] Inflammation, oxidative stress, and maladaptive immune responses further exacerbate this metabolic vascular interface.[5]

Emerging research also implicates early-life exposures, such as maternal obesity and smoking during pregnancy, in programming cardiometabolic risk through developmental epigenetic mechanisms.[15] Collectively, these insights affirm CMS as a systemic disorder driven by both intrinsic genetic risk and extrinsic lifestyle and environmental factors, converging on adipose-driven metabolic dysfunction.

CLINICAL MANIFESTATIONS AND COMPLICATIONS

The clinical spectrum of CMS extends across metabolic and cardiovascular domains. Obesity, particularly when centrally distributed, significantly increases the risk of T2DM, coronary artery disease, heart failure, arrhythmias, and cerebrovascular events.[2,4] The progression is often insidious, with obesity-related insulin resistance preceding overt hyperglycemia and dyslipidemia.

Cardiovascular disease remains the leading cause of morbidity and mortality in CMS. Arterial stiffness, an early marker of vascular aging, is closely associated with hypertension, dyslipidemia, and inflammatory activation, serving as both a surrogate endpoint and a predictor of adverse cardiovascular outcomes.[4] Importantly, studies show that modification of cardiometabolic risk factors can attenuate or reverse vascular stiffening, highlighting its role as a modifiable target.[4]

Beyond CVD, obesity contributes to multiorgan complications including nonalcoholic fatty liver disease, chronic kidney disease, musculoskeletal disorders, and certain cancers.[2,3] Adolescents with obesity exhibit higher fat mass, waist circumference, and blood pressure, translating into elevated lifetime risk of CMS-related outcomes.[15]

Recent pharmacological and interventional advances, including incretin-based therapies, have demonstrated secondary benefits in reducing cardiovascular and renal events.[6,8] Nevertheless, the coexistence of obesity with CMS continues to accelerate premature mortality, underlining the urgency of integrated management.

DIAGNOSIS AND RISK STRATIFICATION

Diagnosis of CMS traditionally requires the presence of three out of five abnormalities: Central obesity, hyperglycemia, dyslipidemia, hypertension, and insulin resistance.[2,6] Anthropometric measures such as BMI and waist circumference remain pragmatic tools but lack sensitivity in distinguishing visceral from subcutaneous fat. The waist-to-height ratio has emerged as a superior predictor of central adiposity and cardiometabolic risk in adolescents.[15]

Advances in precision medicine are reshaping risk stratification. Subclassification of obesity into metabolically healthy versus unhealthy phenotypes, and the identification of intermediate clusters, improves prediction of diabetes and cardiovascular outcomes.[3] Biomarkers including adipokines, inflammatory mediators, and genetic signatures are being studied as tools for individualized risk assessment.[1]

Bibliometric mapping indicates increasing research into visceral adipose tissue, oxidative stress, and nonalcoholic fatty liver disease as mechanistic markers of cardiometabolic disease.[5] Early-life risk factors, such as maternal obesity and gestational diabetes, are also being integrated into predictive models, expanding the scope of stratification to prebirth determinants.[15]

Ultimately, effective diagnosis and risk assessment require a multidimensional approach that combines anthropometry, biochemical markers, and clinical profiling, while acknowledging obesity as a chronic relapsing disease necessitating lifelong surveillance **(Fig. 2)**.[7]

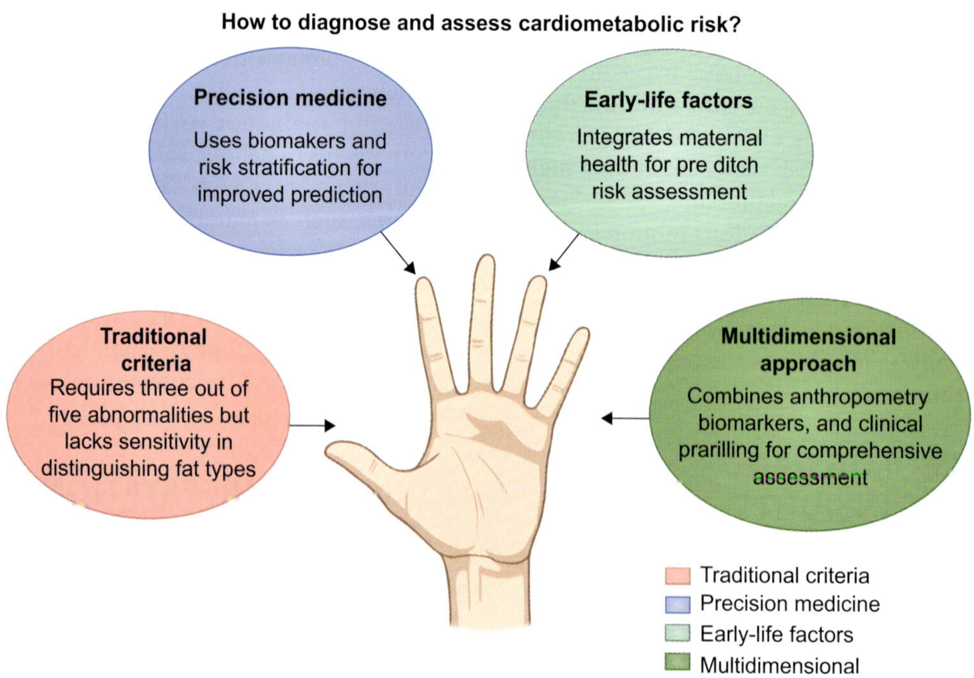

Fig. 2: Framework for diagnosing and assessing cardiometabolic risk. *The 3D illustration highlights four complementary approaches: Traditional criteria, precision medicine, early-life factors, and multidimensional profiling, emphasizing their integration for comprehensive risk assessment.*

MANAGEMENT AND THERAPEUTICS (2025 UPDATE)

Lifestyle interventions remain the cornerstone of obesity and CMS management. Dietary modification, physical activity, and behavioral therapies produce clinically meaningful weight loss of 5–10%, with associated improvements in glycemic control, lipid profiles, and blood pressure.[2,7] However, the chronicity and biological drive to weight regain limit long-term efficacy. Intermittent fasting has emerged as a promising dietary approach, demonstrating reductions in body weight, BMI, total cholesterol, LDL, and diastolic blood pressure, particularly with regimens extending beyond 12 weeks.[14] Alternate day fasting appears superior to time-restricted eating for metabolic improvements, though long-term adherence remains a challenge.[14]

Pharmacotherapy has undergone a paradigm shift. GLP-1 receptor agonists, such as semaglutide and liraglutide, have shown sustained 10–15% weight loss with cardioprotective benefits.[6,9] Tirzepatide, a dual GLP-1/GIP agonist, achieves up to 20% weight loss and favorable effects on glycemia, lipids, and blood pressure.[6] Triple agonists, such as retatrutide, are in advanced trials and demonstrate potential to rival bariatric surgery in efficacy.[12] Systematic reviews highlight that emerging pharmacotherapies consistently reduce body weight by 7–24% across phase 2 and 3 trials, with incretin-based agents dominating the therapeutic landscape **(Table 2)**.[9]

Surgical approaches, including Roux-en-Y gastric bypass and sleeve gastrectomy, remain the most effective interventions for sustained weight loss and remission of CMS, but access, cost, and perioperative risk limit their applicability.[7] Increasingly, multimodal strategies integrating pharmacotherapy with lifestyle and, where indicated, surgery are advocated to maximize outcomes.[10] Importantly, early and continuous treatment is critical, as delays in therapy allow progression of cardiometabolic complications that may become irreversible.[8]

Future management paradigms will likely involve precision-based approaches, tailoring therapy to genetic risk, obesity subphenotypes, and early-life exposures. The transition from a weight-centric to a risk-centric model of obesity management is already underway, with emphasis on preventing downstream cardiovascular and metabolic events rather than focusing solely on weight reduction.[1,3]

FUTURE DIRECTIONS AND RESEARCH NEEDS

Despite therapeutic advances, significant challenges remain. Research continues to be disproportionately skewed toward populations of European ancestry, limiting generalizability of genetic findings and pharmacological efficacy.[1] Longitudinal studies are needed to clarify the durability of novel therapies, particularly incretin-based multi-agonists, in preventing cardiovascular and renal outcomes.[9,12]

Greater emphasis must be placed on developmental origins of health and disease, integrating prenatal and early childhood factors into preventive strategies.[15] Public health initiatives require urgent scaling, with policies targeting ultraprocessed food consumption, sedentary behaviors, and obesogenic environments.[7] Moreover, digital health interventions, artificial intelligence-based risk models, and remote monitoring hold promise in delivering personalized, scalable care.[5]

Future research should prioritize diversity, long-term safety, and patient-centered outcomes, alongside trials that integrate pharmacotherapy, lifestyle, and bariatric

TABLE 2: Therapeutic advances in obesity management within CMS (2025 Update).

Therapy	*Key outcomes*	*Effect size/Evidence*	*Source(s)*
Lifestyle interventions	5–10% WL; improved glycemia, lipids, BP	Short–medium term efficacy, relapse common	2,7
Intermittent fasting (ADF and TRE)	↓ BW (–3.7 kg), ↓ BMI (–1.0 kg/m²), ↓ LDL, ↓ DBP	ADF > TRE; long-term trials needed	14
GLP-1 RAs (semaglutide and liraglutide)	10–15% WL; CV and renal protection	Multiple phase 3 trials	6,9
Dual agonist (tirzepatide)	Up to 20% WL; ↓ HbA1c, ↓ BP, improved lipids	Phase 3 trials, broad efficacy	6
Triple agonists (retatrutide)	Potentially ≥20% WL; under investigation	Phase 2–3 trials	12
Bariatric surgery	Most effective for sustained WL and CMS remission	Limited by cost, access, and perioperative risk	7,10

Note: This table highlights therapeutic strategies in 2025, spanning lifestyle, pharmacotherapy, and surgery, with emphasis on clinical outcomes in CMS.

surgery into multimodal frameworks. Addressing stigma and inequities in access will be equally critical to ensure global translation of scientific advances.

CONCLUSION

Obesity lies at the heart of CMS, amplifying the risks of diabetes, CVD, and premature mortality. Insights from 2025 underscore its multifactorial pathophysiology, early-life origins, and systemic consequences. Advances in pharmacotherapy, particularly incretin-based multi-agonists, offer unprecedented opportunities to rival surgical outcomes, while intermittent fasting and lifestyle interventions remain valuable adjuncts. Yet, the persistence of rising prevalence highlights the need for early, sustained, and multimodal treatment strategies. An integrative, precision-driven approach that spans prevention, diagnosis, and management is essential to reduce the global cardiometabolic burden in the years ahead.

REFERENCES

1. Dash S. Obesity and Cardiometabolic Disease: Insights From Genetic Studies. Can J Cardiol. 2025;41(9):1715-26.
2. Janić M, Janež A, El-Tanani M, et al. Obesity: Recent Advances and Future Perspectives. Biomedicines. 2025; 13(2):368.
3. Sarzani R, Landolfo M, Di Pentima C, et al. Adipocentric origin of the common cardiometabolic complications of obesity in the young up to the very old: pathophysiology and new therapeutic opportunities. Front Med (Lausanne). 2024:11:1365183.
4. De la Maza-Bustindui NS, León-Álvarez M, Ponce-Acosta C, et al. Impact of cardiometabolic risk factors and its management on the reversion and progression of arterial stiffness. npj Cardiovasc Health. 2025;2(1).
5. Yang H, Zhang T, Wang D, et al. A Systematic Bibliometric Analysis of Cardiovascular Disease Risk in Obesity (2014–2024). JMDH. 2025;18:3233-55.
6. Sattar N, García-Pérez L, Rodríguez A, et al. Tirzepatide and cardiometabolic parameters in obesity: Summary of current evidence. Diabetes Obes Metab. 2025;27(10):5386-92.
7. Ahmed SK, Mohammed RA. Obesity: Prevalence, causes, consequences, management, preventive strategies and future research directions. Metabolism Open. 2025;27: 100375.
8. Christensen S, Nelson C. Chronicity of obesity and the importance of early treatment to reduce cardiometabolic risk and improve body composition. Obes Pillars. 2025;15: 100175.
9. Kokkorakis M, Chakhtoura M, Rhayem C, et al. Emerging pharmacotherapies for obesity: A systematic review. Pharmacol Rev. 2025;77(1):100002.
10. Papamargaritis D, le Roux CW, Holst JJ, et al. New therapies for obesity. Cardiovasc Res. 2024;119(18):2825-42.
11. Coral DE, Smit F, Farzaneh A, et al. Subclassification of obesity for precision prediction of cardiometabolic diseases. Nat Med. 2025;31(2):534-43.
12. Liu D, Chen Y. A New Era in Obesity Treatment: The Evolution of Antiobesity Medications (AOMs) Based on Clinical Trials. J Diabetes. 2025;17(6):e70115.
13. Lozano M, Vallejo-Ortega J, Marín N, et al. Determinants of overweight and obesity and other cardiometabolic risks in adolescents: a Spanish longitudinal birth study. Pediatr Res. 2025. [Online ahead of print]
14. Wang B, Wang C, Li H. The impact of intermittent fasting on body composition and cardiometabolic outcomes in overweight and obese adults: a systematic review and meta-analysis of randomized controlled trials. Nutr J. 2025;24(1):120.
15. Dhondge RH, Agrawal S, Patil R, et al. A Comprehensive Review of Metabolic Syndrome and Its Role in Cardio-vascular Disease and Type 2 Diabetes Mellitus: Mechanisms, Risk Factors, and Management. Cureus. 2024;16(8):e67428.

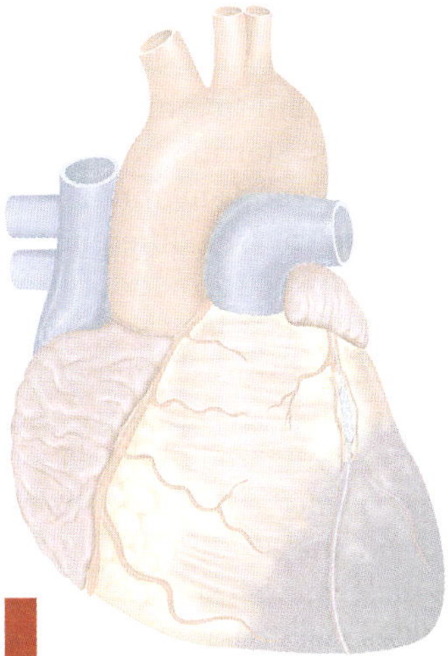

37

CHAPTER

Obesity with Diabetes, Outcome Data: Is it Different in Women?

Vitull K Gupta, Meghna Gupta, Manpreet Singh Brar, Chandi Garg

INTRODUCTION

India, the largest country in South Asia, is undergoing an epidemiological transition resulting in an explosion of noncommunicable diseases (NCDs) making NCDs a grave public health issue.[1] Out of all NCDs, obesity and type 2 diabetes mellitus (T2DM) represent the two most important global public health challenges of the 21st century. According to the World Health Organization (WHO) data,[2] among global population, 2.5 billion adults (43%) are overweight and 890 (16%) million adults are obese. Indian Council of Medical Research (ICMR)–India Diabetes (INDIAB) study[1] documented an alarming prevalence of generalized obesity (254 million) and abdominal obesity (351 million) among adults in India. Only recently, the Lancet Commission on Clinical Obesity has defined obesity as "clinical obesity," obesity associated with illness, and "preclinical obesity," obesity without evidence of any illness.[3] Evidence suggests that Asian Indians have a distinct susceptibility to obesity-related metabolic disorders at a lower body mass index (BMI) and some people with obesity have no cardiometabolic risk factors. Considering this evidence, different subtypes or phenotypes of obesity are being described in the Asian Indian population including 43.3% metabolically obese nonobese (MONO), 28.3% metabolically obese obese (MOO), 26.6% metabolically healthy nonobese (MHNO), and 1.8% metabolically healthy obese (MHO), and MOO was more common among females.[4]

OBESITY AND T2DM: OUTCOME DATA

Increasing prevalence of obesity and diabetes has been termed as a "21st century epidemic" by WHO. WHO has suggested that obesity is responsible for 44% of diabetes and the prevalence of obesity-related diabetes is suggested to be doubled to 300 million by 2025. This very close and strong relationship between obesity and diabetes has resulted in the term "Diabesity."[5] The evil twins of obesity and diabetes have also been described as a syndemic because both may affect a person simultaneously under the influence of an adverse genetic, social, and economic environment resulting in severe adverse health effects. Globally in all age groups, obesity is considered as the most significant and important risk factor for development and progression of T2DM sharing intertwined nonmodifiable as well as modifiable risk factors, pathophysiological, molecular, and metabolic mechanisms including genetics, ethnicity, body fat distribution, physical activity, diet and nutrition, insulin resistance (IR), dyslipidemia, fatty liver disease, dysfunctional adipose tissue, skeletal muscle dysfunction, homeostatic factors such as adipokines (e.g., TNF-alpha, IL-6, and resistin), systemic inflammation, free fatty acids, and gut microbiome.[5]

With increasing BMI from 18.5 to over 35 kg/m^2, the lifetime risk of developing DM increases from 7 to 70% in men and 12 to 74% in women.[6] A study has documented that the relative risk (RR) for developing DM is 4.6-fold higher for women and 3.5-fold higher for men in overweight adults as compared to their normal weight people. Another study demonstrated 25% increase risk of DM with an increase in BMI of 1 kg/m^2.[7] A hospital-based unmatched case-control study observed a significant positive relationship of obesity with T2DM with a crude odds ratio (OR) of 3.6 ($p = 0.000$, 95% CI: 2.0–6.6) and an adjusted OR of 3.7 ($p = 0.004$, 95% CI: 1.9–7.1) and concluded that obesity is strongly associated with development of T2DM.[8] A large case-control US study observed a statistically significant relationship of BMI and T2DM. In overweight population, an adjusted ORs of 1.6 (95% CI: 1.5–1.8) was observed, an adjusted ORs of 3.2 (95% CI: 2.9–3.5) in obesity I category, and an adjusted ORs of 5.8 (95% CI: 5.3–6.5) in obesity II category was observed concluding an increasing ORs with increasing BMI.[9] A meta-analysis of 18 cohort studies from different regions observed a positive relationship of T2DM with obesity with the overall adjusted RRs of 7.28 for obese subjects and 2.99 for overweight subjects as compared to subjects with normal body weight.[10]

Subanalysis of the US National Survey from 1999 to 2006 documented 80.3% of T2DM patients were having BMI of ≥25 kg/m^2 and observed that the prevalence of T2DM increased with increasing BMI.[11] A Chinese population-based cohort study observed 23% increased risk of development of T2DM with each kg/m^2 increase in BMI. The study also observed a linear relationship of obesity with the risk of development of T2DM in all age groups but much stronger in younger age group.[8,12] A meta-analysis of 12 prospective high-quality cohort studies documented sevenfold higher RR of developing T2DM in obese and threefold higher RR in overweight persons as compared to those with normal weight.[10] Bell et al. conducted a meta-analysis and observed a pooled adjusted RR of 4.03 (95% CI: 2.66–6.09) for incident T2DM in MHO adults and RR of 8.93 (6.86–11.62) in metabolically unhealthy obese adults as compared to healthy normal-weight adults.[13] A comprehensive meta-analysis established a strong positive linear relationship between risk of T2DM and BMI documenting a RR of 1.72 (95% CI: 1.65–1.81) for every 5-unit increase in BMI.[14]

A systematic review of 50 studies between January 2000 to March 2022 observed a significant association of all body weight indices with T2DM including obesity with OR = 3.05 (95% CI: 2.58, 3.61), overweight OR = 2.38 (95% CI: 1.51, 3.75), and overweight/obesity OR = 2.07 (95% CI: 1.82, 2.34).[15]

OBESITY AND DIABETES OUTCOME DATA: IS THIS DIFFERENT IN WOMEN?

During the last few decades, research into human biological sex differences in the prevalence of diseases, prevention, disease course, and treatment has gained importance, especially after a 2014 NIH mandate requiring the inclusion of sex as a biological variable in the research of all NIH-funded projects. As a result, sex differences in diseases have become an important area of research. Evidence suggests that every aspect of the association between obesity and T2DM including the risk factors, the outcomes, and response to interventions in T2DM is different in women than men. These differences are suggested to be because of multifactorial factors occurring singly or in clusters including genetic, biological, physiological, and hormonal factors. Starting in utero, a lifelong interaction between biological and environmental factors continues, and these biological "sex differences" during their lifetime as well as psychosociocultural processes arising from gender differences lead to greater variations in prevalence, susceptibility, behaviors, presentations, lifestyles, prevention, treatment, and progression of T2DM in women as compared to men.[16]

Most of global data on the prevalence of T2DM in males and females vary depending on the study population and location but suggest that males have a slightly higher prevalence of T2DM than females. A global meta-analysis and systematic review suggested 10.8% predicted T2DM prevalence in males compared to 13.4% in females. Another study reported 7.3% global prevalence of T2DM in males and 5.3% in females. A prevalence of 10.8% in males and 10.2% in females was reported by a study in a different timeframe, and age-adjusted T2DM prevalence of 7.8% in males and 5.7% in females was also reported.[17]

A meta-analysis and narrative review suggested that in both males and females, obesity is a key risk factor for T2DM and the progression of T2DM shows sex-specific patterns that males tend to develop T2DM at a younger age and lower BMI than females. Evidence observed prevalence of higher BMI in females at diagnosis of T2DM as compared to males suggesting that females have greater metabolic reserve to overcome before manifestation of overt diabetes. Studies suggest that visceral fat (central obesity) is a strong predictor of T2DM risk in women, often more than BMI alone as compared to men, and gynoid fat distribution provides a protective effect in premenopausal women which helps maintain better insulin sensitivity.[18]

Sex hormones are a critical factor in influencing the risk of diabetes. Estrogen has a protective effect in premenopausal women as it promotes healthy fat distribution and improves insulin sensitivity. In postmenopausal women, reduction in estrogen promotes a more dangerous visceral fat distribution, reduces insulin sensitivity, and increases the risk of T2DM and CVDs. Women also encounter unique risk factors of developing T2DM later in life such as gestational diabetes and polycystic ovary syndrome (PCOS).[19] Brown adipose tissue (BAT) has been suggested to influence energy metabolism and IR. BAT is found to be more active and has higher prevalence in obesity-related T2DM in females as compared to males which could contribute to lower risk of T2DM in women. In leptin-deficient animals, BAT transplantation led to reversal of obesity, increased adiponectin, decreased IR, and liver steatosis.[19] An analysis of 10 large cohort studies showed that females more often had MHO phenotype with normal blood glucose and without hypertension (HTN) and dyslipidemia as compared to males.[19]

Evidence suggests that differences in symptom presentations of CV events in males and females may contribute to delays in seeking medical attention, misdiagnosis, and poorer outcomes in females. Men generally present with typical symptoms of CV events like chest pain, whereas women generally present with atypical symptoms like shortness of breath, fatigue, nausea, and back pain.[20] Different responses to interventions and diabetes remission have been observed in men and women. Both men and women benefited from weight loss, but weight loss in men may have provided greater relative benefits in glycemic control, whereas slightly higher rates of remission in diabetes were observed in women after bariatric surgery which could be explained on the basis of differences in baseline metabolic profiles or adaptation of body to postsurgical metabolic changes.[21]

Evidence from several meta-analyses and large cohort studies have observed disproportionately increased risk of fatal CHD, stroke, and overall CV mortality in women with obesity and diabetes as compared to men with the same conditions.[16,22] A meta-analysis in *The Lancet Diabetes and Endocrinology* observed 44% higher RR of fatal CHD and a 27% higher RR of stroke in women with diabetes as compared to men.[23] Evidence from a meta-analysis suggested disproportionate increases in the CVD risk in obese diabetic females as the "female advantage" in risk of CVD is eliminated by presence of diabetes and such females are at a higher RR for certain CV events like heart failure than men with T2DM. Obesity and diabetes together differentially and adversely impacted the CV risk in women because women are more likely to have coronary microvascular dysfunction-related angina and myocardial ischemia without any obstructive atherosclerosis as well as heart failure with preserved ejection fraction (HFpEF).[24]

A large meta-analysis exploring the association between obesity and diabetic outcomes in males and females showed that diabetes-related complications are more common in obese females compared to males. The pooled female-to-male RRR showed a 13% more risk of all-cause mortality associated with diabetes in women as compared to men (RRR 1.13, 95% CI: 1.07–1.19; $p<0.001$). The pooled multiple-adjusted RRR showed a 30% more risk of CVD mortality (RRR 1.30, 95% CI: 1.13–1.49; $p<0.001$), 58% more risk of CAD mortality (RRR_{CHD} 1.58, 95% CI: 1.32–1.90; $p<0.001$), and 8% more risk of stroke mortality (RRR_{stroke} 1.08, 95% CI: 1.01–1.15; $p<0.001$) in women as compared to men.[25] A systematic review and meta-analysis of 64 cohort studies including 775,385 subjects and 12,539 fatal and nonfatal strokes observed significantly higher risk of stroke in women with diabetes than men and documented maximum pooled adjusted RR of 2.28 (95% CI: 1.93–2.69) for stroke associated with diabetes in women and 1.83 (1.60–2.08) in men.[22] A retrospective study including 72,980 subjects with T2DM observed 73.5% prevalence of obesity in females as compared to 59.0% in males, 18.8% of the women achieved glycemic control (HbA1c <7%) as compared to 19.9% in men ($p < 0.001$). Study observed higher prevalence of retinopathy (36.0 vs. 26.3%), neuropathy (42.9 vs. 36.9%), and nephropathy (25.0 vs. 23.3%) and 1.8- and 1.6-times higher risk of developing retinopathy and CAD in males as compared to females.[26] Evidence suggests increased susceptibility to metabolic-associated fatty liver disease (MAFLD) in women after menopause because of an increase in cardiometabolic risk factors like obesity and diabetes. However, Wu et al. reported higher risk of heart failure in younger women (age <45 years) with MAFLD as compared to men.[27] A meta-analysis and systematic review of 5,162,654 subjects observed 54% excess risk of CHD death in women with diabetes, which may be because of multifactorial pathogenesis including sex differences in genetic, biological, cultural, and environmental factors along with documented differences in the diagnosis and management of DM and CVD in females as compared to males.[25]

As compared to men, in women with diabetes, the risk factors of low physical activity, HTN, and high alcohol were stronger predictors of myocardial infarction. Moreover, microcirculation, endothelial response, higher atherothrombotic risk, greater prothrombotic activity, and greater fibrin activity were observed in women with diabetes as compared to men. Evidence suggested poor angiogenesis in response to thrombotic insult that resulted in poor development of collateral vessels after chronic total occlusion in diabetic females as compared to males.[28] One meta-analysis showed a stronger positive association with renal cancer mortality and risk of gastric cancer in diabetic women than in men.[29] Another meta-analysis observed increased risk of esophageal cancer and leukemia in diabetic men as compared to women.[30] A meta-analysis exploring differences in the therapeutic efficacy in T2DM treatment and outcomes in males and females observed that different therapeutic interventions such as dietary interventions, oral antidiabetic drugs (OADs), and insulin often had lesser effect on HbA1c levels in women compared to men.[31] Data from TODAY trial observed better glycemic response with thiazolidinediones (TZDs) in obese females with T2DM as compared to nonobese females or obese males. Greater glycemic treatment outcomes were observed in males as compared to females in studies of glucagon-like peptide-1 (GLP-1) receptor agonists.[32] Various studies have consistently observed a relative undertreatment of females compared with males, and women with T2DM show worse control of HbA1c, lipids, and blood pressure than men. Evidence suggests less aggressive use of revascularization procedures for females with diabetes and CAD as compared to males as well as less guideline-based treatment for ACS. Some of the sex differences in the treatment of acute coronary syndrome may be because of more occurrences of atypical symptoms of CAD in females leading to delayed diagnosis.[32]

In women, modifiable socioeconomic factors such as low education, income, employment, social position, and food insecurity were related to a higher risk of obesity and T2DM because these factors contributed to unhealthy lifestyle behaviors and social disparities as compared to men with same socioeconomic factors. A sex-specific meta-analysis of epidemiological studies showed a 40% higher risk of insomnia in women of all ages and observed that short sleep duration, sleep loss, and reduced sleep quality were related to obesity and IR. Studies suggest that pathogenesis of T2DM in men and women is influenced by mismatch between the social rhythms and circadian clock as well as sex-dependent risk factors and gender-dependent social time and body composition.[28]

CONCLUSION

Obesity and T2DM represent two most important global public health challenges of the 21st century, and very close and strong relationship has resulted in the term "diabesity." The last few decades of research into human biological sex differences in the prevalence of diseases, prevention, pathophysiology, disease course, complications, and treatment have gained importance. Current evidence suggests that every aspect of the association between obesity and T2DM is different in women as compared to men. These differences are suggested to be because of multifactorial factors occurring singly or in clusters including genetic, biological, physiological, psychosociocultural, and hormonal factors. An increased understanding and appreciation of sex differences related to association and outcome data between diabetes and obesity has given the importance to early and aggressive screening for risk factors, holistic management including prevention, and targeted interventions tailored to address the distinct risk profiles and psychosociocultural challenges faced by women with diabesity. By acknowledging the existing evidence of sex-based differences, researchers can generate more data on sex differences not only related to obesity and diabetes but all aspects of human biology and healthcare system that can prevent as well as improve outcomes, reduce complications, enhance the quality of life, and reduce all-cause mortality and morbidity, particularly in female population living with obesity and diabetes. Existing evidence and outcome data call for a fundamental shift in clinical practice to a sex and gender sensitive model of care rather than from a one-size-fits-all approach and strive to reduce health disparities and improve well-being of females living with "diabesity." No doubt managing twin evils of obesity and diabetes in women poses incredible challenges and definitely necessitate formation and implementation of sex-specific strategies and national health plans while taking into consideration the cultural, social, economic, and regional differences in India.

REFERENCES

1. Anjana RM, Unnikrishnan R, Deepa M, et al. Metabolic non-communicable disease health report of India: the ICMR-INDIAB national cross-sectional study (ICMR-INDIAB-17). Lancet Diabetes Endocrinol. 2023; 11(7):474-89.
2. World Health Organization. (2025). Obesity and overweight. [online] Available from https://www.who.int/news-room/fact-sheets/detail/obesity-and-overweight. [Last accessed January, 2026].
3. Rubino F, Cummings DE, Eckel RH, et al. Definition and diagnostic criteria of clinical obesity. Lancet Diabetes Endocrinol. 2025;13:221-62.
4. Deepa M, Pradeepa R, Venkatesan U, et al. High prevalence of metabolic obesity in India: the ICMR-INDIAB national study (ICMR-INDIAB-23). Indian J Med Res. 2025;161:461-72.
5. Chandrasekaran P, Weiskirchen R. The role of obesity in type 2 diabetes mellitus—an overview. Int J Mol Sci. 2024;25(3):1882.
6. Garg C, Daley SF. Obesity and type 2 diabetes. Treasure Island: StatPearls Publishing; 2025.
7. Han SJ, Boyko EJ. The evidence for an obesity paradox in type 2 diabetes mellitus. Diabetes Metab J. 2018;42(3):179-87.
8. Ali S, Hussain R, Malik RA, et al. Association of obesity with type 2 diabetes mellitus: a hospital-based unmatched case-control study. Cureus. 2024;16(1):e52728.
9. Ganz ML, Wintfeld N, Li Q, et al. The association of body mass index with the risk of type 2 diabetes: a case-control study nested in an electronic health records system in the United States. Diabetol Metab Syndr. 2014;6:50.
10. Abdullah A, Peeters A, de Courten M, et al. The magnitude of association between overweight and obesity and the risk of diabetes: a meta-analysis of prospective cohort studies. Diabetes Res Clin Pract. 2010;89(3):309-19.
11. Nguyen NT, Nguyen XM, Lane J, et al. Relationship between obesity and diabetes in a US adult population: findings from the National Health and Nutrition Examination Survey, 1999-2006. Obes Surg. 2011;21:351-5.

12. Chen Y, Zhang XP, Yuan J, et al. Association of body mass index and age with incident diabetes in Chinese adults: a population-based cohort study. BMJ Open. 2018;8:e021768.
13. Bell JA, Hamer M, Batty GD. Metabolically healthy obesity and risk of incident type 2 diabetes: a meta-analysis of prospective cohort studies. Obes Rev. 2015;16(2): 504-11.
14. Jayedi A, Soltani S, Motlagh SZ-T, et al. Anthropometric and adiposity indicators and risk of type 2 diabetes: systematic review and dose-response meta-analysis of cohort studies. BMJ. 2022;376:e067516.
15. Issaka A, Paradies Y, Cameron AJ, et al. The association between body weight indices, behavioral factors, and type 2 diabetes mellitus in Africa: a systematic review and meta-analysis of population-based epidemiological studies. Nutr Metab Cardiovasc Dis. 2024;34(1):1-18.
16. Kautzky-Willer A, Leutner M, Harreiter J. Sex differences in type 2 diabetes. Diabetologia. 2023;66:986-1002.
17. Barbier JM, Amiguet M, Vaucher J, et al. Exploring the gender difference in type 2 diabetes incidence in a Swiss cohort using latent class analysis: an intersectional approach. BMJ Public Health. 2024;2:e000472.
18. Mauvais-Jarvis F. Sex differences in energy metabolism: natural selection, mechanisms and consequences. Nat Rev Nephrol. 2024;20(1):56-69.
19. Kautzky-Willer A, Harreiter J, Pacini G. Sex and gender-related differences in the pathophysiology and epidemiology of type 2 diabetes. Endocr Rev. 2016;37(3): 278-301.
20. St. Joseph's/Candler. (2024). How diabetes affects women differently than men. [online] Available from https://www.sjchs.org/resource-hub/blogs/blog-detail/living-smart-blog/2024/04/24/how-diabetes-affects-women-differently-than-men. [Last accessed January, 2026].
21. Arnetz L, Ekberg NR, Alvarsson M. Sex differences in type 2 diabetes: focus on disease course and outcomes. Diabetes Metab Syndr Obes. 2014;7:409-20.
22. Peters SA, Huxley RR, Woodward M. Diabetes as a risk factor for stroke in women compared with men: a systematic review and meta-analysis of 64 cohorts, including 775,385 individuals and 12,539 strokes. Lancet. 2014;383(9933):1973-80.
23. Razzaghi H, et al. The burden of diabetes and its complications in the United States, 2017. Diabetes Care. 2018;41(3):596-601.
24. Fatade YA, Dave EK, Vatsa N, et al. Obesity and diabetes in heart disease in women. Metab Target Organ Damage. 2024;4:22.
25. Wang Y, O'Neil A, Jiao Y, et al. Sex differences in the association between diabetes and risk of cardiovascular disease, cancer, and all-cause and cause-specific mortality: a systematic review and meta-analysis of 5,162,654 participants. BMC Med. 2019;17:136.
26. Pradeepa R, Shreya L, Anjana RM, et al. Sex-based differences in clinical profile and complications among individuals with type 2 diabetes seen at a Private Tertiary Diabetes Care Centre in India. Healthcare (Basel). 2023;11(11):1634.
27. Wu S, Li Y, Zhang Y, et al. Sex and age differences in the association between metabolic dysfunction-associated fatty liver disease and heart failure: a prospective cohort study. Circ Heart Fail. 2024;17:e010841.
28. Ciarambino T, Crispino P, Leto G, et al. Influence of gender in diabetes mellitus and its complication. Int J Mol Sci. 2022;23(16):8850.
29. Huang W, Ren H, Ben Q, et al. Risk of esophageal cancer in diabetes mellitus: a meta-analysis of observational studies. Cancer Causes Control. 2012;23:263-72.
30. Castillo JJ, Mull N, Reagan JL, et al. Increased incidence of non-Hodgkin lymphoma, leukemia, and myeloma in patients with diabetes mellitus type 2: a meta-analysis of observational studies. Blood. 2012;119:4845-50.
31. McGill JB, Vlajnic A, Knutsen PG, et al. Effect of gender on treatment outcomes in type 2 diabetes mellitus. Diabetes Res Clin Pract. 2013;102(3):167-74.
32. Huebschmann AG, Huxley RR, Kohrt WM, et al. Sex differences in the burden of type 2 diabetes and cardiovascular risk across the life course. Diabetologia. 2019;62:1761-72.

38

CHAPTER

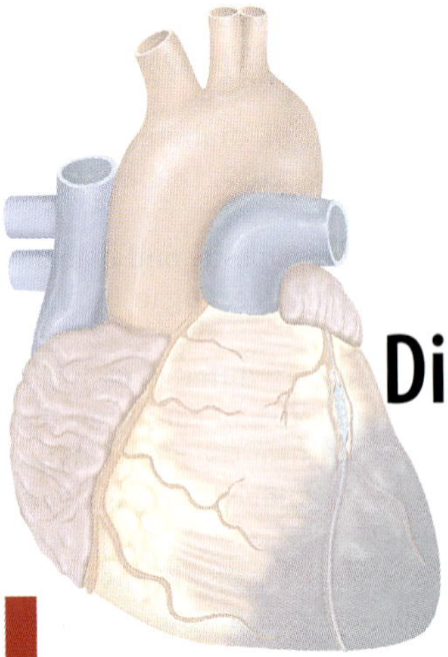

Diabetic Dyslipidemia and its Management

Anil Bhoraskar

INTRODUCTION

A complicated and serious metabolic condition, diabetic dyslipidemia is commonly seen in people with diabetes, especially those with type 2 diabetes mellitus (T2DM). It is distinguished by a unique pattern of abnormalities in lipids that, when combined, raise the risk of atherosclerotic cardiovascular disease (ASCVD), which is the primary cause of mortality for diabetics.

AN OVERVIEW OF DYSLIPIDEMIA IN DIABETES

The three main lipid abnormalities associated with diabetic dyslipidemia are:

1. Hypertriglyceridemia or elevated triglycerides
2. Low amounts of HDL-C or high-density lipoprotein cholesterol
3. A higher frequency of small dense low-density lipoprotein (sdLDL) particles.

Apolipoprotein glycation, elevated triglyceride content in LDL and HDL, and increased susceptibility of LDL to oxidation are among the qualitative changes in addition to the quantitative ones. Normal lipid metabolism is disrupted by insulin resistance and decreased insulin production, which are the primary causes of these abnormalities in people with diabetes. By preventing the hepatic synthesis of very low-density lipoproteins (VLDLs) and encouraging lipoprotein lipase activity, insulin typically controls lipid metabolism; when it malfunctions, VLDL1 particles, sdLDL formation, and HDL catabolism are all elevated. Even in cases when routine assessments of LDL cholesterol levels show normal levels, the overall result is a higher atherogenic lipid profile that dramatically increases cardiovascular risk.

PATHOPHYSIOLOGY

Triglyceride-rich lipoproteins are overproduced, and their clearance is decreased as part of the pathophysiology. Increased insulin resistance causes compensatory hyperinsulinemia, which raises the release of VLDL in the liver in prediabetes and early diabetes. High levels of free fatty acids also promote the production of VLDL in overt type 2 diabetes with relative insulin insufficiency. Despite normal or slightly higher LDL cholesterol levels, small compact LDL particles predominate. These particles are more atherogenic because of their increased capacity to permeate the artery wall and their sensitivity to oxidation. Furthermore, HDL particles become less numerous and less functioning, which exacerbates the lipid imbalance.

CLINICAL IMPLICATIONS AND RISK ASSESSMENT

Cardiovascular Risk

Myocardial infarction and stroke, as well as atherosclerosis, are significantly exacerbated by diabetic dyslipidemia. According to studies, people with diabetes are 2–4 times more likely to develop cardiovascular disease (CVD) than people without the disease.

Risk Stratification

According to recent guidelines, diabetic people should be treated as high or very high cardiovascular risk persons and require rigorous lipid control. For individualized evaluation, risk stratification tools such as the ASCVD risk calculator and QRISK3 are advised.

Screening Recommendations

- Initial lipid profile at diabetes diagnosis
- Annual monitoring
- Earlier screening in children with type 1 diabetes or those with a family history of dyslipidemia.

Indian Perspective

In South Asians, particularly Indians, diabetic dyslipidemia often appears as tiny dense LDL particles and raised triglycerides, even in the absence of significantly elevated LDL-C values. This calls for specialized treatment and screening techniques.

MANAGEMENT STRATEGIES

Lifestyle Modifications

First-line therapy includes:

- Weight loss
- Aerobic exercise
- Diet low in saturated fats and refined carbohydrates
- Smoking cessation
- Moderate alcohol intake.

These interventions improve insulin sensitivity and lipid parameters.

Pharmacologic Therapy

- *Statins:* First-line agents for both primary and secondary prevention. High-intensity statins are preferred in high-risk patients.
- *Ezetimibe:* Add-on therapy to statins for further LDL-C reduction.
- *PCSK9 Inhibitors:* Effective in patients with very high risk or statin intolerance.
- *Fibrates:* Useful in patients with high triglycerides and low HDL-C, especially when combined with statins.
- *Omega-3 fatty acids (EPA):* May reduce triglycerides and inflammation.
- *Bempedoic acid:* A newer agent for statin-intolerant patients.
- *Saroglitazar:* Dual PPAR agonist with benefits on both lipid and glycemic parameters, particularly relevant in Indian patients.

Guideline Highlights

- *ADA/AHA (2024):* LDL-C target <70 mg/dL for primary prevention, <55 mg/dL for secondary prevention.
- *RSSDI (2022):* Emphasizes the unique lipid profile in Indians and recommends a stepwise approach including statins, ezetimibe, fibrates, and newer agents.
- *AACE (2025):* Advocates for personalized therapy using the GRADE framework, focusing on patient-important outcomes.

CONCLUSION

Diabetic dyslipidemia poses a significant risk for ASCVD due to a distinct pattern of lipid abnormalities dominated by hypertriglyceridemia, low HDL cholesterol, and small dense LDL particles. Effective management involves a combination of lifestyle interventions and pharmacotherapy, predominantly statins, tailored to individual risk. Emerging therapies such as PCSK9 inhibitors may further improve outcomes. Early and aggressive treatment is essential to reduce the substantial cardiovascular burden associated with diabetes.

BIBLIOGRAPHY

1. American Diabetes Association. (2024). This infographic is based on recommendations from the ADA's Standards of Care in Diabetes-2024. [online]. Available from https://professional.diabetes.org/sites/dpro/files/2024-03/KDBH-LipidManagement.pdf [Last accessed January, 2026].
2. Banach M, Surma S, Reiner Z, et al. Personalized management of dyslipidemias in patients with diabetes-it is time for a new approach (2022). Cardiovasc Diabetol. 2022;21(1):263.
3. Bereda G. Pathophysiology and Management of Dyslipidaemia. J Sci Tech Res. 2022;43(2):34369-75.
4. C Thambiah S, Lai LC. Diabetic dyslipidaemia. Pract Lab Med. 2021;26:e00248.
5. ESC. (2020). Diabetic dyslipidaemia: which drugs to use. [online] Available from https://www.escardio.org/communities/councils/cardiology-practice/scientific-documents-and-publications/ejournal/volume-19/diabetic-dyslipidaemia-which-drugs-to-use/ [Last accessed January, 2026].
6. Feingold KR, Grunfeld C. (2015). Diabetes and dyslipidemia. [online] Available from https://endotext.org/wp-content/uploads/pdfs/diabetes-and-dislipidemia.pdf [Last accessed January, 2026].

7. Goldberg IJ. Clinical review 124: Diabetic dyslipidemia: causes and consequences. J Clin Endocrinol Metab. 2001;86(3):965-71.
8. Haffner SM; American Diabetes Association. Dyslipidemia management in adults with diabetes. Diabetes Care. 2004;27(Suppl 1):S68-71.
9. Ide S, Maezawa Y, Yokote K. Updates on dyslipidemia in patients with diabetes. J Diabetes Investig. 2023; 14(9):1041-4.
10. Jackson EJ, Willard KE, Ballantyne CM. LDL cholesterol management simplified in adults-lower for longer is better: Guidance from the National Lipid Association. J Clin Lipidol. 2025;19(5):1200-7.
11. Jialal I, Singh G. Management of diabetic dyslipidemia: An update. World J Diabetes. 2019;10(5):280-90.
12. Lee S. (2025). Dyslipidemia Management in Diabetes: Best Practices. [online] Available from https://www.numberanalytics.com/blog/dyslipidemia-management-diabetes-best-practices [Last accessed January, 2026].
13. Martín-Timón I, Sevillano-Collantes C, García-Domínguez M, et al. Update on the Management of Diabetic Dyslipidaemia. EMJ Diabet. 2018;6(1):53-61.
14. Patel SB, Wyne KL, Afreen S, et al. American Association of Clinical Endocrinology Clinical Practice Guideline on Pharmacologic Management of Adults With Dyslipidemia. Endocr Pract. 2025;31(2):236-62.
15. Rhee EJ. Recent dyslipidemia guidelines for patients with diabetes mellitus. Precis Futur Med. 2020;4(4): 133-14025284121.
16. Saboo BD, Agarwal S, Makkar B, et al. RSSDI consensus recommendations for dyslipidemia management in diabetes mellitus. Int J Diabetes Dev Ctries. 2022;42(1):3-28.
17. Vergès B. Pathophysiology of diabetic dyslipidaemia: where are we? Diabetologia. 2015;58(5):886-99.

SECTION 7

Obesity Cardiomyopathy with Heart Failure

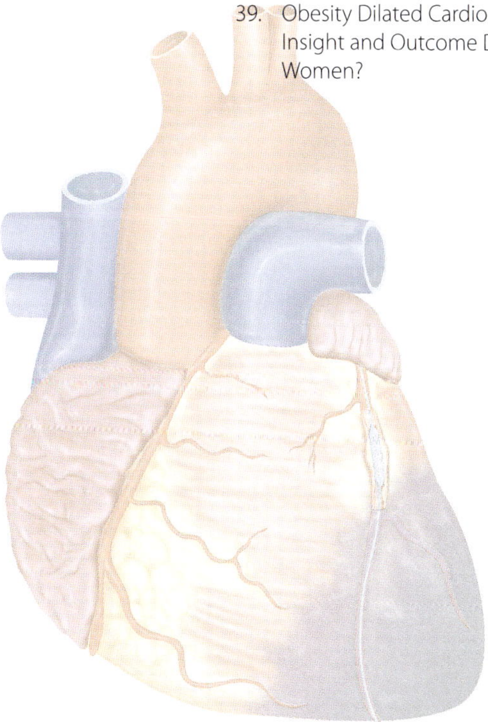

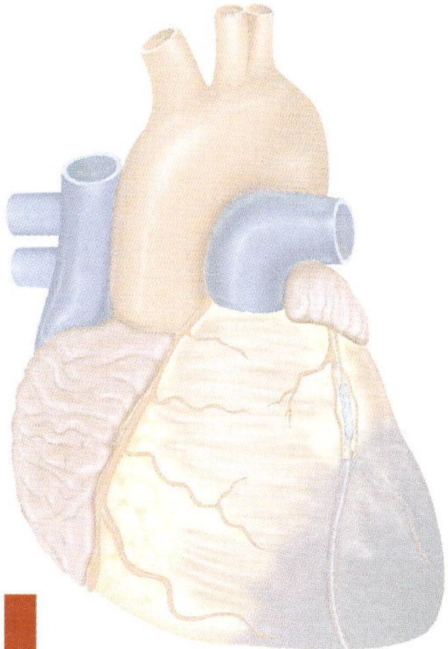

39

CHAPTER

Obesity Dilated Cardiomyopathy: Insight and Outcome Data, is it Different in Women?

Neha Chopra, Shitij Chaudhary, Sandeep Seth

INTRODUCTION

Obesity is a chronic condition characterized by abnormal and/or excessive adipose tissue accumulation, defined as a body mass index (BMI) ≥30 kg/m^2 globally (World Health Organization definition) and ≥25 kg/m^2 for Asian populations.[1] It is becoming a global health issue with 16% of the world's adult population living with obesity, and 43% with overweight, as of 2022.[2] Obesity is associated strongly with incident heart failure (HF), with every 4 kg/m^2 increasing the risk of HF with preserved ejection fraction (HFpEF), and heart failure with reduced ejection fraction (HFrEF) by 1.33- and 1.26-fold, respectively.[3,4] In a subsequent analysis of 5881 participants of the Framingham cohort, the risk of HF in men and women increased by 5% and 7%, respectively, per unit increase in BMI, after adjustment for diabetes mellitus, hypercholesterolemia, hypertension, and myocardial infarction.

OBESITY AND DILATED CARDIOMYOPATHY

Dilated cardiomyopathy (DCM) has been defined as "the presence of left ventricular (LV) dilatation and global and/or regional systolic dysfunction unexplained solely by abnormal loading conditions, such as hypertension, valvular heart disease, congenital heart disease, or coronary artery disease."[5] Obesity is being accepted as one of the causes of DCM apart from genetic, toxins, endocrine (Cushing syndrome, pheochromocytoma, etc.), drugs (anthracyclines, tricyclic antidepressants, etc.), postpartum cardiomyopathy, and autoimmune disorders (systemic lupus erythematosus, rheumatoid arthritis, etc.).[6] However, obesity alone as a cause of severe LV systolic dysfunction is rare, and should trigger exclusion of other causes. An improvement in systolic function with bariatric surgery, demonstrated in small studies, may be an indirect clue to the existence of this rare but potentially treatable etiology.[7,8] The pathophysiology of obesity cardiomyopathy involves hemodynamic, metabolic, neurohumoral, and inflammatory mechanisms **(Fig. 1)**.[9,10]

OBESITY DILATED CARDIOMYOPATHY IN WOMEN

There are limited data on the development and outcomes of DCM in obese women. Based on data from a Swedish prospective cohort of 1,388,571 women of childbearing age with a mean BMI of 23.7 kg/m^2, followed up over a median of 16 years, 1699 women developed a cardiomyopathy (0.1%; 5.9 per 100,000 observation years).[11] Of these, 481 women (28.3%) developed a DCM with an event rate of 2.2 per 100,000 observation years. The others were diagnosed with hypertrophic cardiomyopathy (14.5%), alcohol/drug-induced cardiomyopathy (3.6%), and other cardiomyopathies (30.0%). The remaining 374 cases were considered to be pregnancy-related cardiomyopathies and were censored at diagnosis. In this study, the incidence of DCM assumed a U-shaped curve, with the lowest incidence at a BMI of 21 kg/m^2. There was an incremental rise in event rates with increasing BMI, with the highest risk seen in severely obese women with a BMI of 35 to <60 kg/m^2 [event rate 5.8 per 100,000 observation years,

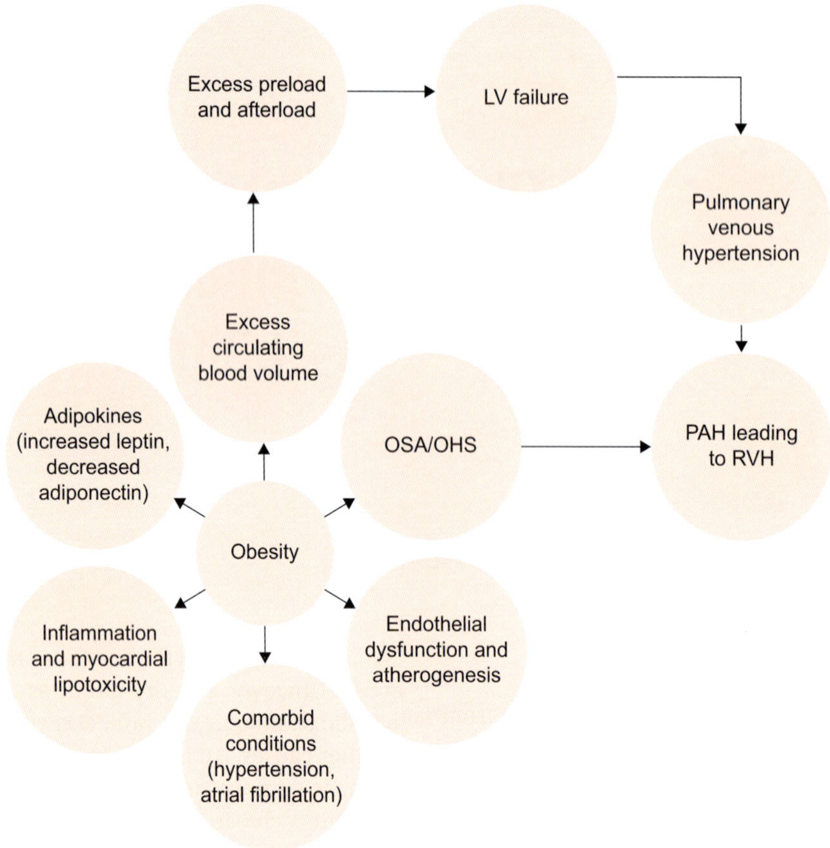

Fig. 1: Pathophysiology of obesity cardiomyopathy.

95% confidence interval (CI), 3.4–9.2]. The adjusted hazard ratio for DCM was around 1.1 per unit increase in BMI. Notably, the risk for DCM also rose in women with BMI <20 kg/m^2. This finding must be interpreted with caution, given the low event rates.

A similar study was conducted by the same investigators among 1,668,893 adolescent Swedish men enlisting for compulsory military service (mean age 18.3 years), followed up for a median of 27 years.[12] A total of 4,447 participants were diagnosed with cardiomyopathy, of which 2631 (59%) were DCM (event rate 5.9 per 100,000 observation years). The incidence of DCM was lowest at a BMI range of 20 to <22.5 kg/m^2, and highest in severely obese men (BMI ≥ 35 kg/m^2) at 24.7 per 100,000 observation years. The adjusted hazard ratio for DCM was around 1.15 per unit increase in BMI. Therefore, women appeared to have slightly lower event rates for DCM compared to men, but showed similar trends with a rise in BMI **(Fig. 2)**. This may be due in part to the shorter duration of follow-up in the study of women. This is also mirrored in previous studies showing a higher prevalence of DCM in men than women (female:male ratios 1:1.9 to 1:4.3).[11,13,14]

In an observational cohort study of 2,294,139 adolescents from Israel, 40% of whom were female, there was a graded increase in mortality risk from cardiomyopathies among other causes, with increasing BMI.[15] During 42,297,007 patient-years of follow-up, the hazard ratios for mortality were 1.5, 2.4, and 4.0 for high-normal (BMI ≥22 to <25 kg/m^2), overweight (BMI ≥25 to <30 kg/m^2), and obese categories (BMI ≥30 kg/m^2). There were only 121 cardiomyopathy-related deaths, and cause-specific and sex-specific distributions were not reported.

A recent retrospective study analyzed 170,924 admissions with DCM from the Nationwide Inpatient Sample of US hospitalizations from 2015 to 2019.[16] The odds ratio for hospitalized obese patients (BMI ≥30 kg/m^2) was 1.82 for DCM (95% CI, 1.79–1.84, $p < 0.001$). The positive association between DCM diagnosis and obesity was driven primarily by the male sex and was insignificant in females. Whether this seemingly contradictory finding is due to the inclusion of only inpatients and other unknown confounders or due to sex-determined differences in adipose tissue biology and myocardial remodeling needs to be studied.

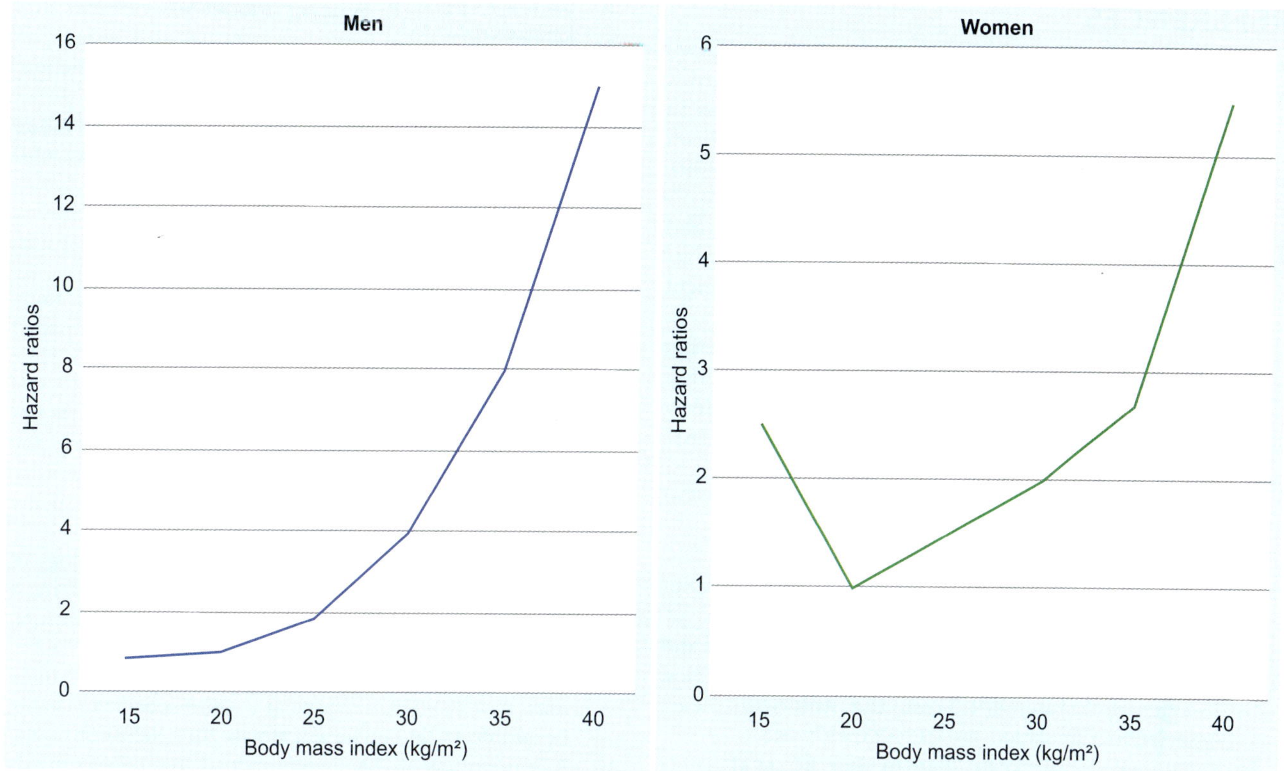

Fig. 2: Changes in adjusted hazard ratio (HR) of dilated cardiomyopathy (DCM) with rising body mass index in men (left) and women (right).

Note: The risk for developing DCM rises with an increment in BMI with a J-shaped curve in men. The risk for development of DCM was lowest in the BMI range of ≥22.5 to <25 kg/m^2. The risk rises in underweight as well as overweight and obese females, with the highest risk seen in severely obese women (BMI ≥35 kg/m^2) (U-shaped curve).

Source: Adapted from Xie SH, Santoni G, Gottlieb-Vedi E, Mattsson F, Lagergren J. Swedish Prescribed Drugs and Health Cohort (SPREDH): cohort profile update. BMJ Open. 2025;15(10):e104455.[11,12]

DISCUSSION

These findings confirm an association between rising BMI and the risk of development of DCM, though the risk may be higher in men. The reasons for this sexual dimorphism are incompletely understood. However, it is important to note that even overweight men and women are at a higher risk of developing DCM at follow-up, compared to normal-weight individuals. This risk may also differ across geographic regions and ethnicities, and the Swedish cohort results may not be generalizable to Asians, for instance. This is especially true given the different definitions of obesity and overweight for Asian populations to account for the differences in body constitution and genetics. Nearly 24% of Indian women are overweight or obese (BMI ≥25 kg/m^2), and 57% have abdominal obesity (abnormal waist-hip ratio), compared to 23% and 48% of Indian men, as per data from the National Family Health Survey-5 (2019–2021). Hence, there is a need for large prospective cohort studies to evaluate cardiomyopathy risk with a change in BMI among Asian-men and women. While newer therapies such as tirzepatide and semaglutide have been shown to improve cardiovascular outcomes in patients with obesity and HFpEF, there is a lack of data in obese patients with HFrEF, and it could be a potential area for future research.

CONCLUSION

There are limited data for sex-based differences in the risk of development and outcomes of DCM in obese patients, with a few studies indicating a higher risk with increasing BMI, more so in men than women. The mechanistic basis of this difference is not fully understood and needs to be studied further. There is also scope for larger prospective studies including patients of other ethnicities.

REFERENCES

1. Kittleson MM, Benjamin EJ, Blumer V, et al. 2025 ACC Scientific Statement on the Management of Obesity in Adults With Heart Failure: A Report of the American College of Cardiology. J Am Coll Cardiol. 2025;86(20): 1953-75.
2. World Health Organization. (2025). Obesity and overweight. [Online]. Available from https://www.who.int/news-room/fact-sheets/detail/obesity-and-overweight [Last accessed January, 2026].
3. Ho JE, Enserro D, Brouwers FP, et al. Predicting heart failure with preserved and reduced ejection fraction: The International Collaboration on Heart Failure Subtypes. Circ Heart Fail. 2016;9(6):10.1161/CIRCHEARTFAILURE.115.003116 e003116.
4. Kenchaiah S, Evans JC, Levy D, et al. Obesity and the risk of heart failure. N Engl J Med. 2002;347(5):305-13.
5. Arbelo E, Protonotarios A, Gimeno JR, et al. 2023 ESC Guidelines for the management of cardiomyopathies. Eur Heart J. 2023;44(37):3503-626.
6. Bozkurt B, Colvin M, Cook J, et al. Current Diagnostic and Treatment Strategies for Specific Dilated Cardiomyopathies: A Scientific Statement From the American Heart Association. Circulation. 2016;134(23):e579-646.
7. Ramani GV, McCloskey C, Ramanathan RC, et al. Safety and efficacy of bariatric surgery in morbidly obese patients with severe systolic heart failure. Clin Cardiol. 2008;31(11):516-20.
8. Vest AR, Patel P, Schauer PR, et al. Clinical and echocardiographic outcomes after bariatric surgery in obese patients with left ventricular systolic dysfunction. Circ Heart Fail. 2016;9(3):e002260.
9. Albakri A. Obesity cardiomyopathy: a review of literature on clinical status and meta-analysis of diagnostic and clinical management. Med Clin Arch. 2018;2(3).
10. Ren J, Wu NN, Wang S, et al. Obesity cardiomyopathy: evidence, mechanisms, and therapeutic implications. Physiol Rev. 2021;101(4):1745-807.
11. Robertson J, Lindgren M, Schaufelberger M, et al. Body mass index in young women and risk of cardiomyopathy: a long-term follow-up study in Sweden. Circulation. 2020; 141(7):520-9.
12. Robertson J, Schaufelberger M, Lindgren M, et al. Higher body mass index in adolescence predicts cardiomyopathy risk in midlife. Circulation. 2019;140(2):117-25.
13. Bagger JP, Baandrup U, Rasmussen K, et al. Cardiomyopathy in western Denmark. Br Heart J. 1984;52(3):327-31.
14. Codd MB, Sugrue DD, Gersh BJ, et al. Epidemiology of idiopathic dilated and hypertrophic cardiomyopathy: a population-based study in Olmsted County, Minnesota, 1975-1984. Circulation. 1989;80(3):564-72.
15. Twig G, Ben-Ami Shor D, Furer A, et al. Adolescent body mass index and cardiovascular disease-specific mortality by midlife. J Clin Endocrinol Metab. 2017;102(8): 3011-20.
16. Antonopoulos AS, Panagiotopoulos I, Terentes-Printzios D, et al. Relationship between obesity and hypertrophic or dilated cardiomyopathy: the role of sex. Clin Obes. 2024;14(6):e12692.

SECTION 8

Obesity with Arrhythmia

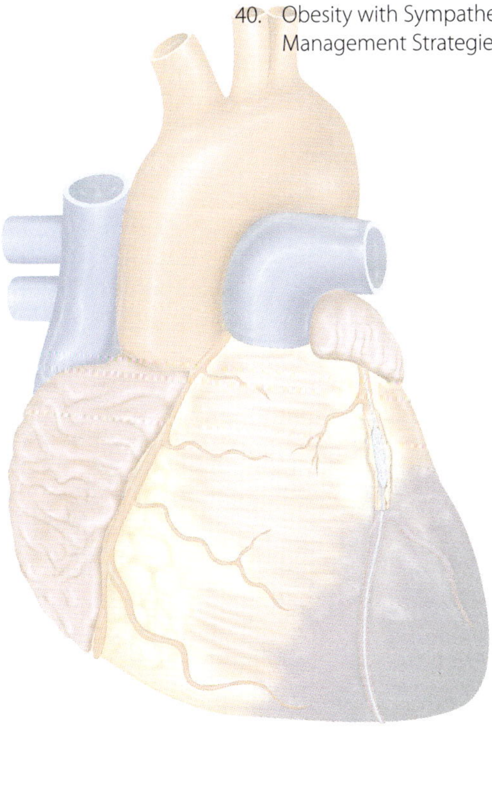

40

CHAPTER

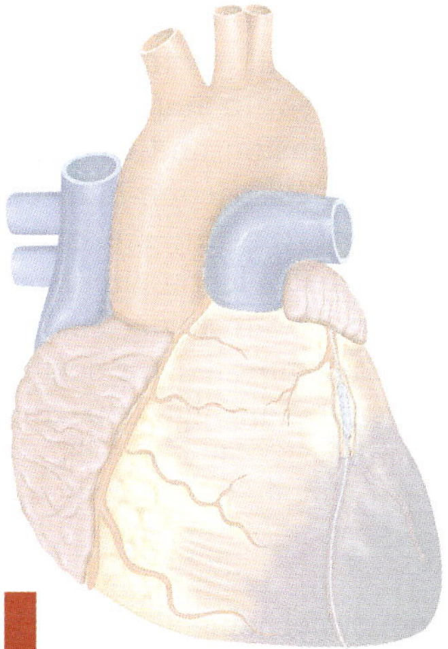

Obesity with Sympathetic Overdrive: Management Strategies

Sarita Rao, K Roshan Rao, Praveen Jaswal, Achukatla Kumar

INTRODUCTION

Obesity is a major global public health problem that increases the risk of multiple noncommunicable diseases such as diabetes, hypertension, and cardiovascular diseases. The new, evidence-based definition distinguishes "clinical obesity," a chronic, systemic disease state directly caused by excess adiposity, from "preclinical obesity," a condition of excess adiposity without current organ dysfunction or limitations in daily activities but with increased future health risk as per the Lancet Commission 2025. The Endocrine Society of India defines obesity as a chronic, relapsing, and progressive disease defined by excessive adiposity that may impair health.[1]

Globally, the prevalence of overweight and obesity has been steadily increasing in recent decades. The WHO estimates that over 1.9 billion adults are overweight, with >650 million classified as obese. This trend is driven by complex interactions between lifestyle, socioeconomic, and environmental factors, including urbanization, dietary changes, and reduced physical activity.[2,3] As per the NFHS-5 Indian data, 23% of women and 22.1% of men are overweight as per the BMI criterion. The preliminary finding on the status of abdominal obesity reveals that 40% of women and 12% of men are abdominally obese in the country.[4,5]

It is a complex condition that involves metabolic, hormonal, and neural factors. One key neural component implicated in obesity-related health risks is "sympathetic overdrive," a state of heightened activity of the sympathetic nervous system (SNS), which regulates involuntary bodily functions such as heart rate, blood pressure, and energy metabolism.[6]

Sympathetic overdrive refers to an abnormal increase in sympathetic nerve activity (SNA), often measured using muscle sympathetic nerve activity (MSNA), plasma norepinephrine levels, or heart rate variability indices. This heightened sympathetic tone is not merely a marker, but also plays a causal role in the pathophysiology of obesity-related cardiovascular and metabolic diseases.[6,7] SNS overactivation in obesity contributes to increased blood pressure, insulin resistance, and dyslipidemia, which are critical components of metabolic syndrome and major cardiovascular risk factors.

Evidence indicates that obesity and overweight states are consistently associated with increased sympathetic nerve traffic. Grassi et al. conducted a meta-analysis of 45 microneurographic studies involving 1,438 obese or overweight individuals, demonstrating significantly elevated MSNA compared with normal weight controls. This sympathetic overactivity correlates positively with BMI, waist-to-hip ratio, blood pressure, and lipid abnormalities, but not directly with insulin or glucose levels.[7] This suggests that sympathetic overdrive reflects the severity of obesity and its cardiovascular risk profile, independent of glycemic control.

Importantly, sympathetic overdrive is not uniform across all metabolic conditions. For example, in type 2 diabetes mellitus (T2DM), sympathetic activation is significantly increased, whereas in T1DM, sympathetic activity is comparable to that in healthy controls.[6] This distinction underscores the interplay between insulin resistance, hyperinsulinemia, and sympathetic regulation. In T2DM, plasma insulin levels are strongly correlated with SNA, suggesting that hyperinsulinemia may drive

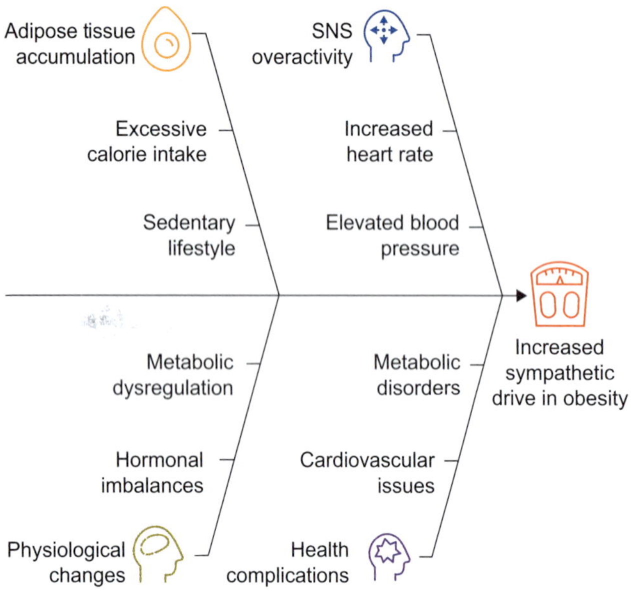

Fig. 1: Causes of increased sympathetic drive in obesity.

sympathetic overactivation, which in turn exacerbates the cardiovascular risk.[6]

Figure 1 summarizes the multifactorial contributors to heightened SNS activity in individuals with obesity. Key upstream factors include adipose tissue accumulation, excessive caloric intake, sedentary lifestyle, metabolic dysregulation, hormonal imbalances, and physiological changes. These pathophysiological mechanisms culminate in SNS overactivity, increased heart rate, and elevated blood pressure, further causing metabolic disorders, cardiovascular issues, and health complications.

Obstructive sleep apnea (OSA), a condition highly prevalent in obese individuals, further amplifies sympathetic overdrive through intermittent hypoxia and sleep fragmentation. These events activate peripheral chemoreflexes, resulting in persistent sympathetic excitation that contributes to hypertension and metabolic dysfunction.[8-10] OSA-related sympathetic activation is a critical mediator linking obesity to cardiovascular morbidity. The SNS's role in OSA is supported by evidence that treatment with continuous positive airway pressure (CPAP) reduces sympathetic activity and improves blood pressure control.[8,9]

At the molecular level, intermittent hypoxia triggers oxidative stress, inflammation, and activation of hypoxia-inducible factors, which collectively promote sympathetic excitation and metabolic derangements.[8] These mechanisms contribute to endothelial dysfunction, insulin resistance, and lipid abnormalities, thereby increasing cardiovascular risk.

Adipose tissue-derived hormones, particularly leptin, further integrate obesity and sympathetic overdrive. Leptin levels increase proportionally with adiposity and stimulate SNS, promoting hypertension and vascular dysfunction. Notably, sex differences exist; leptin-induced sympathetic activation and hypertension are more pronounced in males, whereas in females, leptin stimulates aldosterone production, contributing to hypertension via mineralocorticoid receptor activation. This sexual dimorphism in sympathetic regulation highlights the complexity of obesity-related cardiovascular risks.[11,12]

PATHOPHYSIOLOGY

There are multiple neurohumoral mechanisms by which obesity can activate the SNS. Neural mechanisms include direct activation of the SNA in response to activation of higher cerebral centers by hunger or feeding, and renal afferent nerve activation mediated by perirenal fat accumulation and kidney compression.

Autonomic Nervous System Dysregulation

In healthy persons, the sympathetic and parasympathetic systems operate in balance to regulate blood pressure, energy expenditure, and overall metabolic homeostasis. Obesity disrupts this equilibrium, producing a characteristic pattern of autonomic dysfunction marked by *reduced parasympathetic (vagal) tone and heightened SNS activity*. The loss of vagal modulation weakens gut-brain signaling, blunts satiety responses, and promotes excessive food intake. At the same time, impaired baroreflex sensitivity and exaggerated chemoreflex activity further shift baseline autonomic control toward sympathetic dominance.[13]

Importantly, this autonomic imbalance is *regionally selective rather than generalized*. Sympathetic activity is particularly elevated in the kidneys and skeletal muscle vasculature, where it drives sodium retention, vascular resistance, and elevations in blood pressure. In contrast, cardiac sympathetic tone often remains unchanged or even suppressed, reflecting a redistribution of sympathetic output rather than uniform overactivity. This selective pattern is central to the cardiovascular complications of obesity.[14]

A key mediator of this process is *leptin*. In the obese state, chronic hyperleptinemia is accompanied by *selective leptin resistance*. While leptin's normal anorectic and thermogenic effects are blunted, its sympathoexcitatory actions—especially on renal nerves—remain intact. The consequence is sustained renal sympathetic activation, persistent sodium retention, and the development of hypertension. OSA, common in obesity, further exacerbates sympathetic overactivity. Recurrent hypoxia activates peripheral chemoreceptors, producing chronic sympathetic excitation that extends into the daytime and aggravates blood pressure dysregulation.[15]

Taken together, autonomic dysregulation in obesity represents a maladaptive state. Sympathetic overdrive contributes directly to hypertension and cardiovascular risk, yet fails to enhance energy expenditure because thermogenic pathways remain resistant. This paradoxical pattern sustains weight gain while simultaneously accelerating cardiometabolic complications.[16]

Hypothalamic Regulation, Leptin Resistance, and Adrenergic Activation

Leptin, secreted by adipocytes in proportion to fat mass, normally acts on the hypothalamic arcuate nucleus (ARC) to regulate appetite and energy expenditure. Its binding to long-form leptin receptors (ObRb) activates proopiomelanocortin (POMC) neurons, leading to stimulation of melanocortin-4 receptors (MC4R) in downstream autonomic centers, which increases SNA in various organs, particularly the kidney and brown adipose tissue.[11]

Under normal physiology, leptin reduces appetite and increases energy expenditure by stimulating sympathetic outflow to brown adipose tissue. However, in obesity, circulating leptin levels are persistently elevated due to increased fat mass. Despite this hyperleptinemia, obese individuals often exhibit *selective leptin resistance*—the metabolic actions of leptin (such as appetite suppression and thermogenesis) are blunted, yet its ability to activate sympathetic nerves, particularly those innervating the kidney, remains intact.[17]

This *differential leptin signaling* explains the paradox: While obesity persists because leptin fails to regulate energy balance, sympathetic excitation of the renal system continues, driving sodium retention, increased arterial pressure, and ultimately *hypertension.*[18]

Animal studies (diet-induced obese rabbits, Bardet–Biedl syndrome mouse models) and human data demonstrate that the renal sympathetic nerves are particularly susceptible to leptin-mediated overdrive. Renal denervation experiments further confirm the kidney's central role in obesity-induced hypertension.[19]

At the molecular level, the resistance to leptin in obesity appears to be region-specific within the brain. For example, the *ARC* becomes resistant due to impaired leptin receptor signaling and increased expression of SOCS3 (suppressor of cytokine signaling 3). In contrast, other hypothalamic and brainstem regions that regulate cardiovascular function remain leptin sensitive, allowing continued sympathetic activation.[20]

Role of Insulin Resistance, Inflammation, and Adipokine Imbalance

Hyperinsulinemia, a hallmark of insulin resistance, further increases the central sympathetic drive, augmenting vascular resistance and sodium retention.[21] Insulin may also impair the baroreflex sensitivity, thereby reducing the ability to modulate blood pressure fluctuations.

The adipokine profile in obesity favors sympathetic overactivity. Elevated leptin maintains SNS activation, whereas reduced adiponectin removes vasodilatory and insulin-sensitizing effects.[22] Low-grade inflammation, driven by increased tumor necrosis factor-α (TNF-α) and interleukin-6 (IL-6) from adipose tissue, can also activate hypothalamic pathways that enhance sympathetic discharge.[22]

Interactions between the SNS and renin–angiotensin–aldosterone system (RAAS) further sustain hypertension. Adipose tissue expresses RAAS components that contribute to both systemic and local angiotensin II and aldosterone production.[21] These hormones not only cause vasoconstriction and sodium retention but also stimulate central sympathetic outflow. Endothelin-1, another vasoconstrictor that is elevated in obesity, adds to the pressor load.[21] Obesity-related sympathetic overdrive results from the interplay of preserved hypothalamic leptin–MC4R signaling, insulin resistance, dysregulated adipokines, chronic inflammation, and RAAS activation, forming a sustained neurohumoral stimulus for hypertension and metabolic dysfunction.[21]

Sleep Disorders (Obstructive Sleep Apnea)

Obstructive sleep apnea is highly prevalent in individuals with obesity and represents a potent, independent driver of SNS activation. The condition is characterized by recurrent upper airway collapse during sleep, leading to intermittent hypoxia, hypercapnia, repeated arousals, and marked intrathoracic pressure swings. These physiological stressors stimulate peripheral chemoreceptors, which in turn augment central sympathetic outflow. Importantly, this sympathetic activation is not limited to sleep but frequently persists during the daytime, resulting in sustained elevations of SNS tone that contribute to resistant hypertension. Beyond neural effects, OSA promotes oxidative stress, systemic inflammation, and endothelial dysfunction, all of which accelerate vascular remodeling and compound the cardiovascular burden of obesity.[23]

Renal Mechanisms and the Renin–Angiotensin–Aldosterone System

The kidneys play a pivotal role in the pathogenesis of obesity-induced hypertension. Elevated renal sympathetic traffic increases sodium and water reabsorption, reduces renal blood flow, and stimulates renin release. This activates the RAAS, further enhancing vasoconstriction and fluid retention. Over time, these changes blunt the renal pressure natriuresis relationship, such that normal blood pressure levels require chronically higher sympathetic activity. Thus, the kidney is both a target and an amplifier of sympathetic overdrive.[24]

Gut Hormone Dysregulation

Obesity is also characterized by impaired secretion of key gut hormones involved in appetite and autonomic regulation. Normally, cholecystokinin (CCK), peptide YY (PYY), and glucagon-like peptide-1 (GLP-1) promote satiety and vagal activity, while ghrelin stimulates hunger and is suppressed after meals. In obesity, PYY and GLP-1 levels are reduced, ghrelin suppression is blunted, and vagal responses are impaired. These abnormalities sustain hyperphagia and diminish vagal modulation of SNS tone. Thus, gut-brain axis dysfunction indirectly contributes to sympathetic overdrive and weight gain.[25]

MANAGEMENT

Incretins

Incretin hormones, particularly GLP-1 and GIP, are gut-derived peptides released in response to nutrient intake that regulate satiety, insulin secretion, and glucose metabolism. Beyond their metabolic actions, incretin-based therapies improve autonomic balance in obesity by reducing SNS activity and enhancing parasympathetic tone. GLP-1 receptor agonists slow gastric emptying, suppress appetite via hypothalamic pathways, and improve baroreflex sensitivity, thereby attenuating renal sympathetic drive and lowering blood pressure. Similarly, GIP, through central and pancreatic effects, supports insulin secretion and may contribute to restoring autonomic stability. Together, incretin therapies not only promote weight loss and glycemic control but also counteract *sympathetic overdrive,* reducing cardiometabolic risk in obesity.[26]

Large cardiovascular outcome trials have demonstrated that incretin-based therapies not only attenuate sympathetic overdrive but also reduce major adverse clinical events. In the *SELECT trial,* semaglutide significantly lowered the composite incidence of cardiovascular death, nonfatal myocardial infarction, and nonfatal stroke compared with placebo in individuals with overweight or obesity.[27] Similarly, the *LEADER trial* showed that liraglutide reduced cardiovascular mortality and major cardiovascular events in high-risk patients with type 2 diabetes over a follow-up of nearly 4 years.[28] More recently, the *SUMMIT trial* demonstrated that tirzepatide, a dual GLP-1 and GIP receptor agonist, improved outcomes in patients with heart failure and obesity, resulting in a 38% lower risk of hospitalization, treatment intensification, and cardiovascular death at 1 year. Importantly, many of these benefits are linked to improvements in autonomic balance, with reductions in sympathetic activation and enhanced parasympathetic tone, which in turn translate into reduced morbidity and mortality in obese individuals with or without diabetes.[29]

Emerging Therapies in Obesity and Sympathetic Overdrive

In addition to incretin-based therapies, recent advances have identified alternative neuroendocrine pathways involved in the pathogenesis of obesity, offering new therapeutic targets. Among these, the *hypothalamic leptin-melanocortin signaling pathway* is particularly well characterized. Within this system, *POMC neurons* in the *ARC* produce α-melanocyte-stimulating hormone (α-MSH), which acts on the MC4R to suppress appetite and enhance energy expenditure. In contrast, *agouti-related peptide (AgRP)* functions as an inverse agonist of MC4R, antagonizing α-MSH and promoting food intake. Dysregulation of this pathway contributes to impaired satiety and reduced thermogenesis, which also influences autonomic balance. Importantly, many of the emerging therapies targeting these pathways not only promote weight reduction but may also modulate *sympathetic overdrive*, thereby addressing both metabolic and cardiovascular risk in obesity **(Table 1)**.[30]

Melanocortin-4 Receptor Agonists

Setmelanotide, a selective MC4R agonist, has been approved by the FDA for the chronic management of hypothalamic obesity resulting from genetic deficiencies in *POMC, PCSK1*, or *LEPR*. In a phase II clinical trial (NCT04725240), the drug was evaluated in 18 patients with MRI-confirmed hypothalamic damage and obesity (mean BMI 38 kg/m^2). Participants received escalating doses over 16 weeks, with the primary endpoint defined as achieving at least a 5% reduction in BMI. At study completion, *89% of patients met this endpoint,* with an average BMI reduction of 15%, accompanied by significant improvements in self-reported appetite scores. The most frequently observed

Table 1: List of clinical trials evaluating emerging therapies targeting obesity and sympathetic overdrive.

Drug class	*Intervention (trial)*	*Mean weight loss*	*Common side effects*	*Potential impact on sympathetic overdrive*
GLP-1/GIP/GCGR agonist[31]	Retatrutide, 1–12 mg weekly for 26 weeks (NCT04881760)	~17.5%	Nausea (27%), ↓appetite (18%), diarrhea (13%), vomiting (10%), constipation (9%)	Potent weight loss with improvements in glucose metabolism; expected to reduce renal sympathetic activation and blood pressure similar to GLP-1 analogs
Melanocortin-4 receptor agonist[32]	Setmelanotide, 1–3 mg daily for 16 weeks (NCT04725240)	~15% BMI reduction	Nausea (61%), vomiting (33%), skin hyperpigmentation (33%), diarrhea (22%), abdominal pain (17%)	Directly targets leptin–melanocortin pathway; by restoring satiety signaling, it may normalize hypothalamic control of autonomic output and attenuate sympathetic overdrive
Nonpeptide oral GLP-1 receptor agonist[33]	Orforglipron, 12–45 mg daily for 26 weeks (NCT05051579)	~12.6%	Nausea (42%), vomiting (29%), constipation (19%), diarrhea (16%), GERD (13%)	Oral GLP-1 agonist may improve accessibility; similar to injectables, reduces sympathetic tone via improved baroreflex function and satiety regulation
Long-acting amylin receptor agonist[34]	Cagrilintide, 0.3–4.5 mg weekly for 26 weeks (NCT03856047)	~10.8%	Nausea (47%), constipation (21%), fatigue (20%), injection-site erythema (17%), vomiting (8%)	Enhances satiety and delays gastric emptying; indirectly reduces sympathetic activity linked to overeating and weight gain
Activin receptor type 2B monoclonal antibody[35]	Bimagrumab, 10 mg/kg every 4 weeks for 48 weeks (NCT03005288)	~6.5%	Diarrhea (41%), muscle spasms (41%), nausea (11%), lipase elevation (11%), hypertension (8%)	Promotes lean mass preservation while reducing fat mass; may improve metabolic efficiency and lower sympathetic drive associated with visceral adiposity

side effects included nausea, vomiting, diarrhea, and skin hyperpigmentation.[32]

Beyond weight reduction, MC4R agonism also impacts autonomic regulation. The melanocortin system plays a central role in hypothalamic control of energy expenditure and sympathetic outflow. By restoring satiety signaling and reactivating melanocortin pathways, setmelanotide may *normalize hypothalamic-autonomic circuits,* potentially mitigating obesity-associated *sympathetic overdrive* and its downstream cardiovascular risks.[32]

Triple Receptor Agonists

Recent preclinical and clinical studies highlight the therapeutic potential of *triple receptor agonists,* which simultaneously target the *glucagon receptor (GcGR), glucose-dependent insulinotropic polypeptide (GIP) receptor*, and *GLP-1 receptor*. Activation of the GcGR enhances energy expenditure and stimulates nonshivering thermogenesis through the cyclic AMP (cAMP) pathway in brown adipose tissue. GIP receptor agonism, particularly in combination with GLP-1 receptor activation, prevents weight gain, augments leptin-mediated appetite suppression, and reduces food intake via hypothalamic signaling.[36]

The investigational triagonist *retatrutide* was evaluated in a phase II randomized placebo-controlled trial (NCT04881760) involving 338 adults with obesity (mean BMI 37.3 kg/m^2). After 24 weeks, patients receiving retatrutide achieved a mean weight loss of 17.5% at the highest dose (12 mg) and 7.2% at the lowest dose (1 mg), compared with only 1.2% in the placebo group. Secondary outcomes included improvements in cardiometabolic risk markers such as reversal of prediabetes, reductions in blood pressure and LDL cholesterol, and decreased need for antihypertensive therapy.[31]

In addition to profound metabolic benefits, triple receptor agonists are expected to influence autonomic regulation. By reducing adiposity, improving leptin sensitivity, and enhancing hypothalamic signaling, retatrutide may alleviate obesity-related sympathetic overdrive, leading to improved blood pressure control and reduced cardiovascular burden.

Tirzepatide, a once-weekly dual GIP/GLP-1 receptor agonist, produces marked, dose-dependent weight loss in adults with obesity. In the 72-week SURMOUNT-1 trial (n = 2,539, BMI ≥30 kg/m^2 or ≥27 kg/m^2 with comorbidity, no diabetes), mean reductions from baseline (–3.1% placebo) were –15.0, –19.5, and –20.9% with 5, 10, and 15 mg, respectively; 91, 96, and 96% achieved ≥5% loss, while 55,

69, and 78% lost ≥10%; and 27, 45, and 57% lost ≥20%.[37,38] Comparable gradients were observed in SURMOUNT-2 (T2D, BMI ≥27 kg/m^2): -12.8, -14.7, and -13.0% versus -3.2% placebo at 72 weeks, with 33–51% attaining ≥15% loss.[37] Pooled dose-stratified meta-analyses (26–72 weeks, 9,800 participants) confirm mean relative weight losses of 15–21% at the 10–15 mg range, exceeding semaglutide 2.4 mg by ≈6.5% points in head-to-head SURMOUNT-5 (-20.2 vs. -13.7%, $p < 0.001$).[39] Responder analyses show 55–78% achieve ≥10% and 25–35% ≥15% loss across populations; number-needed-to-treat for ≥10% reduction is 1.6–1.8 versus placebo.[40,41]

Weight loss is maintained only with continued therapy. SURMOUNT-4's randomized withdrawal phase demonstrated that switching to placebo after 36 weeks of open-label 15 mg induced rapid regain (≈0.3% week^{-1}), producing a 19.4% difference in mean weight change by week 88 versus participants who continued tirzepatide (-5.5 vs. -24.9%, $p < 0.001$). This establishes tirzepatide as a chronic, not short-course, pharmacologic strategy requiring escalation to the maximal tolerated dose (commonly 10–15 mg) and indefinite treatment for sustained effect.[42]

Adverse events are chiefly gastrointestinal, dose-related, and concentrated during titration: Nausea 17–31%, diarrhea 15–23%, and vomiting 6–13% with 10–15 mg, leading to discontinuation rates of 4–7 versus 1% placebo.[37] Pooled RCT data (up to 3 years) do not show a statistically significant increase in acute pancreatitis versus placebo (0.2–0.4%); however, composite biliary events (cholelithiasis, cholecystitis) are modestly elevated (HR ≈1.3, 95% CI 1.0–1.7), mandating surveillance in high-risk individuals.[37,43] Cardiometabolic safety is favorable with no excess MACE signal and possible numeric benefit, but definitive cardiovascular outcome trials are ongoing.[44]

Nonpeptide Glucagon-like Peptide-1 Receptor Agonists

The *GLP-1 receptor* is a G-protein-coupled receptor that mediates its metabolic effects primarily through the cAMP signaling pathway. However, receptor activation also triggers β-arrestin recruitment, which promotes receptor internalization and desensitization, thereby limiting its therapeutic efficacy. Novel *nonpeptide GLP-1 receptor agonists* have been developed to preferentially activate the cAMP pathway while minimizing β-arrestin signaling. This mechanism prolongs receptor sensitivity and enhances the durability of GLP-1-mediated actions on satiety, glucose regulation, and weight loss.[45]

Orforglipron is the first oral nonpeptide GLP-1 receptor agonist evaluated in a phase II placebo-controlled trial (NCT05051579) involving 235 adults with obesity (mean BMI 37.9 kg/m^2). Over 36 weeks of treatment, the primary endpoint of weight reduction at 26 weeks was achieved, with participants experiencing *8.6–12.6% weight loss,* depending on dose, compared with minimal change in the placebo group.[33]

Beyond its weight-reducing effects, orforglipron has potential implications for *sympathetic overdrive.* By reducing adiposity, improving satiety signaling, and enhancing baroreflex sensitivity, this agent may indirectly attenuate sympathetic activation, supporting cardiovascular protection in obese individuals.

Amylin Receptor Agonists

Amylin is a peptide hormone cosecreted with insulin from pancreatic β-cells in response to nutrient intake. Acting through receptors in the brainstem and hypothalamus, amylin promotes satiety, delays gastric emptying, suppresses glucagon secretion, and enhances energy expenditure, thereby contributing to postprandial glucose control and weight regulation.[46]

Pramlintide, a short-acting amylin analog, is currently used as an adjunct in types 1 and 2 diabetes to improve postprandial glycemic control and facilitate modest weight loss.[47]

Cagrilintide, a next-generation long-acting amylin receptor agonist, was evaluated in a phase II trial (NCT03856047) involving 703 patients with obesity (mean baseline BMI 37.8 kg/m^2). Participants received weekly escalating doses (0.3–4.5 mg) of cagrilintide, or daily liraglutide (0.6–3 mg), for 26 weeks. The primary endpoint, percentage weight reduction, showed that the cagrilintide group achieved *6.0–10.8% weight loss,* compared with *9.0% in the liraglutide group and 3.0% with placebo.*[34] Beyond weight reduction, amylin receptor agonists may also influence autonomic function. By enhancing satiety signaling and reducing postprandial metabolic load, these agents could indirectly *lower sympathetic drive,* contributing to improved cardiovascular and metabolic outcomes in obesity.

Activin Type 2 Receptor Monoclonal Antibody

The *activin type 2 receptor (ActRII)* is a regulator of skeletal muscle growth and brown adipose tissue metabolism. Preclinical studies demonstrated that inhibiting this receptor improves insulin sensitivity and lowers the risk of metabolic dysfunction-associated steatotic liver disease. These findings were extended to humans, where administration of *bimagrumab,* a monoclonal antibody against ActRII, produced favorable metabolic effects.[35,48]

In a phase II placebo-controlled trial (NCT03005288) including 75 participants with obesity (mean BMI 32.9 kg/m^2, average fat mass 34.7 kg), patients received bimagrumab or placebo every 4 weeks for 48 weeks. At study completion, the bimagrumab group achieved a 20.1% reduction in body fat mass, accompanied by a 3.6% gain in lean mass, 9.0 cm reduction in waist circumference, and 6.5% decrease in body weight.[35] Beyond these metabolic improvements, ActRII blockade may also indirectly modulate sympathetic overdrive. By reducing visceral adiposity, enhancing muscle mass, and improving metabolic efficiency, bimagrumab could help rebalance autonomic function, thereby lowering sympathetic activation and mitigating cardiovascular risk in obesity.[48]

Renal Sympathetic Denervation and Obesity-associated Sympathetic Overdrive

Obesity is strongly associated with heightened renal SNA, which contributes to sodium retention, impaired pressure natriuresis, and the development of resistant hypertension. Excessive sympathetic drive in obesity is further amplified by mechanisms such as leptin resistance, baroreflex impairment, and OSA, all of which disproportionately elevate renal sympathetic outflow compared to other vascular territories. This selective renal activation is a central link between obesity, hypertension, and cardiovascular risk.[18]

Renal sympathetic denervation (RDN), a minimally invasive catheter-based therapy, directly disrupts efferent and afferent sympathetic fibers along the renal arteries. By doing so, RDN attenuates renal norepinephrine spillover, reduces sodium reabsorption, and improves blood pressure regulation. Importantly, modern sham-controlled trials and registry studies have demonstrated that RDN produces sustained reductions in blood pressure across diverse patient groups, including those with resistant hypertension—a phenotype commonly associated with obesity.[49,50]

In the context of obesity with sympathetic overdrive, RDN represents a promising adjunctive strategy. By selectively reducing renal sympathetic tone, it may not only improve blood pressure control but also mitigate obesity-related cardiometabolic complications, such as left ventricular hypertrophy, vascular remodeling, and progression of chronic kidney disease. As such, RDN provides a mechanistically targeted intervention that addresses one of the core autonomic disturbances driving obesity-related cardiovascular morbidity.

CONCLUSION

Obesity with sympathetic overdrive represents a maladaptive state where excess adiposity drives autonomic imbalance, fueling hypertension, insulin resistance, and cardiovascular risk. Modern management now extends beyond weight loss alone to specifically target this dysregulation. Incretin-based therapies, novel receptor agonists, and emerging biologics show dual benefits in reducing weight and attenuating sympathetic drive, while device-based approaches like renal denervation provide nonpharmacological options for resistant hypertension. Together, these strategies highlight a paradigm shift in obesity care addressing both metabolic burden and autonomic dysfunction to reduce morbidity and mortality.

REFERENCES

1. Madhu SV, Nitin K, Sambit D, et al. ESI clinical practice guidelines for the evaluation and management of obesity in India. Indian J Endocrinol Metab. 2022;26(4):295-318.
2. Global Burden of Disease 2019 Cancer Collaboration, Kocarnik JM, Compton K, et al. Cancer incidence, mortality, years of life lost, years lived with disability, and disability-adjusted life years for 29 cancer groups from 2010 to 2019: a systematic analysis for the Global Burden of Disease Study 2019. JAMA Oncol. 2022;8(3):420-44.
3. Sadali UB, Kamal KKBN, Park J, et al. The global prevalence of overweight and obesity among nurses: a systematic review and meta-analyses. J Clin Nurs. 2023;32(23-24):7934-55.
4. National Family Health Survey. National Family Health Survey (NFHS-5)- 2019-21. [online] Available from https://www.nfhsiips.in/nfhsuser/nfhs5.php. [Last accessed January, 2026].
5. Tripathi S, Pathak VK, Lahariya C. Key findings from NFHS-5 India report: observing trends of health indicators between NFHS-4 and NFHS 5. J Fam Med Prim Care. 2023;12(9):1759-63.
6. Grassi G, Biffi A, Dell'Oro R, et al. Sympathetic neural abnormalities in type 1 and type 2 diabetes: a systematic review and meta-analysis. J Hypertens. 2020;38(8):1436-42.
7. Grassi G, Biffi A, Seravalle G, et al. Sympathetic neural overdrive in the obese and overweight state. Hypertension. 2019;74(2):349-58.
8. Arnaud C, Bochaton T, Pépin JL, et al. Obstructive sleep apnoea and cardiovascular consequences: pathophysiological mechanisms. Arch Cardiovasc Dis. 2020;113(5):350-8.
9. Seravalle G, Grassi G. Sleep apnea and hypertension. High Blood Press Cardiovasc Prev. 2022;29(1):23-31.
10. Mansukhani MP, Kara T, Caples SM, et al. Chemoreflexes, sleep apnea, and sympathetic dysregulation. Curr Hypertens Rep. 2014;16(9):476.

11. Rahmouni K. Leptin-induced sympathetic nerve activation: signaling mechanisms and cardiovascular consequences in obesity. Curr Hypertens Rev. 2010;6(2):104-9.
12. Rahmouni K. Obesity, sympathetic overdrive and hypertension: the leptin connection. Hypertension. 2010; 55(4):844-5.
13. Messina G, De Luca V, Viggiano A, et al. Autonomic nervous system in the control of energy balance and body weight: personal contributions. Neurol Res Int. 2013;2013:639280.
14. Borovac JA, D'Amario D, Bozic J, et al. Sympathetic nervous system activation and heart failure: current state of evidence and the pathophysiology in the light of novel biomarkers. World J Cardiol. 2020;12(8):373-408.
15. Bell BB, Rahmouni K. Leptin as a mediator of obesity-induced hypertension. Curr Obes Rep. 2016;5(4):397-404.
16. Kalil GZ, Haynes WG. Sympathetic nervous system in obesity-related hypertension: mechanisms and clinical implications. Hypertens Res. 2012;35(1):4-16.
17. Obradovic M, Sudar-Milovanovic E, Soskic S, et al. Leptin and obesity: role and clinical implication. Front Endocrinol. 2021;12:585887.
18. Hall JE, Hildebrandt DA, Kuo J. Obesity hypertension: role of leptin and sympathetic nervous system. Am J Hypertens. 2001;14(6 Pt 2):103S-15S.
19. Rahmouni K, Fath MA, Seo S, et al. Leptin resistance contributes to obesity and hypertension in mouse models of Bardet-Biedl syndrome. J Clin Invest. 2008;118(4):1458-67.
20. Asgari R, Caceres-Valdiviezo M, Wu S, et al. Regulation of energy balance by leptin as an adiposity signal and modulator of the reward system. Mol Metab. 2025;91: 102078.
21. Chrysant SG. Pathophysiology and treatment of obesity-related hypertension. J Clin Hypertens. 2019;21(5):555-9.
22. Guarino D, Nannipieri M, Iervasi G, et al. The role of the autonomic nervous system in the pathophysiology of obesity. Front Physiol. 2017;8:665.
23. Van Eyck A, Van Hoorenbeeck K, De Winter BY, et al. Sleep disordered breathing and autonomic function in overweight and obese children and adolescents. ERJ Open Res. 2016;2(4):00038-2016.
24. DeMarco VG, Aroor AR, Sowers JR. The pathophysiology of hypertension in patients with obesity. Nat Rev Endocrinol. 2014;10(6):364-76.
25. Lean MEJ, Malkova D. Altered gut and adipose tissue hormones in overweight and obese individuals: cause or consequence? Int J Obes (Lond). 2016;40(4):622-32.
26. Nauck MA, Meier JJ. Incretin hormones: their role in health and disease. Diabetes Obes Metab. 2018;20 Suppl 1:5-21.
27. Deanfield J, Lincoff AM, Kahn SE, et al. Semaglutide and cardiovascular outcomes by baseline and changes in adiposity measurements: a prespecified analysis of the SELECT trial. Lancet. 2025;406(10516):2257-68.
28. Marso SP, Baeres FMM, Bain SC, et al. Effects of liraglutide on cardiovascular outcomes in patients with diabetes with or without heart failure. J Am Coll Cardiol. 2020;75(10):1128-41.
29. American College of Cardiology [Internet]. A Study of Tirzepatide (LY3298176) in Participants With Heart Failure With Preserved Ejection Fraction (HFpEF) and Obesity. [online] Available from https://www.acc.org/latest-in-cardiology/clinical-trials/2024/11/15/15/13/http%3a%2f%2fwww.acc.org%2flatest-in-cardiology%2fclinical-trials%2f2024%2f11%2f15%2f15%2f13%2fsummit. [Last accessed November, 2025].
30. Wen X, Zhang B, Wu B, et al. Signaling pathways in obesity: mechanisms and therapeutic interventions. Signal Transduct Target Ther. 2022;7:298.
31. Jastreboff AM, Kaplan LM, Frías JP, et al. Triple-hormone-receptor agonist retatrutide for obesity—a phase 2 trial. N Engl J Med. 2023;389(6):514-26.
32. Roth CL, Scimia C, Shoemaker AH, et al. Setmelanotide for the treatment of acquired hypothalamic obesity: a phase 2, open-label, multicentre trial. Lancet Diabetes Endocrinol. 2024;12(6):380-9.
33. Eli Lilly and Company. (2023). A Phase 2 Study of Once-Daily LY3502970 Compared With Placebo in Participants Who Have Obesity or Are Overweight With Weight-Related Comorbidities. [online] Available from https://clinicaltrials.gov/study/NCT05051579. [Last accessed January, 2026].
34. Lau DCW, Erichsen L, Francisco AM, et al. Once-weekly cagrilintide for weight management in people with overweight and obesity: a multicentre, randomised, double-blind, placebo-controlled and active-controlled, dose-finding phase 2 trial. Lancet Lond Engl. 2021;398 (10317):2160-72.
35. Heymsfield SB, Coleman LA, Miller R, et al. Effect of bimagrumab vs placebo on body fat mass among adults with type 2 diabetes and obesity: a phase 2 randomized clinical trial. JAMA Netw Open. 2021;4(1):e2033457.
36. Wen J, Nadora D, Truong A, et al. Next generation dual GLP-1/GIP, GLP-1/glucagon, and triple GLP-1/GIP/glucagon agonists: a literature review. Nutr Metab Cardiovasc Dis. 2025;35(12):104213.
37. Jastreboff AM, Aronne LJ, Ahmad NN, et al. Tirzepatide once weekly for the treatment of obesity. N Engl J Med. 2022;387(3):205-16.
38. Garvey WT, Batterham RL, Bhatta M, et al. Two-year effects of semaglutide in adults with overweight or obesity: the STEP 5 trial. Nat Med. 2022;28(10):2083-91.
39. Aronne LJ, Horn DB, le Roux CW, et al. Tirzepatide as compared with semaglutide for the treatment of obesity. N Engl J Med. 2025;393(1):26-36.
40. Tan B, Pan XH, Chew HSJ, et al. Efficacy and safety of tirzepatide for treatment of overweight or obesity. A systematic review and meta-analysis. Int J Obes (Lond). 2023;47(8):677-85.
41. Lin F, Yu B, Ling B, et al. Weight loss efficiency and safety of tirzepatide: a systematic review. PloS One. 2023;18(5): e0285197.
42. Aronne LJ, Sattar N, Horn DB, et al. Continued treatment with tirzepatide for maintenance of weight reduction in adults with obesity: the SURMOUNT-4 randomized clinical trial. JAMA. 2024;331(1):38-48.

43. Zeng Q, Xu J, Mu X, et al. Safety issues of tirzepatide (pancreatitis and gallbladder or biliary disease) in type 2 diabetes and obesity: a systematic review and meta-analysis. Front Endocrinol. 2023;14:1214334.
44. Nauck MA, D'Alessio DA. Tirzepatide, a dual GIP/GLP-1 receptor co-agonist for the treatment of type 2 diabetes with unmatched effectiveness regrading glycaemic control and body weight reduction. Cardiovasc Diabetol. 2022;21(1):169.
45. Sonoda N, Imamura T, Yoshizaki T, et al. β-Arrestin-1 mediates glucagon-like peptide-1 signaling to insulin secretion in cultured pancreatic β cells. Proc Natl Acad Sci USA. 2008;105(18):6614-9.
46. Mietlicki-Baase EG. Amylin-mediated control of glycemia, energy balance, and cognition. Physiol Behav. 2016;162: 130-40.
47. Ryan G, Briscoe TA, Jobe L. Review of pramlintide as adjunctive therapy in treatment of type 1 and type 2 diabetes. Drug Des Devel Ther. 2009;2:203-14.
48. Nunn E, Jaiswal N, Gavin M, et al. Antibody blockade of activin type II receptors preserves skeletal muscle mass and enhances fat loss during GLP-1 receptor agonism. Mol Metab. 2024;80:101880.
49. Bangalore S, Maqsood MH, Bakris GL, et al. Renal denervation—radiofrequency vs. ultrasound: insights from a mixed treatment comparison meta-analysis of randomized sham controlled trials. J Hypertens. 2025;43(2):325-35.
50. Kumar D, Loshak H. (2022). Renal Denervation for People With Hypertension: CADTH Horizon Scan. [online] Available from http://www.ncbi.nlm.nih.gov/books/NBK595358/. [Last accessed January, 2026].

41

CHAPTER

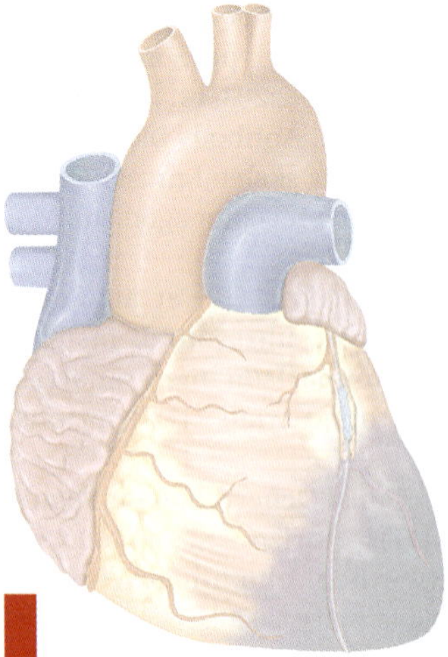

Outcome Data in Obesity Patients with Arrhythmias: Is it Different?

Harinder K Bali, Navdeep S Sidhu

INTRODUCTION

Obesity, often underappreciated in the past, has been an area of rigorous scientific research in the recent decades, with a growing realization of it being a metabolically active organ and its association with adverse outcomes such as decreased exercise capacity, poor quality of life, and curtailed longevity.[1] It is characterized by excessive and/or abnormal adiposity, with or without abnormal fat distribution or function. Obesity is traditionally defined in terms of body mass index (BMI); with age, sex, and ethnicity specific cut-offs (e.g., for adults WHO guidelines: BMI 25–29.9 kg/m^2 overweight/preobesity, BMI ≥30 kg/m^2 obesity; Indian Guidelines: BMI 23–24.9 kg/m^2 overweight, BMI ≥25 kg/m^2 obesity).[2,3] However, in the light of newer evidence, there has been increased stress in updated guidelines[4,5] on combining BMI with other anthropometric measures such as waist circumference, waist-hip ratio, and waist-height ratio to better detect adiposity/obesity and for better assessment of cardiovascular (CV) risk.

OBESITY AND CARDIOVASCULAR DISEASE

While obesity has a negative impact on the health of various body organs and is a risk factor for many diseases including chronic kidney disease and cancer; nearly two-thirds of obesity-related deaths are due to cardiovascular disease (CVD).[6] Obesity contributes to increased disease burden of CVD not only through fostering the development of CV risk factors [insulin resistance/type 2 diabetes mellitus (T2DM), arterial hypertension, dyslipidemia, obstructive sleep apnea (OSA)] but also through direct deleterious effects on CV structure and function independent of other risk factors. The major CVDs related to obesity include atherosclerotic cardiovascular disease (ASCVD), heart failure, venous thromboembolism (VTE), arrhythmias (especially atrial fibrillation [AF], sudden cardiac death [SCD]), and valvular heart disease (particularly aortic valvular stenosis).[7,8] In this chapter, we intend to discuss the relationship between obesity and arrhythmias, with special focus on clinical outcomes of obese patients with arrhythmias.

OBESITY AND ARRHYTHMIAS

Several studies have shown an association between obesity and arrhythmias, with most strong association with AF and SCD.[9-11] Obesity-related ectopic fat deposition, particularly epicardial adipose tissue (EAT), is considered central to the development of structural and electrical remodeling resulting in the genesis of cardiac arrhythmias. Obesity-related CV risk factors (such as hypertension, T2DM, OSA, and dyslipidemia) and the hemodynamic changes [such as increased circulating blood volume, left atrial (LA) dilatation, left ventricular (LV) hypertrophy, and LV diastolic dysfunction] are also thought to play a contributory role **(Flowchart 1)**.[12] The molecular mechanisms of arrhythmogenesis have been postulated to involve lipotoxicity, inflammation, oxidative stress, fibrosis, autonomic imbalance, and ion channel modulation.[13]

Flowchart 1: The genesis of obesity related arrhythmias.[12]

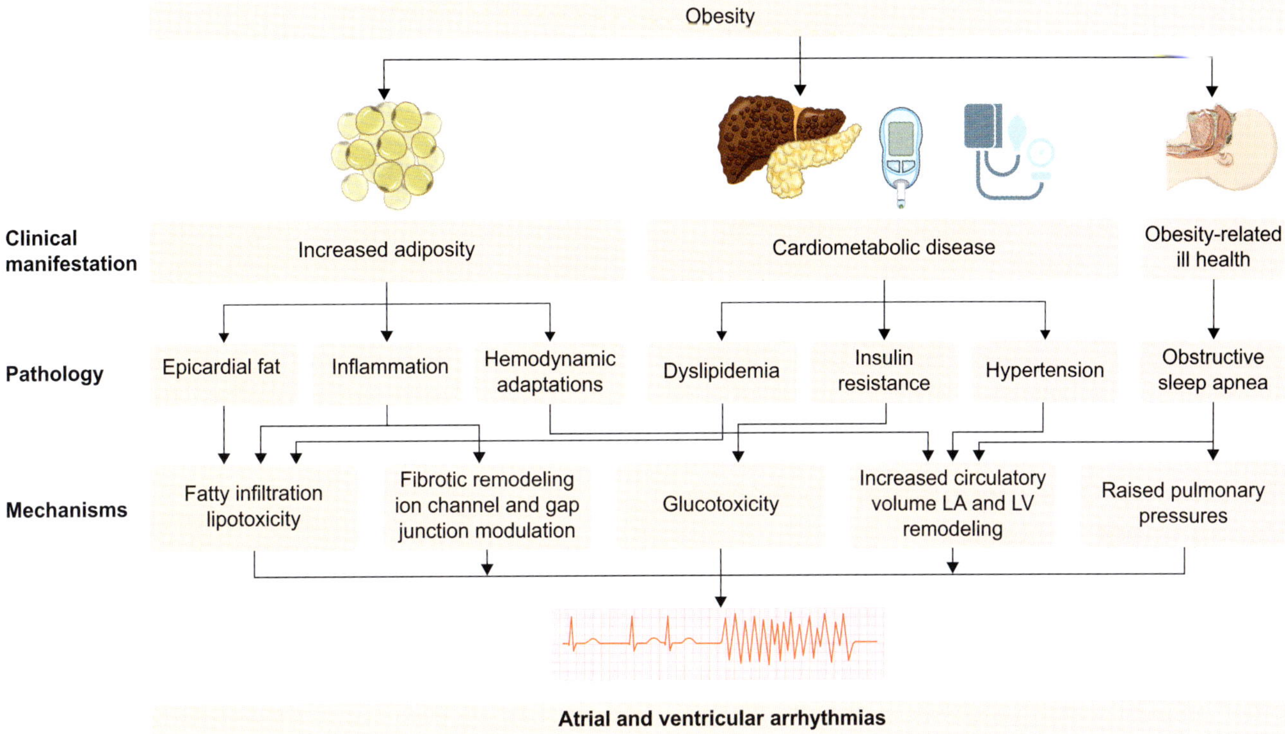

Source: Used original from Patel et al.'s[12] study under Creative Commons CC BY 4.0 license.

OBESITY AND ATRIAL FIBRILLATION

The Framingham Heart Study has shown that obesity increases the risk of new-onset AF by 50%.[13] Similarly, in a large meta-analysis of 51 studies, a 5-unit increase in BMI conferred a 30% increased rate of AF incidence.[10] This dose-response relationship between obesity and incident AF has also been shown for other anthropometric measures of obesity beyond BMI.[11] Obesity has also been linked with a higher risk of progression from paroxysmal to permanent AF in longitudinal cohort studies and this risk persists despite adjustment of other AF risk factors.[15,16] There is ample evidence to suggest that, in obese patients with AF, lifestyle management and weight loss are associated with decreased burden of AF and reversal of cardiac structural and electric remodeling.[13]

Obesity Paradox in Atrial Fibrillation

Studies evaluating the relation between obesity and adverse outcomes in patients with AF have shown mixed results. A post hoc analysis of the AFFIRM study showed that overweight and obese patients had a lower all-cause and CV mortality as compared to normal weight patients, a phenomenon which came to be known as *obesity paradox*.[17] However, this was challenged by a large prospective cohort study by Overvad et al., which showed a higher incidence of composite end point of ischemic stroke, thromboembolism, or death in overweight and obese patients at a median follow-up of 4.9 years.[18] The post hoc analyses of the direct oral anticoagulants (DOACs) trials (ARISTOTLE, ROCKET-AF, ENGAGE-AF TIMI-48) have revealed that obesity is associated with better outcomes (such as stroke, systemic embolism, and mortality).[13,19] Again, these results were countered by the findings of an observational, multicentric, prospective FANTASIIA registry which showed that obesity had no impact on the prognosis,[20] and by a recent meta-analysis of observational data that revealed better outcomes in obese AF patients.[21] Also, a latest meta-analysis by Nteli et al. has shown a J-shaped relation between BMI and AF prognosis in recently hospitalized patients, where a BMI value outside the normal range was associated with poorer prognosis.[22] The discordant data in obese AF patients also extend to the bleeding outcomes. Whereas, in the ENGAGE AF-TIMI 48 trial, the risk of bleeding outcomes was enhanced with increasing BMI values, the data from recent meta-analysis has shown lower rates of major as well as intracranial bleeding in obese patients.[19,21]

The reasons for these conflicting findings in relation to obesity and AF are incompletely understood. Broadly, the post hoc or subgroup analyses from randomized trials are in favor of the obesity paradox, whereas the data from observational/cohort studies are discordant. The possible explanations may include an earlier and generally more rigorous treatment of obese patients with a better tolerance to various medications and the presence of greater metabolic reserve to endure the catabolic stress of cardiac diseases.[13] Statistical flaws such as selection bias/confounders or underpowered analyses may also play a role. It has also been argued that the predominant use of BMI as a measure of obesity may not be ideal in these studies and EAT volume may be a better predictor of AF risk and outcomes.[23]

The Effect of Obesity on Atrial Fibrillation Management Strategies

The management of AF is centered on rate control, rhythm control (pharmacological or catheter ablation), and anticoagulation. Obesity can influence these management strategies by altering the pharmacokinetic and pharmacodynamic properties of drugs (differences in volume of distribution/elimination kinetics, altering the targets like sodium ion channels) and by altering the outcomes after catheter ablation of AF.

- Obesity is associated with a requirement of larger doses of vitamin K antagonists (warfarin) to achieve the desired international normalized ratio (INR) levels and also a longer time to reach the target INR levels. This is partly explained by a positive correlation between plasma vitamin K levels and triglyceride concentrations, which are commonly elevated in the obese patients.[24]
- The pharmacokinetics and pharmacodynamics of DOACs, which are being increasingly used instead of warfarin, are less influenced by body weight and obesity. The current evidence supports the use of standard doses of DOACs in the obese patients. Also, the effectiveness and safety of DOACs in overweight and obese patients have been shown to be equivalent or better than that of warfarin.[13]
- The volume of distribution and CV effects (in terms of heart blood pressure and cardiac output) of β-blockers (propranolol, nebivolol, and labetalol) have not been shown to differ appreciably between the normal-weight and obese individuals, when used in similar doses.[25]
- In a retrospective study of intravenous (IV) diltiazem for rate control in AF, weight-based strategy was shown to be associated with a higher proportion of patients achieving a heart rate of <100 beats per minute.[26]
- Obesity has been shown to be associated with decreased effectiveness of class I antiarrhythmic drugs such as flecainide, but a similar therapeutic response to class III drugs such as amiodarone and sotalol, despite altering the pharmacokinetics of highly lipophilic amiodarone.[13]
- Excess adipose tissue, particularly EAT, is linked with decreased delivery of electrical energy to the heart during electrical cardioversion and lower rates of electrical cardioversion in obese AF patients underscoring the need of using higher electrical energies in this population.[27]
- Obesity has been associated with many negative outcomes during and after AF ablation including higher exposure to ionizing radiation during the procedure, longer hospital stays with more in-hospital complications, higher healthcare costs, and higher rates of AF recurrence with associated need for repeat procedures.[13,28]

OBESITY AND VENTRICULAR ARRHYTHMIAS

There is ample evidence to suggest the association of obesity and ventricular arrhythmias and SCD. Increased weight was associated with an increased risk of SCD during 26 years of follow-up in the Framingham Heart Study, particularly in males.[9] In a large autopsy-based study of 2,661 consecutive victims of SCD from Finland, obesity-related cardiomyopathy was the most common cause of nonischemic SCDs followed by alcoholic cardiomyopathy, hypertensive heart disease, and idiopathic fibrotic cardiomyopathy.[29] In a meta-analysis of 14 prospective studies by Aune et al.,[30] a nonlinear J-shaped association was noted between BMI and SCD with the lowest rates of SCD in normal range weight subgroup. There was a minor increase in SCD in the underweight subgroup, and in the overweight, obese, and severely obese subgroups, the rate of SCD was increased by 14%, 60%, and 2–3 times, respectively.[30]

The postulated mechanisms related to the elevated risk of SCD in obesity are related to the occurrence of adverse structural and electrical remodeling including ventricular hypertrophy, intramyocardial/epicardial adiposity, fibrosis, late potentials, QT prolongation, QRS fragmentation, and premature ventricular complexes.[7]

Severe obesity is associated with reduced chances of successful resuscitation following an in-hospital cardiac arrest;[31] however, in survivors of SCD, there is a suggestion of the obesity paradox, although the results are inconsistent. In a multicentric retrospective cohort study by Sung et al., obesity was associated with worse in-hospital mortality and poorer neurological outcomes in patients resuscitated from cardiogenic arrest.[32] However, another retrospective multihospital study by Matinrazm et al. showed that higher BMI was associated with lower rates of all-cause mortality in SCD survivors.[33]

CONCLUSION

Obesity is associated with numerous adverse CV outcomes including ASCVD, heart failure, VTE, aortic valve disease, and arrhythmias including AF and SCD. Although there is unequivocal evidence for the association of obesity with increased risk of AF and SCD; some authors have proposed the existence of obesity paradox with better outcomes in obese patients with AF and SCD. Nevertheless, the results of existing studies are conflicting and larger, more powered studies are needed to confirm or refute the existence of obesity paradox in arrhythmias.

REFERENCES

1. Rubino F, Puhl RM, Cummings DE, et al. Joint International Consensus Statement for Ending Stigma of Obesity. Nat Med. 2020;26(4):485-97.
2. WHO Expert Consultation. Appropriate body-mass index for Asian populations and its implications for policy and intervention strategies. Lancet. 2004;363(9403):157-63.
3. Misra A, Chowbey P, Makkar BM, et al.; Consensus Group. Consensus statement for diagnosis of obesity, abdominal obesity and the metabolic syndrome for Asian Indians and recommendations for physical activity, medical and surgical management. J Assoc Physicians India. 2009;57:163-70.
4. Rubino F, Cummings DE, Eckel RH, et al. Definition and diagnostic criteria of clinical obesity. Lancet Diabetes Endocrinol. 2025;13(3):221-62.
5. Misra A, Vikram NK, Ghosh A, et al.; India Obesity Commission Members. Revised definition of obesity in Asian Indians living in India. Diabetes Metab Syndr. 2025;19(1):102989.
6. Powell-Wiley TM, Poirier P, Burke LE, et al. Obesity and cardiovascular disease: a scientific statement from the American Heart Association. Circulation. 2021;143(21):e984-1010.
7. Koskinas KC, Van Craenenbroeck EM, Antoniades C, et al.; ESC Scientific Document Group. Obesity and cardiovascular disease: an ESC clinical consensus statement. Eur Heart J. 2024;45(38):4063-98.
8. Savarese G, Schiattarella GG, Lindberg F, et al. Heart failure and obesity: translational approaches and therapeutic perspectives. A scientific statement of the Heart Failure Association of the ESC. Eur J Heart Fail. 2025;27(7):1273-93.
9. Hubert HB, Feinleib M, McNamara PM, et al. Obesity as an independent risk factor for cardiovascular disease: a 26-year follow-up of participants in the Framingham Heart Study. Circulation. 1983;67(5):968-77.
10. Wang TJ, Parise H, Levy D, et al. Obesity and the risk of new-onset atrial fibrillation. JAMA. 2004;292(20):2471-7.
11. Tedrow UB, Conen D, Ridker PM, et al. The long- and short-term impact of elevated body mass index on the risk of new atrial fibrillation the WHS (Women's Health Study). J Am Coll Cardiol. 2010;55(21):2319-27.
12. Patel KHK, Reddy RK, Sau A, et al. Obesity as a risk factor for cardiac arrhythmias. BMJ Med. 2022;1(1):e000308.
13. Sha R, Baines O, Hayes A, et al. Impact of obesity on atrial fibrillation pathogenesis and treatment options. J Am Heart Assoc. 2024;13(1):e032277.
14. Camm CF, Lacey B, Massa MS, et al. Independent effects of adiposity measures on risk of atrial fibrillation in men and women: a study of 0.5 million individuals. Int J Epidemiol. 2022;51(3):984-95.
15. Tsang TS, Barnes ME, Miyasaka Y, et al. Obesity as a risk factor for the progression of paroxysmal to permanent atrial fibrillation: a longitudinal cohort study of 21 years. Eur Heart J. 2008;29(18):2227-33.
16. Thacker EL, McKnight B, Psaty BM, et al. Association of body mass index, diabetes, hypertension, and blood pressure levels with risk of permanent atrial fibrillation. J Gen Intern Med. 2013;28(2):247-53.
17. Badheka AO, Rathod A, Kizilbash MA, et al. Influence of obesity on outcomes in atrial fibrillation: yet another obesity paradox. Am J Med. 2010;123(7):646-51.
18. Overvad TF, Rasmussen LH, Skjøth F, et al. Body mass index and adverse events in patients with incident atrial fibrillation. Am J Med. 2013;126(7):640.e9-17.
19. Boriani G, Ruff CT, Kuder JF, et al. Relationship between body mass index and outcomes in patients with atrial fibrillation treated with edoxaban or warfarin in the ENGAGE AF-TIMI 48 trial. Eur Heart J. 2019;40(19):1541-50.
20. Bertomeu-Gonzalez V, Moreno-Arribas J, Esteve-Pastor MA, et al. FANTASIIA Study Investigators. Association of body mass index with clinical outcomes in patients with atrial fibrillation: a report from the FANTASIIA registry. J Am Heart Assoc. 2020;9(1):e013789.
21. Grymonprez M, Capiau A, De Backer TL, et al. The impact of underweight and obesity on outcomes in anticoagulated patients with atrial fibrillation: a systematic review and meta-analysis on the obesity paradox. Clin Cardiol. 2021;44(5):599-608.
22. Nteli M, Nteli D, Moysidis DV, et al. Prognostic impact of body mass index in atrial fibrillation. J Clin Med. 2024;13(11):3294.
23. Pyman E, Ernault AC, Kumar Patel KH, et al. Subepicardial adipose tissue as a modulator of arrhythmias. Heart Rhythm. 2025;22(4):1110-8.
24. Self TH, Wallace JL, Sakaan S, et al. Effect of body weight on dose of vitamin K antagonists. South Med J. 2015;108(10):637-43.
25. Cheymol G, Poirier JM, Carrupt PA, et al. Pharmacokinetics of beta-adrenoceptor blockers in obese and normal volunteers. Br J Clin Pharmacol. 1997;43(6):563-70.

26. Ward SM, Radke J, Calhoun C, et al. Weight-based versus non-weight-based diltiazem dosing in the setting of atrial fibrillation with rapid ventricular response. Am J Emerg Med. 2020;38(11):2271-6.
27. Voskoboinik A, Moskovitch J, Plunkett G, et al. Cardioversion of atrial fibrillation in obese patients: results from the cardioversion-BMI randomized controlled trial. J Cardiovasc Electrophysiol. 2019;30(2):155-61.
28. Wong CX, Sullivan T, Sun MT, et al. Obesity and the risk of incident, post-operative, and post-ablation atrial fibrillation: a meta-analysis of 626,603 individuals in 51 studies. JACC Clin Electrophysiol. 2015;1(3):139-52.
29. Hookana E, Junttila MJ, Puurunen VP, et al. Causes of nonischemic sudden cardiac death in the current era. Heart Rhythm. 2011;8(10):1570-5.
30. Aune D, Schlesinger S, Norat T, et al. Body mass index, abdominal fatness, and the risk of sudden cardiac death: a systematic review and dose-response meta-analysis of prospective studies. Eur J Epidemiol. 2018;33(8):711-22.
31. Shahreyar M, Dang G, Waqas Bashir M, et al. Outcomes of in-hospital cardiopulmonary resuscitation in morbidly obese patients. JACC Clin Electrophysiol. 2017;3(2):174-83.
32. Sung CW, Huang CH, Chen WJ, et al. Obese cardiogenic arrest survivors with significant coronary artery disease had worse in-hospital mortality and neurological outcomes. Sci Rep. 2020;10(1):18638.
33. Matinrazm S, Ladejobi A, Pasupula DK, et al. Effect of body mass index on survival after sudden cardiac arrest. Clin Cardiol. 2018;41(1):46-50.

SECTION 9

Obesity and Cardiolipidology

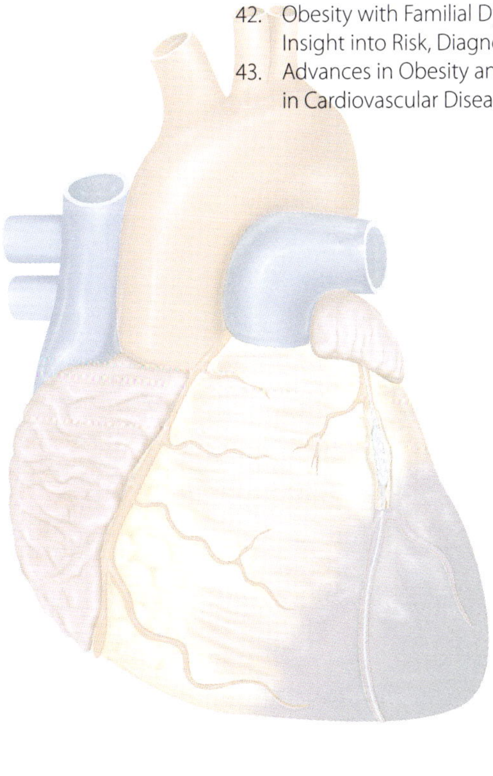

42

CHAPTER

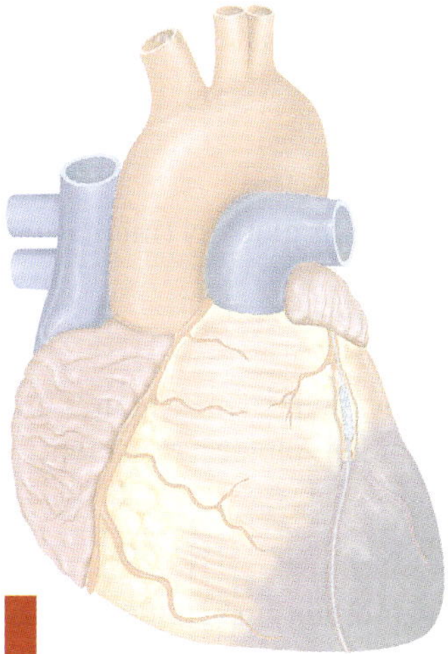

Obesity with Familial Dyslipidemia: Insight into Risk, Diagnosis, and Management

SN Routray, Sura Kishore Mishra

INTRODUCTION

Obesity and familial dyslipidemias together form one of the most powerful combinations driving early and aggressive atherosclerotic cardiovascular disease (ASCVD). While obesity independently fosters an atherogenic environment through insulin resistance, hepatic steatosis, and increased inflammation, familial dyslipidemias such as familial hypercholesterolemia (FH), familial combined hyperlipidemia (FCHL), and familial hypertriglyceridemia (FHTG), expose individuals to lifelong elevated levels of atherogenic lipoproteins. When these conditions coexist, their synergy accelerates vascular injury, worsens metabolic disturbances, and complicates therapy. Evidence from the 2025 ESC/EAS update on dyslipidemia management underscores the urgent need to reclassify risk in patients with both obesity and familial lipid disorders, emphasizing earlier and more aggressive intervention.

Recent data further show that obesity often masks the diagnosis of familial dyslipidemia, as clinicians frequently attribute abnormal lipids solely to lifestyle factors, which delay genetic evaluation and family screening.

This article provides a 2025 update on risk, diagnosis, and evidence-based management of obesity coexisting with familial dyslipidemia.

PATHOPHYSIOLOGY

Obesity-driven Metabolic Disturbances

Obesity promotes key metabolic changes, including:

- *Insulin resistance* reduces LPL activity, thereby increasing triglycerides[1]
- *Enhanced hepatic VLDL production* due to increased free fatty acid flux from enlarged adipose depots[2]
- *Formation of small dense LDL particles*, highly atherogenic and predominant in obesity-associated dyslipidemia.[1]
- *Reduced HDL-C* due to impaired cholesterol efflux and HDL particle maturation[2]

These create the classic phenotype: ↑*TG*, ↓*HDL-C*, ↑*LDL-C*, which is characteristically found in obese individuals.

Genetic Lipid Disorders: Lifelong Lipid Toxicity

In contrast, familial dyslipidemias result from inherited defects:

- *FH* → LDLR/ApoB/PCSK9 mutation → very high LDL-C from birth[1]
- *FCHL* → polygenic origin with ↑ApoB and mixed hyperlipidemia[1]

- *FHTG* → hepatic overproduction of TG-rich VLDL and impaired TG clearance[3]
- *Polygenic hypercholesterolemia* → multiple small-effect variants impair LDL clearance.[1]

Together, these disorders produce sustained elevation in atherogenic lipoproteins, significantly increasing ASCVD risk.

Obesity + Familial dyslipidemia = Exponential risk

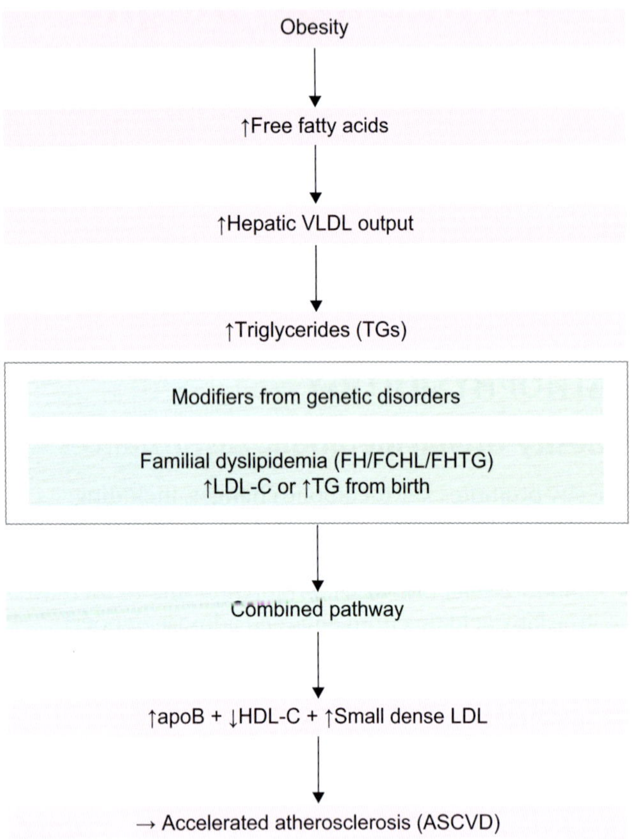

The *2024 cohort on overweight and lipid phenotype* demonstrates how obesity aggravates lipid abnormalities in genetically predisposed individuals:

- Overweight and obese patients show *significantly higher TG and lower HDL-C* across FH, FCHL, and polygenic groups.
- Non-HDL-C is also significantly higher in overweight/obese compared to normal-weight patients.[1]

Obesity also worsens ApoB overproduction and inflammatory cytokine release, further destabilizing the lipid profile.

The *FH obesity cohort* confirms that obesity in FH increases hypertension, insulin resistance, metabolic syndrome prevalence, and coronary plaque burden.[4]

EPIDEMIOLOGY AND RISK PROFILE (2025 UPDATES)

Prevalence Trends

- *Obesity:* Over *1 billion individuals* globally (increasing yearly).
- *FH: 1 in 250* individuals globally.
- *FCHL: 1–2%* prevalence.
- *FHTG:* Approximately *1%* prevalence. These figures are consistent across multiple epidemiologic assessments.[3]

Mortality Implications

The cohort study on obesity and mortality in hyperlipidemia showed:

- *BMI and waist-to-height ratio have a U-shaped association with mortality.*
- *Weight-adjusted waist index (WWI)* shows a linear relationship with mortality—the best predictor of risk.
- Mortality increases sharply in obese individuals with hyperlipidemia.[5]

Thus, central adiposity, not weight alone, is the critical determinant in familial dyslipidemia.

CLINICAL DIAGNOSIS

Distinguishing Obesity-driven versus Familial Dyslipidemia

Diagnosing familial dyslipidemia in obese individuals is challenging because obesity itself can mimic or distort inherited patterns.

Features Suggesting Familial Dyslipidemia Despite Obesity

- LDL-C persistently *>190 mg/dL* despite lifestyle changes[6] 2025
- Triglycerides *>250–500 mg/dL*, unresponsive to diet (suspicious for FHTG or FCHL)
- Strong family history of premature ASCVD
- Tendon xanthomas/corneal arcus at a young age (classic FH findings)[1]
- Elevated ApoB (>130 mg/dL), characteristic of FCHL.[1]

Laboratory Markers (2025 Standards)

European Society of Cardiology/European Atherosclerosis Society (ESC/EAS) 2025 recommends the following panel:

- *Lipid profile:* LDL-C, TG, HDL-C, and non-HDL-C.[6]
- ApoB (better reflects atherogenic particle number)

- Lp(a) once in lifetime
- Genetic testing if FH or FCHL is suspected.

ApoB and non-HDL-C outperform LDL-C in identifying FCHL and mixed dyslipidemia, especially in obesity.[1]

Emerging Biomarkers

Recent research identifies *miR-33b* as a potential combined biomarker of hypercholesterolemia and obesity:

- Higher serum levels correlate with elevated LDL-C and obesity markers
- Regulates cholesterol efflux pathways (ABCA1)
- May predict early lipid dysregulation.[7]

Pediatric Diagnosis

The pediatric dyslipidemia guidelines emphasize **(Table 1)**:

- Universal screening at *9–11 years*
- Targeted screening earlier in high-risk children (obesity, family history).
- Non-HDL-C as a stronger and reliable screening tool[8]
  Early diagnosis prevents decades of LDL exposure.

Step 1: Lipid profile (LDL-C, HDL-C, TG, Non-HDL-C)

↓

Step 2: Rule out secondary causes (thyroid, renal, drugs)

↓

Step 3: ApoB and Non-HDL-C (Better reflect atherogenicity)

↓

Step 4: Apply genetic criteria
(DLCN (Dutch lipid clinical network for FH, apoB for FCHL, TG-pattern for FHTG)

↓

Step 5: ASCVD risk stratification (Very high/high/moderate)

↓

Step 6: Target therapy based (on risk category and phenotype)

TABLE 1: Definition of dyslipidemia based on NHLBI guideline-recommended cutoff points for lipid levels in children and adolescents.

Category	*Low (mg/dL)*	*Acceptable (mg/dL)*	*Borderline-high (mg/dL)*	*High (mg/dL)*
TC		<170	170–199	≥200
LDL-C		<110	110–129	≥130
Non-HDL-C		<120	120–144	≥145
TG (year):				
0–9		<75	75–99	≥100
10–19		<90	90–129	≥130
HDL-C	<40	>45	40–45	

(HDL-C: high-density lipoprotein cholesterol; LDL-C: low-density lipoprotein cholesterol; NHLBI: National Heart, Lung, and Blood institute; Non-HDL-C: non-high-density lipoprotein cholesterol; TC: total cholesterol; TG: triglyceride)

MANAGEMENT STRATEGIES IN 2025

Optimal management requires combining lifestyle, pharmacotherapy, and novel biologics.

Lifestyle Modification (Foundational Therapy)

Weight reduction of 5–15% improves metabolic markers:

- ↓TG by 20–30%
- ↑HDL-C by 5–10%
- ↓ApoB modestly
- Improved insulin resistance.

The Mediterranean diet, with reduced refined carbohydrates, is especially beneficial for FCHL and FHTG.[2]

Pharmacologic Therapy (Fig. 1)

Statins

- First-line in FH, FCHL, and mixed dyslipidemia.
- High-intensity statins ↓lower LDL-C by 50–60%.
- ESC/EAS recommends target LDL-C: *<55 mg/dL for very high risk* (FH + obesity + risk factors).[6]

Ezetimibe

- Adds 15–20% LDL-C reduction
- Useful in obesity due to increased cholesterol absorption.

PCSK9 Inhibitors

- Alirocumab/evolocumab reduces LDL-C by 60%
- However, a 2024 multicenter analysis found:
  - LDL-C control declines over time due to non-adherence and missed doses[9]
  - Inclisiran (PCSK9 siRNA) mitigates this by requiring dosing only twice yearly

Triglyceride-lowering Agents

Crucial in patients with FCHL and especially FHTG:

- Fibrates (↓TG by 30–50%)
- Omega-3 fatty acids
- ApoC-III inhibitors (emerging)
- ANGPTL3 inhibitors (evinacumab)

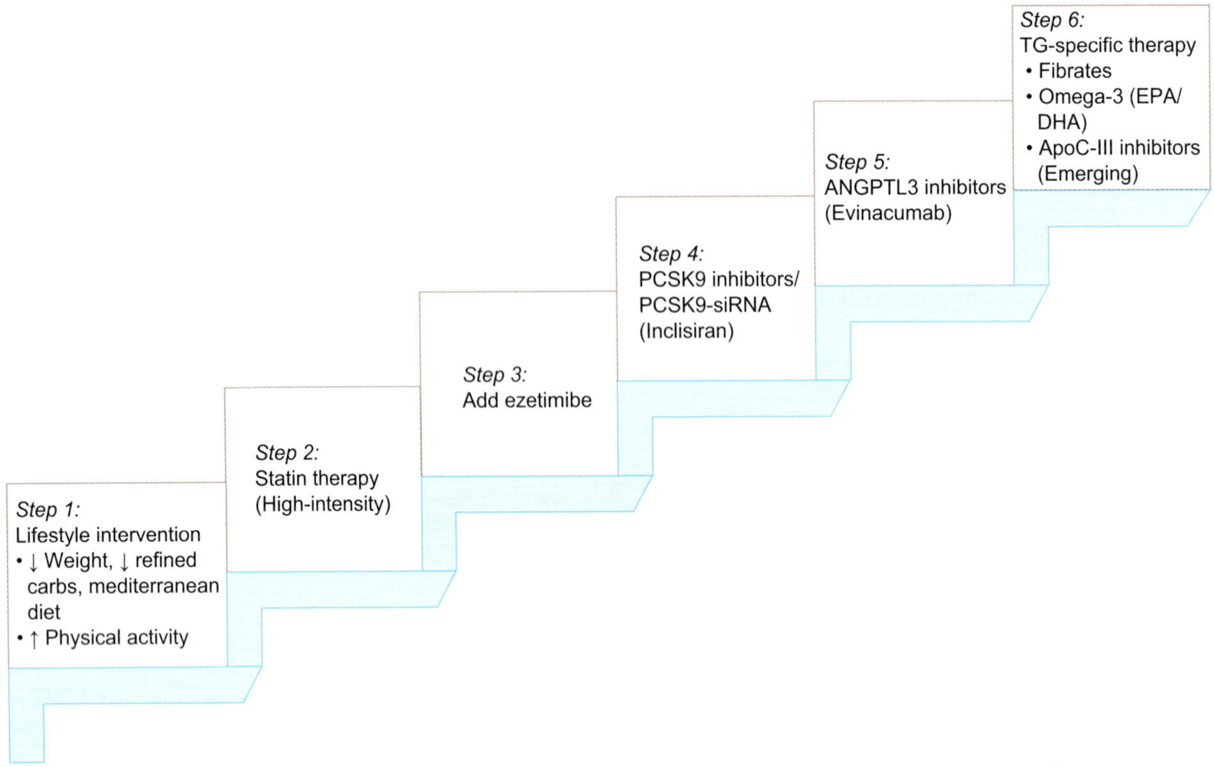

Fig. 1: Management Ladder (2025).

Familial hypertriglyceridemia requires early aggressive therapy to prevent pancreatitis.[3]

Advanced Therapies in 2025

Novel therapeutics include:

- *ANGPTL3 inhibition* for severe mixed dyslipidemias
- *Gene therapy* targeting LDLR/PCSK9 (research phase)
- *ApoC-III inhibitors* for severe hypertriglyceridemia.

These therapies bypass traditional pathways and are especially useful in genetically driven dyslipidemias complicated by obesity.

Special Populations

FCHL with Obesity

Obesity significantly increases TG, non-HDL-C, and ApoB levels in FCHL, requiring early combination therapy.[1]

FHTG with Obesity

Obesity increases VLDL production, amplifying TG levels into the pancreatitis risk range.

Management includes:

- Very low-fat diet
- Absolute alcohol avoidance
- Fibrates + omega-3s
- Emergency plasmapheresis for extreme TG >1,500 mg/dL.[3]

FH with Obesity

- Obesity increases CAD risk and reduces therapeutic efficacy.
- Aggressive LDL-C lowering with statin + ezetimibe ± PCSK9 inhibitors is recommended.[4]

CONCLUSION

The coexistence of obesity and familial dyslipidemia represents a highly dangerous cardiometabolic phenotype. Obesity significantly aggravates lipid abnormalities intrinsic to FH, FCHL, and FHTG, resulting in higher triglycerides, lower HDL-C, increased small dense LDL, and persistent metabolic inflammation. These changes dramatically accelerate ASCVD progression and raise mortality risk.

2025 advances emphasize:

- Earlier screening (including children)
- Prioritizing non-HDL-C, ApoB, and emerging biomarkers like miR-33b

- Unified aggressive therapy using statins, ezetimibe, PCSK9 inhibitors, and triglyceride-lowering agents
- Novel biologics for resistant lipid disorders
- Weight reduction as a central therapeutic pillar

Timely identification and comprehensive management can substantially reduce premature cardiovascular events, mortality, and metabolic complications in this high-risk group.

REFERENCES

1. Formisano E, Proietti E, Borgarelli C, et al. The impact of overweight on lipid phenotype in different forms of dyslipidemia: a retrospective cohort study. J Endocrinol Invest. 2024;47(12):3111-8.
2. Dakal TC, Xiao F, Bhusal CK, et al. Lipids dysregulation in diseases: core concepts, targets and treatment strategies. Lipids Health Dis. 2025;24(1):61.
3. Daley SF, Cusick AS, Reilly E. Familial Hypertriglyceridemia. In: StatPearls [Internet]. Treasure Island (FL): StatPearls Publishing; 2025.
4. Elshorbagy A, Vallejo-Vaz AJ, Barkas F, et al. Overweight, obesity, and cardiovascular disease in heterozygous familial hypercholesterolaemia: the EAS FH Studies Collaboration registry. Eur Heart J. 2025;46(12):1127-40.
5. Zhang Y, Yao Y. The association between obesity indicators and mortality among individuals with hyperlipidemia: evidence from the NHANES 2003–2018. Lipids Health Dis. 2025;24(1):20.
6. Mach F, Koskinas KC, Roeters van Lennep JE, et al. 2025 Focused Update of the 2019 ESC/EAS Guidelines for the management of dyslipidaemias. Eur Heart J. 2025;46(42):4359-78. Erratum in: Eur Heart J. 2025: ehaf1036
7. Masoumi-Ardakani Y, Eghbalian M, Fallah H, et al. Exploring serum miR-33b as a novel diagnostic marker for hypercholesterolemia and obesity: insights from a pilot case-control study. BMC Endocr Disord. 2025;25(1):27.
8. Kim SE. Dyslipidemia in Children and Adolescents: Current Insights and Updated Treatment Approaches. Pediatr Gastroenterol Hepatol Nutr. 2025;28(3):148.
9. Formisano E, Vignati A, Bertolini A, et al. Decline in LDL-C control in patients with dyslipidemia treated with PCSK9-inhibitors: The role of obesity in LDL-C target achievement. J Clin Lipidol. 2025;19(5):1374-84.

43

CHAPTER

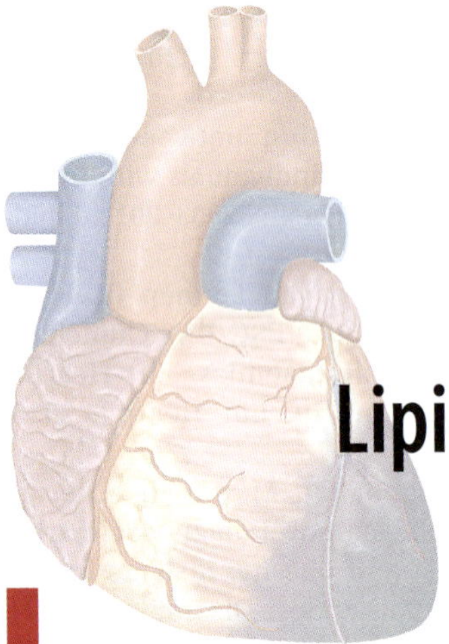

Advances in Obesity and Lipid Management in Cardiovascular Disease

Asha Mahilmaran

INTRODUCTION

Obesity is widely prevalent and is on the increase worldwide especially in countries with developing economies. The most common preceding risk factor of insulin resistance (IR), diabetes mellitus (DM), dyslipidemia, hypertension, and dyslipidemia are obesity. Its significance is often overlooked, and management of obesity has remained casual over time. Obesity causes an atherogenic lipid profile characterized by elevated triglycerides (TGLs), non-high-density lipoprotein (non-HDL), apoprotein B (ApoB), small dense low-density lipoprotein (LDL), and low levels of HDL and this is one of the pathophysiological mechanisms of enhanced cardiovascular (CV) risk.[1] CV disease is a leading cause of mortality in obese individuals and a simultaneous two-pronged treatment of weight reduction and management of lipids is likely to reduce the CV risk. Adiposity is associated with chronic inflammation which promotes the macrophage-mediated uptake of LDL and progression of atherosclerosis. Early intervention to control body weight with lifestyle changes and drugs to control the lipid abnormalities is the key to success in controlling atherosclerotic cardiovascular disease (ASCVD) risk in patients who are obese.

MEASUREMENT OF OBESITY INDICES

Obesity and overweight are widely prevalent, 39–49% of adults worldwide are affected. There are several indices to measure obesity. The most used is the body mass index (BMI). Based on BMI, weight is classified as normal 18.5–24.9, 25–29.9 as overweight, class I obesity 30–34.9, class II obesity 35–39.9, class III obesity >40. In Asians, a revised cut-off of 23 as normal and 23–24.9 as overweight and >25 as obesity is recommended. The major disadvantage of BMI is that it does not assess visceral fat and muscle mass. There are other indices such as waist circumference (WC), waist-hip ratio (WHR), waist-to-height ratio (WHtR), body adiposity index (BAI), and body round index (BRI). The WHR and BRI have been found to be better predictors of CV risk in a 17-year longitudinal study.[2]

LIPID ABNORMALITIES IN OBESITY

Triglycerides

The free fat in the body is predominantly stored in adipocytes. In obese individuals 50% of free fatty acid (FFA) is stored in adipose tissue in comparison to 25% in nonobese individuals. Dietary excess of refined carbohydrates and saturated fat results in large amounts of FFA and glycerol made available in the liver, promoting increased TGL-rich VLDL production and release. Also, obesity is associated with IR with impairment of the lipolysis of TGL mediated by insulin resulting in excess FFA by degradation of TGL in visceral adipose tissue and this FFA is made available in liver for VLDL production. There is also increased FFA delivery to liver through intestinal absorption carried by chylomicron remnants. FFA synthesis is also stimulated in liver by IR. All these effects lead to an increased VLDL production by liver **(Fig. 1)**. The increased circulating VLDL reaches adipose tissue where it is acted upon by lipoprotein lipase which converts the TGL to FFA and glycerol. Inside the fat cells,

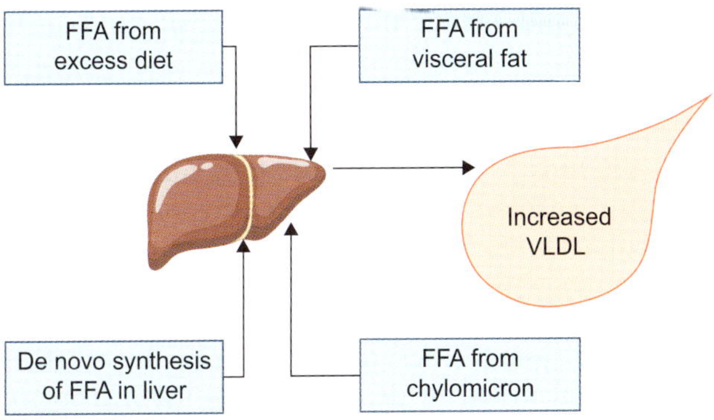

Fig. 1: Mechanism of increased VLDL production from liver in obesity.

TGL is excreted by cholesterol ester transfer protein (CETP) and carried by HDL. The TGL-rich HDL is acted upon by lipoprotein lipase which releases TGL into blood causing hypertriglyceridemia, which is one of the key abnormalities in lipids in obesity. There is an increase in ApoC-III levels in an insulin-resistant state in obesity and this results in decreased clearance of TGL-rich lipoproteins. There is also a decreased activity of lipoprotein lipase which is stimulated normally by insulin which is a key enzyme in TGL clearance. Thus, a combination of increased production and decreased clearance results in high TGL levels in obesity. Genetic factors, hormonal disorders, IR and DM, as well as excessive alcohol consumption plays a role in the TGL elevation. There is an accumulation of TGL in ectopic fat locations such as liver, pericardial, perivascular, and perirenal areas. The relationship between TGL and ectopic fat deposition has been found to be inverted U-shaped with an increase at levels of TGL between 150 and 350 mg/dL[2]. Studies have shown that there is a strong correlation between increased BMI and increased TGL levels and incident DM in young individuals.[3]

High-density Lipoprotein

A strong correlation between increased BMI and low HDL levels has been reported. The low HDL usually is accompanied by high TGL levels. The combination of weight loss and increased physical activity has been shown to increase HDL levels and improve CV protection.[4,5] A state of chronic inflammation with proinflammatory adipokines such as leptin, resistin, and cytokines such as tumor necrosis factor (TNF), interleukin-6, and interleukin-1 (IL-1) are associated with obesity and this results in dysfunctional HDL which loses its protective scavenger action. There is a downregulation of ATP-binding cassette transporter A1 (ABCA1) and scavenger receptor B1 in a proinflammatory state, thereby impeding the reverse transport action of HDL. In obese individuals, the action of cholesteryl ester transfer protein (CETP) is increased in adipocytes which take up TGL-rich lipoproteins and this TGL-rich HDL is acted upon by lipase enzyme and causes hydrolysis of TGL and converts HDL into smaller particles which are excreted by kidneys resulting in lower levels of HDL.

Low-density Lipoprotein

The major abnormality in LDL in obesity is a mild increase in LDL-C levels. The reason for increased atherogenicity in obesity is the composition of LDL which includes a predominance of small dense LDL and there is an increase in LDL particle number. The small dense LDL molecules stay in the circulation for prolonged time due to diminished uptake by LDL receptors, they enter the arterial wall more readily as they are easily oxidized and bind to proteoglycans in the arterial wall.

Chylomicron Remnants

A postprandial absorption of excess cholesterol is accompanied by release of large chylomicrons which do not penetrate vascular wall. Chylomicrons undergo lipolysis to form chylomicron remnants which are rich in cholesterol. They also acquire ApoE through exchange from HDL and become smaller particles which penetrate vascular endothelium and are highly atherogenic. Chylomicron remnants promote platelet activation, plasminogen activator inhibitor-1, smooth cell proliferation, and activation of vascular adhesion molecules which are the basis for elevated CV risk.[6]

ADIPOKINES AND CYTOKINES—ROLE IN OBESITY

The combination of obesity, postprandial hyperlipidemia, and IR stimulate the inflammatory pathways which play an important role in atherosclerosis progression.

Adiponectin increases catabolism of TGL by upregulation of lipoprotein lipase and downregulation of ApoC-III. Adiponectin levels are decreased in obesity. Adiponectin also increases production of ApoA-1 and ABCA1 in liver. This results in elevated TGL levels and low HDL levels. The levels of resistin are increased in obese individuals and increases hepatic VLDL production and decrease HDL and ApoA-1.[7]

Cytokines such as TNF and IL-1 increase FFA by promoting lipolysis in adipocytes. They also have inhibitory action on lipoprotein lipase, which clears TGL-rich lipoproteins. They also decrease ApoA-1 production, they decrease transfer of cholesterol from cell to HDL by decreasing ABCA1 and ABCG1. The activity of LCAT is also decreased which converts cholesterol to cholesterol ester in HDL, a process which is required for formation of normally functioning HDL.[7,8]

Combined the derangement in adipokines and cytokines result in the typical atherogenic pattern in obesity featuring increased TGL and low and less functional HDL levels.[9,10]

ATHEROGENIC DYSLIPIDEMIA IN OBESITY

Obesity is associated with a combination of adverse lipid changes referred to as adiposopathic dyslipidemia. Obesity is also associated with lower socioeconomic class and low education. This double jeopardy can increase CV mortality 1.5–3 times in overweight and obese individuals in comparison to individuals with normal BMI.[6] Dyslipidemia is widely prevalent in obesity to the tune of about 60%. The atherogenic lipid components elevated in obesity are predominantly an increase in TGLs, increase in ApoB, remnant lipids, non-HDL, a mild increase in LDL and lowering of HDL levels. The atherogenicity is mainly due to an increase in small dense LDL and an increase in LDL particle number which enter the vascular endothelium in a ready fashion and are quickly oxidized by the chronic inflammatory milieu in obese individuals and is the major mechanism underlying the progression of atherosclerosis and elevated CV risk **(Fig. 2)**.[10]

CARDIOVASCULAR RISK ASSOCIATED WITH OBESITY

Obesity has been linked to an increase in several CV outcomes. There is increased risk of CAD, hypertension, stroke, heart failure, heart failure with preserved ejection fraction (HFpEF) in particular, atrial fibrillation (AF), pulmonary and venous thromboembolism, and aortic stenosis.

Obesity is an important and independent risk factor of HFpEF, it is one of the key variables in the HFpEF score. There is a state of chronic inflammation which promotes cardiac fibrosis, stiffening of ventricles, ventricular hypertrophy, excess pericardial fat which lead to an increased left ventricular pressure. There are also neurohormonal changes with stimulation of renin-angiotensin system (RAS) and aldosterone by excess of leptin. The increased incidence of hypertension in obesity also leads to increased incidence of LVH, AF, and HFpEF **(Fig. 3)**.[11]

MANAGEMENT OF DYSLIPIDEMIA OF OBESITY

The management of dyslipidemia associated with obesity should begin with diet, lifestyle changes, and drugs which tackle obesity and lipid abnormalities. In severe obesity, use of bariatric surgery also impacts the CV risk factors in obesity.

Diet

Dietary calorie restriction and increased soluble fiber intake decreases TGL and LDL levels. There have been

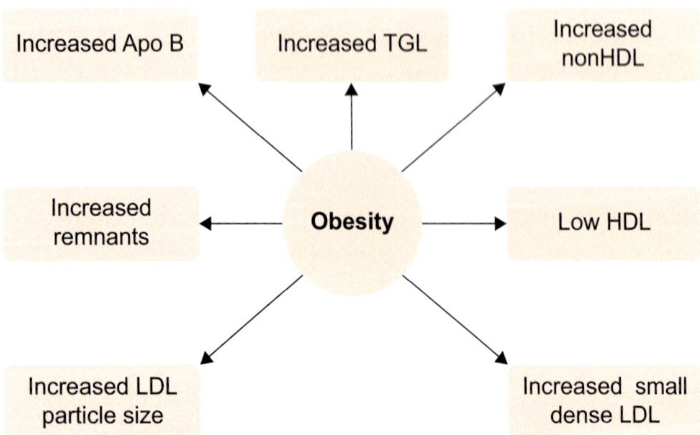

Fig. 2: Lipid abnormalities in obesity.

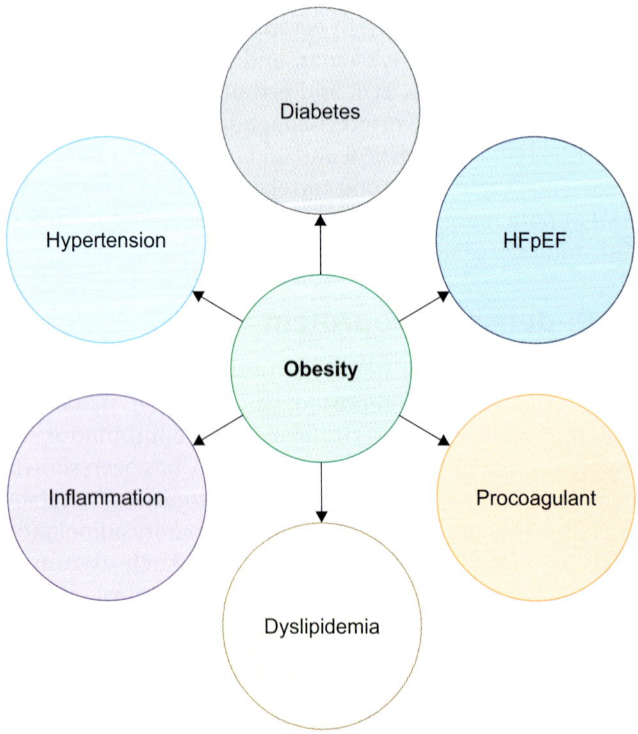

Fig. 3: Cardiovascular risk in obesity.

several diet plans which have been used in the management of obesity. Ketogenic diets decrease TGL but increase LDL levels. Diets high in saturated fat increase LDL levels, but lower TGL levels. Low carbohydrate diet decreases TGL and increases HDL levels.[11]

Physical Activity

Physical exercise can cause weight loss. Even small weight loss by 5% can improve lipid parameters by decreasing TGL and improving HDL. But, only weight loss is not likely to address all the lipid abnormalities in obesity and often, drugs are required.

DRUGS USED IN WEIGHT REDUCTION

The drugs used in obesity for weight reduction can be categorized as follows:

- Absorption inhibitors such as orlistat
- Appetite suppressants such as phentermine
- Combination medications, which combine different ingredients such as naltrexone/bupropion
- GLP-1 receptor antagonists—semaglutide, liraglutide, and tirzepatide.

Individuals with BMI > 30 and BMI >27 kg/m^2 with comorbidities are candidates for pharmacotherapy.

Orlistat

Orlistat is a lipase inhibitor acting on gastric and pancreatic lipases. The action of lipases is breakdown of dietary TGL, converting it into FFA and monoglycerides which are readily absorbed. Orlistat prevents this hydrolysis of TGL which results in less absorption of FFA.[12]

Phentermine

It is a sympathomimetic amine that increases norepinephrine and dopamine and suppresses appetite. A modest weight loss of 5–10% is produced but the major drawback is potential for substance abuse. A combination drug of phentermine/topiramate can result in greater weight reduction at lower doses and better safety.[13]

Naltrexone/Bupropion Combination

The combination acts on hypothalamic pro-opiomelanocortin neurons, and causes decreased appetite. Weight loss is in the range of 5–9%. In addition to headache, vomiting, and dizziness, the main concern is an increase in suicidal thoughts as adverse effect to this drug, which has relegated its use.[13]

Glucagon-like Peptide-1 Receptor Agonists (GLP-1 Analogs)

This class of drugs causes weight loss, blood pressure reduction, and control sugar levels. They decrease the ASCVD risk, benefit in HFpEF, and are beneficial in renal disorders as well. They act at the hypothalamic level increasing satiety, reducing appetite, and slowing gastric emptying.

There are three molecules which have shown benefit, (1) liraglutide, (2) semaglutide, and dual GLP-1 and glucose-dependent insulinotropic polypeptide receptor agonist (GLP-1/GIPRAS) (3) tirzepatide.

1. Liraglutide given as subcutaneous daily injection
2. Semaglutide—daily oral and weekly subcutaneous injectable forms are available.
3. Tirzepatide—weekly subcutaneous injection

The weight loss by these three drugs varies from 9% with liraglutide,15% with semaglutide, and the maximal loss is noted with tirzepatide which can be up to 20% in a year. Liraglutide is used as subcutaneous injection in the dose of 3 mg daily. Semaglutide, oral 14 mg daily, injectable once weekly dose of 2.4 mg and tirzepatide once weekly dose of 15 mg are the dose schedules used in treatment of obesity.

Clinical trials such as Satiety and Clinical Adiposity Liraglutide Evidence (SCALE), Semaglutide Treatment Effect in people with Obesity (STEP), Semaglutide Effects on Cardiovascular Outcomes in People with Overweight or Obesity (SELECT), and SURMOUNT-1 trial with tirzepatide have shown significant weight loss and CV benefits in obese individuals, even without diabetes. Semaglutide has been shown to be beneficial in the management of obesity-related HFpEF in the STEP-HFpEF and STEP-HFpEF DM trials in nondiabetics and diabetics respectively (**Box 1**).

The major side effects are predominantly gastrointestinal such as nausea, diarrhea, constipation and usually seen in the first few months during initiation and dose adjustments. There is a reported increased incidence of gallstones and biliary diseases. Elevation of pancreatic enzymes has been observed but pancreatitis per se, not

BOX 1: Effects of GLP-1 analogs on cardiometabolic protection.

- Improvement in cardiometabolic variables
- Improvement in glycemic control
- Decreases systolic and diastolic blood pressure levels
- Improvement in dyslipidemia
- Protects renal damage by increasing adiponectin/adenosine monophosphate-activated kinase and prevents renal inflammation, fibrosis, and albuminuria

increased. There is no increase in thyroid cancer. The effect on mental health has been noted to be generally positive, but mood disturbances also have been reported.[14-24]

Sodium-glucose Transporter-2 inhibitors

Sodium-glucose transporter-2 (SGLT2) inhibitors are not primary obesity drugs but in diabetic population, their effect causes weight loss and has CV and renal benefits and reduce heart failure mortality and hospitalization for heart failure. They have an important role in the treatment of obesity-induced HFpEF.[22]

BARIATRIC SURGERY

Bariatric surgery is recommended in patients with morbid obesity, BMI >40 kg/m^2 and produces greater weight loss than medications. GLP-1 analogs have also been used in conjunction with bariatric surgery as priming with the drugs for few months decreases the surgical risk and improves the cardiometabolic profile.[23]

MANAGEMENT OF DYSLIPIDEMIA

Atherosclerotic cardiovascular disease is the major disease-causing morbidity and mortality in obese individuals and optimal lipid management along with weight reduction therapies are required to decrease the elevated CV risk.

Statins are the front-line drugs to decrease ASCVD risk and in the Cholesterol Treatment Trialists (CTT) collaborative study, the benefit of statins in reducing CV risk was present in at all BMI levels. Statins lower C-reactive protein, an inflammation marker often elevated in obesity.[24]

Ezetimibe acts by inhibiting absorption of cholesterol from intestine by to Nieman–Pick C1-like 1 cholesterol transporter protein in the intestinal epithelial cells. In a study by Takase et al., ezetimibe decreased visceral fat, increased adiponectin, and decreased IR.[25]

Ezetimibe decreases postprandial hyperlipidemia characterized by elevated TGL, remnant chylomicrons, and small dense LDL after a fatty meal often seen in obese individuals, METS. The combination of ezetimibe with simvastatin was more effective in decreasing apolipoprotein B, TGL, and improving HDL levels.

Fibrates have failed to show consistent CV benefit and increased risk of cholelithiasis and generally are not considered with statins unless the TGL level is >500 mg/dL, when it may be used to prevent pancreatitis.[25-27]

Omega-3 fatty acids decrease TGL and inflammation in obese individuals and they also have benefit in CAD and decrease incidence of arrhythmias. They also decrease IR and increase adiponectin levels.[28]

The Further Cardiovascular Outcomes Research with PCSK9 Inhibition in Subjects with Elevated Risk (FOURIER) trial subanalysis showed that higher BMI >30 kg/m^2 to be an independent high CV risk factor, and evolocumab was effective in decreasing the MACE in obese individuals. High BMI individuals >35 kg/m^2 had larger benefit than individuals with 30–35 kg/m^2 and benefit was seen >30 kg/m^2.[29]

CONCLUSION

Obesity is increasing worldwide and close to half the adult population are overweight or obese. Obesity is an important CV risk factor and associated comorbid conditions of hypertension, DM, IR, atherogenic dyslipidemia of increased TGL, small dense LDL and low HDL, CKD, and OSA. There can be an increased risk of polycystic ovarian syndrome, cancer, and osteoarthritis. BMI is the most familiar obesity index which is well studied but other newer indices such as WHR, WHtR, and BRI have greater predictive value on CV risk. The management of obesity and dyslipidemia needs a multifaceted approach of weight reduction through a combination of diet, exercise, behavioral modification, and drugs especially GLP-1 analogs. Bariatric surgery is reserved for morbid obesity and often in conjunction with GLP-1 analogs. The treatment of associated dyslipidemia is essential, and statins are the cornerstone of therapy, ezetimibe, PCSK9 inhibitors, and omega-3 fatty acids have additional role to tackle residual risk. An early and aggressive comprehensive approach is the need of the hour to address the burgeoning problem of obesity and lipid disorders.

REFERENCES

1. Bays HE, Kirkpatrick C, Maki KC, et al. Obesity, dyslipidaemia, and cardiovascular disease: A joint expert review from the Obesity Medicine Association and the National Lipid Association 2024. Obes Pillars. 2024; 10:100108.
2. Zamaneh F, Hassannejad R, Nouri F, et al The long-term association of nine anthropometric obesity indices with cardiovascular diseases and mortality. Sci Rep. 2025;15(1):35609.
3. Zou Y, Sheng G, Yu M, et al. The association between triglycerides and ectopic fat obesity:An inverted U-shaped curve. Plos One. 2020;15(11):e0243068.
4. Garbuzova EV, Shcherbakova LV, Rymar OD, et al. Triglycerides, Obesity and Education Status Are Associated with the Risk of Developing Type 2 Diabetes in Young Adults, Cohort Study. J Pers Med. 2023;13(9):1403.
5. Nurmohamed NS, Ditmarsch M, Kastelein JJP. Cholesteryl ester transfer protein inhibitors: from high-density lipoprotein cholesterol to low-density

lipoprotein cholesterol lowering agents? Cardiovasc Res. 2022;118(14):2919-31.
6. Anitha R, Prema GS, Padmini O. Comparison of Body Mass Index (BMI) with High Density Lipoprotein (HDL) levels in obese people. J Evid Based Med Healthc. 2016;2(48): 8412-6.
7. Bacchetti T, Morresi C, Simonetti O, et al. Effect of Diet on HDL in Obesity. Molecules. 2024;29(24):5955.
8. Philip J, Hagan K, Shahid I, et al. Unfavorable Social Determinants of Health and Obesity: A Double Jeopardy for Premature Mortality. JACC Adv. 2025;4(11 Pt 1):102154.
9. Feingold KR. Obesity and Dyslipidemia. In: Feingold KR, Adler RA, Ahmed SF, et al., (Eds). Endotext [Internet]. South Dartmouth (MA): MDText.com, Inc.; 2000.
10. Gugliucci A. The chylomicron saga: time to focus on postprandial metabolism. Front Endocrinol (Lausanne). 2024;14:1322869.
11. Klop B, Castro Cabezas M. Chylomicrons: A key biomarker and risk factor for cardiovascular disease and for understanding of obesity. Curr Cardiovasc Risk Rep. 2012;6:27-34.
12. Blagov A, Rufanov K, Irina K, et al. The Significance of Lipoproteins in the Development of Obesity. Front Biosci (Schol Ed). 2024;16(1):8.
13. Masuda D, Yamashita S. Postprandial Hyperlipidemia and Remnant Lipoproteins. J Atheroscler Thromb. 2017;24(2):95-109.
14. Cohen JB, Gadde KM. Weight Loss Medications in the Treatment of Obesity and Hypertension. Curr Hypertens Rep. 2019;21(2):16.
15. Taha MB, Yahya T, Satish P, et al. Glucagon-Like Peptide 1 Receptor Agonists: A Medication for Obesity Management. Curr Atheroscler Rep. 2022;24(8):643-54.
16. Ghusn W, Hurtado MD. Glucagon-like Receptor-1 agonists for obesity: Weight loss outcomes, tolerability, side effects, and risks. Obes Pillars. 2024;12:100127.
17. Celletti F, Farrar J, De Regil L. World Health Organization Guideline on the Use and Indications of Glucagon-Like Peptide-1 Therapies for the Treatment of Obesity in Adults. JAMA. 2025.
18. Peterson SC, Barry AR. Effect of Glucagon-like Peptide-1 Receptor Agonists on All-cause Mortality and Cardiovascular Outcomes: A Meta-analysis. Curr Diabetes Rev. 2018;14(3):273-9.
19. Kang YM, Giugliano RP, Keech AC, et al. Obesity-Associated Cardiovascular Risk and Benefit From PCSK9 Inhibition: A Prespecified Analysis From FOURIER. J Am Coll Cardiol. 2025:S0735-1097(25)10005-3.
20. Grant CH, Bell S. Obesity and Chronic Kidney Disease: The Dual Epidemic in Cardiovascular Health. Eur Cardiol. 2025;20:e28.
21. Kim MS, KimWJ, Khera AV, et al. Association between adiposity and cardiovascular outcomes: an umbrella review and meta-analysis of observational and Mendelian randomization studies. Eur Heart J. 2021;42(34):3388-403.
22. Rosengren A. Obesity and cardiovascular health: the size of the problem. Eur Heart J. 2021;42(34):3404-6.
23. Rodrigues MM, Falcão LM. Pathophysiology of heart failure with preserved ejection fraction in overweight and obesity - Clinical and treatment implications. Int J Cardiol. 2025;430:133182.
24. Butler J, Shah SJ, Petrie MC, et al. Semaglutide versus placebo in people with obesity-related heart failure with preserved ejection fraction: a pooled analysis of the STEP-HFpEF and STEP-HFpEF DM randomised trials. Lancet. 2024;403(10437):1635-48.
25. Takase H, Dohi Y, Okado T, et al. Effects of ezetimibe on visceral fat in the metabolic syndrome: a randomised controlled study. Eur J Clin Invest. 2012;42(12):1287-94.
26. Hiramitsu S, Miyagishima K, Ishii J, et al. Effect of ezetimibe on lipid and glucose metabolism after a fat and glucose load. J Cardiol. 2012;60(5):395-400.
27. Rosen JB, Jimenez JG, Pirags V, et al. Consistency of effect of ezetimibe/simvastatin compared with intensified lipid-lowering treatment strategies in obese and non-obese diabetic subjects. Lipids Health Dis. 2013;12:103.
28. Jerab D, Blangero F, da Costa PCT, et al. Beneficial Effects of Omega-3 Fatty Acids on Obesity and Related Metabolic and Chronic Inflammatory Diseases. Nutrients. 2025;17(7):1253.
29. Formisano E, Vignati A, Bertolini A, et al. Decline in LDL-C control in patients with dyslipidemia treated with PCSK9-inhibitors: The role of obesity in LDL-C target achievement. J Clin Lipidol. 2025;19(5):1374-84.

44

CHAPTER

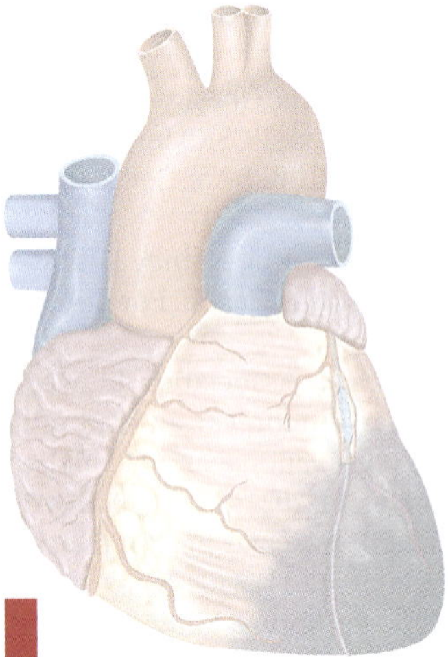

Management Update: Navigating the Complex Triad of Obesity, Hypertriglyceridemia, and Elevated Lipoprotein(a)

Manisha Arora, Anshul Jain

INTRODUCTION: A CONVERGENCE OF CARDIOMETABOLIC RISK FACTORS

The global pandemic of obesity has profoundly reshaped the landscape of cardiovascular disease (CVD), acting as a potent accelerant for traditional and emerging risk factors. Among the most challenging presentations is the triad of obesity, hypertriglyceridemia (HTG), and elevated lipoprotein(a) [Lp(a)]. This confluence of metabolic and genetic dyslipidemia represents a particularly high-risk phenotype, demanding a sophisticated and multipronged management approach. While obesity and HTG are well-established, modifiable risk factors, Lp(a) stands apart as a largely genetically determined, independent causal risk factor for atherosclerotic cardiovascular disease (ASCVD).[1] The management for this complex patient population is not just about intensifying existing therapies but about strategically integrating novel agents and redefining therapeutic targets in an era of precision medicine. We have made an attempt to provide a comprehensive review of the latest evidence, guidelines, and emerging strategies for managing this high-risk patient cohort.

UNDERSTANDING THE PATHOPHYSIOLOGY

The interplay between these three conditions is intricate and synergistic. Obesity, particularly visceral adiposity, drives insulin resistance and chronic low-grade inflammation. This leads to increased hepatic synthesis of triglyceride-rich lipoproteins (TRLs), such as very-low-density lipoprotein (VLDL), and impaired TRL clearance, resulting in HTG. The elevated triglycerides (TGs) also promote the formation of small, dense LDL particles, which are highly atherogenic.

Meanwhile, Lp(a), a modified LDL particle, is a silent but powerful contributor to ASCVD risk.[2] The Lp(a) particle consists of an LDL-like component and a unique glycoprotein, apolipoprotein(a) [apo(a)], which is structurally similar to plasminogen. This similarity contributes to its prothrombotic and proinflammatory properties. Unlike other lipids, Lp(a) levels are largely unaffected by diet, exercise, or most conventional lipid-lowering therapies. However, there is sufficient evidence that high Lp(a) carries a worse prognosis in presence of sedentary lifestyle and increased LDLc in a logarithmic manner. The challenge lies in the fact that Lp(a) amplifies the risk conferred by other lipid abnormalities, including HTG.

MANAGEMENT: A STAGED AND PERSONALIZED APPROACH

The management of this triad requires a stepwise approach, prioritizing lifestyle interventions, followed by targeted pharmacological therapy.

Foundational Therapy: Lifestyle Modification

The cornerstone of management remains aggressive lifestyle intervention, a critical first step often underutilized.

For this patient population, it is not merely a "nice to have" but a "must-do."

- *Weight loss:* Losing even a modest amount of weight (5–10% of body weight) can significantly reduce fasting and postprandial TG levels by increasing lipoprotein lipase (LPL) activity and decreasing apoC-III levels.
- *Dietary adjustments:* A heart-healthy diet is essential. This includes:
  - *Drastic reduction of refined carbohydrates and added sugars:* Fructose and sucrose intake are potent drivers of hepatic VLDL synthesis.
  - *Limitation of saturated and trans fats:* These contribute to obesity and insulin resistance.
  - *Emphasis on polyunsaturated fatty acids (PUFAs):* Particularly omega-3 fatty acids, which have a direct TG-lowering effect.
  - *Alcohol restriction:* Alcohol consumption can dramatically increase TG levels, especially in susceptible individuals.
- *Physical activity:* Regular aerobic exercise not only promotes weight loss but also directly improves insulin sensitivity and TRL metabolism, helping to clear TGs from the bloodstream.

Pharmacological Interventions

The current therapeutic landscape offers a range of options, from well-established drugs to cutting-edge novel agents.

Targeting Hypertriglyceridemia

- *Statins:* While primarily targeting LDL-C, statins can reduce TG levels by 15–30% by decreasing hepatic VLDL production. They remain the first-line therapy to reduce ASCVD risk, as the primary goal is always to address the highest risk factor.
- *Fibrates:* Agents like fenofibrate are highly effective at lowering TG by activating PPAR-alpha, which promotes fatty acid oxidation and increases LPL activity. The ACC/AHA and ESC/EAS guidelines continue to support their use in patients with severe HTG (TG > 500 mg/dL) to prevent pancreatitis, as well as in those with persistent moderate HTG on statins to reduce residual ASCVD risk.[2]
- *Prescription omega-3 fatty acids:* High-dose (4 g/day) icosapent ethyl (a purified EPA) has been a significant development. The REDUCE-IT trial demonstrated a substantial reduction in major adverse cardiovascular events (MACE) in statin-treated patients with elevated TG and established ASCVD or diabetes with risk factors.[3] This has cemented its role in managing residual risk. Other omega-3 preparations (EPA/DHA combinations) also lower TGs but have not shown the same robust cardiovascular outcomes benefit.
- *Niacin:* Extended-release niacin can reduce plasma TG by 20–50%, but its clinical efficacy and safety are questionable.[4]

Targeting Elevated Lp(a)

This is the most challenging and rapidly evolving area of lipid management.

- *Current therapies:* The lack of effective conventional therapies for Lp(a) has been a major unmet need. Statins, ezetimibe, and fibrates have a negligible or even slightly detrimental effect on Lp(a) levels. PCSK9 inhibitors (e.g., evolocumab and alirocumab) offer a modest Lp(a) reduction of 20–30%, which while helpful, is often insufficient for very high Lp(a) levels.
- *Emerging therapies:* The future lies in the targeted RNA-based therapies.
  - *Antisense oligonucleotides (ASOs):* Pelacarsen, an ASO targeting apo(a) mRNA, has demonstrated profound and sustained Lp(a) lowering (up to 80%) in clinical trials. It is currently in a phase 3 trial (Lp(a)HORIZON) to definitively assess its impact on MACE. This therapy represents a paradigm shift, moving from indirect risk reduction to direct Lp(a) modification.[5]
  - *Small-interfering RNA (siRNA):* Olpasiran and zodasiran are siRNAs that also target apo(a) mRNA, showing similar robust Lp(a) reductions. Their less frequent dosing schedule (quarterly or biannually) is a key advantage for patient compliance.[6]

Targeting Obesity and Metabolic Syndrome

- *GLP-1 receptor agonists (GLP-1RAs):* Originally for diabetes, GLP-1RAs like semaglutide and liraglutide have emerged as potent antiobesity medications. Beyond weight loss, they directly improve lipid metabolism by reducing TG production and enhancing clearance, leading to significant TG reductions. This class of drugs is a game changer for patients with this triad, as it simultaneously addresses the root cause of HTG (obesity/insulin resistance) while also providing ASCVD benefits.[7]
- *Dual and triple agonists:* The development of dual (e.g., tirzepatide) and future triple agonists (GIP/GLP-1/glucagon) will further enhance weight loss and metabolic control, offering a powerful tool for managing the obesity-driven component of the dyslipidemia.

PROPOSED THERAPEUTIC ALGORITHM

A proposed algorithm for managing this complex patient is shown further, although this is not a substitute for clinical judgment yet a strategic guide.

- *Step 1: Baseline assessment*: Measure fasting lipids, Lp(a) (at least once), and assess for secondary causes.
- *Step 2: Lifestyle first*: Implement aggressive dietary and exercise counseling.
- *Step 3: Statin therapy*: Initiate high-intensity statin therapy to address the primary ASCVD risk.
- *Step 4: Addressing residual risk*:
    - *Persistent HTG (TG >150 mg/dL):* If TG remain elevated despite lifestyle and statins, consider adding high-dose icosapent ethyl.
    - *Elevated Lp(a):* If Lp(a) is >100 nmol/L (>50 mg/dL), consider a PCSK9 inhibitor as a next step. Monitor ongoing clinical trials for the imminent availability of targeted Lp(a) therapies.
- *Step 5: Obesity management*: For patients with obesity and this triad, the use of a GLP-1RA or a dual/triple agonist is strongly recommended to simultaneously address weight, HTG, and overall metabolic risk. This is often the most effective single step for this phenotype.
- *Step 6: Refractory cases*: For patients with very high Lp(a) and recurrent events despite optimal therapy, lipoprotein apheresis remains an option, though it is resource intensive.[8]

LIMITATIONS AND FUTURE DIRECTIONS

Despite significant advances, key questions and limitations remain:

- *Evidence for Lp(a) lowering:* While pelacarsen and other RNA therapies are highly effective at reducing Lp(a) levels, their impact on hard cardiovascular outcomes is still being investigated in phase 3 trials.
- *Cost and accessibility:* The high cost of newer therapies (e.g., PCSK9i, GLP-1RAs, and RNA-therapies) poses a major barrier to widespread adoption, especially in resource-limited healthcare systems.
- *Treatment burden:* The use of multiple medications (statin, ezetimibe, icosapent ethyl, PCSK9i/RNA-therapy, and GLP-1RA) can lead to reduced patient adherence.

The future of managing this triad will be defined by the results of ongoing trials and the potential for combination therapies. The development of single molecules that target multiple pathways (e.g., dual agonists that also affect lipid metabolism) and the eventual approval of dedicated Lp(a)-lowering agents will streamline management and provide cardiologists with unprecedented tools to combat this complex and lethal combination of risk factors.

CONCLUSION

The management of patients with obesity, HTG, and elevated Lp(a) has evolved from a reactive, stepwise approach to a proactive, precision-based strategy. The convergence of targeted pharmacological agents with powerful metabolic therapies offers new hope for a patient group historically at high residual risk. As we move into the mid-2020s, the cardiologist's armamentarium is expanding, allowing for a more complete and effective assault on this perilous triad. It is our responsibility to stay at the forefront of this knowledge, personalizing treatment strategies to mitigate risk and improve long-term cardiovascular outcomes for our patients.

REFERENCES

1. 2025 Focused Update of the 2019 ESC/EAS Guidelines for the management of dyslipidaemias: Developed by the task force for the management of dyslipidaemias of the European Society of Cardiology (ESC) and the European Atherosclerosis Society (EAS). Eur Heart J. 2025; 4359-78.
2. Rao SV, O'Donoghue ML, Ruel M, et al. 2025 ACC/AHA/ACEP/NAEMSP/SCAI Guideline for the Management of Patients with Acute Coronary Syndromes: A Report of the American College of Cardiology/American Heart Association Joint Committee on Clinical Practice Guidelines. Circulation. 2025;151(13):e771-e862.
3. Sayah N, Bhatt DL, Miller M, et al. Icosapent ethyl following acute coronary syndrome: the REDUCE-IT trial. Eur Heart J. 2024;45(13)1173-6.
4. Zimodro JM, Rizzo M, Gouni-Berthold I. Current and Emerging Treatment Options for Hypertriglyceridemia: State-of-the-Art Review. Pharmaceuticals. 2025;18(2):147.
5. Cho L, Nicholls SJ, Nordestgaard BG, et al. Design and Rationale of Lp(a)HORIZON Trial: Assessing the Effect of Lipoprotein(a) Lowering with Pelacarsen on Major Cardiovascular Events in Patients with CVD and Elevated Lp(a). Am Heart J. 2025;287:1-9.
6. Kosmas CE, Bousvarou MD, Tsamoulis D, et al. Novel RNA-Based Therapies in the Management of Dyslipidemias. Int J Mol. Sci. 2025;26(3):1026.
7. Mahar MU, Mahmud O, Ahmed S, et al. The Effects of Tirzepatide on Lipid Profile: A Systematic Review and Meta-Analysis of Randomized Controlled Trials. J Obes Metab Syndr. 2024;33(4):348-59.
8. Schettler VJJ. Lipoprotein apheresis: Current overview and future outlook in clinical practice. Transfus Apher Sci. 2025;64(5):104209.

SECTION 10

Obesity with Aortic Disease

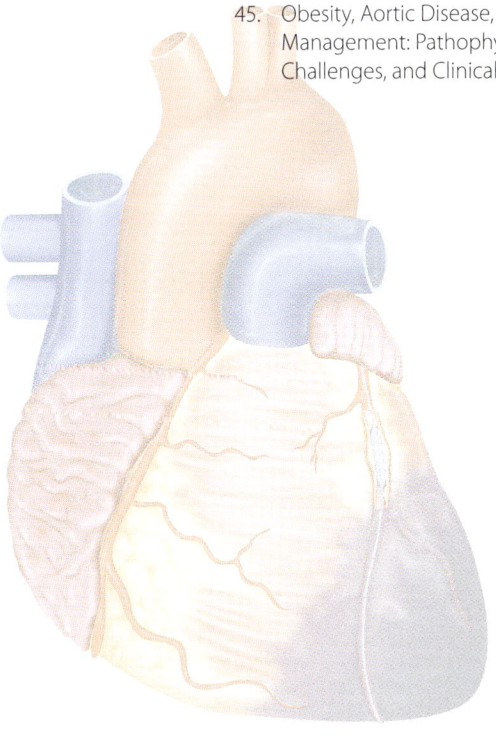

45

CHAPTER

Obesity, Aortic Disease, and Interventional Management: Pathophysiology, Technical Challenges, and Clinical Solutions

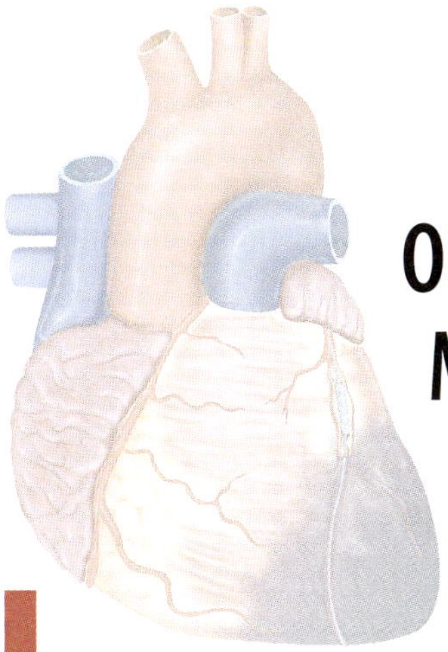

Anil Dhall, Nikhil Chaudhari, Varinder S Bedi

INTRODUCTION

The global obesity epidemic has coincided with rising incidence of aortic disease, particularly abdominal and thoracic aortic aneurysm and acute aortic dissection.[1,2,3] While obesity has not been formally recognized as a traditional risk factor for aortic disease in some guidelines, mounting evidence from epidemiologic and mechanistic studies establishes obesity—especially central adiposity—as a causal contributor to aortic wall degeneration, dilation, and predisposition to dissection.[1,4,5] Paradoxically, mildly obese patients undergoing aortic repair often experience lower perioperative mortality than their nonobese counterparts, an observation termed the "obesity paradox."[6] However, this paradox masks significant interventional complexity: obesity substantially increases technical difficulty and risk of access site complications, fluoroscopic challenges, acute kidney injury (AKI), and respiratory morbidity in both open and endovascular repair.[7-9]

This article provides a comprehensive review of how obesity influences aortic disease biology and interventional outcomes, with particular emphasis on practical solutions for managing large-bore vascular access in morbidly obese patients and optimizing perioperative outcomes across open and endovascular aortic repair.

OBESITY, PERIVASCULAR ADIPOSE TISSUE, AND AORTIC DISEASE

Pathophysiology

Adipose Tissue Dysfunction and Aortic Wall Remodeling

Obesity results not only in excess fat accumulation but also in transformation of adipose tissue from a physiologically benign storage depot to a pathologically inflamed, dysfunctional endocrine organ.[1] Perivascular adipose tissue (PVAT), which encases the aorta and major vessels, undergoes hypertrophy and inflammatory infiltration in obesity, shifting from anti-inflammatory/anticontractile function to proinflammatory, pro-oxidant activity.[1,5]

Obese PVAT secretes elevated levels of TNF-α, IL-6, MCP-1, and leptin while reducing adiponectin, collectively promoting:

- Elastin fiber fragmentation and collagen deposition within the aortic media.[1,5]
- Upregulation of matrix metalloproteinases (MMP-2, MMP-9) and downregulation of tissue inhibitors (TIMPs).[1]
- Smooth muscle cell phenotypic switching and apoptosis.[5]
- Endothelial dysfunction and oxidative stress via increased NADPH oxidase activity.[1,5]

These pathologic changes are present in both abdominal and thoracic aortic aneurysms, rendering obesity a systemic proaneurysmal state.[1,5] Central obesity and visceral fat volume show stronger associations with aortic diameter and AAA presence than BMI alone, highlighting the importance of regional fat distribution.[10,11]

Epidemiology: Risk of Abdominal Aortic Aneurysms and Thoracic Aortic Aneurysms/Dissection

Multiple meta-analyses confirm that obesity is positively associated with AAA prevalence and growth. A dose-response meta-analysis of over 14,000 AAA patients showed that each increment in BMI increased AAA risk, with the relationship being nonlinear and strongest for central obesity markers (waist circumference, waist-to-hip ratio).[11] Central obesity independently predicts AAA presence even after adjustment for overall BMI.[10]

For thoracic aortic disease, evidence is less robust but consistent: obesity and central adiposity are associated with larger ascending aortic diameters in nonsyndromic populations, and obesity is recognized as an independent risk factor for acute aortic dissection incidence alongside hypertension, age, and smoking.[4,12]

INTERVENTIONAL CHALLENGES AND SPECIFIC SOLUTIONS: LARGE-BORE VASCULAR ACCESS IN MORBID OBESITY

Epidemiology and Risk of Access-site Complications

Large-bore femoral access (16–24 F sheaths) is central to EVAR, TEVAR, and fenestrated/branched endografting. Morbid obesity (BMI ≥ 35–40 kg/m^2) dramatically elevates the risk of access-related complications.[13,14]

A pivotal study reported nearly 15-fold higher odds of access-site complications after percutaneous closure in morbidly obese versus non-obese patients.[13] In an EVAR cohort, obese patients undergoing total percutaneous femoral access experienced 50% groin hematoma versus 7.7% in nonobese patients using identical pre-closure techniques, with significantly higher rates requiring vascular repair.[15]

Key anatomic and physiologic factors contributing to access failure in morbid obesity:

- Increased skin-to-artery distance (often 8–10+ cm).[14]
- Loss of palpable landmarks, necessitating alternative guidance modalities.[14]
- Unreliable fluoroscopic visualization of bony landmarks.[14]

High incidence of inadvertent SFA/profunda cannulation, increasing bleeding risk.[14]

Retroperitoneal hemorrhage risk due to high or low arterial punctures.[14]

Ultrasound-guided Femoral Access: Evidence and Technique

Ultrasound-guided (US-guided) femoral access has emerged as a critical safety standard, particularly in morbidly obese patients.[14,16] Multiple studies across coronary intervention, structural heart procedures, and EVAR settings demonstrate that US-guided access reduces:

- Inadvertent venous puncture
- Number of access attempts
- Time to successful puncture
- Overall vascular complications.

Compared with landmark-guided puncture alone.[16,17]

Practical US-guided access technique in morbid obesity:

- *Probe selection:* High-frequency linear probe (7–13 MHz) when feasible; shift to lower-frequency curvilinear probe for very deep vessels to maintain real-time visualization.[14,16]
- *Vessel identification and measurement:* Systematically identify the common femoral artery (CFA), its bifurcation, SFA, and profunda relative to the femoral head. Measure CFA diameter; a minimum of 6–7 mm is typically required for safe large-bore access.[18]
- *Puncture strategy:* Employ micropuncture needle under continuous US guidance, confirming intraluminal position and avoiding posterior wall penetration before upsizing to access needle and sheath.[14,16]
- *Anatomic planning:* Preprocedural CTA or duplex should quantify CFA diameter, degree of calcification, tortuosity, and prior interventions to guide access strategy before the procedure.[14,18]

Percutaneous versus Surgical Access in Morbid Obesity

Total percutaneous access with preclosure (e.g., double ProGlide/ProStyle or plug-based devices) has become standard for many large-bore procedures, reducing operative time, length of stay, and wound infection compared with surgical cut-down **(Fig. 1)**.[18,19]

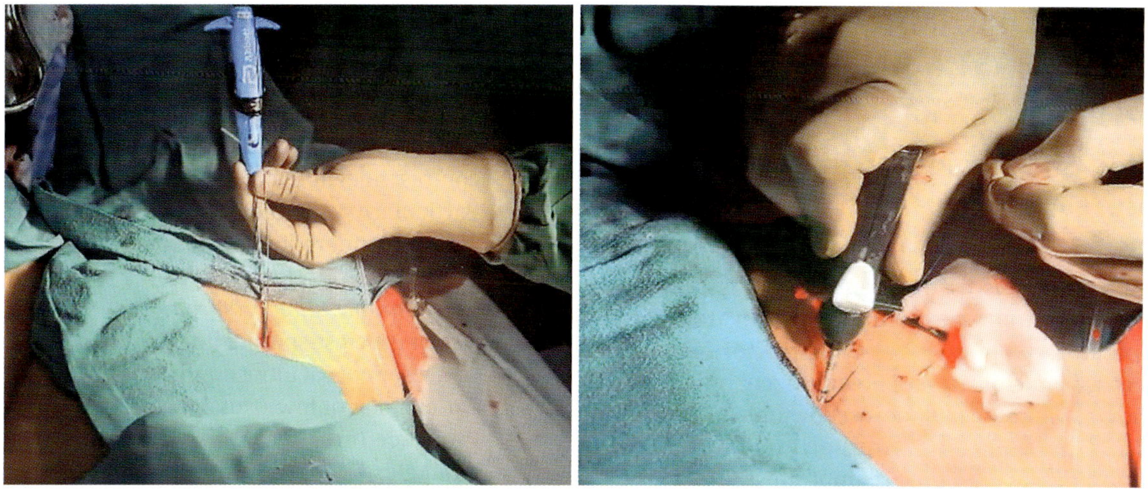

Fig. 1: ProGlide percutaneous CFA access closure in EVAR patient.

However, morbid obesity remains a recognized risk factor for percutaneous closure failure. An EVAR comparison study found that obese patients in the percutaneous group experienced significantly more hematomas and required vascular repair more frequently than nonobese patients, particularly those with CFA stenosis > 50% or heavy anterior calcification.[15]

Current Evidence-based Recommendations

Default approach: US-guided percutaneous access with preclosure in most obese patients, provided CTA/US confirm adequate CFA diameter (≥ 6–7 mm) and limited anterior calcification.[18,19]

- Indications for surgical cut-down or hybrid access:
  - Morbid obesity combined with > 50% CFA stenosis or circumferential heavy calcification.[15,18]
  - Multiple prior groin surgery with scarring.[15]
  - Anticipated very large-bore sheaths (≥ 22 F).[15]
  - Failed percutaneous access attempt.[19]
- *Alternative:* Iliac conduits—in combined morbid obesity with small/tortuous iliac arteries, consideration of surgical iliac conduits provides controlled, safe access, particularly advantageous for complex TEVAR or thoracoabdominal aortic repair.[4,5,20]

Management of Access-site Complications

Access-site complications post-EVAR/TEVAR include hematoma requiring transfusion, pseudoaneurysm, arteriovenous fistula, retroperitoneal hemorrhage, arterial dissection/thrombosis, and limb ischemia.[21] Overall vascular complication rates in large-bore procedures range from 12 to 22%, with morbid obesity consistently identified as an independent risk factor.[21,22]

Mitigation Strategies

- Standardized preoperative assessment:
  - *CTA quantification of femoral/iliac arteries:* Minimal diameter, calcification pattern, bifurcation level relative to femoral head.[14,18]
  - Duplex confirmation in cases of unclear anatomy.
- Intraoperative technique:
  - Routine US-guided access with low threshold to abandon percutaneous approach if CFA anatomy is hostile.[14,18]
  - Customized preclose protocols (e.g., double-suture technique, adjunctive plug in very large sheaths).[19,22]
  - Meticulous hemostasis and pressure application postsheath removal.
- Postoperative surveillance:
  - Early duplex ultrasound in high-risk groins (within 24–48 hours).[22]
  - Serial clinical and duplex follow-up at 1 week, 1 month, and 3 months.[22]
  - Low threshold for intervention if pseudoaneurysm, hematoma expansion, or limb ischemia develops.[22]
- *Institutional support:* Recent data highlight that structured "vascular access teams" and formal training pathways improve vascular access quality and reduce complications across patient groups, including the obese.[23]

FLUOROSCOPIC IMAGING, RADIATION, AND CONTRAST MANAGEMENT IN OBESITY

Imaging Challenges and Radiation Exposure

Obesity poses unique challenges to fluoroscopic imaging. Thick subcutaneous tissue attenuates X-rays, requiring higher tube output and resulting in elevated patient and operator radiation dose with risk of X-ray tube overheating.[4,24] Obesity is a recognized independent determinant of prolonged fluoroscopy time during EVAR/TEVAR and thus cumulative radiation exposure.[4,24,25]

Suboptimal image quality compromises visualization of endograft markers, branch vessels, and dissection entry tears, necessitating steeper angulations and higher magnification, particularly for arch work or fenestrated/branched endografts.[4,24]

Higher contrast volumes are required, amplifying risk of AKI—already elevated in obese TEVAR patients.[4,5,26]

Practical Solutions to Optimize Imaging and Minimize Radiation

- *Preprocedural planning with high-quality 3D CTA:*
    - Meticulous 3D reconstruction to identify optimal working projections, branch vessel locations, and anatomy-specific challenges before the case.[4,24]
    - Reduces "exploratory" angiography and contrast use during procedure.
- *Low-dose, pulsed fluoroscopy:*
    - Tight collimation and avoidance of unnecessary magnification.[25]
    - Adherence to ALARA (as low as reasonably achievable) principles.[25]
- *Image fusion and advanced guidance:*
    - Real-time CTA-fluoroscopy overlay and intravascular ultrasound (IVUS) reduce reliance on contrast injections.[4,24]
    - Particularly valuable in obese, renally vulnerable patients undergoing fenestrated/branched EVAR or complex TEVAR **(Fig. 2)**.
- *Contrast-minimization protocols:*
    - Use of contrast-sparing imaging modalities (IVUS, transesophageal ultrasound).[4]
    - Iso-osmolar or low-osmolar contrast agents.[4,5]
    - Preprocedure hydration and renal-protective strategies (avoiding hypotension, judicious fluid management).[5,26]
- *X-ray tube management:*
    - Operator awareness of heat unit accumulation; proactive management to avoid automatic shutdown during prolonged complex cases in very large patients.[24]

RESPIRATORY, HEMODYNAMIC, AND RENAL MANAGEMENT

Anesthetic and Ventilatory Challenges

Obesity, particularly when combined with obstructive sleep apnea (OSA), reduces functional residual capacity, impairs diaphragmatic excursion, and increases oxygen consumption, predisposing to hypoxemia and difficult ventilation during prolonged TEVAR and open aortic repair.[4,5] General anesthesia and supine positioning worsen atelectasis and venous congestion.[4,5]

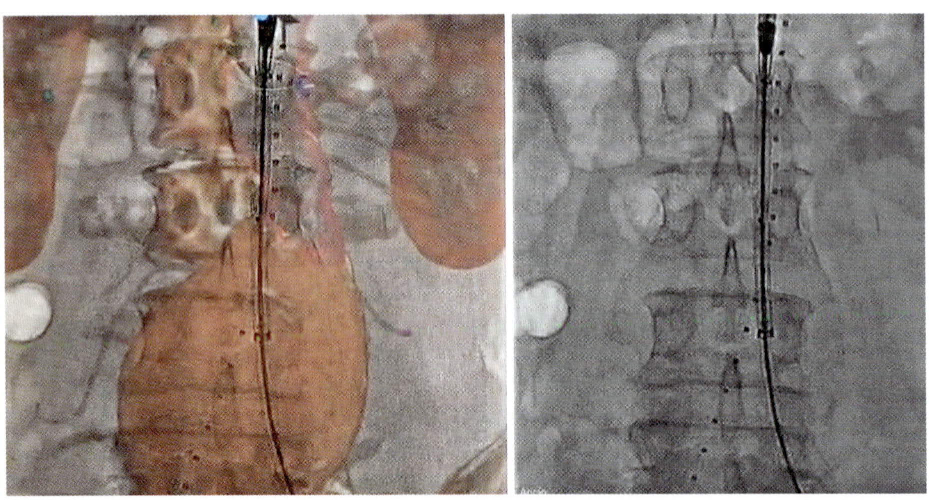

Fig. 2: EVAR guidance software, providing real time CTA image overlay during fluoroscopy for guidance of stent graft positioning.

Blood pressure measurement becomes unreliable with standard noninvasive cuffs on large obese arms; intraarterial monitoring is mandatory in complex thoracic and arch work.[4,5] Hemodynamic swings during rapid pacing (for stent deployment) or during circulatory arrest in arch surgery may be poorly tolerated in obese patients with limited cardiopulmonary reserve.[5,27]

- *Practical strategies:*
    - Preoperative OSA screening and CPAP optimization[5,27]
    - Early arterial line placement (radial or femoral).[4,5]
    - Transesophageal echocardiography or other real-time monitoring to guide volume status and LV function.[4,5]
    - Protective ventilation with moderate PEEP, lung recruitment maneuvers, and careful fluid balance during extensive thoracic/thoracoabdominal repair to balance spinal cord perfusion and pulmonary congestion.[5,26,28]

Acute Kidney Injury Prevention

Acute kidney injury occurs more frequently after TEVAR in obese patients, likely due to increased contrast volume, hemodynamic instability, and underlying metabolic/renal disease.[5,26] Goal-directed hemodynamic optimization is paramount to maintain renal perfusion during TEVAR while managing the hypotensive environment required for safe stent deployment.[4,5,26]

- AKI prevention:
    - Meticulous contrast minimization (as discussed earlier in the text).
    - Avoidance of hypotension; dynamic indices of intravascular volume responsiveness should guide fluid therapy in obese patients.[4,5,26]
    - Consideration of renal replacement therapy or pharmacologic agents if severe AKI develops.[5]

ACUTE TYPE A AORTIC DISSECTION IN OBESE PATIENTS: SURGICAL STRATEGY

Recent series demonstrate that acute type A aortic dissection (ATAAD) surgery in obese patients carries increased respiratory complications, longer ventilation times, and more wound problems.[29,30] However, surgical strategy significantly mitigates this risk.

A retrospective Chinese study of obese ATAAD patients undergoing total arch replacement with triple branched stent graft found that "partial upper sternotomy (PUS)" was superior to full sternotomy (FS) in reducing:

- Thoracic drainage (472.7 ± 115.5 mL vs. 572.9 ± 87.6 mL at 48 h; $p < 0.001$)[29]
- Red blood cell transfusion (503.3 ± 145.6 mL vs. 697.1 ± 179.4 mL; $p < 0.001$)[29]
- Mechanical ventilation time (40.1 ± 12.7 h vs. 47.3 ± 13.7 h; $p = 0.034$)[29]
- Incidence of pulmonary infection (33.3% vs. 60.0%; $p = 0.032$)[29]
- Incidence of hypoxemia (6.7% vs. 25.7%; $p = 0.041$)[29]
- Sternal dehiscence (0 vs. 17.1%; $p = 0.027$)[29]

In-hospital mortality and long-term survival were similar between groups, underscoring safety.[29] These findings support tailored operative strategies—particularly PUS in high-BMI patients—to reduce bleeding, transfusion, and respiratory morbidity without compromising repair quality.[29,30]

EVAR AND TEVAR OUTCOMES IN OBESITY: COMPARATIVE ANALYSIS

TEVAR Outcomes in Obesity

A 2024 systematic review and meta-analysis of 10 high-quality studies (7,849 patients) found that obesity is associated with "higher overall mortality" after TEVAR [OR = 1.49, 95% CI (1.02–2.17), $p = 0.04$], particularly 30-day mortality and in type B aortic dissection.[5,31] However, specific complications (stroke, spinal ischemia, neurologic events, endoleaks, wound issues, renal failure) were not significantly increased, though patients with complications had higher BMI **(Figs. 3A and B)**.[5,31]

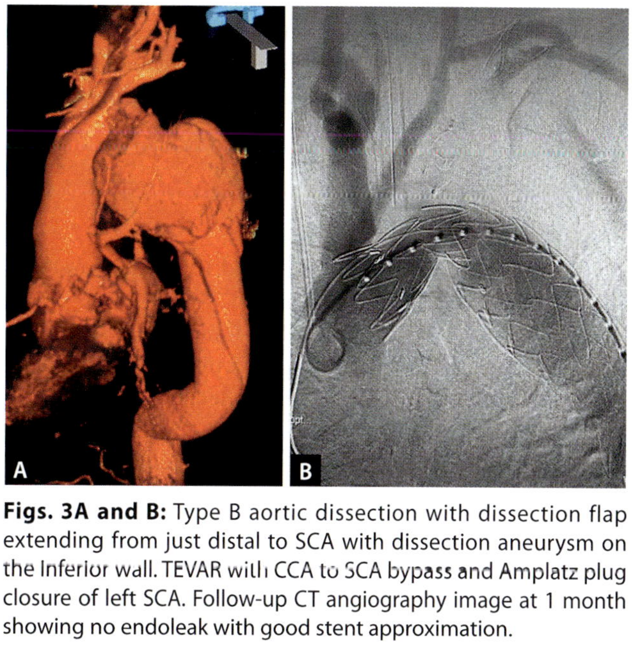

Figs. 3A and B: Type B aortic dissection with dissection flap extending from just distal to SCA with dissection aneurysm on the Inferior wall. TEVAR with CCA to SCA bypass and Amplatz plug closure of left SCA. Follow-up CT angiography image at 1 month showing no endoleak with good stent approximation.

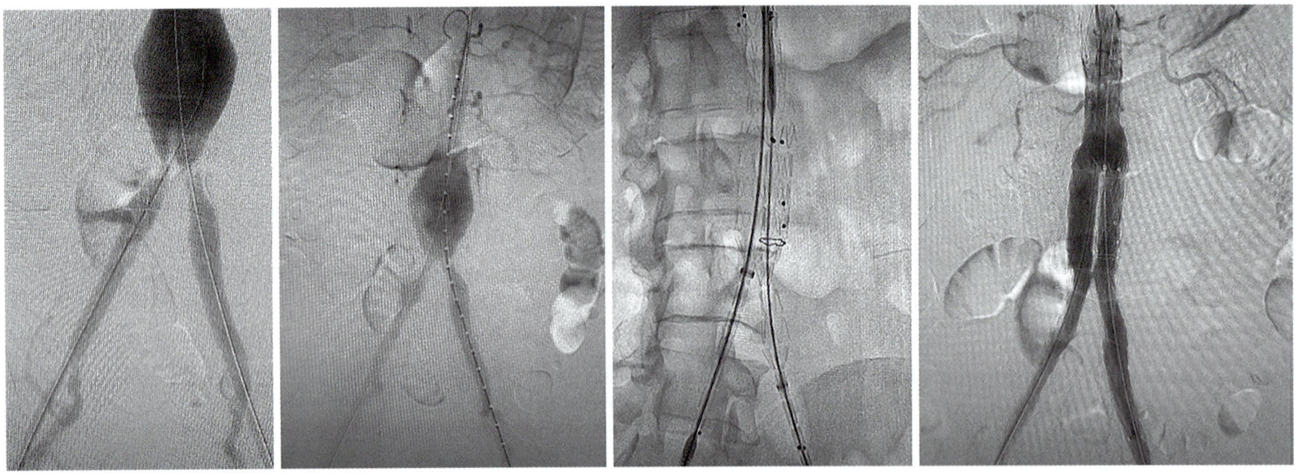

Fig. 4: These DSA images of the abdomen display infra-renal fusiform abdominal aortic aneurysm (AAA) with that shows bi-modular stent graft deployed infra renal renally with extension graft to B/L Iliac artery with good contrast across the stent graft and B/L iliac arteries.

Conclusions from TEVAR data: Obesity is a higher-risk but not contraindicated for TEVAR. Meticulous perioperative management is essential.[5,31]

- *Spinal cord ischemia risk:* TEVAR carries inherent paraplegia risk requiring careful blood pressure management.

EVAR Outcomes: The Obesity Paradox

In contrast, EVAR outcomes in obese patients are generally favorable, with the "obesity paradox" evident. A meta-analysis of AAA surgery reported lower or similar 30-day mortality in obese versus nonobese patients after EVAR, particularly in the overweight-to-mildly obese range (BMI 25–31 kg/m^2).[8,32] Despite higher rates of wound infection and renal dysfunction, obese EVAR patients often fare better than nonobese counterparts.[8,32]

This favorable profile supports EVAR as the preferred approach for obese AAA patients when anatomy permits, effectively mitigating laparotomy-related respiratory and wound complications inherent to open repair **(Figs. 3 and 4)**.[8]

Mechanistic Differences Explaining Divergent Outcomes

The divergence between TEVAR and EVAR outcomes in obesity reflects:

- *Procedural duration:* TEVAR (3–6 hours) versus EVAR (1.5–3 hours) with prolonged supine positioning in morbid obesity causing severe atelectasis.
- *Sheath size requirements:* TEVAR (20–24 F) versus EVAR (14–18 F), increasing access complication risk.
- *Radiation exposure:* TEVAR requires 2–3× higher fluoroscopy time, amplifying AKI risk via contrast requirements.
- *Physiologic stress:* TEVAR involves near-total aortic exclusion with hemodynamic instability; EVAR allows partial perfusion.

FENESTRATED AND BRANCHED ENDOGRAFTING IN OBESE PATIENTS

Fenestrated and branched endografts extend endovascular solutions to juxtarenal and thoracoabdominal aneurysms but substantially increase procedural complexity, fluoroscopy time, and contrast exposure.[33] Despite higher baseline comorbidities, recent series demonstrate that obese patients undergoing fenestrated/branched EVAR achieve similar intraoperative technical success and, in some studies, even decreased postoperative mortality compared to nonobese controls **(Fig. 5)**.[33]

- Key technical considerations for obese patients:
  - Meticulous 3D planning with image fusion and careful device sizing.[4,33]
  - Contrast minimization and renal protection protocols.[4,5,33]
  - Team-based planning involving anesthesia, ICU, and surgical specialists.[33]
  - Consideration of staged interventions and dedicated vascular access teams.[33]

GLP-1 RECEPTOR AGONISTS AND AORTIC PROTECTION: EMERGING THERAPEUTIC STRATEGY

Emerging evidence suggests that GLP-1 receptor agonists (e.g., liraglutide, semaglutide) may slow aortic dilatation progression in obese and diabetic patients.[34,35] A 24-month CTA-based study showed that GLP-1 RA therapy was

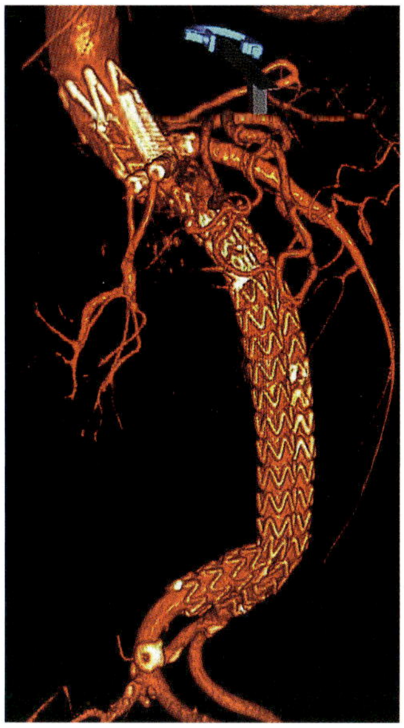

Fig. 5: This image describes a volume-rendered 3D CT aortogram demonstrates an infrarenal endovascular aortic repair with a modular bifurcated stent-graft extending from just below the renal arteries to the aortic bifurcation, with both iliac limbs in situ, a fenestration to SMA and chimney to B/L renal arteries.

independently associated with significantly reduced progression of ascending aortic dilatation compared with standard care (0.36 mm vs. 1.05 mm), independent of blood pressure and HbA1c changes.[34]

Mechanistically, GLP-1 RAs downregulate MMP-2/MMP-9, increase TIMP-1, reduce oxidative stress, and modulate adipose tissue inflammation, potentially attenuating the PVAT-mediated pathogenic loop.[34,35] While prospective imaging-based trials remain limited, these agents represent a promising adjunct to medical management for high-risk obese diabetic patients with mild aortic dilatation.[34,35]

Clinical implications: Preoperative GLP-1 RA optimization (6+ months) may reduce aortic remodeling and narrow the mortality gap observed in TEVAR obese patients.

PERIOPERATIVE OPTIMIZATION AND LONG-TERM MANAGEMENT STRATEGY

Prehabilitation and Weight Loss

Severely obese patients undergoing AAA repair experience higher postoperative mortality, prolonged hospital stays, and increased costs, largely due to thromboembolism, infection, and renal complications.[8,36] Preoperative weight loss, whether through lifestyle intervention, pharmacotherapy, or bariatric surgery, reduces perioperative risk.[8,36]

Moderate preoperative physical activity in AAA patients is beneficial, reducing cardiac, renal, and respiratory complications while maintaining safety.[36,37] A prospective randomized trial showed that community exercise programs significantly improved peak oxygen consumption (VO_2) and triglyceride levels, impacting perioperative mortality.[37]

Comprehensive Risk Factor Management

Long-term care of obese aortic patients should integrate:

- Targeted weight reduction through diet, exercise, GLP-1 RAs, and, where appropriate, bariatric surgery.[6,34,35]
- Aggressive blood pressure control, statin therapy, smoking cessation, and glycemic optimization.[4,38]
- Structured imaging surveillance with intervals tailored to aortic size, growth rate, and overall risk profile.[4,38]
- Sleep apnea screening and treatment, which may reduce aortic wall stress via reduced nocturnal hypertensive surges.[4]

CLINICAL SUMMARY AND KEY RECOMMENDATIONS

Obesity significantly modifies aortic disease risk and treatment outcomes, with distinct patterns between EVAR and TEVAR. Central adiposity drives perivascular inflammation, MMP activation, and aortic wall degeneration, increasing AAA/TAA/dissection prevalence. EVAR demonstrates the "obesity paradox" (lower 30-day mortality in BMI 25–35), while TEVAR carries higher overall mortality (OR 1.49) despite similar complication rates **(Figs. 6A and B)**.

Key interventional challenges and solutions:

- *Vascular access:* Ultrasound-guided puncture reduces failures by 70%; selective surgical cut-down or iliac conduits indicated for BMI ≥ 40 or hostile CFA anatomy.
- *Imaging optimization:* 3D CTA fusion + IVUS minimizes contrast volume, reducing AKI risk in TEVAR.
- *ATAAD surgery:* Partial upper sternotomy reduces mechanical ventilation time (40 vs. 47h), pulmonary infections (33% vs. 60%), and sternal dehiscence (0% vs. 17%) versus full sternotomy.
- *GLP-1 modulation:* Semaglutide/liraglutide slow aortic dilatation (0.36 vs. 1.05 mm/24 months); preoperative optimization (6+ months) may benefit high-risk obese patients.
- *Institutional factors:* Dedicated access teams, vascular surgery specialists, and enhanced monitoring eliminate most obesity-related complications.

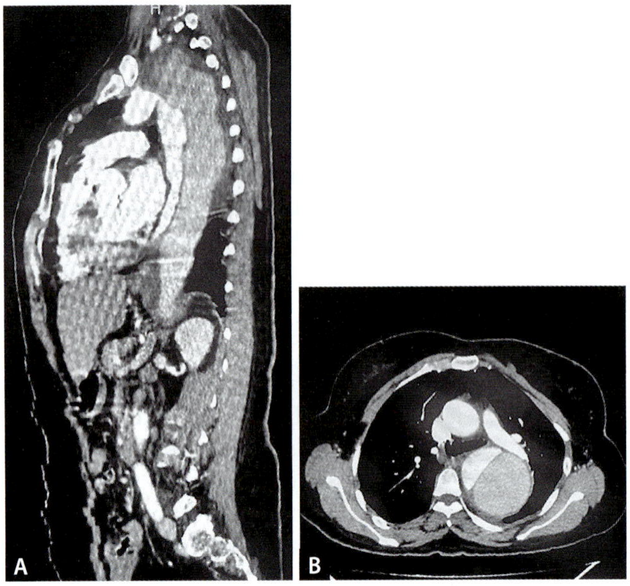

Figs. 6A and B: These images describe a contrast-opacified aorta containing a linear intimal flap that separates a high-attenuation true lumen from a variably opacified false lumen, with relative compression of the true lumen s/o aortic dissection.

Evidence-Based Recommendations

- *EVAR in obesity:* Class I (strong recommendation). Preferred approach for infrarenal AAA regardless of BMI < 40 with ultrasound-guided percutaneous access.
- *TEVAR in obesity:* Class IIa (reasonable). Proceed in high-volume centers (> 25 cases/year) with US-guided access, contrast minimization, and enhanced respiratory/renal monitoring.
- *ATAAD in obesity:* Partial upper sternotomy recommended over full sternotomy to reduce respiratory complications.
- *Absolute contraindications (Class III):* BMI > 45 + hostile thoracic anatomy, uncontrolled OSA (AHI > 50), or Class III obesity with connective tissue disorder.

CONCLUSION

Obesity—especially central adiposity—is a causal contributor to aortic aneurysm and dissection through PVAT dysfunction, chronic inflammation, and hemodynamic overload. It substantially increases the technical difficulty and perioperative risk of aortic interventions but does not preclude successful repair when managed with meticulous planning and tailored approaches.

The interventional challenges posed by obesity—vascular access complexity, imaging constraints, respiratory compromise, renal dysfunction, and wound healing impairment—are addressable through structured protocols: ultrasound-guided access, liberal use of surgical cut-down or iliac conduits in hostile anatomy, contrast and radiation minimization, enhanced perioperative monitoring, and selective minimally invasive surgical strategies (e.g., partial upper sternotomy for obese ATAAD patients).

Emerging pharmacologic therapies (GLP-1 agonists) and integrated prehabilitation pathways offer adjunctive benefit. Future research should define optimal perioperative protocols tailored to obesity class and phenotype, and prospective trials should evaluate structured weight-loss and metabolic interventions as disease-modifying therapy in obese aortic patients. Integration of weight-loss strategies, GLP-1 optimization, and tailored vascular access techniques into comprehensive aortic disease programs will enable safe and effective management of this challenging population.

REFERENCES

1. Lu F, Wang L, Pan A. Obesity and the obesity paradox in abdominal aortic aneurysm. Front Endocrinol (Lausanne). 2024;15:1410369.
2. Xie LF, He J, Wu QS, et al. Do obese patients with type A aortic dissection benefit from total arch repair through partial upper sternotomy? Front Cardiovasc Med. 2023;10:1086738.
3. Jelic S, Lederer DJ, Adams T, et al. Vascular inflammation in obesity and sleep apnea. Circulation. 2010;121:1014-21.
4. Poirier P, Giles TD, Bray GA, et al. Obesity and cardiovascular disease: pathophysiology, evaluation, and effect of weight loss: an update of the 1997 American Heart Association scientific statement on obesity and heart disease from the obesity Committee of the Council on nutrition, physical activity, and metabolism. Circulation. 2006;113:898-918.
5. Kuzmik GA, Sang AX, Elefteriades JA. Natural history of thoracic aortic aneurysms. J Vasc Surg. 2012;56:565-71.
6. Naiem AA, Gohel MS, Sutton AJ, et al. Systematic review and meta-analysis evaluating the impact of obesity on outcomes of abdominal aortic aneurysm treatment. J Vasc Surg. 2022;75(4):1450-5.e3.
7. Li J, Zhang Y, Huang H, et al. The effect of obesity on the outcome of thoracic endovascular aortic repair: a systematic review and meta-analysis. Peer J. 2024;12:e17246.
8. Naazie IN, Chaikof EL, Almasri TN, et al. Association of body mass index with outcomes after thoracic endovascular aortic repair in the vascular quality initiative. J Vasc Surg. 2022;75(2):439-47.
9. Zakko J, Scali S, Beck AW, et al. Percutaneous total endovascular aortic repair outcomes in extremely obese patients. J Endovasc Ther. 2014;60(4):921-8.
10. Cheng Z, Wang L, Pan A, et al. Central obesity markers and abdominal aortic aneurysm presence: systematic review and meta-analysis. Front Cardiovasc Med. 2023;10:1044560.

11. Galyfos G, Geropapas GI, Kerasidis S, et al. The effect of body mass index on major outcomes after vascular surgery. J Vasc Surg. 2017;65(4):1193-207.
12. Isselbacher EM, Preventza O, Hamilton Black J, et al. 2022 AHA/ACC/AATS Guideline for the Management of Thoracic Aortic Disease. Circulation. 2022;146(10):e334-e482.
13. Mussa FF, Horton JD, Moridzadeh R, et al. Acute aortic dissection and intramural hematoma: a systematic review. JAMA. 2016;316(7):754-63.
14. Schneider DB, Dimick JB, Risucci D, et al. Percutaneous femoral artery access during endovascular aortic aneurysm repair in the Vascular Quality Initiative. J Vasc Surg. 2020;71(5):1585-94.
15. De Vos H, Fontaine V, Van Herzeele I, et al. Total percutaneous access versus surgical access in endovascular aortic aneurysm repair. J Endovasc Ther. 2016;23(1):115-22.
16. Shermak MA, Deaton DH, McDaniel MD, et al. Ultrasound-guided femoral artery access improves rate of access-related complications. J Vasc Surg. 2008;48(5):1186-90.
17. Yei K, Lim G, Keeling WB, et al. Six-step approach for optimizing ultrasound-guided femoral artery puncture. Catheter Cardiovasc Interv. 2024;103(3):e456-e462.
18. Malas MB, Hutton LC, Arepally GM, et al. Percutaneous access: success predicted by vessel diameter in endovascular abdominal aortic repair. Vasc Med Rev. 2012;23(2):67-74.
19. Hoel AW, Fairman RM, Johnson MS, et al. Large-bore vascular closure: new devices and techniques. Interv Cardiol Rev. 2019;14(1):6-12.
20. Hajibandeh S, Hajibandeh M, Antoniou GA, et al. Endovascular abdominal aortic aneurysm repair: risk factors and mitigation strategies. Eur J Vasc Endovasc Surg. 2024;67(2):142-54.
21. Schanzer A, Messina L, Dillavou E, et al. Femoral vascular access-site complications in the cardiac catheterization laboratory. Cardiology. 2016;18(4):12-9.
22. Sohail MR, Karamanos E, Timaran CH, et al. Large-bore vascular closure device outcomes: SAFE-VEIN study. Catheter Cardiovasc Interv. 2024;103(4):527-36.
23. Rushton M, Singh R, Tiwari V, et al. Vascular access specialist teams versus standard practice in endovascular aortic repair. BMJ Open. 2024;14(7):e082631.
24. Pelosi P, Croci M, Ravagnan I, et al. The effects of body mass on lung volumes, respiratory mechanics, and gas exchange during general anesthesia. Anesth Analg. 1998;87(3):654-60.
25. Radiological Society of North America. Fluoroscopy time and radiation dose in endovascular procedures. AJNR Am J Neuroradiol. 2012;33(11):2043-9.
26. Suneja M, Kumar AB. Obesity and perioperative acute kidney injury: focused review. J Crit Care. 2014;29(4):694.e1-694.e6.
27. Choban PS, Flancbaum L. The impact of obesity on surgical outcomes. J Am Coll Surg. 1997;185(6):593-603.
28. Prowle JR, Peake SL, Bellomo R, et al. Fluid management for the prevention and attenuation of acute kidney injury. Nat Rev Nephrol. 2014;10(1):37-47.
29. Xie LF, He J, Wu QS, et al. Total arch replacement through partial upper sternotomy in obese patients with acute aortic dissection. Eur J Cardiothorac Surg. 2023;63(1):ezad012.
30. Aizawa K, Suzuki T, Masuda H, et al. Obesity as a risk factor for young onset acute aortic dissection. Kyobu Geka. 2013;66(6):437-44.
31. Li J, Zhang Y, Huang H, et al. Obesity and outcomes of thoracic endovascular aortic repair: meta-analysis. PeerJ. 2024;12:e17246.
32. Badran A, Kamal A, Fatima S, et al. Elective thoracic aortic aneurysm surgery in a tertiary center. Cureus. 2023;15(5):e39102.
33. Borghese O, Serino A, Piazza M, et al. Obesity is not associated with adverse outcomes following fenestrated and branched endovascular aortic repair. Ann Vasc Surg. 2023;95:42-9.
34. Chen X, Wang Y, Liu J, et al. GLP-1 receptor agonists are associated with reduced ascending aortic dilatation progression in type 2 diabetes. Circulation. 2025;151(18):1742-52.
35. Yoshida T, Kadam S, Smith PW. Liraglutide attenuates angiotensin II-induced aortic dissection. J Hypertens. 2024;42(3):412-24.
36. Kocher A, Coti I, Laufer G, et al. Minimally invasive aortic valve replacement through an upper hemisternotomy: the Vienna technique. Eur J Cardiothorac Surg. 2018;53(Suppl 1):ii29–ii31.
37. Inoue Y, Minatoya K, Seike Y, et al. Early results of total arch replacement under partial sternotomy. Gen Thorac Cardiovasc Surg. 2018;66(5):327-33.
38. Deschka H, Erler S, Machner M, et al. Surgery of the ascending aorta, root remodelling and aortic arch surgery with circulatory arrest through partial upper sternotomy: results of 50 consecutive cases. Eur J Cardiothorac Surg. 2013;43(3):580-4.

SECTION 11

Obesity with Stroke: Clinical Insight and Management

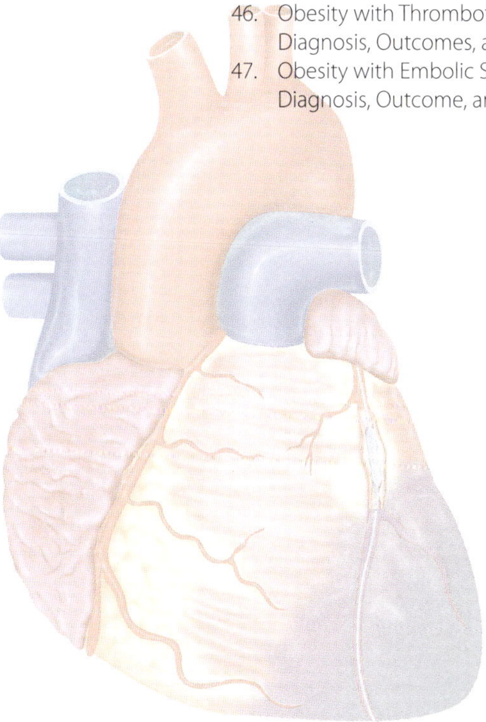

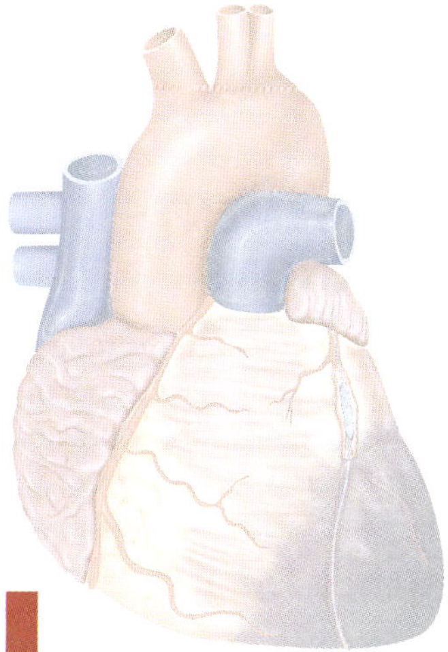

46

CHAPTER

Obesity with Thrombotic Stroke: Clinical Insights, Diagnosis, Outcomes, and Clinical Management

Lovelina Singh

INTRODUCTION

Obesity is a chronic and complex disease marked by excessive fat. By 2025, obesity will affect more than a quarter of adults in many countries and is a major cause of cardiovascular and cerebrovascular problems. Ischemic (thrombotic) stroke is closely linked to obesity through several mechanisms that promote atherothrombosis, thrombosis, and metabolic dysfunction. Therefore, tackling obesity is critical for preventing both primary and secondary strokes.[1-6]

PATHOPHYSIOLOGY—MECHANISMS LINKING OBESITY TO THROMBOSIS

Adipose Tissue as Endocrine Organ[7-11]

Adipocytes and nearby support cells release adipokines (such as leptin, adiponectin, and resistin), cytokines (such as IL-6 and TNF-α), and chemokines. Visceral fat is especially active and inflammatory. The chronic release of these substances leads to endothelial activation, the recruitment of white blood cells, and oxidative stress, all of which promote the formation and instability of atherosclerotic plaques.[7-11]

Prothrombotic and Hypofibrinolytic State[1,4,5]

Obesity increases levels of fibrinogen, factor VII, factor VIII, von Willebrand factor, and plasminogen activator inhibitor-1 (PAI-1). Higher PAI-1, mainly produced by fat tissue, reduces plasmin generation and fibrinolysis. This results in persistent blood clots and a greater risk of arterial and venous thrombosis. Endothelial dysfunction and heightened platelet activity (partially driven by leptin) further increase the risk of clotting.[7-14]

Insulin Resistance, Dyslipidemia, and Atherogenesis

Insulin resistance, predominant in obesity, leads to atherogenic dyslipidemia, characterized by high triglycerides, low HDL, and small-dense LDL particles. This is coupled with glycation and oxidative stress, which promote plaque development. The combination of lipid-driven atherosclerosis and a prothrombotic environment raises the chances of clot formation in the brain's arteries.[24-30]

Hemodynamic Contributors and Cardiac Sources

Obesity boosts blood volume and heart output, leads to high blood pressure, and increases the risk of atrial enlargement and atrial fibrillation. Atrial fibrillation can occur without symptoms and is often overlooked as a source of cardio embolism in obese patients. Obstructive sleep apnea (OSA), common among those with obesity, worsens nighttime low oxygen levels, increases sympathetic activation, raises blood pressure, and causes arrhythmias in the atria.[15,16]

EPIDEMIOLOGY AND CLINICAL PATTERNS

Large population studies and stroke registries from 2020 to 2024 show consistent links between excess weight and a higher risk of ischemic stroke, earlier age at first stroke, and a higher rate of vascular health issues. Central obesity measurements (waist circumference, waist-hip ratio) predict stroke risk better than BMI alone.

Age and Demographics

Obese individuals typically experience ischemic strokes about 8–12 years earlier than those with normal weight in many studies. Socioeconomic and ethnic factors influence this pattern; disadvantaged groups with high levels of obesity often bear a greater early stroke burden.

Stroke Subtypes and Patterns

Obesity is most closely tied to strokes caused by large artery atherosclerosis and small vessel disease (associated with hypertension and diabetes). Though less common, cerebral venous thrombosis and paradoxical embolism (related to venous thromboembolism) are still important, especially in severely obese patients who are less mobile.

RISK STRATIFICATION AND BIOMARKERS

Thorough risk assessment should consider more than just BMI. Important factors include body measurements (waist circumference, waist-height ratio), metabolic profiles, inflammatory markers, blood clotting tests, and imaging for atherosclerotic buildup.

Laboratory and Biomarker Panel

Essential tests: Fasting glucose, HbA1c, lipid profile, kidney and liver function tests, full blood count, CRP/hs-CRP, fibrinogen, and D-dimer. Specialized tests may be needed: PAI-1, thrombin generation tests, antiphospholipid antibodies, and thrombophilia tests for younger patients or unusual cases.

Imaging and Vascular Evaluation

Neuroimaging: Noncontrast CT for urgent evaluation; CT angiography (CTA), or MR angiography (MRA) for checking vessel blockages and plaque; MRI using diffusion-weighted imaging for early detection of infarcts. Carotid ultrasound and high-resolution vessel wall MRI may help find risky plaques and internal bleeding in obese patients with atherosclerosis.

ACUTE CLINICAL MANAGEMENT—PRACTICAL CONSIDERATIONS

Managing acute ischemic stroke in obese patients follows standard protocols for treatment and support, with specific logistical and dosing considerations noted in the following text.

Prehospital and Emergency Triage

Quick identification (using FAST or BE-FAST screening) is vital. Prehospital notifications should address body size issues that could impact airway management, imaging table weight limits, and the need for extra staff during transfers.

IV Thrombolysis (Alteplase)

The weight-based dose (0.9 mg/kg, max 90 mg) should use the patient's actual measured weight upon arrival. In severely obese patients, getting an accurate weight is crucial; if that is not available, achieve the best estimate and document why. Be aware of possible differences in how the drug works in such cases, but stick to guideline dosing.[20,21]

Mechanical Thrombectomy[22,23]

Mechanical thrombectomy works well for large-vessel blockages regardless of BMI. Planning for the procedure should account for access challenges, weight limits of tables and instruments, and the possibility of longer procedural time. Early mobilization after the procedure should weigh the need to reduce the risk of blood clots against safety at the procedure site.[22,23]

Periprocedural Anticoagulation and VTE Prevention

Preventing blood clots in immobilized stroke patients is essential. Medication for prevention (like low-molecular-weight heparin or unfractionated heparin) should consider weight; LMWH dosing often relies on weight. Mechanical prevention (such as intermittent pneumatic compression) should be added for patients at high risk of bleeding.

SECONDARY PREVENTION—DETAILED STRATEGIES

Antiplatelet and Anticoagulant Therapy

Antiplatelet treatment is necessary for noncardioembolic ischemic strokes (aspirin, clopidogrel; short-term dual antiplatelet therapy in select minor stroke/TIA cases). For cardioembolic strokes (like those stemming from AF or thrombus in the left atrial appendage), long-term anticoagulation is required. Direct oral anticoagulants (DOACs) are usually effective, but little data exists for patients with extreme body weight (>120 kg or BMI >40). In such cases, it may be best to discuss options and consider using warfarin with INR monitoring.

Lipid and Blood Pressure Management

High-dose statin therapy should be given for atherosclerotic ischemic strokes unless contraindications exist. Blood pressure targets should follow guidelines (for many, this means lowering to below 130/80 mm Hg). Weight loss efforts often lead to significant improvements in blood pressure and lipid levels.

Glycemic Management and Metabolic Therapies

Aim for optimal glycemic control based on individualized targets for hemoglobin A1c, considering comorbid conditions and frailty. Evidence supports the use of GLP-1 receptor agonists (like semaglutide) for weight loss and reducing cardiovascular risk; these drugs can be included in a multidisciplinary secondary prevention plan, taking into account any contraindications and cost or access issues.

Weight Management Interventions

A stepped-care approach is suggested:

- *Lifestyle changes:* Structured diet plans, progressive exercise suited to individual abilities, and support for behavioral changes.
- *Medications:* Consider GLP-1 receptor agonists and other approved weight-loss drugs for suitable patients.
- *Metabolic/bariatric surgery:* For patients who meet criteria (like BMI ≥40 or BMI ≥35 with related health issues) following assessment by multiple specialists—this surgery has been linked to long-term reductions in cardiovascular events.[35-40]

Sleep Apnea Treatment[15,16]

Routine screening for OSA in obese stroke survivors is essential. Continuous positive airway pressure (CPAP) improves sleep, helps control blood pressure, and may decrease the chance of future cardiovascular events; support for adherence is critical.

REHABILITATION, FUNCTIONAL RECOVERY, AND COMPLICATIONS[17,18]

Obese stroke survivors face specific rehabilitation challenges like mobility limitations, risk of pressure ulcers, the need for specialized equipment (such as bariatric beds and hoists), and a higher prevalence of health problems that can slow recovery. Rehabilitation programs should include early mobilization, VTE prevention, nutritional assessment to support safe weight loss without hindering recovery, and psychological support for depression and motivation.[29-39]

Functional Outcome Predictors

Factors indicating poorer recovery include higher initial BMI (especially class II–III obesity), uncontrolled diabetes, severe stroke (high NIHSS), and social factors such as limited support and access to rehabilitation services.[17-19]

Pressure Injury and Skin Care

Preventing pressure ulcers with protocols, frequent repositioning, and team-based wound care is vital for obese patients who have mobility challenges.

SPECIAL POPULATIONS AND CONSIDERATIONS

Considerations include elderly obese patients, young adults with strokes related to obesity, women (focusing on pregnancy-related risks), and ethnic groups exhibiting different fat distribution patterns. Young obese adults experiencing strokes should undergo extensive evaluations for causes (including thrombophilia and heart sources) due to their higher lifetime risk.

HEALTH SYSTEMS, EQUITY, AND IMPLEMENTATION

Implementing obesity-focused secondary prevention requires system-level integration. Specialized clinics should combine neurology, cardiometabolic medicine, nutrition, sleep medicine, and behavioral health. Equity issues include access to new treatments and surgery for obesity, which vary both globally and within countries.[38,39]

RESEARCH GAPS AND FUTURE DIRECTIONS

Key research priorities include:

- Randomized trials examining weight-loss treatments (both drug and surgical) focusing on stroke recurrence and functional outcomes.
- Pharmacokinetic and outcome research for DOACs in individuals with severe obesity.
- Biomarker-focused risk assessment (such as PAI-1, adipokine panels, and thrombin generation).
- Studies on integrating metabolic and stroke secondary prevention methods.
- Long-term studies on the effects of GLP-1 receptor agonists on the rates of recurrent strokes.

CONCLUSION

Use comprehensive measures of body fat (like waist circumference and waist-height ratio) during risk assessment. Guarantee prompt treatment for acute strokes; obesity does not prevent reperfusion—use precise weight for dosing. Regularly screen for OSA and provide treatment as needed. Initiate early prevention of blood clots, paying attention to weight-based dosing. Begin or continue recommended antiplatelet/anticoagulant therapy based on the stroke type. Refer eligible patients for multidisciplinary services for weight management; consider GLP-1 receptor agonists and bariatric surgery when suitable. Adjust rehabilitation programs and resources to meet the requirements of obese survivors. Monitor and tackle social factors that impact access to metabolic therapies and long-term rehabilitation.[38,39]

REFERENCES

1. Bushnell CD, Kernan WN, Sharrief AZ, et al. Guidelines for the primary prevention of stroke: A guideline for healthcare professionals. Stroke. 2024;55(1):e1-e60.
2. Steinberger J. Obesity and cardiovascular disease: Pathophysiology, evaluation, and effect of weight loss. Circulation. 2014;129(7):e71-99.
3. Lavie CJ, Laddu D, Arena R, et al. The obesity paradox and cardiovascular diseases: A fresh perspective. Prog Cardiovasc Dis. 2017;60(5-6):521-8.
4. Strazzullo P, D'Elia L, Cairella G, et al. Excess body weight and incidence of stroke: Meta-analysis of prospective studies. Stroke. 2010;41(5):e418-26.
5. O'Donnell MJ, Xavier D, Liu L, et al. Risk factors for ischemic and intracerebral hemorrhagic stroke in 22 countries (INTERSTROKE). Lancet. 2010;376(9735):112-23.
6. Abdelaal M, le Roux CW, Docherty NG. Morbidity and mortality associated with obesity. Ann Transl Med. 2017;5(7):161.
7. Samad F, Ruf W. Inflammation, obesity, and thrombosis. Blood. 2013;122(20):3415-22.
8. Lau DC, Dhillon B, Yan H, et al. Adipokines: Molecular links between obesity and atherothrombosis. Am J Physiol Heart Circ Physiol. 2005;288:H2031-41.
9. De Taeye BM. Adipocyte-derived PAI-1 contributes to hypercoagulability in obesity. J Clin Invest. 2005;115(5):1318-24.
10. Bouchard L. Plasma PAI-1 levels in obesity: Clinical relevance. J Thromb Haemost. 2020;18(8):2078-90.
11. Mertens I, Van Gaal L. Obesity, haemostasis and the fibrinolytic system. Obes Rev. 2002;3(2):85-101.
12. Mesnier J. Obesity phenotypes and risk of ischemic stroke. Stroke. 2021;52(3):912-9.
13. Emerging Risk Factors Collaboration. Diabetes mellitus, fasting glucose, and risk of stroke. Lancet. 2010;375(9733):2215-22.
14. Wang Y, et al. Obesity and risk of stroke in adults: A systematic review and meta-analysis. J Stroke Cerebrovasc Dis. 2014;23(7):1990-8.
15. Howard VJ, et al. Sleep apnea and risk of stroke. Stroke. 2006;37(9):2300-5.
16. Redline S, Yenokyan G, Gottlieb DJ, et al. Obstructive sleep apnea-hypopnea and incident stroke. Am J Respir Crit Care Med. 2010;182(2):269-77.
17. Kim Y, et al. Body mass index and functional outcomes after ischemic stroke. Stroke. 2020;51(3):912-9.
18. Andersen KK, et al. Influence of BMI on stroke incidence and outcomes. Stroke. 2010;41(7):e181-6.
19. Oesch L, Tatlisumak T, Arnold M, et al. Obesity paradox in stroke: Myth or reality? Int J Stroke. 2017;12(4):369-76.
20. Kernan WN, Ovbiagele B, Black HR, et al. Guidelines for the prevention of stroke in patients with stroke and TIA. Stroke. 2014;45(7):2160-236.
21. Powers WJ, Rabinstein AA, Ackerson T, et al. 2019 Update to acute ischemic stroke guidelines. Stroke. 2019;50: e344-418.
22. Goyal M, Menon BK, van Zwam WH, et al. Endovascular thrombectomy after large vessel stroke: Meta-analysis. Lancet. 2016;387(10029):1723-31.
23. Saver JL, Goyal M, van der Lugt A, et al. Time to treatment and outcomes with endovascular therapy. JAMA. 2016;316(12):1279-88.
24. Coutinho JM. Cerebral venous thrombosis in obese patients. Stroke. 2010;41(10):e88-93.
25. Tripolino C. Dyslipidemia, small dense LDL and stroke risk. Nutr Metab Cardiovasc Dis. 2021;31(4):1083-9.
26. Eckel RH. Obesity and type 2 diabetes: Pathophysiologic mechanisms. Lancet. 2005;365:1415-28.

27. Boulanger M, Scherer PE. Adipose tissue, inflammation and vascular disease. Circ Res. 2019;124:1788-806.
28. Petersen KF, Shulman GI. Pathogenesis of insulin resistance. N Engl J Med. 2022;387(22):2054-66.
29. Grundy SM, Cleeman JI, Daniels SR, et al. Metabolic syndrome and cardiovascular disease. Circulation. 2005;112:2735-52.
30. Fox CS. Waist circumference and stroke risk. Stroke. 2007;38:1055-61.
31. Yatsuya H. Cardiovascular risk and waist-hip ratio. Atherosclerosis. 2010;212(1):316-21.
32. Koton S, Rexrode KM. Trends in incidence of ischemic stroke by obesity status. Neurology. 2013;81(17):1582-9.
33. Shen L. Obesity and long-term mortality after stroke. Neurology. 2017;88(15):1514-20.
34. Cani PD. Gut microbiota, endotoxemia, and stroke risk in obesity. Nat Rev Cardiol. 2019;16:259-72.
35. Blüher M. Obesity: Global epidemiology and pathogenesis. Nat Rev Endocrinol. 2019;15(5):288-98.
36. Wilding JPH, Batterham RL, Calanna S, et al. Once-weekly semaglutide in adults with overweight or obesity. N Engl J Med. 2021;384:989-1002.
37. Marso SP, Bain SC, Consoli A, et al. Semaglutide and cardiovascular outcomes. N Engl J Med. 2016;375:1834-44.
38. Sjöström L. Bariatric surgery and reduction in cardiovascular events. JAMA. 2012;307(1):56-65.
39. Adams TD, Gress RE, Smith SC, et al. Long-term mortality after gastric bypass. N Engl J Med. 2007;357:753-61.
40. Virani SS. Heart disease and stroke statistics—2023 update. Circulation. 2023;147:e102-e103.

47

CHAPTER

Obesity with Embolic Stroke: Clinical Insights, Diagnosis, Outcome, and Management

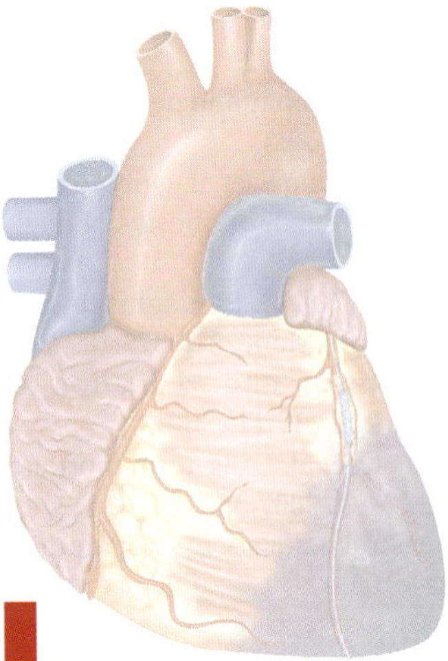

Vinit Suri

INTRODUCTION

Obesity has been described as "the great humbler" because many investigators have anticipated finding an easy cure only to learn that it is stubbornly difficult to treat. Worldwide, stroke is the second leading cause of death and obesity is the second leading preventable cause of death after tobacco. Obesity is a significant risk factor for multiple cardiovascular diseases, such as coronary disease, coronary death, congestive heart failure, and stroke.

Individuals are classified as overweight if their body mass index (BMI) is between 25 and 30 kg/m^2, obese if it is between 30 and 40 kg/m^2, and morbidly obese if it is >40 kg/m^2. BMI has been criticized because it does not differentiate between fatness, obesity, and adiposity measurement. Other methods, including waist circumference and central and peripheral fat mass, have also been proposed for an alternative diagnosis, though BMI continues to be most widely used for the classification of obesity. For every 1 unit increase in BMI (≈7 pounds for a human of average height), the risk for ischemic stroke increases ≈5% and the risk seems to be nearly linear starting with a still-normal BMI of ≈20 kg/m^2. Obesity is widely accepted and known as a cardiocerebrovascular risk factor, so it is recommended that adequate body weight control (BMI <25 kg/m^2) is maintained as primary prevention, as well as a secondary prevention of stroke.

Obesity has long been known to increase the risk of various cardiovascular diseases, and its role in causing atrial fibrillation is undisputed. There are multiple mechanisms, including structural remodeling of the heart, epicardial adipose tissue (EAT), and inflammatory markers secreted by the fatty tissues which may lead to atrial fibrillation and hence cardioembolic stroke in obese adult population. Atrial fibrillation in obese individuals is the most common cause of embolic stroke. The causal relationship between obesity and atrial fibrillation is also evident because studies over the years have reported a positive role of weight loss in treating and preventing atrial fibrillation in obese patients.

OBESITY AND ISCHEMIC STROKE

Four important concepts[1] emerge from research on the relationship between obesity and stroke risk. First, compared with BMI, measures of central obesity are better predictors of stroke. Second, the relative risk for stroke associated with obesity seems to be higher for middle-aged individuals compared with older individuals. Third, the association is true for both ischemic and intraparenchymal hemorrhage, but it is more consistently demonstrated for the former. Finally, the association between obesity and increased risk for stroke is actually explained by the presence of hypercholesterolemia, hypertension, and diabetes mellitus in obese individuals.

There is a debate whether obesity itself is a risk factor for ischemic stroke or whether metabolic syndrome which is a consequence of obesity defines the risk. Hence, there has been a recent concept that classifies individuals into six phenotypes based on the BMI and metabolic health: Metabolically healthy normal weight (MHNW), metabolically healthy overweight (MHOW), metabolically healthy obese (MHO), metabolically unhealthy normal weight (MUNW), metabolically unhealthy overweight (MUOW), and metabolically unhealthy obese (MUO),[2] whether MHOW/obese increases the cardiocerebrovascular risk is a substantial debate. However, a recent meta-analysis of eight prospective cohorts revealed that MHO is positively associated with an elevated risk of stroke.[3]

However, obesity is widely accepted and known as a cardiocerebrovascular risk factor, so it is recommended that adequate body weight control (BMI <25 kg/m^2) is maintained as primary prevention as well as secondary prevention.

OBESITY AND CARDIOEMBOLIC STROKE

Cardioembolic stroke can be caused by various cardiac disorders including atrial fibrillation, vegetations, atrial or ventricular clots and tumors, patent foramen ovale, and aortic arch atheromas of which atrial fibrillation is one of the most important causes. There are a variety of risk factors in turn predisposing for atrial fibrillation. Modifiable factors include smoking, hypertension, diabetes mellitus, sedentary lifestyle, and obesity and nonmodifiable factors include genetic predisposition.

Obesity is a well-known risk factor for multiple systemic conditions such as metabolic syndrome, type 2 diabetes mellitus, and sleep-related disorders. In addition, it contributes directly to the development of various cardiovascular disorders such as hypertension, myocardial infarction, and, more notably, atrial fibrillation. Several mechanisms have been suggested in obesity-driven AF, including cardiac adiposity, inflammation, fibrosis, oxidative stress, ion channel remodeling, and autonomic dysfunction.[4] These mechanisms promote the development of AF triggers and substrate, ultimately leading to increased AF vulnerability. Obesity causes hemodynamic changes that alter cardiac morphology and physiology. Obesity causes a high output state due to an increase in total blood volume, which causes an increased cardiac output and filling pressures leading to left ventricular enlargement. Obesity hypoventilation syndrome and OSA can also increase pulmonary artery pressures leading to right ventricular hypertrophy which causes concentric hypertrophy and left ventricular diastolic dysfunction, eventually leading to systolic dysfunction in turn leading to a significant increase in left atrium pressure, and increase in left atrial wall thickness, left atrial enlargement, insufficient left atrial emptying, dysfunction of the left atrium, and ultimately atrial fibrillation. Gene expression of all renin–angiotensin–aldosterone system (RAAS) components, including aldosterone, increases in obese patients, and aldosterone causes atrial fibrosis and conduction pathway disturbances, a risk factor for atrial fibrillation. EAT is adipose tissue surrounding the heart, located between the myocardium and the visceral pericardium, and meta-analysis suggests that it is more predominant in patients with atrial fibrillation than in healthy controls.[5] EAT is a better predictor of atrial fibrillation than other measures of adiposity, such as BMI, waist circumference, waist-to-hip ratio, and intrathoracic fat. Apart from providing a fat cushion to the myocardium, EAT secretes cytokines such as vascular endothelial growth factor-1, interleukins, transforming growth factor-β, metalloproteinase 1–13, tissue necrosis factor-α, CRP, monocyte chemoattractant protein-1, and adipokines such as adiponectin, leptin, resistin, visfatin, and omentin, all of which are involved in atrial remodeling. In long-term obesity, there is greater EAT and, therefore, a greater risk of developing fibrosis, which provides a substrate for reentry circuits in the myocardium. Apart from causing fibrosis, EAT infiltration may also separate myocardial fibers, thus disrupting the normal conduction pathway.

OBESITY AND STROKE PARADOX

There is a phenomenon called "The Obesity Paradox" which states that patients with an elevated BMI may present with better clinical outcomes after a heart failure and after stroke. This means that even though obesity leads to higher complications and risk of suffering from multiple diseases and complications, high adiposity can provide a protective role in stroke resulting in reduced mortality and better outcomes when stroke does occur.

The obesity paradox can be explained by the protective effect of a major endocrine organ known as adipose tissue, which secretes soluble tumor necrosis factor-alpha (TNF-α)-receptors and neutralizes the impact of TNF-α in the human biological system and inflammatory responses. Overweight and obese patients have higher lipoproteins and lipids serum levels, and these play an important role in detoxifying and binding lipopolysaccharides and are related to inflammatory cytokines cascade blocking. Further, these molecules impede the inflammatory state after a stroke episode. There are other potential explanations for the paradox. Obese stroke patients, compared with low or normal-weight patients, may experience stroke subtypes associated with lower recurrence risk (like small artery disease) or receive more aggressive therapy. Alternatively, the paradox may simply reflect a survival bias; obese patients who have survived until their event may be somehow healthier individuals or have metabolically benign obesity. A 12-month longitudinal observational study on patients with documented atrial fibrillation concludes that mortality in obese patients was inversely related to high BMI.[6]

MANAGEMENT OF CARDIOEMBOLIC STROKE IN OBESITY

Management of cardioembolic stroke in obese individuals includes lifestyle modification, risk factor management, weight loss, rate and rhythm control, and anticoagulation.

Weight Loss

Studies have shown the positive effect of weight loss and risk factor management on atrial fibrillation progression and recurrence. For example, the supervised obesity reduction trial for AF ablation (SORT-AF)[7] demonstrated that well-structured weight-loss programs were beneficial for obese patients with atrial fibrillation who underwent ablation by decreasing the recurrences in adult population suffering from persistent atrial fibrillation. A randomized control trial of 150 Australian adults reported a decrease in atrial fibrillation disease burden, symptom severity, and disease recurrence in the intervention group undergoing weight reduction compared to the control group.[8] Furthermore, sustained weight control and metabolic bariatric surgery have shown a reduced atrial fibrillation disease burden in the long term.

Vitamin K Antagonists

A patient's high BMI can change the pharmacodynamics and pharmacokinetics of warfarin. Anticoagulation is one of the pillars of atrial fibrillation management to minimize thromboembolic risk. Patients with high BMI (>40 kg/m^2) should preferentially be treated with warfarin rather than direct oral anticoagulants (DOACs) even though these individuals have a significantly higher warfarin requirement than patients with lower BMI. A meta-analysis confirmed that the dose of warfarin required to achieve an international normalized ratio within the therapeutic range was positively associated with body weight and recommended that obese and morbidly obese patients may benefit from an increase in warfarin dose of 30–50%.[9] Plasma vitamin K is positively correlated with triglyceride concentrations and, therefore, warfarin dose. This may explain why the optimal warfarin dose increases with weight. In addition, obese and morbidly obese patients prescribed warfarin needed a longer median time to achieve a therapeutic international normalized ratio, a higher average daily dose, and mean discharge dose than healthy-weight patients. Together, this evidence indicates that BMI status should be considered during the initiation of warfarin therapy.

Direct Oral Anticoagulants

Direct oral anticoagulants are increasingly recommended over warfarin for stroke prevention in patients with AF. However, there is only minimal clinical trial data of DOACs in patients with high BMI. The International Society on Thrombosis and Haemostasis does not support the use of DOACs in patients with a BMI of >40 kg/m^2 or >120 kg/m^2.[10] Evidence about the impact of obesity on safety and the effectiveness of anticoagulants is limited. A systematic review including 13 studies found no indication that obesity is related to inferior DOAC effectiveness or safety.[11] These findings support the recommendation that a standard fixed dose of DOACs is adequate for healthy-weight and obese patients. However, further research is required to conclusively determine optimal dosing in morbidly obese patients.

Effect of Obesity on Rate Control

The therapeutic goal of rate control is to regulate heart rate to ≤80 beats per minute at rest. β-blockers are used to slow the heart rate in patients with AF. Lipophilicity of a drug can alter its pharmacokinetics in obese patients. Sotalol, a markedly hydrophilic β-blocker, showed similar pharmacokinetic parameters in obese and lean patients, whereas lipophilic β-blocker propranolol had a lower volume of distribution in obese patients. Total volume of distribution at steady state for labetalol and nebivolol (lipophilic β-blockers) was larger in obese than in healthy-weight subjects and positively related to weight. However, when accounting for body weight, volume of distribution (per kilogram) is slightly but not significantly smaller in obese patients. These results suggest lipophilic β-blockers preferentially diffuse into lean tissue over adipose tissue, in contrast to other lipophilic drugs that commonly show increased distribution volume and prolonged elimination half-life in obese patients. Thus, additional factors to lipid solubility are possibly involved in β-blockers' pharmacokinetics in obese patients.

A study on diltiazem blocker for rate control management of AF with a rapid ventricular response also confirmed the impact of obesity on rate control drugs.[12] In this study, obese patients receiving a weight-based dose were significantly more likely to achieve a heart rate <100 beats per minute than those administered a fixed dose. In addition, the distribution and clearance of digoxin, a positive inotropic cardiac glycoside, were seemingly unaffected by obesity. However, no studies to date report on digoxin effectiveness in obese versus healthy-weight patients with AF.

Effect of Obesity on Rhythm Control

- Direct cardioversion is commonly used as a means of converting AF to sinus rhythm. Both pharmacologic and electrical cardioversion failure was demonstrated to be more frequent in obese patients. Patients with higher BMI have shown lower success rates with cardioversion. Due to adiposity, the lower success rate likely results from reduced energy delivery to the heart. It has been suggested to use more powerful defibrillators to increase the success rates of cardioversion in morbidly obese patients. The probable reason may be that obese patients have more EAT, intrathoracic fat, and visceral adipose tissue, which block energy delivery to the heart.
- *Pharmacologic rhythm control strategies:* Class I AADs are commonly used for rhythm control by inhibiting sodium channels to reduce cardiac excitability and abnormal automaticity. Class I AADs primarily block fast sodium channels, which are responsible for rapid depolarization of phase 0 of the cardiac action potential. For every 2.5-unit increment of BMI, there is a reduced effectiveness of class I AADs in patients with obesity. Flecainide, a class Ic AAD, reduces peak sodium current by inhibiting voltage-gated sodium channels. Obesity effects interchamber differences in sodium current density and β-subunit expression and hence flecainide shows reduced efficacy in AF in obese patients. Class III AADs block potassium channels, leading to increased APD and ERP, increased cardiac wave-length, and prevention of reentry. Amiodarone is a class III AAD used for the treatment of AF and ventricular arrhythmias. Amiodarone and its metabolite, N-desethylamiodarone, have high lipophilicity and particularly accumulate in adipose tissue. There is evidence that amiodarone clearance is affected by BMI and is reduced by 22.3% when BMI is >25 kg/m^2, thus resulting in significantly higher serum concentration in obese patients.

The European Society of Cardiology guidelines[13] recommend class I AADs over class III AADs for patients with AF but with no mention of specific recommendations for obese patients with AF. On the basis of the current evidence of AAD in obese individuals, one should select class III AAD for obese patients with AF, since class III AADs may show higher efficacy in the obese patient subgroup over class I. Further randomized clinical trials are required to establish clear AAD guidance in obese patients.

Effect of Obesity on AF after Cardiac Surgery

Postoperative AF (POAF) is the most common complication after cardiac surgery. The occurrence of POAF is multifactorial, and obesity is recognized as an independent risk factor. Recently, meta-analyses have found that EAT was associated with POAF. The underlying mechanism of POAF is not fully elaborated. EAT has an abundance of ganglionic plexi, which may contribute to postsurgery autonomic imbalance and initiate POAF. In obesity, EAT also undergoes disequilibrium between excessive oxidative stress and protective adipokine levels, promoting POAF susceptibility. Obesity-mediated structural remodeling, including increased cardiac fibrosis, left ventricular hypertrophy, and LA dilatation, may also trigger POAF because they are independent risk factors of AF.

CONCLUSION

- Obesity mediates AF by structural and electrical remodeling, including adiposity, neurohormonal changes, inflammation, fibrosis, and oxidative stress.
- Obesity can also affect AF treatment success through alterations in drug pharmacokinetics and target expression or function. Preference for using DOAC and class III AADs for obese patients with AF, since they retain similar efficacy in obesity.
- Obese patients with AF are more likely to experience reduced catheter ablation outcomes, comorbidities, and POAF.
- Although the obesity paradox has been postulated in AF, weight loss is a demonstrated beneficial measure in reducing AF burden and postablation recurrence.
- In addition, EAT, a key mediator of obesity-linked AF, provides a promising therapeutic target, both pharmacologically and in ablation.

REFERENCES

1. Kernan WN, Inzucchi SE, Sawan C, et al. Obesity: a stubbornly obvious target for stroke prevention. Stroke. 2013;44:278-86.
2. Stefan N, Häring HU, Hu FB, et al. Metabolically healthy obesity: epidemiology, mechanisms, and clinical implications. Lancet Diabetes Endocrinol. 2013;1:152-62.
3. Ma LZ, Sun FR, Wang ZT, et al. Metabolically healthy obesity and risk of stroke: a meta-analysis of prospective cohort studies. Ann Transl Med. 2021;9:197.
4. Gupta V, Munjal JS, Jhajj P, et al. Obesity and atrial fibrillation: a narrative review. Cureus. 2022;14(11):e31205.

5. Gaeta M, Bandera F, Tassinari F, et al. Is epicardial fat depot associated with atrial fibrillation? A systematic review and meta-analysis. Europace. 2017;19:747-52.
6. Rodríguez-Reyes H, Lara-Vaca S, Ochoa-Guzmán A, et al. Obesity paradox and 12 month outcome in patients with atrial fibrillation. Arch Med Res. 2021;52:233-9.
7. Gessler N, Willems S, Steven D, et al. Supervised obesity reduction trial for AF ablation patients: results from the SORT-AF trial. Europace. 2021;23:1548-58.
8. Abed HS, Wittert GA, Leong DP, et al. Effect of weight reduction and cardiometabolic risk factor management on symptom burden and severity in patients with atrial fibrillation: a randomized clinical trial. JAMA. 2013;310:2050-60.
9. Self TH, Wallace JL, Sakaan S, et al. Effect of body weight on dose of vitamin K antagonists. South Med J. 2015;108:637-43.
10. Antiarrhythmic and DOAC dosing in obesity. (2019). [online] Available from https://www.acc.org/latest-in-cardiology/articles/2019/07/03/08/22/antiarrhythmic-and-doac-dosing-in-obesity. [Last accessed April, 2022].
11. Proietti M, Guiducci E, Cheli P, et al. Is there an obesity paradox for outcomes in atrial fibrillation? A systematic review and meta-analysis of non-vitamin K antagonist oral anticoagulant trials. Stroke. 2017;48:857-66.
12. Ward SM, Radke J, Calhoun C, et al. Weight-based versus non-weight-based diltiazem dosing in the setting of atrial fibrillation with rapid ventricular response. Am J Emerg Med. 2020;38:2271-6.
13. Hindricks G, Potpara T, Dagres N, et al. 2020 ESC Guidelines for the diagnosis and management of atrial fibrillation developed in collaboration with the European Association for Cardio-Thoracic Surgery (EACTS): the Task Force for the diagnosis and management of atrial fibrillation of the European Society of Cardiology (ESC) developed with the special contribution of the European Heart Rhythm Association (EHRA) of the ESC. Eur Heart J. 2021;42:373-498.

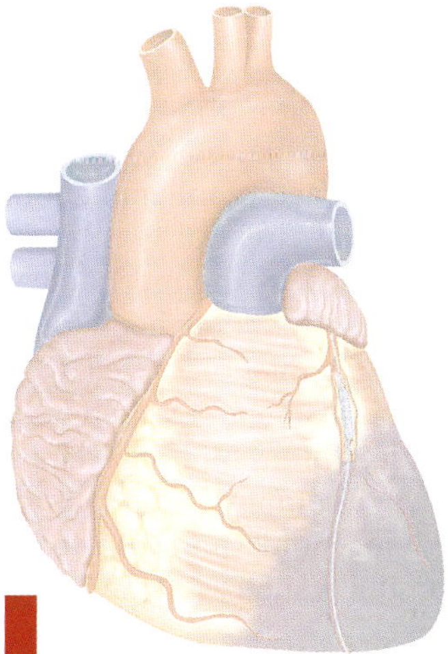

48

CHAPTER

Obesity in Hemorrhagic Stroke: Clinical Insights, Diagnosis, Outcome and Management

Joy Dev Mukherji, Mukesh Kumar, Vaibhav Deorari, Nilesh Jadhao

INTRODUCTION

Definition of Hemorrhagic Stroke

Hemorrhagic stroke is a disorder characterized by the abrupt onset of focal neurological symptoms caused by the rupture of intracranial blood vessels. This condition involves spontaneous bleeding into the brain parenchyma [intracerebral hemorrhage (ICH)], the subarachnoid space [subarachnoid hemorrhage or (SAH)], or the intraventricular space. It is a devastating subtype of acute stroke, accounting for about 35% of all strokes globally, with ICH comprising 29% and SAH about 6%.[1] Unlike ischemic stroke, which results from vessel occlusion, hemorrhagic stroke is caused by vessel rupture. It carries a disproportionately high risk of early mortality and long-term disability, with a 1-month case fatality rate of around 40%.[2]

Hemorrhagic strokes are classified based on the site of bleeding and underlying pathophysiology **(Fig. 1)**.[3]

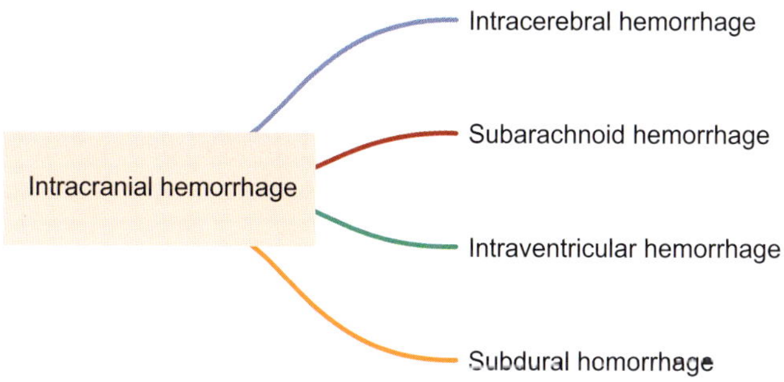

Fig. 1: Common types of intracranial hemorrhage.

- *ICH:* This is bleeding directly into the brain tissue. It can be categorized based on location (e.g., lobar, putaminal, and thalamic) or cause, such as arteriolosclerosis-related (often linked to hypertension) or cerebral amyloid angiopathy (CAA)-related bleeds. It is the most common and dangerous type of hemorrhagic stroke.
- *SAH:* This involves bleeding into the space between the pia mater and the arachnoid mater surrounding the brain. About 85% of spontaneous SAH cases are due to a ruptured intracranial aneurysm.
- *Other intracranial hemorrhages:* These include primary intraventricular hemorrhage (IVH), which is rare, and spontaneous subdural hemorrhage (SDH).

Prevalence and Impact of Obesity

Obesity, defined as a body mass index (BMI) of 30 kg/m^2 or higher, has reached epidemic proportions globally. In India alone, over 135 million people are affected by obesity. The prevalence in India varies significantly by gender, region, and socioeconomic status, with rates ranging from 11.8 to 31.3%.[4] For instance, a 2015–2016 survey showed obesity prevalence in Punjab was 27.8% for men and 31.3% for women, while in Jharkhand it was 11.1 and 10.3%, respectively.[5]

Obesity is a major risk factor for a range of chronic noncommunicable diseases (NCDs), including hypertension, type 2 diabetes mellitus, dyslipidemia, coronary artery disease, and certain cancers. It is associated with low-grade chronic inflammation, endothelial dysfunction, and hormonal dysregulation, which collectively contribute to vascular damage and heightened cardiovascular risk. The economic and health burden is immense, with obesity being a leading cause of morbidity and mortality worldwide.

Why Focus on the Intersection

The intersection of obesity and intracranial hemorrhage is significant due to several compelling reasons. Obesity is a key contributor to hypertension, which is the primary risk factor for ICH. By promoting systemic inflammation, insulin resistance, and endothelial dysfunction, obesity elevates blood pressure, thereby increasing the risk of hemorrhagic stroke.[6,7] Furthermore, as the global prevalence of obesity rises, a greater number of patients presenting with ICH are also obese, creating unique clinical challenges. These patients often have multiple comorbidities, complex physiological alterations affecting drug metabolism, and difficulties in clinical management, from airway control to surgical intervention.[8]

Paradoxically, some studies suggest that obese patients with stroke may have better outcomes than their nonobese counterparts, a phenomenon termed the "obesity paradox". Investigating this paradox is crucial for understanding the complex interplay between adipose tissue, inflammation, and stroke prognosis, which could guide nutritional management and therapeutic strategies.[9] Given the high mortality and disability associated with ICH and the growing obesity epidemic, a focused examination of their intersection is essential for improving prevention, acute management, and long-term outcomes for this high-risk population.

PATHOPHYSIOLOGY

Mechanisms of Hemorrhagic Stroke

Spontaneous hemorrhagic stroke results from the rupture of an intracranial blood vessel. The underlying mechanisms vary by stroke subtype:[3]

- *ICH:* The most common cause is the rupture of small and deep-penetrating arterioles damaged by chronic hypertension. This damage, known as arteriolosclerosis, manifests as lipohyalinosis, microaneurysms (Charcot–Bouchard aneurysms), microatheroma, or fibrinoid necrosis. These weakened vessels, particularly in the basal ganglia, thalamus, pons, and cerebellum, are prone to rupture under high pressure. Another major cause, especially for lobar ICH in the elderly, is CAA, where amyloid protein deposition weakens cortical and leptomeningeal arteries.
- *SAH:* The predominant cause is the rupture of a saccular ("berry") aneurysm, typically located at the bifurcation of large arteries in the circle of Willis. The exact cause of aneurysm formation is not fully understood but involves genetic factors, inflammation, and biomechanical stress on the vessel wall.

The initial brain injury is caused by the mechanical compression of brain tissue by the expanding hematoma and the resulting increase in intracranial pressure (ICP). This leads to reduced cerebral perfusion and ischemia in the surrounding tissue. Secondary brain injury develops over hours to days and is driven by a complex inflammatory cascade, perihematomal edema, and the neurotoxic effects of blood breakdown products such as hemoglobin and thrombin.

Obesity-related Vascular Changes

Obesity induces a state of chronic, low-grade inflammation, and endothelial dysfunction, which are central to its impact on vascular health.

- *Endothelial dysfunction:* In obesity, there is a decrease in nitric oxide (NO) bioavailability, which impairs vasodilation. This is coupled with increased oxidative stress and upregulation of proinflammatory cytokines, which damage the endothelium. Normal perivascular adipose tissue (PVAT) helps dilate blood vessels, but in obesity, PVAT becomes dysfunctional and releases adipo-cytokines that reduce vasorelaxation. This dysfunction contributes to vascular remodeling, increased arterial stiffness, and atherosclerosis.[7]
- *Structural vascular changes:* Obesity is associated with alterations in both large and small arteries. Studies on subcutaneous resistance arteries in obese individuals show increased media thickness and media-to-lumen ratio, indicating vascular remodeling. The aorta in individuals with obesity shows disorganized extracellular matrix, significantly increased collagen deposits, and a thinner tunica media, which can lead to increased aortic stiffness.[6]
- *Hypertension pathogenesis:* The vascular changes are key drivers of obesity-related hypertension. Mechanisms include activation of the sympathetic nervous system and the renin-angiotensin-aldosterone system (RAAS), increased renal sodium reabsorption, and insulin resistance. This sustained hypertension is a primary driver of the arteriolosclerosis that leads to deep ICH.[6]

The "Obesity Paradox" in Stroke

The "obesity paradox" is a counterintuitive phenomenon where overweight or obese patients with certain chronic

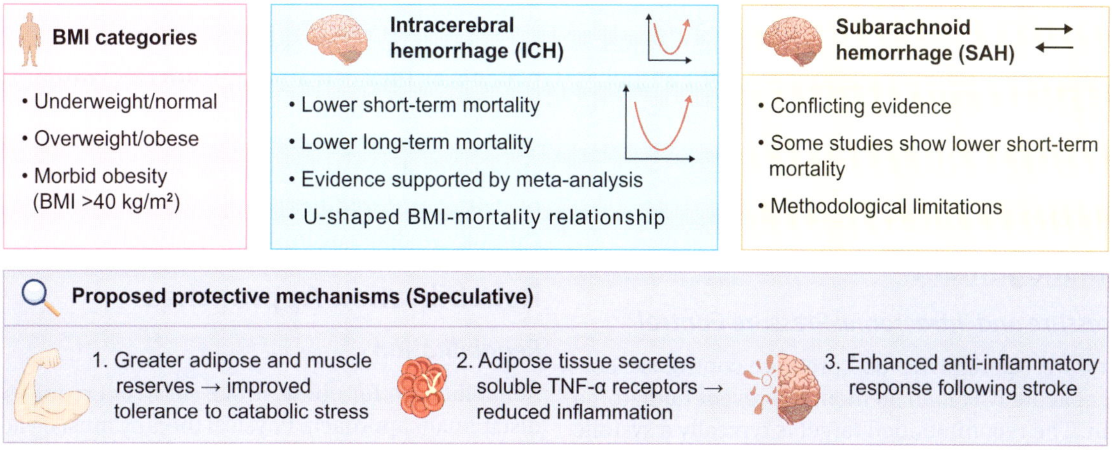

Fig. 2: The obesity paradox in stroke outcomes.

diseases, including stroke, exhibit better outcomes, and lower mortality compared to their normal-weight or underweight counterparts **(Fig. 2)**. Several studies have identified this paradox in ICH. A meta-analysis of six studies found that obesity was significantly associated with lower short-term (in-hospital or 30-day) and long-term mortality after ICH. Some studies found that while obesity was protective, morbid obesity (BMI >40 kg/m^2) was associated with higher mortality, suggesting a U-shaped relationship. The evidence for an obesity paradox in SAH is less clear, with studies showing conflicting results. Two studies found a protective effect of obesity on short-term SAH mortality, but these were limited by methodological shortcomings.[10] The reasons for the paradox are not fully understood and remain speculative.[9,11] The proposed reasons could be obese patients have larger adipose and muscle mass reserves, which may help them tolerate the catabolic and inflammatory stress of critical illness better than leaner individuals. Also, adipose tissue secretes soluble TNF-α receptors that may neutralize proinflammatory cytokines, dampening the harmful systemic inflammation that follows a stroke. Obese patients may mount a more robust anti-inflammatory response in the days following a stroke.

CLINICAL PRESENTATION

The classic symptoms of ICH, such as sudden neurological deficits, headache, nausea, vomiting, and altered consciousness, are expected to be similar regardless of body habitus. Similarly, for SAH, the hallmark symptom is a sudden, severe "thunderclap" headache. However, one study noted that vertigo was more prevalent in female stroke patients.

DIAGNOSTIC WORKUP

Imaging (CT/MRI Considerations in Obese Patients)

Neuroimaging is the cornerstone of diagnosing intracranial hemorrhage. Noncontrast computed tomography (CT) is the primary imaging modality for acute stroke to quickly differentiate between ischemic and hemorrhagic types. It is highly sensitive for detecting acute blood. Magnetic resonance imaging (MRI) can provide more detailed information about the hemorrhage, including its age and potential underlying causes.

Laboratory and Biomarker Profiles

Obese patients are more likely to have associated metabolic abnormalities, such as dyslipidemia (elevated LDL and triglycerides, low HDL) and hyperglycemia. Markers of inflammation, such as C-reactive protein, may be elevated in obese individuals and have been linked to ICH severity.

Challenges in Diagnosis Related to Obesity

Obesity presents several challenges in the clinical assessment and diagnosis of critically ill patients, which are applicable to those with intracranial hemorrhages. Physical examination can be difficult in obese patients. Assessing for subtle neurological signs may be hampered by body habitus. Noninvasive blood pressure measurement can be inaccurate due to difficulties in finding an appropriately sized cuff. Diagnostic imaging can be challenging. Many CT and MRI scanners have weight and bore size limitations, which can prohibit or delay imaging for morbidly obese patients. The quality of portable bedside radiographs is often poor in obese individuals. Abdominal and pelvic ultrasonography quality can also be limited by extensive adipose tissue.

MANAGEMENT STRATEGIES

Acute Management

Blood Pressure and Intracranial Pressure Control

Blood pressure: Aggressive blood pressure control is a cornerstone of acute ICH management to prevent hematoma expansion. The recommended target is typically a systolic blood pressure of <140 mm Hg. Continuous intravenous antihypertensives are often used.[6]

Intracranial pressure: Management of elevated ICP is critical. This includes head elevation, osmotic therapy (e.g., mannitol), and potentially sedation and mechanical ventilation to control $PaCO_2$. ICP monitoring via an external ventricular drain may be necessary.

Surgical Considerations in Obese Patients

Surgical evacuation of the hematoma is considered for patients with large cerebellar hemorrhages (>3 cm) or certain superficial lobar hematomas (>30 mL) who are experiencing neurological decline.[12] But morbidly obese patients present significant surgical and anesthetic challenges. Airway management is more difficult due to anatomical factors such as a short, thick neck, and excess pharyngeal tissue. Furthermore, surgical positioning can be difficult, and prolonged surgery times increase the risk of complications like pressure injuries. Anesthetic drug dosing must be carefully adjusted based on ideal or lean body weight to avoid overdose or prolonged effects.

Secondary Prevention

Lifestyle Interventions

It is considered as the first-line approach for managing obesity and its related risk factors. Various comprehensive lifestyle programs that recommend a reduced-calorie diet, increased physical activity, and behavioral support for at least 6–12 months. Not only weight reduction but long-term strategies are needed for weight maintenance. These interventions should be individualized based on the patient's preferences and capabilities.[13]

Pharmacotherapy

For patients with ICH, strict control of hypertension is paramount for secondary prevention. Antihypertensive drug regimens based on ACE inhibitors, ARBs, and calcium channel blockers are often preferred in obese patients as they can also improve insulin sensitivity and have neutral or beneficial metabolic effects.[6] Weight-loss medications may be considered as an adjunct to lifestyle changes in eligible patients (e.g., BMI $\geq$30 kg/m^2 or $\geq$25 kg/m^2 with comorbidities), but their use post-ICH must be carefully weighed against potential risks.[14]

Rehabilitation Approaches

Rehabilitation

Rehabilitation for obese stroke survivors requires a multidisciplinary approach. Physical therapy must be adapted to account for limited mobility and potential musculoskeletal comorbidities. Early mobilization is crucial to prevent complications like VTE. Respiratory physiotherapy, including coughing exercises and incentive spirometry, is important to prevent pulmonary complications.

Psychosocial Support and Counseling

Patients with obesity often experience anxiety and depression, which can be exacerbated after a stroke. Psychosocial support and counseling are critical components of recovery, addressing both the psychological impact of the stroke and the challenges of managing obesity.

COMPLICATIONS AND SPECIAL CONSIDERATIONS

Medical Complications in Obese Stroke Patients

Obese critically ill patients have an increased risk of many complications. About 70% of morbidly obese individuals have OSA, which heightens perioperative respiratory issues such as atelectasis, hypoventilation, aspiration, and ventilator-associated pneumonia. They are also prone to VTE (DVT and PE) due to immobility, venous stasis, and a hypercoagulable state, requiring both mechanical and pharmacologic prophylaxis. Obesity raises infection risks, including sepsis and surgical site infections, from poor wound healing and chronic inflammation. Drug dosing is complex because of altered pharmacokinetics: Use IBW for drugs such as propofol, fentanyl, and some antibiotics, and TBW for heparin and vancomycin.[15]

Bariatric Surgery and Stroke Risk/ Management

Bariatric surgery is the most effective treatment for severe obesity and significantly improves or resolves comorbidities such as hypertension and diabetes. A meta analysis of 17 studies showed that bariatric surgery was associated with a remarkable reduction in the risk of cerebrovascular events, including both ischemic and hemorrhagic stroke.[16] For patients who have had bariatric surgery, clinicians should be aware of potential long-term nutritional deficiencies that could impact recovery.

OUTCOMES AND PROGNOSIS

Impact of Obesity on Acute Outcomes

The impact of obesity on acute outcomes in ICH is complex, largely due to the "obesity paradox". Multiple large and retrospective studies have found that obesity and morbid obesity are associated with lower in-hospital and 30-day mortality after ICH. One meta-analysis showed a significant association between obesity and lower short-term mortality.[17,18] Despite the survival advantage, obesity is associated with a higher rate of medical complications during hospitalization. Obese ICH patients have higher rates of pulmonary, renal, and venous thromboembolic (VTE) complications.[10] They are also more likely to require mechanical ventilation and have a longer ICU and hospital length of stay.

Long-term Outcomes

The obesity paradox extends to long-term outcomes. Studies have shown that overweight and obese patients have lower long-term mortality after ICH compared to normal-weight individuals. A meta-analysis confirmed a significant association between obesity and reduced long-term mortality. The relationship with functional disability is also paradoxical. Some studies report that a higher BMI is associated with better functional recovery at 3 and 12 months, as measured by the modified Rankin Scale (mRS). However, this association can be attenuated or disappear after adjusting for initial neurological severity, suggesting that obese patients may simply present with less severe strokes.[9] Some evidence suggests a lower risk of recurrent stroke in overweight and obese patients compared to their normal-weight counterparts.

Influence of Obesity on Recovery and Rehabilitation

Obese patients face unique challenges during recovery and rehabilitation. Limited mobility, joint pain (e.g., osteoarthritis), and decreased exercise tolerance can hinder participation in physical therapy. Basic nursing care, such as changing posture, wound dressing, and preventing pressure sores, is more difficult and labor-intensive in obese patients. These patients are at a higher risk for pressure sores due to their weight and compromised circulation in dependent areas. After an ICH, implementing lifestyle changes for weight loss can be challenging due to physical disability and potential cognitive or emotional changes.

CONCLUSION

- Hemorrhagic stroke results from the rupture of intracranial vessels, leading to bleeding within or around the brain; it causes high early mortality and disability. Major subtypes are ICH and SAH.
- Obesity triggers chronic inflammation, endothelial dysfunction, and arterial stiffness, all of which increase cerebrovascular vulnerability.
- The "obesity paradox" suggests lower short- and long-term mortality among obese ICH patients, though mechanisms remain unclear.
- Obese stroke patients face higher risks of respiratory, thromboembolic, and infectious complications.
- Secondary prevention focuses on lifestyle modification, hypertension control, and weight management through tailored programs.
- Rehabilitation requires multidisciplinary adaptation for limited mobility and comorbidities.

REFERENCES

1. Hsu SP, Kang JH, Hung TH, et al. Postdischarge participation and functional outcomes across three common stroke subtypes based on the exploratory retrospective study. Sci Rep. 2025;15(1):35432.
2. González-Pérez A, Gaist D, Wallander MA, et al. Mortality after hemorrhagic stroke: data from general practice (The Health Improvement Network). Neurology. 2013;81(6):559-65.
3. Morais Filho AB, Rego TL, Mendonça LL, et al. The physiopathology of spontaneous hemorrhagic stroke: a systematic review. Rev Neurosci. 2021;32(6):631-58.
4. Ahirwar R, Mondal PR. Prevalence of obesity in India: A systematic review. Diabetes Metab Syndr. 2019;13(1):318-21.
5. International Institute for Population Sciences (IIPS) and ICF. National Family Health Survey (NFHS-4), 2015–16: India. Mumbai: IIPS; 2017.
6. Seravalle G, Grassi G. Obesity and hypertension. Pharmacol Res. 2017:122:1-7.
7. Engin A. Endothelial dysfunction in obesity and therapeutic targets. Adv Exp Med Biol. 2024:1460:489-538.
8. Marik P, Varon J. The obese patient in the ICU. Chest. 1998;113(2):492-8.
9. Wang Z, Wang J, Wang J, et al. The obesity paradox in intracerebral hemorrhage: a systematic review and meta-analysis. Front Endocrinol (Lausanne). 2023;14:1255538.

10. Rautalin I, Kaprio J, Korja M. Obesity paradox in subarachnoid hemorrhage: a systematic review. Neurosurg Rev. 2020;43(6):1555-63.
11. Artham SM, Lavie CJ, Milani RV, et al. The obesity paradox: impact of obesity on the prevalence and prognosis of cardiovascular diseases. Postgrad Med. 2008;120(2):34-41.
12. Cobis AY, Bisri DY, Rachman IA. Perioperative management of hemorrhagic stroke in morbidly obese patients: A narrative review. Surg Neurol Int. 2025;16:401.
13. Semlitsch T, Stigler FL, Jeitler K, et al. Management of overweight and obesity in primary care—A systematic overview of international evidence-based guidelines. Obes Rev. 2019;20(9):1218-30.
14. Semlitsch T, Stigler FL, Jeitler K, et al. Management of overweight and obesity in primary care—A systematic overview of international evidence-based guidelines. Obes Rev. 2019;20(9):1218-30.
15. Bajwa SJ, Sehgal V, Bajwa SK. Clinical and critical care concerns in severely ill obese patient. Indian J Endocrinol Metab. 2012;16(5):740-8.
16. Cai Z, Zhang Q, Jiang Y, et al. Bariatric Surgery and the Risk of Cerebrovascular Events: a Meta-analysis of 17 Studies Including 3,124,063 Subjects. Obes Surg. 2022;32(11):3523-32.
17. Andersen KK, Olsen TS. The obesity paradox in stroke: lower mortality and lower risk of readmission for recurrent stroke in obese stroke patients. Int J Stroke. 2015;10(1):99-104.
18. Forlivesi S, Cappellari M, Bonetti B. Obesity paradox and stroke: a narrative review. Eat Weight Disord. 2021;26(2):417-23.

49

CHAPTER

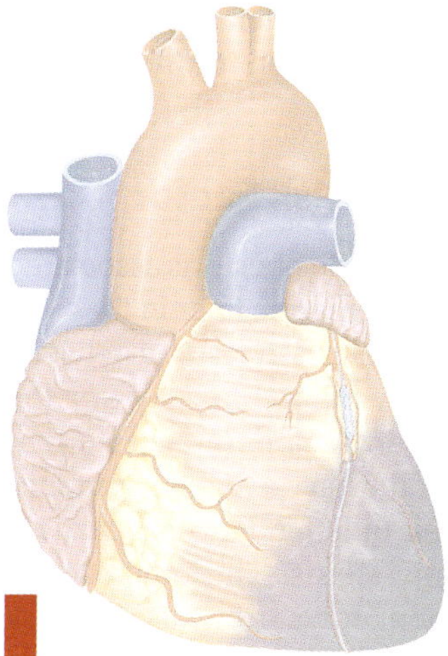

Obesity and Dementia: A Comprehensive Clinical Chapter

Lovelina Singh

INTRODUCTION

Dementia is a term for several diseases that affect memory, thinking, and the ability to perform daily activities. The illness gets worse over time. It mainly affects older people, but not all people will get it as they age.

Things that increase the risk of developing dementia include:

- Age (more common in those 65 or older)
- High blood pressure (hypertension)
- High blood sugar (diabetes)
- *Being overweight or obese*
- Smoking
- Drinking too much alcohol
- Being physically inactive
- Being socially isolated
- Depression

Dementia is a syndrome that can be caused by a number of diseases which over time destroy nerve cells and damage the brain, typically leading to deterioration in cognitive function (i.e., the ability to process thought) beyond what might be expected from the usual consequences of biological aging. While consciousness is not affected, the impairment in cognitive function is commonly accompanied, and occasionally preceded, by changes in mood, emotional control, behavior, or motivation.

Dementia has physical, psychological, and social and economic impacts, not only for people living with dementia, but also for their careers, families, and society at large. There is often a lack of awareness and understanding of dementia, resulting in stigmatization and barriers to diagnosis and care.[1]

Dementia is a growing global public health challenge, marked by cognitive decline, memory deficits, and behavioral changes. In 2019, the global prevalence of dementia reached 57.4 million people, and this figure is projected to triple by 2050, rising to approximately 152.8 million cases. Concurrently, dementia-related deaths have escalated, nearly tripling from 0.56 million in 1990 to 1.62 million in 2019, with its global economic burden reaching an estimated $948 billion in 2016.[2]

Obesity and dementia represent two of the most important converging health crises of the 21st century. Dementia currently affects >55 million people worldwide, and projections estimate that this number will rise to 153 million by 2050 as global populations age and survival improves. Obesity, on the other hand, has tripled since the 1970s and now affects >650 million adults globally. The two conditions share not only similar epidemiological trajectories but also overlapping biological pathways, risk factors, and social determinants. Increasingly, clinicians are faced with older adults who present with both cognitive decline and obesity—or who demonstrate complex body composition phenotypes such as sarcopenic obesity, cachexia, or unintentional weight loss in the context of early neurodegenerative change.

Understanding the intricate bidirectional relationship between obesity and dementia is essential for prevention, diagnosis, and management. Evidence accumulated over the last two decades has established midlife obesity as a major modifiable risk factor for later life Alzheimer's disease (AD), vascular dementia (VaD), and mixed dementia. In contrast, late life obesity displays a different, often confusing pattern known as the "obesity paradox," in which higher body mass index (BMI) may appear protective for outcomes such as mortality or dementia incidence. This paradox has led to debate and confusion among clinicians and policymakers. However, deeper analyses suggest that reverse causality, survival bias, and the limitations of BMI as a measurement tool explain most of this phenomenon.

EPIDEMIOLOGY

Global Rise of Obesity and Dementia

Obesity prevalence continues to rise across all world regions, including low- and middle-income countries where dual malnutrition burdens now coexist. Parallel to this, dementia prevalence has increased not merely because of aging populations but also because of improved survival from cardiovascular diseases, diabetes, and cancer—conditions which themselves interact with metabolic health. Thus, epidemiologically, obesity and dementia occupy the same risk environment.

Obesity is a significant modifiable risk factor for dementia. This study aims to quantify the global impact of obesity on dementia burden and examine how national strategies for managing overweight/obesity and dietary factors influence dementia prevalence and mortality, with a focus on sex-specific differences. We used data from the Global Burden of Disease (GBD) and World Health Organization (WHO) to evaluate the association between obesity age-standardized prevalence rate (ASPR) and dementia age-standardized mortality rate (ASMR) across 161 countries.[1] A two-step multivariate analysis adjusted for socioeconomic and lifestyle factors was performed. Temporal trends in dementia were analyzed based on the presence of national obesity management strategies and varying dietary scores. A 1% increase in national obesity prevalence was associated with a 0.36% increase in dementia mortality in males and 0.12% in females. A 1% increase in national obesity ASPR was associated with an increase in ASPR of dementia by 0.26% for males and 0.05% for females. Males exhibited a higher susceptibility to obesity-related dementia. Countries with national obesity management strategies showed a significantly greater reduction in dementia mortality, particularly among females ($p = 0.025$). Higher dietary scores were associated with a more significant decrease in dementia prevalence across both sexes. Rising obesity prevalence is linked to increased dementia burden globally, with males being more vulnerable to this relationship. National management of overweight/obesity and healthier dietary habits may help mitigate the dementia burden, emphasizing the need for integrated public health interventions.[3-6]

Midlife Obesity as Causal Risk Factor

Studies consistently show that midlife obesity is associated with a 30–70% increased risk of dementia later in life. This association is strongest when obesity is measured between ages 40 and 65.[3] Large prospective cohorts from the United States, Scandinavia, and Asia demonstrate that individuals with obesity in midlife have a higher incidence of AD, VaD, and mixed dementia independent of education, smoking, and socioeconomic status. The relationship persists even after adjustment for cardiovascular risk factors, suggesting that obesity has independent effects on neurodegeneration.

Obesity in middle age might increase the risk of dementia at older ages, whereas obesity in old age could reduce the dementia risk. An understanding of the association of BMI (measured in kg/m^2) with dementia is a public health priority because the number of people affected by dementia worldwide is expected to rise from 30 million in 2010, to 106 million in 2050, and the prevalence of obesity is also increasing worldwide. In England, the prevalence of obesity has almost doubled between 1993 and 2010, and the global burden of obesity in 2008 was estimated to be 1.46 billion overweight adults (BMI $\geq$25 kg/m^2) and 502 million obese adults (BMI $\geq$30 kg/m^2).[4-6]

Late-life Obesity and Obesity Paradox[5]

Late-life obesity behaves differently. When BMI is measured over age 70, the association with dementia risk weakens substantially. Some studies report a neutral association, while others suggest mild protective effects. However, this protective effect is likely artefactual. Individuals with preclinical dementia commonly experience unintentional weight loss years before formal diagnosis. This reverse causation makes late-life underweight look like a high-risk state and late-life obesity appear beneficial. Another factor is survival bias: those obese individuals who survive into older age may represent biologically resilient subgroups.

Fat Distribution and Visceral Adiposity[5,6]

BMI is a crude measure that does not capture differences in fat distribution, especially visceral adiposity, which is metabolically active and strongly associated with inflammation, insulin resistance, and cardiovascular risk. Studies using CT or MRI-derived abdominal fat measures consistently show that visceral fat predicts cognitive decline better than BMI or waist circumference alone. Women, particularly postmenopausal women, appear more vulnerable to the cognitive effects of central obesity.

Central obesity in midlife increases risk of dementia independent of diabetes and cardiovascular comorbidities. 50% of adults have central obesity; therefore, mechanisms linking central obesity to dementia need to be unveiled.

It has been known for some time that a centralized distribution of fat is linked with numerous health risks. The abdominal distribution of body fat, referred to as central obesity, is an independent and more potent risk factor for type 2 diabetes, insulin resistance, coronary heart disease, stroke, and mortality than total body obesity. Indeed, individuals with a healthy weight but with a centralized distribution of adipose tissue have a much higher risk of disease and death. This may be attributable in part to the role of intraabdominal fat, also known as visceral adiposity, on metabolic abnormalities, which increases risk of diabetes and cardiovascular disease. Visceral fat is more metabolically active than subcutaneous fat and is thought to have a stronger influence on adipocytokine production and insulin resistance.[5]

Recent population-based research shows that obesity contributes to cognitive impairment. Obesity, as measured by BMI, particularly in middle age, increases the risk of dementia, AD, and neurodegenerative changes. However, it remains unknown whether distribution of adiposity plays a similar role in dementia risk as it does with cardiovascular disease and diabetes.

Sarcopenic Obesity

Sarcopenic obesity is one of the most important phenotypes bridging obesity and dementia risk. It is defined by the coexistence of excess fat mass and low muscle mass and/or strength. Sarcopenia contributes to frailty, reduced mobility, and systemic inflammation. Because muscle is metabolically active tissue and produces myokines beneficial to brain health, its loss worsens metabolic flexibility and accelerates cognitive decline. Sarcopenic obesity predicts dementia far more strongly than obesity alone.[7,8]

PATHOPHYSIOLOGICAL MECHANISMS LINKING OBESITY TO DEMENTIA

Metabolic Syndrome and Vascular Brain Injury

Obesity frequently coexists with metabolic syndrome, diabetes, hypertension, and dyslipidemia. These conditions lead to cerebrovascular damage through mechanisms such as endothelial dysfunction, arterial stiffness, atherosclerosis, and impaired cerebral autoregulation. White-matter hyperintensities, small-vessel disease, lacunar infarcts, and microbleeds are common radiological findings in obese individuals with cognitive impairment. These lesions strongly correlate with gait disturbances, executive dysfunction, and slowed information processing.

Insulin Resistance as Core Mechanism

The brain is highly dependent on glucose for energy, and insulin plays a key role in neuronal survival, synaptic plasticity, and memory consolidation. Insulin resistance interferes with these processes. Furthermore, impaired insulin signaling increases amyloid-β production, reduces its clearance, and facilitates tau hyperphosphorylation. AD has therefore been conceptualized as "type 3 diabetes," though this description oversimplifies a complex disease process.[4,6]

Chronic Inflammation[4,9]

Adipose tissue is metabolically active and secretes a variety of inflammatory mediators, including IL-6, TNF-α, and CRP. These molecules disrupt the blood-brain barrier, activate microglia, and promote neuroinflammation. Chronic inflammation is a unifying mechanism in both metabolic disorders and neurodegenerative diseases. Visceral fat is the most potent source of inflammatory cytokines.[4,9]

Changes in Brain Morphology and Connectivity

Neuroimaging studies show that individuals with obesity have smaller hippocampal volumes, reduced total brain volume, and poorer white-matter integrity.[9,10] Longitudinal studies reveal that obesity accelerates age-related brain atrophy. Diffusion tensor imaging shows reduced fractional anisotropy in key white-matter tracts associated with memory, attention, and executive function.

Sarcopenic Obesity Mechanisms

Muscle tissue secretes myokines such as brain-derived neurotrophic factor (BDNF) and irisin, which support neurogenesis and synaptic plasticity. Loss of muscle mass reduces these protective signals. Sarcopenic individuals often have reduced physical activity, poor balance, and frailty—factors linked to dementia progression.

DIAGNOSTIC APPROACH

History-taking

A detailed clinical history must capture weight trajectory, the timing of any weight loss relative to cognitive change, appetite variation, activity level, sleep patterns, depression, and comorbid conditions. Unintentional weight loss, even before overt cognitive deficits appear, raises suspicion for early neurodegeneration.

Cognitive Evaluation[9,10]

Standard tools include MMSE, MoCA, ACE-III, and detailed neuropsychological batteries. Executive dysfunction, psychomotor slowing, and attention deficits may be more prominent in obesity-linked vascular cognitive impairment. AD typically presents with episodic memory loss and then spreads to visuospatial and language deficits.

Anthropometry and Body Composition[5,9]

Beyond BMI, waist circumference, waist-hip ratio, and body composition (DXA or BIA) help identify visceral adiposity and sarcopenia. Grip strength, gait speed, and chair-rise tests provide insights into frailty and muscle function.

Laboratory Assessment

This includes HbA1c, fasting insulin, lipid panel, thyroid function, vitamin D/B12, inflammatory markers, and markers of liver function to detect nonalcoholic fatty liver disease, which independently contributes to cognitive decline.

Neuroimaging[7,8]

MRI is the imaging modality of choice. It helps differentiate AD, frontotemporal dementia, Lewy body dementia, and VaD. Obesity-associated imaging findings include reduced hippocampal volume, white-matter hyperintensities, and deep-brain microstructural changes.

MANAGEMENT STRATEGIES

Prevention in Midlife[2,3]

Midlife is the optimal window for intervention. A weight loss of 5–10% through diet and physical activity improves insulin sensitivity, reduces cardiovascular risk, and may reduce dementia risk decades later. A Mediterranean diet rich in fruits, vegetables, fish, and monounsaturated fats has strong observational evidence supporting its neuroprotective effect.

Management in Older Adults with Mild Cognitive Impairment

In early stages of cognitive decline, weight management requires careful balance. Moderate, intentional weight loss may improve metabolic health but must not lead to muscle loss. Resistance training is essential for protecting brain health through increased BDNF and improved cerebral blood flow.

Advanced Dementia

Unintentional weight loss is common and associated with poor prognosis. Primary goals include maintaining comfort, preventing malnutrition, supporting hydration, and optimizing swallowing safety.

GLP-1 Receptor Agonists[10]

Drugs such as liraglutide and semaglutide have demonstrated neuroprotective properties in preclinical studies. Observational human studies show reduced dementia risk in diabetics treated with GLP-1 agonists. However, large clinical trials have not yet confirmed disease-modifying effects in AD.

Sarcopenic Obesity Treatment

Treatment focuses on preserving muscle mass: high-protein diets, resistance training, vitamin D optimization, and avoidance of sedating medications.

CONCLUSION[1,2]

Public health strategies must emphasize prevention of obesity early in life while simultaneously addressing malnutrition and frailty in older adults. Policies should include improved urban walkability, healthier school food systems, early screening for metabolic disorders, and social support systems that prevent loneliness—a powerful risk factor for both obesity and dementia.

REFERENCES

1. GBD Collaborators. Estimation of the global prevalence of dementia in 2019 and forecasted prevalence in 2050:

an analysis for the Global Burden of Disease Study 2019. Lancet Pub Health. 2022;7(2):e105-e125.
2. Livingston G, Huntley J, Sommerlad A, et al. Dementia prevention, intervention, and care: 2020 report of the Lancet Commission. Lancet. 2020;396(10248):413-46.
3. Whitmer RA, Sidney S, Selby J, et al. Midlife cardiovascular risk factors and risk of dementia in late life. Neurology. 2005;64(2):277-81.
4. Pedditzi E, Peters R, Beckett N. The risk of overweight/obesity in mid-life and late life for the development of dementia: a systematic review and meta-analysis of longitudinal studies. Age Ageing. 2016;45(1):14-21.
5. Qizilbash N, Gregson J, Johnson ME, et al. BMI and risk of dementia in two million people over two decades: a retrospective cohort study. Lancet Diabetes Endocrinol. 2015;3(6):431-6.
6. Tolppanen AM, Ngandu T, Kåreholt I, et al. Midlife and late-life body mass index and late-life dementia: results from a prospective population-based cohort. J Alzheimers Dis. 2014;38(1):201-9.
7. Buchman AS, Wilson RS, Bienias JL, et al. Change in body mass index and risk of incident Alzheimer disease. Neurology. 2005;65(6):892-7.
8. Prado CM, Wells JC, Smith SR, et al. Sarcopenic obesity: A critical appraisal of the current evidence. Clin Nutr. 2012;31(5):583-601.
9. Debette S, Beiser A, Hoffmann U, et al. Visceral fat is associated with lower brain volume in healthy middle-aged adults. Ann Neurol. 2010;68(2):136-44.
10. Yoon S, et al. Obesity. 2021;29:882-90.

SECTION 12

Obesity and Kidney

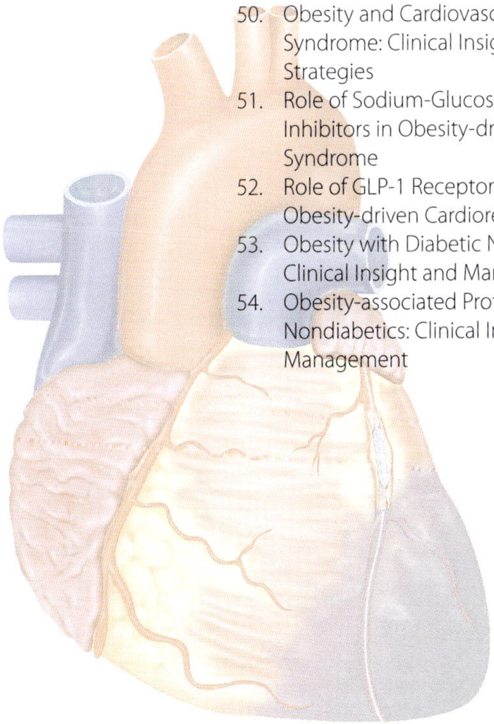

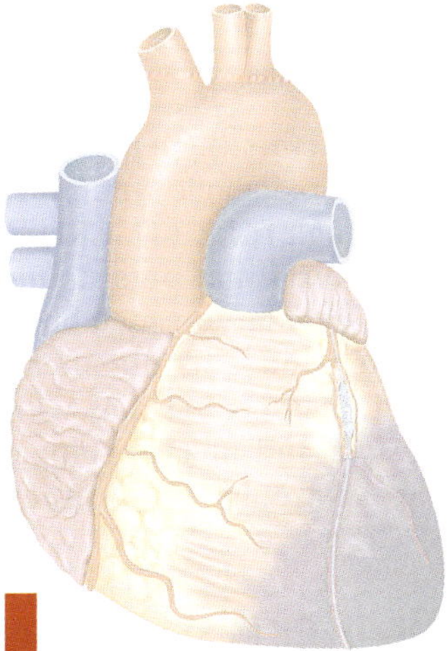

CHAPTER 50

Obesity and Cardiovascular-Kidney-Metabolic Syndrome: Clinical Insight and Management Strategies

Dinesh Khullar, Narinder Pal Singh, Raghav Khullar, Anish Kumar Gupta

INTRODUCTION

Cardiovascular-kidney-metabolic (CKM) syndrome describes the interconnected pathophysiology linking metabolic risk factors—most notably obesity—with chronic kidney disease (CKD) and the cardiovascular system, leading to a substantially higher risk of cardiovascular disease (CVD), early mortality, multisystem involvement, and increased healthcare utilization and costs. Rather than distinct cardiorenal or cardiometabolic entities, CKM syndrome reflects their overlap, wherein excess and dysfunctional adiposity promotes insulin resistance, inflammation, kidney dysfunction, and heightened cardiovascular risk, particularly heart failure. Despite its public health urgency and disproportionate impact across populations, CKM syndrome also presents a major therapeutic opportunity through interventions that simultaneously target obesity, metabolic abnormalities, kidney disease, and cardiovascular risk. This chapter will emphasize obesity as the cornerstone of CKM pathophysiology and provide a clear definition of CKM syndrome, a pragmatic staging framework to limit disease progression, risk prediction approaches relevant to CKM health, and evidence-based strategies for prevention and management of obesity-associated CKM-related adverse outcomes.

OBESITY: A COMPONENT OF CARDIOVASCULAR-KIDNEY-METABOLIC SYNDROME

Cardiovascular-kidney-metabolic syndrome is best understood as a systemic disorder and syndrome rather than a single disease, reflecting the interconnected pathophysiology of metabolic risk factors (notably obesity and diabetes), CKD, and CVD with a wide spectrum of severity and clinical consequences including heart failure, atrial fibrillation, coronary heart disease, stroke, and peripheral artery disease, and reflects a continuum of risk leading to multiorgan dysfunction and adverse cardiovascular outcomes.[1]

Pathogenetically, the majority of CKM syndrome factors stem from an excess and dysfunction of adipose tissue, particularly visceral and ectopic body fat. Excess visceral adipose tissue, which is frequently accompanied by ectopic fat deposition in normally lean tissues (e.g., liver, heart, skeletal muscle, pancreas, and kidney), is associated with the development of insulin resistance, systemic inflammation, and oxidative stress that contribute to the development of metabolic risk factors and CKD. A consequence of dysfunctional adipose tissue is impaired glucose tolerance and subsequent hyperglycemia, which increase the likelihood of metabolic risk factors and can occur even in those with normal BMI.

EPIDEMIOLOGY OF OBESITY ASSOCIATED CARDIOVASCULAR-KIDNEY-METABOLIC SYNDROME

Globally, 43% of adults are overweight and 16% are obese, with obesity prevalence reaching 20%–30%.[2] In India, CKM risk factors are highly prevalent and occur at lower body mass index (BMI) thresholds. NFHS-5 data show 13%–14% general obesity and 40%–58% abdominal obesity, while nearly one-third of adults have metabolic syndrome.[3] The ICMR-INDIAB study reports 11.4% diabetes, 35.5%

hypertension, and >80% dyslipidemia, with CKD affecting 13%–17% of the population.[4,5] CVD now accounts for about 26% of all deaths, highlighting the growing burden of CKM risk in India.[5]

Individuals are classified as overweight at a BMI of 23.0–24.9 kg/m² and obese at a BMI ≥25.0 kg/m², while central (abdominal) obesity—an important determinant of CKM syndrome—is defined by a waist circumference ≥90 cm in men and ≥80 cm in women.[6,7]

STAGING OF CARDIOVASCULAR-KIDNEY-METABOLIC SYNDROME (FLOWCHART 1)

Stage 0: No CKM Risk Factors (Absence of Excess Adiposity, Metabolic Risk Factors, and CKD)

Stage 0 CKM describes individuals with no cardiometabolic risk factors, normal anthropometric and metabolic parameters, and no CKD or CVD, with an emphasis on primordial prevention to maintain ideal cardiovascular health from early life.

Stage 1: Excess or Dysfunctional Adiposity (Hyperglycemia or Prediabetes)

Individuals with excess or dysfunctional adiposity—defined by overweight/obesity, central obesity, or prediabetes—without other metabolic risk factors or CKD. Criteria include BMI ≥23 kg/m² (in Asians), waist circumference ≥80/90 cm (in Asians) in women/men or fasting glucose 100–124 mg/dL or HbA1c 5.7%–6.4%.[7] Visceral and ectopic fat drive insulin resistance and inflammation.[8]

Stage 2: Metabolic Risk Factors and Kidney Disease

Characterized by metabolic risk factors [hypertension, hypertriglyceridemia (≥135 mg/dL), metabolic syndrome, and diabetes] and/or moderate-high risk CKD. CKD is defined by low eGFR or albuminuria that persists for ≥3 months, most often occurs secondary to metabolic risk factors, especially hypertension and diabetes.[9] These interrelated conditions increase CVD risk, with management focused on lifestyle and pharmacologic interventions to prevent cardiovascular and kidney disease progression.

Stage 3: Subclinical CVD in CKM Syndrome

Characterized by subclinical CVD in individuals with excess or dysfunctional adiposity, metabolic risk factors, or CKD, identified by subclinical atherosclerotic cardiovascular disease (ASCVD) (most commonly elevated coronary artery calcium or nonobstructive coronary disease) or subclinical heart failure detected by elevated cardiac biomarkers and/or abnormal cardiac imaging in the absence of symptoms; it also includes those with high predicted CVD risk or very high-risk CKD (KDIGO G4–G5),[9] representing a high-risk stage where early preventive therapy can effectively delay progression to overt CVD, kidney failure, and mortality.

Stage 4: Clinical CVD in CKM Syndrome with and without Kidney Failure

It refers to established clinical CVD (coronary heart disease, heart failure, stroke, peripheral artery disease, or atrial fibrillation) in individuals with excess/dysfunctional adiposity, other CKM risk factors, or CKD. It is classified

Flowchart 1: Staging of cardiovascular-kidney-metabolic syndrome.

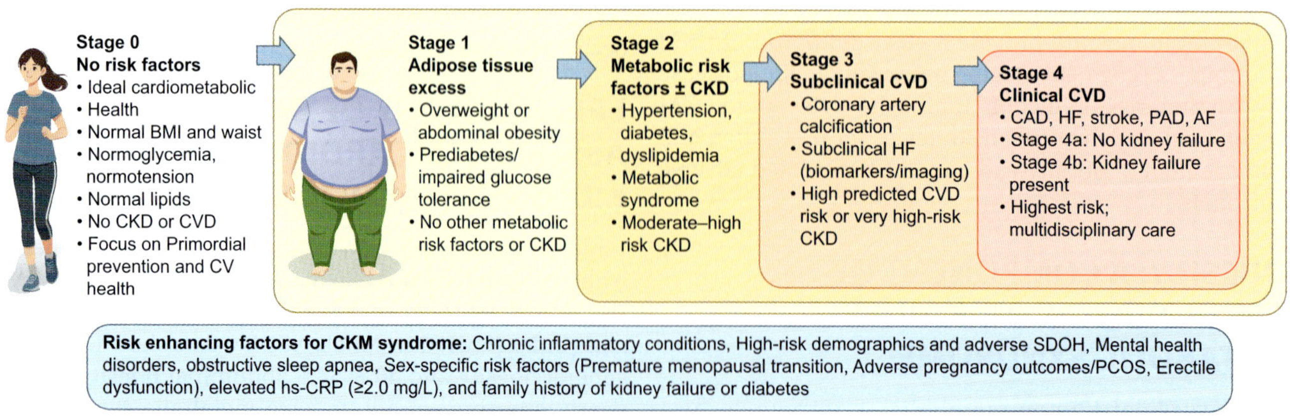

as 4a (without kidney failure) and 4b (with kidney failure) due to distinct management needs and represents a very high-risk stage requiring coordinated multidisciplinary care.[1]

SCREENING

The CKM staging framework enables stratification of individuals across the spectrum of syndromic severity, creating opportunities for timely preventive interventions to slow, halt, or reverse disease progression. A key emphasis is the early identification of individuals in the preclinical phase, with the aim of delaying or preventing the development of overt CVD and kidney failure. CKM screening broadly encompasses two domains: Biological risk factors and social determinants of health (SDOH). Biological screening includes assessment of metabolic risk, kidney function, and, in appropriate clinical contexts, evaluation for subclinical atherosclerosis or cardiac dysfunction. Screening for SDOH or economic, social, environmental, and psychosocial factors that influence health behaviors, access to care, and disease outcomes. Integrating SDOH into CKM assessment supports more effective, equitable, and real-world-relevant care. Screening approach across early life and adulthood is summarized in **Table 1**.

PREVENTION AND MANAGEMENT (FLOWCHART 2)

Management of CKM syndrome across all stages emphasizes multidisciplinary care and systematic integration of SDOH. Preventive strategies dominate stages 0–3, aiming to delay or prevent CVD, while stage 4 focuses on optimal CVD management in the presence of cardiometabolic and kidney disease.[1]

Stage 1: Excess or Dysfunctional Adiposity

Management prioritizes weight reduction to prevent metabolic risk. Both BMI and waist circumference should be assessed, with abdominal obesity identifying individuals at higher metabolic risk, particularly in those with overweight or mild obesity. Lifestyle modification targeting ≥5% weight loss is recommended, with greater benefit from larger reductions.[1,10,11] Pharmacotherapy and bariatric surgery may be considered when lifestyle measures are insufficient. Metformin can be used in individuals with persistent prediabetes to reduce progression to diabetes.

TABLE 1: Screening of obesity-associated CKM syndrome.[1]

Period	*Screening*	*Comments*
Early life (<21 years)	• Overweight/obesity	• Annual screening using age- and sex-specific CDC growth charts
	• Blood pressure	• Start at 3 years, annually if no risk factors • Every visit if obesity, diabetes, kidney disease, or structural heart disease
	• Mental and behavioral health/SDOH	• Screen all children
	• Lipid profile (fasting)	• Once at 9–11 years and again at 17–21 years • Start at ≥2 years if family history of premature CVD or severe hypercholesterolemia
	• Glycemia and liver enzymes (FPG/OGTT/HbA1c, ALT)	• Start at 9–11 years • Repeat every 2–3 years if normal in children with obesity • Repeat every 2–3 years in overweight children with additional risk factors
Adulthood (≥21 years)	• SDOH	• Screen all adults
	• Anthropometry	• BMI and waist circumference annually
	• Metabolic syndrome components	• Stage 2 CKM: Annually, Stage 1 CKM/prior GDM: every 2–3 years, Stage 0 CKM: Every 3–5 years
	• MASLD (advanced fibrosis)	• FIB-4 every 1–2 years in diabetes, prediabetes, or ≥2 metabolic risk factors
	• Kidney assessment	• UACR + serum creatinine/cystatin C (annually in ≥Stage 2 CKM and more often with higher KDIGO risk)
	• ASCVD risk refinement	• CAC scoring in intermediate 10-year risk
	• Subclinical HF	• Echo and/or cardiac biomarkers in selected high-risk groups

Flowchart 2: Management algorithm for patients with CKM syndrome stage 1 to stage 3.

CKM syndrome stage 1–3 at risk for CVD

↓

Physical activity, eat better, quit tobacco, sleep well, weight control, cholesterol control, manage blood sugar and blood pressure
Screening for social determinant of health

↓

Interdisciplinary care model:
High risk CKM patient referral to specialists

Stage 1
Excess or Dysfunctional Adiposity
- Strategies to overcome and prevent obesity (weight loss)
- Interdisciplinary care (dietician, pharmacy, mental health/community health worker):
- Intensive lifestyle intervention
- Pharmacotherapies (BMI ≥30 kg/m^2)
  – Bariatric surgery (BMI ≥40 kg/m^2)

Stage 2
Established CKM Risk Factors
Presence of MetS affects intensive lifestyle intervention targeting multifactorial risk control
Pharmacological management of MetS

Hypertriglyceridemia
- Lifestyle modification
- Statin therapy
- *TG* ≥500 mg/dL: Fibrates
- TG ≥135–499 mg/dL and patients with diabetes/additional risk factors: EPA

Hypertension
- Lifestyle modification
- Target BP: <130/80 mm Hg
- Optimize ACEi/ARBs, consider MRAs for RH
- Avoid CCB in HFrEF

Chronic kidney disease
- UACR >30 mg/g: ACEi/ARBs
- HFrEF: ARNi
- With/without diabetes: SGLT2i
- DKD with residual albuminuria (AUCR >30 mg/g) on ACEi/ARBs: Finerenone (in background of SGLT2i)

Diabetes
- Lifestyle modification
- Statin therapy
- Ezetimibe for high-risk patients
- Comorbid condition
  – BMI ≥35 kg/m^2: GLP-1 RA
  – HbA1c ≥9% or on high dose of high insulin: GLP-1 RA
  – CKD: consider SGLT2i

Metformin coutilization:
  – HbA1c ≥7.5% or on insulin: metformin and cardioprotective antihyperglycemic agents
  – HbA1c <7.5%: cardioprotective antihyperglycemic agents (continue metformin if already using)

Stage 3
Subclinical CVD or high-risk CKD
- Subclinical atherosclerosis
  – CAC >0: Statin
  – CAC>100: Aspirin (in low bleed risk)
  – Other agents based on CKM profile: PCSK9i, GLP-1RA, icosapent ethyl
- Subclinical HF
  – EF <40%: ACEi/ARBs, β blocker
  – In diabetes: SGLT2i

Stage 2: Metabolic Risk Factors and CKD

Care focuses on comprehensive control of metabolic abnormalities and kidney disease to prevent progression to subclinical or overt CVD.

Stage 3: Subclinical CVD or High-risk CKD

Preventive therapies should be intensified in individuals with subclinical atherosclerosis, advanced CKD, or high predicted cardiovascular risk to avert clinical CVD and kidney failure.

Stage 4: Established CVD with CKM (Flowchart 3)

Management at stage 4 CKM focuses on optimizing cardiovascular care and strengthening secondary prevention in patients with established CVD alongside metabolic risk factors, CKD, or both. Annual assessment of BMI and waist circumference is advised. Intentional weight loss (5%–10%) improves metabolic control and

Flowchart 3: Management algorithm for patients with CKM syndrome stage 4.

CKM syndrome stage 4 with existing CVD

↓

Cardiovascular health: Physical activity, eat better, quit tobacco, sleep well, weight control, cholesterol control, manage blood sugar and blood pressure
Screening for social determinant of health using validated tools
Interdisciplinary care model: High risk CKM patient referral to the specialists

↓

HF: GDMT
ASCVD: Aspirin and statin, consider addition of ezetimibe and PCSK9i as per LDL levels/goals/risk of ASCVD

↓

Management of Excess/Dysfunctional adiposity
- Strategies to overcome and prevent obesity (weight loss)
- Interdisciplinary care (dietician, pharmacy, mental health/community health worker):
  - Intensive lifestyle intervention
  - Pharmacotherapies (BMI ≥30 kg/m^2)
  - Bariatric surgery (BMI ≥40 kg/m^2)

Management of other CKM Risk Factors
Presence of MetS affects intensive lifestyle intervention targeting multifactorial risk control
Pharmacological management of uncontrolled MetS components

Hypertriglyceridemia
- Lifestyle modification
- Statin therapy
- TG ≥500 mg/dL: Fibrates
- TG ≥135–499 mg/dL and patients with diabetes/additional risk factors: EPA

Hypertension
- Lifestyle modification
- Target BP: <130/80 mm Hg
- Optimize ACEi/ARBs, consider MRAs for RH
- Avoid CCB in HFrEF

Chronic kidney disease
- With albuminuria, UACR >30 mg/g: ACEi/ARBs
- HFrEF: ARNi
- With/without diabetes: SGLT2i
- DKD with residual albuminuria (AUCR >30 mg/g) on
- ACEi/ARBs: Finerenone (used in background of SGLT2i)

Diabetes
- Lifestyle modification
- If HbA1c ≥7.5% or patient on insulin: metformin and cardioprotective antihyperglycemic agents

In patients with ASCVD
- To reduce in MACE events: Either SGLT2i or GLP1-RA
- To reduce hospitalization rate: SGLT2i

Comorbid condition: GLP-1 RA/SGLT2i based on
- BMI ≥35 kg/m^2: GLP-1 RA
- HbA1c ≥9% or on high dose of high insulin: GLP-1 RA
- *CKD:* consider SGLT2i
- Concomitant HF: SGLT2i

In patients with heart failure:
To reduce MACE events and hospitalization rate:
SGLT2i SGLT2i in all HF patients along with:
- BMI ≥35 kg/m^2: add GLP-1 RA
- HbA1c ≥9% or on high dose of high insulin: add GLP-1 RA
- Diabetes with multiple co-morbidities: add GLP-1 RA
- Albuminuria: consider adding finerenone

functional status, particularly in heart failure, while greater weight loss (>10%) may confer additional cardiovascular benefit.[12,13]

All individuals with ASCVD should receive antiplatelet therapy and high-intensity statins. Additional LDL-cholesterol-lowering agents should be used in those at very high cardiovascular risk or when LDL-cholesterol targets are not achieved. Heart failure management should follow contemporary guideline-directed medical therapy (GDMT), with particular emphasis on β-blockers, angiotensin receptor-neprilysin inhibitors (ARNI), mineralocorticoid receptor antagonists (MRA), and SGLT2 inhibitors in patients with heart failure with reduced ejection fraction.

Therapies that slow kidney disease progression and lower cardiovascular mortality, particularly SGLT2 inhibitors, are recommended for all patients with CKD and heart failure irrespective of ejection fraction, diabetes status, or baseline albuminuria, and may be initiated down to an eGFR of 20 mL/min/1.73 m^2 and continued until kidney replacement therapy is required.[14,15] When metformin and SGLT2 inhibitors cannot be used because of reduced eGFR or decompensated heart failure, GLP-1 receptor agonists offer effective glycemic control, remain effective despite declining kidney function, and are generally safe in advanced CKD.[16]

Finerenone is a nonsteroidal MRA may be added in patients with diabetes and CKD receiving maximally tolerated renin–angiotensin system blockade, with or without SGLT2 inhibitors, to further reduce cardiovascular and renal events.[17,18] In HFrEF, ARNI are favored over ACE inhibitors or ARBs, with dose reduction of sacubitril–valsartan considered when eGFR is <30 mL/min/1.73 m^2; these agents are also linked to slower kidney function decline, fewer renal adverse events, and improved blood pressure control across the eGFR range.[19] ACE inhibitors or ARBs may still be continued in advanced CKD with HFrEF, provided close monitoring for hyperkalemia is ensured. In patients prone to hyperkalemia, use of oral potassium binders such as patiromer or sodium zirconium cyclosilicate can help sustain RAAS inhibitor therapy safely.

OBESITY, METABOLIC SYNDROME, AND CARDIOVASCULAR DISEASE

Initial management should emphasize lifestyle intervention, including behavioral change, moderate calorie reduction, and regular physical activity. These efforts are best delivered through a coordinated multidisciplinary team.

When lifestyle measures alone are insufficient, adjunctive therapies such as antiobesity medications (for BMI ≥27 kg/m^2) and metabolic surgery (for BMI ≥35 kg/m^2) may be employed to achieve greater weight reduction and cardiometabolic benefit. Incretin-based therapies—including GLP-1 receptor agonists and dual or triple incretin agonists—should be favored due to their robust effects on weight loss and metabolic risk factor improvement. Emerging evidence from the SELECT trial suggests that high-dose semaglutide reduces cardiovascular events in individuals with obesity and established CVD, supporting its potential role as first-line therapy in this population.[20]

CONCLUSION

Despite major advances in understanding obesity and its role in CKM syndrome, effective implementation in clinical practice remains limited. Strengthening obesity prevention and treatment is therefore a clinical and public health priority. This requires better training of health professionals, wider use of structured obesity care tools, improved patient access to lifestyle, pharmacologic, and surgical therapies, and greater reliance on multidisciplinary care models. Policy support and investment in early-stage CKM obesity management are essential and are likely to reduce long-term morbidity, mortality, and healthcare costs while improving patient quality of life.

REFERENCES

1. Ndumele CE, Rangaswami J, Chow SL, et al. Cardiovascular-Kidney-Metabolic Health: A Presidential Advisory from the American Heart Association. Circulation. 2023;148(20):1606-35.
2. World Health Organization. (2025). Obesity and Overweight. [online] Available from https://www.who.int/news-room/fact-sheets/detail/obesity-and-overweight [Last accessed January, 2026].
3. Gupta RD, Tamanna N, Siddika N, et al. Obesity and abdominal obesity in Indian population: Findings from a nationally representative study of 698,286 participants. Epidemiologia (Basel). 2023;4:163-72.
4. Anjana RM, Unnikrishnan R, Deepa M, et al. Metabolic non-communicable disease health report of India: the ICMR-INDIAB national cross-sectional study (ICMR-INDIAB-17). Lancet Diabetes Endocrinol. 2023;11(7):474-89.
5. Talukdar R, Ajayan R, Gupta S, et al. Chronic kidney disease prevalence in India: A systematic review and meta-analysis from community-based representative evidence between 2011 to 2023. Nephrology (Carlton). 2025;30:e14420.
6. Kalra A, Jose AP, Prabhakaran P, et al. The burgeoning cardiovascular disease epidemic in Indians – Perspectives on contextual factors and potential solutions. Lancet Reg Health Southeast Asia. 2023;12:100156.
7. Grundy SM, Cleeman JI, Daniels SR, et al. Diagnosis and management of the metabolic syndrome: an American Heart Association/National Heart, Lung, and Blood Institute Scientific Statement. Circulation. 2005;112(17):2735-52.
8. Powell-Wiley TM, Poirier P, Burke LE, et al. Obesity and cardiovascular disease: a scientific statement from the American Heart Association. Circulation. 2021; 143:e984-1010.
9. Kidney Disease: Improving Global Outcomes (KDIGO) CKD Work Group. KDIGO 2024 Clinical Practice Guideline for the Evaluation and Management of Chronic Kidney Disease. Kidney Int. 2024;105(4S):S117-314.
10. Gallagher C, Corl A, Dietz WH. Weight can't wait: a guide to discussing obesity and organizing treatment in the primary care setting. Obesity (Silver Spring). 2021;29:821-4.
11. George Washington University Milken Institute School of Public Health. (2020). Guideline for the Management of Obesity in the Primary Care Setting. Strategies to Overcome & Prevent (STOP) Obesity Alliance. [online] Available from https://stoppublichealth9.drupal.gwu. edu/sites/g/files/zaxdzs4356/files/2022-02/

wcw-guide-for-the-management-of-obesity-in-the-primary-care-setting.pdf [Last accessed January, 2026].
12. McDowell K, Petrie MC, Raihan NA, et al. Effects of intentional weight loss in patients with obesity and heart failure: a systematic review. Obes Rev. 2018;19:1189-204.
13. Doumouras AG, Wong JA, Paterson JM et al. Bariatric surgery and cardiovascular outcomes in patients with obesity and cardiovascu lar disease: a population-based retrospective cohort study. Circulation. 2021;143:1468-80.
14. Nuffield Department of Population Health Renal Studies Group; SGLT2 inhibitor Meta-Analysis Cardio-Renal Trialists' Consortium. Impact of diabetes on the effects of sodium glucose co-transporter-2 inhibitors on kidney outcomes: collaborative meta-analysis of large placebo-controlled trials. Lancet. 2022;400:1788-801.
15. Vaduganathan M, Docherty KF, Claggett BL, et al. SGLT-2 inhibitors in patients with heart failure: a comprehensive meta-analysis of five randomised controlled trials. Lancet. 2022;400:757-67.
16. Rangaswami J, Bhalla V, de Boer IH, et al. Cardiorenal protection with the newer antidiabetic agents in patients with diabetes and chronic kidney disease: a scientific statement from the American Heart Association Circulation. 2020;142:e265-86 [Correction in: Circulation. 2020;142:e304; Circulation. 2021;143:e1019-20].
17. Khullar D, Gupta AK, Singh K. Finerenone: Will It Be a Game-changer? Card Fail Rev. 2024;10:e19.
18. Agarwal R, Filippatos G, Pitt B, et al. Cardiovascular and kidney outcomes with finerenone in patients with type 2 diabetes and chronic kidney disease: the FIDELITY pooled analysis. Eur Heart J. 2022;43:474-84.
19. Zhang H, Huang T, Shen W, et al. Efficacy and safety of sacubitril-valsartan in heart failure: a meta-analysis of randomized controlled trials. ESC Heart Fail. 2020;7:3841-50.
20. Lincoff AM, Brown-Frandsen K, Colhoun HM, et al. Semaglutide and Cardiovascular Outcomes in Obesity without Diabetes. N Engl J Med. 2023;389(24):2221-32.

51 CHAPTER

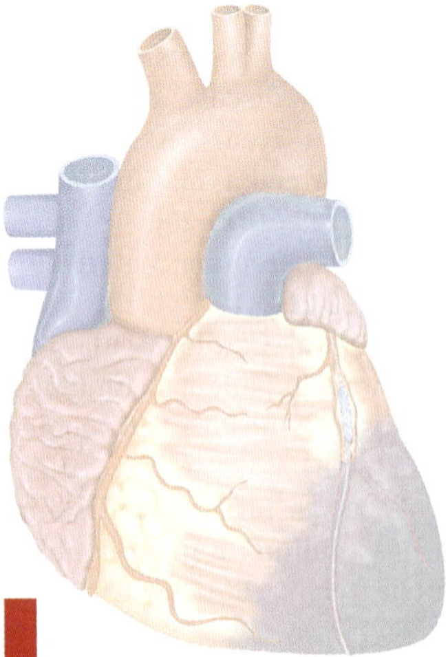

Role of Sodium-Glucose Cotransporter-2 Inhibitors in Obesity-driven Cardiorenal Syndrome

Pallavi Prasad

INTRODUCTION

Overweight and obesity, particularly excess intra-abdominal adiposity, are strongly associated with a spectrum of cardiometabolic disorders, including type 2 diabetes mellitus (DM), dyslipidemia, hypertension, atherosclerotic cardiovascular disease, and heart failure. Obesity-related cardiomyopathy has been described as a distinct clinical entity, typically characterized by eccentric left ventricular hypertrophy, preserved ejection fraction, and diastolic dysfunction, frequently accompanied by right ventricular dysfunction independent of obstructive sleep apnea. These structural and functional cardiac abnormalities, together with metabolic dysregulation and renal involvement, highlight the intricate interplay between obesity, cardiovascular disease, and chronic kidney disease (CKD) within the cardiorenal-metabolic continuum.

Sodium-glucose cotransporter-2 (SGLT2) inhibitors, initially developed as glucose-lowering agents, have emerged as pleiotropic therapies with benefits extending well beyond glycemic control. By inhibiting renal glucose and sodium reabsorption, SGLT2 inhibitors induce glucosuria, natriuresis, and mild osmotic diuresis, leading to sustained reductions in blood glucose, blood pressure, body weight, and adiposity. Despite modest weight loss, these agents favorably modulate insulin sensitivity, fuel utilization, inflammatory pathways, and myocardial and renal energetics, while conferring substantial cardiovascular and renal protection across a broad range of patients, including those without diabetes. Large cardiovascular and renal outcome trials have demonstrated their efficacy in heart failure with both reduced and preserved ejection fraction and in CKD, irrespective of diabetic status. This chapter will describe the role of SGLT2 inhibitors in obesity-driven cardiorenal syndrome, integrating mechanistic insights with clinical evidence to define their therapeutic relevance in this evolving clinical entity.

EPIDEMIOLOGY OF OBESITY AND CHRONIC RHINOSINUSITIS

Obesity is a chronic multisystem disease characterized by excess adiposity that adversely affects health. According to the World Health Organization, approximately one in eight individuals worldwide was living with obesity in 2022.[1] Obesity frequently coexists with DM, CKD, and heart failure (HF), forming a tightly interrelated cardio-renal-metabolic continuum.[2]

Among patients with type 2 diabetes mellitus (T2DM), over 90% are overweight or obese, and more than half have three or more concomitant cardio-renal-metabolic conditions. Increasing body mass index (BMI) is associated with a 5–7% higher risk of incident HF per unit increase, with a stronger association observed for heart failure with preserved ejection fraction (HFpEF) than for reduced ejection fraction (HFrEF).[3] Findings from the Framingham Heart Study and pooled cohort analyses involving over 50,000 participants have consistently demonstrated a robust link between elevated BMI and HFpEF.[3]

Population-based studies also demonstrate that obesity is independently associated with the development and progression of CKD. Higher BMI is linked to an increased risk of proteinuria, accelerated decline in estimated glomerular filtration rate, and progression to kidney failure, even in individuals without pre-existing kidney disease.[4]

ROLE OF SODIUM-GLUCOSE COTRANSPORTER-2 INHIBITORS IN OBESITY/METABOLIC SYNDROME

Sodium-glucose cotransporter 2 inhibitors are antihyperglycemic agents that lower plasma glucose concentrations by blocking renal reabsorption of glucose and sodium, thereby promoting urinary glucose loss. Treatment with SGLT2 inhibitors results in the excretion of approximately 60–100 g of glucose per day, leading to improvements in glycemic control, reductions in HbA1c and blood pressure, and modest decreases in body weight and adiposity.[5]

Although weight reduction is a consistent finding with SGLT2 inhibitor therapy, the magnitude of weight loss remains limited, largely due to compensatory physiological mechanisms that act to preserve body weight. Network metanalysis show a decrease in body weight of 1.5–2 kg with SGLT2i in patients with diabetes, which is sustained over a 4-year period if taken regularly. When combined with drugs with other mechanisms of action, especially GLP-1 receptor agonists, the weight loss is more pronounced since the counter-regulatory increase in appetite due to caloric loss is also inhibited by the action of GLP-1 agonists.

In nondiabetic obese patients, both SGLT2i alone and in combination have been shown to decrease weight by an average of 2–4 kg, although the number of studies is fewer than in those with diabetes.

Sodium glucose cotransporter 2 inhibitors exert direct metabolic effects by lowering circulating glucose concentrations, which in turn suppress insulin secretion and increase glucagon levels, accompanied by a paradoxical rise in endogenous glucose production. Several mechanisms have been proposed to explain this compensatory increase in glucose output, including an elevated glucagon-to-insulin ratio, direct inhibition of SGLT2 in pancreatic α-cells leading to enhanced glucagon release, upregulation of hepatic gluconeogenesis, and activation of a kidney–liver neural axis that stimulates hepatic glucose production.[6]

This increase in endogenous glucose production may partially offset the glucose-lowering effect of SGLT2 inhibitors and contribute to a low risk of hypoglycemia. Consequently, the cardiorenal benefits of SGLT2 inhibitors may arise from the combined effects of effective glycemic reduction while preserving metabolic safety through avoidance of hypoglycemic episodes.[6]

MECHANISM OF ACTION OF SODIUM-GLUCOSE COTRANSPORTER-2 INHIBITORS IN OBESITY DRIVEN CARDIORENAL SYNDROME

The potential mechanisms underlying the cardiorenal benefits of SGLT2 inhibitors are multifactorial:[6]

- *Renal effects:* SGLT2 inhibitors block glucose and sodium reabsorption in the proximal tubule, increasing urinary glucose excretion, and producing mild osmotic diuresis.
- *Tubuloglomerular feedback:* Reduced proximal sodium and glucose reabsorption restores tubuloglomerular feedback and attenuates glomerular hyperfiltration.
- *Hemodynamic benefits:* Natriuresis and diuresis lower blood pressure and cardiac preload/afterload, partly mediated by inhibition of sodium–hydrogen exchanger-3 and reduced sympathetic activity.
- *Erythropoiesis and oxygen delivery:* Induction of a hypoxia-like state stimulates erythropoiesis, potentially improving tissue oxygenation.
- *Metabolic modulation:* Reduction in insulin secretion with improvement in β-cell function and peripheral insulin sensitivity.
- *Cardiac effects:* Improvement in myocardial energy metabolism and attenuation of adverse cardiac remodeling, partly through inhibition of sodium–hydrogen exchanger-1 in cardiomyocytes.
- *Anti-inflammatory and cytoprotective actions:* Suppression of inflammation, oxidative stress, and apoptosis, with enhancement of autophagy.
- *Renal metabolic protection:* Reversal of tricarboxylic acid cycle intermediate accumulation and oxidative stress in the renal cortex, consistent with reduced glomerular injury.
- *Fuel utilization shift:* Chronic therapy promotes lipolysis, fatty acid oxidation, and ketogenesis, shifting energy utilization from carbohydrates to fatty acids and ketone bodies.
- *Ketone-mediated organ efficiency:* Liver-derived ketone bodies act as energy-efficient substrates for the heart and kidneys, enhancing myocardial and renal epithelial function.
- *Molecular signaling pathways:* Activation of the AMPK–SIRT1–PGC-1α axis and inhibition of mTOR signaling improves mitochondrial function, redox balance, and cellular stress responses.

- *Adipose tissue effects:* Reduction in adipose tissue inflammation and increased brown adipose tissue activity demonstrated in experimental models.

EVIDENCE FOR USE OF SODIUM-GLUCOSE COTRANSPORTER-2 INHIBITORS IN CARDIORENAL SYNDROMES

A network meta-analysis of 38 randomized clinical trials demonstrated that, compared with placebo, SGLT2 inhibitors produced significant improvements in multiple cardiometabolic parameters in adults with T2DM. These included reductions in glycated hemoglobin (0.6–0.9%), fasting plasma glucose (1.1–1.9 mmol/L), body weight (1.6–2.5 kg), systolic blood pressure (2.8–4.9 mm Hg), and diastolic blood pressure (1.5–2.0 mm Hg), along with modest increases in high-density lipoprotein cholesterol (0.05–0.07 mmol/L).[7]

Cardiovascular outcome data further support the clinical benefits of SGLT2 inhibitors. A meta-analysis encompassing three major cardiovascular outcome trials and 34,322 patients with T2DM showed an 11% reduction in major adverse cardiovascular events, with benefits largely confined to individuals with established atherosclerotic cardiovascular disease. In contrast, a consistent 23% reduction in cardiovascular death or hospitalization for heart failure was observed irrespective of baseline atherosclerotic disease status.[8] Notably, these heart failure benefits extend to patients without diabetes, including those with heart failure and reduced ejection fractions.[9] Early initiation of SGLT2 inhibitors following episodes of worsening heart failure in patients with T2DM has also been associated with substantial reductions in cardiovascular mortality and recurrent heart failure hospitalizations.[10]

Evidence for efficacy in heart failure with preserved ejection fractions has emerged from large, randomized trials. The EMPEROR-Preserved trial demonstrated that empagliflozin significantly reduced the composite endpoint of cardiovascular death or hospitalization for heart failure in patients with HFpEF, regardless of diabetic status.[11] Similarly, the DELIVER trial showed that dapagliflozin lowered the risk of worsening heart failure or cardiovascular death in patients with left ventricular ejection fraction >40%.[12]

Renal outcome trials have consistently shown that SGLT2 inhibitors reduce the risk of kidney disease progression in patients with T2DM. The DAPA-CKD trial was stopped early because of a pronounced reduction in kidney-related outcomes, benefits that were evident in both diabetic and nondiabetic participants.[13] The EMPA-KIDNEY trial further expanded this evidence base by demonstrating cardiorenal protection with empagliflozin across a broad CKD population, including patients with significant albuminuria and estimated glomerular filtration rates as low as 20 mL/min/1.73 m^2.[14]

Limitation

There are no dedicated studies for obesity related cardiorenal syndromes. Directed studies in this area may be able to better define the role of SGLT2 inhibitors in this field.

CONCLUSION

Sodium-glucose cotransporter 2 inhibitors are useful drugs for moderate weight loss in obesity, in heart failure, both reduced and preserved ejection fraction, and in albuminuric CKD. Their use in obesity driven cardiorenal syndrome derives from their role in each of the above illnesses. Further studies are needed to delineate the exact role of SGLT2 inhibitors in patients with obesity-driven cardiorenal syndrome.

REFERENCES

1. World Health Organization. Obesity and overweight. WHO Fact Sheet; 2025. [Online] Available from https://www.who.int/news-room/fact-sheets/detail/obesity-and-overweight [Last accessed January, 2026].
2. Ndumele CE, Rangaswami J, Chow SL, et al. Cardiovascular-Kidney-Metabolic Health: A Presidential Advisory From the American Heart Association. Circulation. 2023;148(20):1606-35.
3. Meems LMG, van Veldhuisen DJ, Sattar N, et al. Heart failure and obesity: novel insights leading to new treatment paradigms. Nat Rev Cardiol. 2025;23(2):87-99.
4. Sanz RL, Inserra F, García Menéndez S, et al. Metabolic Syndrome and Cardiac Remodeling Due to Mitochondrial Oxidative Stress Involving Gliflozins and Sirtuins. Curr Hypertens Rep. 2023;25(6):91-106.
5. Pereira MJ, Eriksson JW. Emerging Role of SGLT-2 Inhibitors for the Treatment of Obesity. Drugs. 2019;79(3):219-30.
6. Gao YM, Feng ST, Wen Y, et al Cardiorenal protection of SGLT2 inhibitors-Perspectives from metabolic reprogramming. EBioMedicine. 2022;83:104215.
7. Zaccardi F, Webb DR, Htike ZZ, et al. Efficacy and safety of sodium-glucose co-transporter-2 inhibitors in type 2 diabetes mellitus: systematic review and network meta-analysis. Diabetes Obes Metab. 2016;18(8):783-94.

8. Zelniker TA, Wiviott SD, Raz I, et al. SGLT2 inhibitors for primary and secondary prevention of cardiovascular and renal outcomes in type 2 diabetes: a systematic review and meta-analysis of cardiovascular outcome trials. Lancet. 2019;393(10166):31-9.
9. Packer M, Anker SD, Butler J, et al. Cardiovascular and renal outcomes with empagliflozin in heart failure. N Engl J Med. 2020;383(15):1413-24.
10. Bhatt DL, Szarek M, Steg PG, et al. Sotagliflozin in patients with diabetes and recent worsening heart failure. N Engl J Med. 2021;384(2):117-28.
11. Anker SD, Butler J, Filippatos G, et al. Empagliflozin in heart failure with a preserved ejection fraction. N Engl J Med. 2021;385(16):1451-61.
12. Williams DM, Evans M. Dapagliflozin for heart failure with preserved ejection fraction: will the DELIVER Study deliver? Diabetes Ther. 2020;11(10):2207-19.
13. Heerspink HJL, Stefánsson BV, Correa-Rotter R, et al. Dapagliflozin in patients with chronic kidney disease. N Engl J Med. 2020;383(15):1436-46.
14. Almaimani M, Sridhar VS, Cherney DZI. Sodium-glucose cotransporter 2 inhibition in non-diabetic kidney disease. Curr Opin Nephrol Hypertens. 2021;30(5):474-81.

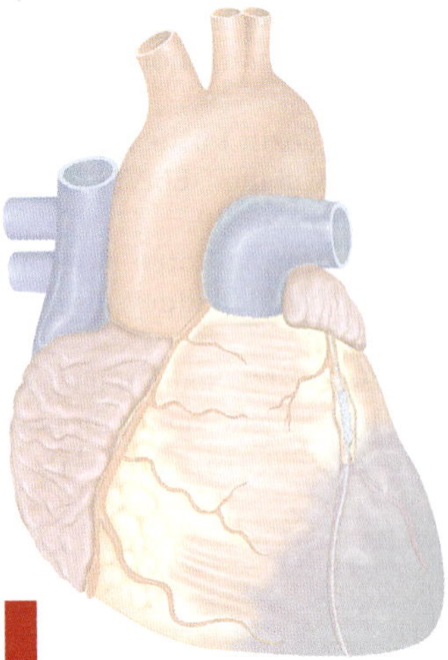

52

CHAPTER

Role of GLP-1 Receptor Agonists in Obesity-driven Cardiorenal Disease

Priti Meena

INTRODUCTION

Obesity-associated cardiovascular-kidney-metabolic (CKM) disease is now increasingly recognized as one of the important contributors to significant morbidity and mortality worldwide.[1] A complex interplay of excess adiposity, insulin resistance, diabetes mellitus, and chronic kidney disease (CKD) along with hypertension and lipid disorders plays important role in amplifying risk across the cardiovascular and renal domains. This integrated construct has been formalized as CKM syndrome, emphasizing that heart, kidney, and metabolic dysfunction rarely occur in isolation in contemporary practice.

In this context, glucagon-like peptide 1 receptor agonists (GLP-1 RAs) are now taking spotlight as an important disease-modifying agents. Originally developed as glucose-lowering agents for T2 diabetes mellitus (T2DM), GLP-1 RAs have now demonstrated substantial benefits on body weight, atherosclerotic CV events, heart failure, and kidney outcomes.[2] Importantly, these pleiotropic effects extend beyond the glycemic control alone, supported by a growing body of clinical evidence. Large outcome trials and meta-analyses now show consistent reductions in major adverse CV events, and improved composite kidney outcomes, in people with T2DM as well as, increasingly, in individuals with obesity without diabetes.

The GLP-1 RAs are generating considerable interest within the nephrology community as they simultaneously address upstream drivers (obesity, insulin resistance, and dyslipidemia) and downstream manifestations (albuminuria, eGFR decline, HF, and atherosclerotic disease).[3] Their role is complementary to, not competitive with, sodium-glucose cotransporter-2 inhibitors (SGLT2i) and nonsteroidal mineralocorticoid receptor antagonists (MRAs), which primarily target hemodynamic and fibrotic pathways. Integrating GLP-1 RAs into nephrology practice therefore requires a nuanced understanding of mechanisms, trial evidence, guideline recommendations, and real-world implementation challenges.

This chapter reviews mechanistic and clinical data on GLP-1 RAs in obesity-driven cardiorenal disease, focusing on pathophysiological links between obesity, CKD and cardiovascular disease, and practical application in nephrology practice and future directions.

PATHOPHYSIOLOGICAL LINKS BETWEEN OBESITY, KIDNEY DISEASE, AND CARDIOVASCULAR DISEASE

Obesity drives development and the progression of both CKD and cardiovascular diseases through complex hemodynamic, metabolic, inflammatory, and structural pathways.[2] Early hyperfiltration due to altered tubuloglomerular feedback and RAAS activation leads to progressive glomerulosclerosis and GFR decline. Adipose tissue-derived adipokines and cytokines promote insulin resistance, endothelial dysfunction, lipotoxicity, and fibrosis in both the kidney and myocardium. Obesity independently increases HFpEF risk through adipose tissue-driven inflammation, aldosterone excess, natriuretic peptide deficiency, neurohormonal activation, and adverse cardiac remodelling.[4] Visceral and epicardial fat promote concentric LV remodeling, elevated filling pressures, microvascular inflammation, collagen deposition, and myocardial fibrosis. HFpEF with obesity is associated with worse prognosis with increased risk for recurrent hospitalization and mortality. The role of CKD is well established in worsening HF through neurohormonal activation, anemia, and congestion, establishing a maladaptive cardiorenal cycle. Chronic inflammation, oxidative stress, and AGE accumulation accelerate renal and myocardial fibrosis, while atherogenic dyslipidemia markedly increases systemic atherosclerotic burden. Within this complex milieu, GLP-1 RAs exert pleiotropic effects that address multiple pathophysiological nodes simultaneously.

A BRIEF ON PHARMACOLOGY GLP-1RAs

Glucagon-like peptide 1 is an incretin hormone produced by L-cells of the intestine and released after meals. It contributes to maintaining glucose balance by enhancing insulin secretion only when glucose levels are elevated, reducing glucagon output, and slowing gastric emptying, which together promote early satiety and help lower food intake. Because native GLP-1 is rapidly broken down by dipeptidyl peptidase 4 (DPP-4), its biological half-life is extremely short typically under 2–3 minutes. To overcome this limitation, GLP-1RAs are developed as synthetic analogs that partially or fully resemble the natural peptide but are structurally modified to resist DPP-4–mediated degradation. These modifications allow sustained receptor activation and support once-daily, twice-daily, or even once-weekly dosing, depending on the formulation used. GLP-1 signals through the GLP-1 receptor, which is widely distributed across several organs, including pancreatic β-cells, the gastrointestinal system, kidneys, cardiovascular tissues, and various regions of the central nervous system. Clinically used GLP-1 RAs include exenatide, lixisenatide, and longer-acting agents such as liraglutide, dulaglutide, and semaglutide **(Table 1)**.

More recently, multiagonist molecules that combine GLP-1 agonism with GIP, glucagon or amylin receptor activity (e.g., tirzepatide) have also shown even greater weight-loss and metabolic benefits. A triple agonist retatrutide (targeting GLP-1R, GIPR, and GCGR) has also shown beneficial role in diabetes control and weight reduction.

TABLE 1: Combined overview of commonly used GLP-1 receptor agonists.

GLP-1RA	*Half-life*	*Dose*	*HbA1c reduction*
Exenatide	2.4 hours	5–10 µg BID SC	+
Liraglutide	11–13 hours	0.6–1.8 mg QD SC	++
Lixisenatide	2–4 hours	10–20 µg QD SC	+
Albiglutide	6–8 hours	30–50 mg QW SC	
Dulaglutide	108–112 hours	0.75–1.5 mg QW SC	++
Exenatide ER	2 weeks	2 mg QW SC	++
Semaglutide (SC)	6–7 days	0.25–0.5 mg QW SC	++
Oral semaglutide	24 hours	3–7 mg QD PO	+

MECHANISMS OF CARDIORENAL PROTECTION

Although the exact mechanisms underlying the renoprotective effects of GLP-1RAs are yet to be elucidated, it is increasingly evident that these benefits arise from both direct renal actions and indirect systemic effects mediated through extra-renal GLP-1 receptor–expressing tissues. Clinical evidence from the FLOW trial, as well as posthoc analyses of multiple cardiovascular outcome trials, consistently demonstrates that GLP-1RAs significantly reduce kidney injury in patients with T2DM. GLP-1R expression in the kidney is modest, it is detectable in juxtaglomerular cells, vascular smooth muscle, endothelial cells, and possibly podocytes. Experimental data further support the presence of direct renoprotective mechanisms, including suppression of inflammatory signaling pathways, reduced activation of receptor for advanced glycation end-products, attenuation of oxidative stress, mitigation of renal fibrosis, and restoration of immune dysregulation, accompanied by reductions in circulating inflammatory biomarkers. Beyond these direct effects, GLP-1RAs exert important indirect renal benefits through improvements in glycemic control, body weight, and blood pressure modulation through actions on the central nervous system and vasculature. The importance of intrinsic GLP-1 receptor signaling in renal protection is further supported by preclinical studies demonstrating that genetic deletion of GLP-1R leads to spontaneous renal injury in both diabetic and nondiabetic animal models, with exaggerated inflammation, oxidative stress, and accelerated progression of diabetic kidney disease.

The GLP-1RAs produce glycemic lowering with HbA1c reductions of approximately 0.8–1.5%, alongside weight loss mediated by central appetite suppression and delayed gastric emptying reaching ~15% with semaglutide 2.4 mg weekly and up to 20–22% with dual GIP/GLP-1 agonism using tirzepatide. These effects are accompanied by improvements in insulin sensitivity, hepatic steatosis, triglycerides, and non-HDL cholesterol, thereby alleviating key CKM drivers such as hyperglycemia, hyperinsulinemia, dyslipidemia, and ectopic fat accumulation. In parallel, GLP-1 RAs exert favorable hemodynamic actions through natriuresis and diuresis via reduced proximal tubular sodium reabsorption, modest systolic blood pressure lowering (2–5 mm Hg), and attenuation of glomerular hyperfiltration through modulation of tubuloglomerular feedback and arteriolar tone, leading to consistent reductions in albuminuria and slower eGFR decline.[5] Beyond atherosclerotic risk modification, they improve endothelial function, reduce arterial stiffness and inflammatory biomarkers, and may exert direct myocardial effects by improving energetics, reducing lipotoxicity, and limiting fibrosis.[6]

IMPORTANT CLINICAL TRIALS

LEADER

It was a double blinded, RCT comparing liraglutide versus placebo comprising 9,340 patients with a median follow-up of 3.8 years.[7] The primary outcomes were CV benefits. Liraglutide group was found to be superior to placebo group. The rate of death from any cause was lower in the liraglutide group. Kidney secondary outcomes showed reductions in new-onset macroalbuminuria and a favorable trend in composite renal endpoints.

SUSTAIN-6

SUSTAIN-6 established Semaglutide's cardiovascular safety in T2DM who were at high CV risk and showed a significant reduction in nonfatal stroke.[8] The trial also reported greatly reduced new-onset macroalbuminuria and an improvement in composite kidney outcomes, raising early interest in potential renoprotective effects.

The FLOW Trial

This double-blind, placebo-controlled trial randomized over 3,500 individuals with T2DM and CKD characterized by albuminuria and reduced eGFR.[9] All participants received maximal tolerated RAAS blockade; SGLT2i use was permitted but relatively low at baseline. Semaglutide once weekly dosing reduced the primary composite outcome by 24% and kidney-specific composite outcomes by ~21% when compared with placebo. Annual eGFR decline was slower with semaglutide by >1 mL/min/1.73 m^2/year, and albuminuria was significantly reduced.

META-ANALYTIC EVIDENCE FOR CARDIORENAL OUTCOMES

In a meta-analysis by Chen et al., that included 17,996 RCT participants,[10] use of GLP-1RAs in CKD patients were significantly associated with a reduced risk of the composite kidney outcomes and all-cause mortality. In another meta-analysis of 85,373 participants with T2DM, GLP-1RAs reduced composite kidney outcome and all-cause death.[11]

Recommendations

KDIGO diabetes management in CKD guidelines had recommended using GLP-1 RAs in T2DM with CKD patients for CV benefits who have not attained glycemic targets despite other agents in particular, metformin and SGLT2i, or who cannot use those agents.[12] Therefore, GLP-1 RAs should be considered in addition to SGLT2i and RAAS blockade in T2DM with CKD, particularly when albuminuria and obesity are present. In obesity with HFpEF or ASCVD, with or without diabetes, GLP-1 RA such as semaglutide 2.4 mg can be used as a core therapy, SGLT2i and RAAS blockers should be added in cases with CKD, diabetes or HF indications exist. Dual GIP/GLP-1 agonists such as tirzepatide, which have shown substantial renal benefit in posthoc analyses may further expand therapeutic possibilities, pending dedicated CKD outcome trials.

PRACTICAL CONSIDERATIONS FOR NEPHROLOGISTS

Patient Selection

Ideal candidates for GLP-1 RA therapy from a nephrology perspective include:

- T2DM with CKD (eGFR ≥25–30 mL/min/1.73 m^2), particularly with obesity and albuminuria
- Obese individuals with ASCVD or HFpEF, irrespective of diabetes status
- Patients with CKM syndrome in whom weight loss and ASCVD risk reduction are priority goals.

Agent Choice and Dosing

- For combined glucose and cardiorenal indications in T2DM with CKD, long-acting agents with proven CV and kidney benefits such as liraglutide, dulaglutide, or semaglutide are preferred.
- For more aggressive weight loss and potential extra-cardiorenal benefit, dual agonists (e.g. tirzepatide) are promising, although kidney outcome data remain scare.

Safety and Tolerability

- Gastrointestinal adverse events (nausea, vomiting, and diarrhea) are the most common and dose-limiting; they can usually be managed with slow titration and dietary advice. Gallbladder disease risk is modestly increased, particularly with substantial weight loss; clinicians should monitor for biliary symptoms.
- Concerns about pancreatitis and pancreatic cancer have not been confirmed in large trials and meta-analyses, although vigilance is warranted in patients with prior pancreatitis.
- Retinopathy worsening has been reported in rapid glycemic improvement settings with semaglutide; careful retinal monitoring is advisable in patients with proliferative diabetic retinopathy.
- *Advanced CKD and dialysis:* Data remain limited for eGFR <25 mL/min/1.73 m^2 and in dialysis patients; cautious use and individualized risk-benefit assessment are necessary.

CONCLUSION

The CKM disease associated with obesity represents a complex scenario for management and associated with significant mortality and morbidity. Traditional approaches focused primarily on glycemic control and blood pressure are no longer sufficient to address the complex interplay between adiposity, insulin resistance, atherosclerosis, HF, and CKD. GLP-1RAs, by targeting multiple upstream and downstream mechanisms, offer a powerful avenue to reduce cardiorenal risk in this high-risk population. For nephrologists, GLP-1 RAs are a potential agent for CKM management that can be combined with SGLT2i, RAAS blockade, and MRAs when appropriate. Careful patient selection, titration, monitoring, and multidisciplinary collaboration are essential to maximize benefit and minimize adverse events.

REFERENCES

1. Sebastian SA, Padda I, Johal G. Cardiovascular-Kidney-Metabolic (CKM) syndrome: A state-of-the-art review. Curr Probl Cardiol. 2024;49(2):102344.
2. Yu JH, Park SY, Lee DY, et al. GLP-1 receptor agonists in diabetic kidney disease: current evidence and future directions. Kidney Res Clin Pract. 2022;41(2):136-49.
3. Jiang Z, Wang Y, Zhao X, et al. Obesity and chronic kidney disease. Am J Physiol Endocrinol Metab. 2023;324(1):E24-E41.
4. Borlaug BA, Jensen MD, Kitzman DW, et al. Obesity and heart failure with preserved ejection fraction: new insights and pathophysiological targets. Cardiovasc Res. 2023;118(18):3434-50.
5. Lee B, Holstein-Rathlou NH, Sosnovtseva O, et al. Renoprotective effects of GLP-1 receptor agonists and SGLT-2 inhibitors-is hemodynamics the key point? Am J Physiol Cell Physiol. 2023;325(1):C243-C256.
6. Park B, Bakbak E, Teoh H, et al. GLP-1 receptor agonists and atherosclerosis protection: the vascular endothelium takes center stage. Am J Physiol Heart Circ Physiol. 2024;326(5):H1159-76.
7. Marso SP, Daniels GH, Brown-Frandsen K, et al; LEADER Steering Committee; LEADER Trial Investigators. Liraglutide and Cardiovascular Outcomes in Type 2 Diabetes. N Engl J Med. 2016;375(4):311-22.
8. Marso SP, Bain SC, Consoli A, et al; SUSTAIN-6 Investigators. Semaglutide and Cardiovascular Outcomes in Patients with Type 2 Diabetes. N Engl J Med. 2016;375(19):1834-44.
9. Perkovic V, Tuttle KR, Rossing P, et al; FLOW Trial Committees and Investigators. Effects of Semaglutide on Chronic Kidney Disease in Patients with Type 2 Diabetes. N Engl J Med. 2024;391(2):109-21.
10. Chen JY, Hsu TW, Liu JH, et al. Kidney and cardiovascular outcomes among patients with CKD receiving GLP-1 receptor agonists: a systematic review and meta-analysis of randomized trials. Am J Kidney Dis. 2025;85(5):555-69.e1.
11. Badve SV, Bilal A, Lee MMY, et al. Effects of GLP-1 receptor agonists on kidney and cardiovascular disease outcomes: a meta-analysis of randomised controlled trials. Lancet Diabetes Endocrinol. 2025;13(1):15-28.
12. de Boer IH, Khunti K, Sadusky T, et al. Diabetes Management in Chronic Kidney Disease: A Consensus Report by the American Diabetes Association (ADA) and Kidney Disease: Improving Global Outcomes (KDIGO). Diabetes Care. 2022;45(12):3075-90.

53

CHAPTER

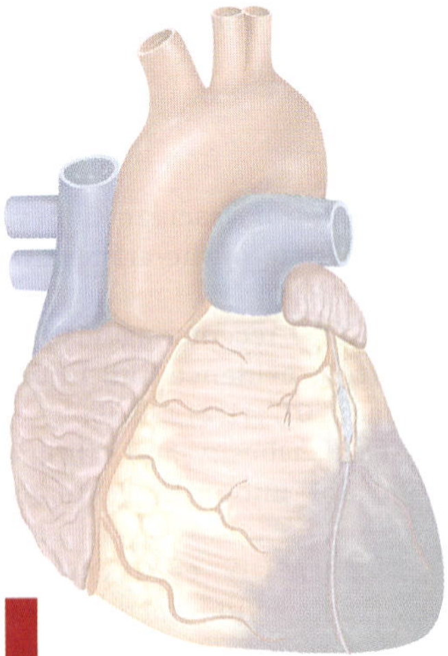

Obesity with Diabetic Nephropathy: Clinical Insight and Management

Vineet Behera, Jayakrishan Pillai, Suman Kumar

INTRODUCTION

The convergence of obesity and diabetes—commonly termed "diabesity"—has emerged as a major driver of chronic kidney disease (CKD) globally. Obesity accelerates diabetic nephropathy (DN) progression through intertwined metabolic disturbances—hypertension, dyslipidemia, insulin resistance—and through direct renal injury pathways. India faces a dual epidemic: Skyrocketing rates of obesity (with millions affected by general/ abdominal obesity) and diabetes, leading to a dramatic rise in DN and making it a leading cause of end-stage kidney disease.

EPIDEMIOLOGY OF OBESITY AND DIABETIC NEPHROPATHY

The World Health Organization (WHO) reports a tripling of global obesity since 1975, with over 1.9 billion adults overweight and 650 million obese by 2016. Obesity itself increases CKD risk independent of diabetes. Obesity is a major driver of the escalating DN epidemic in India, with studies showing high prevalence (around 44%) of kidney disease in type 2 diabetes.[1]

Obesity increases type 2 diabetes risk by nearly six times in India; it significantly raises diabetes odds (e.g., 27% higher in men, 5% in women), with over 50% of Indian adults having it. Obesity also increases the risk and prevalence of DN in India, with studies showing higher rates in obese/overweight diabetic patients (around 68%) versus leaner ones (around 32%). As a corollary, 60% of DN patients are obese or overweight, with figures sometimes exceeding 80% (overweight/obese combined) in DN groups compared to lower rates in diabetic patients without kidney issues.[1,2]

PATHOPHYSIOLOGY: OBESITY AND DIABETIC NEPHROPATHY

Obesity aggravates DN through metabolic, hemodynamic, inflammatory, hormonal, and structural pathways, as shown in **Figure 1**.[3-6]

- Glomerular hyperfiltration and hemodynamic stress: Both obesity and diabetes cause early increases in GFR and glomerular capillary pressure through increased proximal tubular sodium reabsorption, tubuleglomerular feedback-mediated afferent arteriolar dilation, and impaired autoregulation.[4]
- Renin–angiotensin–aldosterone system (RAAS) and sympathetic nervous system activation: Visceral adiposity increases RAAS activity, sympathetic tone, and physical renal compression, producing hypertension and glomerular hypertension, which accelerate DN progression.[3]
- Adipokines and inflammation: Obesity is a chronic low-grade inflammatory state. Key features include macrophage infiltration in adipose tissue and kidney, overproduction of TNF-α, IL-6, MCP-1, and NADPH oxidase-mediated oxidative stress.[5]
- Lipotoxicity and renal lipid accumulation: Lipid deposition within glomeruli and interstitium ("foam cells") is frequently observed in obesity-related renal injury.[4,6]
- Oxidative stress and mitochondrial dysfunction: Hyperglycemia, adipokine dysregulation, and RAAS

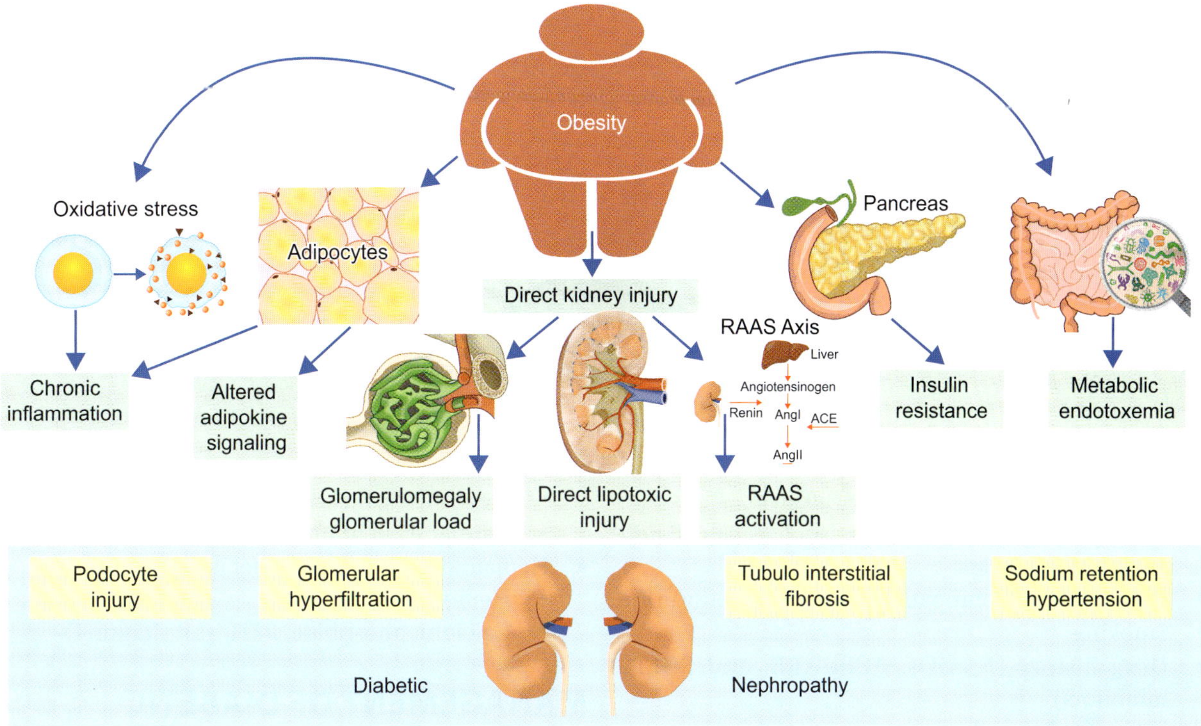

Fig. 1: Pathophysiology of diabetic nephropathy in obesity.

activation increase ROS production and impair mitochondrial function, driving podocyte loss and fibrosis.[3,5]

RISK FACTORS OF DIABETIC NEPHROPATHY IN OBESITY

Diabetic nephropathy and obesity share several common risk factors that interact to accelerate renal injury and metabolic dysfunction, as given in **Figure 2**. Insulin resistance is a central link, leading to hyperglycemia, hyperinsulinemia, and glomerular hyperfiltration. Poor glycemic control promotes advanced glycation end-product formation, oxidative stress, and mesangial expansion, contributing to progressive kidney damage. Hypertension, frequently present in obese individuals with diabetes, increases intraglomerular pressure and accelerates proteinuria and nephron loss. Dyslipidemia, characterized by elevated triglycerides and LDL cholesterol, causes renal lipotoxicity and endothelial dysfunction. Both conditions are associated with chronic low-grade inflammation, driven by adipokines and proinflammatory cytokines, which promotes fibrosis and glomerulosclerosis. Activation of the RAAS further worsens glomerular hypertension and albuminuria.[4,6]

MONITORING AND EARLY DETECTION

Monitoring and management of CKD due to DN in obese patients must be stage-specific and proactive. In early CKD (stages 1 and 2), emphasis is on intensive glycemic control, weight reduction, blood pressure management, and reduction of albuminuria. Moderate CKD (stages 3 and 4) requires close monitoring of eGFR, albuminuria, electrolytes, anemia, and bone-mineral disorders, with dose adjustment of drugs and avoidance of nephrotoxins. Advanced CKD (stage 5) focuses on dialysis planning and transplant evaluation. Special issues include accelerated cardiovascular risk, difficult volume control, insulin resistance, and challenges in vascular access. Regular multidisciplinary follow-up is essential to slow progression and improve outcomes.

CLINICAL ASSESSMENT OF OBESE PATIENTS WITH DIABETIC NEPHROPATHY

- History:
  - Diabetes type, duration, and control of diabetes
  - Detailed dietary habits including carbohydrates and fat consumed

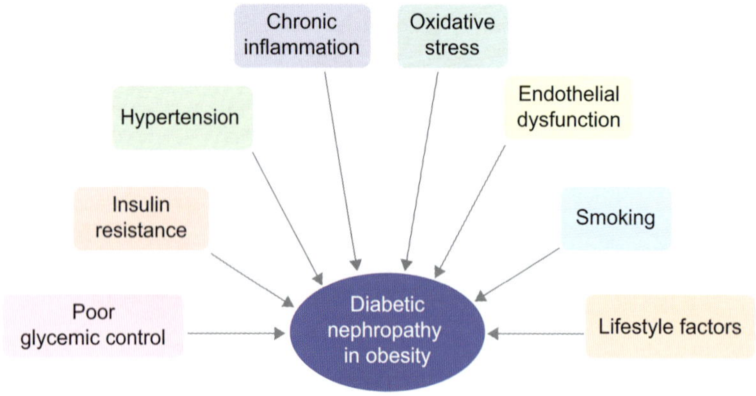

Fig. 2: Risk factors of diabetic nephropathy in obesity.

  - Physical activity and sedentary lifestyle
  - History of other renal diseases such as calculi and glomerulonephritis
  - Symptoms of nephropathy: Edema and frothy urine
  - Smoking
  - Drug history (NSAIDs, ACEi/ARB, and SGLT2 inhibitors)
  - Features of complications of diabetes—retinopathy, neuropathy, and CVD
  - Metabolic complications of obesity
- Physical examination:
  - Height, weight, and BMI
  - Waist circumference
  - Waist–hip ratio
  - Skin fold thickness
  - Blood pressure (including orthostatic BP)
  - Edema
  - Signs of fluid overload
  - Acanthosis nigricans, features of insulin resistance
  - Diabetic retinopathy

Laboratory Evaluation of Obese Patients with Diabetic Nephropathy[3,5]

- Glycemic status:
  - Fasting plasma glucose, postprandial glucose
  - HbA1c
- Renal assessment:
  - Serum creatinine, urea, and eGFR
  - Urine albumin–creatinine ratio (UACR)
  - Urine routine and microscopy
  - 24-hour urine protein
  - Ultrasound of the kidneys
- Metabolic profile:
  - Lipid profile
  - Serum uric acid
  - Electrolytes, bicarbonate
  - Cardiac evaluation—ECG, 2D ECHO, and stress test
- Hematological and bone metabolism:
  - Hemoglobin
  - Calcium, phosphate, PTH, and vitamin D

MANAGEMENT OF DIABETIC NEPHROPATHY IN OBESITY

Weight Reduction[5]

Weight reduction is a key therapeutic strategy in obese patients with DN, as it improves insulin resistance, reduces blood pressure, and decreases glomerular hyperfiltration and albuminuria. Lifestyle measures form the foundation, while pharmacotherapy may be added, including GLP-1 receptor agonists. Orlistat (120 mg three times daily) may be used selectively. Bariatric surgery is considered in morbid obesity (BMI ≥35 kg/m^2 with comorbidities), leading to sustained weight loss and improvement in glycemic control.

Lifestyle Modification

Lifestyle management is fundamental in DN with obesity and complements pharmacological therapy. A balanced diet with low glycemic index foods, reduced saturated fats, sodium restriction (<2 g/day), and moderate protein intake (~0.8 g/kg/day) is recommended. Regular physical activity (at least 150 minutes per week of moderate exercise) improves glycemic control, blood pressure, and lipid profile.

Glycemic Control

- KDIGO recommends individualized HbA1c targets of <6.5%.

- Antidiabetics
  - Metformin (if eGFR ≥30 mL/min/1.73 m^2)
  - Sulfonylureas—glipizide and gliclazide—are safe in CKD, but carry the risk of hypoglycemia.
  - DPP4 inhibitors—Sitagliptin and vildagliptin—may need dose modification in advanced CKD. Linagliptin may be used at the full dose.
  - SGLT2i—moderate hypoglycemic effect
- Insulin—short-acting insulin + long-acting analogs (basal-bolus regimen) or mixed insulin (split-mix regimen)—may be used in patients with poor glycemia control, with close monitoring for risk of hypoglycemia.

Blood Pressure Management

KDIGO recommends a BP target <130/80 mm Hg for patients with diabetes and CKD.[7] Apart from ACE inhibitors or ARB, other antihypertensives such as calcium channel blockers, diuretics, beta-blockers, and others may be used based on the patient profile.[8]

Renin–angiotensin–aldosterone System Blockade

Renin–angiotensin–aldosterone system blockade is a cornerstone in the management of DN in obese patients by reducing intraglomerular hypertension and proteinuria.[9,10] ACE inhibitors and ARBs decrease efferent arteriolar resistance, thereby lowering albuminuria and slowing CKD progression, independent of blood pressure reduction. Commonly used drugs include enalapril (5–20 mg/day), ramipril (2.5–10 mg/day), losartan (50–100 mg/day), and telmisartan (40–80 mg/day).

SGLT2 Inhibitors

SGLT2 inhibitors play a key role in managing DN in obese patients by reducing renal glucose reabsorption, improving glycemic control, and promoting natriuresis.[9,11] They lower intraglomerular pressure, reduce albuminuria, and slow CKD progression independent of glucose lowering. Common agents include empagliflozin (10–25 mg once daily), dapagliflozin (10 mg once daily), and canagliflozin (100–300 mg once daily), with dose adjustment based on eGFR.

Nonsteroidal Mineralocorticoid Receptor Antagonists

Nonsteroidal mineralocorticoid receptor antagonists (ns-MRAs) are effective adjuncts in DN, particularly in obese patients with residual albuminuria despite ACE inhibitor or ARB therapy.[10] They selectively block mineralocorticoid receptor-mediated inflammation and fibrosis, reducing renal and cardiovascular injury. Finerenone is the primary agent, prescribed at 10–20 mg once daily, with dosing guided by eGFR and serum potassium levels.

GLP-1 Analogs

GLP-1 receptor agonists play an important role in managing DN in obese patients by improving glycemic control and promoting weight loss.[8] They reduce insulin resistance, lower albuminuria, and may slow kidney disease progression through anti-inflammatory and hemodynamic effects. Common agents include liraglutide (0.6–1.8 mg subcutaneously daily), semaglutide (0.25–1 mg weekly), and dulaglutide (0.75–1.5 mg weekly). Benefits include significant weight reduction, improved HbA1c, blood pressure lowering, and proven cardiovascular risk reduction.

Lipid Management

Lipid management is essential in DN with obesity to reduce accelerated cardiovascular and renal risk.[12] Dyslipidemia contributes to endothelial dysfunction, renal lipotoxicity, and progression of kidney disease. Statins are first-line therapy, with commonly used agents including atorvastatin (10–40 mg/day) and rosuvastatin (5–20 mg/day), adjusted for renal function. In patients with persistent hypertriglyceridemia, ezetimibe (10 mg/day) or fenofibrate (dose adjusted) may be added cautiously **(Fig. 3)**.

DIALYSIS

Dialysis in patients with DN and obesity presents unique challenges and requires individualized planning. Initiation of dialysis is based on standard indications such as uremic symptoms, refractory fluid overload, hyperkalemia, or declining nutritional status, rather than eGFR alone.[13] Hemodialysis (HD) is commonly used but is often complicated by difficult vascular access due to obesity, diabetes-related vascular disease, and higher rates of catheter dependence, access failure, and infection. Peritoneal dialysis (PD) offers advantages such as better hemodynamic stability and avoidance of vascular access,[14] but may be limited by reduced peritoneal membrane efficiency, increased risk of mechanical complications, and challenges in achieving adequate clearance in obese patients. Both modalities carry higher risks of cardiovascular events, infections, and malnutrition.

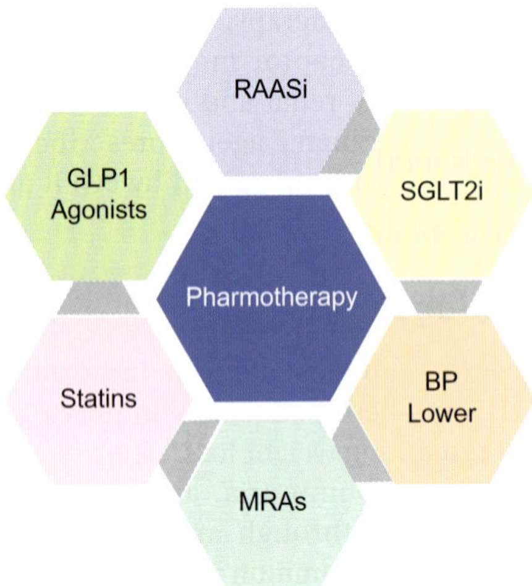

Fig. 3: Pharmacological agents in diabetic nephropathy and obesity.

KIDNEY TRANSPLANT

Kidney transplantation is the preferred renal replacement therapy in DN,[15] but obesity poses important challenges. Obese diabetic patients have higher risks of perioperative complications, including wound infections, delayed graft function, and thrombosis. Cardiovascular disease is common and requires meticulous pretransplant evaluation. Obesity is associated with longer waiting times, technical difficulties during surgery, and increased risk of posttransplant diabetes and infections. Immunosuppressive drug dosing and wound healing may be problematic. Weight reduction, including lifestyle measures or bariatric surgery, is often required before listing. Despite these issues, transplantation offers superior survival and quality of life compared with long-term dialysis in this population.

CONCLUSION

Emerging themes include adipose-renal axis as a therapeutic target[6] (adipokines, adipose inflammation), lipotoxicity modulation via SREBP inhibitors and lipid-lowering interventions, precision obesity metrics (ABSI, WWI, and BRI) for individualized DN risk prediction, anti-inflammatory and antifibrotic therapies targeting TNF-α, IL-6, MCP-1, TGF-β pathways, bariatric metabolic surgery as renal-protective therapy in severe obesity, and other *novel* therapeutic targets such as endothelin receptor antagonists, anti-inflammatory/antifibrotic agents, and next-generation incretin polyagonists.

REFERENCES

1. Viswanathan V, Mirshad R. The burden of diabetic nephropathy in India: need for prevention. Diabetic Nephropathy. 2023;3(2):25-8.
2. Maric-Bilkan C. Obesity and diabetic kidney disease. Med Clin North Am. 2013;97(1):59-74.
3. Amann K, Benz K. Structural renal changes in obesity and diabetes. Semin Nephrol. 2013;33:23-33.
4. Maric C, Hall JE. Obesity, metabolic syndrome and diabetic nephropathy. Contrib Nephrol. 2011;170:28-35.
5. Moosaie F, Ghaemi F, Mechanick JI, et al. Obesity and diabetic complications: a study from the Nationwide Diabetes Report of the National Program for Prevention and Control of Diabetes (NPPCD-2021) implications for action on multiple scales. Prim Care Diabetes. 2022;16(3):422-9.
6. Câmara NO, Iseki K, Kramer H, et al. Kidney disease and obesity: epidemiology, mechanisms and treatment. Nat Rev Nephrol. 2017;13(3):181-90.
7. Murty MS, Pandey R, Behera S, et al. Plasma renin-guided therapy in patients of primary hypertension on antihypertensives: a prospective cohort study. J Assoc Physicians India. 2022;70(8):11-2.
8. Sharma I, Liao Y, Zheng X, et al. New pandemic: obesity and associated nephropathy. Front Med. 2021;8:673556.
9. Katsiki N, Anagnostis P, Kotsa K, et al. Obesity, metabolic syndrome and the risk of microvascular complications in patients with diabetes mellitus. Curr Pharm Des. 2019;25(18):2051-9.
10. Behera V, Chauhan R, Sinha S, et al. Anaphylactic shock secondary to intravenous iron sucrose in chronic kidney disease. Indian J Hematol Blood Transfus. 2015;31(3):391-3.
11. Zhang W, Liu Y. The obesity-related indices are useful for predicting diabetic nephropathy in patients with type II diabetes mellitus. Endocrinol Diabetes Metab. 2025;8:e70087.
12. Shekhawat VS, Behera V, Nayak AK, et al. Evaluation of the prevalence and pattern of dyslipidemia in newly detected type 2 diabetes mellitus patients and nondiabetic controls. J Mar Med Soc. 2024;26(3):392-7.
13. Kidney Disease: Improving Global Outcomes (KDIGO) Diabetes Work Group. KDIGO 2022 Clinical Practice Guideline for diabetes management in chronic kidney disease. Kidney Int. 2022;102(5S):S1-27.
14. Behera V, Ahmad S, Sinha S, et al. Tunneled dialysis catheter insertion in external jugular vein by nephrologists. Indian J Nephrol. 2025;35(1):46.
15. Dash SC, Nair R, Behera V. Kidney transplantation: the journey across a century. Med J Armed Forces India. 2023;79(6):631-7.

54

CHAPTER

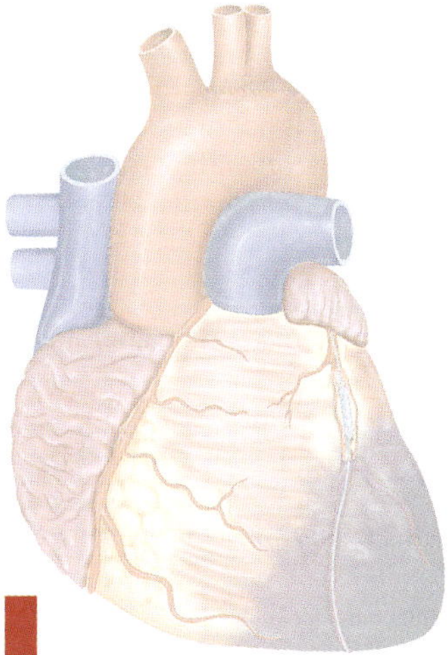

Obesity-associated Proteinuria in Nondiabetics: Clinical Insight and Management

Divya Bajpai

INTRODUCTION

Obesity [defined as body mass index (BMI) ≥30 kg/m^2 and ≥25 kg/m^2 for Western and Asian populations, respectively] has now been declared by the World Health Organization (WHO) and has now emerged as a major preventable epidemic affecting over a billion individuals worldwide.[1] It is associated with expansive morbidity and wide-ranging complications on end organs, including kidneys.[2] Raised BMI is strongly associated with high risk of new-onset chronic kidney disease (CKD).[3] Association of obesity with diabetes, popularly known as "diabesity," has gained much attention, where concurrence of obesity predisposes to diabetic nephropathy and progressive kidney failure.[4] However, proteinuria (defined as excretion of abnormally high levels of proteins in urine) is a significant consequence of obesity, even in nondiabetic individuals, predicting adverse cardiovascular and renal outcomes. In this chapter, we explore obesity-associated proteinuria in nondiabetic patients, focusing on its epidemiology, pathophysiology, diagnostic challenges, and management.

EPIDEMIOLOGY

Are the obese more likely to have proteinuria?

Cohort and cross-sectional studies indicate that the prevalence of proteinuria in obese individuals is significantly higher than that of their nonobese counterparts, even after adjusting for diabetes and controlling blood pressure.[5,6] Data from NHANES (2003–2020) involving 59,717 adults suggests that 40% of obese US adults had albuminuria.[7] After adjusting for socioeconomic status, obese individuals had a 36% higher odds of albuminuria compared to normal-weight individuals.[7] In a cohort of 218 obese patients undergoing bariatric surgery at a New York City hospital, proteinuria was found in 21% and albuminuria in 19.7%.[8] In obese individuals, glomerular hyperfiltration precedes the development of proteinuria and hypertension. Thus, a "higher-normal" glomerular filtration rate can predict susceptible populations prone to develop proteinuria.[9,10]

Does weight loss lead to regression in proteinuria?

Evidence from clinical trials shows that intentional weight loss, whether through lifestyle modifications or surgery, reduces proteinuria. In a systematic review of trials involving 522 subjects, weight loss decreased proteinuria by 1.7 g [95% confidence interval (CI): 0.7–2.6 g] and 14 mg [95% CI: 11–17 mg]. This was independent of blood pressure control and was observed across all modalities of weight-loss interventions.[11] This reduction in proteinuria is documented as early as 4–12 weeks after starting a weight-loss program.[12] Weight loss attenuates the activity of the renin–angiotensin–aldosterone system and reduces adipocyte-derived cytokines, such as TNF-α.[13,14] This, in turn, alleviates the glomerular hyperfiltration which precedes the decline in proteinuria.[13]

Does obesity increase the risk of kidney failure?

Large-scale epidemiologic studies have demonstrated obesity as one of the strongest independent risk factors for both the onset and progression of CKD.[3] There appears to be a dose-response relationship between BMI and CKD risk, with risk steeply increasing once BMI crosses 25 kg/m^2.[15,16]

Herrington et al. analyzed a cohort of over 1.4 million adults from England. They recorded a higher risk of incident CKD with each additional unit of BMI over 25, regardless of diabetes or hypertension.[17] They estimated that since 2000, up to 39% of advanced CKD in women and 26% in men aged 40 years to 79 years resulted from being overweight or obese.[17] Hsu et al. followed over 300,000 adults and demonstrated a graded increase in risk of end-stage kidney disease (ESKD) with a 6-fold higher risk when BMI is over 35 kg/ m^2.[18]

Are these risks similar in children and adolescents?
One in five children globally is obese, and the rate of rise of childhood obesity is higher than that of adult obesity.[19] A case-control study involving 112 overweight and obese patients aged 7–16 years demonstrated significantly higher blood pressure, creatinine, and 24-hour urine protein values in the overweight and obese groups.[20] In a 25-year follow-up study of 1.2 million adolescents, being overweight at the age of 17 years was associated with a 3.4-fold higher risk of nondiabetic kidney failure in adulthood.[21]

Obesity-related Glomerulopathy (Box 1)

Obesity-related glomerulopathy (ORG) is a distinct histopathological diagnosis characterized by clinical obesity (as defined by BMI cut-offs), kidney biopsy evidence of oligonephronia (low glomerular density) and glomerulomegaly (glomerular hypertrophy), with or without focal segmental glomerular sclerosis (FSGS).[22,23] It differs from primary FSGS in having a more indolent course, preserved albumin levels, milder foot-process effacement, and fewer glomeruli with FSGS lesions.[23,24] Nevertheless, ORG is closely associated with kidney dysfunction, with up to 30% patients developing chronic kidney disease and 10% progressing to ESKD.[23]

BOX 1: Kidney biopsy in an obese nondiabetic patient with proteinuria.

As mentioned in the text, a kidney biopsy is not mandatory in all patients for the initial diagnosis. Patients with persistent proteinuria >1 g/day despite treatment would merit a kidney biopsy.

Red flags mandating early kidney biopsy are:
- Patients with nephrotic syndrome (edema, serum albumin <3 g/dL, UPCR >3 g/g, dyslipidemia)
- Rapidly increasing proteinuria, even if <3 g/g
- Active urinary sediment (presence of red blood cell casts or significant microscopic hematuria)
- Substantial and rapid decline in eGFR with or without new onset of hypertension
- Presence of positive serology for lupus, hepatitis, or vasculitis. Systemic signs or symptoms suggest the same
- Persistent hypocomplementemia
- Mild obesity with disproportionate proteinuria

Kidney biopsy findings:
Light microscopy (LM)—kidney biopsies in obese patients often reveal:
- Glomerulomegaly (glomerular diameter >200–220 µm)
- Oligonephronia (low glomerular density)
- With or without focal segmental glomerular sclerosis (FSGS). FSGS is usually a perihilar variant due to "wear-and-tear" at the vascular pole of the glomerulus caused by hyperfiltration.

These features are required for the diagnosis of obesity-related glomerulopathy (ORG).[22] Not all patients with obesity-induced proteinuria have ORG.
- *Mesangial expansion:* Mild increase in the mesangial matrix (less pronounced than in diabetic nephropathy)

Immunofluorescence (IF): In nondiabetic obese individuals, immunofluorescence is typically negative. Nonspecific trapping of IgM or C3 can occur in areas of segmental sclerosis

Electron microscopy (EM): Segmental effacement is seen involving <50% of podocyte foot processes. Podocyte hypertrophy is seen—absence of electron-dense deposits

PATHOPHYSIOLOGY

Mechanisms involving multiple hemodynamic, metabolic, and inflammatory pathways converge on glomerular and tubular structures **(Flowchart 1)**.

Hemodynamic Stress and Renin-Angiotensin-Aldosterone System Activation

- *Increased filtration load:* Obesity-related increased metabolic demand increases cardiac output and total blood volume, thereby increasing renal plasma flow. This is also compounded by the renin-angiotensin-aldosterone system (RAAS) and sympathetic activation by visceral adipocytes.
- *Increased intraglomerular pressure:* Obesity causes hyperinsulinemia, leading to increased proximal tubular sodium reabsorption and reduced sodium delivery to the macula dense. This causes deactivation of tubuloglomerular feedback (TGF) and afferent arteriolar vasodilation, further increasing intraglomerular pressure.[25]
- *Podocyte stress* results in a higher single-nephron glomerular filtration rate (GFR), referred to as glomerular hyperfiltration.[5,16,26] While initially adaptive, persistent glomerular hyperfiltration eventually leads to maladaptation and glomerulomegaly. As podocytes are terminally differentiated cells, they become stretched and eventually detach, leading to FSGS lesions. This podocyte stress causes protein

Flowchart 1: Pathophysiology of obesity-related kidney injury.

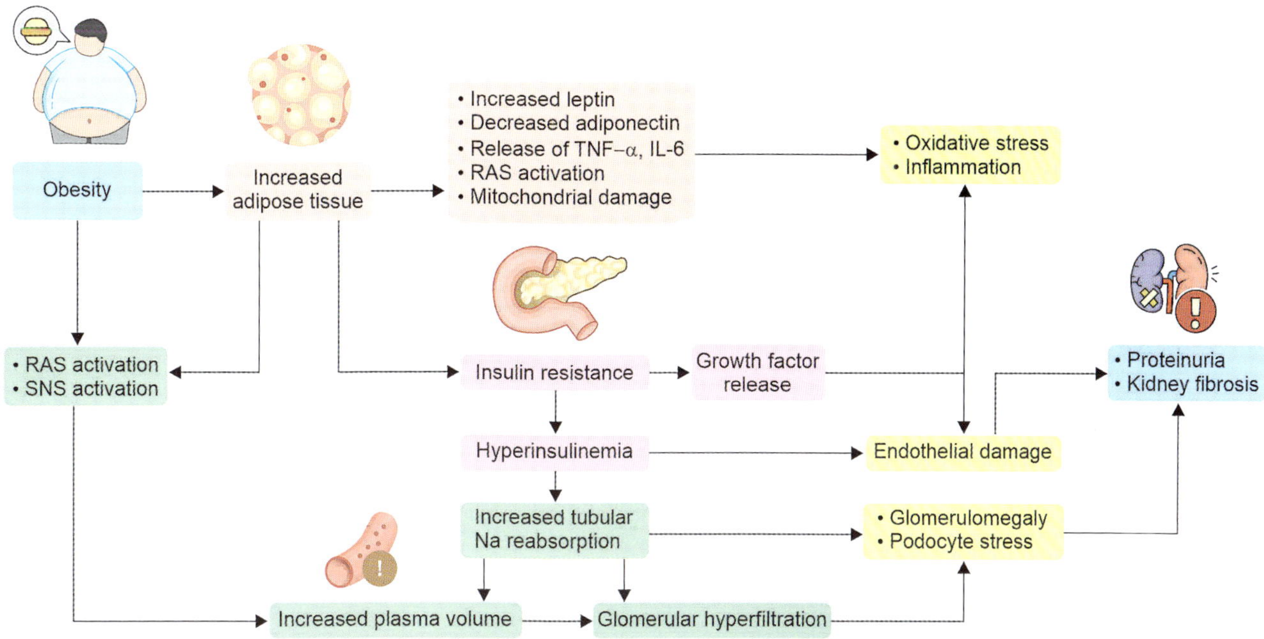

(IL-6: interleukin 6; Na: sodium; RAS: renin angiotensin system; SNS: sympathetic nervous system; TNF: tissue necrosis factor)

leakage and progressive kidney injury.[6,26] These mechanisms, though exacerbated in diabetes, can occur independently of the same.

Adipokine Dysregulation and Lipotoxicity

Visceral adipose tissue is an active endocrine organ that secretes proinflammatory cytokines (IL-6 and TNF-α) and adipokines. Insulin resistance, dyslipidemia, and ectopic lipid accumulation in renal tissue augment the kidney damage.

- *Inflammatory stress:* In obesity, leptin is elevated, which stimulates TGF-β production. Fat accumulation in the renal sinus also triggers local inflammation and oxidative stress.[26,27]
- *Adiponectin:* Obesity leads to a deficiency of adiponectin, which is a key protective molecule against podocyte oxidative stress. This causes mitochondrial damage, endothelial dysfunction, and mesangial expansion, resulting in proteinuric kidney injury.[27]
- *Renal fibrosis:* Chronic inflammatory and oxidative stress leads to higher collagen turnover and matrix accumulation, culminating in renal fibrosis.[5,28]

Clinical Phenotypes and Approach to Diagnosis

The majority of patients with obesity-associated proteinuria are often asymptomatic till advanced stages of kidney injury. This "silent" presentation highlights the importance of routine screening **(Flowchart 2)**.

Clinical Features

- *Raised BMI:* In the Western population, the cut-offs for overweight and obesity are BMI >25 kg/m^2 and ≥30 kg/m^2, respectively. Asians have higher visceral fat and hence lower cut-offs of >23 kg/m^2 and ≥25 kg/m^2, respectively.
- *Higher waist circumference (WC):* WC thresholds used for identifying health risks in Western populations are 102 cm for men and 88 cm for women. For Asian populations, these are redefined as 90 cm for men and 80 cm for women.
- *Albuminuria:* Persistent moderately increased albuminuria, defined as urine albumin-to-creatinine ratio (UACR) >30 mg/g, is often an early feature.
- *Proteinuria:* Persistent proteinuria is defined as urine protein-to-creatinine ratio (PCR) >150 mg/g.
- *Nonnephrotic range proteinuria:* Urine PCR is usually between 300 mg/g and 3,500 mg/g. Nephrotic-range proteinuria (>3,500 mg/g) is rare. Nephrotic syndrome is uncommon even in patients with heavy proteinuria. The presence of nephrotic syndrome points toward an alternative pathology.
- *Renal function:* In early stages, eGFR may be normal or even elevated due to glomerular hyperfiltration. If untreated, there is a slow, progressive decline in eGFR.

Flowchart 2: Approach toward diagnosis of obesity-associated proteinuria.

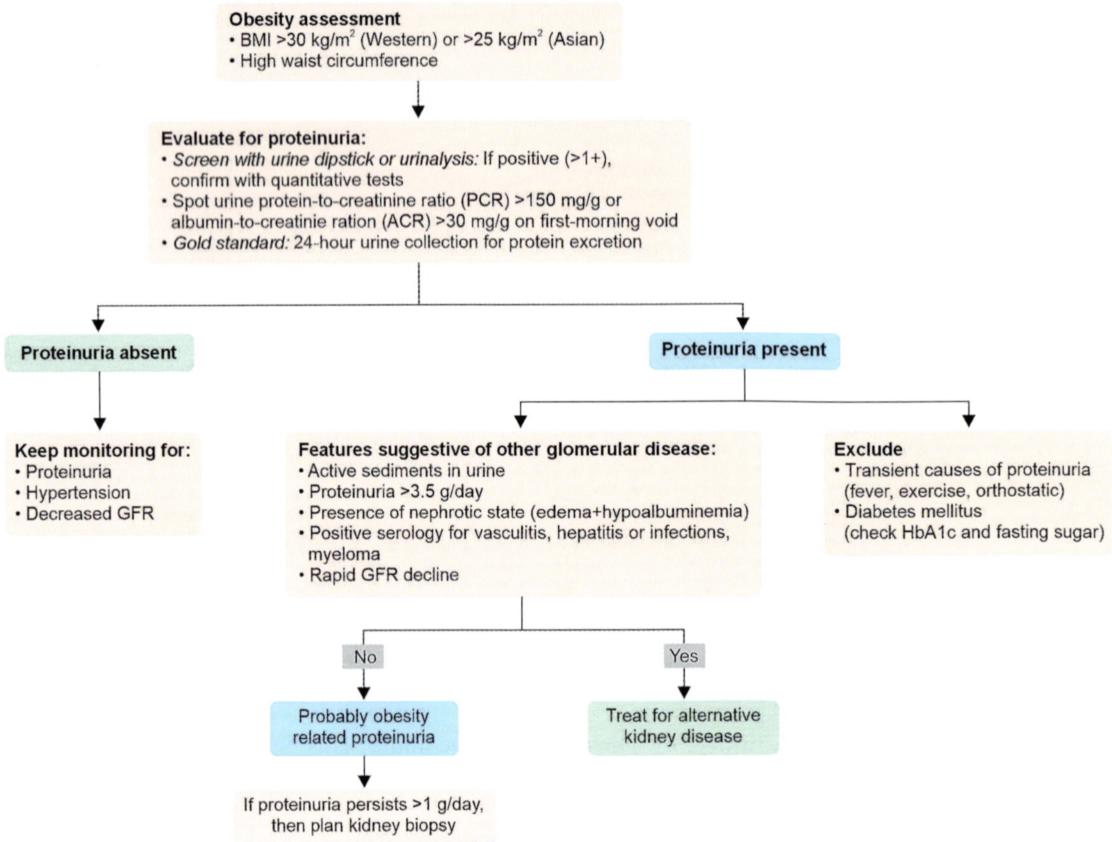

The course is indolent compared to other portonephrotic kidney diseases.

- *Hypertension:* Hypertension is usually present, specifically in later stages of the disease.
- *Absence of active urinary sediment:* The urine examination does not show cellular elements such as red blood cells (RBCs), white blood cells (WBCs), and casts (e.g., RBC casts).
- *Features of cardiometabolic dysfunction:* Commonly, patients have dyslipidemia, cardiovascular, or peripheral vascular disease.

Histopathological features: Kidney biopsy is not mandatory for the diagnosis of obesity-related proteinuria. Patients with long-standing obesity with a BMI ≥30 kg/m^2 and an indolent course with subnephrotic proteinuria with no active sediments, normal eGFR, and negative serology for lupus, hepatitis, and vasculitis can be managed initially without a kidney biopsy. However, for patients with persistent proteinuria >1 g/day, biopsy should be planned if the risks do not outweigh the benefits. Red flags mandating a kidney biopsy and biopsy findings are given in **Table 1**.

Pitfalls in Kidney Function Assessment in Obesity

Obesity complicates the accurate assessment of kidney function, as most eGFR equations, such as the CKD-EPI equation, were developed for populations with standard body composition. Serum creatinine is a byproduct of muscle mass, which can be significantly decreased in some patients with obesity and CKD (referred to as sarcopenic obesity).[16] This low muscle mass can lead to falsely high eGFR and mask significant renal impairment. Cystatin C is touted as more accurate because it is independent of muscle mass. Still, it is significantly affected by adipose tissue and inflammation present in obesity, leading to an underestimation of eGFR. Equations combining creatinine and cystatin C are more accurate. Another problem is that the indexing of eGFR to 1.73 m^2 in an obese individual with a BSA higher than 2 m^2 can lead to an inappropriate decline in the estimated GFR. GFR calculations using 24-hour urinary creatinine clearance can be used; however, it is cumbersome.[16]

TABLE 1: Differences between obesity-related glomerulopathy and primary FSGS.

Clinical parameter	*Obesity-related glomerulopathy*	*Primary FSGS*
Body mass index	Always ≥30 kg/m^2	Might be normal
Proteinuria level	0.5–1.5 g/day	Variable but can be >3–3.5 g/day
Nephrotic syndrome (edema + low albumin + dyslipidemia)	Rare, even with a high degree of proteinuria	Commonly seen in up to 50%
Serum albumin	More than 3–3.5 g/dL	<3–3.5 g/dL
Progression to kidney failure	Slower progression; indolent course	Faster progression if nonresponsive to treatment
Light microscopy	Glomerulomegaly in 100%, mild sclerosis usually perihilar	Minimal glomerulomegaly, prominent segmental sclerosis
Foot process effacement	Usually <50%	Usually >50%
Response to RAAS blockade	Proteinuria improves up to 60%	Variable response
Response to steroids	No response	Standard treatment
Comorbidities	Diabetes and hypertension	Viral infections and drugs

Pitfalls in Proteinuria Assessment in Obesity

In patients with sarcopenic obesity, muscle mass is generally low, which leads to lower urinary creatinine excretion. Thus, assessing urine albumin-creatinine ratio (UACR) or urine protein-creatinine ratio (UPCR) in such patients may lead to an overestimation of proteinuria.[16] Also, while on treatment, if the patient gains muscle mass, UACR would improve due to increased creatinine excretion. Proteinuria estimation using 24-hour urinary protein is recommended.

DIFFERENTIAL DIAGNOSIS

It is crucial to distinguish obesity-associated proteinuria from other causes of proteinuria.

- *Primary FSGS:* Differences in **Table 1**
- *Hypertensive nephrosclerosis:* Presence of hyaline arteriosclerosis and shrunken glomeruli with long-standing hypertension and proteinuria <1.5 g/day
- *Occult diabetic nephropathy:* Prominent mesangial expansion, thickened glomerular capillaries, and occasionally Kimmelstiel-Wilson lesions.

MANAGEMENT

Lifestyle Modifications for Weight Loss: Diet and Exercise

Weight loss is the cornerstone of the management of obesity-related proteinuria. Evidence from randomized controlled trials (RCTs) confirms that calorie restriction and increased physical activity lead to weight loss and improve functional capacity in people living with obesity and CKD.[29] Comprehensive lifestyle interventions, such as the diabetes prevention program (DPP), have shown benefit in the Look AHEAD (Action for Health in Diabetes) study.[30] DPP led to a minimum of 7% weight loss using a low-fat, low-calorie diet with over 150 minutes of exercise per week.[30]

Dietary therapy: Options include the Mediterranean diet or a low-fat diet with energy restriction. The goal is to create an energy deficit by reducing energy intake below energy expenditure.[16] These diets can be consumed on a time-restricted basis (i.e., intermittent fasting). Diet must ensure 1–1.5 g of protein per kilogram of ideal body weight daily in patients with preserved GFR. High protein intake helps build muscle mass and, indirectly, increases calorie expenditure. Regardless of the diet type, the most important predictor of weight loss is dietary adherence. Dietary sodium restriction helps reduce RAAS activation and control blood pressure, thereby decreasing proteinuria associated with obesity.

Exercise: Physical activity, when performed for at least 30 minutes, 5–7 days per week, improves insulin sensitivity, reduces inflammation, helps maintain body weight, and improves cardiovascular health.[31] It is the most critical determinant of maintaining lean muscle mass during the period of active weight loss.[32] As the effect of exercise is dose dependent, it should always be combined with a calorie-restricted diet to achieve weight loss. The type of exercise must be determined by age, comorbidities, and personal preferences, and combining both aerobic and resistance exercises yields the best results.

Bariatric Surgery for Obesity

Bariatric surgery is a potent intervention for durable weight loss and improves metabolic health, especially in patients with a BMI over 30 kg/m^2. Surgical interventions significantly reduce the UACR in obese individuals in over 50% of patients and can also reverse early histological features of ORG.[33] An RCT evaluating 5-year outcomes of bariatric surgery in diabetic patients reported that combining bariatric surgery with intensive medical therapy improved long-term outcomes.[34]

PHARMACOLOGICAL INTERVENTIONS

Antiobesity Medications

Candidates for antiobesity drug therapy are individuals who have not lost at least 5% of their weight despite 3–6 months of comprehensive lifestyle interventions and have a BMI ≥30 kg/m^2, or BMI 27–29.9 kg/m^2 and ≥1 weight-related comorbidities, or central adiposity plus >1 weight-related comorbidities.

Glucagon-like peptide 1 (GLP-1)-based therapies: GLP1-based drugs are the first-line choice due to evidence on improved cardiovascular outcomes. These include GLP-1 receptor agonists (GLP1- RA)—semaglutide, liraglutide, and glucose-dependent insulinotropic polypeptide (GIP) /GLP-1 dual receptor agonist—tirzepatide.

Semaglutide: In the landmark FLOW trial semaglutide, given 1 mg subcutaneously (SC) every week, reduced the risk of major kidney adverse events (a composite of eGFR decline, ESRD, and renal death) by 24% in diabetic patients with CKD.[35] A similar effect was seen in obese patients without diabetes in the SELECT trial. At a dose of 2.4 mg SC per week, the cardiovascular benefit was observed independent of the magnitude of weight loss.[36]

Liraglutide: It is indicated at 3 mg subcutaneously daily for the treatment of obesity in adults with or without diabetes. In the SCALE maintenance study, liraglutide, along with diet and exercise, induced significant weight loss over 56 weeks and showed improvements in some cardiovascular disease-risk factors.[37]

Tirzepatide: It is a dual-acting GLP-1 and GIP receptor agonist with significant efficacy for weight reduction in individuals with obesity.[38,39] The weight-related benefits of tirzepatide were found to be greater in nondiabetics.[39] It is initially administered subcutaneously once weekly at a dose of 2.5 mg per week for 4 weeks, then increased. It is also FDA approved for the treatment of severe obstructive sleep apnea in adults with obesity.

Precautions for GLP-1-based therapies: Gastrointestinal side effects (e.g., nausea and diarrhea) are common and can be mitigated over time by starting at a low dose and slowly escalating, eating slowly and in small meals, and limiting high-fat foods. They are contraindicated in pregnancy, personal or family history of medullary thyroid cancer or multiple endocrine neoplasia 2A or 2B, severe inflammatory bowel disease, gastroparesis, and history of pancreatitis.

Alternative Antiobesity Drugs

Other antiobesity drugs include:

- Phentermine-topiramate and naltrexone-bupropion works by reducing appetite and metabolism.
- Orlistat alters fat digestion.
- Phentermine—sympathomimetic drug

Combining medications with different mechanisms of action improves efficacy and tolerability.

Interventions for Proteinuria Reduction and Kidney Protection

In patients with obesity with or without CKD, higher degrees of albuminuria are associated with a more rapid decline in kidney function. Thus, albuminuria reduction is a primary treatment goal in overweight or obese patients.

Blood Pressure Control

A patient-level meta-analysis of RCTs suggests that targeting BP <130/80 mm Hg is associated with albuminuria reduction and better kidney outcomes.[40] Lifestyle modifications such as reduction in salt intake (<2,000 mg of sodium per day), enhanced dietary potassium, consuming more fruits, vegetables, legumes, and low-fat dairy products, and less sweets, sugar-sweetened beverages, and animal proteins (DASH diet), abstinence from alcohol, exercise, and weight loss are effective in controlling blood pressure. In patients with albuminuria, the choice of antihypertensives is dictated by their impact on albuminuria.

Renin-angiotensin System Inhibitors

Angiotensin-converting enzyme (ACE) inhibitors and angiotensin II receptor blockers (ARBs) have an antialbuminuric effect by reducing the intraglomerular pressure, which is significantly increased in obesity. Thus, these should be offered to all patients with obesity-related proteinuria, with or without hypertension.[41] It is essential to watch for hyperkalemia and eGFR decline while on RAS inhibition.

Mineralocorticoid receptor antagonists provide additional albuminuria reduction when added to RAS inhibitors.[42] Spironolactone and eplerenone can cause hyperkalemia, especially in patients with reduced GFR. The nonsteroidal MRA finerenone is a newer alternative that effectively slows the progression of kidney disease and has a lower risk of hyperkalemia.[43]

SGLT2 Inhibitors

SGLT2 inhibitors have shown renoprotective effects in nondiabetic kidney disease patients with proteinuria. Major mechanisms include natriuresis, leading to a reduction in intravascular volume, which is raised in obesity. This normalizes the increased tubuloglomerular feedback and thereby reduces intraglomerular pressure (i.e., reduces glomerular hyperfiltration) by constricting the afferent arteriole. As glomerular hyperfiltration is central to obesity-induced proteinuria, these are indicated in nondiabetic proteinuric patients.[44] In such patients, the antiproteinuric effects of SGLT2i appear BMI dependent, with higher reductions in overweight/obese patients, suggesting normalization of hyperfiltration states.[45]

Monitoring and Multidisciplinary Care

Long-term monitoring is warranted given the relapsing-remitting nature of the disease. Regular assessment of anthropometric parameters of obesity, home blood pressure control, urine protein excretion, renal function, and metabolic parameters (e.g., dyslipidemia and insulin resistance) is recommended. Any worsening in proteinuria or GFR should prompt escalation of therapy. A multidisciplinary team, including a primary physician, nurse educator, dietitian, physiotherapist, psychologist, nephrologist, endocrinologist, cardiologist, and bariatric surgeons, is required for comprehensive monitoring. The team must follow a nonjudgmental "stigma-free" approach.

CONCLUSION

Obesity-associated proteinuria in nondiabetic patients represents a growing health crisis that is potentially preventable. It has significant implications for kidney and cardiovascular outcomes. Early detection, comprehensive risk assessment, and implementation of evidence-based treatment will help mitigate disease progression. A multidisciplinary team with an empathetic approach will improve patient outcomes across the lifespan.

REFERENCES

1. World Health Organization. (2025). Obesity and overweight. [online] Available from https://www.who.int/news-room/fact-sheets/detail/obesity-and-overweight [Last accessed January, 2026].
2. Hoey H, Roche E. Obesity: a triple pandemic, the trillion dollar disease: Prevention is imperative. Glob Pediatr. 2024;7:100141.
3. Kovesdy CP, Furth SL, Zoccali C, et al. World Kidney Day Steering Committee. Obesity and kidney disease: hidden consequences of the epidemic. J Nephrol. 2017;30(1):1-10.
4. Zaman SB, Hossain N, Rahman M. Associations between Body Mass Index and Chronic Kidney Disease in Type 2 Diabetes Mellitus Patients: Findings from the Northeast of Thailand. Diabetes Metab J. 2018;42(4):330-7.
5. Verde L, Lucà S, Cernea S, et al. The Fat Kidney. Curr Obes Rep. 2023;12(2):86-98.
6. Snyder S, Turner GA, Turner A. Obesity-related kidney disease. Prim Care. 2014;41(4):875-93.
7. Batool A, Habib H, et al. Prevalence of Albuminuria in US Adults with Obesity and Its Possible Impact on CKD Screening: A Cross-Sectional Analysis of NHANES Data, 2003-2020: SA-PO1077. J Am Soc Nephrol. 2024;35(10S):10.
8. Rosenstock JL, Pommier M, Stoffels G, et al. Prevalence of Proteinuria and Albuminuria in an Obese Population and Associated Risk Factors. Front Med. 2018;5:122.
9. Cortinovis M, Perico N, Ruggenenti P, et al. Glomerular hyperfiltration. Nat Rev Nephrol. 2022;18(7):435-51.
10. Hall JE, Mouton AJ, da Silva AA, et al. Obesity, kidney dysfunction, and inflammation: interactions in hypertension. Cardiovasc Res. 2021;117(8):1859-76.
11. Afshinnia F, Wilt TJ, Duval S, et al. Weight loss and proteinuria: systematic review of clinical trials and comparative cohorts. Nephrol Dial Transplant. 2010;25(4):1173-83.
12. Ezequiel DGA, Costa MB, Chaoubah A, et al. Weight loss improves renal hemodynamics in patients with metabolic syndrome. Braz J Nephrol. 2012;34:36-42.
13. Gong X, Zeng X, Fu P. The impact of weight loss on renal function in individuals with obesity and type 2 diabetes: a comprehensive review. Front Endocrinol. 2024;15:1320627.
14. Praga M, Morales E. Weight loss and proteinuria. Contrib Nephrol. 2006;151:221-9.
15. Yun HR, Kim HW, Chang TI, et al. Increased risk of chronic kidney disease associated with weight gain in healthy adults: insight from metabolic profiles and body composition. Front Med. 2021;8:705881.
16. Furth SL, Colhoun HM, Kanbay M, et al. The relationship between obesity and chronic kidney disease: conclusions from a Kidney Disease: Improving Global Outcomes (KDIGO) Controversies Conference. Kidney Int. 2025;S0085-2538(25)00774-4.

17. Herrington WG, Smith M, et al. Body-mass index and risk of advanced chronic kidney disease: Prospective analyses from a primary care cohort of 1.4 million adults in England. PLoS One. 2017;12(3):e0173515.
18. Hsu C Yuan, McCulloch CE, Bankhead C, et al. Body mass index and risk for end-stage renal disease. Ann Intern Med. 2006;144(1):21-8.
19. Zhang X, Liu J, Ni Y, et al. Global Prevalence of overweight and obesity in children and adolescents: a systematic review and meta-analysis. JAMA Pediatr. 2024;178(8): 800-13.
20. Renda R. The Glomerular Filtration Rate and Proteinuria in Obese Children. Iranian J Pediatr. 2017:e65040.
21. Vivante A, Golan E, Tzur D, et al. Body mass index in 1.2 million adolescents and risk for end-stage renal disease. Arch Intern Med. 2012;172(21):1644-50.
22. Martínez-Montoro JI, Morales E, Cornejo-Pareja I, et al. Obesity-related glomerulopathy: Current approaches and future perspectives. Obes Rev. 2022;23(7):e13450.
23. Lee-Boey JS, Tan JK, Lim ZF, et al. Obesity-related glomerulopathy: How it happens and future perspectives. Diabet Med. 2025;42(6):e70042.
24. Kambham N, Markowitz GS, Valeri AM, et al. Obesity-related glomerulopathy: an emerging epidemic. Kidney Int. 2001;59(4):1498-509.
25. Chagnac A, Herman M, Zingerman B, et al. Obesity-induced glomerular hyperfiltration: its involvement in the pathogenesis of tubular sodium reabsorption. Nephrol Dial Transplant. 2008;23(12):3946-52.
26. Hall JE, Mouton AJ, da Silva AA, et al. Obesity, kidney dysfunction, and inflammation: interactions in hypertension. Cardiovasc Res. 2021;117(8):1859-76.
27. Lin L, Tan W, Pan X, et al. Metabolic syndrome-related kidney injury: a review and Update. Front Endocrinol. 2022;13:904001.
28. Yazıcı D, Demir SÇ, Sezer H. Insulin resistance, obesity, and lipotoxicity. Adv Exp Med Biol. 2024;1460:391-430.
29. Conley MM, McFarlane CM, Johnson DW, et al. Interventions for weight loss in people with chronic kidney disease who are overweight or obese. Cochrane Database Syst Rev. 2021;3(3):CD013119.
30. Wing RR, Bolin P, Brancati FL, et al. Look AHEAD Research Group, cardiovascular effects of intensive lifestyle intervention in type 2 diabetes. N Engl J Med. 2013;369(2):145-54.
31. Piercy KL, Troiano RP, Ballard RM, et al. The Physical Activity Guidelines for Americans. JAMA. 2018;320(19):2020-8.
32. Villareal DT, Aguirre L, Gurney AB, et al. Aerobic or resistance exercise, or both, in dieting obese older adults. N Engl J Med. 2017;376(20):1943-55.
33. Colquitt JL, Pickett K, Loveman E, et al Surgery for weight loss in adults. Cochrane Database Syst Rev. 2014;2014(8):CD003641.
34. Schauer PR, Bhatt DL, Kirwan JP, et al. Bariatric Surgery versus Intensive Medical Therapy for Diabetes: 5-year Outcomes. N Engl J Med. 2017;376(7):641-51.
35. Perkovic V, Tuttle KR, Rossing P, et al. Effects of Semaglutide on Chronic Kidney Disease in Patients with Type 2 Diabetes. N Engl J Med. 2024;391(2):109-21.
36. Lincoff AM, Brown-Frandsen K, Colhoun HM, et al. Semaglutide and cardiovascular outcomes in obesity without diabetes. N Engl J Med. 2023;389(24):2221-32.
37. Wadden TA, Hollander P, S Klein, et al. Weight maintenance and additional weight loss with liraglutide after low-calorie-diet-induced weight loss: the SCALE Maintenance randomized study. Int J Obes. 2013;37(11):1443-51.
38. Jastreboff AM, le Roux CW, Stefanski A, et al. Tirzepatide for Obesity Treatment and Diabetes Prevention. N Engl J Med. 2025;392(10):958-71.
39. Cerchi E, Santo PA do E, de Oliveira MC, et al. Effects of tirzepatide on weight management in patients with and without diabetes: a systematic review and meta-analysis. Int J Obes. 2025;49(12):2415-25.
40. Jafar TH, Stark PC, Schmid CH, et al. Progression of chronic kidney disease: the role of blood pressure control, proteinuria, and angiotensin-converting enzyme inhibition: a patient-level meta-analysis. Ann Intern Med. 2003;139(4):244-52.
41. Hall JE, Mouton AJ, da Silva AA, et al. Obesity, kidney dysfunction, and inflammation: interactions in hypertension. Cardiovasc Res. 2021;117(8):1859-76.
42. Navaneethan SD, Nigwekar SU, Sehgal AR, et al. Aldosterone antagonists for preventing the progression of chronic kidney disease: a systematic review and meta-analysis. Clin J Am Soc Nephrol CJASN. 2009;4(3):542-51.
43. Bakris GL, Agarwal R, Chan JC, et al. Effect of finerenone on albuminuria in patients with diabetic nephropathy: a randomized clinical trial. JAMA. 2015;314(9):884-94.
44. Zelniker TA, Wiviott SD, Raz I, et al. SGLT2 inhibitors for primary and secondary prevention of cardiovascular and renal outcomes in type 2 diabetes: a systematic review and meta-analysis of cardiovascular outcome trials. Lancet Lond Engl. 2019;393(10166):31-9.
45. Romagnani P. SGLT2 inhibitors in CKD: are they really effective in all patients? Nephrol Dial Transplant Off Publ Eur Dial Transpl Assoc-Eur Ren Assoc. 2025;40(10):1838-42.

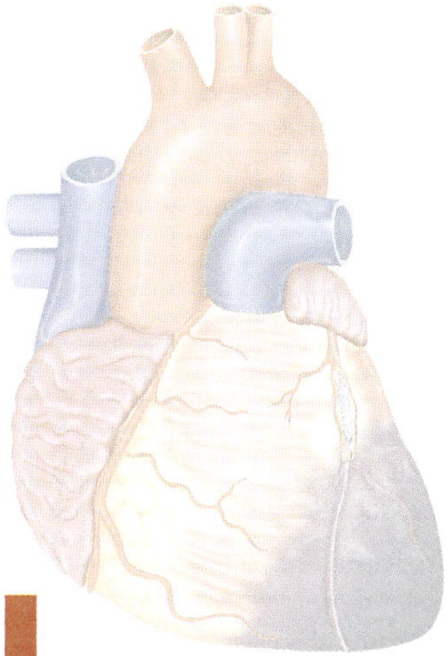

55

CHAPTER

Obesity with Renovascular Disease: Clinical Insight and Management

Dinesh Khullar, Kulwant Singh, Abhishek

INTRODUCTION

As obesity and metabolic syndrome become more prevalent, increasing numbers of patients present with overlapping obesity, hypertension, diabetes, CKD, and possible renovascular disease, carrying important clinical and public-health implications. Obesity independently drives albuminuria, accelerates GFR decline, and increases progression to ESRD, while also worsening traditional atherosclerotic risk factors, thereby raising the likelihood of renovascular disease such as atherosclerotic renal artery stenosis.[1] Renovascular disease is a leading cause of secondary hypertension and contributes significantly to ischemic damage in the kidneys.[2] Populations with high obesity prevalence, including rapidly transitioning countries like India, therefore represent a high-risk group for both metabolic and renovascular kidney disease, emphasizing the need for weight control, optimal management of metabolic risk factors, and early detection strategies to reduce overall renovascular disease burden. This review provided updated clinical insights and management strategies for obesity-associated renovascular disease.

EPIDEMIOLOGY OF RENOVASCULAR DISEASE (TABLE 1)

Atherosclerotic renovascular disease (ARVD) is the leading cause of renovascular pathology, typically involving large-artery narrowing, and occurs in about 6–7% of adults over 65.[3] Its prevalence is similar across racial groups, and outcomes after revascularization are comparable. ARVD is strongly associated with traditional cardiovascular risk factors—especially peripheral artery disease, where rates can reach 14–40%. Many lesions remain hemodynamically insignificant until stenosis exceeds 70–80%. Renovascular hypertension accounts for about 0.1–5% of all hypertension cases, with higher rates (14–24%) in patients with resistant hypertension.[3] Historically, ARVD frequently progressed before the widespread use of statins. In contrast, fibromuscular dysplasia (FMD) is a nonatherosclerotic disease primarily affecting middle-aged women; the renal arteries are involved in most cases, and hypertension is a common presentation. A significant proportion of patients with multifocal or focal FMD require intervention. Less common causes of renovascular disease include aneurysm, dissection, external compression, infarction, mid-aortic coarctation, stent graft-related obstruction, allograft inflow issues, and anatomical variants.

MECHANISM OF OBESITY ASSOCIATED POSTSTENOTIC KIDNEY HEMODYNAMIC (FLOWCHART 1)

Obesity significantly alters renal hemodynamics and worsens outcomes in renovascular disease.[9] Excess adiposity activates the renin–angiotensin–aldosterone system (RAAS) and sympathetic pathways, leading to sodium retention, expansion of extracellular volume, and glomerular hyperfiltration.[10] Increased proximal tubular sodium reabsorption further amplifies this cycle. Although early obesity may transiently preserve renal blood flow and GFR in the stenotic kidney, it simultaneously intensifies

TABLE 1: Types of renovascular disease.

Type of renovascular disease	*Definition*
Renal artery stenosis (RAS)	A condition characterized by *significant narrowing of one or both of renal arteries*, leading to reduced blood flow to the kidneys. This reduction activates the RAAS, causing *renovascular hypertension* and potentially progressive renal dysfunction. The most common cause is *atherosclerosis*, while *fibromuscular dysplasia (FMD)* is a nonatherosclerotic cause.[4]
Renal artery thrombosis	A condition in which a *blood clot forms within the renal artery*. This can lead to *acute kidney injury, renal infarction, severe flank pain,* and potential permanent damage if not promptly treated. It may arise from emboli, trauma, or hypercoagulable states.[5]
Renal vein thrombosis	This disorder involves the formation of a *thrombus in the major renal veins or its* tributaries. The resulting venous congestion increases intrarenal pressure and may cause *hematuria, flank pain, and proteinuria*. It is commonly associated with *nephrotic syndrome* or hypercoagulability.[6]
Renal artery aneurysm	A *focal dilation or outpouching of the renal artery* that exceeds twice the diameter of a normal renal artery. While many aneurysms are asymptomatic, larger ones pose risks of *rupture, dissection, hypertension, or distal embolization*. Causes include atherosclerosis, fibromuscular dysplasia, trauma, or connective tissue disorders.[7]
Atheroembolic renal disease	A systemic atherosclerotic complication in which *cholesterol crystals break off from plaques in major arteries (e.g., aorta)* and embolize to the small renal arteries and arterioles. This leads to *progressive renal ischemia, inflammation, and kidney failure*, often occurring after vascular procedures or anticoagulation therapy.[8]

oxidative stress, inflammation, and microvascular dysfunction, accelerating fibrosis and long-term renal injury. These adverse effects extend to the contralateral kidney, where obesity-driven hyperfiltration and hypertrophy promote glomerulosclerosis and eventual decline in overall renal function.[10]

Leptin, produced by adipose tissue, normally suppresses appetite and insulin secretion, but in obesity a state of leptin resistance develops, reducing its satiety effect while preserving actions that promote salt retention, vasoconstriction, hypertension, and increased cardiovascular and kidney disease risk. Adiponectin, in contrast, has anti-inflammatory and insulin-sensitizing effects and provides protection against atherosclerosis.[11-13]

Renovascular hypertension: Existing experimental studies of swine models showed that obesity amplifies renovascular hypertension.[14] Mechanisms include high-fat dietary effects, increased sympathetic activity driven by altered adipokines (high leptin, low adiponectin), kidney compression from visceral fat causing impaired pressure natriuresis, and enhanced tubular sodium reabsorption. Obesity also activates the RAAS through increased aldosterone and angiotensinogen production from adrenal and adipose tissues. Thus, obesity-related hypertension can worsen damage in the nonstenotic kidney in individuals with coexisting renal artery stenosis.

Microvascular remodeling: Obesity causes microvascular remodeling with dysregulated angiogenesis and increased VEGF-driven neovascularization, but these new vessels are often unstable and prone to loss, especially in injured tissues.[15,16] In renal artery stenosis, obesity can accelerate microvascular rarefaction in the poststenotic kidney, worsening tissue injury through increased oxidative stress, inflammation, and endothelial dysfunction. Obesity also impairs endothelium-dependent vasodilation due to disrupted NO/ET-1 balance and elevated thromboxane activity.[17] Overall, obesity exacerbates microvascular dysfunction and hemodynamic impairment in the ischemic kidney.

Inflammation: Obesity creates an inflammatory and oxidative environment driven largely by visceral adipose tissue. Early macrophage infiltration and adipocyte-derived cytokines such as TNF-α, IL-6, and leptin sustain systemic inflammation.[18] Leptin further amplifies cytokine production and oxidative stress through ROS generation and NAD(P)H oxidase activation, while reduced adiponectin levels in obesity diminish antioxidant protection, insulin sensitizing, anti-inflammatory, antifibrogenic, antiatherogenic, and cardioprotective.[19,20] Additionally, ectopic lipid accumulation in the kidney (fatty kidney) can injure mesangial cells, podocytes, and tubular cells, doubling the risk of renal parenchymal damage.

Insulin resistant: Multiple endocrine, inflammatory, and cellular disturbances in obesity contribute to insulin resistance (IR), which is increasingly recognized as a driver of kidney disease. Because insulin acts on all

Flowchart 1: Mechanism of obesity associated poststenotic kidney hemodynamic.

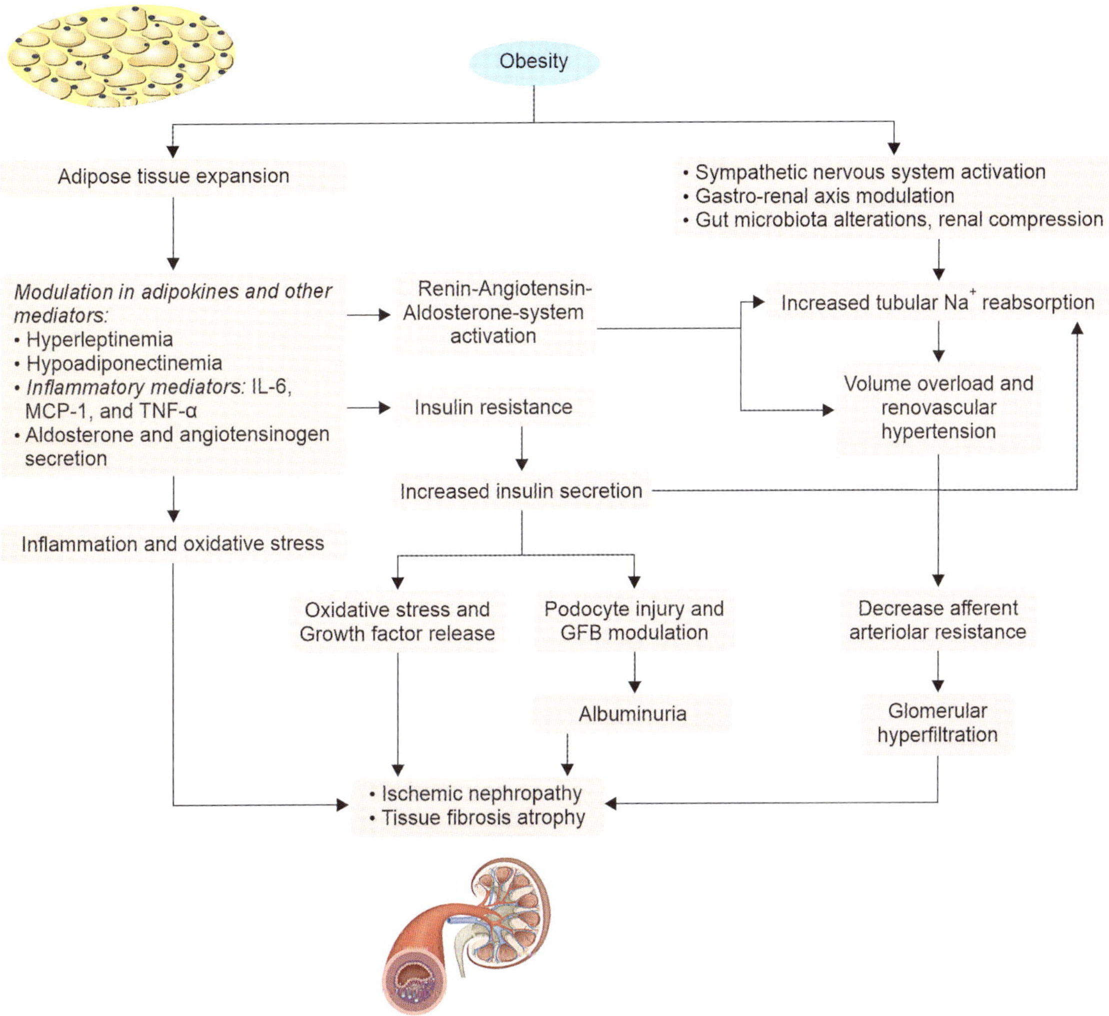

nephron segments, especially podocytes, which have the highest density of insulin receptors—IR can impair podocyte function, glomerular permeability, and insulin-mediated renal vasodilation. Experimental models show that podocyte IR leads to albuminuria, early glomerular changes, and reduced cell viability, effects worsened by low adiponectin levels. IR can also arise independently of obesity or diabetes, such as in uremia, and is associated with loss of insulin-mediated GFR regulation and higher CKD prevalence even in mildly overweight individuals.[17,21]

INTERVENTIONS IN OBESITY ASSOCIATED RENOVASCULAR DISEASE (TABLE 2)

Management options include lifestyle modifications, medical management, percutaneous procedures, and surgical revascularization. The primary objectives are to achieve blood pressure control, maintain renal function, and minimize treatment-related complications and adverse effects.

Lifestyle modifications: Obesity worsens outcomes in renovascular disease, making lifestyle modification, and weight reduction essential first-line strategies.[22] Weight loss can reduce hyperfiltration, improve podocyte survival, and enhance endothelial function, while selected patients may benefit from medications or bariatric surgery.

RAAS inhibitors: When weight control is inadequate, therapies that target obesity-related mechanisms become important. RAAS blockade using ACEIs or ARBs can reduce proteinuria, improve insulin sensitivity, and correct adipokine imbalance, making them useful adjuncts in obese patients with kidney disease.[1,23]

TABLE 2: Indications for renal revascularization.[3]

Clinical populations	• Unilateral RAS with characteristic syndromes • Fibromuscular dysplasia with hypertension • *High-risk clinical syndromes:* Rapidly progressive hypertension, rapid fall in eGFR, flash pulmonary edema • Bilateral RAS with declining renal function • Single functioning kidney with RAS
Special populations	• Renal transplant renal artery stenosis (with/without calcineurin inhibitors) • Recurrent pulmonary edema with bilateral atherosclerotic RAS • Progressive loss of GFR due to occlusive RAS without other kidney disease • Aortic disease requiring renal protection during endovascular repair • LV assist device patients • Radiation-induced RAS with symptoms • Vasculitides or external vascular compression (e.g., Takayasu arteritis) • Children with mid-aortic syndrome or fibromuscular variants
Features suggesting benefit from revascularization	• Recent onset/worsening hypertension (<1 year) • No proteinuria • Evidence of RAS-mediated RAAS activation • Hyperreninemia • Lateralized renal vein renin in unilateral disease • Younger age • Imaging showing progressive renal artery occlusion • Resistant hypertension despite therapy • Angiotensin-dependent GFR

Microvascular-stabilizing therapies: Because obesity aggravates microvascular rarefaction in the stenotic kidney, proangiogenic options—such as VEGF or angiopoietin-1—may help repair microvascular networks, though safety concerns and practical challenges limit their clinical use.[24,25] Statins may also help by stabilizing microvessels and reducing inflammation and oxidative stress.[26]

Bariatric surgery: Most of the available evidence linking bariatric surgery to benefits in renovascular disease is indirect and suggests that the substantial and sustained weight loss achieved after surgery favorably modifies key vascular risk factors. Bariatric surgery leads to significant reductions in blood pressure, attenuation of systemic and renal inflammation, improvement in endothelial and microvascular function, and suppression of excessive RAAS activation, all of which are central mechanisms in the development and progression of renovascular pathology and renovascular hypertension.[27-29]

Insulin-sensitizing therapeutic strategies: Emerging therapies that improve insulin sensitivity show promise in reducing renal injury in experimental obesity, but these targeted strategies require further study before being applied clinically.[30]

Percutaneous or surgical intervention: Balloon angioplasty and stenting help open narrowed vessels, though repeated treatment may be required. Stent placement is recommended when standard percutaneous transluminal renal angioplasty (PTRA) fails to produce a satisfactory angiographic result, when early restenosis occurs after the procedure, or when a renal artery dissection develops during PTRA.[31] Clinical factors associated with poor outcomes following PTRA or stent placement include a small kidney size (<8 cm), markedly elevated serum creatinine levels (>3.0–4.0 mg/dL), the presence of another underlying cause of renal impairment such as diabetes or amyloidosis, long-standing essential hypertension, chronic renal dysfunction, and widespread atherosclerotic disease. Surgical revascularization procedures like endarterectomy or aortorenal and extra-anatomic bypass are typically chosen when percutaneous interventions fail or when patients have challenging vascular anatomy or coexisting aortic aneurysms.[31]

CONCLUSION

Obesity and metabolic syndrome substantially amplify the burden of renovascular disease by accelerating atherosclerosis, promoting renovascular hypertension, and worsening renal ischemic injury through hemodynamic, inflammatory, microvascular, and metabolic pathways. Obesity-driven activation of the RAAS, sympathetic nervous system, adipokine imbalance, insulin resistance, and chronic inflammation not only aggravate injury in the poststenotic kidney but also accelerate hyperfiltration and structural damage in the contralateral kidney, hastening progression to ESKD. Effective management of obesity-associated renovascular disease therefore requires a comprehensive, multifaceted approach that prioritizes weight reduction and lifestyle modification, optimal medical therapy including RAAS blockade and statins, and careful patient selection for revascularization procedures. Bariatric surgery, although supported largely by indirect evidence, emerges as a powerful risk-modifying strategy by improving blood pressure control, reducing systemic and renal inflammation, restoring endothelial and microvascular function, and attenuating RAAS overactivation. Integrating metabolic control with vascular and renal protection strategies is essential to reduce disease progression, improve long-term renal and cardiovascular outcomes, and address the growing public health impact of obesity-related renovascular disease, particularly in high-risk and rapidly transitioning populations.

REFERENCES

1. Zhang X, Lerman LO. Obesity and renovascular disease. Am J Physiol Renal Physiol. 2015;309(4):F273-9.
2. Nair R, Vaqar S. Renovascular Hypertension. In: StatPearls. Treasure Island (FL): StatPearls Publishing; 2025.
3. Sarafidis PA, Theodorakopoulou M, Ortiz A, et al. Atherosclerotic renovascular disease: a clinical practice document by the European Renal Best Practice (ERBP) board of the European Renal Association (ERA) and the Working Group Hypertension and the Kidney of the European Society of Hypertension (ESH). Nephrol Dial Transplant. 2023;38(12).2835-50.
4. Bokhari MR, Bokhari SRA. Renal Artery Stenosis. In: StatPearls. Treasure Island (FL): StatPearls Publishing; 2025.
5. Poggiali E, Ferrari MG, Botti C, et al. Renal artery thrombosis. A case of acute flank pain in a patient with a new onset of renal failure and atrial fibrillation. Acta Biomed. 2023;94(3):e2023140.
6. Mazhar HR, Aeddula NR. Renal Vein Thrombosis. In: StatPearls. Treasure Island (FL): StatPearls Publishing; 2025.
7. González J, Esteban M, Andrés G, et al. Renal artery aneurysms. Curr Urol Rep. 2014;15(1):376.
8. Singh NP, Gupta AK, Kaur G. Atheroembolic renal disease. Indian J Nephrol. 2020;30:1-2.
9. Hall JE, Brands MW, Dixon WN, et al. Obesity-induced hypertension. Renal function and systemic hemodynamics. Hypertension. 1993;22:292.
10. Monica TJ, Houben AJH, Peter W, et al. The link between adipose tissue renin-angiotensin-aldosterone system signaling and obesity-associated hypertension. Physiology. 2017;32(3):197-209.
11. Kieffer TJ, Habener JF. The adipoinsular axis: effects of leptin on pancreatic beta-cells. Am J Physiol Endocrinol Metab. 2000;278:E1-E14.
12. Tesauro M, Mascali A, Franzese O, et al. Chronic kidney disease, obesity, and hypertension: the role of leptin and adiponectin. Int J Hypertens. 2012;943605:1-7.
13. Shargorodsky M, Boaz M, Goldberg Y, et al. Adiponectin and vascular properties in obese patients: is it a novel biomarker of early atherosclerosis? Int J Obes. 2009;33:553-8.
14. Zhang X, Li ZL, Woollard JR, et al. Obesity-metabolic derangement preserves hemodynamics but promotes intrarenal adiposity and macrophage infiltration in swine renovascular disease. Am J Physiol Renal Physiol. 2013;305:F265-76.
15. Iliescu R, Chade AR. Progressive renal vascular proliferation and injury in obese Zucker rats. Microcirculation. 2010;17:250-8.
16. Schrijvers BF, Flyvbjerg A, Tilton RG, et al. A neutralizing VEGF antibody prevents glomerular hypertrophy in a model of obese type 2 diabetes, the Zucker diabetic fatty rat. Nephrol Dial Transplant. 2006;21:324-9.
17. Jonk AM, Houben AJ, de Jongh RT, et al. Microvascular dysfunction in obesity: a potential mechanism in the pathogenesis of obesity-associated insulin resistance and hypertension. Physiology (Bethesda). 2007;22:252-60.
18. Weisberg SP, McCann D, Desai M, et al. Obesity is associated with macrophage accumulation in adipose tissue. J Clin Invest. 2003;112:1796-808.
19. Yamagishi SI, Edelstein D, Du XL, et al. Leptin induces mitochondrial superoxide production and monocyte chemoattractant protein-1 expression in aortic endothelial cells by increasing fatty acid oxidation via protein kinase A. J Biol Chem. 2001;276:25096-100.
20. Gustafsson S, Lind L, Soderberg S, et al. Oxidative stress and inflammatory markers in relation to circulating levels of adiponectin. Obesity (Silver Spring). 2013;21:1467-73.
21. Qatanani M, Lazar MA. Mechanisms of obesity-associated insulin resistance: many choices on the menu. Genes Dev. 2007;21:1443-55.
22. Chagnac A, Weinstein T, Herman M, et al. The effects of weight loss on renal function in patients with severe obesity. J Am Soc Nephrol. 2003;14:1480-6.
23. Sharma AM. Is there a rationale for angiotensin blockade in the management of obesity hypertension? Hypertension. 2004;44:12-9.
24. Lerman LO, Chade AR. Angiogenesis in the kidney: a new therapeutic target? Curr Opin Nephrol Hypertens. 2009;18:160-5.
25. Iliescu R, Fernandez SR, Kelsen S, et al. Role of renal microcirculation in experimental renovascular disease. Nephrol Dial Transplante. 2010;25:1079-87.
26. Chade AR, Zhu X, Mushin OP, et al. Simvastatin promotes angiogenesis and prevents microvascular remodeling in chronic renal ischemia. FASEB J. 2006;20:1706-8.

27. Morales E, Porrini E, Martin-Taboada M, et al. Renoprotective role of bariatric surgery in patients with established chronic kidney disease. Clin Kidney J. 2020;14(9):2037-46.
28. Schiavon CA, Bersch-Ferreira AC, Santucci EV, et al. Effects of bariatric surgery in obese patients with hypertension: The GATEWAY Randomized Trial (Gastric Bypass to Treat Obese Patients With Steady Hypertension). Circulation. 2018;137(11):1132-42.
29. Zhang T, Wang Y, Zhang X, et al. The impact of bariatric surgery on renal function: a retrospective analysis of short-term outcomes. Obes Surg. 2021;31(8):3476-82.
30. Belin de Chantemele EJ, Ali MI, Mintz JD, et al. Increasing peripheral insulin sensitivity by protein tyrosine phosphatase 1B deletion improves control of blood pressure in obesity. Hypertension. 2012;60:1273-9.
31. Bhalla V, Textor SC, Beckman JA, et al. Revascularization for renovascular disease: A scientific statement from the American Heart Association. Hypertension. 2022;79(8):e128-43.

56

CHAPTER

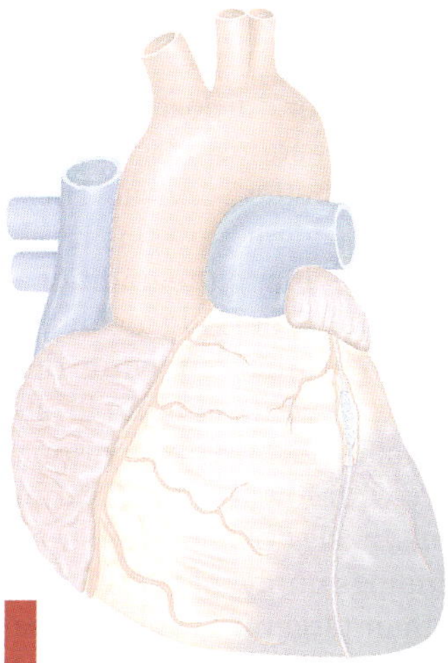

Obesity in Dialysis Patients: Clinical Insight and Management

Dinesh Khullar, Manu Prakash, Deepak Kumar Panigrahi

INTRODUCTION

Obesity is a multidimensional risk factor for developing chronic kidney disease (CKD) and CKD progression. Traditionally, kidney failure including dialysis population was associated with malnutrition and protein-energy wasting (PEW); however, obesity is now increasingly prevalent among patients initiating dialysis therapy, prevalence rising from ~36.8% to >40% over a decade, making obesity one of the most common comorbid conditions in the dialysis population.[1] Moreover, extrapolating cardiovascular risk paradigms from the general population to dialysis patients may be misleading as dialysis population exhibits a distinct epidemiology and risk-factor profile. This chapter focuses on obesity in dialysis patients, underlying mechanisms of the obesity paradox, clinical implications across dialysis modalities and management strategies relevant to patient care.

MISCLASSIFICATION OF BODY MASS INDEX IN DIALYSIS

In dialysis patients, BMI is an imprecise marker of obesity, as it fails to differentiate fat from muscle mass, ignores fat distribution, and is confounded by fluid overload, resulting in underrecognition of masked obesity and sarcopenia. An accurate assessment of obesity should be based on body composition and functional measures. Techniques such as bioelectrical impedance analysis (BIA) can estimate fat and lean mass, waist-to-height ratio or waist circumference can measure central adiposity and metabolic risk, and functional assessments using handgrip strength and gait speed can identify sarcopenia. Dual-energy X-ray absorptiometry (DEXA) provides the most detailed evaluation but has limited routine availability. Interventions should focus on preserving muscle mass and function while reducing excess, particularly visceral, adiposity over time rather than relying on BMI at a single time point.[2,3]

ADIPOSITY IN DIALYSIS: GOOD OR BAD?

A growing body of evidence has paradoxically shown inverse associations between conventional cardiovascular risk factors and survival in dialysis patients, a phenomenon termed as reverse epidemiology. Several observational studies report a paradoxical association in dialysis populations and obesity is often linked with better survival, known as the *obesity paradox, a subset of reverse epidemiology.*[4-9] Understanding the reverse epidemiology of obesity in dialysis populations is critical, as it is currently premature to advocate for excess adiposity as being beneficial or intentional weight loss as being dangerous. Optimal weight targets should be individualized by clinicians with careful supervision and follow-up. Weight loss strategies must prioritize preservation of lean muscle mass through regular exercise and adequate protein intake.

THE PROTECTIVE MECHANISMS BY WHICH OBESITY MAY AFFECT SURVIVAL

The mechanisms of reverse epidemiology of obesity are not well understood. Reverse epidemiology challenges conventional views by demonstrating an inverse relationship between obesity and mortality in dialysis patients, contrasting sharply with patterns seen in the general population. This phenomenon reflects not the absence of an association, but a true reversal, where low BMI confers higher risk and greater adiposity appears protective. Such findings suggest the presence of unique pathophysiological conditions in maintenance dialysis and similar populations that predispose individuals with low BMI to worse outcomes, while obesity may offer survival advantages.[10]

More stable hemodynamic status in obese patients: Overweight and obese patients associate with higher baseline blood pressure, which may allow better hemodynamic tolerance to afterload-reducing therapies. As a result, obese patients may be more likely to tolerate survival-benefiting antihypertensive agents such as angiotensin-converting enzyme inhibitors.[11,12] Some theories suggest adipose tissue acts as a buffer against metabolic demands of chronic illness, reduces risk of malnutrition and hence cachexia while on dialysis. Additionally, it provides cardiovascular protection via favorable response to volume overload and rates of ultrafiltration therapy thereby preventing intradialytic hypotension and attenuate the degree of sympathetic nerve and RAS activities.[13]

Alteration in tumor necrosis factor-α (TNF-α) receptors and neuroendocrine profile in obesity: In heart failure and dialysis, elevated TNF-α contributes to poor outcomes, while adipose-derived soluble TNF receptors may counteract its harmful effects.[14]

Overnutrition versus undernutrition: The impact of obesity on outcomes depends on the time frame and competing risks. While overnutrition drives long-term cardiovascular mortality in populations with longer life expectancy, undernutrition remains a dominant cause of morbidity and death in settings with shorter survival. In maintenance hemodialysis (MHD) patients, who face a very high short-term mortality risk, the immediate protective effects of better nutritional reserves may outweigh the long-term cardiovascular harms of obesity, resulting in an apparent survival advantage.[10]

Malnutrition-inflammation complex syndrome (MICS): MICS are a strong predictor of adverse outcomes in dialysis patients. Proinflammatory cytokine activation in CKD promotes anorexia, muscle wasting, hypoalbuminemia, and atherosclerosis, thereby increasing mortality risk. The apparent protective association of obesity in dialysis patients may largely reflect the adverse impact of MICS in underweight individuals, who are more vulnerable to infection and inflammatory complications.[10]

Should Maintenance Hemodialysis Patients Gain Weight in Order to Live Longer?

In dialysis care, it is uncertain whether purposeful weight gain can safely improve nutritional status and whether such gain in weight translates into better survival. These questions are unanswered yet as weight gain has rarely been studied as a primary outcome due to the traditional view that obesity is undesirable. Emerging evidence suggests otherwise, with small studies showing that appetite stimulation can improve weight, albumin levels, and inflammation without major harm. Observational data consistently link obesity with lower mortality and higher survival in MHD patients, likely driven by the strong influence of MICS.[10] These findings imply that addressing MICS may be more critical than targeting conventional cardiovascular risk factors in this population. Although reverse epidemiology challenges traditional cardiovascular paradigms, it warrants objective evaluation, as similar survival patterns may exist in other high-risk groups. With improving dialysis care and longer survival, this paradox may eventually diminish, reverting toward traditional risk relationships, as seen after kidney transplantation (**Table 1**).

TABLE 1: Possible complications of obesity in dialysis patients.[15]

Aspect	*MHD*	*PD*
Dialysis feasibility	Technically feasible but logistically challenging therapy for obese patients	Not a contraindication with modern PD techniques
Vascular access/ catheter issues	Deeper vessels, difficult cannulation, cause reduced long-term access survival	Catheter malfunction due to visceral fat/ omentum; migration or blockage
Dialysis adequacy	May require more frequent sessions for longer time	May need longer dwell times or more exchanges
Infection risk	Increase risk of calciphylaxis-related infections	Increased peritonitis and exit-site infections
Procedural challenges	Difficult central venous catheter placement	Higher risk of hernias and dialysate leaks
Metabolic concerns	Difficulty achieving dry weight; intradialytic hypotension	Glucose absorption causing weight gain and metabolic effects
Comorbidities	OSA, PHTN, and HFpEF increase dialysis complications	Due to glucose load, metabolic syndrome may be worsened
Resource requirements	There is need for specialized equipment and additional staff	Need for careful catheter placement and care for exit-site

(MHD: maintenance hemodialysis; PD: peritoneal dialysis; PHTN: pulmonary hypertension)

Additionally, from prospective transplant perspective, obesity poses high anesthetic and recovery risk with higher rates of rejection linked with high BMI individuals, slow metabolism needing immunosuppression dose adjustments. Obese patients on peritoneal dialysis (PD) may pose the surgical wound complications, especially if they have suffered with PD catheter-related infections.

MANAGEMENT OF OBESITY IN DIALYSIS PATIENTS AND CHALLENGES

The effects of obesity vary across CKD stages **(Table 2)**. In predialysis patients, obesity accelerates CKD progression and weight loss is recommended. In contrast, obesity is associated with improved survival in dialysis patients but limits access to kidney transplantation. Therefore, weight loss in dialysis remains controversial and is often suggested only for transplant-eligible patients. Weight reduction is difficult to achieve in this group, with unclear or absent clinical benefit. Moreover, growing concerns regarding bariatric surgery further complicate decisions on optimal weight-loss strategies in wait-listed dialysis patients.[16]

Observational data consistently show better survival among obese dialysis patients compared with those with lower BMI,[4-9] and unintentional weight loss is linked to adverse outcomes. However, these findings do not imply that deliberately maintaining or promoting higher BMI is advisable. Intentional weight reduction, particularly in individuals with severe obesity, may still confer clinical benefits especially it aim is to gain lean muscle mass. This situation parallels observations in the hemodialysis population where higher BP appears protective in observational studies, yet interventional trials demonstrate improved outcomes with blood pressure control. Importantly, evidence evaluating the effects of intentional weight loss in patients with ESRD remains limited.

Weight reduction may also enhance access to kidney transplantation or improve post-transplant outcomes in comorbid obese dialysis patient. Many transplant centers impose BMI thresholds, between 30 and 35 kg/m^2, which restrict transplant eligibility for obese individuals.[17] Moreover, obese kidney transplant recipients experience higher rates of delayed graft function and few of them increased risk of graft loss, however, overall mortality does not differ significantly from nonobese recipients. Moreover, survival after transplantation is consistently superior across all BMI categories including obese and severely obese patients compared with dialysis patients who remain on the waiting list.

Glucagon-like peptide-1 receptor agonists (GLP-1RAs) (incretin-based therapies), and newer dual agonists GLP-1, and GIP receptors (Tirzepatide) demonstrate a transformative shift in the treatment of overweight and obesity, allowing a substantial proportion of patients to achieve weight reductions of 20% or more.[18] Of note, trails including the participants with CKD excluded transplant recipients and many excluded CKD patients with eGFR <30 mL/min. Dialysis and transplant are not listed as contraindications to using GLP-1RAs plus other peptides although there is lack of data especially in dialysis patients on dialysis.[19] The two strong indicators in dialysis population being fitness for transplant from all aspects and improvement in sleep apnea in these patients. Some studies have supported benefit of semaglutide in MHD patients with type 2 diabetes. KDIGO recommends in its guidelines the use of GLP-1RA in patients with CKD (including dialysis) and diabetes type 2 not controlled by metformin and SGLT2 inhibitors. But, more data and RCTs are needed for evidence-based benefit and validation.

Lifestyle modification-based weight management strategies (diet restriction and exercise) are effective, and intensive weight loss program including utilizing very low calorie diet (VLCD) or low calorie diet (LCD) along with physical activity is beneficial in a modest decrease of 3–10% in weight.[20-22]

In sarcopenic obesity, therapeutic strategies should prioritize preservation of muscle mass while reducing excess adiposity. Randomized trials demonstrate that intradialytic resistance training program improves muscle volume, strength, and physical performance. Combining resistance exercise with anabolic agents has been shown to increase lean body mass and reduce fat mass, although

TABLE 2: Paradox of being obese across the CKD.[16]

Predialysis	*Dialysis*	*Transplantation*
• Obesity increases risk of CKD progression • Partially reversed by weight loss – Weight loss is recommended – Strict control to avoid malnutrition – *Bariatric surgery:* Improve clinical parameters	• Obesity has survival advantages • Partially offset by weight loss – Weight loss required for being waitlisted transplantation – Strict control to avoid malnutrition – *Bariatric surgery:* High morbidities, conflicting results	• Obese patients may be excluded from kidney transplantation • Survival disadvantages may be reversed by weight loss – Weight loss is recommended – Strict control to avoid malnutrition – *Bariatric surgery:* High morbidities, but overall favorable results

issues regarding hepatotoxicity limit the use of some oral androgens, favoring alternative delivery routes for future research.

CONCLUSION

While higher BMI is associated with improved survival in hemodialysis patients, to date the concept of excess adiposity being inherently protective remains debated. BMI alone is an inadequate and unreliable marker of obesity, and greater emphasis should be placed on body composition. Moreover, unintentional weight loss predicts poor outcomes, intentional weight reduction in stable obese dialysis patients may be justified, particularly to improve transplant waitlist and long-term survival. Interventions targeting preservation of muscle mass and reduction of visceral fat may offer the greatest benefit in this population. Optimal weight targets should be patient centric with careful supervision and follow-up. Weight loss strategies must prioritize preservation of lean muscle mass through regular physical exercise and adequate protein intake. More data is strongly needed to support relatively novel medical therapies in dialysis patients such as GLP1-RA, GIPs, and combinations.

REFERENCES

1. Friedman AN. Obesity in patients undergoing dialysis and kidney transplantation. Adv Chronic Kidney Dis. 2013;20:128-34.
2. Gracia-Iguacel C, Qureshi AR, Avesani CM, et al. Subclinical versus overt obesity in dialysis patients: more than meets the eye. Nephrol Dial Transplant. 2013;28 Suppl 4:iv175-181.
3. Kittiskulnam P, Chertow GM, Kaysen GA, et al. Misclassification of Obesity by Body Mass Index Among Patients Receiving Hemodialysis. Am J Kidney Dis. 2016;67(4):709-11.
4. Fleischmann E, Teal N, Dudley J, et al. Influence of excess weight on mortality and hospital stay in 1346 hemodialysis patients. Kidney Int. 1999;55(4):1560-7.
5. Port FK, Ashby VB, Dhingra RK, et al. Dialysis dose and body mass index are strongly associated with survival in hemodialysis patients. J Am Soc Nephrol. 2002;13(4):1061-6.
6. Park J, Ahmadi SF, Streja E, et al. Obesity paradox in end-stage kidney disease patients. Prog Cardiovasc Dis. 2014;56(4):415-25.
7. Leavey SF, McCullough K, Hecking E, et al. Body mass index and mortality in 'healthier' as compared with 'sicker' haemodialysis patients: Results from the Dialysis Outcomes and Practice Patterns Study (DOPPS). Nephrol Dial Transplant. 2001;16:2386-94.
8. Leavey SF, Strawderman RL, Jones CA, et al. Simple nutritional indicators as independent predictors of mortality in hemodialysis patients. Am J Kidney Dis. 1998;31:997-1006.
9. Wong JS, Port FK, Hulbert-Shearon TE, et al. Survival advantage in Asian American end-stage renal disease patients. Kidney Int. 1999;55:2515-23.
10. Kalantar-Zadeh K. Causes and consequences of the reverse epidemiology of body mass index in dialysis patients. J Ren Nutr. 2005;15(1):142-7.
11. Horwich TB, Fonarow GC, Hamilton MA, et al. The relationship between obesity and mortality in patients with heart failure. J Am Coll Cardiol. 2001;38:789-95.
12. Fonarow GC, Chelimsky-Fallick C, Stevenson LW, et al. Effect of direct vasodilation with hydralazine versus angiotensin converting enzyme inhibition with captopril on mortality in advanced heart failure: The Hy-C trial. J Am Coll Cardiol. 1992;19:842-50.
13. Baker C, Palmer BF, Clegg DJ. Novel Hypothesis for the "Obesity Paradox" in ESKD Subjects on Dialysis. Clin J Am Soc Nephrol. 2025;20(12):1807-9.
14. Feldman AM, Combes A, Wagner D, et al. The role of tumor necrosis factor in the pathophysiology of heart failure. J Am Coll Cardiol. 2000;35:537-44.
15. Diwan TS, Cuffy MC, Linares-Cervantes I, et al. Impact of obesity on dialysis and transplant and its management. Semin Dial. 2020;33(3):279-85.
16. Piccoli GB, Moio MR, Fois A, et al. The Diet and Haemodialysis Dyad: Three Eras, Four Open Questions and Four Paradoxes. A Narrative Review, Towards a Personalized, Patient-Centered Approach. Nutrients. 2017;9(4):372.
17. Hossain M, Woywodt A, Augustine T, et al. Obesity and listing for renal transplantation: weighing the evidence for a growing problem. Clin Kidney J. 2017;10(5):703-8.
18. Abasheva D, Ortiz A, Fernandez-Fernandez B. GLP-1 receptor agonists in patients with chronic kidney disease and either overweight or obesity. Clin Kidney J. 2024;17(Suppl 2):19-35.
19. Furth SL, Colhoun HM, Kanbay M, et al. The relationship between obesity and chronic kidney disease: conclusions from a Kidney Disease: Improving Global Outcomes (KDIGO) Controversies Conference. Kidney Int. 2025:S0085-2538(25)00774-4.
20. Kramer H, Tuttle KR, Leehey D, et al. Obesity management in adults with CKD. Am J Kidney Dis. 2009;53(1):151-65.
21. Position of the American Dietetic Association: very-low-calorie weight loss diets. J Am Diet Assoc. 1990;90(5):722-6.
22. Kittiskulnam P, Johansen KL. The obesity paradox: A further consideration in dialysis patients. Semin Dial. 2019;32(6):485-9.

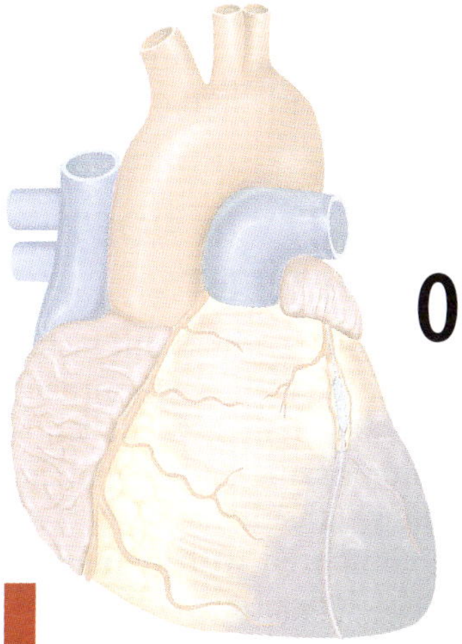

57 CHAPTER

Obesity in Postkidney Transplant Patients: Clinical Insight and Management

Yashendu Sarda, Narayan Prasad

INTRODUCTION

Obesity has emerged as a major global public health challenge and has become an increasingly important determinant of post-transplant outcomes.[1] It represents a distinct and multifactorial clinical entity in post-kidney transplant recipients. While many patients undergo transplantation with preexisting overweight or obesity, a considerable proportion experience significant weight gain after transplantation, specifically within the first 1–2 years.[2]

Early identification and targeted management of obesity are essential components of comprehensive post-kidney transplant care. A strong interrelationship between obesity, cardiovascular disease, and long-term graft outcomes has been shown. However, evidence-based recommendations remain limited, and many therapeutic strategies are extrapolated from the general population, with unique considerations related to graft function, immunosuppressive drug interactions, and long-term safety.[3] This chapter discusses an up-to-date on obesity in post-kidney transplant recipients, addressing its clinical insides and current management approaches with special focus on minimizing cardiovascular risk and optimizing long-term graft survival.

EPIDEMIOLOGY AND BURDEN

Obesity poses a significant health challenge in the post-transplant period. The literature has shown that around one-third of patients were overweight or obese at the time of kidney transplantation,[4] and additional weight gain frequently occurred thereafter, specifically during the first 1–2 years.[2,5,6] Younger age, female sex, higher pretransplant body weight, low physical activity, and greater cumulative corticosteroid exposure have been identified as key predictors of post-transplant weight gain.[7]

Obesity has significant clinical implications and strongly linked with an increased risk of metabolic syndrome, NODAT, hypertension, and dyslipidemia, resulting in increased CV morbidity and mortality.[2,3,8] CVD remains the leading cause of death with a functioning graft, and obesity acts as a central modifiable risk factor amplifying this risk.[1]

From a kidney allograft perspective, obese patients are at a higher risk of delayed graft function, acute rejection, and poor long-term graft survival due to increased proteinuria secondary to glomerular hyperfiltration injury.[9,10] Additionally, obesity adversely influences peritransplant outcomes and has been associated with higher intraoperative surgical risk, perioperative anesthesia-related complications, and immediate post-transplant complications of poor wound healing, wound gaping, incisional hernias, and seromas.[11]

PATHOPHYSIOLOGY

The development of obesity after kidney transplantation is a multifactorial process resulting from the complex interplay between immunosuppressive therapy, metabolic recalibration following restoration of kidney function, lifestyle factors, and altered body composition. Unlike obesity in the general population, post-kidney transplant obesity occurs in a unique biological milieu shaped by chronic kidney disease-related metabolic adaptations and long-term immunosuppression.

Immunosuppressive agents play a central role in post-transplant weight gain. Corticosteroids promote increased appetite, adipogenesis, insulin resistance, and preferential accumulation of visceral fat. Calcineurin inhibitors are toxic to islet cells of pancreas, thereby leading to glucose intolerance and impaired insulin secretion, while mammalian target of rapamycin (mTOR) inhibitor is associated with dyslipidemia and altered adipocyte metabolism. This may allow to predispose transplant recipients to weight gain and cardiometabolic dysregulation.[5,8] Restoration of kidney function after transplantation leads to reversal of the catabolic state associated with advanced uremia. Improved appetite, normalization of taste perception, resolution of chronic inflammation, and correction of metabolic acidosis collectively result in an anabolic state, particularly in the early post-transplant period.[5] When not accompanied by proportional increases in physical activity, this metabolic shift favors fat accumulation rather than lean muscle gain. Physical inactivity further amplifies post-transplant obesity risk. Fear of graft injury, postsurgical deconditioning, sarcopenia related to prolonged pre-transplant illness, and lack of structured rehabilitation programs contribute to reduced energy expenditure. Thus, majority of transplant recipients develop sarcopenic obesity which is strongly associated with insulin resistance and CV risk.[7]

Adipose tissue itself acts as an active endocrine organ, secreting pro-inflammatory cytokines and adipokines that promote systemic inflammation, endothelial dysfunction, and activation of the renin–angiotensin–aldosterone system. In the transplanted kidney, these mechanisms contribute to glomerular hyperfiltration, proteinuria, and progressive graft injury, particularly in the setting of obesity-related metabolic stress.[9]

MANAGEMENT OF OBESITY IN POST–KIDNEY TRANSPLANT PATIENTS

Management of obesity in post–kidney transplant recipients requires a structured multidisciplinary approach aimed at achieving sustained weight control while preserving graft function and minimizing cardiometabolic complications. Although kidney transplantation confers a clear survival advantage compared with remaining on dialysis across all body mass index (BMI) categories, obesity in the post-transplant setting is associated with increased cardiometabolic risk, surgical complications, and healthcare utilization, warranting active long-term management rather than passive observation **(Fig. 1)**.[6,7,12]

GENERAL PRINCIPLES OF WEIGHT MANAGEMENT

Weight management strategies in transplant recipients should emphasize gradual, intentional, and sustainable weight loss, rather than rapid or aggressive reductions in body weight. Observational studies in patients with ESKD and transplant candidates have shown that unintentional weight loss, specifically losses exceeding 5 kg of dry weight or ≥10% of baseline body weight, is associated with increased mortality and adverse post-transplant outcomes.[13-15] Consequently, the rate and quality of weight loss are as important as the absolute magnitude of weight reduction. Although current transplantation guidelines

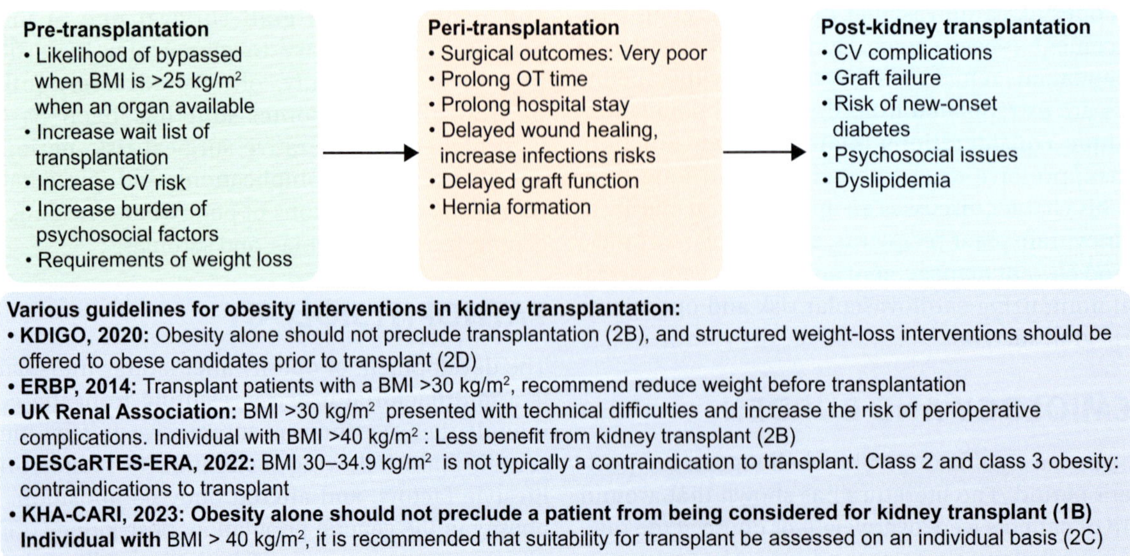

Fig. 1: Obesity and kidney transplantation: Clinical implications and various guidelines for obese patients.

do not consider obesity an absolute contraindication, obese candidates continue to face significant barriers to deceased donor listing and organ allocation[16-20] **(Fig. 1)**.

Early intervention is critical, as the first 1–2 years following transplantation represents a high-risk period for excessive weight gain due to immunosuppressive therapy, reversal of uremic catabolism, and reduced physical activity.

Lifestyle and Behavioral Interventions

Lifestyle modification should be recommended to all patients. Dietary interventions should focus on to achieve a modest caloric deficit while ensuring adequate protein intake to preserve lean body mass. Extreme caloric restriction should be avoided, as it may exacerbate muscle loss and worsen metabolic outcomes.[12]

After surgical recovery and stabilization of graft function, physical activity should be encouraged. A combination of aerobic and resistance exercise is recommended to improve cardiovascular fitness, enhance insulin sensitivity, and counter steroid-related muscle loss while addressing barriers such as fear of graft injury and post-transplant deconditioning to improve adherence.[12,21]

Pharmacological Therapy

There is lack of robust transplant-specific randomized controlled trials (RCTs) on post–kidney transplant obese patients. Therefore, pharmacotherapy should be considered adjunctive to lifestyle interventions and reserved for carefully selected individuals.

Metformin may be considered in stable transplant recipients with preserved graft function and insulin resistance or new-onset diabetes after transplantation (NODAT), provided contraindications such as advanced graft dysfunction or recurrent infections are absent. Renal function and GI tolerance should be monitored routinely.[2]

Emerging observational data suggest that GLP-1 RAs may be used safely in selected kidney transplant recipients; however, careful monitoring and follow-up are required for GI adverse effects and potential alterations in immunosuppressant absorption. As there is lack of transplant-specific RCTs, currently their use should be individualized and guided by overall cardiometabolic risk.[12,22,23]

SGLT2 inhibitors represent an evolving therapeutic option. However, evidence in kidney transplant recipients remains limited. Their use should be restricted to stable patients with adequate graft function and low infection risk, with vigilant monitoring for volume depletion and genitourinary infections.[12]

Bariatric Surgery

Bariatric surgery may be considered in selected post-kidney transplant recipients with severe or refractory obesity who fail to achieve meaningful weight loss with conservative measures. Evidence from systematic reviews and meta-analyses suggests that bariatric surgery can achieve sustained weight reduction and improvement in metabolic parameters without adversely affecting graft survival when appropriately timed and carefully monitored.[24-27]

Bariatric surgery, including laparoscopic sleeve gastrectomy and Roux-en-Y bypass surgery, may safely reduce obesity-related morbidity in such a population. However, the choice of bariatric procedure is critical in transplant recipients due to its impact on drug absorption. Restrictive procedures, particularly sleeve gastrectomy, are generally preferred over malabsorptive techniques because of a more predictable effect on immunosuppressant pharmacokinetics. Nevertheless, significant changes in immunosuppressant exposure have been reported even after sleeve gastrectomy, underscoring the need for close therapeutic drug monitoring in the perioperative and long-term postoperative periods.[28,29] Studies have also reported nutritional deficiencies of iron, folic acid, vitamin B_{12}, zinc, and vitamin D, and oxalate nephropathy has been reported as a complication post surgery due to enteric hyperoxaluria.[30]

CONCLUSION

The relationship between obesity and kidney transplant outcomes is multifaceted; however, obese patients who receive a kidney transplant have better survival compared with those who remain on dialysis.

Higher BMI is associated with increased perioperative complexity in kidney transplantation, with obese recipients experiencing a greater risk of delayed graft function and graft failure compared with nonobese patients. These adverse outcomes are thought to result from altered pharmacokinetics of immunosuppressive drugs, a chronic low-grade inflammatory milieu characteristic of obesity, and a higher prevalence of cardiovascular comorbidities.

Despite these challenges and the ongoing debate surrounding the obesity paradox, obesity alone should not be a reason to deny transplantation. Evidence from multiple studies and meta-analyses assessing both short- and long-term outcomes including surgical wound complications, duration of hospitalization, readmissions, cardiovascular events, new-onset diabetes after transplant, rejection episodes, graft survival, and patient survival generally indicates more favorable outcomes in recipients with normal BMI compared with those who are obese.[31]

REFERENCES

1. Lentine KL, Costa SP, Weir MR, et al. Cardiac disease evaluation and management among kidney and liver transplantation candidates. Circulation. 2012;126:617-63.
2. Kasiske BL, Snyder JJ, Gilbertson D, et al. Diabetes mellitus after kidney transplantation in the United States. Am J Transplant. 2003;3:178-85.
3. Cashion AK, Hathaway DK, Stanfill A, et al. Pre-transplant predictors of weight gain after kidney transplantation. Clin Transplant. 2014;28:1271-8.
4. Kidney Disease: Improving Global Outcomes (KDIGO) Transplant Work Group. KDIGO clinical practice guideline for the care of kidney transplant recipients. Am J Transplant. 2009;9 Suppl 3:S1-155.
5. Misra A, Chowbey P, Makkar BM, et al. Consensus statement for diagnosis of obesity, abdominal obesity and the metabolic syndrome for Asian Indians and recommendations for physical activity, medical and surgical management. J Assoc Physicians India. 2009;57:163-70.
6. Lentine KL, Delos Santos R, Axelrod D, et al. Obesity and kidney transplant candidates: how big is too big for transplantation? Am J Nephrol. 2012;36:575-86.
7. Nicoletto BB, Fonseca NK, Manfro RC, et al. Effects of obesity on kidney transplantation outcomes: a systematic review and meta-analysis. Transplantation. 2014;98(2):167-76.
8. Clunk JM, Lin CY, Curtis JJ. Variables affecting weight gain in kidney transplant recipients. Am J Kidney Dis. 2001;38:349-53.
9. Praga M, Hernández E, Herrero JC, et al. Influence of obesity on the appearance of proteinuria and renal insufficiency after unilateral nephrectomy. Kidney Int. 2000;58(5):2111-8.
10. Gore JL, Pham PT, Danovitch GM, et al. Obesity and outcome following renal transplantation. Am J Transplant. 2006;6(2):357-63.
11. Modlin CS, Flechner SM, Goormastic M, et al. Should obese patients lose weight before receiving a kidney transplant? Transplantation. 1997;64(4):599-604.
12. Gadwal S, Madipalli RT, Sharma S, et al. Obesity in renal transplantation. Indian J Transplant. 2024;18:3-8.
13. Molnar MZ, Streja E, Kovesdy CP, et al. Associations of body mass index and weight loss with mortality in transplant-waitlisted maintenance hemodialysis patients. Am J Transplant. 2011;11:725-36.
14. Harhay MN, Ranganna K, Boyle SM, et al. Association between weight loss before deceased donor kidney transplantation and post-transplantation outcomes. Am J Kidney Dis. 2019;74:361-72.
15. Harhay MN, Chen X, Chu NM, et al. Pre-kidney transplant unintentional weight loss leads to worse post-kidney transplant outcomes. Nephrol Dial Transplant. 2021;36:1927-36.
16. Chadban SJ, Ahn C, Axelrod DA, et al. KDIGO Clinical Practice Guideline on the Evaluation and Management of Candidates for Kidney Transplantation. Transplantation. 2020;104(4S1 Suppl 1):S11-S103.
17. Abramowicz D, Cochat P, Claas FH, et al. European renal best practice guideline on kidney donor and recipient evaluation and perioperative care. Nephrol Dial Transplant. 2015;30:1790-7.
18. Dudley C, Harden P. Renal Association Clinical Practice Guideline on the assessment of the potential kidney transplant recipient. Nephron Clin Pract. 2011;118 (Suppl 1):c209-24.
19. Oniscu GC, Abramowicz D, Bolignano D, et al. Management of obesity in kidney transplant candidates and recipients: A clinical practice guideline by the DESCARTES working group of ERA. Nephrol Dial Transplant. 2021;37:i1-15.
20. Campbell S, Pilmore H, Gracey D, et al. KHA-CARI guideline: recipient assessment for transplantation. Nephrology (Carlton). 2013;18(6):455-62.
21. Dombrowski SU, Knittle K, Avenell A, et al. Long-term maintenance of weight loss with non-surgical interventions in obese adults. BMJ. 2014;348:g2646.
22. Drucker DJ. The expanding landscape of GLP-1 medicines. Nat Med. 2026;32(1):47-57.
23. Alicic RZ, Neumiller JJ, Tuttle KR. GLP-1 receptor agonists and next-generation metabolic hormone therapies in chronic kidney disease. Nat Rev Nephrol. 2026.
24. Lee Y, Raveendran L, Lovrics O, et al. The role of bariatric surgery on kidney transplantation: A systematic review and meta-analysis. Can Urol Assoc J. 2021;15(10):E553-E562.
25. Ku E, McCulloch CE, Roll GR, et al. Bariatric surgery prior to transplantation and risk of early hospital re-admission, graft failure, or death following kidney transplantation. Am J Transplant. 2021;21(11):3750-57.
26. Pencovich N, Long JJ, Smith BH, et al. Outcomes of Kidney Transplantation in Patients That Underwent Bariatric Surgery: A Systematic Review and Meta-analysis. Transplantation. 2024;108(2):346-56.
27. Modanlou KA, Muthyala U, Xiao H, et al. Bariatric surgery among kidney transplant candidates and recipients: analysis of the United States renal data system and literature review. Transplantation. 2009;87(8):1167-73.
28. Yemini R, Nesher E, Winkler J, et al. Bariatric surgery in solid organ transplant patients: Long-term follow-up results of outcome, safety, and effect on immunosuppression. Am J Transplant. 2018;18:2772-80.
29. Chan G, Hajjar R, Boutin L, et al. Prospective study of the changes in pharmacokinetics of immunosuppressive medications after laparoscopic sleeve gastrectomy. Am J Transplant. 2020;20(2):582-8.
30. Troxell ML, Houghton DC, Hawkey M, et al. Enteric oxalate nephropathy in the renal allograft: an underrecognized complication of bariatric surgery. Am J Transplant. 2013;13(2):501-9.
31. Lafranca JA, IJermans JN, Betjes MG, Dor FJ. Body mass index and outcome in renal transplant recipients: A systematic review and metaanalysis. BMC Med. 2015;13:111.

58

CHAPTER

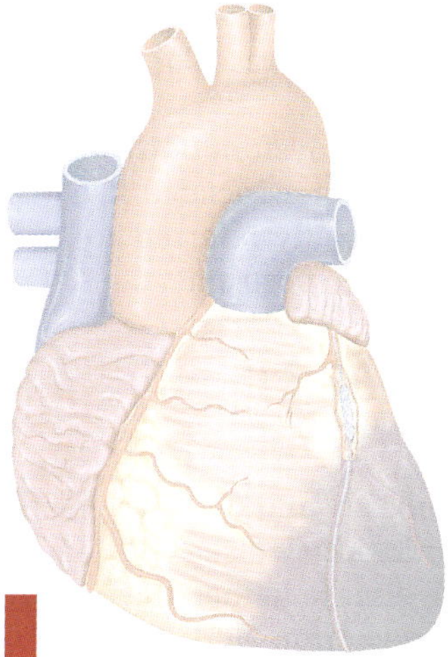

Obesity and Cardiovascular-Kidney-Metabolic Relationship

Manisha Sahay

INTRODUCTION

Obesity and cardiovascular-kidney-metabolic (CKM) health are closely interconnected. CKM syndrome refers to the diseases involving the heart (cardiovascular system), kidneys, and metabolism, including conditions, such as diabetes, high blood pressure, lipid disorders, and kidney disease. The concept of CKM is assuming importance as the burden of diabetes, heart disease, and chronic kidney disease (CKD) is increasing globally. Obesity is a risk factor for diabetes, heart disease, and CKD. ICMR-INDIAB study shows adult obesity rates vary by region, with obesity prevalence roughly between 11.8% and 31.3%, and central obesity even higher (16.9–36.3%).[1]

The treatment of end-stage kidney disease (ESKD) is either dialysis or transplantation. About 2 lakh people in India develop ESKD annually. However, only 20,000 undergo a renal transplant. Others are initiated on dialysis. Dialysis is expensive, uses a huge quantity of water, and generates massive quantities of biomedical waste. Quality of life on dialysis is suboptimal, and the cardiovascular risk is high. Similarly, the treatment of end-stage heart failure is expensive. Hence, prevention is a cheaper and more effective alternative, which is also associated with a better quality of life.

WHAT IS OBESITY?

Obesity is characterized by excess body fat accumulation, which has negative effects on health.[2] Obesity is traditionally measured using body mass index (BMI):

- BMI ≥30 = Obesity. In India, however, BMI ≥25 is classified as obesity.

TABLE 1: Obesity staging and risk calculator.

BMI (kg/m²)	*Category*
<18.5	Underweight
18.5–24.9 18.5–22.9	• Normal • Asian normal
25–29.9 23–25	• Overweight • Asian overweight
30–34.9 25–29.9	• Obesity Class I • Asian
35–39.9 >30–34.9	• Obesity Class II • Asian
≥40 >35	• Obesity Class III • Asian
≥50 ≥45	• Super obesity • Super obesity in Asians

- BMI 25–29.9 = Overweight; however, in our country BMI ≥25 is classified as overweight **(Table 1)**.

In India, it is also important to measure visceral obesity as visceral fat is inversely related to cardiovascular health as compared to subcutaneous fat. Thus, an individual may be overall falling in the normal weight category by BMI criteria but may still have high visceral fat and may be metabolically obese. This is the typical thin, fat Indian phenotype and is called the "Y-Y" paradox. Clinical studies now emphasize that measures of abdominal obesity, such as the Body Roundness Index (BRI) or waist circumference, are stronger predictors of advanced CKM syndrome and frailty than traditional BMI alone **(Box 1) (Table 2)**.[3]

Obesity increases inflammation, insulin resistance, and strain on organs.

DEFINITION OF CARDIOVASCULAR-KIDNEY-METABOLIC

Cardiovascular-kidney-metabolic is a novel concept, and it refers to the integrated approach for assessing the health of the cardiovascular system, kidneys, and metabolic function (mainly glucose regulation, lipid profile, and body weight). This provides a holistic approach and emphasizes that the three entities should not be treated in silos but should be addressed together as the risk factors. Screening tests and management are broadly similar for all three entities.

Cardiovascular-kidney-metabolic recognizes that heart disease, kidney disease, diabetes, hypertension, dyslipidemia, and obesity are not isolated conditions, but part of a continuum of risk. CKM is a spectrum that ranges from optimal health to advanced cardiovascular or kidney failure.[4,5]

When CKM syndrome (CKM dysfunction) occurs together with metabolic dysfunction-associated steatotic liver disease (MASLD), it is broadly referred to as a cardiorenal-metabolic-liver disease spectrum.

BOX 1: Waist circumference (important for CKM risk).

- Cut-off for high risk
- Men >102 cm (40 inch)
  - Asian men >90 cm
- Women > 88 cm (35 inch)
- Asian women >80 cm

TABLE 2: Obesity risk stage [Edmonton obesity staging system (EOSS) simplified].

Stage	Description
0	No risk factors, normal metabolic laboratories
1	Mild risk (slightly elevated cholesterol and BP)
2	Diagnosed with metabolic disease (diabetes and HTN)
3	Organ damage present (kidney disease and heart disease)
4	Severe disability/failure from obesity

WHY THE CKM APPROACH IS IMPORTANT?

Metabolic diseases such as obesity and diabetes greatly increase the risk of heart and kidney disease. Damage in one system can accelerate disease in the others. Early identification allows for prevention and slowing of progression.

CARDIOVASCULAR-KIDNEY-METABOLIC CLASSIFICATION (STAGES OF CARDIOVASCULAR-KIDNEY-METABOLIC HEALTH)

A commonly used model is the five-stage CKM spectrum, moving from no disease to advanced heart/kidney failure **(Table 3)**.

PATHOGENESIS OF CARDIOVASCULAR-KIDNEY-METABOLIC IN OBESITY

Obesity is considered a major risk factor for CKM disorders. It influences all three systems:

1. *Cardiovascular system:* Excess fat causes higher blood pressure, elevated cholesterol/triglycerides, and

TABLE 3: Classification of CKM syndrome.

CKM Stage	Description	Key indicators
CKM Stage 0—healthy	No risk factors, optimal metabolic profile	Normal BP, glucose, lipids, and kidney function
CKM Stage 1—risk present	Presence of risk factors without disease	Overweight/obesity, family history, sedentary lifestyle, smoking
CKM Stage 2—early metabolic dysfunction	Metabolic abnormalities present	Prediabetes, elevated BP, dyslipidemia, fatty liver, and insulin resistance
CKM Stage 3—established disease	Diagnosed with metabolic or kidney/cardiovascular disease	Type 2 diabetes, hypertension, CKD Stage 1–3, dyslipidemia requiring treatment
CKM Stage 4—advanced disease	Significant organ damage or complications	CKD stage 4–5, heart failure, MI/stroke history
CKM Stage 5—end-stage disease	Advanced failure requiring intensive care	Dialysis, transplant, and advanced heart failure

Note: Some groups Stages 4 and 5 together as "Advanced CKM disease."

thereby contributes to an increased risk of heart attack and stroke. Fat tissue releases inflammatory chemicals that damage blood vessels, especially the visceral fat, which acts as a metabolically active tissue that secretes pro-inflammatory cytokines and adipokines, leading to systemic inflammation, endothelial dysfunction, and oxidative stress. Kidney impairment results in hypertension, which is an important cause of heart disease, which may manifest as left ventricular hypertrophy or heart failure. Obesity also contributes to atherosclerosis, which can result in coronary artery disease. Adipose deposits around the heart (pericardial and epicardial fat) can cause local inflammation and structural remodeling, predisposing individuals to heart failure and arrhythmias, such as atrial fibrillation.

2. *Kidney health:* Obesity can lead to CKD by increasing workload on the kidneys, causing glomerular hyperfiltration (overworking the filtration system), increased intraglomerular hypertension, and worsening systemic hypertension. Diabetes is also the harbinger of kidney strain.
3. *Metabolic function:* Obesity is strongly associated with Insulin resistance, nonalcoholic fatty liver disease, and Metabolic syndrome (high blood sugar, high BP, abnormal lipids, and abdominal obesity). Insulin resistance is the precursor of prediabetes, which in turn leads to diabetes.

Thus, each condition can worsen the others. This is why modern healthcare considers them together as CKM disorders instead of separate conditions. Obesity is a central driver of CKM disease. Managing weight reduces the risk of progression of heart disease, kidney disease, and metabolic disorders, such as diabetes.[0-0]

CLINICAL EVALUATION OF CARDIOVASCULAR-KIDNEY-METABOLIC AND OBESITY

Screening for CKD should be mandatory at all levels of care, i.e., primary, secondary, and tertiary health care. It should be driven by health care workers, which includes not only the health care professionals but also the nursing staff, ASHA workers, and Anganwadi workers. They should be trained to recognize CKM and to initiate diet, lifestyle measures, and organ protective treatment (mentioned under management). They should also be trained to recognize the red flags for referral to tertiary care hospitals. Screening starts with measurement of BMI, waist circumference, and blood pressure.

- *Calculate BMI:*
  - BMI = Weight (kg)/height (m^2)
- Waist circumference
- Assessment of the severity of obesity

LABORATORY INVESTIGATIONS OF CARDIOVASCULAR-KIDNEY-METABOLIC AND OBESITY

- Blood glucose, HbA1c
- Lipid profile (HDL/LDL and triglycerides)
- Kidney function (eGFR and creatinine)
- Urine albumin-creatinine ratio (ACR)
- Liver enzymes (ALT/AST, for fatty liver)
- Heart evaluation when needed (ECG and echo), stress test in select cases.

MANAGEMENT OF CARDIOVASCULAR-KIDNEY-METABOLIC AND OBESITY

Diet Counseling for Cardiovascular-Kidney-Metabolic and Obesity

Meals should be balanced with emphasis on whole foods. Portion control is important.

Principles

- 45–55% calories from complex carbohydrates (whole grains and vegetables).
- 25–35% from healthy fats (nuts, seeds, and olive oil).
- 15–25% from lean proteins (fish, legumes, poultry, and tofu). If the patient has CKD, protein should be 0.8 g/kg/day instead of 1 g/kg/day for others.
- Increase fiber intake (25–35 g/day) for satiety and metabolic health.
- Reduce added sugar, salt, deep-fried foods, and refined carbohydrates.
- *Hydration goal:* 2–3L water/day (unless restricted medically, e.g., in advanced CKD patients with fluid overload).

Physical Activity

The patient should be counseled to undertake 150–300 min/week of activity. This should include aerobics or cardio, along with muscle strengthening and balance.[9] Weekly exercise routine with types of physical activities and their respective durations are discussed in **Table 4**.

The physical activity should be started slowly, and then the intensity should be increased gradually.

Lifestyle Changes

- Sugary beverages (soft drinks, juices, sweetened tea) should be avoided as far as possible.
- Home-cooked meals are preferred to ordering or consuming food from outside.
- Track calories or steps using apps/wearable

- Eat slowly and stop at *80% full.*
- Weigh yourself weekly to monitor progress
- Aim for 5,000–8,000 daily steps, gradually to 10,000.
- Alcohol should be restricted to ≤2 standard drinks per day for men and ≤1 for women. 1 standard drink = ~14 g pure alcohol, equal to 350 mL beer (5% alcohol), 150 mL wine (12% alcohol), or 45 mL spirits/hard liquor (40% alcohol). In most cases of CKD, e.g., >CKD 3, CHF, hypertension, and MASLD, complete alcohol abstinence is recommended.
- Tobacco in all forms should be stopped.
- Sleep is important, and less quantity of sleep has been shown to be associated with obesity. An average of 7–9 hours of nightly sleep is recommended.
- Daily screen time should be restricted to <2 h/day. Screen time, especially late at night, should be curtailed.
- Stress releases inflammatory hormones. Stress-relieving methods include meditation, breathing exercises, and pursuing different hobbies.

Pharmacological Management of Cardiovascular-Kidney-Metabolic Syndrome

The goal is to improve glycemic control, optimize blood pressure and lipid levels, weight reduction, and renal-cardiovascular protection. The major therapeutic advancement of the last decade has been the availability of organ-protective drugs that protect the heart and kidneys and improve metabolism.[9-12]

TABLE 4: Physical activity.

Activity	Frequency and duration
Brisk walking/cycling	30–45 minutes × 5 days/week
Strength training (resistance training/isometric exercises)	2–3 days/week (full body)
Flexibility/yoga	2–3 days/week
High-intensity interval training (optional)	1–2 sessions/week

Antidiabetic Agents (with Cardiorenal Benefits) (Table 5)

Metformin is the first-line agent. However, if GFR <30 mL/min/1.73 m^2, it is contraindicated. SGLT2i are essential for CKM and should be initiated if GFR >20 mL/min/1.73 m^2. These are cardio and renoprotective as highlighted in major landmark trials like CREDENCE, DAPA-CKD < EMPA Kidney, DECLARE TIMI, CANVAS, and EMPAREG. These are specifically indicated when diabetes, insulin resistance, or metabolic dysregulation is present, but can be used in nondiabetic patients with CKD as well. GLP1Ra are also renoprotective and cardioprotective and can be used in patient's intolerance to SGLT2i. Renal protection has been demonstrated in diabetic kidney disease patients in the FLOW trial. They also have significant benefits in reducing weight. They are not recommended in nondiabetic patients. DPP4 can be used, but most need to dose adjustment with low GFR. Linagliptin and teneligliptin can be used in regular doses.

Antihypertensive Therapy

Most guidelines recommend controlling BP to <130/80 mm Hg (KDIGO recommends Systolic BP <120 mm Hg). The various drugs recommended for BP control in CKM are shown in **Table 6**.

Lipid-lowering Therapy

It is indicated for dyslipidemia and/or CV protection. Statins are indicated in all diabetics with CKD with age >18 years and those with CVD for CV risk reduction **(Table 7)**.

TABLE 5: Antidiabetic drugs.

Class	Examples	Key benefits
SGLT2 inhibitors	Empagliflozin 10 mg/day, dapagliflozin 10 mg/day, canagliflozin 100 mg/day	↓ CKD progression, ↓ HF hospitalization, glycemic control, weight loss
GLP-1 receptor agonists	Semaglutide 1 mg SC weekly, liraglutide, dulaglutide	Weight loss, ↓ major CV events, and good for obesity
Metformin	Metformin 1gm bd if GFR >60 500 mg BD if GFR 30–60 mL/min/1.73 m^2	First-line for T2DM; improves insulin sensitivity
DPP-4 inhibitors	Sitagliptin 100 mg/day, linagliptin 5 mg/day, and vildagliptin	Moderate glucose control; weight-neutral
Insulin	Long/short-acting insulin Insulin analogs	Used in advanced/uncontrolled hyperglycemia

Note: SGLT2 inhibitors and GLP-1 RAs are preferred when diabetics have CKM due to cardiorenal benefits.

TABLE 6: Antihypertensive drugs in CKM.

Class	*Examples*	*Indication/benefits*
ACE inhibitors	Enalapril 40 mg/day, ramipril 20 mg/day, lisinopril	First line in CKD with albuminuria; protects the kidneys
ARBs	Losartan 100 mg/day, telmisartan 80 mg/day, valsartan	Alternative to ACEI; renoprotective
Calcium channel blockers	Amlodipine 10 mg OD, diltiazem 90 mg/day	Add-on when BP is uncontrolled
Diuretics	Thiazide (HCTZ), loop (furosemide)	Used for edema, BP control
Beta blockers	Metoprolol and carvedilol	Used in heart failure, post-MI

Note: ACEI/ARB are cornerstone drugs in CKM patients with hypertension and kidney involvement.

TABLE 7: Antihyperlipidemic drugs in CKM.

Class	*Examples*	*Benefits*
Statins	Atorvastatin and rosuvastatin	First-line for LDL lowering; strong CV protection
Ezetimibe	Ezetimibe	Add-on if statin insufficient
PCSK9 inhibitors	• *Evolocumab* 140 mg SC every 2 weeks *or* 420 mg monthly • *Alirocumab* 75–150 mg SC every 2 weeks • *Inclisiran* 284 mg day 0, then at 3 months, then every 6 months, no renal dose modification required for PCSK9i	For high-risk patients not controlled on statins

Note: Targets usually: LDL <70 mg/dL in high-risk CKM patients.

Antiobesity/Weight-loss Pharmacotherapy

Pharmacotherapy can be used along with diet and lifestyle measures when BMI is ≥30 kg/m^2 or if BMI is ≥27 kg/m^2 with comorbidities **(Table 8)**.

Cardiovascular Protection

These drugs are used in moderate to advanced stages of CKM or if CVD is present **(Table 9)**.

Renoprotection in Obesity and Cardiovascular-Kidney-Metabolic

Renoprotective strategies include RAASi, SGLT2i, and nonsteroidal mineralocorticoid receptor antagonists such as finerenone **(Table 10)**.

TABLE 8: Antiobesity drugs in CKM.

Drug	*Mechanism/benefit*
• GLP-1 agonists (semaglutide and liraglutide) • Oral semaglutide 3, 7, 14 mg/day • SC semaglutide 1 mg weekly	Significant weight loss + CV benefit
GLP-GIP agonist (tirzepatide)	15–20% weight loss,
Orlistat	Reduce fat absorption
Phentermine-topiramate/ bupropion-naltrexone	Appetite suppression (varies by country approval)

TABLE 9: Drugs for Cardiovascular protection.

Group	*Examples*	*Purpose*
Antiplatelets	Aspirin, Clopidogrel	Secondary prevention of MI/stroke, not for primary prevention
Heart failure drugs	ACEI/ARB, beta-blockers, and MRAs (spironolactone), finerenone, and ARNI	HF management
Anticoagulants	Apixaban and warfarin	Used for AF or clot risk

PHARMACOTHERAPY OF OBESITY AND CARDIOVASCULAR-KIDNEY-METABOLIC

The drug treatment in obesity and CKM can be simplified by choosing drugs according to the stage of CKM **(Table 11)**.

Surgical Management of Cardiovascular-Kidney-Metabolic and Obesity

Cardiovascular-kidney-metabolic patients may require weight loss surgery in certain situations.

TABLE 10: Drugs for renoprotection in CKM.

Drug/group	Benefits
ACEI/ARB	Reduce proteinuria and CKD progression
SGLT2 inhibitors	Strong kidney protection
Finerenone (MRA)	Reduces CKD progression in diabetes with albuminuria

TABLE 11: Drug treatment in obesity and CKM.

CKM stage	Main pharmacological focus
Stage 1 (risk)	Lifestyle + statins can be considered if dyslipidemia
Stage 2 (metabolic dysfunction)	Metformin, SGLT2i/GLP-1 RA, antihypertensives as required
Stage 3 (established disease)	Add ACEI/ARB, statins, and weight loss agents
Stage 4–5 (advanced CKD/CVD)	Multidrug regimen; HF/renal-specific therapy

TABLE 12: Types of bariatric surgery.

Type of surgery	Procedure	Advantages	Disadvantages/complications	Indications
Roux-en-Y gastric bypass (RYGB)	Creation of a small gastric pouch + bypass of a portion of the small intestine (jejunum). Combines restriction + malabsorption	Rapid and sustained weight loss; improvement in type 2 DM; reduces GERD; improves metabolic risk factors	Dumping syndrome; micronutrient deficiencies (iron, B_{12}, and calcium); complex procedure; risk of anastomotic leak	BMI ≥35 or ≥30 with comorbidities (diabetes, HTN, sleep apnea). Good for severe GERD and uncontrolled diabetes
Sleeve gastrectomy (SG)	About 75–80% of the stomach is removed, tubular "sleeve" is left. Restrictive procedure	Simpler procedure; good weight loss; fewer nutrient deficiencies; no intestinal bypass; less dumping	Risk of GERD worsening; irreversible; long-term dilation possible; risk of leak	BMI ≥35 or ≥30 with comorbidities. Preferred for high-risk patients or as the first stage in super obesity.
Adjustable Gastric Banding (AGB/LAP-BAND)	Band placed around the upper stomach, creating a small pouch. Restrictive only	Reversible; adjustable; lower surgical risk; minimal malabsorption	Slower and less weight loss; foreign body complications (band erosion/slippage); frequent follow-up required	BMI ≥35 or ≥30 with comorbidities. For patients, preferring a reversible/less invasive option
Biliopancreatic diversion with duodenal switch (BPD-DS)	Sleeve gastrectomy + bypass large portion of the intestine. Strong malabsorption	Most effective for long-term weight loss; excellent remission of diabetes; good metabolic effect	High risk of malnutrition, vitamin deficiency, diarrhea; technically complex; frequent follow-ups essential	Super obesity or severe metabolic disease requiring maximum weight reduction
Mini gastric bypass/one-anastomosis gastric bypass (OAGB)	Creation of a long gastric pouch + loop anastomosis to the jejunum. Restrictive + malabsorptive	Weight loss comparable to RYGB; simpler surgery; strong diabetes remission	Bile reflux risk; marginal ulcers; vitamin/mineral deficiency	Similar to RYGB: BMI ≥ 35 or ≥30 with comorbidities
Intragastric balloon (endoscopic)	Balloon placed in the stomach endoscopically to create fullness. Temporary (6 months)	Minimally invasive; reversible; no cutting or bypass; short recovery.	Temporary weight loss; nausea/vomiting common; balloon deflation complication	BMI 30–35 with failed lifestyle therapy or bridge before surgery.

Indications for Bariatric Surgery

- BMI ≥40 kg/m^2 (Asians BMI ≥35 kg/m^2)regardless of comorbidities.
- BMI ≥35 kg/m^2 (Asians BMI ≥30 kg/m^2 with obesity-related comorbidities such as:
  - Type 2 diabetes
  - Hypertension
  - Dyslipidemia
  - Obstructive sleep apnea
  - Nonalcoholic fatty liver disease
    - BMI 30–34.9 only if uncontrolled diabetes/metabolic syndrome (selected cases).

- Failed conservative management (diet/exercise/medication).
- Motivated patients with the ability to follow postoperative care.

Bariatric surgery is of multiple types and has its own advantages and disadvantages **(Table 12)**.

Thus, sleeve gastrectomy and RYGB are most commonly performed. RYGB is considered the best for GERD and diabetes control. Sleeve is simpler and is associated with fewer nutrient deficiencies. Banding has the advantage of being reversible but is less effective. Duodenal switch is the most effective but is associated with the highest risk of nutrient deficiency. Mini bypass is a simpler alternative to RYGB with strong outcomes.[13-15]

CONCLUSION

Obesity is a known risk factor for *CKD*. However, in patients with *CKD5 on dialysis,* higher BMI is associated with improved survival. This is called the *obesity paradox.* This may result from better nutritional status and energy reserves in obese patients or reverse causality, i.e., sicker patients lose weight, making low BMI appear riskier.

Also, inflammation and cachexia lead to worse outcomes in nonobese CKD patients. Management should focus on *preserving muscle mass, individualizing weight goals, and avoiding malnutrition,* rather than aiming for aggressive weight loss in all.[16]

REFERENCES

1. Anjana RM, Deepa M, Pradeepa R, et al. Prevalence of diabetes and prediabetes in 15 states of India: results from the ICMR–INDIAB population-based cross-sectional study. Lancet Diabetes Endocrinol. 2017;5(8):585-96.
2. Bala C, Roman G, Hancu N. Lancet Diabetes & Endocrinology Commission on diagnosis of clinical obesity- possible implications on clinical practice. Rom J Diabetes Nutr Metab Dis. 2025;32(1):1-4.
3. Misra A, Chowbey P, Makkar BM, et al. Consensus statement for diagnosis of obesity, abdominal obesity and the metabolic syndrome for Asian Indians and recommendations for physical activity, medical and surgical management. J Assoc Physicians India. 2009;57:163-70.
4. American Heart Association. 2023 AHA Scientific Statement: Cardiovascular-Kidney-Metabolic Health: A Presidential Advisory from the AHA. Circulation. 2023;148(14):e1-23.
5. Agarwal R, Light RP. Interaction between heart and kidney in cardiorenal syndrome. Clin J Am Soc Nephrol. 2008;3(3):551-60.
6. Hall JE, do Carmo JM, da Silva AA, et al. Obesity, kidney dysfunction, and hypertension: mechanistic insights. Hypertension. 2019;73(2):235-47.
7. De Boer IH, Khunti K, Sadusky T, et al. Diabetes, kidney disease, and cardiovascular outcomes: A narrative review. Kidney Int. 2022;102(6):1080-90.
8. Petramala L, Gigante A, Sarlo F, et al. Relevance of obesity-related organ damage and metabolic syndrome classification in cardiovascular and renal risk stratification in patients with essential hypertension. Front Cardiovasc Med. 2024;11:1369090.
9. KDIGO 2022 Clinical Practice Guideline for Diabetes Management in Chronic Kidney Disease. Kidney Int. 2022;102(4S):S1-127.
10. American Diabetes Association Professional Practice Committee. 11. Chronic Kidney Disease and Risk Management: Standards of Care in Diabetes-2025. 2025;48(Suppl_1):S239-51.
11. Arnett DK, Blumenthal RS, Albert MA, et al. 2019 ACC/AHA Guideline on the Primary Prevention of Cardiovascular Disease: A Report of the American College of Cardiology/American Heart Association Task Force on Clinical Practice Guidelines. Circulation. 2019;140(11):e596-e646.
12. Bajaj HS, Punthakee Z. Management of obesity and diabetes: an overview. Can J Diabetes. 2021;45(7):620-7.
13. Gadde KM, Martin CK, Berthoud HR, et al. Pharmacological and surgical treatment of obesity. Nat Rev Endocrinol. 2018;14:597-622.
14. De Luca M, Angrisani L, Himpens J, et al. Indications for surgery for obesity and weight-related diseases: IFBSO Recommendations 2020. Obes Surg. 2020;30:2071-5.
15. Brethauer SA, Kim J, el Chaar M, et al. ASMBS clinical issues committee systematic review of sleeve gastrectomy. Surg Obes Relat Dis. 2015;11(6):1276-86.
16. Kalantar-Zadeh K, Rhee CM, Chou JA, et al. The obesity paradox in kidney disease: how to reconcile it with obesity management. Kidney Int Rep. 2017;2(2):271-81.

SECTION 13

Obesity and Sexual Dysfunction

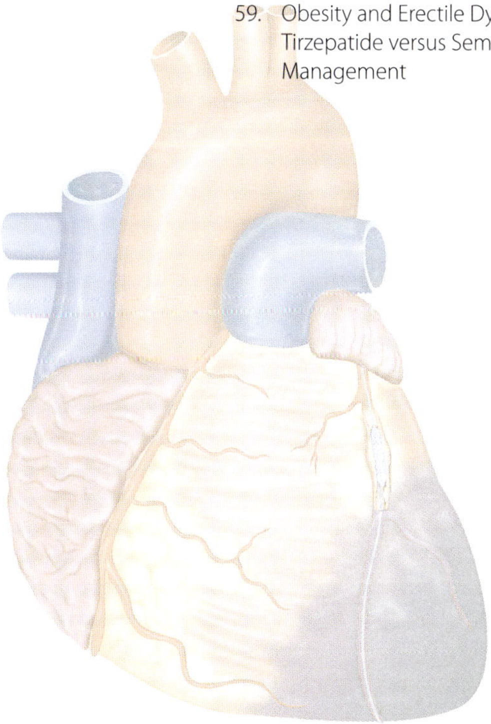

CHAPTER 59

Obesity and Erectile Dysfunction Tirzepatide versus Semaglutide: Management

Deepak K Jumani

INTRODUCTION

Obesity significantly increases the risk of erectile dysfunction (ED) through various mechanisms, including hormonal imbalance, endothelial dysfunction, inflammation, insulin resistance, and psychological factors. Key factors are oxidative stress, leptin resistance, and reduced testosterone levels, often stemming from abdominal obesity.

Studies have shown that the risk and severity of ED increase with higher body mass index (BMI) and waist circumference. Excess weight can disrupt the hormonal balance, damage blood vessels, and lead to systemic inflammation, all of which interfere with a man's ability to get and maintain an erection.

Weight loss through lifestyle changes like a healthy diet and regular exercise, and in some cases, bariatric surgery or certain medications, can improve erectile function by mitigating these underlying issues.

HOW OBESITY CONTRIBUTES TO ERECTILE DYSFUNCTION

- *Hormonal imbalance:* Excess fat, especially visceral fat, can lead to a decrease in testosterone levels and an increase in estrogen, with the formation of an enzyme aromatase thus disrupting the hormonal balance required for sexual function.
- *Endothelial dysfunction:* Obesity contributes to endothelial dysfunction, a condition where the lining of blood vessels is damaged. This impairs blood flow, which is crucial for achieving an erection.
- *Insulin and leptin resistance:* Both insulin and leptin resistance are common in obesity and are linked to inflammation, which negatively affects vascular and erectile health.
- *Inflammation and oxidative stress:* The increased adipose tissue in obesity promotes chronic inflammation and oxidative stress, creating an internal environment that is harmful to the blood vessels and erectile tissues.
- *Psychological factors:* The psychological impacts of obesity, such as depression and poor body image, can also contribute to sexual dysfunction.

Losing weight improves more than ED.

The good news is that once you make the lifestyle changes you need to safely and permanently lose unhealthy, excess weight, your erections improve and so do many other aspects of your health. Switching to a whole-foods, fresh diet, and adding plenty of exercise to your daily regimen brings you benefits such as:

- Reduced risk for heart attack or stroke
- Reduced risk for diabetes
- Improved blood glucose levels
- Reduced risk for arthritis

Achieving and maintaining a healthy weight also gives you a confidence boost, which may make it easier to achieve and maintain a healthy erection, too. Physicians can help their patients to imbibe habits that improve your overall health and your erections, such as:

- Quit smoking.
- Reduce alcohol use.
- Limit unhealthy fats and processed foods.
- Add in more fresh vegetables, fruits, and high-quality protein.
- Develop a sustainable exercise regimen.

DIABETES AND OBESITY: A UNIQUE LINK

Diabetes (DM) as well as obesity, due to their increasing incidence, were recognized as epidemic by the World Health Organization.[2] Obesity is an important environmental factor involved not only in the etiopathogenesis of the most common worldwide type of DM—type 2 diabetes (T2D)—but also in the development of its complications. Increasing scientific evidence points also to the role of obesity and overweight in type 1 diabetes (T1D). On one hand, weight gain may be considered as a complication of insulin treatment, but on the other, it reveals significant pathophysiological impact on various stages of the disease.

Overweight and obesity are very strongly correlated with T2D. Obesity is the most important culprit of insulin resistance, which appears early in the disease, and is primarily compensated by hyperinsulinemia.[1]

Diabetes can lead to many severe complications among others: cardiovascular diseases (CVDs), nephropathy, retinopathy, and microangiopathy leading in example to limp amputations.[3] Such complications as CVD, apnea, and obstructive sleep seem to be especially related with obesity and diabetes.[4] Gaining more weight in T2D increases the risk of cardiometabolic complications, which are the main reason of morbidity in T2D.[4]

MECHANISMS INVOLVING WEIGHT LOSS IN OBESITY AND DIABETES

Weight loss can effectively reduce hyperglycemia in diabetes, primarily by improving insulin sensitivity, restoring pancreatic beta-cell function, and reducing systemic inflammation. This occurs through several interconnected physiological mechanisms that are disrupted by obesity.

MECHANISMS BEHIND IMPROVED GLUCOSE CONTROL

- Enhanced insulin sensitivity weight loss directly improves how the body's tissues respond to insulin, a condition known as insulin sensitivity.
    - *Reduced free fatty acids:* Obesity is characterized by high levels of free fatty acids circulating in the blood, which interfere with insulin signaling in the liver and muscles. Losing weight reduces these fatty acid levels, enabling insulin to work more effectively.
    - *Decreased adipose tissue inflammation:* Excess body fat, particularly visceral fat, is linked to a state of chronic, low-grade inflammation. Immune cells in adipose tissue secrete pro-inflammatory cytokines such as TNF-α and IL-6, which disrupt the insulin signaling pathway in other organs. Weight loss diminishes this inflammation, restoring proper insulin function.
- *Restored pancreatic beta-cell function*: Weight loss can help restore the function of the pancreatic beta-cells, which produce insulin.
    - *Reduced glucolipotoxicity:* In obese individuals, high levels of glucose and fat can create a toxic environment for beta-cells, impairing their ability to secrete insulin. By lowering blood glucose and free fatty acid levels, weight loss alleviates this "glucolipotoxicity," allowing the beta-cells to recover.
    - *Decreased pancreatic fat:* Studies have shown an inverse relationship between the amount of fat in the pancreas and insulin secretion. Weight loss helps reduce intra-pancreatic fat, which has been associated with improved beta-cell function.
    - *Earlier insulin peak:* In type 2 diabetes, the insulin response to a meal is often delayed. Weight loss can shift the insulin secretion peak to an earlier, more effective time, leading to better control of postprandial (after-meal) blood sugar.
- *Reversed leptin resistance*: Obese individuals often develop resistance to the hormone leptin, which is produced by fat cells and helps regulate appetite. This causes the brain to think the body is starving, leading to overeating and further weight gain.
    - Weight loss can increase the body's sensitivity to leptin, helping to correct the brain's signaling and restore a normal appetite response. This reduces overall food intake, contributing to better glycemic control.
- *Reduced ectopic fat accumulation:* When fat-storing capacity is overwhelmed, excess lipids spill over and accumulate in other organs such as the liver and muscle, a process known as ectopic fat deposition.
    - Weight loss reduces this ectopic fat, which is a major driver of insulin resistance, especially in the liver. This can significantly improve hepatic insulin sensitivity and reduce overall blood sugar.[5]

CLINICAL EVIDENCE

Numerous studies have demonstrated the direct link between weight loss and improved glycemic control:

- The Diabetes Remission Clinical Trial (Direct)[6] showed that intensive weight management in people with type 2 diabetes led to remission in 46% of participants after 1 year.

- Other studies have found that losing as little as 5–10% of body weight can significantly lower blood sugar levels and, for some, prevent prediabetes from progressing to diabetes.

Recent advances in management of diabetes have revolutionized the outcomes of therapeutic targets which not only include reduction of hyperglycemia but also considerable reduction of weight.

Two such molecules which have recently bombarded in pharma market are tripeptide and semaglutide. Both these molecules have a unique effect on body weight. Infect these molecules have dual therapeutic effects, viz., controlling diabetes and obesity thus reducing the burden of the complications of both diabetes and obesity mainly improvement of erectile issues in men and also curb cardiovascular disease.

Tirzepatide and Semaglutide: Tirzepatide (Mounjaro and Zepbound) and semaglutide (Ozempic, Rybelsus, and Wegovy) are both incretin-mimetic drugs used to treat type 2 diabetes and aid in weight loss, but they differ in their mechanism of action, efficacy, side effects, and approved uses.

EFFICACY FOR WEIGHT LOSS AND BLOOD SUGAR

Clinical studies show tirzepatide generally has a greater effect on weight reduction and blood sugar control than semaglutide, likely due to its dual-receptor action **(Table 1)**.

MECHANISM OF ACTION

The primary difference is how they mimic incretin hormones to regulate appetite and blood sugar.

- *Tirzepatide:* A dual agonist that activates both the GLP-1 (glucagon-like peptide-1) and GIP (glucose-dependent insulinotropic polypeptide) receptors. This dual action may lead to greater effects on insulin secretion and appetite suppression.

TABLE 1: Comparison of tirzepatide and semaglutide with respect to average weight loss and HbA1c reduction observed in clinical trials.

Measure	Tirzepatide	Semaglutide
Average weight loss	Up to 15–21% in clinical trials, depending on dosage	Typically, around 15% in clinical trials
HbA1c reduction	Decreases by 2.0–2.5%, depending on dosage	Decreases by 1.5–2.0%

- *Semaglutide:* A single agonist that activates only the GLP-1 receptor. It mimics the natural GLP-1 hormone to control blood sugar and reduce appetite.
- *Side effects:* Both medications share similar gastrointestinal side effects, which tend to be more frequent when starting treatment or increasing the dose.
- *Common side effects:* Nausea, vomiting, diarrhea, and constipation are the most common for both drugs.
- *Side effect severity:* Higher doses of tirzepatide may increase the risk of gastrointestinal issues. However, some reports suggest tirzepatide's dual-action mechanism may cause milder symptoms for some patients compared to semaglutide.
- *Cardiovascular risks:* Semaglutide has been shown to reduce cardiovascular risks such as heart attack and stroke in patients with existing heart disease. Tirzepatide's cardiovascular outcomes are still being studied.
- *Boxed warning:* Both drugs carry an FDA Boxed Warning for the potential risk of thyroid C-cell tumors, based on animal studies.
- *Other differences*
    - *Cost:* While costs vary, some analysts suggest that tirzepatide may be more cost-effective for weight loss in the long run due to its higher efficacy.
    - *Administration:* Most formulations of both drugs are once-weekly subcutaneous injections. An oral tablet version of semaglutide (Rybelsus) is available for type 2 diabetes.
    - *Pediatric use:* As of October 2025, only semaglutide (Wegovy) is approved for weight loss in children aged 12 years and older.
- There is growing evidence that tirzepatide (Mounjaro, Zepbound) and semaglutide (Ozempic, Rybelsus, and Wegovy) can improve or lower the risk of ED in patients with diabetes and obesity. This effect is not a direct, immediate treatment for ED but rather a positive secondary outcome resulting from the drugs' primary functions—weight loss and metabolic improvements.
- *How GLP-1 agonists improve erectile function:* Erectile dysfunction in patients with obesity and type 2 diabetes often stems from poor cardiovascular health and impaired nerve function caused by high blood sugar and excess weight. Tirzepatide and semaglutide address these underlying causes through several mechanisms:
    - *Significant weight loss:* A reduction in body weight, especially visceral fat, is linked to improved endothelial function, hormonal balance, and sexual health.

   - *Improved metabolic health:* By regulating blood glucose and insulin levels, these drugs can prevent nerve and blood vessel damage that impairs penile blood flow and sensation.
   - *Enhanced vascular function:* GLP-1 agonists have been shown to have protective effects on blood vessels by reducing inflammation and oxidative stress, which leads to better blood flow essential for an erection.
   - *Increased testosterone levels:* Weight loss, in general, can help increase testosterone levels, which are often low in obese men with or without diabetes. Some studies show that GLP-1 agonists can also help boost testosterone.
- *Comparative efficacy for erectile dysfunction:* While both drugs offer benefits, tirzepatide's dual mechanism of action may provide a slight advantage in managing ED for patients with type 2 diabetes.
   - *Tirzepatide:* A 2025 study found that men with type 2 diabetes on tirzepatide had a 33% lower risk of developing ED compared to those on injectable semaglutide. The researchers suggest this is due to tirzepatide's superior weight loss and overall metabolic benefits, which have downstream effects on vascular and neurohormonal health.
   - *Semaglutide:* Some research, including a 2023 study of diabetic patients, has shown that long-term use of GLP-1 agonists like semaglutide can boost erectile function. However, a 2024 study on young, non-diabetic obese men found a slightly increased risk of ED, though the overall incidence was low (1.47%). This suggests that the relationship between these drugs and ED can be complex and may depend on a patient's underlying health status.
- Tirzepatide,[7] a novel dual glucose-dependent insulinotropic polypeptide (GIP) and glucagon-like peptide-I (GLP-I) receptor agonist, may provide more than simply glycemic management for men with type 2 diabetes (T2D), according to a recent study published in the Journal of Diabetes and Its Complications. Compared to other frequently prescribed diabetic drugs, tirzepatide may considerably lower the chance of developing ED, according to research from the University of South Florida lead by Kevin Cowart of the Taneja College of Pharmacy.
- Data from the TriNetX global health research network,[8] spanning the months of May 2022 through May 2025, were examined in the retrospective cohort study. Male patients with T2D who had no prior history of ED and were between the ages of 18 and 70 made up the study cohort. Three distinct propensity score-matched comparisons between tirzepatide and injectable semaglutide, dulaglutide, and sitagliptin were carried out by the researchers.
- A diagnosis of ED or the start of phosphodiesterase type 5 (PDE-5) inhibitor therapy, which is frequently used to treat ED, was the main outcome evaluated.

The following noteworthy findings came from the study:
- In every comparison, using tirzepatide was linked to a noticeably lower risk of ED.
- Compared to men using sitagliptin, those receiving tirzepatide had a 30% lower risk of developing ED (RR: 0.70).
- The following noteworthy findings came from the study:
- Tirzepatide users had a 33% lower risk of ED than semaglutide users (RR: 0.67).
- Tirzepatide was associated with a 45% lower risk of ED than dulaglutide (RR: 0.55). The results of every comparison were statistically significant.
- The study is the first to look at the connection between incident ED and tirzepatide use in males with type 2 diabetes, according to the authors. According to the authors, tirzepatide's superior metabolic effects, which include better glycemic management and increased weight reduction, may be crucial in improving neurohormonal and vascular health and lowering the risk of ED.
- DPP-4 inhibitor sitagliptin has not been connected to a lower incidence of ED before. The comparison thus emphasizes tirzepatide's wider physiological advantages. The study emphasizes that erectile function, a major quality-of-life issue for many men with type 2 diabetes, may be impacted by the metabolic enhancements linked to tirzepatide.
- In order to confirm their results and learn more about the underlying mechanisms—particularly the vascular, hormonal, and neurogenic pathways that may mediate the effect of tirzepatide on erectile function—the authors recommend conducting additional randomized controlled studies. They also advise determining whether patients already receiving GLP-I receptor agonist medication respond differently to PDE-5 inhibitors.
- The study contributes to the increasing amount of data demonstrating tirzepatide's broader advantages in the treatment of diabetes, indicating that its use may have a good effect on men's sexual health in addition to glycemic and weight results, the authors concluded.

OTHER MODALITIES TO TREATING ERECTILE DYSFUNCTION RELATED TO OBESITY

- *Lifestyle changes:* A cornerstone of treatment involves weight loss through a healthy diet and regular physical activity. Even a modest weight loss can significantly improve erectile function.
- *Medications:* For men with insulin resistance, medications like metformin may be beneficial in conjunction with phosphodiesterase 5 (PDE5) inhibitors (such as sildenafil, tadalafil vardenafil, or avanafil).
- *Bariatric surgery:* For some individuals, bariatric surgery can lead to substantial weight loss and a notable improvement in ED.
- *Addressing comorbidities:* Managing obesity-related conditions such as high blood pressure and high cholesterol is important for overall health and can indirectly help with ED.

CONCLUSION

For a holistic approach to treat Erectile Dysfunction Counselling on Lifestyle modification for lifetime is mandatory. weight loss, plant-based food, nutrition intervention, adequate sleep, quitting alcohol, smoking or any substance of abuse and reducing stress through any means forms the first line therapy for managing ED.

Tirzepatide or semaglutide are not primary line of treatment for ED: These drugs are not a first-line treatment for ED and should not be used as a substitute for standard ED medications such as PDE5 inhibitors (e.g., sildenafil, tadalafil) when a rapid effect is desire. While tirzepatide or semaglutide may be beneficial, other interventions such as lifestyle changes, counseling, or traditional ED medications may be necessary. Some individuals have anecdotally reported a reduced sex drive or ED after starting these medications.

REFERENCES

1. Pulgaron ER, Delamater AM. Obesity and type 2 diabetes in children: epidemiology and treatment. Curr Diab Rep. 2014;14(8):508.
2. Chobot A, Górowska-Kowolik K, Sokołowska M, et al. Obesity and diabetes—Not only a simple link between two epidemics. Diabetes Metab Res Rev. 2018;34(7): e3042.
3. Reinehr T. Type 2 diabetes mellitus in children and adolescents. World J Diabetes. 2013;4(6):270-81.
4. Wilding JP. The importance of weight management in type 2 diabetes mellitus. Int J Clin Pract. 2014;68(6):682-91.
5. Baranwal M. Medical dialogues: Tirzepatide tied to Lower risk of erectile dysfunction in men with type 2 DM. 2025.
6. Leslie WS, Ford I, Sattar N, et al. The Diabetes Remission Clinical Trial (DiRECT): protocol for a cluster randomised trial. BMC Fam Pract. 2016;17:20.
7. Cowart K, Murphy C, Carris N. Association of tirzepatide with erectile dysfunction in people with type 2 diabetes. J Diabetes Complications. 2025;39(10):109116.
8. Cowart K, Murphy C, Carris N. Association of tirzepatide with erectile dysfunction in people with type 2 diabetes. J Diabetes Complications. 2025;39(10):109116.

SECTION 14

Obesity and Women

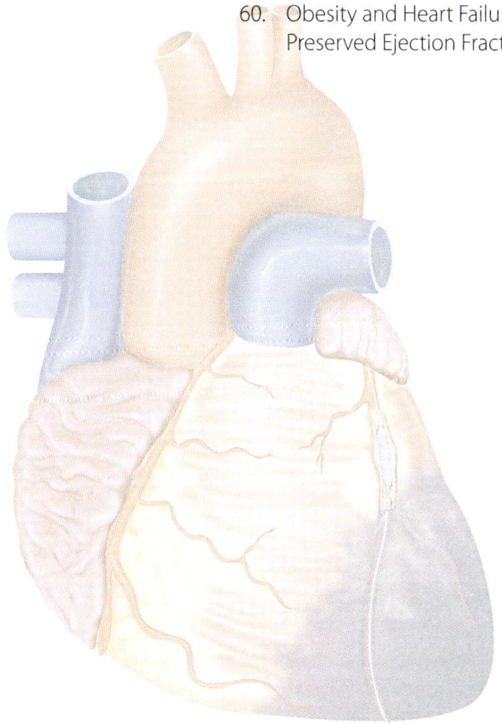

60

CHAPTER

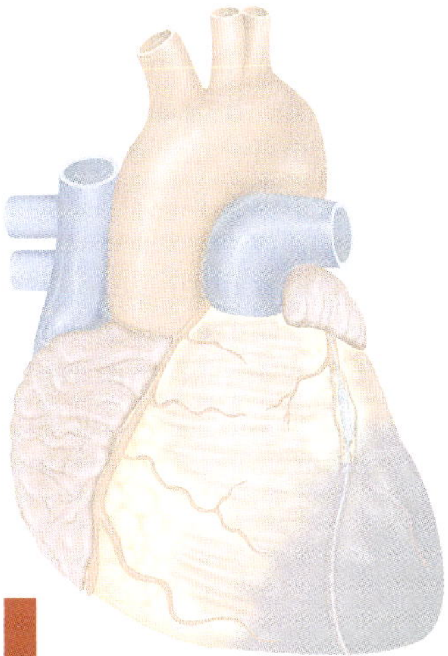

Obesity and Heart Failure with Preserved Ejection Fraction in Women

Shibba Takkar Chhabra, Manuhaar, Prerna Goyal, Abhishek Garg

INTRODUCTION

Obesity is a chronic systemic inflammatory state that produces hemodynamic, metabolic, and hormonal derangements that adversely affect the cardiovascular system.[1] Excess adiposity is a major, independent risk factor for the development of heart failure with preserved ejection fraction (HFpEF).[2] Obese individuals commonly exhibit subclinical abnormalities in left ventricular (LV) structure and diastolic function even when LV ejection fraction (EF) is preserved.[3] Women demonstrate distinct epidemiology and pathophysiology of obesity-related HFpEF, influenced by sex hormones, fat distribution, and female-specific exposures such as pregnancy-related disorders and menopause.[4] Obesity-related HFpEF in women poses a unique diagnostic and therapeutic challenge because symptoms overlap with other obesity-associated conditions, natriuretic peptide levels are often falsely low, and echocardiographic interpretation may be confounded by body habitus. Therapeutically, women exhibit variable drug responses, greater intolerance to polypharmacy, and limited inclusion of women in pivotal HFpEF trials, underscoring the need for sex-specific approaches. This chapter summarizes epidemiology, mechanisms, clinical phenotype, and evidence-based management—emphasizing contemporary randomized trials and major guideline recommendations with a special focus on women.

EPIDEMIOLOGY

Globally as well as in India, the prevalence of overweight and obesity continues to rise. Contemporary cohort studies indicate that the majority of patients with HFpEF are overweight or obese [body mass index (BMI) $\geq$25 kg/m^2], and increasing BMI is more strongly associated with HFpEF than with HFrEF. Sex-specific analyses reveal a disproportionately higher burden and lifetime risk of HFpEF in women as compared to men, along with distinct comorbidity profiles.[5-7]

In Asian populations, obesity is strongly associated with HFpEF, even at lower BMI thresholds, due to a higher proportion of visceral adiposity. The I-PRESERVE subanalysis reported a greater incidence of HFpEF among Asian women compared with Western cohorts. In India, data from the Trivandrum Heart Failure Registry and other regional cohorts demonstrate an increasing prevalence of HFpEF among obese, middle-aged, and postmenopausal women, with hypertension and diabetes as the predominant comorbidities. These findings underscore the disproportionate burden of HFpEF in South Asian women.[8]

PATHOPHYSIOLOGY—KEY MECHANISMS

Obesity contributes to HFpEF through multiple interrelated mechanisms. Hemodynamically, increased circulating volume and cardiac preload promote concentric LV remodeling and increase myocardial stiffness. Adipose-driven inflammatory mediators induce systemic and microvascular endothelial inflammation and impair myocardial energetics. In parallel, obesity-driven neurohormonal activation, notably aldosterone and mineralocorticoid receptor axis, exacerbates myocardial fibrosis and diastolic dysfunction[9] **(Flowchart 1)**.

Flowchart 1: Pathophysiologic links between obesity and HFpEF in women.

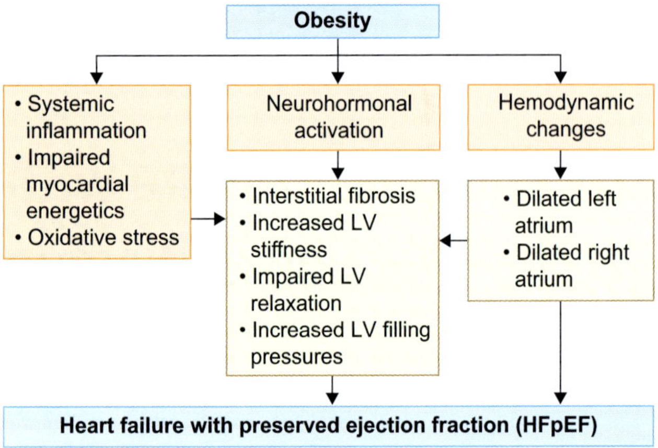

TABLE 1: Distinctive risk factors and pathophysiology of HFpEF in women and men.

Domain	*Women*	*Men*
Risk factors	Older age, obesity, menopause, hypertensive disorders of pregnancy	More often CAD, diabetes, and hypertension
Hormonal milieu	Estrogen deficiency, androgen excess postmenopause	Testosterone-related risk modulation
Fat distribution	More subcutaneous and pericardial fat, ↑ inflammatory profile	More visceral adiposity
Functional impact	Greater vascular stiffness, concentric remodeling	Mixed remodeling, more ischemic burden

In women, postmenopausal hormonal alterations characterized by estrogen deficiency and relative androgen excess, combined with sex-specific patterns of adipose distribution (higher subcutaneous and pericardial fat), further amplify vascular stiffening and diastolic dysfunction[10] **(Table 1)**.

DIAGNOSIS

The diagnosis of obesity-related HFpEF in women requires an integrative, multimodal approach that combines clinical evaluation, biomarker assessment, and advanced imaging. Clinical features include exertional dyspnea, exercise intolerance, and signs of congestion, which often overlap with obesity-associated respiratory or deconditioning syndromes.

Furthermore, natriuretic peptide levels are frequently reduced in obese individuals, leading to underdiagnosis. Therefore, echocardiography remains the cornerstone diagnostic modality, with emphasis on diastolic indices: *E*/*e*′ ratio, left atrial volume index, and tricuspid regurgitation velocity. Cardiopulmonary exercise testing and invasive hemodynamic assessment during exercise can reveal early HFpEF physiology. Advanced modalities such as cardiac magnetic resonance imaging provide additional insights into myocardial structure and function, facilitating the detection of diffuse interstitial fibrosis and quantification of adipose tissue.

MANAGEMENT

Treatment is directed toward alleviating symptoms, improving exercise tolerance and quality of life (QoL), reducing heart failure (HF) hospitalizations, and addressing associated comorbidities.[11] Therapeutic strategies are inherently multimodal, encompassing lifestyle/weight-loss interventions, evidence-based pharmacotherapy, optimization of comorbid conditions, and consideration of device-based or advanced therapies in selected patients **(Flowchart 2)**. Key recent randomized trials and evolving guideline recommendations are summarized and tabulated in **Table 2**.

Lifestyle and Nonpharmacologic Therapies

- *Structured exercise training and cardiac rehabilitation:* High-intensity interval training has been shown to improve peak oxygen uptake, exercise capacity, symptoms, and QoL in patients with HFpEF. The *OptimEx-CLIN* trial demonstrated significant functional gains and enhanced diastolic reserve with supervised exercise interventions.[19,20]
- *Dietary modification:* Sodium restriction and Dietary Approaches to Stop Hypertension (DASH) type diets have been shown to improve diastolic function and ventricular-arterial coupling, particularly in hypertensive HFpEF phenotypes.
- *Weight-loss interventions:* Substantial weight reduction (medical or surgical) favorably remodels hemodynamics, reducing resting and exercise pulmonary capillary wedge pressure, mean pulmonary artery (PA) pressure, and systemic blood pressure (BP). Referral to multidisciplinary obesity clinics is recommended for patients with a BMI ≥35 kg/m^2.
- *Pharmacologic weight-loss agents:* Glucagon-like peptide-1 (GLP-1) receptor agonists and dual glucose-dependent insulinotropic polypeptide (GIP)/GLP-1 receptor agonists have demonstrated clinically

Flowchart 2: Therapeutic algorithm for obesity-related HFpEF.

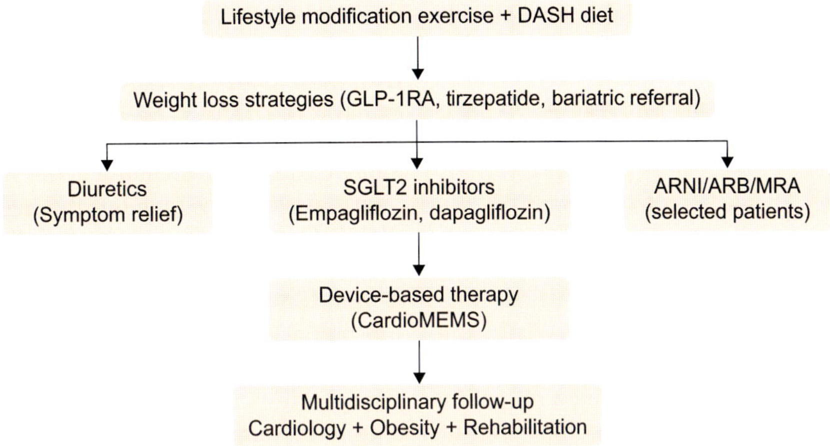

TABLE 2: Summary of major randomized trials in HFpEF.

Trial	*Population*	*Key findings*	*Implications*
TOPCAT[12]	HFpEF, spironolactone	Reduced HF hospitalizations (regional heterogeneity)	MRA in selected patients
PARAGON-HF[13]	HFpEF, sacubitril/valsartan versus valsartan	Trend to reduced events, benefit in women, and EF 45–57%	Consider ARNI, especially in women
EMPEROR-Preserved[14]	HFpEF, empagliflozin	↓CV death/HF hospitalization (21%)	SGLT2i foundational therapy
DELIVER[15]	HFmrEF/HFpEF, dapagliflozin	↓ Worsening HF/CV death	Broad benefit across EF spectrum
STEP-HFpEF[16]	Obesity + HFpEF, semaglutide	↓ symptoms, ↑exercise tolerance, major weight loss	GLP-1 RA promising
SURMOUNT-1[17]	Obesity (some with CV disease)	20% weight loss with tirzepatide	Emerging therapy for obesity-related HFpEF
NuSH (pilot)[10]	Obese HFpEF	Nutrition + supervised exercise	Improved peak VO_2 and reduced NT-proBNP (pilot)

meaningful weight loss and improvement in HFpEF symptoms in obesity-enriched HFpEF cohorts.

PHARMACOLOGIC THERAPIES: CONTEMPORARY EVIDENCE AND RECOMMENDATIONS

SGLT2 Inhibitors (Class IIA–I Recommendation in Contemporary Guidelines for HFpEF)

Large randomized outcome trials have established the efficacy of SGLT2 inhibitors across the full spectrum of EF. In *EMPEROR-Preserved* (empagliflozin), a 21% relative risk reduction was observed in the composite of CV death or HF hospitalization (driven primarily by a decrease in HF hospitalizations). Similarly, *DELIVER* (dapagliflozin) demonstrated a significant reduction in the composite of worsening HF or CV death among patients with mildly reduced and preserved EF. Benefits were consistent irrespective of diabetes status and were broadly maintained across sex subgroups. Collectively, these trials now form the cornerstone of guideline-directed pharmacologic therapy for HFpEF.[14,15]

Angiotensin Receptor–Neprilysin Inhibitor

PARAGON-HF trial evaluated sacubitril-valsartan versus valsartan in patients with EF ≥45%. Although the primary composite endpoint narrowly missed statistical significance, predefined subgroup analyses suggested greater benefit among women and in those with EF at the lower end of the preserved range. Emerging mechanistic and post-hoc data support selective use of angiotensin receptor–neprilysin inhibitors (ARNIs) in HFpEF, particularly in women and patients with mildly reduced-to-preserved transition range after individualized risk–benefit assessment.[13]

Mineralocorticoid Receptor Antagonists

TOPCAT trial assessed spironolactone in HFpEF, yielding heterogeneous outcomes across regions. While the overall primary composite endpoint was not significantly reduced, the Americas cohort demonstrated a reduction in HF hospitalizations. Mineralocorticoid receptor antagonists (MRAs) may be considered in appropriately selected HFpEF patients, particularly those with elevated natriuretic peptides, evidence of congestion, or features suggesting an aldosterone-driven phenotype, with careful monitoring of renal function and serum potassium.[12]

Diuretics and Blood Pressure Management

Loop diuretics remain the mainstay for symptomatic relief of congestion in HFpEF. Optimal BP control mitigates disease progression and event risk. Current recommendations endorse a target BP <130/80 mm Hg in most patients, often requiring combination therapy along with management of comorbid contributors such as sleep apnea, obesity, and resistant hypertension.[21]

Hemodynamic Monitoring and Device-based Strategies

Ambulatory PA pressure monitoring systems, such as *CardioMEMS*, have demonstrated reductions in HF hospitalizations among patients with recurrent decompensation, including HFpEF subgroups. Device-based monitoring can be considered in carefully selected patients with refractory congestion despite optimal medical therapy.[22]

WEIGHT-LOSS PHARMACOTHERAPY AND HFpEF: RANDOMIZED EVIDENCE

Lifestyle and Behavioral Interventions

The *NuSH* (nutrition and lifestyle in HFpEF) pilot trial demonstrated that structured dietary counseling combined with supervised physical activity improved exercise tolerance and reduced NT-proBNP levels in obese women with HFpEF, reinforcing the benefits of lifestyle-focused interventions.[18]

Incretin-based Therapies (GLP-1 and Dual GIP/GLP-1 Agonists)

Recent trials have reshaped the landscape of obesity pharmacotherapy in HFpEF. The *SURMOUNT-1* and *SUMMIT* programs evaluated tirzepatide in obese populations, including HFpEF patients. Both trials demonstrated approximately 20% mean weight reduction, substantial improvements in Kansas City Cardiomyopathy Questionnaire (KCCQ) scores, and exercise capacity. Tirzepatide is now emerging as a promising option for obesity-driven HFpEF, though long-term cardiovascular outcome data remain pending.[16,17] Similarly, *STEP-HFpEF* trials evaluated semaglutide in patients with obesity-related HFpEF, reporting significant improvements in symptoms, physical limitations, KCCQ scores, and exercise capacity, alongside robust and sustained weight loss. Importantly, the safety of GLP-1/GIP agents in patients with established HFpEF requires continued evaluation, especially regarding lean mass changes and potential effects on sarcopenia.[16]

Prior weight-loss medications, including orlistat, bupropion/naltrexone, and topiramate/phentermine, achieved only modest efficacy in obesity control and have restricted use in HFpEF in the absence of dedicated CV outcome data.

INTEGRATION WITH GUIDELINE RECOMMENDATIONS

The *2025 ACC Guideline on Obesity and HF* underscores the importance of phenotype-driven management in obesity-related HFpEF, designating *SGLT2 inhibitors* as foundational therapy across the HFpEF spectrum, also endorsing supervised weight-loss interventions and GLP-1/GIP receptor agonists for selected patients, and calls for sex-specific trial enrollment and mandates long-term safety surveillance.[23]

Similarly, the *2023 ACC Expert Consensus Decision Pathway on HFpEF* advocates a multidisciplinary phenotype-guided approach; rigorous management of comorbidities (hypertension, obesity, atrial fibrillation, diabetes, and sleep-disordered breathing) alongside tailored pharmacologic strategies. The document highlights SGLT2 inhibitors as first-line therapy for most patients with HFpEF, while recognizing the selective utility of ARNI, MRAs, and diuretics for distinct clinical phenotypes.

SPECIAL CONSIDERATIONS IN WOMEN

Obesity and HFpEF during pregnancy represent a critical intersection of metabolic and cardiovascular vulnerability. Obese women are predisposed to hypertensive disorders of pregnancy, preeclampsia, and gestational diabetes, all of which confer an increased risk of developing HFpEF in later life. Pregnancy-related hemodynamic stresses can precipitate decompensation in obese women with latent diastolic dysfunction. Early recognition and vigilant hemodynamic monitoring during pregnancy are therefore essential. Key women-centric considerations include:

- *Comprehensive hormonal and reproductive assessment (notably history of preeclampsia and gestational diabetes, menopausal timing, and prior or ongoing hormone replacement therapy):* These factors collectively influence lifetime CV risk and HFpEF susceptibility.
- *Phenotype-targeted therapy:* Women with obesity-driven HFpEF have pathophysiologic distinctions (increased plasma volume, heightened pericardial restraint, and greater right ventricular involvement), which impact diuretic strategies, device candidacy, and the potential responses to MR blockade and ARNI therapy.
- *Weight-loss therapies:* Incretin-based therapies have been shown to enhance symptoms, functional capacity, and QoL in women with obesity-related HFpEF. A multidisciplinary involvement (cardiology, endocrinology, and nutrition) is recommended before initiation, particularly in women with advanced HF or at risk for sarcopenia.[17]

RESEARCH GAPS AND FUTURE DIRECTIONS

While incretin-based agents offer substantial symptomatic and metabolic benefits, continued evaluation of long-term safety in HFpEF populations is essential, particularly concerning changes in lean body mass and potential impact on sarcopenia. Ongoing and forthcoming trials are expected to clarify the net clinical benefit and optimal integration of these agents into guideline-directed therapy for obesity-related HFpEF.[16] Future research should prioritize sex-specific mechanistic studies to explain the biological basis for differential drug responses, and phenotype-adaptive randomized trials that can match current therapies to biological subtypes (e.g., aldosterone-driven, obesity-inflammatory, and pulmonary vascular).

CONCLUSION

Obesity-related HFpEF represents a distinct clinical and pathophysiologic phenotype, disproportionately affecting women, particularly South Asian populations. The confluence of visceral adiposity, metabolic dysregulation, and hormonal alterations underlies its unique trajectory and therapeutic challenges in women. Despite advances in understanding its mechanisms, diagnostic ambiguity and therapeutic inertia pose major barriers to improving outcomes in this population. Given the diagnostic challenges in obese women, a comprehensive, multiparametric strategy integrating clinical, hemodynamic, and imaging data is essential for accurate diagnosis and phenotypic characterization. Public health efforts addressing obesity, hypertension, and diabetes remain foundational to disease prevention. Ultimately, a paradigm shift from symptom management to pathophysiology-directed care will be essential to mitigate the rising global burden of obesity-related HFpEF in women.

REFERENCES

1. Kitzman DW, Shah SJ. The HFpEF obesity phenotype: the elephant in the room. J Am Coll Cardiol. 2016;68:200-3.
2. Kenchaiah S, Evans JC, Levy D, et al. Obesity and the risk of heart failure. N Engl J Med. 2002;347:305-13.
3. Wong CY, O'Moore-Sullivan T, Leano R, et al. Alterations of LV myocardial characteristics associated with obesity. Circulation. 2004;110:3081-7.
4. Kittleson MM, Panjrath GS, Amancherla K, et al. 2023 ACC expert consensus decision pathway on management of heart failure with preserved ejection fraction: a report of the American College of Cardiology Solution Set Oversight Committee. J Am Coll Cardiol. 2023;81(18):1835-78.
5. Du J, Liu J, Wang X, et al. The role of estrogen in the sex difference for the risk factors of heart failure with preserved ejection fraction. Biol Direct. 2025;20(1):28.
6. Haass M, Kitzman DW, Anand IS, et al. Body mass index and adverse cardiovascular outcomes in heart failure patients with preserved ejection fraction: results from the Irbesartan in Heart Failure with Preserved Ejection Fraction (I-PRESERVE) trial. Circ Heart Fail. 2011;4(3):324-31.
7. Savji N, Meijers WC, Bartz TM, et al. The association of obesity and cardiometabolic traits with incident HFpEF and HFrEF. JACC Heart Fail. 2018;6(8):701-9.
8. Tadic M, Cuspidi C. Heart failure and the obesity paradox. Obesity and Diabetes: Scientific Advances and Best Practice. Cham: Springer International Publishing; 2020. pp. 427-35.
9. Ebong IA, Goff Jr DC, Rodriguez CJ, et al. Mechanisms of heart failure in obesity. Obes Res Clin Pract. 2014;8(6):e540-8.

10. Redfield MM, Jacobsen SJ, Borlaug BA, et al. Age-and gender-related ventricular-vascular stiffening: a community-based study. Circulation. 2005;112(15):2254-62.
11. Mueller S, Winzer EB, Duvinage A, et al. Effect of high-intensity interval training, moderate continuous training, or guideline-based physical activity advice on peak oxygen consumption in patients with heart failure with preserved ejection fraction: a randomized clinical trial. JAMA. 2021;325(6):542-51.
12. Pitt B, Pfeffer MA, Assmann SF, et al. Spironolactone for heart failure with preserved ejection fraction. N Engl J Med. 2014;370(15):1383-92.
13. Solomon SD, McMurray JJV, Anand IS, et al. Angiotensin–neprilysin inhibition in heart failure with preserved ejection fraction. N Engl J Med. 2019;381(17):1609-20.
14. Anker SD, Butler J, Filippatos G, et al. Empagliflozin in heart failure with a preserved ejection fraction. N Engl J Med. 2021;385(16):1451-61.
15. Solomon SD, McMurray JJV, Claggett B, et al. Dapagliflozin in heart failure with mildly reduced or preserved ejection fraction. N Engl J Med. 2022;387(12):1089-98.
16. Kosiborod MN, Abildstrøm SZ, Borlaug BA, et al. Semaglutide in patients with heart failure with preserved ejection fraction and obesity. N Engl J Med. 2023;389(12):1069-84.
17. Kim SE, Yoo B-S. Obesity and heart failure with preserved ejection fraction: focus on new drugs and future direction in medical treatment. Korean J Intern Med. 2025;40(3):357-70.
18. Czernichow S, Rassy N, Carette C, et al. Nutritional and functional outcomes in trials of nutrient-stimulated hormone-based therapy: a systematic mapping review. Obes Rev. 2025;26(5):e13890.
19. Hummel SL, Seymour EM, Brook RD, et al. Low-sodium DASH diet improves diastolic function and ventricular–arterial coupling in hypertensive heart failure with preserved ejection fraction. Circ Heart Fail. 2013;6(6):1165-71.
20. Suchy C, Massen L, Rognmo O, et al. Optimising exercise training in prevention and treatment of diastolic heart failure (OptimEx-CLIN): rationale and design of a prospective, randomised, controlled trial. Eur J Prev Cardiol. 2014;21(2_suppl):18-25.
21. Obokata M, Reddy YNV, Melenovsky V, et al. Uncoupling between intravascular and distending pressures leads to underestimation of circulatory congestion in obesity. Eur J Heart Fail. 2022;24(2):353-61.
22. Alam A, Van Zyl J, Nayyar N, et al. Improvement in metabolic co-morbidities after implantation of CardioMEMS in patients with heart failure with preserved ejection fraction phenotype. J Clin Med. 2021;10(19):4308.
23. Gilbert O, Gulati M, Gluckman TJ, et al. 2025 Concise Clinical Guidance: an ACC Expert Consensus Statement on medical weight management for optimization of cardiovascular health: a report of the American College of Cardiology Solution Set Oversight Committee. J Am Coll Cardiol. 2025;86(7):536-55.

61

CHAPTER

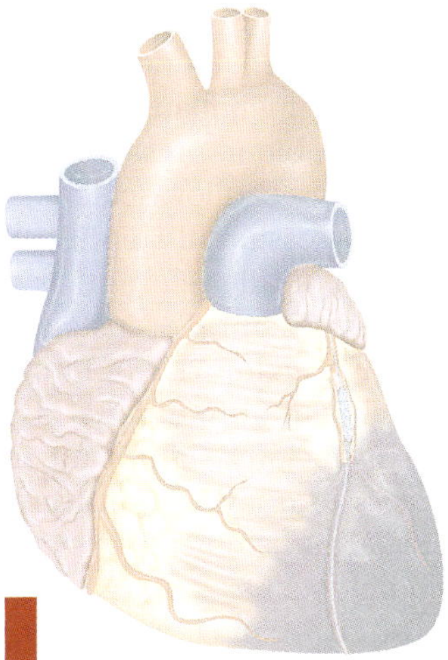

Obesity and Heart Failure with Preserved Ejection Fraction in Women: Management Strategies

Shubham Srivastava, Harshit Khare, Roopali Khanna

INTRODUCTION

Heart failure (HF) is one of the leading causes of morbidity and mortality worldwide, with an estimated lifetime risk of 20% at the age of 40 years.[1] While the incidence of HF seems to be similar over the past three decades, there has been an increase in the incidence of heart failure with preserved ejection fraction (HFpEF) subset.[2-3] HFpEF now makes up around half of all HF cases,[4] carrying a prognosis comparable to heart failure with reduced ejection fraction (HFrEF)[5] but often remains underdiagnosed, leading to extensive use of healthcare resources. Surveillance data show that rates of hospitalization for HF are increasing over time, due to an increase in HFpEF, which occurs more frequently in women.[6] Traditional risk factors, such as diabetes, obesity, hypertension, and tobacco use, impact the risk of HF more in women than in men. Women presenting with acute decompensated HF are approximately twice as likely as men to exhibit preserved left ventricular function, or HF with preserved ejection fraction, with obesity emerging as a significant risk factor in this population.[7] The difficulty of identifying and managing HFpEF becomes even more pronounced in women patients. While treatment for HF may offer comparable benefits across sexes, the underrepresentation of women in HF clinical trials—combined with the higher prevalence of HFpEF among women—has contributed to a limited evidence base regarding optimal therapeutic strategies for women with HF. Therefore, there is a critical need for evidence-based diagnostic and therapeutic algorithms tailored to this population.

PATHOPHYSIOLOGY AND THE PREVALENCE

The increasing prevalence of obesity in the present era has predisposed the aging population to the risk of HFpEF, particularly in women, affecting around 60–80% of them with HFpEF.[8] This risk appears to be more closely associated with increases in visceral adipose tissue—a hallmark of central obesity—which is more strongly linked to cardiometabolic stressors, including insulin resistance, hypertension, and diabetes mellitus.[9-11] The lifetime risk of HFpEF is nearly double that of HFrEF among women (10.7% vs. 5.8%), whereas the lifetime risk of HFpEF and HFrEF is similar among men.[6] Data from the ARIC (Atherosclerosis Risk In Communities) study of HF-related hospitalizations in four US communities between 2005 and 2014 show that average event rates for the first HFpEF hospitalization were higher among women than among men.[6]

Although the exact mechanisms underlying sex-specific differences in HFpEF prevalence remain incompletely understood, several hypotheses have emerged. As discussed above, the development of HFpEF is strongly influenced by comorbidities, particularly obesity and diabetes, which act as central drivers of systemic microvascular inflammation.[12] This inflammatory state leads to decreased nitric oxide bioavailability, reduced cyclic guanosine monophosphate signaling, altered titin phosphorylation, and increased myocardial fibrosis, ultimately impairing cardiomyocyte function and diastolic relaxation. In addition to systemic inflammation, excess adipose tissue contributes directly to disease progression through several mechanisms—enhanced pericardial restraint; accelerated coronary atherosclerosis mediated by epicardial fat; worsening renal dysfunction due to perirenal fat; capillary rarefaction and impaired tissue perfusion from adipose-derived vasoconstrictors; abnormal pulmonary diffusion and ventilation; and impaired skeletal muscle perfusion and mitochondrial dysfunction.[13] Together, these interrelated processes establish the multifactorial pathophysiologic substrate of HFpEF.

HEART FAILURE DIAGNOSTIC CRITERIA

The main clinical signs and symptoms used to diagnose HF, as enumerated in the Framingham study, included both major and minor criteria. The major criteria mentioned included orthopnea, elevated jugular venous pressure, and positive hepatojugular reflux, as well as the presence of rales, an S3 gallop, acute pulmonary edema, and significant cardiomegaly. The minor criteria included dyspnea on exertion, nocturnal cough, pedal edema, heart rate >120 beats per minute, and hepatomegaly or pleural effusion. To make the diagnosis of HF, at least two or more major criteria or one major criterion and two minor criteria were required.[14]

The Universal Definition of HF provides clinicians with a more pragmatic framework for incorporating all signs and symptoms of a patient that point to the presence of HF.[15] It also includes one of the following: (1) Natriuretic peptides levels and (2) evidence for either pulmonary or systemic congestion.

The current European Society of Cardiology guidelines recommend that a diagnosis of HFpEF should be based on the presence of one of the three following features: (1) Clinical features and signs consistent with a diagnosis of HF; (2) Preserved LV systolic function with an LVEF of >50%; and (3) Objective evidence of cardiac structural and/or functional abnormalities consistent with the presence of LV diastolic dysfunction/raised LV filling pressures, including raised natriuretic peptides.[16]

Compared to men, women face a higher attributable risk from traditional risk factors such as hypertension, diabetes, and obesity. In addition, they have unique sex-specific risk factors that may play an important role in HFpEF. These include early menopause, central obesity/visceral adiposity, and complications during pregnancy such as polycystic ovary syndrome, preeclampsia, gestational diabetes, or repeated miscarriages. HFpEF is more common in older women, particularly after menopause, when estradiol levels decline. Estradiol supports cardiovascular health by regulating inflammation, oxidative stress, endothelial function, and nitric oxide signaling. Its decline after menopause leads to adverse shifts in body composition, blood pressure, and lipid metabolism, all of which increase cardiovascular risk and play a central role in the progression of HFpEF.[17-19] A detailed pregnancy history is clinically relevant, as it can provide prognostic insight into HFpEF. For instance, preeclampsia has been linked to a higher risk of future HFpEF hospitalizations, independent of traditional risk factors.[20] This association is especially significant in populations with limited access to quality healthcare, including underrepresented racial and ethnic groups and individuals of lower socioeconomic status.

Women with HFpEF often experience more pronounced dyspnea and tend to report poorer overall health status.[21] Physical examination, however, does not differ much between the two genders with HFpEF.

GENDER-RELATED VARIATIONS IN DIAGNOSING HFpEF

While the universal definition of HF aids clinicians, diagnosing HFpEF can be challenging since echocardiograms may lack clear abnormalities, and natriuretic peptide levels can be normal, particularly in obesity. In such cases, clinical scoring systems such as H_2FPEF[22] **(Fig. 1)** and HFA-PEFF[23] may support diagnosis.

However, the gender differences become more apparent on echocardiographic evaluation, as women tend to have more prominent and concentric LV remodeling, besides having higher grades of diastolic dysfunction when compared to male patients with HFpEF.[24] These findings suggest that the pathophysiologic substrate of

H_2	Heavy (BMI >30 kg/m²)	→	2
	Hypertensive (on 2 or more anti-hypertensives)	→	1
F	Atrial fibrillation	→	3
P	Pulmonary hypertension (PASP >35 mm Hg)	→	1
E	Elder (age >60 years)	→	1
F	Filling pressures raised (E/e' >9 on Doppler)	→	1
H_2FPEF score >6 is highly diagnostic of HFpEF			

Fig. 1: Heart failure with preserved ejection fraction (HFpEF) score.

HFpEF may differ between sexes, potentially contributing to variations in clinical presentation, disease progression, and therapeutic response.[25] While the use of similar cutoffs for normal LV ejection fraction can lead to a substantial underestimation of left ventricular function in women, cardiac biomarkers such as natriuretic peptides may be more reliable for excluding HFpEF in women. However, normal thresholds and comorbidities still influence accuracy.[26]

MANAGEMENT STRATEGY

Management of HFpEF[27] includes:

- Identification and early control of various risk factors contributing to HFpEF, such as hypertension, diabetes, and obesity, along with management of other prevalent comorbidities in this subset, such as atrial fibrillation, renal dysfunction, underlying coronary artery disease, and obstructive sleep apnea.
- Emphasizing the role of other non-pharmacological preventive strategies that target the above-mentioned risk factors at the root level. Such strategies include maintaining a healthy lifestyle, cultivating regular exercise habits, and maintaining a balanced diet to achieve an age- and gender-appropriate weight. More recently, implantable pulmonary artery monitors have been developed to track patients who require intensification of therapy.
- Pharmaceutical therapies include loop diuretic agents to treat symptoms of congestion, along with disease-modifying agents such as SGLT2is and RAAS antagonists to reverse the LV remodeling.

PREVENTION OF TRADITIONAL RISK FACTORS

In 2010, the AHA introduced Life's Simple 7 to promote cardiovascular health through seven key factors—a healthy diet, regular physical activity, maintaining a normal BMI, avoiding smoking, and keeping blood pressure, fasting glucose, and cholesterol within normal ranges. This framework was later updated to the Life's Essential 8, which includes sleep health. These straightforward measures should be reinforced by primary care physicians, obstetricians/gynecologists, cardiologists, and other specialists throughout a woman's life to help prevent traditional risk factors that contribute to HFpEF.[28]

MANAGEMENT OF COMORBIDITIES

Complex interactions among multiple risk factors and a susceptible phenotype often cause HFpEF. A brief overview of these dynamics is provided in **Table 1**.

TABLE 1: HFpEF-related comorbidities and their management.

Comorbidities	*Strategies for management*
Obesity	• Weight loss by diet and exercise • Use GLP-1 analog for achieving early and rapid weight loss
Hypertension	• Target BP <130/80, using diuretics or RAAS inhibitors. Rule out secondary hypertension
Coronary artery disease	• Symptom-targeted medical therapy and revascularization as per guidelines
Atrial fibrillation	• Rate vs. rhythm control strategy guided by symptoms • Beta-blockers, non-dihydropyridine calcium channel blockers, or digoxin • Anticoagulation unless contraindicated
Type II diabetes mellitus	• Target HbA1c <7 • Use SGLT2i and GLP-1 analogs
Chronic kidney disease	For reducing progression of renal impairment, may use— • ARNi (eGFR should be >30 mL/min/m^2) or • SGLT2i (eGFR should be >20 mL/min/m^2)
Sleep apnea	• Polysomnography • Weight loss • Seek OSA specialist referral if required

REHABILITATION

Lifestyle modification and cardiac rehabilitation are key non-pharmacological strategies in the care of HFpEF. Since obesity and a sedentary lifestyle have been linked to poorer outcomes in HFpEF,[29] numerous studies have examined the effect of weight loss (via caloric restriction or bariatric surgery) on the incidence of HF events.[30] Even the 2019 ACC/AHA Guideline on the Primary Prevention of Cardiovascular Disease recommends a comprehensive lifestyle approach that includes self-monitoring of diet, exercise, and physical activity to achieve a healthy weight. The recommendations also advocate 150 minutes of aerobic exercise per week, with at least 30 minutes of daily physical activity or exercise.[31]

Engaging in regular physical activity, particularly isotonic exercise, improves exercise tolerance and quality of life, with women potentially experiencing greater gains due to lower baseline functional capacity.[32] Nonetheless, poor adherence remains a significant barrier, emphasizing the importance of tailored interventions to improve program uptake and long-term participation. Implementation of supervised exercise training (SET) has been shown to help improve exercise capacity and reduce morbidity.

THERAPEUTIC STRATEGIES AND OUTCOMES (FLOWCHART 1)

Diuretic agents form the first line of therapy targeting congestive symptoms in these subsets of HF and have been given a Class 1 recommendation in both recent ESC and ACC HF guidelines.

While beta-blockers are a major pillar of therapy in HFrEF subsets, in HFpEF, their role is limited to specific conditions, such as a history of myocardial infarction, CAD, or AF with a rapid ventricular rate.

Several clinical trials, including ACE-I/ARB and ARNI, have not demonstrated significant improvement in their primary endpoints in this patient population. Both the TOP-CAT[33] and PARAGON-HF[34] trials in patients with HFpEF (EF >45%) failed to meet their primary endpoints, although TOP-CAT showed a reduction in HF hospitalizations with spironolactone.

Sodium-glucose cotransporter-2 inhibitors (SGLT2i), initially developed for diabetes management, have demonstrated significant cardiovascular benefits in patients with HFpEF, as shown in the EMPEROR-PRESERVED and DELIVER trials.[35-36]

An emerging therapeutic option is the glucagon-like peptide-1 receptor agonist (GLP-1 RA). The SUMMIT trial,[37] including 731 patients with HF, an ejection fraction >50%, and obesity (BMI >30), reported that treatment with tirzepatide (administered subcutaneously up to 15 mg/week) led to a 38% relative risk reduction in cardiovascular mortality and worsening HF over a follow-up period of approximately 100 weeks. Like tirzepatide, another drug from this class that has shown a beneficial role in the HFpEF subset is semaglutide. It has shown promising results in STEP-HFpEF in improving functional status and reducing HHF in these patients.[38]

SEX-RELATED DISPARITIES IN GUIDELINE-DIRECTED MEDICAL THERAPY FOR HFpEF

Important sex-specific differences exist in the therapeutic response of patients with HFpEF. Sex differences in treatment response remain an active area of research. Subgroup analyses from major trials have begun to elucidate sex-specific responses. In the EMPEROR-PRESERVED trial, women experienced a 25% relative risk reduction in the primary outcome compared to 19% in men, although this difference did not reach statistical significance. Similarly, in the DELIVER trial, the relative risk reduction was 23% in women versus 15% in men **(Table 1)**. These findings, although exploratory, raise the hypothesis that the cardioprotective effects of SGLT2i may be more pronounced in women. Despite these findings, sex-stratified analysis remains underpowered in most studies, and none of the current guidelines provide sex-specific recommendations.

While SGLT2 inhibitors remain the cornerstone of therapy for both women and men, provided there are no contraindications, additional consideration should be given to the use of sacubitril/valsartan[20] and spironolactone[21] across the full range of LVEF in women. The more favorable response observed in women at relatively higher EF levels may be explained by their tendency to have smaller LV chambers, which predispose them to higher LVEF than men.[22] In practical terms, an LVEF of 50–55% may represent an abnormally low value for women compared with men, which could help explain their different responses to neurohormonal therapies.

Flowchart 1: Treatment algorithm for guideline-directed medical therapy in HFpEF. Green color identifies a Class 1 therapy from clinical practice guidelines, yellow color indicates a Class 2b therapy.

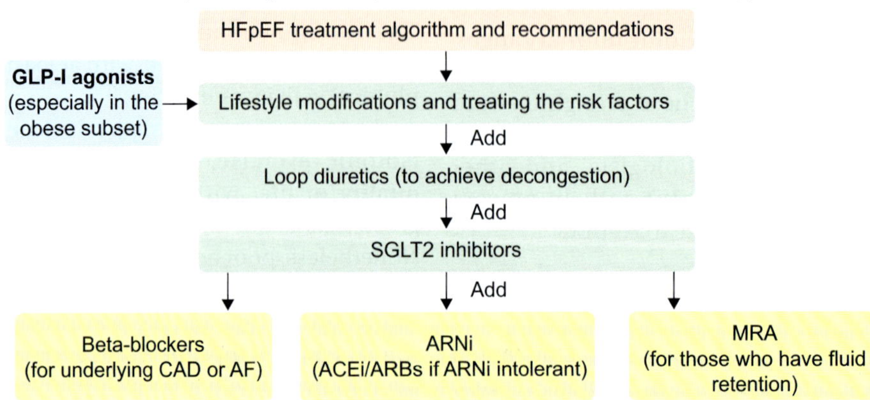

LIMITATIONS/KNOWLEDGE GAPS AND FUTURE DIRECTIONS

In recent years, progress has been made in distinguishing LVDD from HFpEF, but important gaps remain in understanding how LVDD progresses to HFpEF, particularly with potential sex-specific mechanisms. While common risk factors such as hypertension, diabetes, and obesity are especially relevant in women, additional factors unique to or more prevalent in women, such as pregnancy-related complications, may be underrecognized. Further challenges include the lack of clear definitions of HFpEF phenotypes, limited integration of noninvasive imaging and biomarkers into risk stratification, and underutilization of advanced technologies such as artificial intelligence to enhance diagnosis. Standardizing diagnostic criteria are, therefore, essential to enable early identification, guide targeted therapies, and improve outcomes in HFpEF.

CONCLUSION

Heart failure with preserved ejection fraction disproportionately affects women, with obesity, diabetes, and hypertension acting as major drivers of disease risk and progression. Female-specific factors such as pregnancy complications, early menopause, and estrogen deficiency further amplify vulnerability, yet women remain underrepresented in clinical trials, limiting sex-specific insights and treatment strategies. Non-pharmacological measures—including weight management, exercise, and lifestyle optimization—remain cornerstones of prevention and management, while emerging therapies such as SGLT2 inhibitors and GLP-1 receptor agonists have shown promise in improving outcomes, particularly among women with obesity. The current barriers in extending these therapeutic strategies to women with HFpEF include limited representation of women in the HFpEF trials, high burden of undiagnosed disease in them, and lack of understanding of gender-specific mechanisms and pathophysiologic derangement, warranting specific recommendations. Addressing these gaps through more inclusive research and personalized approaches is essential to improve early detection, targeted treatment, and overall outcomes for women with HFpEF.

REFERENCES

1. Lloyd-Jones DM, Larson MG, Leip EP, et al. Lifetime risk for developing congestive heart failure: the Framingham Heart Study. Circulation. 2002;106:3068-72.
2. Gerber Y, Weston SA, Redfield MM, et al. A contemporary appraisal of the heart failure epidemic in Olmsted County, Minnesota, 2000 to 2010. JAMA Intern Med. 2015;175:996-1004.
3. Tsao CW, Lyass A, Enserro D, et al. Temporal trends in the incidence of and mortality associated with heart failure with preserved and reduced ejection fraction. J Am Coll Cardiol Heart Fail. 2018;6:678-85.
4. Virani SS, Alonso A, Benjamin EJ, et al. Heart disease and stroke statistics-2020 update: a report from the American Heart Association. Circulation. 2020;141:e139-e596.
5. Shah KS, Xu H, Matsouaka RA, et al. Heart failure with preserved, borderline, and reduced ejection fraction: 5-year outcomes. J Am Coll Cardiol. 2017;70:2476-86.
6. Chang PP, Wruck LM, Shahar E, et al. Trends in hospitalizations and survival of acute decompensated heart failure in four US Communities (2005–2014): ARIC study community surveillance. Circulation. 2018;138:12-24.
7. Lam CSP, Arnott C, Beale AL, et al. Sex differences in heart failure. Eur Heart J. 2019;40:3859-68c.
8. Obokata M, Reddy YN, Pislaru SV, et al. Evidence supporting the existence of a distinct obese phenotype of heart failure with preserved ejection fraction. Circulation. 2017;136:6-19.
9. Rao VN, Zhao D, Allison MA, et al. Adiposity and incident heart failure and its subtypes: MESA (Multi-Ethnic Study of Atherosclerosis). JACC Heart Fail. 2018;6:999-1007.
10. Sorimachi H, Obokata M, Takahashi N, et al. Pathophysiologic importance of visceral adipose tissue in women with heart failure and preserved ejection fraction. Eur Heart J. 2021;42:1595-605.
11. Rao VN, Fudim M, Mentz RJ, et al. Regional adiposity and heart failure with preserved ejection fraction. Eur J Heart Fail. 2020;22:1540-50.
12. Paulus WJ, Tschope C. A novel paradigm for heart failure with preserved ejection fraction: comorbidities drive myocardial dysfunction and remodeling through coronary microvascular endothelial inflammation. J Am Coll Cardiol. 2013;62:263-71.
13. Kitzman DW, Lam CSP. Obese heart failure with preserved ejection fraction phenotype: from pariah to central player. Circulation. 2017;136: 20-3.
14. McKee PA, Castelli WP, McNamara PM, et al. The natural history of congestive heart failure: the Framingham study. N Engl J Med. 1971;285:1441-6.
15. Bozkurt B, Coats AJ, Tsutsui H, et al. Universal definition and classification of heart failure: a report of the Heart Failure Society of America, Heart Failure Association of the European Society of Cardiology, Japanese Heart Failure Society and Writing Committee of the Universal Definition of Heart Failure: Endorsed by the Canadian Heart Failure Society, Heart Failure Association of India, Cardiac Society of Australia and New Zealand, and Chinese Heart Failure Association. Eur J Heart Fail. 2021;23(3):352-80.
16. McDonagh TA, Metra M, Adamo M, et al. 2021 ESC Guidelines for the diagnosis and treatment of acute and chronic heart failure: Developed by the task Force for the diagnosis and treatment of acute and chronic heart failure

of the European Society of Cardiology (ESC) with the special contribution of the Heart Failure Association (HFA) of the ESC. Eur Heart J. 2021;42(36):3599-726.
17. Gökçe M, Karahan B, Erdöl C, et al. Left ventricular diastolic function assessment by tissue Doppler echocardiography in relation to hormonal replacement therapy in postmenopausal women with diastolic dysfunction. Am J Ther. 2003;10:104-11.
18. Coppi F, Cavalletti A, Pagnoni G, et al. Pulmonary hypertension in patients with Sjögren's syndrome: Gender differences in cardiovascular risk factors and instrumental data. Int J Cardiol. 2025;428:133131.
19. Sabbatini AR, Kararigas G. Menopause-related estrogen decrease and the pathogenesis of HFpEF: JACC Review Topic of the Week. J Am Coll Cardiol. 2020;75:1074-82.
20. Williams D, Stout MJ, Rosenbloom JI, et al. Preeclampsia predicts risk of hospitalization for heart failure with preserved ejection fraction. J Am Coll Cardiol. 2021;78:2281-90.
21. Tibrewala A, Yancy CW. Heart failure with preserved ejection fraction in women. Heart Fail Clin. 2019;15:9-18.
22. Reddy YNV, Carter RE, Obokata M, et al. A simple, evidence-based approach to help guide diagnosis of heart failure with preserved ejection fraction. Circulation. 2018;138:861-70.
23. Pieske B, Tschope C, de Boer RA, et al. How to diagnose heart failure with preserved ejection fraction: the HFA-PEFF diagnostic algorithm: a consensus recommendation from the Heart Failure Association (HFA) of the European Society of Cardiology (ESC). Eur J Heart Fail. 2020;22:391-412.
24. Sotomi Y, Hikoso S, Nakatani D, et al. Sex differences in heart failure with preserved ejection fraction. J Am Heart Assoc. 2021;10:e018574.
25. Sugimoto T, Dulgheru R, Bernard A, et al. Echocardiographic reference ranges for normal left ventricular 2D strain: results from the EACVI NORRE study. Eur Heart J Cardiovasc Imaging. 2017;18:833-40.
26. Cediel G, Codina P, Spitaleri G, et al. Gender-related differences in heart failure biomarkers. Front Cardiovasc Med. 2020;7:617705.
27. Kittleson M, Panjrath G, Amancherla K, et al. 2023 ACC Expert Consensus Decision Pathway on Management of Heart Failure with Preserved Ejection Fraction: A Report of the American College of Cardiology Solution Set Oversight Committee. JACC. 2023;81(18)1835-78.
28. Lloyd-Jones DM, Allen NB, Anderson CA, et al. Life's essential 8: updating and enhancing the American Heart Association's construct of cardiovascular health: a presidential advisory from the American Heart Association. Circulation. 2022;146(5):e18-43.
29. Pandey A, LaMonte M, Klein L, et al. Relationship between physical activity, body mass index, and risk of heart failure. J Am Coll Cardiol. 2017;69:1129-42.
30. Persson CE, Bjorck L, Lagergren J, et al. Risk of heart failure in obese patients with and without bariatric surgery in Sweden-a registry-based study. J Card Fail. 2017;23:530-7.
31. Arnett DK, Blumenthal RS, Albert MA, et al. 2019 ACC/AHA guideline on the primary prevention of cardiovascular disease: a report of the American College of Cardiology/American Heart Association Task Force on Clinical Practice Guidelines. J Am Coll Cardiol. 2019;74:e177-e232.
32. Ji H, Gulati M, Huang TY, et al. Sex differences in association of physical activity with all-cause and cardiovascular mortality. J Am Coll Cardiol. 2024;83(8):783-93.
33. Pitt B, Pfeffer MA, Assmann SF, et al. Spironolactone for heart failure with preserved ejection fraction. N Engl J Med. 2014;370(15):1383-92.
34. Solomon SD, McMurray JJ, Anand IS, et al. Angiotensin–neprilysin inhibition in heart failure with preserved ejection fraction. N Engl J Med. 2019;381(17):1609-20.
35. Solomon SD, McMurray JJV, Claggett B, et al. Dapagliflozin in heart failure with mildly reduced or preserved ejection fraction. N Engl J Med. 2022;387:1089-98.
36. Anker SD, Butler J, Filippatos G, et al. Empagliflozin in heart failure with a preserved ejection fraction. N Engl J Med. 2021;385:1451-61.
37. Packer M, Zile MR, Kramer CM, et al. Tirzepatide for heart failure with preserved ejection fraction and obesity. N Engl J Med. 2025;392(5):427-37.
38. Verma S, Butler J, Borlaug BA, et al., on behalf of the STEP-HFpEF Trial Committees and Investigators. Efficacy of Semaglutide by Sex in Obesity-related Heart Failure with Preserved Ejection Fraction: STEP-HFpEF trials. J Am Coll Cardiol. 2024;84:773-85.

SECTION 15

Obesity, Heart Failure, and Echocardiography

62
CHAPTER

Three-dimensional Echocardiography in the Assessment of Obesity Heart Failure with Preserved Ejection Fraction

Yaser Ahmad, Navin C Nanda, HK Chopra

INTRODUCTION

Heart failure (HF) is an increasingly common clinical entity that can be classified by the left ventricular ejection fraction (LVEF), with about half of patients with HF having heart failure with preserved ejection fraction (HFpEF). Accurate calculation of LVEF is crucial, as this parameter guides diagnostic and treatment decisions. A mainstay for calculating LVEF is echocardiography, a noninvasive imaging modality.

Heart failure with preserved ejection fraction is defined as having an LVEF of ≥50%, while heart failure with reduced ejection fraction (HFrEF) is defined as having an LVEF of ≤40%. Patients with an LVEF of between 41 and 49% are defined as having heart failure with "mid-range" LVEF (HFmrEF).[1] The diagnosis of HFpEF, including the obesity phenotype, also requires evidence of increased LV filling pressures during rest or activity.[2]

While a two-dimensional transthoracic echocardiogram (2DTTE) can be used to calculate LVEF, this method makes geometric assumptions of the left ventricle (LV) that can lead to variability in measurements and underestimation of values, compared to the gold standard, cardiac magnetic resonance imaging (cMRI).[3] Three-dimensional transthoracic echocardiography (3DTTE) circumvents these geometric assumptions and can provide more accurate estimations of LVEF.[4]

In addition, 3DTTE assessment of right ventricular ejection fraction (RVEF), which is more reliable than 2DTTE, demonstrates decreased values in a significant number of patients with HFpEF.[5,6] In HFpEF patients, RVEF becomes impaired due to elevated LV filling pressures, development of pulmonary hypertension, and progressive remodeling of the RV.[7]

Also, 3DTTE assessment of speckle tracking echocardiography (STE) has advantages over the 2DTTE modality in the assessment of LV global longitudinal strain (GLS). Lastly, increased left-sided filling pressures lead to left atrial (LA) enlargement, another hallmark of HFpEF, and 3DTTE assessment of LA size is more accurate than 2DTTE.

INCREMENTAL VALUE OF THREE-DIMENSIONAL TRANSTHORACIC ECHOCARDIOGRAPHY OVER TWO-DIMENSIONAL TRANSTHORACIC ECHOCARDIOGRAM

Left ventricular ejection fraction is a common parameter derived from echocardiograms and is crucial in guiding management of cardiac pathologies. 2DTTE can be used to measure LVEF, but it has high intra- and interobserver variability, and its accuracy depends highly on image quality and sonographer expertise and experience.[8,9] A commonly used method to calculate LV volume using 2DTTE is the modified Simpson's biplane rule.[10] This method is a summation of disks that requires tracing of the LV endocardial border and is limited by a commonly made assumption that the LV is ellipsoid in shape.[11] Furthermore, in some instances, 2DTTE fails to capture the true apex of the LV, leading to foreshortening and an underestimation in volume.[12] Off-axis imaging can also lead to inaccurate measurements.[13]

Three-dimensional transthoracic echocardiography, on the other hand, uses a matrix array to image the entire LV in the data set, eliminating the geometric assumptions made by 2DTTE. It also has lower intra- and interobserver variability. In a 2012 meta-analysis, 3DTTE was compared to 2DTTE. 3DTTE underestimated ventricle volume about half as often as 2DTTE in comparison to cMRI.[14] LVEF assessment by 3DTTE also correlates well with cMRI.[15] **Figure 1** demonstrates calculation of LV volume and LVEF using 3DTTE.

In addition to LVEF, previous research has shown that the LV remodels itself in response to disease states. LV dilatation and increased sphericity are associated with decreases in LVEF.[16] Maffessanti et al. developed an approach to quantify LV shape using 3DTTE and demonstrated that LV conicity was directly correlated with LV volume and LVEF. This underscores the potential 3DTTE has to assess cardiac remodeling in pathological disease states, such as HF, as well as in response to pharmacologic treatment.[17]

In addition, 3DTTE-measured parameters hold predictive potential. For instance, Medvedofsky et al. compared the 2DTTE- and 3DTTE-measured LVEF prognostic value. They retrospectively studied inpatients referred for 2DTTE. They found that 3DTTE-calculated LVEF was a superior predictor of cardiovascular mortality.[9] A similar study by Stanton et al. demonstrated that the 3DTTE-measured LVEF had a stronger association than 2DTTE with clinical outcomes such as mortality.[18]

Two-dimensional transthoracic echocardiogram also faces obstacles in assessing the RV, including the RV's irregular geometry and asymmetric remodeling. The pyramidal dataset used in 3DTTE avoids these roadblocks.[19] 3DTTE volumetric assessment of the RV correlates highly with cMRI, although it does have greater margins of error and can lead to underestimation of RV volume.[20,21] The use of contrast enhancement can make 3DTTE assessment of the RV more accurate.[22]

Artificial Intelligence

Artificial intelligence, or computerized systems performing tasks that traditionally required human intelligence, can make an impact on the field of echocardiography. 3DTTE

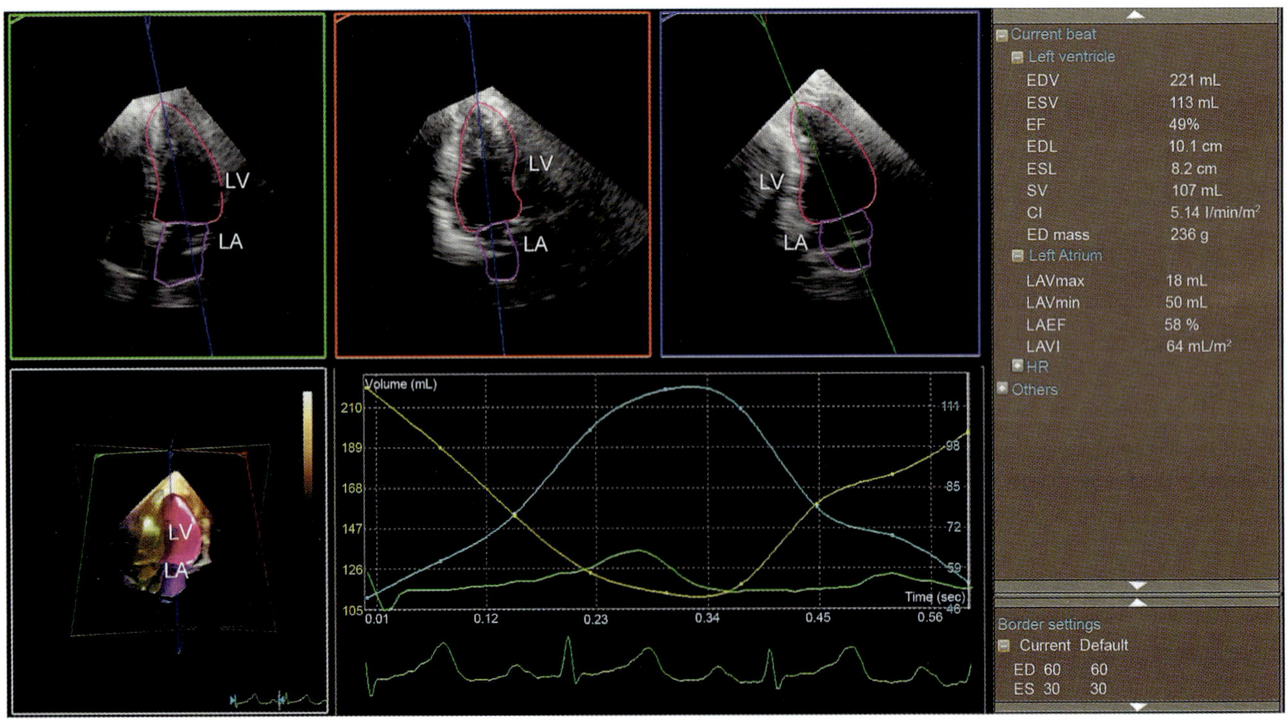

Fig. 1: Calculation of left ventricular ejection fraction/volume (yellow curve) and left atrial volume (blue curve) using three-dimensional transthoracic echocardiography. (LA: left atrium; LV: left ventricle)
Courtesy: Navin C Nanda.

may benefit from automated volumetric measurements more than 2DTTE, because 3DTTE is free from the approximation process that is used in 2DTTE (modified Simpson's biplane rule).[23] By automating 3DTTE, there is increased reproducibility and faster image acquisition/reporting.[24] For instance, studies have shown that deep learning models can calculate LV GLS in a fraction of the time as compared to manual, while also decreasing variability.[25] Additionally, machine learning software can automate 3D quantification of the RV volume and function, leading to accurate measurements, less variability, and faster results **(Table 1)**.[26]

SPECKLE TRACKING ECHOCARDIOGRAPHY

Myocardial fibers are arranged in a complex three-dimensional array. STE is a technique used to measure myocardial strain during contraction and relaxation.

Table 1: Advantages and limitations of 2D and 3D transthoracic echocardiography.

Modality	Advantages	Limitations
2DTTE	Widely available, cost-effective	Reader- and operator-dependent, more variability, underestimation of volume
3DTTE	Less variability, stronger prognostic value	Less available, less accurate in individuals with larger ventricles[14]

(2DTTE: two-dimensional transthoracic echocardiogram; 3DTTE: three-dimensional transthoracic echocardiogram)

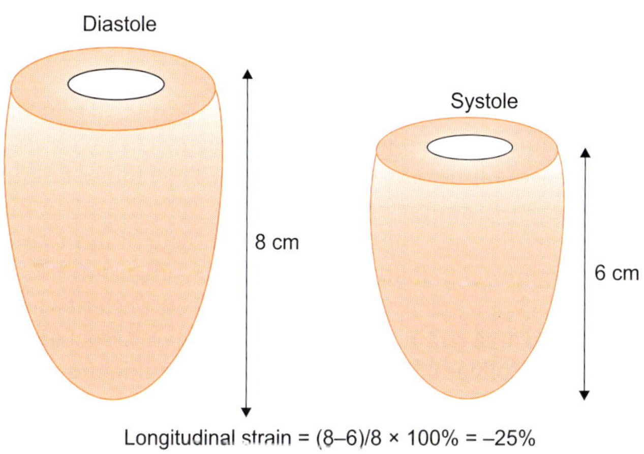

Fig. 2: Longitudinal strain. Refers to the base to LV apex longitudinal shortening during systole and can be expressed as a percentage.
Courtesy: Siemens Ultrasound.

Base-to-LV apex longitudinal shortening during systole is referred to as LV GLS **(Fig. 2)**. This is achieved by interaction of the ultrasound probe and myocardium that forms grayscale images, consisting of small dots, known as speckles, which are tracked throughout the cardiac cycle. STE-measured GLS can allow for detection of subtle changes in LV function, even before changes in LVEF are noted by conventional 2DTTE, thus allowing for early diagnosis and treatment of cardiac pathologies.[27] In general, 2DSTE faces the same limitations as conventional 2DTTE. These include geometric assumptions, foreshortened views, and inability to capture motion in the third dimension.[28] 3DSTE, on the other hand, circumvents these limitations and has a promising role in providing insight into the diagnosis and treatment of HF. **Figure 3**

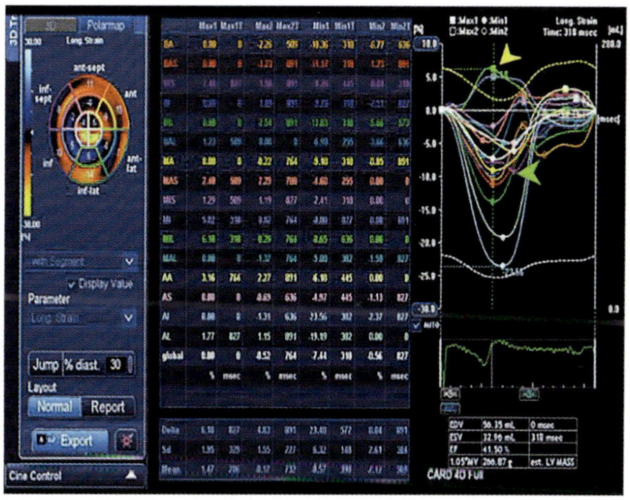

Fig. 3: Three-dimensional (3D) spectral tracking echocardiography. An example of the display of information by commercial software. The graph on the right side of the figure displays longitudinal strain values from a single cardiac cycle. Different myocardial segments are denoted by different colors of the curves. The dotted vertical green line indicates end-systole. As normal longitudinal strain is denoted by a negative sign, normal longitudinal strain curves would be plotted below the baseline with negative values, and they would peak in end-systole. However, in this example, some curves are abnormal. For instance, the light green curve (yellow arrowhead) representing the midinferolateral segment (MIL) of the left ventricle is located above the baseline, indicative of wall thinning during systole. The peak strain value can be read from the graph, and in this case, is abnormal at around +6%. Also, the purple curve (green arrowhead) representing the basal inferoseptal segment peaks way beyond end-systole and during diastole, indicating postsystolic thickening. This finding is frequently associated with myocardial ischemia. All the values and curves shown in the illustration were obtained using 3D echocardiography.
Source: Reproduced with permission from Nanda NC (Ed). Comprehensive Textbook of Echocardiography. New Delhi and London: Jaypee Brothers Medical Publishers; 2025.

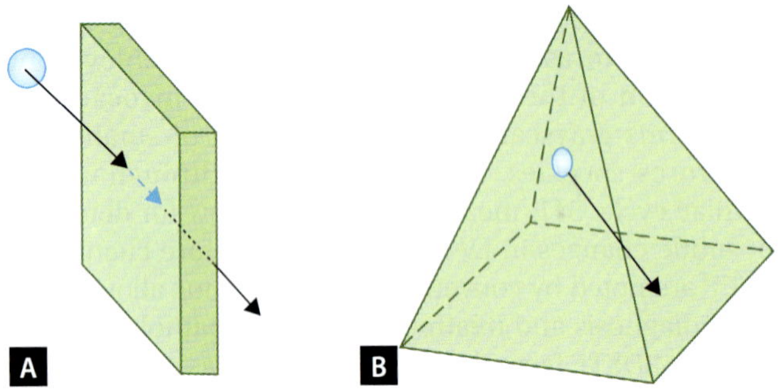

Figs. 4A and B: Advantage of three-dimensional (3D) speckle tracking echocardiography over the two-dimensional (2D) technique. (A) As 2D echocardiography represents only a thin slice through the cardiac structures, it is easy for the speckle particle to move out of the scanning plane as the heart moves, making it difficult or impossible to track the same speckle during the cardiac cycle. (B) On the other hand, with the 3D technique, a much larger pyramidal-shaped section is obtained, making it more difficult for the speckle particle to move out of the 3D dataset.
Courtesy: Toshiba Medical Systems Europe BV.

demonstrates 3DSTE, while **Figures 4A and B** demonstrate the advantages of 3DSTE over 2DSTE.

With regards to the LV, Medvedofsky et al. compared 2D and 3D calculations of GLS. They found that 3DSTE-calculated GLS was a better predictor of mortality than 3DTTE-calculated LVEF, 2DTTE-calculated LVEF, and also 2DSTE-calculated GLS.

Speckle tracking echocardiography assessment of the RV has been shown to be helpful in the diagnosis of HFpEF. 2DSTE is limited, however, by foreshortened views and out-of-plane motion of speckles.[5] In a 2021 study by Meng et al., 81 patients with HFpEF underwent both 2DSTE and 3DSTE. 2DSTE was used to calculate the 2D right ventricular longitudinal strain of free wall (RVFWLS). 3DSTE was employed to calculate the 3D-RVFWLS. They found that patients with endpoint events (HF hospitalization or death) had a lower 3D-RVFWLS, while 2D-RVFWLS was not different, highlighting the superior role of 3DSTE over 2DSTE in predicting outcomes related to HFpEF.

Area Strain

A novel parameter that can be calculated with 3DSTE, but not 2SDSTE, is area strain. With contraction of the LV, the surface area of the endocardium decreases, as a result of longitudinal shortening, circumferential shortening, and radial thickening **(Figs. 5 and 6)**. Area strain combines the effect of both longitudinal and circumferential shortening and hence would be expected to be superior to either alone. Given the physiology of area strain, its value is closely tied

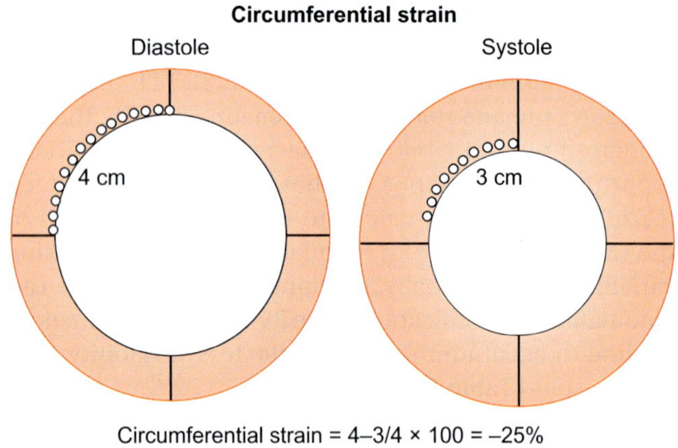

Fig. 5: Circumferential strain. Represents the amount of shortening of the short axis of the left ventricular wall during systole and can be expressed as a percentage.
Courtesy: Toshiba Medical Systems Europe BV.

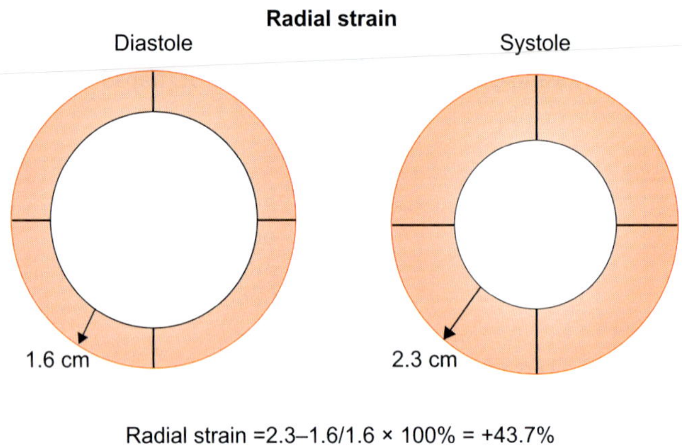

Fig. 6: Radial strain. Refers to myocardial thickening perpendicular to the wall's surface during contraction of the left ventricle and can be expressed as a percentage.
Courtesy: Toshiba Medical Systems Europe BV.

to wall motion and LVEF. Kleijn et al. performed 3DSTE on 140 patients and validated area strain against both the wall motion score index (WMSI) and LVEF. They found strong correlation between area strain and WMSI and LVEF. With regard to variability, they noted excellent intra- and interoperative reliability when calculating area strain.[29]

Wen et al. performed 3DSTE in 160 patients and calculated area strain. Using American Heart Association/American College of Cardiology HF staging guidelines, they stratified patients by the following: Control group, stage A (at risk for HF), stage B (pre-HF), stage C (symptomatic HF), and stage D (advanced HF).[2] GLS and LVEF were not statistically different between the control group and patients with stage A HF. However, area strain was indeed statistically different between the two, underlining its utility in early detection of cardiac pathology. Increased sensitivity of area strain could be explained by the fact that the endocardium is highly susceptible to ischemia, and therefore, it is expected that it would be affected prior to LVEF.[30]

Similarly, Luo et al. studied 149 patients, including those with HFpEF, HFrEF, and normal EF with 3DSTE. They were able to measure area strain of the endocardial surface throughout the cardiac cycle. 3DSTE images were acquired, and subsequent datasets were analyzed by 3D-wall motion tracking software. They found that LV global area strain measured by 3DSTE had strong correlation with LVEF.[31]

LEFT VENTRICLE TORSION

Torsion refers to the wringing motion of the LV, as its myofibers contract, as a result of the opposing rotations of the LV base and apex.[32] This pattern of rotation is demonstrated in **Figure 7**. 2DSTE can also be used to analyze torsion of the LV.[33] LV torsion has been demonstrated to be correlated with LVEF using 2DSTE, but less so than GLS.[34] Common barriers to analyzing LV torsion with 2DSTE include dropout of ultrasound data, reverberations, and losing speckles that are being tracked because of out-of-plane movement.[35]

In contrast, 3DSTE tracks speckles within the much larger pyramidal volume scan, compared to razor-thin 2DSTE sections, thereby circumventing the limitation of 2DSTE.[36] However, lower temporal and spatial resolution may impact measurements by 3DSTE.[37] In a study by Minatoguchi et al., 3DSTE was used to calculate global torsion (average torsion from the three myocardial layers), which was preserved in patients with HFpEF.[38] Using cMRI, LV torsion has been shown to be decreased in patients with HFrEF.[39]

There appear to be effects of aging on torsion. Kaku et al. found that LV torsion was lowest in children and adolescents, increased with age, and then there was a decrease in basal rotation with further aging, while apical rotation increased.[37] As we age, there is decreased LV GLS, likely due to progressive subendocardial pathologies. An increase in LV torsion with age helps compensate for this to maintain cardiac output.[40] Napp et al. used 3DTTE to demonstrate that LV rotational parameters decreased as body weight increased.[41]

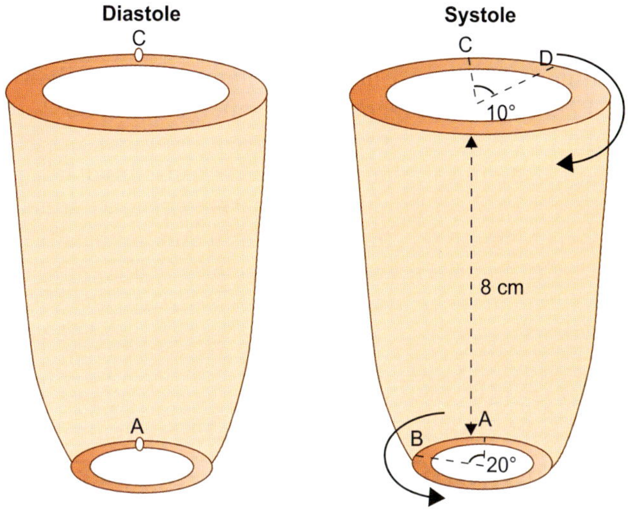

Fig. 7: Differential rotational movements of left ventricular apex and the base. In the normal individual, the apex rotates more than the base. By convention, counterclockwise motion is assigned a positive (+) sign and clockwise motion a negative (–) sign. In the above example, the apex rotates 20° in counterclockwise direction from end-diastole (point A) to end-systole (point B); hence, the rotation of the apex will be +20°. As the base rotates at the same time 10° clockwise from point C to D, the rotation of the base will be –10°. "Twist" is calculated as the algebraic difference in the rotation of the apex and base; in other words, how far apart a point in the apex and base moves from each other. In the above example, the twist will be apex rotation (20°) minus base rotation (–10°), that is, 20 – (–10) = +30°. Twist can be calculated for any point in the myocardium compared to a reference basal point. "Torsion" is a way of adjusting for the distance of a point of interest from the reference point in the base, as it is expected that the twist will be higher for the segments farther away from the base. Torsion = twist/the distance from the base or distance between any two points that are evaluated. In the above example, the torsion, calculated between apex and base, would be 30/8 = 3.75°/cm. As would be expected, the middle portion of the left ventricle would not show any rotation.

Courtesy: Toshiba Medical Systems Europe BV.

Left Atrium

While traditionally much of the focus in HF has been on the LV, in recent years, attention has shifted to LA size and function. In advanced HF, LA enlargement and loss of function can lead to worsening symptoms.[42] LA enlargement is seen in around 50–66% of patients with HFpEF, including the obesity phenotype.[13] In particular, LA size and function can serve as a marker for LV diastolic dysfunction, which is an essential component of HFpEF.[43] LA volume indexed to body surface area is an indirect measure of LV filling pressures.[44] 3DTTE-measured left atrial parameters have been shown to be strongly correlated to the gold standard, cMRI.[45-47] In contrast, 2DTTE is generally less accurate. One explanation for this is the asymmetric enlargement and foreshortening of the LA, which makes assumptions required to calculate volumes using the biplane methods more invalid.[48,49] A systematic review by Mahmod et al.

compared 2DTTE-measured LA parameters to cMRI. They found that 2DTTE significantly underestimated LA volume and had worse intra- and interoperator variability. 2DTTE missed a diagnosis of LA enlargement in 38% of patients.[44] Factors such as increased body mass index seen in the obesity phenotype may also affect image quality with 2DTTE, making measurements inaccurate.[50] However, this could affect 3DTTE estimations also, likely to a lesser degree. **Figure 1** demonstrates calculation of left atrial volume using 3DTTE.

LIMITATIONS OF THREE-DIMENSIONAL TRANSTHORACIC ECHOCARDIOGRAPHY AND THREE-DIMENSIONAL SPECKLE TRACKING ECHOCARDIOGRAPHY

Three-dimensional speckle tracking echocardiography has lower temporal and spatial resolution, which can make speckle tracking difficult.[51] 3DSTE image acquisition entails patient breath holding, which can be difficult. In addition, multibeat acquisition can make 3DSTE difficult in patients with irregular rhythms.[52] Furthermore, in 3DTTE, it can be difficult to trace the endocardial border, due to a lack of standardized guidelines on tracing, low contrast, operator subjectivity, and signal dropout, making measurements such as LVEF inaccurate.[53-56]

CONCLUSION

Three-dimensional transthoracic echocardiography and 3DSTE are robust imaging modalities that circumvent limitations of 2DTTE and 2DSTE in HFpEF, especially the obesity phenotype. However, 3D image quality needs to be improved before it can replace 2DTTE. Artificial intelligence holds value in reducing analysis time and making quantitative assessments less variable.[57] This would be true for both 2D and 3DTTE assessment of LV, RV, and LA function. There is also potential in combining 3DSTE with other imaging modalities. For instance, coupling 3DSTE with dobutamine stress echocardiography would allow for prompt identification of abnormalities in regional contractility. There is also potential in virtual reality models using 3DTTE-derived images to create 3D visualizations of cardiac structures using virtual reality headsets.[58] In summary, the future of 3D echocardiography, both 3DTTE and 3DSTE, in the evaluation of HFpEF, including the obesity phenotype, appears bright and will continue to make an increasingly significant impact on patient care.

REFERENCES

1. Dunlay SM, Roger VL, Redfield MM. Epidemiology of heart failure with preserved ejection fraction. Nat Rev Cardiol. 2017;14(10):591-602.
2. Heidenreich PA, Bozkurt B, Aguilar D, et al. 2022 AHA/ACC/HFSA guideline for the management of heart failure: a report of the American College of Cardiology/American Heart Association Joint Committee on Clinical Practice Guidelines. Circulation. 2022;145(18):e895-1032.
3. Morbach C, Lin BA, Sugeng L. Clinical application of three-dimensional echocardiography. Prog Cardiovasc Dis. 2014;57(1):19-31.
4. Wu VC, Takeuchi M. Three-dimensional echocardiography: current status and real-life applications. Acta Cardiol Sin. 2017;33(2):107-18.
5. Meng Y, Zhu S, Xie Y, et al. Prognostic value of right ventricular 3D speckle-tracking strain and ejection fraction in patients with HFpEF. Front Cardiovasc Med. 2021;8:694365.
6. Melenovsky V, Hwang SJ, Lin G, et al. Right heart dysfunction in heart failure with preserved ejection fraction. Eur Heart J. 2014;35(48):3452-62.
7. Mohammed SF, Hussain I, AbouEzzeddine OF, et al. Right ventricular function in heart failure with preserved ejection fraction. Circulation. 2014;130(25):2310-20.
8. Monaghan MJ. Role of real time 3D echocardiography in evaluating the left ventricle. Heart. 2006;92(1):131-6.
9. Medvedofsky D, Maffessanti F, Weinert L, et al. 2D and 3D echocardiography-derived indices of left ventricular function and shape: relationship with mortality. JACC Cardiovasc Imaging. 2018;11(11):1569-79.
10. Kim W-JC, Beqiri A, Lewandowski AJ, et al. Beyond Simpson's rule: accounting for orientation and ellipticity assumptions. Ultrasound Med Biol. 2022;48(12):2476-85.
11. Foley TA, Mankad SV, Anavekar NS, et al. Measuring left ventricular ejection fraction - techniques and potential pitfalls. Eur Cardiol. 2012;8(2):108-14.
12. Jenkins C, Moir S, Chan J, et al. Left ventricular volume measurement with echocardiography: a comparison of left ventricular opacification, three-dimensional echocardiography, or both with magnetic resonance imaging. Eur Heart J. 2009;30(1):98-106.
13. Omar AMS, Bansal M, Sengupta PP. Advances in echocardiographic imaging in heart failure with reduced and preserved ejection fraction. Circ Res. 2016;119(2):357-74.
14. Dorosz JL, Lezotte DC, Weitzenkamp DA, et al. Performance of 3-dimensional echocardiography in measuring left ventricular volumes and ejection fraction: a systematic review and meta-analysis. J Am Coll Cardiol. 2012;59(20):1799-808.
15. Nazir MS, Okafor J, Murphy T, et al. Echocardiography versus cardiac MRI for measurement of left ventricular ejection fraction in individuals with cancer and suspected cardiotoxicity. Radiol Cardiothorac Imaging. 2024;6(1):e230048.

16. Lewis RP, Sandler H. Relationship between changes in left ventricular dimensions and the ejection fraction in man. Circulation. 1971;44(4):548-57.
17. Maffessanti F, Lang RM, Corsi C, et al. Feasibility of left ventricular shape analysis from transthoracic real-time 3-D echocardiographic images. Ultrasound Med Biol. 2009;35(12):1953-62.
18. Stanton T, Jenkins C, Haluska BA, et al. Association of outcome with left ventricular parameters measured by two-dimensional and three-dimensional echocardiography in patients at high cardiovascular risk. J Am Soc Echocardiogr. 2014;27(1):65-73.
19. Randazzo M, Maffessanti F, Kotta A, et al. Added value of 3D echocardiography in the diagnosis and prognostication of patients with right ventricular dysfunction. Front Cardiovasc Med. 2023;10:1263864.
20. Sugeng L, Mor-Avi V, Weinert L, et al. Multimodality comparison of quantitative volumetric analysis of the right ventricle. JACC Cardiovasc Imaging. 2010;3(1):10-8.
21. Shimada YJ, Shiota M, Siegel RJ, et al. Accuracy of right ventricular volumes and function determined by three-dimensional echocardiography in comparison with magnetic resonance imaging: a meta-analysis study. J Am Soc Echocardiogr. 2010;23(9):943-53.
22. Medvedofsky D, Mor-Avi V, Kruse E, et al. Quantification of right ventricular size and function from contrast-enhanced three-dimensional echocardiographic images. J Am Soc Echocardiogr. 2017;30(12):1193-202.
23. Yoon YE, Kim S, Chang HJ. Artificial intelligence and echocardiography. J Cardiovasc Imaging. 2021;29(3):193-204.
24. Barbieri A, Pepi M. Three-dimensional echocardiography based on automation and machine learning principles and the renaissance of cardiac morphometry. J Clin Med. 2022;11(15):4357.
25. Dulal S, Wasan R, Wuni G, et al. Use of artificial intelligence in echocardiography. Comprehensive Textbook of Echocardiography (2 Volumes), 3rd edition. New Delhi: Jaypee Brothers Medical Publishers (P) Ltd; 2025. p. 13.
26. Genovese D, Rashedi N, Weinert L, et al. Machine learning-based three-dimensional echocardiographic quantification of right ventricular size and function: validation against cardiac magnetic resonance. J Am Soc Echocardiogr. 2019;32(8):969-77.
27. Mihos CG, Liu JE, Anderson KM, et al. Speckle-tracking strain echocardiography for the assessment of left ventricular structure and function: a scientific statement from the American Heart Association. Circulation. 2025;152(10):e96-109.
28. Urbano-Moral JA, Patel AR, Maron MS, et al. Three-dimensional speckle-tracking echocardiography: methodological aspects and clinical potential. Echocardiography. 2012;29(8):997-1010.
29. Kleijn SA, Aly MF, Terwee CB, et al. Three-dimensional speckle tracking echocardiography for automatic assessment of global and regional left ventricular function based on area strain. J Am Soc Echocardiogr. 2011;24(3):314-21.
30. Wen H, Liang Z, Zhao Y, et al. Feasibility of detecting early left ventricular systolic dysfunction using global area strain: a novel index derived from three-dimensional speckle-tracking echocardiography. Eur J Echocardiogr. 2011;12(12):910-6.
31. Luo XX, Fang F, Lee AP, et al. What can three-dimensional speckle-tracking echocardiography contribute to evaluate global left ventricular systolic performance in patients with heart failure? Int J Cardiol. 2014;172(1):132-7.
32. Rüssel IK, Götte MJW, Bronzwaer JG, et al. Left ventricular torsion: an expanding role in the analysis of myocardial dysfunction. JACC Cardiovasc Imaging. 2009;2(5):648-55.
33. Yildiz M, Oktay AA, Stewart MH, et al. Left ventricular hypertrophy and hypertension. Prog Cardiovasc Dis. 2020;63(1):10-21.
34. Lima MSM, Villarraga HR, Abduch MCD, et al. Global longitudinal strain or left ventricular twist and torsion? Which correlates best with ejection fraction? Arq Bras Cardiol. 2017;109(1):23-9.
35. Kim HK, Sohn DW, Lee SE, et al. Assessment of left ventricular rotation and torsion with two-dimensional speckle tracking echocardiography. J Am Soc Echocardiogr. 2007;20(1):45-53.
36. Zhang L, Zhang J, Han W, et al. Three-dimensional rotation, twist and torsion analyses using real-time 3d speckle tracking imaging: feasibility, reproducibility, and normal ranges in pediatric population. PLoS One. 2016;11(7):e0158679.
37. Kaku K, Takeuchi M, Tsang W, et al. Age-related normal range of left ventricular strain and torsion using three-dimensional speckle-tracking echocardiography. J Am Soc Echocardiogr. 2014;27(1):55-64.
38. Minatoguchi S, Yoshizane T, Tanaka R, et al. Left ventricular torsion in hypertension and hypertensive heart failure 3-dimensional speckle tracking echocardiography assessment. Circ Rep. 2019;1(2):78-86.
39. Gao Y, Li B, Ma Y, et al. Myocardial mechanical function measured by cardiovascular magnetic resonance in patients with heart failure. J Cardiovasc Magn Reson. 2024;26(2):101111.
40. Hung CL, Gonçalves A, Shah AM, et al. Age- and sex-related influences on left ventricular mechanics in elderly individuals free of prevalent heart failure: the ARIC study (atherosclerosis risk in communities). Circ Cardiovasc Imaging. 2017;10(1):e004510.
41. Napp J, Gelbrich G, Sahiti F, et al. 3D echocardiography derived reference values and determinants of left ventricular twist and torsion from the population-based STAAB cohort study. Sci Rep. 2025;15(1):4524.
42. Bandera F, Mollo A, Frigelli M, et al. Cardiac imaging for the assessment of left atrial mechanics across heart failure stages. Front Cardiovasc Med. 2022;8:750139.
43. Linden K, Goldschmidt F, Laser KT, et al. Left atrial volumes and phasic function in healthy children: reference values

using real-time three-dimensional echocardiography. J Am Soc Echocardiogr. 2019;32(8):1036-45.e9.

44. Mahmod M, Bull S, Kailayanathan T, et al. Left atrial volume quantification by transthoracic echocardiography versus cardiovascular magnetic resonance: a systematic review and meta-analysis. Int J Cardiovasc Imaging. 2025;41(9):1657-69.
45. Li J, Wang Y, Zhao C, et al. Incremental value of three-dimensional echocardiography for evaluating left atrial function in patients with coronary slow flow phenomenon: a case control study. Cardiovasc Ultrasound. 2020;18(1):6.
46. Keller AM, Gopal AS, King DL. Left and right atrial volume by freehand three-dimensional echocardiography: in vivo validation using magnetic resonance imaging. Eur J Echocardiogr. 2000;1(1):55-65.
47. Artang R, Migrino RQ, Harmann L, et al. Left atrial volume measurement with automated border detection by 3-dimensional echocardiography: comparison with magnetic resonance imaging. Cardiovasc Ultrasound. 2009;7:16.
48. Heo R, Hong G-R, Kim Y-J, et al. Automated quantification of left atrial size using three-beat averaging real-time three dimensional echocardiography in patients with atrial fibrillation. Cardiovasc Ultrasound. 2015;13(1):38.
49. Hoit BD. Assessment of echocardiographic left atrial size: how accurate do we need to be? JACC Cardiovasc Imaging. 2012;5(8):778-80.
50. Ellenberger K, Jeyaprakash P, Sivapathan S, et al. The effect of obesity on echocardiographic image quality. Heart Lung Circ. 2022;31(2):207-15.
51. Nabeshima Y, Seo Y, Takeuchi M. A review of current trends in three-dimensional analysis of left ventricular myocardial strain. Cardiovasc Ultrasound. 2020;18(1):23.
52. Muraru D, Niero A, Rodriguez-Zanella H, et al. Three-dimensional speckle-tracking echocardiography: benefits and limitations of integrating myocardial mechanics with three-dimensional imaging. Cardiovasc Diagn Ther. 2018;8(1):101-17.
53. Cosyns B, Haberman D, Droogmans S, et al. Comparison of contrast enhanced three dimensional echocardiography with MIBI gated SPECT for the evaluation of left ventricular function. Cardiovasc Ultrasound. 2009;7(1):27.
54. Papachristidis A, Galli E, Geleijnse ML, et al. Standardized delineation of endocardial boundaries in three-dimensional left ventricular echocardiograms. J Am Soc Echocardiogr. 2017;30(11):1059-69.
55. Hammoude A. Endocardial border identification in two-dimensional echocardiographic images: review of methods. Comput Med Imaging Graph. 1998;22(3):181-93.
56. Naser N, Stankovic I, Neskovic A. The reliability of automated three-dimensional echocardiography-HeartModel[A.I.] versus 2D echocardiography Simpson methods in evaluation of left ventricle volumes and ejection fraction in patients with left ventricular dysfunction. Med Arch. 2022;76(4):259-66.
57. Italiano G, Fusini L, Mantegazza V, et al. Novelties in 3D transthoracic echocardiography. J Clin Med. 2021;10(3):408.
58. Lang RM, Addetia K, Narang A, et al. 3-dimensional echocardiography: Latest developments and future directions. JACC Cardiovasc Imaging. 2018;11(12):1854-78.

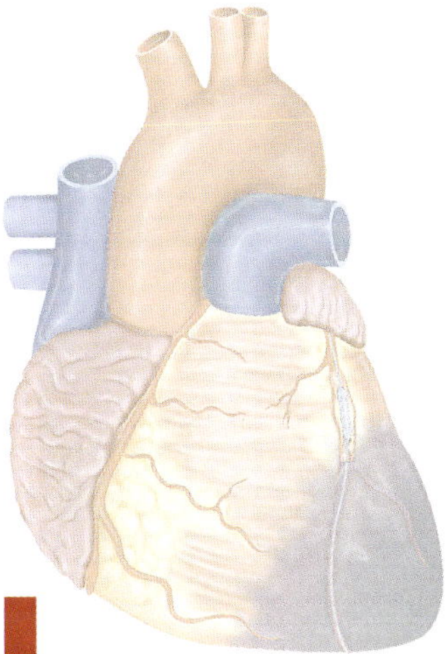

CHAPTER 63

Echocardiographic Assessment of Epicardial Adipose Tissue in Cardiovascular Disease and Associated Risk Factors

Yaser Ahmad, Vaidehi Mendpara, Vijayadithyan Jaganathan, Navin C Nanda, HK Chopra

INTRODUCTION

Epicardial adipose tissue (EAT) is a layer of fatty tissue between the myocardium and visceral layer of the pericardium. It is supplied by the same microcirculation as the contiguous myocardium.[1]

Functionally, EAT cushions the heart, offers thermal regulation, and provides the myocardium energy. However, in pathological states, the EAT secretes bioactive substances such as pro-inflammatory cytokines, adipokines, and reactive oxygen species, which may exert harmful paracrine effects on the myocardium and coronary arteries.[2] EAT thickness, as measured by two dimensional transthoracic echocardiography (2DTTE), correlates with several cardiac disease entities and associated cardiovascular risk factors. This chapter focuses on these issues.

ECHOCARDIOGRAPHIC IDENTIFICATION AND ASSESSMENT

Epicardial adipose tissue is regularly assessed using 2DTTE. It is most commonly identified as an echoic layer, with or without echolucencies, or occasionally as a completely anechoic layer overlying the right ventricle in the parasternal long axis **(Fig. 1A)** and parasternal short axis **(Fig. 1B)** views taken at the level of mid chordae/papillary muscles.[3] Maximum measurements perpendicular to the right ventricular wall are taken at the end of systole in both views over three cardiac cycles and averaged.[4] There is no consensus in the literature over normal measurements but in general, measurements >7 mm in males and >6.5 mm in females are considered abnormal. 2DTTE-measured EAT thickness is highly reproducible, with studies demonstrating excellent interobserver and intraobserver reproducibility, supporting its use in clinical practice.[5]

Two-dimensional transthoracic echocardiography allows for differentiation between EAT and the pericardial adipose tissue layer, which is located anterior to the EAT and is between the parietal and visceral layers of the pericardium, which is the same anatomic location in which pericardial effusions form **(Fig. 2)**.[6] Lastly, the paracardiac adipose tissue layer is located outside the parietal pericardium **(Fig. 3)**.[7]

Due to its wide availability and high reproducibility, 2DTTE is a robust technique to analyze the EAT. Other imaging modalities such as cardiac magnetic resonance imaging (MRI) and computed tomography (CT) can be used to characterize EAT, and their general advantages and disadvantages are detailed in **Table 1** here.

EPICARDIAL ADIPOSE TISSUE AND CARDIOVASCULAR DISEASE

Atherosclerosis

Coronary Artery Disease

Coronary artery disease (CAD) is a primary cause of cardiovascular morbidity and mortality and can be caused by atherosclerosis, which is driven by inflammation.[11,12] It is postulated that the pro-inflammatory substances secreted by the EAT in pathological states contribute to CAD. For instance, Jehn et al. performed beside 2DTTE

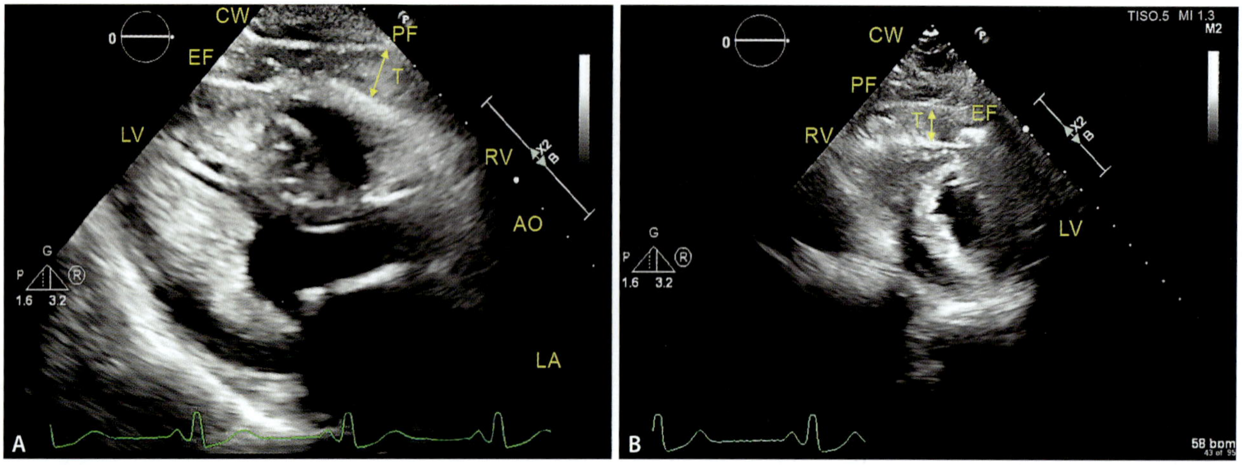

Figs. 1A and B: (A) Two-dimensional transthoracic echocardiographic assessment of epicardial adipose tissue (EF). Maximal thickness (T) of EF is 13 mm. Parasternal long axis view; (B) Two-dimensional transthoracic echocardiographic assessment of epicardial adipose tissue (EF). Maximal thickness (T) of EF is 14 mm. Parasternal short axis view. Abbreviations as in Figure 1A.
(AO: aorta; CW: chest wall; LA: left atrium; LV: left ventricle; RV: right ventricle; PF: pericardial fat pad)

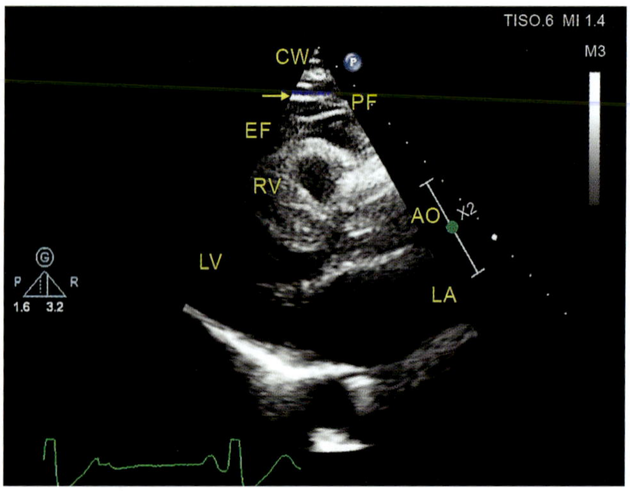

Fig. 2: Two-dimensional transthoracic echocardiographic assessment of epicardial adipose tissue (EF) with incidental small pericardial effusion (asterisks). Parasternal long axis view. Arrow points to paracardiac fat. Abbreviations as in Figure 1A.

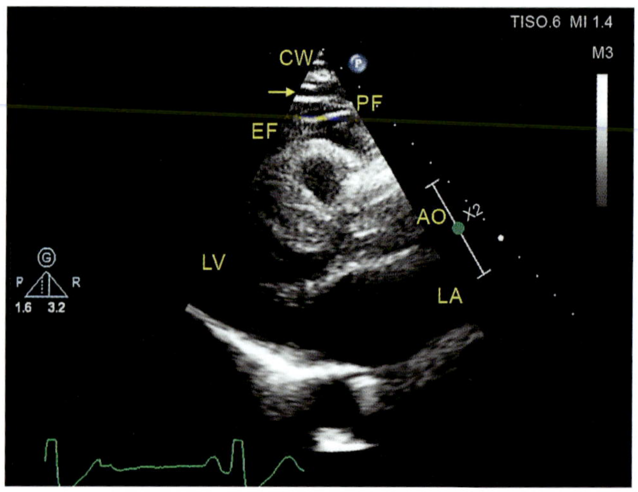

Fig. 3: Two-dimensional transthoracic echocardiographic assessment of epicardial adipose tissue (EF) in another patient. Parasternal short axis view. Arrow points to paracardiac fat. Abbreviations as in Figure 1A.

TABLE 1: Modality and technique with their advantages and limitations.

Modality	*Technique*	*Advantages*	*Limitations*
2DTTE	Linear thickness	Cost effective, highly reproducible	Linear and not volumetric, difficult to use in individuals with poor cardiac windows[8]
CT	Volumetric quantification	Excellent spatial resolution, potential for automation[9]	Radiation exposure, cost, requires greater expertise, cancer potential
MRI	T1-weighted fat segmentation	Highly precise, no radiation, may not require contrast agents	High operational costs, claustrophobic, may be incompatible with certain implanted hardware/devices[10]

(2DTTE: two-dimensional transthoracic echocardiography; CT: computed tomography; EAT: epicardial adipose tissue; MRI: magnetic resonance imaging) on consecutive patients presenting to the hospital with chest pain. They noted that an increase in EAT thickness by 1 mm resulted in doubling the odds of having obstructive CAD (defined in this study as requiring coronary revascularization therapy within 90 days of presentation).[13] Similar findings were demonstrated by Shambu et al., who performed 2DTTE on 503 patients undergoing coronary angiography. They noted a relationship between increase in linear thickness of the EAT and worsening coronary obstruction, measured using the Gensini score, a widely used scoring system for degree of coronary obstruction in CAD.[14,15] The calculation of the Gensini score divides coronary obstruction into the following reductions in lumen diameter: 1–25%, 26–50%, 51–75%, 76–90%, 91–99%, and 100%.[16] Meenakshi et al. also performed 2DTTE on patients admitted for coronary angiography. They too noted that an increased EAT thickness was associated with severity of CAD, as measured by the Gensini score.[17]

Morales-Portano et al. studied 107 patients who underwent 2DTTE and coronary angiography for suspected CAD. Increasing EAT thickness correlated with major adverse cardiovascular events (MACEs) during the follow-up period, highlighting EAT's predictive value.[18]

In a 2023 cohort of patients undergoing coronary angiography, an echocardiographic EAT thickness of ≥0.55 cm marked individuals at higher risk for future CAD progression, independent of traditional risk factors. Those who developed progression had noticeably greater baseline EAT thickness.[19]

Myocardial Infarction

Paracrine effects from the EAT can result in vascular plaque instability, contributing to acute coronary syndrome.[20] In a cohort of 159 patients with ST-segment elevation myocardial infarction (STEMI) undergoing primary percutaneous coronary intervention, EAT was measured using 2DTTE. EAT positively correlated with angiographic CAD severity. EAT thickness ≥5.45 mm delineated a high-risk phenotype, which predicted a moderate or high SYNTAX score, high thrombus burden, and no-reflow.[21]

Similarly, Tahindi et al. measured EAT thickness using 2DTTE in 200 patients undergoing coronary angiography for stable angina or acute coronary syndrome and reported that increased EAT thickness was independently linked to acute myocardial infarction.[22]

After an acute myocardial infarction, there is growing evidence that the EAT affects cardiac remodeling and fibrosis and can influence the development of heart failure.[23]

Coronary Microvascular Dysfunction

Coronary microvascular dysfunction (CMD) can result in myocardial ischemia despite normal coronary angiography.[24] Inflammation is theorized to drive endothelial dysfunction and subsequently influence development of CMD, as a result of microvascular ischemia.[25] Mahmoud et al. measured EAT thickness via 2DTTE in 399 patients who underwent coronary angiography and did not require coronary revascularization. They noted greater EAT thickness in patients with CMD. This study suggests that EAT thickness may be a robust piece of data that can help diagnose CMD.[26]

Kalçık et al. enrolled 200 patients diagnosed with CMD and 200 control patients and performed 2DTTE to calculate EAT thickness. They too noted that increased EAT thickness was associated with CMD compared to the control group. Increased EAT is thought to result in local and paracrine inflammatory effects, contributing to the vascular inflammation central to CMD.[27]

Atrial Fibrillation

Atrial fibrillation (AF) is one of the most common types of cardiac arrythmia and is a leading cause of morbidity and mortality worldwide. The EAT is thought to influence the development of AF due to paracrine mediators that promote atrial fibrosis and remodeling.[28] Zhang et al. recruited 136 patients with paroxysmal AF, persistent AF, and normal sinus rhythm. Using 2DTTE, they noted that EAT thickness at the base of the right ventricle was independently associated with atrial fibrillation.[29] Increased 2DTTE-measured EAT thickness is also associated with recurrence of AF after catheter ablation.[30]

Heart Failure

Heart Failure with Reduced Ejection Fraction

Heart failure with reduced ejection fraction (HFrEF) is defined as having a left ventricular ejection fraction (LVEF) <50% [individuals with an LVEF between 41 and 49% can be labelled as having heart failure with mildly reduced ejection fraction (HFmrEF)].[31] In HFrEF, there is an energy mismatch, as the failing heart tries to meet its metabolic needs, resulting in consumption of adipose tissue. This catabolic state is thought to affect the EAT and result in decreased thickness.[32] For instance, Rossi et al. studied patients using 2DTTE with either HFrEF or heart failure with preserved ejection fraction (HFpEF). They found that EAT thickness was decreased in patients with HFrEF, supporting the theory of a catabolic state.[33]

Heart Failure with Preserved Ejection Fraction

In an aging population, the prevalence of HFpEF continues to increase. The relationship between the EAT and HFpEF is a highly studied area. Due to its location, the EAT is thought to mechanically affect the heart and result in constriction physiology. In addition, release of inflammatory mediators results in myocardial remodeling, central to HFpEF.[34] Increased EAT is also thought to result in impaired diastolic dysfunction.[35]

Sidhu et al. studied outpatient patients with either HFpEF or HFrEF. Using 2DTTE, they concluded that EAT thickness was greater in patients with HFpEF compared to HFrEF. Even after accounting for BMI, EAT was significantly thicker in patients with HFpEF. Increased EAT was also associated with decreased left ventricular internal diameters, supporting the theory that increased EAT limits cardiac expansion.[36] Similar findings were reported by Jin et al. who calculated 2DTTE EAT thickness in healthy patients, HFpEF patients, and HFrEF/HFmrEF patients. They concluded that there is increased EAT thickness in patients with HFpEF.[37]

Obesity has been implicated in the development of HFpEF as well lending to a specific "obesity phenotype." This distinct phenotype entails left ventricular diastolic dysfunction, increase in chamber volumes, and increases in overall blood volume.[38] Koepp et al. studied 169 obese patients with HFpEF. They noted that individuals with increased EAT thickness (defined in this study as >9mm) had increased pressures in the right atrium, pulmonary artery, and pulmonary capillaries. In addition, patients with increased EAT had decreased peak oxygen consumption.[39]

In addition, the occurrence of AF is closely related to HFpEF. The left atrial dilatation and remodeling seen in HFpEF is theorized to promote AF. Conversely, the tachycardia accompanied with AF is thought to lead to fibrosis of the left ventricle.[40] In a study of 110 HFpEF patients, 20 had documented AF. Using 2DTTE, it was noted that patients with AF had significantly increased EAT thickness compared to those patients without AF.[41]

EPICARDIAL ADIPOSE TISSUE AND ASSOCIATED RISK FACTORS

Type 2 Diabetes Mellitus

Type 2 diabetes mellitus (T2DM) is an established cardiovascular risk factor. Song et al. recruited 154 patients with T2DM and divided them based on EAT thickness (either less than or greater than 5 mm) using 2DTTE. They noted that individuals with increased EAT thickness had right ventricular systolic or diastolic dysfunction.[42] Iacobellis et al. performed 2DTTE on 142 subjects with T2DM. They followed up patients for 1 year to assess for development of CAD. They found that increased EAT thickness was a predictor of CAD, highlighting the role of EAT in predicting outcomes, beyond traditional risk factors such as hemoglobin A1c.[43] Similarly, elevated EAT thickness, as measured by 2DTTE, was linked to a higher risk of cardiovascular events and mortality in T2DM patients, especially in men, and offered modest improvement in risk prediction when added to conventional cardiovascular risk factors.[44]

Hypertension

Hypertension is one of the most crucial modifiable risk factors in the development of cardiovascular disease. Erdogan et al. recruited a total of 150 participants with normotension, controlled hypertension, and resistant hypertension. They calculated EAT thickness using 2DTTE. They noted EAT thickness was increased in the resistant hypertension and controlled hypertension groups in comparison to the normotension group.[45] Eroglu et al. compared EAT thickness using 2DTTE in hypertensive patients compared to normotensive patients and also found increased EAT in hypertensive individuals.[46]

Obesity

General

Adipocyte proliferation is thought to result in EAT expansion in obese individuals. Aitken-Buck et al. used 2DTTE to measure EAT thickness and noted increased thickness in individuals with increased body mass index.[47] Park et al. divided a cohort of patients based on BMI less than or greater than 27 kg/m^2. Using 2DTTE, they noted that EAT thickness was increased in the higher BMI group compared to the lower.[48]

Visceral: The accumulation of intra-abdominal, or visceral adipose tissue (VAT), is correlated with risk for cardiovascular disease.[49] Compared to subcutaneous adipose tissue, VAT secretes more inflammatory mediators.[50] Using 2DTTE, Iacobellis et al. noted a strong correlation between EAT thickness and visceral adipose tissue stores.[3]

Obstructive Sleep Apnea

As a result of systemic inflammation and vascular dysfunction, obstructive sleep apnea (OSA) is a major cardiovascular risk factor.[51] Song et al. conducted a meta-analysis comparing EAT thickness in patients with and without OSA. They found EAT thickness to be higher in the OSA group.[52]

NONALCOHOLIC FATTY LIVER DISEASE

Nonalcoholic fatty liver disease (NAFLD), or now more commonly referred to as metabolic dysfunction-associated steatotic liver disease (MASLD), is associated with cardiovascular disease.[53] Iacobellis et al. used 2DTTE to calculate EAT thickness in 62 obese patients with NAFLD compared to 62 obese control patients. They noted increased EAT thickness in the NAFLD patients, highlighting the role of EAT in predicting liver steatosis.[54] Colak et al. also used 2DTTE to conclude that EAT thickness was higher in biopsy-proven NAFLD patients compared to healthy controls.[55] Yilmaz et al. also demonstrated increased EAT thickness using 2DTTE in NAFLD patients compared to a control group of patients.[56]

CHRONIC KIDNEY DISEASE

Chronic kidney disease (CKD), staged by glomerular filtration rates, is strongly associated with cardiovascular disease, especially in later stages. In a meta-analysis by Song et al., they demonstrated increased EAT thickness in the CKD group of patients compared to a control group of patients.[57] Similarly, Yilmaz et al. compared EAT thickness, using 2DTTE, between CKD Stage five patients not on dialysis and healthy controls. They demonstrated the CKD group to have increased EAT thickness.[58]

RHEUMATOID ARTHRITIS

Rheumatoid arthritis (RA) is an autoimmune disease, characterized by systemic inflammation. High levels of inflammation can increase the risk of cardiovascular disease. Dinçer et al. recruited 81 patients with RA and 70 age- and sex-matched healthy controls. Using 2DTTE, they determined EAT thickness to be significantly higher in the group of RA patients.[59] Fatma et al. similarly compared RA patients and healthy controls using 2DTTE and found that EAT thickness was increased in the group of RA patients. They also noted RA patients to have increased incidence of left ventricular diastolic dysfunction.[60] Lima-Martínez et al. compared EAT thickness using 2DTTE in patients with RA on biological disease modifying anti-rheumatic drugs (DMARDs) and non-biological DMARDs. They found that EAT thickness was decreased in individuals treated with biological DMARDs compared to non-biological DMARDs.[61]

HUMAN IMMUNODEFICIENCY VIRUS

Human immunodeficiency virus (HIV) is associated with cardiovascular disease, likely due to dysregulation of the immune system and chronic inflammation, which can lead to endothelial dysfunction.[62] Iacobellis et al. studied patients with HIV who had highly active antiretroviral therapy (HAART) associated lipodystrophy (LDS) compared to those on an HAART without LDS. Using 2DTTE, they noted that EAT thickness was increased in those with LDS compared to those without.[63]

EPICARDIAL ADIPOSE TISSUE AS A THERAPEUTIC TARGET

Due to its prominence in many cardiac diseases and risk factors, the EAT layer is increasingly becoming a therapeutic target. For instance, Song et al. evaluated 27 patients with T2DM, measuring EAT thickness by 2DTTE at baseline and again 6 months after initiating the sodium-glucose cotransporter-2 inhibitor (SGLT-2I), dapagliflozin. They observed a reduction in EAT thickness over the treatment period.[64] Similarly, Iacobellis et al. compared the effects of two glucagon-like peptide-1 (GLP-1) receptor agonists, dulaglutide and semaglutide, on EAT thickness in patients with T2DM and obesity. EAT thickness was measured by 2DTTE at baseline and after 12 weeks of therapy. Both groups showed a reduction in EAT thickness. Interestingly, they also noted a dose-responsive decrease in EAT thickness with higher doses of the GLP-1 receptor agonist.[65] In addition, statins like atorvastatin have been shown to decrease EAT thickness, likely reflecting their pleiotropic cholesterol-independent effects, including anti-inflammatory actions.[66,67] Furthermore, lifestyle modifications and bariatric surgeries have been associated with decreased EAT thickness.[68] In a 6-month low-calorie program, Iacobellis demonstrated that obese individuals who lost weight had a 32% decrease in EAT thickness. Collectively, these therapeutic options highlight EAT as a modifiable risk factor.

CONCLUSION

This chapter summarizes the link between EAT and common disease states and risk factors. In conclusion, EAT is highly intertwined with cardiovascular disease entities and also risk factors associated with cardiovascular disease. Visualizing a large EAT layer should make one suspect underlying coronary artery disease or presence of risk factors associated with cardiovascular disease. 2DTTE is a widely available non-invasive imaging modality that can be used to characterize the EAT layer. Contemporary research is exploring EAT as a therapeutic target and also integration of techniques such as artificial intelligence. However, certain limitations remain, including the absence of standardized cutoffs for normal EAT thickness and the relatively lower imaging resolution of 2DTTE compared with more advanced modalities such as CT and MRI.

REFERENCES

1. Iacobellis G. Epicardial adipose tissue in contemporary cardiology. Nat Rev Cardiol. 2022;19(9):593-606.
2. Villasante Fricke AC, Iacobellis G. Epicardial Adipose Tissue: Clinical Biomarker of Cardio-Metabolic Risk. Int J Mol Sci. 2019;20(23).
3. Iacobellis G, Assael F, Ribaudo MC, et al. Epicardial fat from echocardiography: a new method for visceral adipose tissue prediction. Obes Res. 2003;11(2):304-10.
4. Eroğlu S. How do we measure epicardial adipose tissue thickness by transthoracic echocardiography? Anatol J Cardiol. 2015;15(5):416-9.
5. Iacobellis G, Willens HJ, Barbaro G, et al. Threshold values of high-risk echocardiographic epicardial fat thickness. Obesity (Silver Spring). 2008;16(4):887-92.
6. Iacobellis G, Willens HJ. Echocardiographic epicardial fat: a review of research and clinical applications. J Am Soc Echocardiogr. 2009;22(12):1311-9; quiz 417-8.
7. Konwerski M, Gąsecka A, Opolski G, et al. Role of Epicardial Adipose Tissue in Cardiovascular Diseases: A Review. Biology (Basel). 2022;11(3).
8. Li C, Liu X, Adhikari BK, et al. The role of epicardial adipose tissue dysfunction in cardiovascular diseases: an overview of pathophysiology, evaluation, and management. Front Endocrinol (Lausanne). 2023;14:1167952.
9. West HW, Siddique M, Williams MC, et al. Deep-Learning for Epicardial Adipose Tissue Assessment With Computed Tomography: Implications for Cardiovascular Risk Prediction. JACC Cardiovasc Imaging. 2023;16(6):800-16.
10. Trimarchi G, Carerj ML, Zito C, et al. Epicardial Adipose Tissue: A Multimodal Imaging Diagnostic Perspective. Medicina (Kaunas). 2025;61(6).
11. Ajoolabady A, Pratico D, Lin L, et al. Inflammation in atherosclerosis: pathophysiology and mechanisms. Cell Death & Disease. 2024;15(11):817.
12. Fan W, Si Y, Xing E, et al. Human epicardial adipose tissue inflammation correlates with coronary artery disease. Cytokine. 2023;162:156119.
13. Jehn S, Roggel A, Dykun I, et al. Epicardial adipose tissue and obstructive coronary artery disease in acute chest pain: the EPIC-ACS study. Eur Heart J Open. 2023;3(3):oead041.
14. Shambu SK, Desai N, Sundaresh N, et al. Study of correlation between epicardial fat thickness and severity of coronary artery disease. Indian Heart J. 2020;72(5):445-7.
15. Rampidis GP, Benetos G, Benz DC, Giannopoulos AA, Buechel RR. A guide for Gensini Score calculation. Atherosclerosis. 2019;287:181-3.
16. Dar M, Beig J, Jan I, et al. Prevalence of type 2 diabetes mellitus and association of HbA1c with severity of coronary artery disease in patients presenting as non-diabetic acute coronary syndrome. The Egyptian heart journal : (EHJ) : official bulletin of the Egyptian Society of Cardiology. 2020;72:66.
17. Meenakshi K, Rajendran M, Srikumar S, et al. Epicardial fat thickness: A surrogate marker of coronary artery disease - Assessment by echocardiography. Indian Heart J. 2016;68(3):336-41.
18. Morales-Portano JD, Peraza-Zaldivar J, Suárez-Cuenca JA, et al. Echocardiographic measurements of epicardial adipose tissue and comparative ability to predict adverse cardiovascular outcomes in patients with coronary artery disease. Int J Cardiovasc Imaging. 2018;34(9):1429-37.
19. Con E, Yilmaz A, Suygun H, et al. The relationship between epicardial adipose tissue thickness and coronary artery disease progress. Bratisl Lek Listy. 2023;124(7):545-8.
20. Napoli G, Pergola V, Basile P, et al. Epicardial and Pericoronary Adipose Tissue, Coronary Inflammation, and Acute Coronary Syndromes. J Clin Med. 2023;12(23).
21. El-Naggar HM, Abdel-Maseh JG, Hasan-Ali H, et al. Epicardial fat thickness predicts severe coronary artery disease and high mortality risk among ST-elevation myocardial infarction patients. Echo Res Pract. 2025;12(1):17.
22. Tanındı A, Kocaman SA, Erkan AF, et al. Epicardial adipose tissue thickness is associated with myocardial infarction and impaired coronary perfusion. Anatol J Cardiol. 2015;15(3):224-31.
23. Krauz K, Kempiński M, Jańczak P, et al. The Role of Epicardial Adipose Tissue in Acute Coronary Syndromes, Post-Infarct Remodeling and Cardiac Regeneration. Int J Mol Sci. 2024;25(7).
24. Recio-Mayoral A, Rimoldi OE, Camici PG, et al. Inflammation and microvascular dysfunction in cardiac syndrome X patients without conventional risk factors for coronary artery disease. JACC Cardiovasc Imaging. 2013;6(6):660-7.
25. Hurst T, Olson TH, Olson LE, et al. Cardiac syndrome X and endothelial dysfunction: new concepts in prognosis and treatment. Am J Med. 2006;119(7):560-6.
26. Mahmoud I, Dykun I, Kärner L, et al. Epicardial adipose tissue differentiates in patients with and without coronary microvascular dysfunction. Int J Obes (Lond). 2021;45(9):2058-63.
27. Kalçık M, Yesin M, Güner A, et al. Echocardiographic measurement of epicardial adipose tissue thickness in patients with microvascular angina. Interv Med Appl Sci. 2019;11(2):106-11.
28. Willar B, Tran KV, Fitzgibbons TP. Epicardial adipocytes in the pathogenesis of atrial fibrillation: An update on basic and translational studies. Front Endocrinol (Lausanne). 2023;14:1154824.
29. Zhang QX, Liu ZJ, Liu XH, et al. The Correlation between Epicardial Adipose Tissue Thickness Measured by Echocardiography and P-Wave Dispersion and Atrial Fibrillation. Rev Cardiovasc Med. 2024;25(8):287.
30. Chao TF, Hung CL, Tsao HM, et al. Epicardial adipose tissue thickness and ablation outcome of atrial fibrillation. PLoS One. 2013;8(9):e74926.
31. Heidenreich PA, Bozkurt B, Aguilar D, et al. 2022 AHA/ACC/HFSA Guideline for the Management of Heart Failure: A Report of the American College of Cardiology/

American Heart Association Joint Committee on Clinical Practice Guidelines. Circulation. 2022;145(18):e895-e1032.
32. Cho DH, Park SM. Epicardial Adipose Tissue and Heart Failure, Friend or Foe? Diabetes Metab J. 2024;48(3):373-84.
33. Rossi VA, Nebunu D, Haider T, et al. Diverging role of epicardial adipose tissue across the entire heart failure spectrum. ESC Heart Fail. 2023;10(6):3419-29.
34. Oduah MT, Sundaram V, Reddy YN. Epicardial Fat in Heart Failure with Preserved Ejection Fraction: Bad Actor or Just Lying Around? Card Fail Rev. 2023;9:e06.
35. Li Q, Muhib UR, Ma X, et al. Potential Mechanisms of Epicardial Adipose Tissue Influencing Heart Failure with Preserved Ejection Fraction. Rev Cardiovasc Med. 2024;25(9):311.
36. Sidhu GS, Rabkin SW. Epicardial Fat in Heart Failure with Preserved Ejection Fraction Compared with Reduced Ejection Fraction. J Clin Med. 2024;13(18).
37. Jin X, Hung CL, Tay WT, et al. Epicardial adipose tissue related to left atrial and ventricular function in heart failure with preserved versus reduced and mildly reduced ejection fraction. Eur J Heart Fail. 2022;24(8):1346-56.
38. Obokata M, Reddy YNV, Pislaru SV, et al. Evidence Supporting the Existence of a Distinct Obese Phenotype of Heart Failure With Preserved Ejection Fraction. Circulation. 2017;136(1):6-19.
39. Koepp Katlyn E, Obokata M, Reddy Yogesh NV, et al. Hemodynamic and Functional Impact of Epicardial Adipose Tissue in Heart Failure With Preserved Ejection Fraction. JACC: Heart Failure. 2020;8(8):657-66.
40. Packer M, Lam CSP, Lund LH, et al. Interdependence of Atrial Fibrillation and Heart Failure With a Preserved Ejection Fraction Reflects a Common Underlying Atrial and Ventricular Myopathy. Circulation. 2020;141(1):4-6.
41. Yucel O. Relationship Between Epicardial Adipose Tissue and Atrial Fibrillation in Heart Failure With Preserved Ejection Fraction. Cureus. 2025;17(3):e80827.
42. Song XT, Zhang PY, Fan L, et al. Epicardial adipose tissue and right ventricular function in type 2 diabetes mellitus using two-dimensional speckle tracking echocardiography. Diab Vasc Dis Res. 2022;19(4):14791641221118622.
43. Iacobellis G, Goldberger JJ, Malavazos AE, et al. Epicardial fat thickness in type 2 diabetes outpatient care. Nutr Metab Cardiovasc Dis. 2024;34(3):618-23.
44. Christensen RH, von Scholten BJ, Hansen CS, et al. Epicardial adipose tissue predicts incident cardiovascular disease and mortality in patients with type 2 diabetes. Cardiovasc Diabetol. 2019;18(1):114.
45. Erdogan G, Belen E, Sungur MA, et al. Assessment of epicardial adipose tissue thickness in patients with resistant hypertension. Blood Pressure Monitoring. 2016;21(1).
46. Eroğlu S, Sade LE, Yıldırır A, et al. Association of epicardial adipose tissue thickness by echocardiography and hypertension. Turk Kardiyol Dern Ars. 2013;41(2):115-22.
47. Aitken-Buck HM, Moharram M, Babakr AA, et al. Relationship between epicardial adipose tissue thickness and epicardial adipocyte size with increasing body mass index. Adipocyte. 2019;8(1):412-20.
48. Park JS, Ahn SG, Hwang JW, et al. Impact of body mass index on the relationship of epicardial adipose tissue to metabolic syndrome and coronary artery disease in an Asian population. Cardiovasc Diabetol. 2010;9:29.
49. Mathieu P, Poirier P, Pibarot P, et al. Visceral Obesity. Hypertension. 2009;53(4):577-84.
50. Kahn D, Macias E, Zarini S, et al. Exploring Visceral and Subcutaneous Adipose Tissue Secretomes in Human Obesity: Implications for Metabolic Disease. Endocrinology. 2022;163(11):bqac140.
51. Shamsuzzaman AS, Gersh BJ, Somers VK. Obstructive sleep apnea: implications for cardiac and vascular disease. Jama. 2003;290(14):1906-14.
52. Song G, Sun F, Wu D, et al. Association of epicardial adipose tissues with obstructive sleep apnea and its severity: A meta-analysis study. Nutr Metab Cardiovasc Dis. 2020;30(7):1115-20.
53. Chung GE, Yu SJ, Yoo J-J, et al. Metabolic dysfunction-associated steatotic liver disease increases cardiovascular disease risk in young adults. Scientific Reports. 2025;15(1):5777.
54. Iacobellis G, Barbarini G, Letizia C, et al. Epicardial fat thickness and nonalcoholic fatty liver disease in obese subjects. Obesity (Silver Spring). 2014;22(2):332-6.
55. Colak Y, Karabay CY, Tuncer I, et al. Relation of epicardial adipose tissue and carotid intima-media thickness in patients with nonalcoholic fatty liver disease. Eur J Gastroenterol Hepatol. 2012;24(6):613-8.
56. Yilmaz Y, Kurt R, Gurdal A, et al. Circulating vaspin levels and epicardial adipose tissue thickness are associated with impaired coronary flow reserve in patients with nonalcoholic fatty liver disease. Atherosclerosis. 2011;217(1):125-9.
57. Song G, Qiao W, Liu K, Yu X. Epicardial adipose tissue in patients with chronic kidney disease: a meta-analysis study and trial sequential analysis. Int Urol Nephrol. 2020;52(12):2345-55.
58. Yilmaz Z, İnce H, Aydin E, et al. Relationship Between Epicardial Adipose Tissue and Body Composition as Determined by Multi-Frequency Bioelectrical Impedance Analysis in Patients with Stage 5 Chronic Kidney Disease. Med Sci Monit. 2020;26:e920233.
59. Keleşoğlu Dinçer AB, Şahan HF. Increased epicardial adipose tissue thickness as a sign of subclinical atherosclerosis in patients with rheumatoid arthritis and its relationship with disease activity indices. Intern Emerg Med. 2024;19(4):1015-24.
60. Fatma E, Bunyamin K, Savas S, et al. Epicardial fat thickness in patients with rheumatoid arthritis. Afr Health Sci. 2015;15(2):489-95.
61. Lima-Martínez MM, Campo E, Salazar J, et al. Epicardial fat thickness as cardiovascular risk factor and therapeutic target in patients with rheumatoid arthritis treated with biological and nonbiological therapies. Arthritis. 2014;2014:782850.

62. Afolabi JM, Kirabo A. HIV and Cardiovascular Disease. Circulation Research. 2024;134(11):1512-4.
63. Iacobellis G, Sharma AM, Pellicelli AM, et al. Epicardial adipose tissue is related to carotid intima-media thickness and visceral adiposity in HIV-infected patients with highly active antiretroviral therapy-associated metabolic syndrome. Curr HIV Res. 2007;5(2):275-9.
64. Song XT, Wei YL, Rui YF, et al. Echocardiographic evaluation of the effect of dapagliflozin on epicardial adipose tissue and left ventricular systolic function in type 2 diabetes mellitus. J Diabetes Complications. 2023;37(7):108509.
65. Iacobellis G, Villasante Fricke AC. Effects of Semaglutide Versus Dulaglutide on Epicardial Fat Thickness in Subjects with Type 2 Diabetes and Obesity. J Endocr Soc. 2020;4(4):bvz042.
66. Park JH, Park YS, Kim YJ, et al. Effects of statins on the epicardial fat thickness in patients with coronary artery stenosis underwent percutaneous coronary intervention: comparison of atorvastatin with simvastatin/ezetimibe. J Cardiovasc Ultrasound. 2010;18(4):121-6.
67. Choudhary A, Rawat U, Kumar P, et al. Pleotropic effects of statins: the dilemma of wider utilization of statin. The Egyptian Heart Journal. 2023;75(1):1.
68. Mihăilă MD, Caloian B, Frîngu FI, et al. Beyond Traditional Risk Factors: Integrating Epicardial Adipose Tissue into the Comorbidity Landscape of HFpEF. J Clin Med. 2025;14(17).

64 CHAPTER

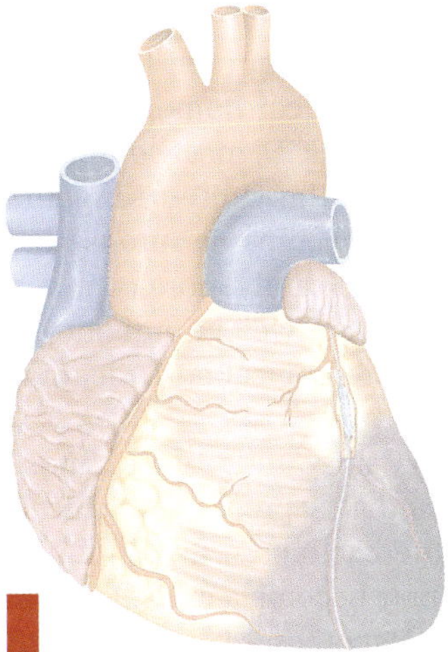

Obesity Review: New Dimensions

Juliana Spanova, Raj Wasan, Nayna Nanda, Navin C Nanda, HK Chopra

INTRODUCTION

Obesity is a chronic medical condition that is expected to affect one-fourth of the world's population by 2035.[1] At present, body mass index (BMI) is the primary tool used to define weight categories; obesity is defined as a BMI of 30 kg/m^2 or greater, while severe class III obesity is defined as a BMI of 40 kg/m^2.[2] However, BMI is a suboptimal indicator of total body fat content, making it a poor predictor of health at the individual level.[3] One study of 21,000 individuals in the United Kingdom considered both BMI and total body fat mass, which was calculated via full-body imaging. This investigation found that approximately one-third of women who fell into the overweight category by BMI fell within the normal range for total body fat mass. Men were similarly miscategorized by the BMI: 1 in 10 men in the overweight category were found to have normal total body fat mass, while one in four men in the overweight category were recategorized into the obese range based on total body fat mass.[4]

However, calculating total body fat mass with imaging is not always an accessible option. One analysis of nineteen thousand patients diagnosed with cardiovascular, renal, or metabolic disease explored the relationship between alternative measurements, including waist circumference and waist-to-height-ratio, with patient outcomes. The study demonstrated that the relationship between waist-to-height-ratio and cardiovascular disease outcomes was linear, with higher ratios having an association with poorer outcomes;[5] a waist-to-height ratio of greater than or equal to 0.5 defines central obesity, which has been associated with increased cardiovascular disease risk in both sexes across ethnic populations.[6] Alternatively, the association between BMI and cardiovascular outcomes in this study was more parabolic and less predictable.[5] This suggests waist-to-height ratio is superior to BMI for estimating cardiovascular risk and may be a useful supplemental tool for clinicians to utilize when more specific imaging modalities are unavailable.

Though some sources contend that the definition of obesity as a disease remains controversial,[3] the World Health Organization (WHO) stresses the importance of viewing obesity as more than a risk factor of excess body weight, but rather as a chronic medical condition that is affected by numerous complex biological, environmental, and psychosocial factors. When we, as health care providers, view obesity as a one-dimensional problem that can be corrected with discipline and a caloric deficit, we fail to acknowledge and address the systemic factors at play, which have contributed to the continually rising prevalence of obesity globally. Furthermore, when obesity is treated as a behavioral risk factor, we see immediate gaps in care for individuals living with obesity—from diagnostic delays and insufficient treatment to missed opportunities to provide well-rounded, comprehensive care.[7]

Provider biases and stereotypes also shape the care that patients with obesity receive. Multiple reviews have demonstrated that weight bias among healthcare providers has remained pervasive over time. Commonly held stereotypes are that obese patients are nonadherent, lack discipline, and are uninterested in their health. These beliefs not only impact the behavior of the clinician, but of the patient as well; obese patients are more likely to avoid seeking care, have less trust in their care team, and have less overall satisfaction with the care they receive.[8] A survey of one-thousand Latin American cardiologists found that though most respondents viewed obesity as a chronic medical illness, significant stigma remained, and many still viewed it as a patient choice.[9] Unfortunately, the perceptions of healthcare professionals—and society as a whole—are challenging to shift. Despite the American Medical Association (AMA) designating obesity a disease in 2013, it is often still viewed as an individual moral failure.[8]

Further complicating the definition of obesity and its risk factors is the variation of body fat distribution between individuals based on sex alone. Men are more likely to have visceral fat, while women are more likely to have increased adiposity in the lower body. Visceral fat specifically promotes inflammatory processes and is associated with negative health outcomes. Visceral fat, adipose infiltration of muscle tissue, and the ratio of liver fat content to normal liver tissue have been associated with accelerated cardiovascular aging in both sexes. Conversely, increased adiposity in the gluteal-femoral region has demonstrated beneficial effects on cardiovascular aging in pre-menopausal women. Increased levels of abdominal subcutaneous fat were shown to have negative effects on cardiovascular aging in males, while in females, it was shown to have neutral to beneficial effects.[4] It is important to keep these variations in mind when implementing obesity-related interventions.

OBESITY, CARDIOVASCULAR DISEASE, AND OTHER COMORBIDITIES

Obesity is associated with atherosclerosis, heart failure with preserved ejection fraction (HFpEF), heart failure with reduced ejection fraction (HFrEF), cardiac arrhythmias, sudden cardiac death (SCD), venous thromboembolism, and valvular abnormalities.[10] One article by the American College of Cardiology (ACC) emphasizes the importance of distinguishing between obesity without metabolic syndrome components versus obesity with metabolic syndrome components (e.g., impaired insulin sensitivity, hypertension, and hyperlipidemia) as distinct phenotypes with different risks. Obesity with metabolic syndrome causes systemic inflammation, impaired glucose sensitivity, and ectopic lipid accumulation. This can lead to cardiac fibrosis, diastolic dysfunction, and ultimately HFpEF.[11,12]

Obesity cardiomyopathy (OCM) refers to the cardiac remodeling that occurs in obese individuals, independent of risk factors, such as hypertension and coronary artery disease (CAD). Due to increased adiposity, there is increased total blood volume and higher stroke volume, resulting in increased hemodynamic burden that leads to left ventricular remodeling and cardiomegaly. This condition has been associated with SCD, most commonly in young men. One study out of the United Kingdom examined the hearts of SCD death victims via autopsy and found that cardiomegaly was significantly more common in obese individuals than in normal-weight individuals, suggesting OCM is a distinct pathological entity leading to SCD.[13]

Furthermore, the heart is surrounded by adipose tissue, and the amount of epicardial fat present is positively associated with coronary atherosclerosis. Evaluation of pericoronary adipose tissue may become a crucial part of CAD evaluation in the future. Hypotheses have suggested that adipose tissue surrounding the coronary arteries can promote plaque formation and lesion instability by causing local inflammation.[14] The ORFAN study, a cohort study of forty-thousand individuals in the United Kingdom, found that coronary inflammation measured by the perivascular fat attenuation index (FAI) score predicted cardiovascular events, particularly in individuals with nonobstructive CAD. This could fundamentally change how cardiologists approach patients with cardiovascular symptoms in the absence of obstructive CAD.[15]

Recent data have demonstrated one approach to attenuating the increased cardiovascular risk in obese individuals with CAD. The FOURIER trial demonstrated that patients who received evolocumab, a PCSK9 inhibitor, in addition to their statin therapy, had a significantly decreased risk of major adverse cardiovascular events (MACE) than those who received statin monotherapy. This beneficial effect was more pronounced in obese individuals, with an absolute risk reduction (ARR) of nearly six percent in patients with a BMI $\geq$35 kg/m^2. The ARR in nonobese individuals was one-quarter that seen in obese individuals. This enhanced effect made obese individuals' risk of MACE similar to patients that did not fall into the obese category, suggesting that PCSK9 therapy, in addition to statin therapy, in obese patients with established CAD may mitigate their increased risk of adverse cardiovascular events.[16]

Interestingly, through mechanisms that are not yet well understood, the obesity paradox has demonstrated that among individuals with established cardiovascular disease, those who are overweight or obese may have more favorable outcomes. One meta-analysis found that of the patients with established CAD, those with a BMI of 25 kg/m^2 or higher had lower all-cause and cardiovascular mortality compared to those who fell into the normal weight or underweight range.[17] Many other studies have shown similar findings over the years. Despite the known effects of obesity on cardiovascular physiology, studies have also found the same pattern in patients with heart failure: Those who fall into the overweight and obese categories have better outcomes. However, this effect disappears at a BMI of 40 kg/m^2 or greater.[18] It is important to acknowledge that the relationship between obesity and cardiovascular disease, including atherosclerosis and heart failure, remains well-established and that treating obesity is key in primary prevention of these issues; however, once the disease process has been established, that is when the obesity paradox comes into play.[17] Furthermore, most of these studies categorize patients based on BMI, which is likely missing true risk factors and not characterizing patients appropriately, and could be contributing to this phenomenon.

Obesity is also a well-established predictor of chronic kidney disease (CKD). A global meta-analysis of more than five million adults showed associations between increased BMI and decline in estimated glomerular filtration rate (eGFR), even with adjustments for comorbidities.[19] The renal tamponade hypothesis states that perinephric and intra-abdominal fat compress the kidneys, negatively affecting kidney function. A pooled analysis of seventeen thousand patients from four HFpEF trials found that waist circumference—not BMI—was associated with sustained decrease in eGFR, end-stage renal disease (ESRD), and death due to renal dysfunction. These results again emphasize the importance of considering body fat distribution rather than solely BMI when considering obesity-related risk factors.[20]

Unique clinical challenges arise in the diagnosis and treatment of concurrent obesity and cardiovascular disease. Electrocardiography (ECG), one of the key diagnostic tests in cardiology, can be affected by numerous factors in an individual with obesity. This includes displacement of the heart from an elevated diaphragm when lying flat due to increased abdominal pressure and increased adiposity in the chest wall, both of which increase the distance from the ECG leads. Therefore, an ECG may falsely show low QRS voltage, a leftward axis, and T-wave flattening in inferior and lateral leads. This results in decreased specificity and an increased false-positive rate of diagnosing inferior myocardial infarction. Transthoracic echocardiography (TTE) is also limited by suboptimal windows due to increased adiposity in the chest wall, posing a diagnostic challenge; for example, it is more difficult to differentiate between subepicardial fat and pericardial effusion in some of these patients. These, and other factors, are often limitations to various stress testing modalities in individuals with obesity. Other imaging modalities, including computerized tomography (CT), coronary angiography, and cardiac magnetic resonance imaging (CMR), also have limitations.[2] Because optimal treatment requires an accurate diagnosis, this must be taken into consideration. Given that patients who are obese are less likely to seek medical care, as previously mentioned, it is even more important that our diagnostics are high-quality and as accurate as possible.

OBESITY: NOVEL THERAPIES

Recently published WHO guidelines on obesity management emphasize the importance of a well-rounded approach to treating patients with obesity that includes sustainable behavior and lifestyle interventions supported by medical and surgical intervention when appropriate. The guidelines also recommend pharmacological intervention with glucagon-like peptide (GLP-1) receptor agonists and glucose-dependent insulinotropic peptide (GIP)/GLP-1 dual agonists for long-term obesity management in the right context. On a global scale, this requires a capable government, an adequate healthcare system, and sufficient funding because these medications can be costly.[7,21]

Since their release in 2005, GLP-1 receptor agonists have had a substantial impact on the management of type 2 diabetes and obesity. Recent data have shown that GLP-1 receptor agonists not only promote weight loss but also decrease major adverse cardiovascular events and all-cause mortality in patients with diabetes, ultimately leading to FDA approval of these drugs for cardiovascular risk reduction.[22] These medications have also been shown to decrease adverse cardiovascular events in individuals with obesity and established coronary atherosclerosis, as well as those with HFpEF.[23] In 2024, the dual GLP-1 and GIP receptor agonist tirzepatide was FDA-approved for patients with obstructive sleep apnea and obesity.[24] Unknowns remain for these medications, including long-term efficacy, as well as safety and efficacy in special populations such as individuals with CKD, cognitive decline, and pregnant women, all of which warrant further research.[7]

Side effects of GLP-1 drugs are a concern. Nutritional deficiencies are also a concern,[25] given that patients have significantly reduced caloric intake from reduced appetite. Baseline dietary patterns in patients with obesity can further increase their risk of nutritional deficiencies before therapy is initiated. When this is compounded with gastrointestinal side effects, nutrient deficiency poses a legitimate concern. Clinicians prescribing these medications should counsel their patients on signs of severe nutrient deficiency, including excess fatigue, hair loss, dermatologic changes, and weakness.[26] **Tables 1 and 2** show novel therapies currently approved for patient use and those in the pipeline.

Availability of an oral formulation of semaglutide will benefit patients who wish to avoid needles and those who are concerned about local skin reactions. The oral formulation will also likely not need to be refrigerated, which could improve accessibility when reliable refrigeration is not an option.[27] Retatrutide has been shown to result in weight loss comparable to that of bariatric surgery, though meta-analyses have demonstrated that this superior efficacy is accompanied by a higher adverse event risk.[28] Cagrilintide monotherapy has similar weight loss effects to semaglutide with a significantly decreased risk of vomiting, which could be a reasonable option for individuals who cannot tolerate GLP-1 receptor agonists due to this side effect.[29] Survodutide may help reverse metabolic dysfunction-associated steatosis (MASH) in addition to promoting weight loss,[30] which could be a good option specifically for patients with this comorbidity. Both cagrilintide-semaglutide and survodutide have been associated with improvement in cardiovascular risk factors, however they have yet to demonstrate comprehensive cardiovascular benefit in dedicated cardiovascular outcomes trials, which are in the works.[31-33]

Maridebart cafraglutide, with its 21-day half-life and monthly (or less) administration schedule, could be beneficial for patients who struggle with adherence to a daily oral drug or a weekly injection. Bimagrumab, when administered in combination with semaglutide, has been shown to minimize or increase lean body mass.[34,35] This is distinct from the weight loss effects of GLP-1 receptor agonists, from which approximately 10–20% of total weight loss comes from muscle mass.[36] The development of these novel medications could facilitate our ability as providers to utilize a more individualized approach to obesity management.

Comparatively, bariatric surgery remains the most effective obesity intervention based on the current available data. Surgical options include Roux-en-Y gastric bypass, laparoscopic sleeve gastrectomy, laparoscopic adjustable gastric band, and biliopancreatic diversion; these surgeries are indicated for individuals who fall into the severe class III obese category or individuals in the class II obese category with a diagnosed comorbidity. A systematic review of six randomized controlled trials (RCTs),[37] with >400 participants from 2024, found that surgery was more efficient than medical treatment for long-term weight loss. Notably, data on the long-term impact of medical management with newer drugs is limited and a rapidly growing area of research. In clinical practice, these therapies are not mutually exclusive, and GLP-1 receptor agonists can be utilized in patients with a suboptimal

TABLE 1: Currently approved novel therapies for obesity.

Generic drug name	*Brand name (USA)*	*Mechanism**	*Method of administration*	*Dosing*	*Efficacy†*	*Side effects‡*
Semaglutide	Wegovy Ozempic (only for diabetic patients)	GLP-1 RA	Subcutaneous injection	0.25 mg weekly initial dose titrated up every 4 weeks; 2.4 mg maintenance dose§	14.9% weight loss at 68 weeks (2.4 mg dose)	Nausea, diarrhea, vomiting, constipation, abdominal pain[41]
Liraglutide	Saxenda Victoza (only for diabetic patients)	GLP-1 RA§	Subcutaneous injection	0.6 mg once daily, titrated up weekly to a maintenance dose of 3.0 mg[42]	8.0% weight loss at 56 weeks	Same as above[43]
Tirzepatide	Zepbound Mounjaro (only for diabetic patients)	GLP-1 RA, GIP-agonist	Subcutaneous injection	2.5 mg once weekly for 4 weeks, increased to 5 mg weekly, then increased by 2.5 mg every 4 weeks as tolerated up to 15 mg once weekly[44]	15% weight loss at 72 weeks (5 mg dose) 20.9% weight loss at 72 weeks (15 mg dose)[45]	Same as above[41]

(GLP-1 RA: glucagon-like peptide-1 receptor agonist; GIP: glucose-dependent insulinotropic polypeptide)

*These drugs act centrally to reduce appetite and hunger, increase satiety, delay gastric emptying, and induce microbiota modulation.[46,47] Patients are also recommended to follow dietary and exercise regimens when taking these drugs.

†The efficacy listed is based on trials in overweight and obese patients without diabetes.

‡These lists are not comprehensive. The FDA website has a comprehensive list of side effects, including rare or serious adverse reactions that have been reported in clinical trials. Decreased food intake may also result in iron deficiency anemia.

§There is now established safety data for the use of semaglutide in obese patients with HFpEF. Less is known about use in HFrEF. Therefore, this therapy requires a shared-decision-making approach in which the potential of GLP-1 receptor agonists further reduce EF and increase the risk of cardiovascular events is discussed. This is particularly a concern with liraglutide.[40]

TABLE 2: Novel therapies for obesity in the pipeline.

Drug name	Mechanism	Method of administration	Dosing	Efficacy*	Side effects	Stage in development
Semaglutide	GLP-1 receptor agonist (RA)	Oral§	25–50 mg once daily	13.6% weight loss at 64 weeks (25 mg dose) 15.1% weight loss at 68 weeks (50 mg dose)	Nausea, diarrhea, vomiting, constipation[27,48]	Studied in phase 3 trials
Retatrutide	GLP-1 RA, GIP RA, and glucagon RA	Subcutaneous injection	1 mg, 4 mg, 8 mg, or 12 mg once weekly	8.7% weight loss at 48 weeks (1 mg dose) 24.2% weight loss at 48 weeks (12 mg dose)	Same as above[49]	Studied in phase 2 trials; phase 3 trials underway
Cagrilintide	Amylin analogue	Subcutaneous injection	0.3–4.5 mg once weekly (starting at 0.3–0.6 mg uptitrated every 2 weeks)[50]	10.8% weight loss at 26 weeks (4.5 mg dose)	Same as above[29]	Studied in phase 2 trials
Cagrilintide-semaglutide	Amylin analog, GLP-1 RA	Subcutaneous injection	2.4 mg/2.4 mg once weekly	20.4% weight loss at 68 weeks	Same as above[32]	Studied in phase 3 trials
Survodutide	GLP-1 RA, glucagon RA	Subcutaneous injection	3.6–6.0 mg once weekly (starting at 0.6 mg, uptitrated every 2–4 weeks)	14.9% weight loss at 48 weeks (4.8 mg dose)	Same as above[51,52]	Phase 2 trials completed; phase 3 trials in progress
Maridebart cafraglutide	GLP-RA, GIP receptor antagonist	Subcutaneous injection	140–420 mg every 4–8 weeks	12.3–16.2% weight loss at 52 weeks (variable dosing regimens)	Same as above; dry heaving[34]	Studied in phase 2 trials
Bimagrumab	Monoclonal antibody targeting activin type II receptor	Intravenous infusion	1–30 mg/kg or 1,200 mg fixed dose once monthly	6.5% weight loss at 48 weeks with 3.6% increase in lean mass (10 mg/kg dosing)†35	Muscle spasms, falls, diarrhea, skin reactions[53‡]	Studied in phase 2 trials
		Subcutaneous injection	52.5–300 mg once weekly[54,55]			Studied in phase 1 trials

*The reported data is based on studies done on populations that are overweight or obese without type 2 diabetes, unless otherwise specified. All clinical trials for these weight loss pharmacotherapies included structured lifestyle intervention counseling, aside from maridebart cafraglutide, which did not explicitly describe lifestyle intervention counseling.[34]

†This data is based off a phase 2 clinical trial of adults with type 2 diabetes and obesity. The data on overweight/obese middle-aged adults without type 2 diabetes is limited.

‡This data is from a trial on patients with inclusion body myositis; other phase 2 trials of populations without inclusion body myositis have reported similar side effect profiles.

§Oral semaglutide has been FDA-approved for the treatment of type 2 diabetes mellitus, under the brand name Rybelsus (USA).[24]

response to bariatric surgery.[38] These medications can also be utilized pre-operatively to optimize patients for surgery and may reduce perioperative complications. Combining surgical treatment with medical treatment may result in more benefits than a monotherapy approach.[39]

Bariatric surgery is an option even for patients with heart failure, though these patients have a greater risk of adverse events following surgery. Encouragingly, down the road, bariatric surgery in patients with HFrEF has been associated with decreased frequency of hospitalizations for HF exacerbations and an improvement in mortality.[40]

CONCLUSION

Obesity is a chronic medical condition that is multifactorial in etiology, affected by genetic, psychosocial, behavioral, and environmental factors. Addressing the worldwide evergrowing obesity epidemic requires an eclectic, multidisciplinary approach on a systemic and local scale, in which cardiologists and primary care physicians play a key role. Pharmacologic options for obesity management have diversified in the past few decades, and many new, more effective medications are on the horizon, which could be key in addressing this global problem.

REFERENCES

1. Worldobesity.Org. World obesity atlas 2023. [Online] Available from https://data.worldobesity.org/publications/WOF-Obesity-Atlas-V5.pdf [Last accessed January, 2026].
2. Bianchettin RG, Lavie CJ, Lopez-Jimenez F. Challenges in cardiovascular evaluation and management of obese patients: JACC state-of-the-art review. J Am Coll Cardiol. 2023;81(5):490-504.
3. Rubino F, Cummings DE, Eckel RH, et al. Definition and diagnostic criteria of clinical obesity. Lancet Diabetes Endocrinol. 2025;13(3):221-62.
4. Losev V, Lu C, Tahasildar S, et al. Sex-specific body fat distribution predicts cardiovascular ageing. Eur Heart J. 2025;46(46):5076-88.
5. Gorter TM, Meems LMG, van Veldhuisen DJ. Cracking the Code of Central Obesity: Are Anthropometrics Enough? J Am Coll Cardiol. 2025;86(20):1802-4.
6. Nadolsky K, Garvey WT, Agarwal M, et al. American Association of Clinical Endocrinology Consensus Statement: Algorithm for the Evaluation and Treatment of Adults with Obesity/Adiposity-Based Chronic Disease - 2025 Update. Endocr Pract. 2025;31(11):1351-94.
7. Celletti F, Farrar J, Regil LD. World Health Organization Guideline on the Use and Indications of Glucagon-Like Peptide-1 Therapies for the Treatment of Obesity in Adults. JAMA. 2025.
8. Peck J. (2025). Weight bias in the hospital: Implicit attitudes shape care. [Online] Available from https://www.medscape.com/viewarticle/weight-bias-hospital-implicit-attitudes-shape-care-2025a1000xmt [Last accessed January, 2026].
9. Forte E, Acevedo M, Mora L, et al. Obesity awareness and management among cardiologists in the Americas. JACC. 2025; 85 (12_Supplement):2681.
10. Sinha SS, Morrow DA, Kapur NK, et al. 2025 Concise Clinical Guidance: An ACC Expert Consensus Statement on the Evaluation and Management of Cardiogenic Shock: A Report of the American College of Cardiology Solution Set Oversight Committee. J Am Coll Cardiol. 2025;85(16):1618-41.
11. Sun P. Metabolic Health Status: A Critical Unaddressed Dimension in Obesity Phenotyping for Heart Failure With Preserved Ejection Fraction. J Am Coll Cardiol. 2025;S0735-1097(25)07773-3.
12. Liu J, Ayada I, Zhang X, et al. Estimating global prevalence of metabolic dysfunction-associated fatty liver disease in overweight or obese adults. Clin Gastroenterol Hepatol. 2022;20(3):e573-82.
13. Westaby J, Dalle-Carbonare C, Ster IC, et al. Obesity cardiomyopathy in sudden cardiac death: a distinct entity? a comparative study. JACC Adv. 2023;2(5): 100414.
14. Shaw LJ, Blankstein R, Chandrashekhar YS. Perivascular fat: multiple differences impacting progress. JACC Cardiovasc Imaging. 2025;18(8):939-41.
15. Chan K, Wahome E, Tsiachristas A, et al. Inflammatory risk and cardiovascular events in patients without obstructive coronary artery disease: the ORFAN multicentre, longitudinal cohort study. Lancet. 2024;403(10444): 2606-18.
16. Kang YM, Giugliano RP, Keech AC, et al. Obesity-Associated Cardiovascular Risk and Benefit From PCSK9 Inhibition: A Prespecified Analysis From FOURIER. J Am Coll Cardiol. 2025;S0735-1097(25)10005-3.
17. Romero-Corral A, Montori VM, Somers VK, et al. Association of bodyweight with total mortality and with cardiovascular events in coronary artery disease: a systematic review of cohort studies. Lancet. 2006; 368(9536):666-78.
18. Aggrawal K, Gupta V, Singh B, et al. Exploring the obesity parADOX: a multisystem review. Am J Med Sci. 2025;370(4):315-20.
19. Furth SL, Colhoun HM, Kanbay M, et al. The relationship between obesity and chronic kidney disease: conclusions from a Kidney Disease: Improving Global Outcomes (KDIGO) Controversies Conference. Kidney Int. 2025; S0085-2538(25)00774-4.
20. Lassen MCH, Ostrominski JW, Claggett BL, et al. Obesity and Risk of Kidney Outcomes in Heart Failure With Preserved Ejection Fraction: A Participant-Level Pooled Analysis of 4 Contemporary Trials. JACC Heart Fail. 2025;13(8):102498.
21. Tucker ME. (2025). Myostatin blocker preserves muscle with GLP-1 treatment. [Online] Available from https://www.medscape.com/viewarticle/myostatin-blocker-preserves-muscle-glp-1-treatment-2025a1000qs4 [Last accessed January, 2025].
22. Sattar N, Lee MMY, Kristensen SL, et al. Cardiovascular, mortality, and kidney outcomes with GLP-1 receptor agonists in patients with type 2 diabetes: a systematic

review and meta-analysis of randomised trials. Lancet Diabetes Endocrinol. 2021;9(10):653-62.

23. Gilbert O, Gulati M, Gluckman TJ, et al. 2025 Concise Clinical Guidance: An ACC Expert Consensus Statement on Medical Weight Management for Optimization of Cardiovascular Health: A Report of the American College of Cardiology Solution Set Oversight Committee. J Am Coll Cardiol. 2025;86(7):536-55.
24. Food and Drug Administration. Approved Drug Products with Therapeutic Equivalence Evaluation. [Online] Available from https://www.fda.gov/drugs/drug-approvals-and-databases/approved-drug-products-therapeutic-equivalence-evaluations-orange-book [Last accessed January, 2026].
25. Mozaffarian D, Agarwal M, Aggarwal M, et al. Nutritional priorities to support GLP-1 therapy for obesity: A joint Advisory from the American College of Lifestyle Medicine, the American Society for Nutrition, the Obesity Medicine Association, and The Obesity Society. Obesity (Silver Spring). 2025;33(8):1475-503.
26. Mozaffarian D, Agarwal M, Aggarwal M, et al. Nutritional priorities to support GLP-1 therapy for obesity: A joint Advisory from the American College of Lifestyle Medicine, the American Society for Nutrition, the Obesity Medicine Association, and The Obesity Society. Obesity (Silver Spring). 2025;33(8):1475-503.
27. Wharton S, Lingvay I, Bogdanski P, et al. Oral semaglutide at a dose of 25 mg in adults with overweight or obesity. N Engl J Med. 2025;393(11):1077-87.
28. Sinha B, Ghosal S. Efficacy and Safety of GLP-1 Receptor Agonists, Dual Agonists, and Retatrutide for Weight Loss in Adults With Overweight or Obesity: A Bayesian NMA. Obesity (Silver Spring). 2025;33(11):2046-54.
29. Dutta D, Nagendra L, Harish BG, et al. Efficacy and Safety of Cagrilintide Alone and in Combination with Semaglutide (Cagrisema) as Anti-Obesity Medications: A Systematic Review and Meta-Analysis. Indian J Endocrinol Metab. 2024;28(5):436-44.
30. Kaya E, Yilmaz Y, Alkhouri N. Survodutide in MASH: bridging the gap between hepatic and systemic metabolic dysfunction. Expert Opin Investig Drugs. 2024;33(12):1167-76.
31. Sanyal AJ, Bedossa P, Fraessdorf M, et al. A Phase 2 Randomized Trial of Survodutide in MASH and Fibrosis. N Engl J Med. 2024;391(4):311-9.
32. Garvey WT, Blüher M, Osorto Contreras CK, et al. Coadministered Cagrilintide and Semaglutide in Adults with Overweight or Obesity. N Engl J Med. 2025;393(7):635-47.
33. Warburg E. (2025). New Antiobesity drugs eagerly anticipated. [Online] Available from https://www.medscape.com/s/viewarticle/new-antiobesity-drugs-eagerly-anticipated-2025a1000xoy [Last accessed January, 2026].
34. Kushner RF, Jastreboff AM, Ryan DH. Current and future medications for obesity treatment. JAMA. 2025;334(17):1551-2.
35. Heymsfield SB, Coleman LA, Miller R, et al. Effect of Bimagrumab vs Placebo on Body Fat Mass Among Adults With Type 2 Diabetes and Obesity: A Phase 2 Randomized Clinical Trial. JAMA Netw Open. 2021;4(1):e2033457. Erratum in: JAMA Netw Open. 2021;4(2):e211376. Erratum in: JAMA Netw Open. 2021;4(3):e212581.
36. Karakasis P, Patoulias D, Fragakis N, et al. Effect of glucagon-like peptide-1 receptor agonists and co-agonists on body composition: Systematic review and network meta-analysis. Metabolism. 2025;164:156113.
37. Ko A, Chang YC, Bahar F, et al. Risk for cancer with glucagon-like peptide-1 receptor agonists and dual agonists: a systematic review and meta-analysis. Ann Intern Med. 2025.
38. Pipek LZ, Moraes WAF, Nobetani RM, et al. Surgery is associated with better long-term outcomes than pharmacological treatment for obesity: a systematic review and meta-analysis. Sci Rep. 2024;14(1):9521.
39. Alabduljabbar K, le Roux CW. Pharmacotherapy before and after bariatric surgery. Metabolism. 2023;148:155692.
40. Vest AR, Schauer PR, Rodgers JE, et al. Obesity and weight loss strategies for patients with heart failure. JACC Heart Fail. 2024;12(9):1509-27.
41. Makary MA. Food and Drug Administration. [Online] Available from https://www.fda.gov/about-fda/fda-commissioner [Last accessed January, 2026].
42. Grunvald E, Shah R, Hernaez R, et al. AGA Clinical Practice Guideline on Pharmacological Interventions for Adults With Obesity. Gastroenterology. 2022;163(5):1198-225.
43. Pi-Sunyer X, Astrup A, Fujioka K, et al. A Randomized, Controlled Trial of 3.0 mg of Liraglutide in Weight Management. N Engl J Med. 2015;373(1):11-22.
44. In: Apovian CM, Aronne L, Powell AG (Eds). Clinical management of obesity. West Islip, NY: Professional Communications, Inc.; 2015.
45. Jastreboff AM, Aronne LJ, Ahmad NN, et al. Tirzepatide once weekly for the treatment of obesity. N Engl J Med. 2022;387(3):205-16.
46. Psaltis JP, Marathe JA, Nguyen MT, et al. Incretin-based therapies for the management of cardiometabolic disease in the clinic: Past, present, and future. Med Res Rev. 2025;45(1):29-65.
47. Gofron KK, Wasilewski A, Małgorzewicz S. Effects of GLP-1 Analogues and Agonists on the Gut Microbiota: A Systematic Review. Nutrients. 2025;17(8):1303.
48. Harris E. Oral Semaglutide Led to Similar Weight Loss as Injection, Company Says. JAMA. 2023;329(23):2011.
49. Jastreboff AM, Kaplan LM, Frías JP, et al. Triple-Hormone-Receptor Agonist Retatrutide for Obesity - A Phase 2 Trial. N Engl J Med. 2023;389(6):514-26.
50. Lau DCW, Erichsen L, Francisco AM, et al. Once-weekly cagrilintide for weight management in people with overweight and obesity: a multicentre, randomised, double-blind, placebo-controlled and active-controlled, dose-finding phase 2 trial. Lancet. 2021;398(10317):2160-72.

51. le Roux CW, Steen O, Lucas KJ, et al. Glucagon and GLP-1 receptor dual agonist survodutide for obesity: a randomised, double-blind, placebo-controlled, dose-finding phase 2 trial. Lancet Diabetes Endocrinol. 2024;12(3):162-73.
52. le Roux CW, Wharton S, Bozkurt B, et al. Survodutide for treatment of obesity: Baseline characteristics of participants in a randomized, double-blind, placebo-controlled, phase 3 trial (SYNCHRONIZE™-1). Diabetes Obes Metab. 2026;28(1):337-46.
53. Hanna MG, Badrising UA, Benveniste O, et al. Safety and efficacy of intravenous bimagrumab in inclusion body myositis (RESILIENT): a randomised, double-blind, placebo-controlled phase 2b trial. Lancet Neurol. 2019;18(9):834-44.
54. Prillaman M. The 'breakthrough' obesity drugs that have stunned researchers. Nature. 2023;613(7942):16-8.
55. Petricoul O, Nazarian A, Schuehly U, et al. Pharmacokinetics and Pharmacodynamics of Bimagrumab (BYM338). Clin Pharmacokinet. 2023;62(1):141-55.

65

CHAPTER

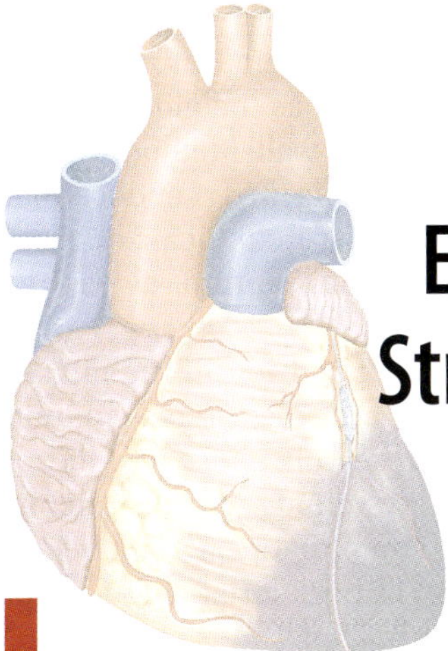

Echocardiography Evaluation of Left Atrial Strain after GLP-1 RA in Obese Heart Failure with Preserved Ejection Fraction

Amrish Agrawal, Omar Hallak, Wael Al Mahmeed, Thair Al Jumaily

INTRODUCTION

The left atrium (LA) plays a critical role in regulating left ventricular filling throughout diastole, particularly by delivering an LA boost toward the end of ventricular diastole. LA dysfunction independently predicts adverse cardiovascular outcomes, including heart failure (HF), myocardial infarction, atrial fibrillation (AF), and mortality.

Obesity, a global health issue affecting nearly half the population,[1] is closely linked to heart failure with preserved ejection fraction (HFpEF), with over half of HFpEF patients being obese. This association persists independently of traditional risk factors such as hypertension and diabetes.

Left atrium remodeling arises from the atrial myocytes' adaptive response to mechanical and metabolic stress, leading to hypertrophy, necrosis, and extracellular matrix changes. These alterations are detectable via echocardiographic techniques, including volumetric and Doppler methods. While LA size and volume remain standard metrics, strain imaging is increasingly valuable for assessing LA function, especially in evaluating HF therapies.

OBESITY AND HEART FAILURE WITH PRESERVED EJECTION FRACTION

Global estimates suggest that 39–49% of the population—around 2.8–3.5 billion people—are overweight or obese. In 2015, elevated body mass index (BMI) contributed to 4 million deaths, with cardiovascular disease (CVD) responsible for over two-thirds of them.[1] Obesity is strongly linked to conditions such as AF, HFpEF, and diastolic dysfunction. Registry data show that 55.7% of HFpEF patients are obese, and 42.5% also have metabolic syndrome.[2] Importantly, obesity remains an independent risk factor for HFpEF, even after adjusting for hypertension and diabetes. Obese individuals with HFpEF often present with additional comorbidities such as AF, hypertension, and chronic kidney disease.[3] This underscores the need for targeted interventions addressing both metabolic and hemodynamic contributors to HFpEF.

Several pathophysiological mechanisms explain this link:

- *Hemodynamic stress:* Excess body mass increases blood volume and cardiac output, promoting LV remodeling and impaired diastolic function.
- *Inflammation:* Adipose tissue drives systemic inflammation, reducing myocardial compliance.
- *Metabolic imbalance:* Insulin resistance and lipid abnormalities contribute to endothelial dysfunction and fibrosis.
- *Neurohormonal activation:* Obesity enhances sympathetic and RAAS activity, further compromising cardiac performance.

ADVANCES IN ECHOCARDIOGRAPHY FOR LEFT ATRIAL FUNCTION ASSESSMENT

Advancements in echocardiography have progressively refined how left atrial function is assessed.[4] Tissue Doppler imaging (TDI), less influenced by loading conditions, introduced A velocity as a marker of LA contractile function, correlating well with Doppler and volumetric measures. However, A velocity requires rhythm to be sinus, prompting the development of the LA function index (LAFI) to assess function even in AF. Left atrial volume index (LAVI) is also commonly used and tends to decrease with HF improvement, though it lacks sensitivity for tracking diastolic dysfunction.

Two-dimensional speckle-tracking echocardiography (2D-STE) allows angle-independent evaluation of myocardial deformation by tracking speckle movement during the cardiac cycle[5] and provides angle-free assessment of the atrial deformation. LA strain (LAS) derived from 2D-STE overcomes many limitations of earlier techniques. Strain reflects tissue deformation, while strain rate captures its temporal change. Both can be measured across the reservoir, conduit, and contractile phases of LA activity, enhancing early detection and prognostic accuracy in diastolic dysfunction.[6]

METHODOLOGY AND PITFALLS IN OBTAINING LEFT ATRIAL STRAIN

The 2018 EACVI/ASE/Industry Taskforce consensus document[6] recommends standardized LAS analysis using apical four-chamber views with high frame rates (50–70 fps). Segmentation of the LA wall is discouraged, as it may inadvertently include noncontractile regions such as the pulmonary veins and appendage, compromising strain accuracy. Biplane imaging remains optional. LA longitudinal strain is referred to as the global longitudinal strain (LA-GLS) of the entire wall. Methodological challenges for LAS include contouring the LA endocardial surface due to the thin LA wall, far-field localization of LA on echo, and mobile interatrial septum, as well as aneurysms.

Left atrial function is categorized into three phases aligned with the left ventricular cycle: Reservoir, conduit, and contraction. During the reservoir phase, the mitral valve is closed, and pulmonary venous return stretches the LA, producing a positive strain that peaks just before mitral valve opening—known as peak atrial longitudinal strain (PALS), a key prognostic marker.

The second phase, conduit phase, follows mitral valve opening, where passive LA emptying into the LV occurs (corresponding to the E wave), influenced by atrial and ventricular compliance. This results in a decline in strain with a negative deflection. The final contractile phase reflects active atrial systole (A wave), producing a second strain deflection—measured as peak atrial contraction strain (PACS), which occurs after the P wave and corresponds to active atrial contraction **(Fig. 1)**.

Strain analysis typically begins at the nadir, coinciding with mitral valve closure and the onset of ventricular systole at the onset of QRS. PALS reflects reservoir

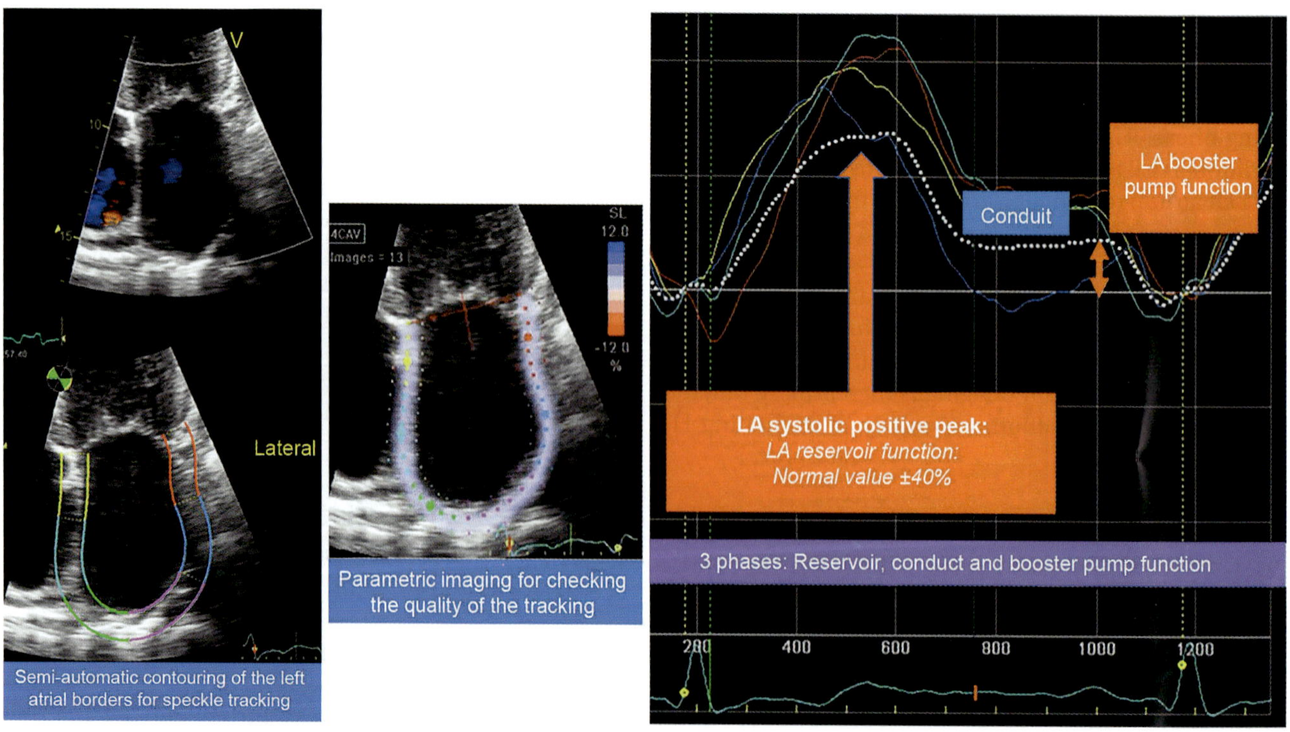

Fig. 1: Example of how to get left atrial strain for quantifying left atrial function.[7]

TABLE 1: Normal values of left atrial reservoir, conduit, and booster strain.[8]

Phasic left atrial strain	*Mean with 95% CI*
Left atrial reservoir strain (PALS)	39.4% (38–40.8)
Left atrial conduit strain (LAS-cd)	23% (20.7–25.2)
Left atrial booster or contractile strain (LAS-ct)	17.4% (16–19)

function, early diastolic strain indicates conduit activity, and PACS captures contractile performance. LAS values depend on image quality, acoustic window clarity, and ECG gating—preferably R-to-R—to minimize arrhythmia-related variability. Reference values for each phase are summarized in **Table 1**.[8]

SUPERIORITY OF LEFT ATRIAL STRAIN IN HEART FAILURE

Heart failure is an important condition that requires careful and detailed evaluation of the function of the left ventricle (LV) and the LA. Current European and American guidelines describe pEF as those with EF >50%. Though LA function is impaired in all subtypes of HF, assessment of diastolic dysfunction is very important in HFpEF and HFmEF, as it is its main pathophysiological mechanism.

Echocardiographic evaluation of diastolic dysfunction involves a complex, multiparametric approach incorporating transmitral flow, tissue Doppler velocities, left atrial volume index (LAVI), and estimated pulmonary artery pressures.[9] However, in advanced stages of dysfunction, the diagnostic utility of LAVI and E/e' ratio diminishes due to saturation effects and altered chamber compliance.

Progressive elevation in left ventricular filling pressures leads to structural and functional deterioration of the LA, including chamber dilatation and impaired contractility. Serial assessment of LAS offers a sensitive method to track disease progression and distinguish between stages of diastolic dysfunction. In early HFpEF, elevated LV pressures impair LA relaxation and reduce PALS. As severity advances, LAVI increases and contributes to the diagnostic framework for diastolic impairment.[9]

Singh et al.[10] found that an LAS cutoff of 19% separates grade III diastolic dysfunction with >90% accuracy, and an LAS threshold of >24% differentiates grade I from grade II or grade III diastolic dysfunction. It has also demonstrated utility in HFpEF patients as it is decreased in the early stages of the disease, being able to predict admissions, cardiovascular mortality, and sudden death.[11]

Atrial fibrillation is common in all categories of HF due to atrial overload, dilatation, and fibrosis. Atrial arrhythmias are common in patients with setting of HFpEF and restrictive cardiomyopathy, particularly in cardiac amyloidosis related to amyloid deposition. In a large cohort of patients with cardiac amyloidosis, Bandera et al.[12] found increased atrial stiffness and reduced left atrial reservoir and contraction function, which was independently associated with reduced clinical outcomes.

IMPACT OF OBESITY ON LEFT ATRIAL FUNCTION

Research has shown that LA enlargement often precedes AF, with BMI emerging as a strong predictor of LA size.[13] Obesity-related factors, such as elevated plasma volume, ventricular diastolic dysfunction, and increased neurohormonal activity, may contribute to LA enlargement and electrical instability.[14] Additionally, recent evidence links adiposity to direct myocardial alterations, possibly due to oxidative stress or inflammation **(Fig. 2)**.[15]

Obesity-induced structural and functional alterations in the LA may be reversible with lifestyle modification, particularly among young adults. In contrast, middle-aged individuals often exhibit more pronounced and potentially irreversible LA remodeling, increasing the risk of arrhythmias and cardiovascular complications, and the impact of lifestyle interventions tends to diminish with age. A study by Larios et al.[16] demonstrated that obese adolescents exhibit strain abnormalities in both the LA and LV, indicating early myocardial stress and subclinical cardiac dysfunction.

Steele et al.[17] evaluated early left atrial and left ventricular function in 331 individuals categorized by normal weight, obesity, and type 2 diabetes mellitus (T2DM). Using advanced echocardiographic modalities, the study demonstrated that both obese and T2DM groups exhibited significantly reduced atrial reservoir, conduit, and booster strain compared to normal-weight controls, despite comparable LA volumes. These findings underscore the adverse impact of obesity on LA function across age groups, with younger individuals showing greater potential for reversibility than middle-aged adults.

Singleton et al.[18] studied older obese HFpEF patients versus healthy controls using MRI cine imaging. They showed HFpEF patients had lower LA reservoir and conduit strain, higher LASt, and lower scores in exercise and quality of life measures compared to controls. LASt emerged as an independent predictor of reduced exercise ability and quality of life, suggesting that targeting LA dysfunction could benefit obese HFpEF patients.

Interestingly, LA function can be restored by weight loss. Aga et al.[19] found that in 77 obese participants and 46 matched controls, obese patients who had

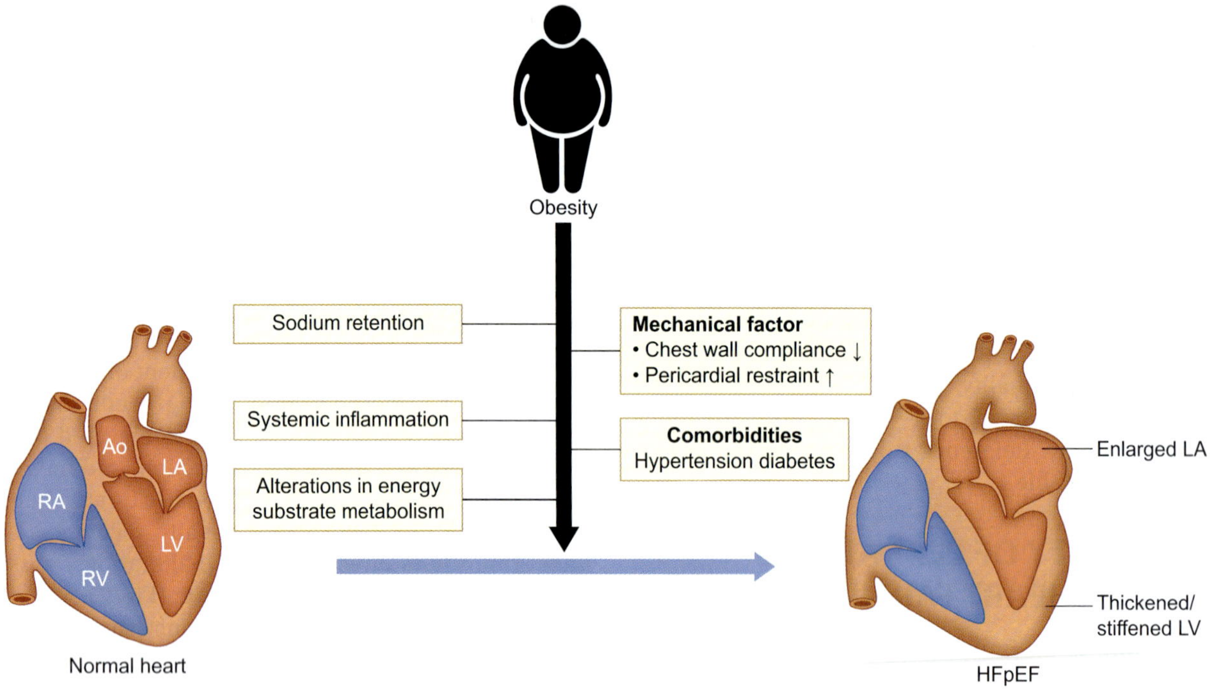

Fig. 2: Pathophysiology of obesity-related heart failure with preserved ejection fraction. (LA: left atrial; LV: left ventricular)
Source: Jung et al.[15]

bariatric surgery showed increased LA reservoir strain on echocardiography 1 year postsurgery. Multivariable analysis showed BMI independently reduced all LAS values, suggesting obesity could lead to HFpEF and that LA dysfunction may be reversible by weight loss. Given the adverse atrial remodeling observed in obesity-related HFpEF, therapeutic strategies targeting both metabolic and cardiac pathways are of growing interest.

CURRENT THERAPEUTIC RECOMMENDATIONS FOR TREATMENT OF HEART FAILURE WITH PRESERVED EJECTION FRACTION

Guideline-directed medical therapy (GDMT) has improved medical outcomes for patients with HFrEF. Class I recommendation medications include a beta blocker, ARNI (if not possible, then ACEi or ARB), mineralocorticoid receptor antagonist, and sodium-glucose cotransporter 2 inhibitors (SGLT2i). All the above drugs have been tested in the setting of HFpEF.

Currently, only SGLT2i carry a class I recommendation in the setting of HFpEF for strong evidence of reduced HF hospitalizations and improved QoL. ARNI are class IIa, and MRA are class IIb recommendation for HFpEF.

As of 2025, glucagon-like peptide-1 receptor agonists (GLP-1 RAs) are not yet included in formal ACC/AHA or ESC guidelines. But they are emerging as a promising adjunct therapy for HFpEF, especially in patients with obesity and type 2 diabetes, and accumulating evidence suggests they may offer incremental benefit in patients with obesity (BMI ≥27) and HFpEF phenotype with metabolic syndrome.[20,21]

DOES GLP-1 RA USE IMPACT HEART FAILURE WITH PRESERVED EJECTION FRACTION OUTCOMES?

The effects of GLP-1 RAs are exerted by binding to GLP-1 receptors distributed across multiple tissues. Beyond their antihyperglycemic properties, they delay gastric emptying and suppress hypothalamic appetite centers, promoting weight loss. Additional benefits include improved endothelial function, enhanced myocardial metabolism, natriuresis, anti-inflammatory effects, and blood pressure reduction. Among these, weight loss is particularly critical in obese HF patients, as excess visceral and epicardial adipose tissue (EAT), along with plasma volume expansion, contributes to significant hemodynamic burden both at rest and during exertion, directly impacting cardiac performance.

A meta-analysis of 22 RCTs[22] that included a considerably larger cohort ($n = 61{,}412$) of T2D patients with or without CVD and patients with CVD alone revealed that treatment with GLP-1 RAs led to improvements in diastolic function [E-wave; standardized mean difference −0.40; 95% CI (−0.60, −0.20); p <0.001], E/A ratio [WMD −0.10; 95% CI (−0.18, −0.02); p = 0.01], E/e' ratio [WMD −0.97; 95% CI (−1.54, −0.41); p <0.001], and E-wave DT [WMD −9.96 ms; 95% CI (−18.52, −1.41 ms); p = 0.02], although LVEF was not affected.

More promising evidence is available regarding GLP-1 RAs in obesity-related HFpEF. The benefits of semaglutide in obese HFpEF patients were established in the landmark STEP-HFpEF trial,[23] where patients receiving semaglutide experienced greater reductions in weight (estimated difference −10.7%; p <0.001) and increases in 6-minute walk test distance (estimated difference +20.3 m; p <0.001) compared with those in the control group. This result was confirmed by the recent pooled analysis of the STEP-HFpEF and STEP-HFpEF DM trials, which included 1,145 patients.[24]

The 2024 JACC HF study[20] evaluated the impact of adding GLP-1 RAs to SGLT2i therapy in patients with HFpEF, type 2 diabetes, and obesity (BMI ≥27). Using a large retrospective cohort from the TriNetX Global Research Network, the study matched 7,044 patients receiving both GLP-1 RA and SGLT2i with 7,044 patients on SGLT2i alone. Over a 12-month follow-up, the combination therapy group showed significantly lower rates of HF exacerbations [hazard ratio (HR) 0.62], all-cause hospitalizations and emergency visits (HR 0.74), and all-cause mortality (HR 0.64), suggesting incremental benefit beyond SGLT2i alone.

A meta-analysis[21] presented during the annual European Society of Cardiology meeting held in Madrid 2025, synthesized data from multiple key trials evaluating GLP-1 RAs in patients with HFpEF, such as SELECT, FLOW, STEP-HFpEF, and STEP-HFpEF DM, focusing on individuals with obesity, type 2 diabetes, and preserved ejection fraction. Across these trials, GLP-1 RAs demonstrated consistent reductions in HF events, inpatient days, and ICU admissions. Notably, the meta-analysis introduced a novel metric assessing the environmental footprint of care, showing that GLP-1 RA therapy may reduce healthcare resource utilization and its associated ecological impact.

IMPACT OF TREATMENT WITH GLP-1 RA ON LEFT ATRIAL STRAIN IN HEART FAILURE WITH PRESERVED EJECTION FRACTION

Emerging evidence suggests that treatment with GLP-1 RAs may positively influence LAS in patients with HFpEF, particularly those with obesity and metabolic dysfunction.[25] Although direct randomized trial data on LAS are limited, mechanistic studies and subgroup analyses from recent meta-analyses, including the 2025 Clinical Research in Cardiology review,[26] indicate that GLP-1 RAs may improve LA compliance and reservoir function by reducing systemic inflammation, improving endothelial function, and promoting weight loss.

What has been directly tested in HFpEF so far:

- In the STEP-HFpEF trial, semaglutide 2.4 mg improves symptoms (KCCQ), 6-minute walk distance, and weight in obesity-related HFpEF, but the parent trials did not report LAS.[27] The prespecified STEP-HFpEF echocardiography substudy showed favorable reverse remodeling after 52 weeks, most notably a reduction in LA volume.
- In the pooled STEP-HFpEF/STEP-HFpEF DM trials,[28] 491 participants underwent echo at baseline and at 52 weeks. The prespecified primary echocardiographic outcome was change in LA volume. Semaglutide attenuated regression of LA remodeling compared to placebo: Estimated mean difference in LA volume change = –6.13 mL (95% CI –9.85 to –2.41; p = 0.0013). Semaglutide also improved transmitral flow (E-wave velocity reduced by 5.63 cm/s; p = 0.0037) and E/e' average (EMD –0.79; borderline p = 0.05) versus placebo. However, LAS was not reported in that echo substudy. Reductions in LA volume and E/e' with semaglutide are directionally consistent with improved LA mechanics, but that is inference (a favorable milieu for strain change). Greater reduction in body weight with semaglutide was associated with greater reduction in LA volume (p interaction = 0.033).
- The clearest human data for LAS come from diabetic cohorts, not HFpEF per se. Katogiannis et al.[29] conducted a 6-month randomized study in 200 T2DM patients on metformin, comparing insulin (control) versus liraglutide versus empagliflozin versus their combination. They measured LA reservoir strain and LV global longitudinal strain by speckle tracking at baseline and 6 months. In the GLP-1 RA arm, LA reservoir strain increased from 30.7% ± 9.3 to 33.9% ± 9.7 (p = 0.011) versus essentially no change in the insulin arm (33.0 ± 8.3 to 32.8 ± 7.4; p = 0.829).

These agents appear to attenuate the adverse remodeling of the LA often seen in HFpEF, which is closely linked to elevated filling pressures and impaired diastolic function. In patients with concurrent AF, GLP-1 RAs were associated with greater reductions in HF hospitalizations, suggesting a potential link between improved LA mechanics and clinical outcomes. While LAS was not a primary endpoint in these studies, the observed benefits on atrial rhythm

TABLE 2: Impact of GLP-1 RAs on left atrial structure and function across HFpEF and metabolic disease cohorts.

Study/population	GLP-1 RA agent	Duration	LA volume change	LA strain change	Notes
STEP-HFpEF echo substudy[28]	Semaglutide 2.4 mg	52 weeks	−6.13 mL versus placebo ($p = 0.0013$)	Not reported	HFpEF, obesity phenotype
Katogiannis et al., T2DM[29]	Liraglutide	6 months	N/A	+3.2% absolute (30.7 → 33.9%) ($p = 0.011$)	Metabolic disease

stability and hemodynamics support further investigation into GLP-1 RA-mediated improvements in atrial function **(Table 2)**.

MECHANISTIC PLAUSIBILITY AND TRANSLATIONAL PATHWAYS

There are several biologically plausible mechanisms through which GLP-1 RAs may improve LAS in patients with HFpEF.[30]

First, GLP-1 RAs promote weight loss and reduce epicardial and pericardial adipose tissue, which in turn lowers cardiac filling pressures and wall stress, thereby alleviating preload and afterload burden on the LA. Second, improvements in left ventricular diastolic function—via enhanced myocardial relaxation and reduced stiffness—may diminish retrograde pressure transmission to the LA, preserving its compliance and reservoir capacity.

Third, preclinical studies suggest that GLP-1 RAs exert antiremodeling and antifibrotic effects through modulation of intracellular signaling pathways, including AMPK/mTOR and PKA/RhoA/ROCK, which may attenuate atrial hypertrophy and fibrosis. Finally, GLP-1 RAs have been shown to improve endothelial function and reduce oxidative stress and systemic inflammation, potentially benefiting atrial microvascular integrity and metabolic homeostasis.

These mechanisms collectively support the hypothesis that GLP-1 RAs may confer direct atrial benefits in HFpEF beyond their metabolic and hemodynamic effects.

CONCLUSION

In conclusion, echocardiographic evaluation of LAS offers a nuanced assessment of atrial function in HFpEF, particularly in obese phenotypes. Emerging data suggest that GLP-1 RAs may favorably influence LA mechanics through weight reduction, improved diastolic function, and anti-inflammatory signaling. While direct evidence in HFpEF remains limited, studies in diabetic populations demonstrate measurable improvements in LA reservoir strain, supporting the hypothesis of atrial remodeling benefits. Future trials incorporating speckle-tracking-derived LAS as a primary endpoint are essential to validate these mechanistic insights and guide personalized therapy in patients with obesity and metabolic dysfunction.

REFERENCES

1. Powell-Wiley TM, Poirier P, Burke LE, et al. Obesity and cardiovascular disease: a scientific statement from the American Heart Association. Circulation. 2021;143:e984-1010.
2. Bae J, Kallenbach L, Nelson D, et al. Obesity and metabolic syndrome in patients with heart failure with preserved ejection fraction: a cross-sectional analysis of the Veradigm Cardiology Registry. BMC Endocr Disord. 2024;24:59.
3. Borlaug B, Jensen M, Kitzman D, et al. Obesity and heart failure with preserved ejection fraction: new insights and pathophysiological targets. Cardiovasc Res. 2022;118:3434-50.
4. Hoit BD. Left atrial size and function: role in prognosis. J Am Coll Cardiol. 2014;63:493-505.
5. Gan G, Ferkh A, Boyd A, et al. Left atrial function: evaluation by strain analysis. Cardiovasc Diagn Ther. 2018;8:29-46.
6. Badano L, Kolias T, Muraru D, et al. Standardization of left atrial, right ventricular, and right atrial deformation imaging using two-dimensional speckle tracking echocardiography: a consensus document of the EACVI/ASE/Industry Task Force to standardize deformation imaging. Eur Heart J Cardiovasc Imaging. 2018;19:591-600.
7. Thomas L, Muraru D, Popescu B, et al. Evaluation of left atrial size and function: relevance for clinical practice. J Am Soc Echocardiogr. 2020;33:934-52.
8. Pathan F, D'Elia N, Nolan MT, et al. Normal ranges of left atrial strain by speckle-tracking echocardiography: a systematic review and meta-analysis. J Am Soc Echocardiogr. 2017;30:59-70.
9. Nagueh SF, Smiseth OA, Appleton CP, et al. Recommendations for the evaluation of left ventricular diastolic function by echocardiography: an update from the American Society of Echocardiography and the European Association of Cardiovascular Imaging. J Am Soc Echocardiogr. 2016;29:277-314.
10. Singh A, Medvedofsky D, Mediratta A, et al. Peak left atrial strain as a single measure for the non-invasive assessment of left ventricular filling pressures. Int J Cardiovasc Imaging. 2019;35:23-32.

11. Fan J, Su B, Zhao X, et al. Correlation of left atrial strain with left ventricular end-diastolic pressure in patients with normal left ventricular ejection fraction. Int J Cardiovasc Imaging. 2020;36:1659-66.
12. Bandera F, Martone R, Chacko L, et al. Clinical importance of left atrial infiltration in cardiac transthyretin amyloidosis. JACC Cardiovasc Imaging. 2021;15:17-29.
13. Wang TJ, Parise H, Levy D, et al. Obesity and the risk of new-onset atrial fibrillation. JAMA. 2004;292:2471-7.
14. Engeli S, Sharma AM. The renin-angiotensin system and natriuretic peptides in obesity-associated hypertension. J Mol Med (Berl). 2001;79:21-9.
15. Jung M-H, Shin M-S. Obesity-related heart failure with preserved ejection fraction: diagnostic and therapeutic challenges. Korean J Int Med. 2023;38(2):157-66.
16. Larios G, Uribe S, Trincado C, et al. Myocardial function, mechanics and work by echocardiography in adolescents with severe obesity. Cardiovasc Endocrinol Metab. 2024;13:e0301.
17. Steele J, Urbina E, Mazur W, et al. Left atrial strain and diastolic function abnormalities in obese and type 2 diabetic adolescents and young adults. Cardiovasc Diabetol. 2020;19:163.
18. Singleton M, Nelson M, Samuel T, et al. Left atrial stiffness index independently predicts exercise intolerance and quality of life in older, obese patients with heart failure with preserved ejection fraction. J Card Fail. 2022;28:567-75.
19. Aga Y, Kroon D, Snelder S, et al. Decreased left atrial function in obesity patients without known cardiovascular disease. Int J Cardiovasc Imaging. 2023;39:471-9.
20. Patel R, Wadid M, Makwana B, et al. GLP-1 receptor agonists among patients with overweight or obesity, diabetes, and HFpEF on SGLT2 inhibitors. JACC Heart Fail. 2024;12:1814-26.
21. Makwana B, et al. Environmental impact of novel anti-obesity medications on healthcare-related greenhouse gas emissions in patients with heart failure with preserved ejection fraction. ESC Congress 2025, abstract 86569.
22. Huixing L, Di F, Daoquan P. Effect of glucagon-like peptide-1 receptor agonists on prognosis of heart failure and cardiac function: a systematic review and meta-analysis of randomized controlled trials. Clin Ther. 2023;45:17-30.
23. Kosiborod M, Abildstrøm S, Borlaug B, et al. Semaglutide in patients with heart failure with preserved ejection fraction and obesity. N Engl J Med. 2023;389:1069-84.
24. Butler J, Shah S, Petrie M, et al. Semaglutide versus placebo in people with obesity-related heart failure with preserved ejection fraction: a pooled analysis of the STEP-HFpEF and STEP-HFpEF DM randomized trials. Lancet. 2024;403:1635-48.
25. Yang H-M. GLP-1 agonists in cardiovascular diseases: mechanisms, clinical evidence, and emerging therapies. J Clin Med. 2025;14(19):6758.
26. Gonzales-Uribe A, Ruiz-Cortez R, Collantes-Silva N, et al. Impact of GLP-1 receptor agonists on cardiovascular outcomes in heart failure with preserved ejection fraction (HFpEF): systematic review and meta-analysis. Clin Res Cardiol. 2025.
27. Kelly AS, Abildstrøm SZ, Borlaug BA, et al. Semaglutide in patients with obesity-related heart failure with preserved ejection fraction. N Engl J Med. 2023;389:1211-21.
28. Solomon SD, Ostrominski JW, Wang X, et al. Effect of semaglutide on cardiac structure and function in patients with obesity-related heart failure. J Am Coll Cardiol. 2024;84:1592-1604.
29. Katogiannis K, Thymis J, Kousathana F, et al. Effects of liraglutide, empagliflozin and their combination on left atrial strain and arterial function. Medicina (Kaunas). 2024;60:395.
30. Jalil J, Gabriclli L, Ocaranza M, et al. New mechanisms to prevent heart failure with preserved ejection fraction using glucagon-like peptide-1 receptor agonism (GLP-1 RA) in metabolic syndrome and in type 2 diabetes: a review. Int J Mol Sci. 2024;25:4407.

66

CHAPTER

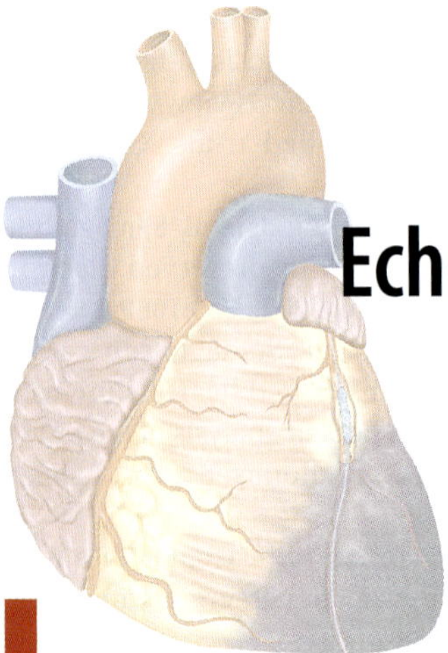

Echocardiographic Evaluation of Atrial Strain Regression by SGLT2 Inhibitors and GLP-1 Receptor Agonists

Aniruddha De

INTRODUCTION

This chapter provides a comprehensive review of advanced echocardiographic assessment of atrial strain parameters in diabetic patients, with particular focus on therapeutic regression induced by sodium-glucose cotransporter-2 (SGLT2) inhibitors and glucagon-like peptide-1 receptor agonist (GLP-1RA). As novel cardioprotective agents, these medications demonstrate significant benefits beyond glycemic control, offering profound implications for cardiovascular risk reduction in diabetic cardiomyopathy.

DIABETES, HEART FAILURE, AND THE ROLE OF ATRIAL STRAIN

Global Diabetes Burden

Diabetes mellitus affects over 9% of the global population, representing a major public health challenge with profound cardiovascular implications. The International Diabetes Federation reports escalating prevalence worldwide, particularly in aging populations.[1]

Early Cardiac Involvement

Diabetic cardiomyopathy manifests early as diastolic dysfunction and atrial remodeling, detectable by advanced imaging modalities before overt clinical heart failure develops. These subclinical changes predict future cardiovascular events.[2,3]

Atrial Strain Assessment

Left atrial strain by speckle tracking echocardiography is emerging as a sensitive marker of atrial function and powerful predictor of adverse outcomes in diabetic patients, offering superior prognostic value compared to conventional parameters.[4]

The intersection of diabetes and cardiovascular disease represents a critical frontier in contemporary cardiology. Recognition of early myocardial dysfunction through advanced imaging techniques enables targeted therapeutic interventions that may prevent progression to symptomatic heart failure. This chapter explores how novel antidiabetic medications are transforming our approach to cardioprotection in this vulnerable population.

PATHOPHYSIOLOGY OF ATRIAL DYSFUNCTION IN DIABETES MELLITUS

The pathophysiological cascade linking diabetes to atrial dysfunction involves multiple interconnected mechanisms. Chronic hyperglycemia induces myocardial fibrosis through advanced glycation end-product accumulation, oxidative stress via mitochondrial dysfunction, and microvascular rarefaction. These processes collectively impair atrial compliance and contractility, establishing a substrate for both functional and structural remodeling.[5,6]

Left atrial remodeling contributes substantially to elevated filling pressures, increases atrial fibrillation risk through electromechanical dissociation, and accelerates progression of heart failure with preserved or mildly reduced ejection fraction. The atrium serves as a barometer of chronic diastolic stress, with impaired reservoir function indicating chronic pressure overload and reduced contractile function suggesting intrinsic myopathic changes.[7]

Clinical Significance

Early detection of LA strain abnormalities through speckle tracking echocardiography can guide timely therapeutic interventions, potentially preventing irreversible structural changes and clinical decompensation.[3]

- *Hyperglycemia:* Sustained elevation in glucose levels initiates metabolic stress
- *Oxidative injury:* Free radical generation damages myocardial tissue
- *Fibrotic remodeling:* Collagen deposition impairs atrial mechanics
- *Clinical manifestation:* Progressive heart failure and arrhythmia risk

SPECKLE TRACKING ECHOCARDIOGRAPHY: PRINCIPLES AND PARAMETERS OF ATRIAL STRAIN

Speckle tracking echocardiography represents a quantum advancement in noninvasive cardiac imaging, quantifying myocardial deformation by tracking natural acoustic markers ("speckles") in a frame-by-frame analysis throughout the cardiac cycle. This angle-independent technique overcomes limitations of Doppler-based methods, providing objective assessment of regional and global myocardial function.[8]

- *Reservoir strain:* LA filling during ventricular systole reflects atrial compliance and conduit function.
- *Conduit strain:* Passive emptying during early diastole indicates LA-LV pressure gradient
- *Contractile strain:* Active atrial contraction in late diastole demonstrates intrinsic function
- *Technical considerations:*
  - High frame rate acquisition (60–90 fps) essential for accurate tracking
  - Optimal image quality requires focused atrial views
  - Semiautomated border detection with manual adjustment
  - Vendor-specific software with evolving standardization

Clinical Application

Normal reference values have been established through multicenter studies, enabling clinical application across diverse populations. Reproducibility metrics demonstrate excellent intra- and interobserver agreement when standardized protocols are followed, supporting integration into routine practice.[9]

SODIUM-GLUCOSE COTRANSPORTER-2 INHIBITORS: MECHANISMS BEYOND GLYCEMIC CONTROL

Initially developed for glucose lowering through renal mechanisms, SGLT2 inhibitors have emerged as transformative cardiovascular therapeutics. Landmark trials including EMPEROR-Reduced, EMPEROR-Preserved, and DAPA-HF demonstrated dramatic reductions in heart failure hospitalizations and cardiovascular mortality across the ejection fraction spectrum, remarkably independent of diabetic status.[10]

- *Natriuresis:* Enhanced sodium and water excretion reduces preload and ventricular filling pressures, decreasing atrial wall stress
- *Hemodynamic effects:* Modest blood pressure reduction and decreased systemic vascular resistance improve cardiac efficiency
- *Metabolic optimization:* Shift toward ketone body utilization enhances myocardial energetics and contractile function
- *Antifibrotic action:* Direct myocardial effects reduce collagen deposition and promote reverse remodeling

"The 2023 European Society of Cardiology guidelines now recommend SGLT2 inhibitors as first-line therapy in heart failure with preserved and mildly reduced ejection fraction, reflecting the paradigm shift in heart failure management."[11]

The pleiotropic mechanisms underlying SGLT2 inhibitor cardioprotection extend far beyond glucose control, encompassing hemodynamic, metabolic, neurohormonal, and direct myocardial effects that collectively improve outcomes across the heart failure spectrum.

GLUCAGON-LIKE PEPTIDE-1 RECEPTOR AGONISTS: CARDIOPROTECTIVE EFFECTS

Glycemic Optimization

Glucagon-like peptide-1 receptor agonists enhance glucose-dependent insulin secretion, suppress inappropriate glucagon release, and slow gastric emptying, achieving excellent glycemic control with low hypoglycemia risk. Weight loss effects further improve metabolic parameters.[12]

Anti-inflammatory Actions

Reduction in systemic inflammatory markers including C-reactive protein and interleukin-6 contributes to vascular protection. Direct effects on immune cell function modulate atherosclerotic plaque stability and reduce vascular inflammation.[13]

Vascular Benefits

Improved endothelial function, reduced arterial stiffness, and antiatherosclerotic effects protect against macrovascular complications. Blood pressure reduction occurs through multiple mechanisms including natriuresis and improved vascular compliance.

Direct Myocardial Effects

Glucagon-like peptide-1 receptors expressed in cardiomyocytes mediate direct protective effects including enhanced myocardial glucose uptake, reduced apoptosis, and improved contractile function. Cardioprotection against ischemia-reperfusion injury has been demonstrated in experimental models.

Major cardiovascular outcomes trials including LEADER, SUSTAIN-6, and REWIND demonstrated significant reductions in major adverse cardiovascular events among high-risk diabetic patients treated with GLP-1RAs. The cardiovascular benefits appear to be a class effect, though magnitude varies across specific agents. Their impact on atrial function and strain parameters represents an active and rapidly evolving area of investigation.[14]

CLINICAL EVIDENCE: IMPACT OF SGLT2 INHIBITOR ON LEFT ATRIAL STRAIN

Emerging clinical evidence demonstrates significant favorable effects of SGLT2 inhibitor therapy on left atrial strain parameters. A prospective observational study by Katogiannis and colleagues enrolled 70 patients with heart failure with mildly reduced ejection fraction and type 2 diabetes mellitus (T2DM), evaluating echocardiographic parameters before and after 6 months of SGLT2 inhibitor therapy with empagliflozin or dapagliflozin.[15,16]

The study revealed statistically significant improvements across all three phases of atrial function: reservoir strain increased by 40.7%, conduit strain improved by 45.9%, and contractile strain enhanced by 34.5%. These changes occurred in parallel with reductions in left atrial volume index and improvements in diastolic function parameters, particularly the E/e2 ratio, which decreased from 13.4 to 10.2, indicating reduced filling pressures.[2,17]

Mechanistic Insights

The improvements in atrial strain correlated strongly with enhanced left ventricular global longitudinal strain (LV GLS), suggesting coordinated reverse remodeling of both chambers. Volume unloading effects reduced atrial wall stress, while metabolic improvements enhanced myocardial contractility.

Clinical Implications

These findings provide objective evidence supporting SGLT2 inhibitors' role in reversing diabetic atrial remodeling and improving overall cardiac mechanics, with potential implications for reducing atrial fibrillation risk and heart failure progression **(Fig. 1)**.

CLINICAL EVIDENCE: GLUCAGON-LIKE PEPTIDE-1 RECEPTOR AGONIST EFFECTS ON ATRIAL AND VENTRICULAR STRAIN

Complementary evidence demonstrates beneficial effects of GLP-1RA therapy on atrial strain parameters. In a randomized controlled trial conducted by Ielapi and colleagues, 200 patients with T2DM were randomized to liraglutide versus insulin therapy, with comprehensive echocardiographic assessment performed at baseline and 6 months.[18]

Liraglutide Monotherapy

Patients receiving liraglutide demonstrated significant improvements in LA reservoir strain (21.3–28.7%, $p < 0.001$) and LA conduit strain (11.2–15.8%, $p < 0.001$) compared to insulin-treated controls who showed minimal change.

Combination Therapy

A subset receiving combination therapy with empagliflozin plus liraglutide showed additive benefits, with LA reservoir strain reaching 31.4% and greater reductions in arterial stiffness measured by pulse wave velocity (8.9–7.2 m/s).[6,19]

Vascular-cardiac Coupling

Improvements in LA strain correlated significantly with reductions in pulse wave velocity and central systolic

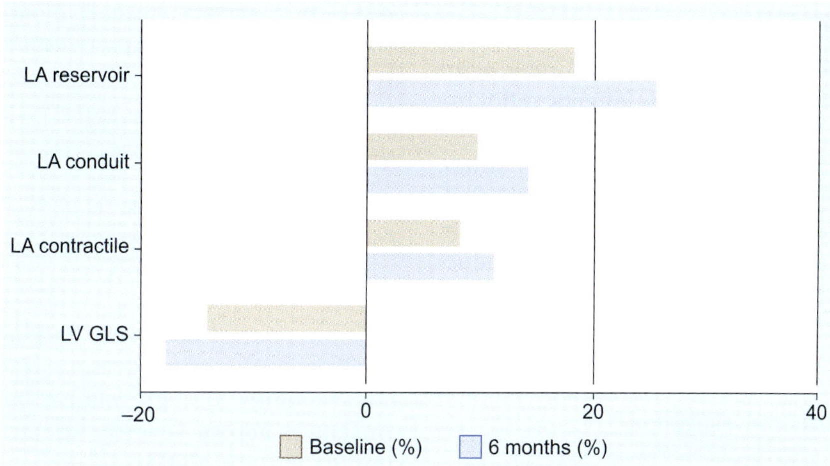

Fig. 1: Comparison of baseline and 6-month values of left atrial reservoir, conduit, and contractile strain, and left ventricular global longitudinal strain (LV GLS).

blood pressure, linking vascular and myocardial benefits through improved ventricular-arterial coupling and reduced atrial afterload.

Additional mechanistic insights emerged from subgroup analyses. Patients with higher baseline inflammatory markers (hs-CRP >3 mg/L) experienced greater improvements in atrial strain, suggesting anti-inflammatory mechanisms contribute to cardiac benefits. Weight loss correlated modestly with strain improvement but did not fully account for the observed effects, indicating direct myocardial actions independent of metabolic improvements.[20]

Synergistic Effects

The superior outcomes with combination therapy suggest complementary mechanisms: SGLT2 inhibitors primarily through hemodynamic and metabolic pathways, and GLP-1RAs through anti-inflammatory and direct myocardial effects. This provides rationale for dual therapy in high-risk patients.

COMPARATIVE EFFECTS OF SGLT2 INHIBITOR AND GLUCAGON-LIKE PEPTIDE-1 RECEPTOR AGONIST ON ATRIAL FUNCTION

Sodium-glucose Cotransporter-2 Inhibitors

- Predominant effects on volume status through natriuresis
- Rapid hemodynamic benefits within days to weeks
- Stronger effects on reducing systemic vascular resistance
- Direct myocardial metabolic effects via ketone utilization
- Consistent benefits across ejection fraction spectrum

Glucagon-like Peptide-1 Receptor Agonists

- Predominant effects on volume status through natriuresis
- Rapid hemodynamic benefits within days to weeks
- Stronger effects on reducing systemic vascular resistance
- Direct myocardial metabolic effects via ketone utilization
- Consistent benefits across ejection fraction spectrum

Volume Effects

Sodium-glucose cotransporter-2 inhibitors produce more pronounced volume unloading, particularly beneficial in hypervolemic states.

Metabolic Impact

Both classes improve myocardial energetics through distinct pathways and ketones versus enhanced glucose utilization.

Combination Therapy

Additive or synergistic benefits suggest complementary mechanisms and potential for superior outcomes.

Anti-inflammatory

Glucagon-like peptide-1 receptor agonist may exert stronger systemic anti-inflammatory effects reducing fibrotic remodeling.

While both drug classes improve LA reservoir strain, SGLT2 inhibitors may exert stronger early effects through volume unloading and vascular resistance reduction, while GLP-1RAs may additionally enhance atrial conduction velocity and demonstrate more gradual but sustained myocardial energetic improvements. Combination therapy appears particularly promising for synergistic cardioprotection, though optimal patient selection and sequencing require further investigation.[21]

ECHOCARDIOGRAPHIC ASSESSMENT OF LEFT VENTRICULAR STRAIN IN DIABETES

Left ventricular global longitudinal strain represents the most sensitive echocardiographic parameter for detecting early systolic dysfunction in diabetic cardiomyopathy. Unlike ejection fraction, which remains preserved until advanced disease stages, LV GLS identifies subclinical abnormalities years before clinical manifestations. Normal LV GLS values exceed –18%, with impairment defined as values greater than –16% in absolute magnitude.[8,22,23]

Subclinical Dysfunction

Left ventricular global longitudinal strain impairment detected in asymptomatic diabetic patients with preserved EF, indicating early cardiomyopathy.

Sodium-glucose Cotransporter-2 Inhibitor Treatment

Six months of empagliflozin or dapagliflozin improves LV GLS by 15–25%, with parallel NT-proBNP reductions.

Glucagon-like Peptide-1 Receptor Agonists Effects

Liraglutide, semaglutide, and dulaglutide improve LV GLS after 6 months, supporting direct myocardial benefits.

Reverse Remodeling

Sustained improvements indicate true reverse remodeling rather than transient hemodynamic effects.

The magnitude of LV GLS improvement with SGLT2 inhibitor and GLP-1RA therapy correlates with baseline strain impairment, NT-proBNP levels, and degree of glycemic control achieved. Patients with more severe baseline dysfunction demonstrate greater absolute improvements, though relative improvements remain consistent across severity spectrum. These findings support early initiation in diabetic patients with any evidence of ventricular dysfunction **(Table 1)**.[24]

TABLE 1: Changes in echocardiographic and biomarker parameters from baseline to post-treatment.

Parameter	*Baseline*	*Post-treatment*
LV GLS (%)	–14.2 ± 2.1	–17.9 ± 2.3
NT-proBNP (pg/mL)	842 ± 321	486 ± 198
LVEF (%)	48 ± 6	52 ± 5
E/e2 ratio	13.6 ± 3.2	10.8 ± 2.4

HEMODYNAMIC AND VASCULAR EFFECTS UNDERLYING ATRIAL STRAIN IMPROVEMENT

Mechanisms of Cardiovascular Benefit

The improvements in atrial strain observed with SGLT2 inhibitor and GLP-1RA therapy reflect complex interactions between hemodynamic, vascular, and direct myocardial effects.

Understanding these mechanisms provides insight into therapeutic efficacy and guides clinical application.[25]

- *Afterload reduction:* Decreased systemic vascular resistance and arterial stiffness reduce LA afterload during reservoir phase.
- *Preload optimization:* Volume unloading via natriuresis decreases atrial wall stress and improves compliance
- *Vascular function:* Improved endothelial function and reduced inflammation enhance overall cardiovascular coupling.
- *Heart failure subtypes:* Early hemodynamic changes differ by heart failure phenotype. In HFrEF and HFmrEF, volume unloading predominates with rapid improvements in filling pressures. In HFpEF, vascular resistance reduction and improved arterial compliance represent primary mechanisms, with more gradual strain improvements reflecting reverse remodeling of chronic pressure overload.[26]
- *Timeline of effects:*
  - SGLT2 inhibitors produce measurable hemodynamic benefits within days, with strain improvements detectable at 3 months and continuing to accrue over 6–12 months. GLP-1RAs demonstrate more gradual effects, with peak strain

improvements at 6–9 months, correlating with weight loss and inflammatory marker reductions.

- The multifaceted hemodynamic and vascular effects of these agents create optimal conditions for myocardial recovery, reducing both the initiating stresses and perpetuating factors that drive progressive atrial remodeling in diabetes.

INTEGRATION OF ATRIAL STRAIN IN CLINICAL PRACTICE AND PROGNOSIS

Left atrial strain assessment has emerged as a powerful prognostic tool in diabetic patients, providing risk stratification beyond traditional echocardiographic parameters. Multiple studies demonstrate that impaired LA reservoir strain independently predicts atrial fibrillation development, heart failure hospitalizations, stroke, and all-cause mortality in diabetic populations.[27,28]

- *2.4x AF risk:* Relative risk increases for new-onset atrial fibrillation with LA reservoir strain <18% in diabetic patients
- *1.8x HF hospitalization:* Hazard ratio for heart failure admission per 5% decrease in LA reservoir strain over 3-year follow-up.
- *64% event-free survival:* Three-year composite endpoint-free survival in patients with preserved LA strain (>23%) on optimal therapy **(Table 2)**.
- *Baseline assessment:* Obtain LA strain in all diabetic patients with suspected cardiac involvement or cardiovascular risk factors.
- *Risk stratification:* Integrate strain values with clinical parameters, biomarkers, and other imaging to determine risk profile.
- *Serial monitoring:* Reassess strain at 6–12 months to evaluate treatment response and guide therapy adjustments.
- *Outcome tracking:* Monitor clinical endpoints including symptoms, exercise capacity, biomarkers, and hospitalizations.

Incorporation of atrial strain assessment into routine echocardiographic protocols is increasingly recommended by expert consensus documents and clinical practice guidelines. Standardized reporting including all three strain phases enhances clinical utility and enables meaningful serial comparisons to guide therapeutic decision-making.[29]

TABLE 2: Normal ranges and abnormal thresholds for left atrial (LA) strain parameters and left ventricular global longitudinal strain (LV GLS).

Strain parameter	*Normal range*	*Abnormal threshold*
LA reservoir strain	23–39%	<18%
LA conduit strain	13–22%	<10%
LA contractile strain	10–17%	<8%
LV GLS	<–18%	>–16%

LIMITATIONS AND CHALLENGES IN ATRIAL STRAIN IMAGING

Technical Variability

Significant variability exists between vendor-specific software platforms, with absolute strain values differing by 10–20% despite similar relative changes. Lack of universal standardization limits comparability across institutions and hampers establishment of unified reference values. Ongoing efforts toward vendor-neutral analysis algorithms show promise but remain incomplete.[30]

Image Quality Dependence

Accurate strain measurement requires high-quality two-dimensional images with clear endocardial definition. Obesity, lung disease, and chest wall abnormalities commonly present in diabetic populations frequently compromise image acquisition. Poor acoustic windows necessitate contrast enhancement or alternative imaging modalities in 15–20% of patients.

Rhythm Considerations

Atrial fibrillation and frequent ectopy significantly affect atrial strain measurement accuracy and interpretation. Averaging across multiple cardiac cycles improves reproducibility but may not fully capture dynamic changes. Strain assessment during sinus rhythm provides most reliable data, though this limitation excludes many high-risk patients.

Clinical Validation Gaps

While prognostic value is established, optimal strain thresholds for therapeutic intervention require validation. Large-scale, multicenter prospective studies with standardized protocols and hard clinical endpoints remain necessary to define treatment targets and demonstrate outcome improvements with strain-guided therapy.

Practical Recommendations

Until complete standardization is achieved, institutions should maintain consistency by using the same vendor platform and analysis software for serial studies in individual patients. Reporting both absolute values and percent changes enhances interpretability and clinical utility.

Despite these limitations, atrial strain imaging provides valuable incremental information beyond conventional parameters. Awareness of technical considerations and appropriate quality control measures enable reliable clinical application in properly selected patients.

DIRECTIONS: NOVEL IMAGING AND THERAPEUTIC STRATEGIES: THE EVOLVING LANDSCAPE

Advanced Imaging Modalities

Three-dimensional speckle tracking echocardiography overcomes geometric assumptions of two-dimensional techniques, providing true volumetric strain assessment. Early validation studies demonstrate improved reproducibility and stronger prognostic associations. Cardiac magnetic resonance strain imaging with feature tracking offers superior tissue characterization, detecting fibrosis and edema that influence mechanical function.[31]

Artificial Intelligence Integration

Machine learning algorithms are being developed for automated atrial border detection, strain calculation, and quality control. AI-based approaches may reduce measurement variability, accelerate analysis workflow, and identify subtle patterns predictive of outcomes. Validation against expert readers and clinical endpoints is ongoing.

Ongoing clinical trials are evaluating long-term effects of SGLT2 inhibitors and GLP-1RAs on atrial remodeling and clinical endpoints including atrial fibrillation and stroke. Emerging combination therapies and novel agents targeting specific pathophysiological pathways promise further advances in preventing and reversing diabetic cardiac remodeling **(Fig. 2)**.[32]

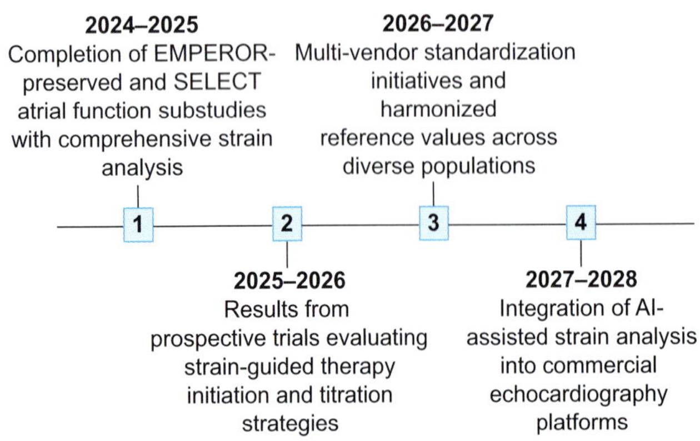

Fig. 2: Roadmap for the evolution of strain-guided cardiometabolic imaging (2024–2028).

The convergence of advanced imaging technologies, precision therapeutics, and personalized medicine approaches will transform our ability to prevent and treat diabetic cardiovascular complications in the coming decade.

CASE STUDIES: ECHOCARDIOGRAPHIC IMPROVEMENT OF ATRIAL STRAIN WITH SGLT2 INHIBITOR AND GLP-1 RECEPTOR AGONIST

Case 1: SGLT2 Inhibitor Monotherapy in HFmrEF

An elderly patient with 12-year history of T2DM, coronary artery disease, and hypertension presented with exertional dyspnea NYHA class II. Baseline echocardiography revealed LVEF 48%, E/e' 14.2, and severely impaired LA reservoir strain of 13%. LV GLS was –13.2%. NT-proBNP measured 986 pg/mL. He was initiated on empagliflozin 10 mg daily in addition to guideline-directed medical therapy.

Baseline Parameters

- *LA reservoir strain:* 13%
- *LA conduit strain:* –6%
- *LA contractile strain:* –7%
- *LA volume index:* 42 mL/m^2
- *LV GLS:* –13.2%

Six-month Follow-up

- *LA reservoir strain:* 35% (marked increase)
- *LA conduit strain:* –19% (+46% increase)
- *LA contractile strain:* –16% (+77% increase)
- *LA volume index:* 33 mL/m^2 (–21% decrease)
- *LV GLS:* –17.8% (+34% improvement)

Clinical status improved to NYHA class I with NT-proBNP declining to 423 pg/mL. This case illustrates substantial reverse remodeling achievable with SGLT2 inhibitor therapy, with coordinated improvements in atrial and ventricular mechanics reflecting comprehensive cardioprotection **(Figs. 3A and B)**.

Case 2: GLP-1 Receptor Agonist with Vascular Effects

A 58-year-old female with 8-year history of type 2 diabetes, obesity (BMI of 34), and metabolic syndrome presented for cardiovascular risk assessment. Despite preserved LVEF of 58%, she demonstrated subclinical cardiac dysfunction with LA reservoir strain of 21% and elevated arterial stiffness (pulse wave velocity 10.4 m/s). Liraglutide

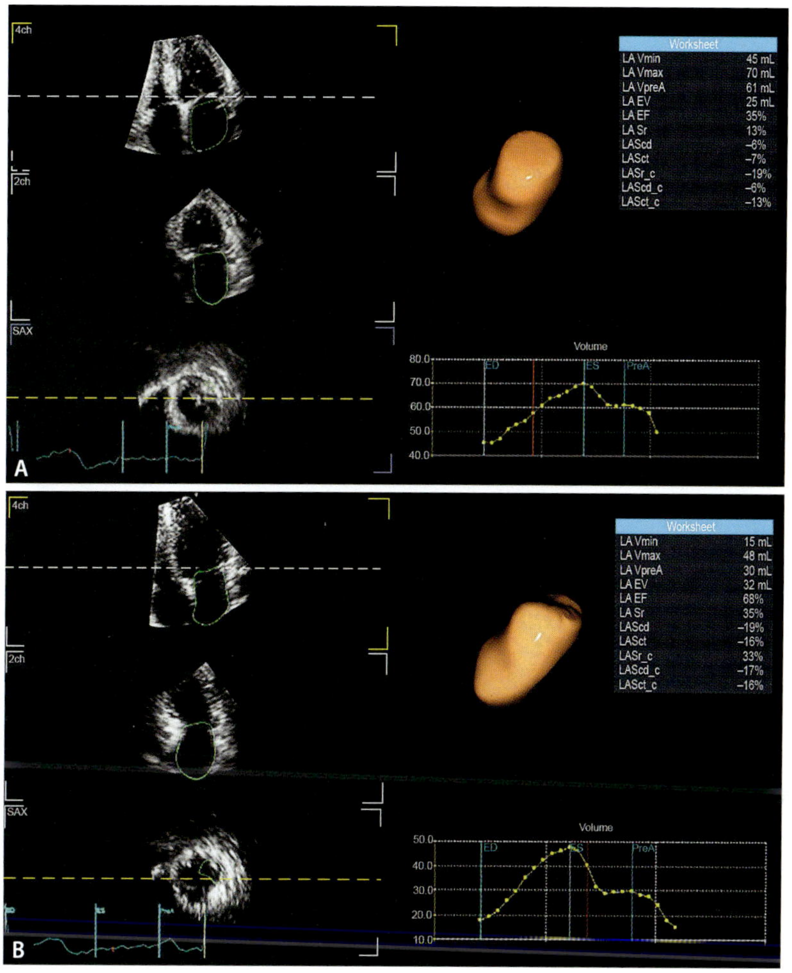

Figs. 3A and B: (A) Before SGLT2 inhibitor therapy and (B) After SGLT2 inhibitor therapy.

1.8 mg daily was initiated for glycemic control and weight management. Six-month follow-up revealed LA reservoir strain improvement to 32%, conduit strain increase from 8% to 24%, and pulse wave velocity reduction to 8.2 m/s. Central systolic blood pressure decreased from 146 to 124 mm Hg. She achieved 9.4 kg weight loss with improved exercise tolerance. This case demonstrates GLP-1RA effects on atrial mechanics correlating with vascular function improvements, highlighting the integrated cardiovascular benefits extending beyond glycemic control **(Figs. 4A and B)**.

SUMMARY OF KEY CLINICAL TRIALS AND META-ANALYSES (FIG. 5)

EMPEROR-Preserved

Empagliflozin reduced HF hospitalizations and CV death in HFpEF (HR: 0.79, $p < 0.001$).

Substudy analysis demonstrated LA strain improvements correlating with clinical benefits, supporting mechanistic link between atrial function and outcomes.[33]

DELIVER

Dapagliflozin showed consistent benefits across HFmrEF and HFpEF spectrum. Echocardiographic substudy revealed improvements in diastolic parameters and atrial remodeling markers, with greater effects in diabetic subgroup.

LEADER and SUSTAIN-6

Glucagon-like peptide-1 receptor agonists (liraglutide and semaglutide) reduced MACE in high-risk T2DM patients. Post hoc analyses linked cardiovascular benefits to improvements in myocardial strain and vascular function parameters.[14]

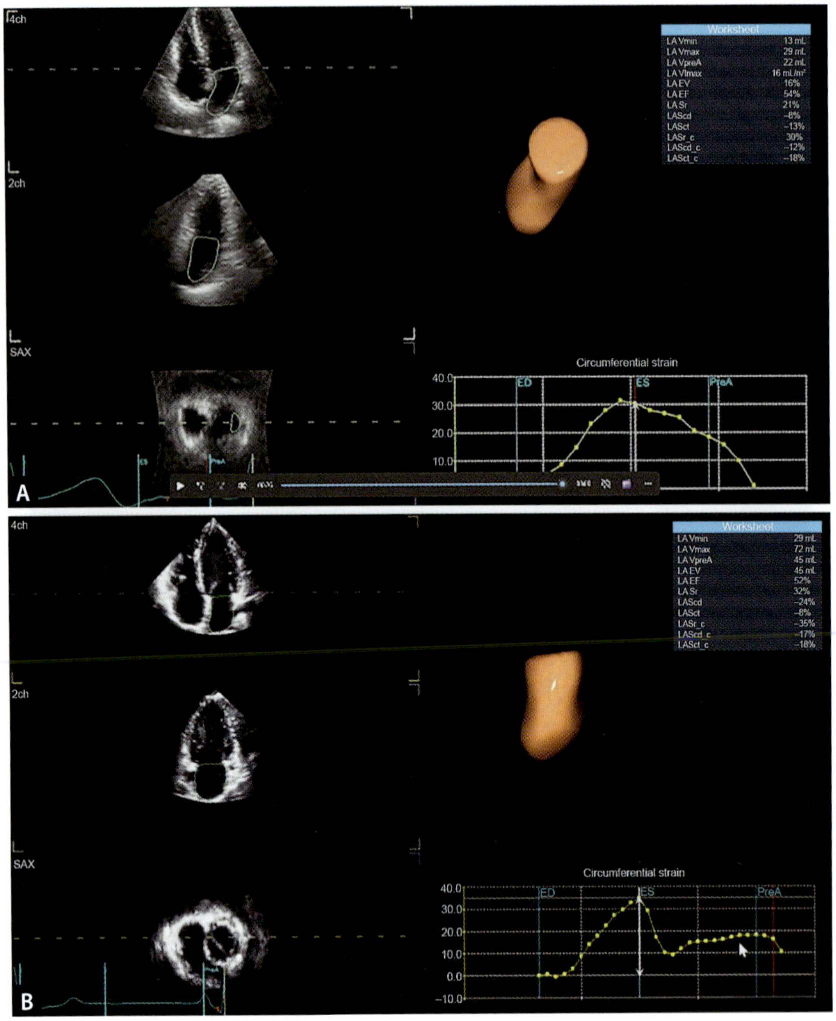

Figs. 4A and B: (A) Before GLP1 receptor agonist therapy and (B) After GLP1 receptor agonist therapy.

Comprehensive meta-analyses synthesizing data from multiple trials provide robust evidence supporting cardioprotective effects of both SGLT2 inhibitors and GLP-1RAs. A 2024 meta-analysis by Basile and colleagues included 18 studies with over 3,200 patients undergoing serial echocardiographic assessment. SGLT2 inhibitor therapy was associated with significant improvements in LA reservoir strain (weighted mean difference +4.2%, 95% CI: 3.1–5.3, $p < 0.001$) and LV GLS (weighted mean difference −2.1%, 95% CI: −2.8 to −1.4, $p < 0.001$). Effects were consistent across diabetic and nondiabetic subgroups, supporting mechanisms independent of glucose lowering.[34]

Combined evidence from these landmark trials and meta-analyses forms the foundation for current guideline recommendations supporting early use of SGLT2 inhibitors and GLP-1RAs in diabetic patients with cardiac involvement, regardless of heart failure phenotype or baseline ejection.[35]

PRACTICAL RECOMMENDATIONS FOR ECHOCARDIOGRAPHIC EVALUATION

Clinical Protocol

Patient Selection

Perform comprehensive echocardiography including speckle tracking strain analysis in all diabetic patients with suspected cardiac involvement, symptoms of dyspnea or exercise intolerance, elevated natriuretic peptides, or established cardiovascular disease.

Image Acquisition

Obtain high frame rate (60–90 fps) apical four-chamber and two-chamber views optimized for atrial visualization. Ensure complete atrial cavity inclusion without foreshortening. Acquire three consecutive cardiac cycles during breath-hold in sinus rhythm.

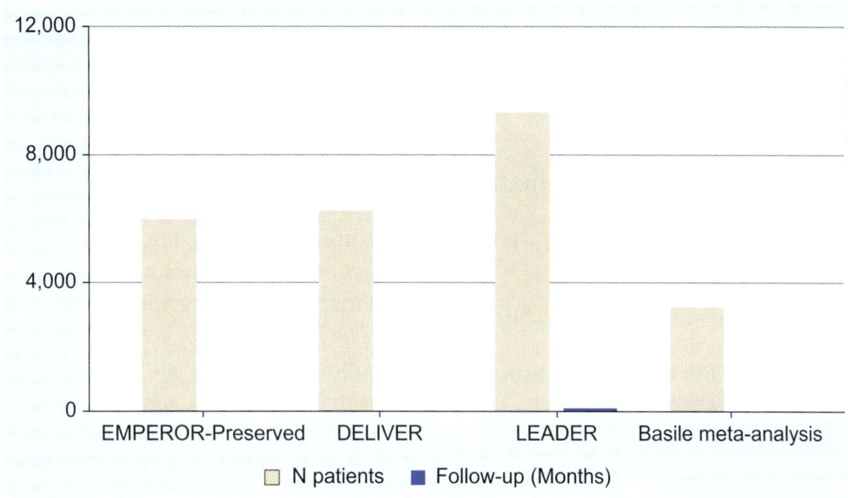

Fig. 5: Major clinical trials and meta-analyses in heart failure with preserved ejection fraction (HFpEF).

TABLE 3: Normal ranges and abnormal threshold values for left atrial (LA) strain parameters and left ventricular global longitudinal strain (LV GLS).

Strain parameter	*Normal range*	*Abnormal threshold*
LA reservoir strain	23–39%	<18%
LA conduit strain	13–22%	<10%
LA contractile strain	10–17%	<8%
LV GLS	<–18%	>–16%

Strain Analysis

Use vendor-specific or vendor-neutral software with standardized protocols. Trace LA endocardial border and adjust region of interest to atrial wall thickness. Measure reservoir, conduit, and contractile strain with quality control verification.

Comprehensive Assessment

Integrate strain findings with LA volume, mitral inflow velocities, tissue Doppler, and LV strain parameters. Calculate E/e2 ratio and estimate filling pressures. Assess for structural abnormalities and valvular disease.

Serial Monitoring

Repeat echocardiography at 6–12 months after therapeutic intervention or with clinical status change. Compare strain values using identical methodology and software version. Document relative and absolute changes **(Table 3)**.

IMPLICATIONS FOR CARDIOLOGY PRACTICE AND PATIENT MANAGEMENT

The accumulating evidence demonstrating beneficial effects of SGLT2 inhibitors and GLP-1RAs on atrial strain parameters has profound implications for contemporary cardiovascular practice. Early identification of atrial dysfunction through speckle tracking echocardiography enables timely initiation of these cardioprotective agents, potentially preventing progression from subclinical remodeling to symptomatic heart failure and atrial fibrillation.[36]

Preventive Paradigm

Shift from reactive treatment of advanced disease to proactive intervention at earliest signs of cardiac involvement. Strain imaging identifies patients who would benefit most from SGLT2 inhibitor/GLP-1RA therapy before irreversible remodeling occurs.

Individualized Therapy

Strain parameters guide selection between monotherapy and combination approaches. Patients with severe baseline impairment may warrant dual SGLT2 inhibitor plus GLP-1RA therapy, while those with mild dysfunction may respond adequately to single-agent therapy.

Treatment Monitoring

Serial strain assessment provides objective evidence of therapeutic efficacy, identifying treatment responders and nonresponders. Lack of improvement prompts investigation of adherence, dosing optimization, or consideration of additional interventions.

Integrated Care

Echocardiographic findings facilitate communication between cardiology and endocrinology, promoting coordinated management. Strain parameters serve as common language for multidisciplinary decision-making and shared treatment goals.

Clinical Decision Algorithm

1. Screen diabetic patients with echocardiography including strain
2. Identify impaired LA reservoir strain (<23%) or LV GLS (> −16%)
3. Initiate SGLT2 inhibitor as first-line therapy per guidelines
4. Consider adding GLP-1RA for high-risk features or inadequate response
5. Reassess at 6 months; optimize therapy based on strain evolution

Surrogate Endpoints

Strain parameters serve as valuable surrogate endpoints in clinical trials evaluating novel therapeutic agents. Improvements in atrial and ventricular strain may predict long-term clinical benefits, enabling more efficient drug development and regulatory approval pathways for cardioprotective diabetes therapies.

CONCLUSION

The convergence of advanced cardiac imaging techniques with novel cardioprotective pharmacotherapies has fundamentally transformed our understanding and management of diabetic cardiovascular disease. Speckle tracking echocardiography, particularly assessment of left atrial strain parameters, provides a sensitive, noninvasive tool for detecting early cardiac involvement and monitoring therapeutic responses in diabetic patients.

- *Robust evidence base:* Multiple clinical trials and meta-analyses demonstrate significant improvements in atrial strain with SGLT2 inhibitor and GLP-1RA therapy.
- *Evolving field:* Ongoing research into combination therapies, novel imaging modalities, and AI-assisted analysis promises continued advancement.
- *Guideline support:* Major society guidelines now recommend SGLT2 inhibitor and GLP-1RA as first-line therapy in diabetic patients with cardiac involvement.
- *Mechanistic understanding:* Pleiotropic effects including hemodynamic, metabolic, anti-inflammatory, and direct myocardial actions explain observed benefits.
- *Prognostic value:* Atrial strain independently predicts atrial fibrillation, heart failure events, and mortality in diabetic populations.
- *Clinical feasibility:* Standardized protocols enable reliable strain assessment in routine echocardiographic practice with excellent reproducibility.

Sodium-glucose cotransporter-2 inhibitors and GLP-1RAs significantly improve atrial strain parameters across all three phases of atrial function and reservoir, conduit, and contractile and reflecting genuine regression of diabetic atrial remodeling rather than mere hemodynamic effects. These improvements correlate with parallel enhancements in left ventricular strain, reductions in natriuretic peptides, and most importantly, reductions in clinical endpoints including heart failure hospitalizations and major adverse cardiovascular events.

The integration of echocardiographic strain assessment into clinical practice enables early detection of subclinical cardiac dysfunction, objective monitoring of therapeutic efficacy, and personalized optimization of cardioprotective therapy. As we move toward precision medicine approaches in cardiovascular care, strain imaging provides quantitative phenotyping that guides individualized management.

REFERENCES

1. International Diabetes Federation. IDF Diabetes Atlas, 10th edition. Brussels: International Diabetes Federation; 2021.
2. Salerno N, Ielapi J, Cersosimo A, et al. Early hemodynamic impact of SGLT2 inhibitors in overweight cardiometabolic heart failure: beyond fluid offloading to vascular adaptation—a preliminary report. Cardiovasc Diabetol. 2025;24:141.
3. Basile P, Guaricci AI, Piazzolla G, et al. Improvement of Left Ventricular Global Longitudinal Strain after 6-Month Therapy with GLP-1RAs Semaglutide and Dulaglutide in Type 2 Diabetes Mellitus: A Pilot Study. J Clin Med. 2023;12:1586.
4. Liao J, Wang L, Duan L, et al. Association between estimated glucose disposal rate and cardiovascular diseases in patients with diabetes or prediabetes: a cross-sectional study. Cardiovasc Diabetol. 2025;24:13.
5. Soysal AU, Raimoglou D, Soysal A, et al. The impact of dapagliflozin on left atrial functions and recurrence in non-diabetic patients in the early post-cryoablation period. J Interv Card Electrophysiol. 2025.
6. Katogiannis K, Thymis J, Kousathana F, et al. Effects of Liraglutide, Empagliflozin and Their Combination on Left Atrial Strain and Arterial Function. Medicina. 2024;60:395.
7. Preda A, Montecucco F, Carbone F, et al. SGLT2 inhibitors: from glucose-lowering to cardiovascular benefits. Cardiovasc Res. 2024;120(5):443-60.
8. Cameli M, Mandoli GE, Lisi E, et al. Left atrial, ventricular and atrio-ventricular strain in patients with subclinical heart dysfunction. Int J Cardiovasc Imaging. 2019 Feb;35(2):249-258.
9. McMurray JJV, Solomon SD, Inzucchi SE, et al. Dapagliflozin in Patients with Heart Failure and Reduced Ejection Fraction. N Engl J Med. 2019;381(21):1995-2008.
10. Wagdy K, Selwanos P. DAPA-HF trial signals the birth of 'diabetic cardiology' and more. Glob Cardiol Sci Pract. 2020;2020(2):e202022.

11. McDonagh TA, Metra M, Adamo M, et al. 2023 Focused Update of the 2021 ESC Guidelines for the diagnosis and treatment of acute and chronic heart failure. Eur Heart J. 2023;44(37):3627-39.
12. Marso SP, Daniels GH, Brown-Frandsen K, et al. Liraglutide and Cardiovascular Outcomes in Type 2 Diabetes. N Engl J Med. 2016;375(4):311-22.
13. Kristensen SL, Rørth R, Jhund PS, et al. Cardiovascular, mortality, and kidney outcomes with GLP-1 receptor agonists in patients with type 2 diabetes: a systematic review and meta-analysis of cardiovascular outcome trials. Lancet Diabetes Endocrinol. 2019;7(10):776-85.
14. Verma S, McGuire DK, Bain SC, et al. Effects of glucagon-like peptide-1 receptor agonists liraglutide and semaglutide on cardiovascular and renal outcomes across body mass index categories in type 2 diabetes: Results of the LEADER and SUSTAIN 6 trials. Diabetes Obes Metab. 2020;22(12):2487-92.
15. El-Saied SB, El-Sherbeny WS, El-Sharkawy SI. Impact of sodium glucose co-transporter-2 inhibitors on left atrial functions in patients with type-2 diabetes and heart failure with mildly reduced ejection fraction. Int J Cardiol Heart Vasc. 2023;50:101329.
16. Savcılıoglu MD, Duzen IV, Tuluce SY, et al. The effects of SGLT-2 inhibitors on echocardiographic indices and antioxidative properties in patients with heart failure with reduced ejection fraction and diabetes mellitus. Eur Rev Med Pharmacol Sci. 2024;28(16):4121-35.
17. Rusali CA, Lupu IC, Rusali LM, et al. Left Atrial Strain-Current Review of Clinical Applications. Diagnostics (Basel). 2025;15(11):1347.
18. Russell-Jones D, Vaag A, Schmitz O, et al. Liraglutide vs insulin glargine and placebo in combination with metformin and sulfonylurea therapy in type 2 diabetes mellitus (LEAD-5 met+SU): a randomised controlled trial. Diabetologia. 2009;52(10):2046-55.
19. Ikonomidis I, Pavlidis G, Thymis J, et al. Effects of Glucagon-Like Peptide-1 Receptor Agonists, Sodium-Glucose Cotransporter-2 Inhibitors, and Their Combination on Endothelial Glycocalyx, Arterial Function, and Myocardial Work Index in Patients With Type 2 Diabetes Mellitus After 12-Month Treatment. J Am Heart Assoc. 2020;9(9):e015716.
20. Morello M, Lindner JR. Left Atrial Strain During Exercise: A Window to Atrioventricular Coupling in Heart Failure. Circ Cardiovasc Imaging. 2024;17(8):e017160.
21. Gourdy P, Darmon P, Dievart F, et al. Combining glucagon-like peptide-1 receptor agonists (GLP-1RAs) and sodium-glucose cotransporter-2 inhibitors (SGLT2is) in patients with type 2 diabetes mellitus (T2DM). Cardiovasc Diabetol. 2023;22(1):79.
22. Ghoreyshi-Hefzabad SM, Jeyaprakash P, Vo HQ, et al. Subclinical systolic dysfunction detected by 2D speckle tracking echocardiography in adults with diabetes mellitus: systematic review and meta-analysis of 6668 individuals with diabetes mellitus and 7218 controls. Int J Cardiovasc Imaging. 2023;39(5):977-89.
23. Voigt JU, Pedrizzetti G, Lysyansky P, et al. Definitions for a common standard for 2D speckle tracking echocardiography: consensus document of the EACVI/ASE/Industry Task Force to standardize deformation imaging. Eur Heart J Cardiovasc Imaging. 2015;16(1):1-11.
24. Tanaka H, Soga F, Tatsumi K, et al. Positive effect of dapagliflozin on left ventricular longitudinal function for type 2 diabetic mellitus patients with chronic heart failure. Cardiovasc Diabetol. 2020;19(1):6.
25. Molnár AÁ, Merkely B. The Added Value of Atrial Strain Assessment in Clinical Practice. Diagnostics (Basel). 2022;12(4):982.
26. Simmonds SJ, Cuijpers I, Heymans S, et al. Cellular and Molecular Differences between HFpEF and HFrEF: A Step Ahead in an Improved Pathological Understanding. Cells. 2020;9(1):242.
27. Javadi N, Bismee NN, Abbas MT, et al. Left Atrial Strain: State of the Art and Clinical Implications. J Pers Med. 2024;14(11):1093.
28. Shah SJ, Borlaug BA, Kitzman DW, et al. Research Priorities for Heart Failure With Preserved Ejection Fraction: National Heart, Lung, and Blood Institute Working Group Summary. Circulation. 2020;141(12):1001-26.
29. Nagueh SF, Sanborn DY, Oh JK, et al. Recommendations for the Evaluation of Left Ventricular Diastolic Function by Echocardiography and for Heart Failure With Preserved Ejection Fraction Diagnosis: An Update From the American Society of Echocardiography. J Am Soc Echocardiogr. 2025;38(7):537-69.
30. Chamberlain R, Shiino K, Scalia GM, et al. Advantage and validation of vendor-independent software for myocardial strain analysis compared to vendor-specific software. Australas J Ultrasound Med. 2020;24(1):48-57.
31. Muraru D, Niero A, Rodriguez-Zanella H, et al. Three-dimensional speckle-tracking echocardiography: benefits and limitations of integrating myocardial mechanics with three-dimensional imaging. Cardiovasc Diagn Ther. 2018;8(1):101-17.
32. Li P, Chen W, Chen R, et al. Long-term effects of SGLT2 inhibitors on arrhythmias: a systematic review and meta-analysis. Front Pharmacol. 2025;16:1558367.
33. Wagdy K, Nagy S. EMPEROR-Preserved: SGLT2 inhibitors breakthrough in the management of heart failure with preserved ejection fraction. Glob Cardiol Sci Pract. 2021;2021(3):e202117.
34. Novo G, Guarino T, Di Lisi D, et al. Effects of SGLT2 inhibitors on cardiac structure and function. Heart Fail Rev. 2023;28(3):697-707.
35. Zhu JJ, Wilding JPH, Gu XS. Combining GLP-1 receptor agonists and SGLT-2 inhibitors for cardiovascular disease prevention in type 2 diabetes: A systematic review with multiple network meta-regressions. World J Diabetes. 2024;15(10):2135-46.
36. Marx N, Federici M, Schütt K, et al. 2023 ESC Guidelines for the management of cardiovascular disease in patients with diabetes. Eur Heart J. 2023;44(39):4043-140. Erratum in: Eur Heart J. 2023;44(48):5060. Erratum in: Eur Heart J. 2024;45(7):518.

67

CHAPTER

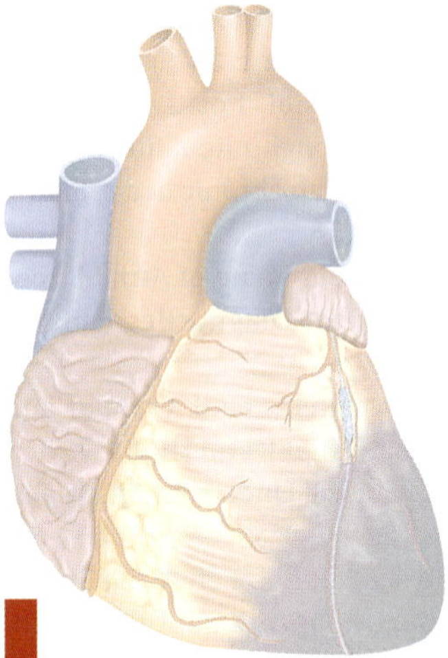

Echocardiographic Evaluation of Left Atrial Remodeling Reversal with GLP-1 RA in HFpEF

Nilufar Fatema

INTRODUCTION

Heart failure with mildly reduced or preserved ejection fraction (HFpEF) constitutes more than half of all heart failure (HF) cases in the world. The prevalence is consistently increasing. Obesity is one of the common factors in this group of patients. Obesity is not only a coexisting factor but also contributes to development and progression of HFpEF. The advancement of treatment, such as mineralocorticoid receptor antagonists and sodium-glucose cotransporter 2 inhibitors, has shown some improvement in clinical outcomes for patients with HFpEF, but there is still a high residual risk of HF. So, there is a need for an alternative treatment option. Glucagon-like peptide-1 receptor agonists (GLP-1 RAs), established as a first-line therapy for type 2 diabetes mellitus (T2DM) in patients with atherosclerotic cardiovascular (CV) disease and obesity,[1] have emerged as a potential treatment for HF. Initial data suggest their efficacy in improving clinical outcomes in HFpEF, but most individual trials contain modest numbers of patients with HFpEF and were not designed with the intent of detecting effects on CV death or worsening HF events. A meta-analysis builds on recent evidence of the efficacy of semaglutide in HFpEF with obesity.[2] The SUMMIT study has shown that the use of tirzepatide in obese patients with HFpEF, once weekly subcutaneous tirzepatide, was superior to placebo in improving the composite endpoint of CV death and HF-related events over 104 weeks of follow-up,[3] and the EXSCEL study has shown the use of exenatide for lowering the CV event.[4] There is no such single evidence of comparison of the efficacy of different GLP-1 RAs on clinical outcomes in patients with HFpEF with obesity or T2DM.

Glucagon-like peptide-1 receptor agonists have shown potential cardiometabolic benefits, but their role in HFpEF remains unclear. Another systematic review and meta-analysis of six randomized controlled trials (RCTs), involving 8,788 patients, evaluated GLP-1 RAs in HFpEF. Studies evaluating GLP-1 RA in combination with glucose-dependent insulinotropic polypeptide (GIP) were also included. The endpoints included CV death, worsening HF events, and their composite, which were analyzed, and the hazard ratios (HRs) with 95% confidence intervals (CIs) were pooled using a random-effects model. GLP-1 RAs significantly reduced the composite outcome of CV death or worsening HF events [HR: 0.68 (0.51–0.89); $p = 0.006$, $I^2 = 47\%$] as well as worsening HF events alone [HR: 0.56 (0.38–0.82); $p = 0.003$, $I^2 = 51\%$]. No significant reduction was observed for CV death alone [HR: 0.86 (0.67–1.12); $p = 0.27$, $I^2 = 0\%$]. GLP-1 RAs reduce worsening HF events and the composite of CV death or worsening HF in HFpEF, particularly in patients with obesity or diabetes. These findings support their role as a promising therapy requiring further HFpEF-focused trials.[1]

The obese patients have physical limitations and suffer from HFpEF. A GLP-1 RA such as semaglutide has a positive impact on primary and secondary outcomes in obese patients. In a meta-analysis of five RCTs with 6,898 patients, the safety and efficacy of semaglutide in obese HF patients were evaluated. Semaglutide was compared with placebo in obese patients with HF, regardless of the baseline ejection fraction (EF), and the primary endpoint was the incidence of CV mortality in a subgroup analysis based on the ejection fraction [HFpEF and HF with reduced EF (HFrEF)]. Semaglutide significantly reduced the overall incidence of CV mortality compared with placebo. More reduction of mortality was observed in HFrEF patients (RR, 0.66; 95% CI, 0.47–0.92; $p = 0.01$) than in HFpEF patients (RR, 0.84; 95% CI, 0.59–1.22; $p = 0.37$). Semaglutide exhibited a significant reduction in CV mortality and improvement in the 6-minute walk distance (MD, 14.83; 95% CI, 4.23–25.43; $p = 0.006$) compared with placebo in both subgroups.[2]

Another meta-analysis showed that GLP-1 RAs have shown promising effects on HF outcomes, particularly in phenotype-specific populations. Six RCTs (n = 1,195) compared GLP-1 RA with placebo in HF patients. Outcomes included changes in left ventricular ejection fraction (LVEF), left ventricular end-diastolic volume (LVEDV), left ventricular end-systolic volume (LVESV), global longitudinal strain (GLS), left ventricular mass, left atrial volume (LAV), and NT-proBNP levels. In patients with HFpEF, GLP-1 RA significantly reduced the LV mass (WMD: –8.6 g; 95% CI, –14.6, –2.6; $p = 0.005$) and LAV (WMD: –5.4 mL; 95% CI, –8.8, –2.0; $p = 0.002$) and lowered NT-proBNP concentration throughout (HR: 0.85; 95% CI, 0.8, 0.9; $p < 0.001$). GLP-1 RA demonstrated phenotype-specific benefits, improving structural remodeling of LA and LV in HFpEF.[5]

In a cohort study, the extent of left atrial (LA) structural and functional reverse remodeling following radiofrequency catheter ablation (RFCA) for atrial fibrillation (AF) was assessed in patients with persistent AF and HFpEF. Thirty consecutive HFpEF patients with persistent AF were prospectively enrolled and planned for RF ablation. Prior to the procedure, transthoracic echocardiography was performed to assess LA structure, LA strain, and LA contractile function. The same evaluation of LA structure and functional parameters was performed postablation at discharge, 1 month, 3 months, 6 months, and 12 months. Baseline data were compared between patients with AF recurrence and nonrecurrence postablation. In patients with persistent AF and HFpEF, RF ablation for AF, with resultant preservation of sinus rhythm, results in the reversal of LA morphologic remodeling and notable improvements in LA reservoir and contractile function.[6]

Kramer et al. showed that the CMR substudy of the SUMMIT trial demonstrated that tirzepatide therapy in obesity-related HFpEF led to reduced LV mass and paracardiac adipose tissue as compared with placebo, and the change in LV mass paralleled weight loss. These physiologic changes may contribute to the reduction in HF events seen in the main SUMMIT trial. The primary endpoint of the study was LV mass, and secondary endpoints included epicardial and pericardial adipose tissue, LV and LA volumes, and LV and LA strains. In the tirzepatide group, the change in LV mass correlated with the change in body weight ($r = 0.34$; $p < 0.02$). The change in LV mass was also associated with change in LV end-diastolic volume ($r = 0.33$; $p < 0.03$) and stroke volume ($r = 0.28$; $p = 0.05$); the change in LA end-systolic volume ($r = 0.42$; $p = 0.003$) and end-diastolic volume ($r = 0.50$; $p < 0.001$), and although not statistically significant, tended to correlate with change in systolic blood pressure ($r = 0.27$; $p = 0.06$).[7]

LEFT ATRIAL REMODELING

Left atrial remodeling refers to structural and functional changes in the left atrium, which can be assessed using echocardiography. This is a significant indicator of CV conditions such as HF and AF. Echocardiography evaluates LA remodeling by measuring LA volume and function, with the left atrial volume index (LAVi) being a key measurement. Advanced techniques such as 3D echocardiography and speckle tracking provide more accurate measurements of LA volume and function, respectively, than traditional 2D methods.

LEFT ATRIAL VOLUME INDEX

This is the standard method for assessing structural remodeling, calculated by indexing the LA volume to body surface area. LAVi normal value: 22 ± 6 mL/m^2, mild enlargement: >28 mL/m^2, moderate enlargement: >34 mL/m^2, severe enlargement: ≥40 mL/m^2.

The LA endocardium was then planimetered manually by the operator at each frame of the cardiac cycle. LA minimum and maximum volume, stroke volume, and ejection fraction were calculated using the following formula: LA volume = (0.85 × LA area 4 chamber × LA area 2 chamber) × [(LA length 2 chamber + LA length 4 chamber)/2][8] **(Figs. 1 to 4)**.

LEFT ATRIAL STRAIN

This measures the functional remodeling and how well the LA contracts and expands. Reduced LA strain is associated with an increased risk of AF and is considered an important prognostic indicator. The precise assessment of LA function was performed by measuring global peak reservoir strain **(Fig. 5)**.

3D ECHOCARDIOGRAPHY

This is an advanced method that provides more accurate and reproducible LA volume measurements compared

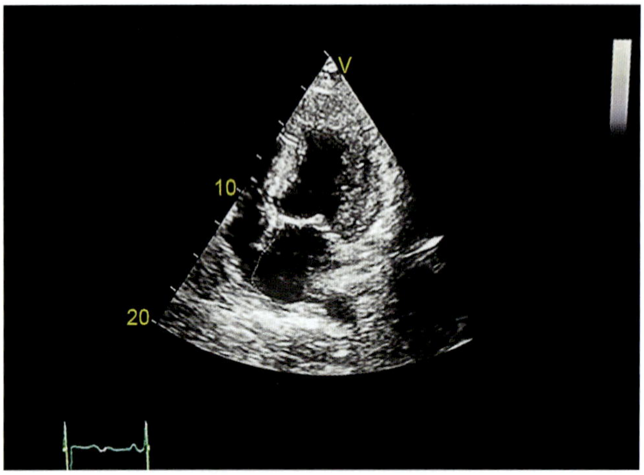

Fig. 1: ECG-gated apical four-chamber view reveals LA area: 19.6 cm^2.

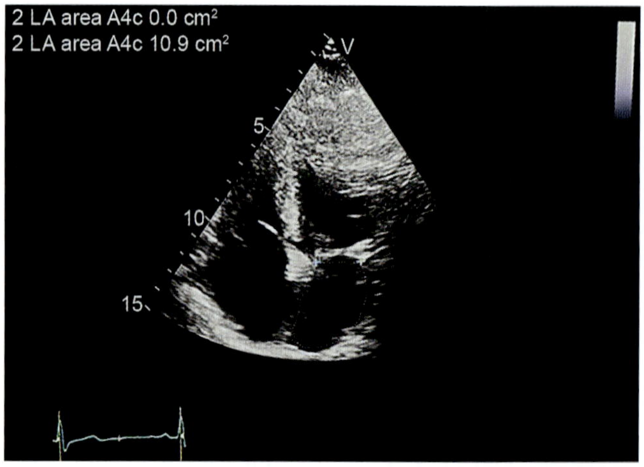

Fig. 4: ECG-gated apical four-chamber view reveals reduced LA area after 6-month treatment with GLP-1 RA.

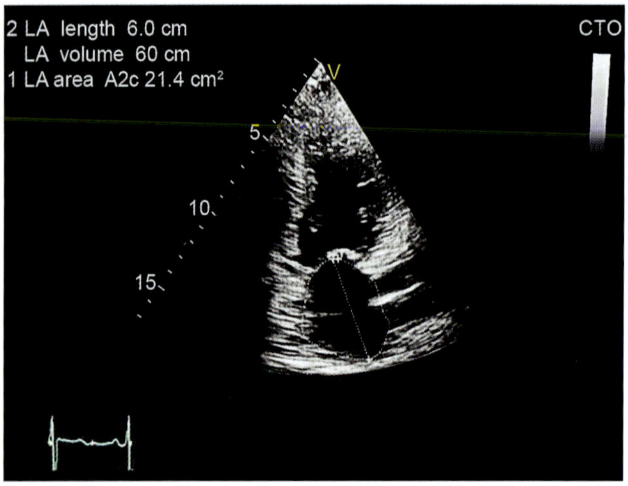

Fig. 2: ECG-gated apical two-chamber view reveals LA area: 21.4 cm^2, LA length: 6.0 cm, LA volume: 60 mL.

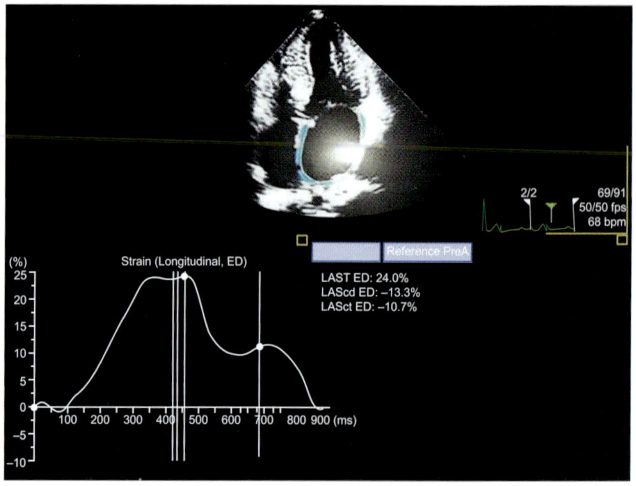

Fig. 5: LA strain imaging in a HFpEF patient.

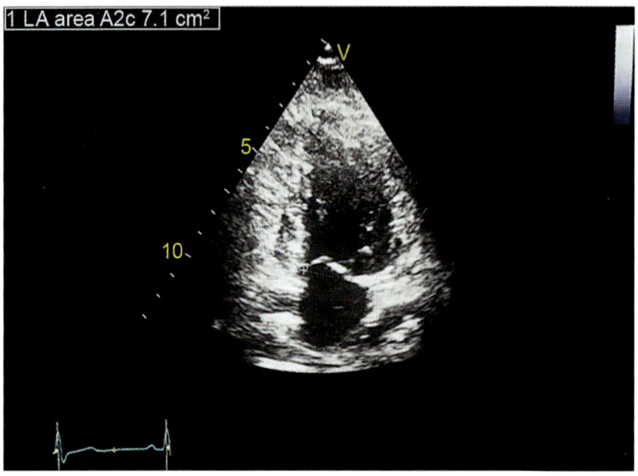

Fig. 3: ECG-gated apical two-chamber view reveals reduced LA area after 6-month treatment with GLP-1 RA.

to 2D methods by avoiding geometric assumptions and foreshortening.

CONCLUSION

Echocardiography is an essential tool for detection of LA remodeling, both functional and morphologic, in HFpEF patients. This remodeling can be reversed with GLP-1 RA in this group. Evaluation of LA remodeling reversal can also be detected by follow-up echocardiography.

REFERENCES

1. Waqas SA, Sohail MU, Saad M, et al. Efficacy of GLP-1 receptor agonists in patients with heart failure and mildly reduced or preserved ejection fraction: a systematic review and meta-analysis. J Card Fail. 2025; 31(7):1076-80.

2. Otmani Z, Elsayed HA, Negmeldin Aly Yassin M, et al. Semaglutide in patients with obesity and heart failure irrespective of their baseline ejection fraction: an efficacy and safety meta-analysis of randomized controlled trials. Cardiol Rev. 2025 [online ahead of print].
3. Zile MR, Borlaug BA, Kramer CM, et al. Effects of tirzepatide on the clinical trajectory of patients with heart failure, preserved ejection fraction, and obesity: The SUMMIT trial. Circulation. 2025;1(10):656-68.
4. Holman RR, Bethel MA, Mentz RJ, et al.; EXSCEL Study Group. Effects of once-weekly exenatide on cardiovascular outcomes in type 2 diabetes. N Engl J Med. 2017;377(13):1228-39.
5. Siddiqui HF, Waqas SA, Batool RM, et al. The effect of GLP-1 receptor agonists on cardiac remodeling in heart failure patients with preserved and reduced ejection fraction: a systematic review and meta-analysis. Heart Fail Rev. 2025;30(5):991-1004.
6. Chen Y, Li M, Wang X, et al. Left atrial reverse remodeling in patients with persistent atrial fibrillation and HFpEF following radiofrequency ablation: prospective evaluation with echocardiographic atrial analysis. Clinics. 2025;80:100730.
7. Kramer CM, Borlaug BA, Zile MR, et al.; The SUMMIT Trial Study Group. Tirzepatide reduces LV mass and paracardiac adipose tissue in obesity-related heart failure: SUMMIT CMR Substudy, J Am Coll Cardiol. 2025;85(7):699-706.
8. Kaminski M, Steel K, Jerosch-Herold M, et al. Strong cardiovascular prognostic implication of quantitative left atrial contractile function assessed by cardiac magnetic resonance imaging in patients with chronic hypertension. J Cardiovasc Magn Reson. 2011;13:42.

CHAPTER 68

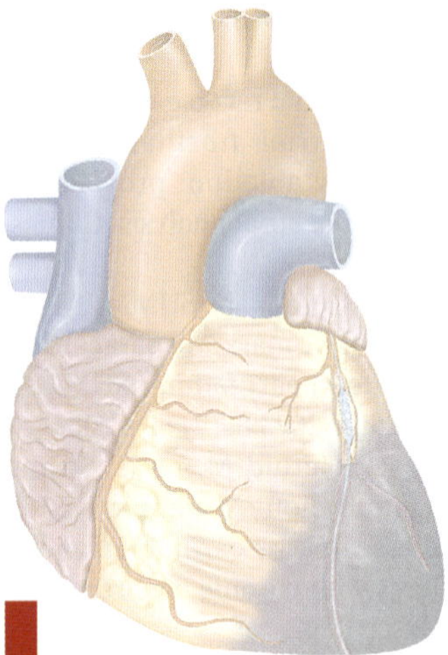

Echocardiographic Evaluation of Obese HFpEF: Remodeling Reversal with GLP-1 RA

Abdirahman Wardhere, Mohamed Nor, Wissam I Khalife, Masood Ahmad

INTRODUCTION

Heart failure with preserved ejection fraction (HFpEF) affects nearly 3 million people in the United States and up to 32 million worldwide,[1] causing substantial morbidity and mortality.[2] HFpEF is associated with multiple comorbidities, and obesity is one of the most common. A distinct phenotype has been proposed for obese patients with HFpEF.[3] Recently, glucagon-like peptide-1 receptor agonists (GLP-1RAs), previously approved for the treatment of diabetes mellitus, have shown cardiovascular benefits in this patient group.[4] This chapter discusses echocardiographic structural changes in obesity-related HFpEF and the role of GLP-1RAs.

OBESITY AND HEART FAILURE WITH PRESERVED EJECTION FRACTION

Obesity contributes to HFpEF by promoting left and right ventricular (RV) remodeling, dysfunction, and cardiac fibrosis[5] **(Fig. 1)**.[3] Excess adipose tissue increases collagen in the extracellular matrix. This stiffens the myocardium and impairs relaxation. Expansion and infiltration of epicardial fat alter cardiac geometry. This process leads to chamber dilation and hypertrophy.[6] Adipose tissue secretes cytokines, including activin A, connective tissue growth factor, insulin-like growth factor, growth differentiation factor-11, transforming growth factor-β, and metalloproteinases. All of these contribute to the development of fibrosis. Adipose tissue also produces angiotensin II and aldosterone, further driving remodeling and increasing LV wall stress.[7]

Epicardial adipose tissue (EAT), located between the myocardium and the visceral pericardium, is more abundant in HFpEF than in other types of heart failure. It is associated with worse outcomes and increased mortality.[8,9] In obese HFpEF patients, higher EAT levels correlate with greater hemodynamic abnormalities, at rest and with exertion. These include higher filling pressures, more severe pulmonary hypertension, and increased pericardial restraint, all of which reduce exercise tolerance.[10] Obesity also raises the risk of sudden cardiac death.[11] Proposed mechanisms include conduction slowing due to hypertrophy, impaired repolarization resulting from potassium current downregulation, calcium-handling abnormalities leading to diastolic calcium leak, and increased fibrosis caused by systemic inflammation.[12]

GLUCAGON-LIKE PEPTIDE-1 RECEPTOR AGONISTS—MECHANISMS OF ACTION

Glucagon-like peptide-1 receptor agonists, synthesized mainly in L cells of the small intestine, augment glucose-dependent insulin secretion from pancreatic islets, delay gastric emptying, and suppress postprandial glucagon secretion, which together improve glycemic control.[13] GLP-1 influences satiety through peripheral mechanisms, such as enteroenteric reflexes and central hypothalamic pathways involved in appetite regulation.[14,15] The ability of GLP-1RAs to attenuate oxidative stress and decrease systemic inflammation represents an important mechanism supporting their therapeutic potential in this patient population.[16] Activation of the GLP-1

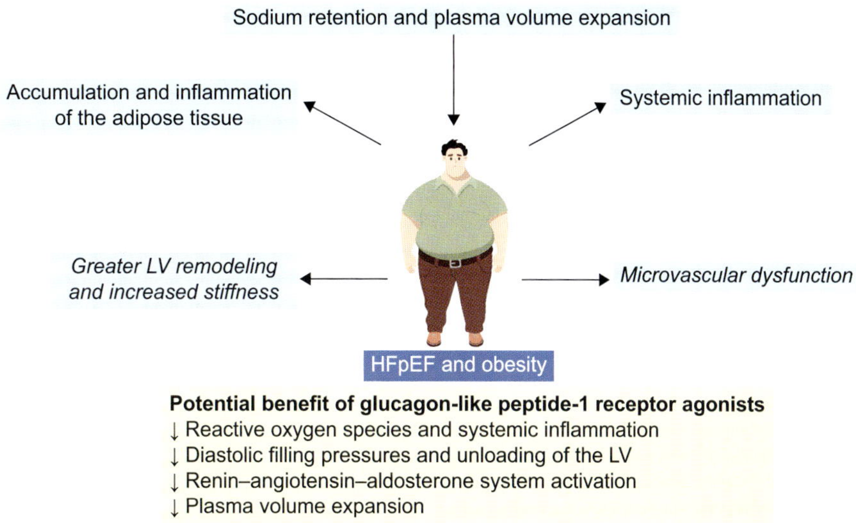

Fig. 1: Obesity and heart failure with preserved ejection fraction (HFpEF). The figure illustrates the clinical features and pathophysiology of obesity and HFpEF, as well as the potential benefits derived from glucagon-like peptide-1 receptor agonists.
Source: Cimino G, et al.[3]

receptor has been shown to shift macrophages from the proinflammatory M1 phenotype to the anti-inflammatory M2 phenotype. This transition is associated with a reduction in inflammatory mediators and an enhancement of tissue repair mechanisms.[17]

ECHOCARDIOGRAPHY IN EVALUATION OF OBESE HFpEF—CARDIAC REMODELING/REVERSE REMODELING WITH GLP-1RA THERAPY

With the abovementioned metabolic and inflammatory effects in mind, obesity-related cardiac remodeling is characterized by notable structural and functional alterations of the heart. In an observational study by Huang et al.,[18] comparing baseline echocardiographic parameters between obese individuals (n = 589) and nonobese controls (n = 100), obesity was associated with significant cardiac structural and functional alterations. Obese participants demonstrated larger left atrial (LA) and ventricular diameters, increased interventricular septal, and posterior wall thickness, and a modest but statistically significant reduction in left ventricular ejection fraction, which nevertheless remained within the normal range. In addition, evidence of diastolic dysfunction was observed among obese patients, characterized by a lower E/A ratio and higher E/e′ ratio. Global longitudinal strain was also significantly reduced in the obese group, suggesting the presence of early subclinical systolic impairment **(Table 1)**. Discrepancies in the assessment of LA size in a lean versus an obese patient of similar height are illustrated in **Figure 2.**[19] In another study, evaluating RV remodeling with significant tricuspid regurgitation, increased RV remodeling with higher end-diastolic and end-systolic areas was reported in obese patients.[20]

Reverse remodeling refers to the regression of pathological, structural, and functional alterations in the heart that occur in response to effective therapy.[21] Echocardiography is effective in assessing these structural and functional changes in patients with HFpEF. However, image acquisition and interpretation may be technically challenging in this population **(Fig. 2)**. In subgroup analyses of the STEP HFpEF program and SUMMIT trials, GLP-1RAs improved cardiac remodeling.[22,23] Out of 1,145 participants, 43% underwent echocardiographic randomization over a 52-week period[22] **(Fig. 3)**.[24,25] Semaglutide reduced LA remodeling, with a significant decrease in LA volume compared to placebo [estimated mean difference (EMD): –6.13 mL; 95% CI: –9.85 to –2.41 mL; P = 0.0013]. Semaglutide also reduced RV enlargement, with lower RV end-diastolic area (EMD: –1.99 cm^2; 95% CI: –3.60 to –0.38 cm^2; P = 0.016) and RV end-systolic areas (EMD: –1.41 cm^2; 95% CI: –2.42 to –0.40 cm^2; P = 0.0064). Improvements were seen in diastolic function, including E-wave velocity (EMD: –5.63 cm/s; 95% CI: –9.42 to –1.84 cm/s; P = 0.0037), E/A ratio (EMD: –0.14; 95% CI: –0.24 to –0.04; P = 0.0075), and E/e′ average (EMD: –0.79; 95% CI: –1.60 to 0.01; P = 0.05). These effects were consistent regardless of whether the individual had diabetes or atrial fibrillation.

TABLE 1: Comparison of selected echocardiographic parameters between normal controls and obese patients.

Echocardiographic parameters Mean ± SD	*Normal controls (n = 100, BMI = 22.80 ± 2.79)*	*Obese group (n = 589, BMI = 37.53 ± 5.40*)*
LA diameter (mm)	32.68 ± 2.88	37.39 ± 3.78*
IVS diameter (mm)	8.82 ± 0.93	9.97 ± 1.09*
LVPW diameter (mm)	8.75 ± 2.41	9.90 ± 2.54*
LV diameter (mm)	45.80 ± 3.08	48.86 ± 4.66*
LVEF (%)	63.88 ± 3.86	62.05 ± 4.06*
E/A ratio	1.44 (1.40–1.54)	1.16 (1.17–1.24)*
E/e' ratio	6.36 (6.22–6.67)	7.30 (7.34–7.64)*
GLS (%)	–21.91 ± 1.89	–19.28 ± 2.79*

Mean ± SD, * = $p < 0.05$

[A: peak late diastolic velocity of mitral inflow; e': early diastolic mitral annular velocity (tissue Doppler, average of septal and lateral); E: peak early diastolic velocity of mitral inflow; GLS: global longitudinal strain; IVS: interventricular septum; LA: left atrial; LVPW: left ventricular posterior wall; LV: left ventricular; LVEF: left ventricular ejection fraction]

Source: Huang J, et al.[18]

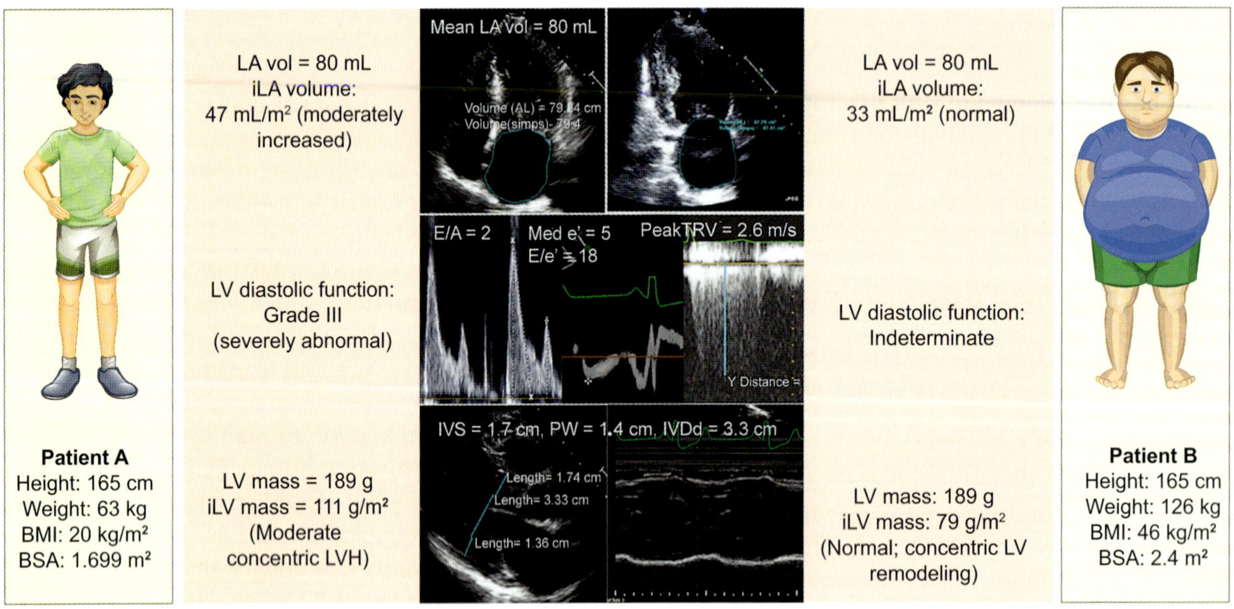

Fig. 2: Imaging pitfalls in obese individuals. Illustration showing discrepancies in assessment of LA volume, diastolic function, and LVH assessment in a lean vs. an obese patient of similar height. [BMI: body mass index; BSA: body surface area (Mosteller formula); i: indexed; IVDd: internal left ventricular diameter in diastole; IVS: interventricular septum; LA: left atrial; LV: left ventricle; LVH: left ventricular hypertrophy; PW: posterior wall; TRV: tricuspid regurgitant velocity]

Source: Singh M, et al.[19]

CARDIAC MAGNETIC RESONANCE IMAGING IN OBESITY WITH HFpEF AND GLP-1RA THERAPY

While a detailed discussion of cardiac magnetic resonance (CMR) imaging findings is beyond the scope of this chapter, a subgroup analysis of the SUMMIT trial[26] demonstrated that tirzepatide significantly reduced LV mass compared to placebo (mean –11 g; 95% CI: –19 to –4; $P = 0.004$). Tirzepatide also reduced paracardiac adipose tissue volume by 45 mL compared to placebo (95% CI: –69 to –22; $P < 0.001$). Additionally, a recent meta-analysis of STEP-HFpEF and SUMMIT trials showed GLP-1RA led to favorable reverse cardiac remodeling in HFpEF patients, with significant reductions in LV mass [weighted mean difference (WMD): –8.6 g; 95% CI: –14.6 to –2.6; $p = 0.005$]

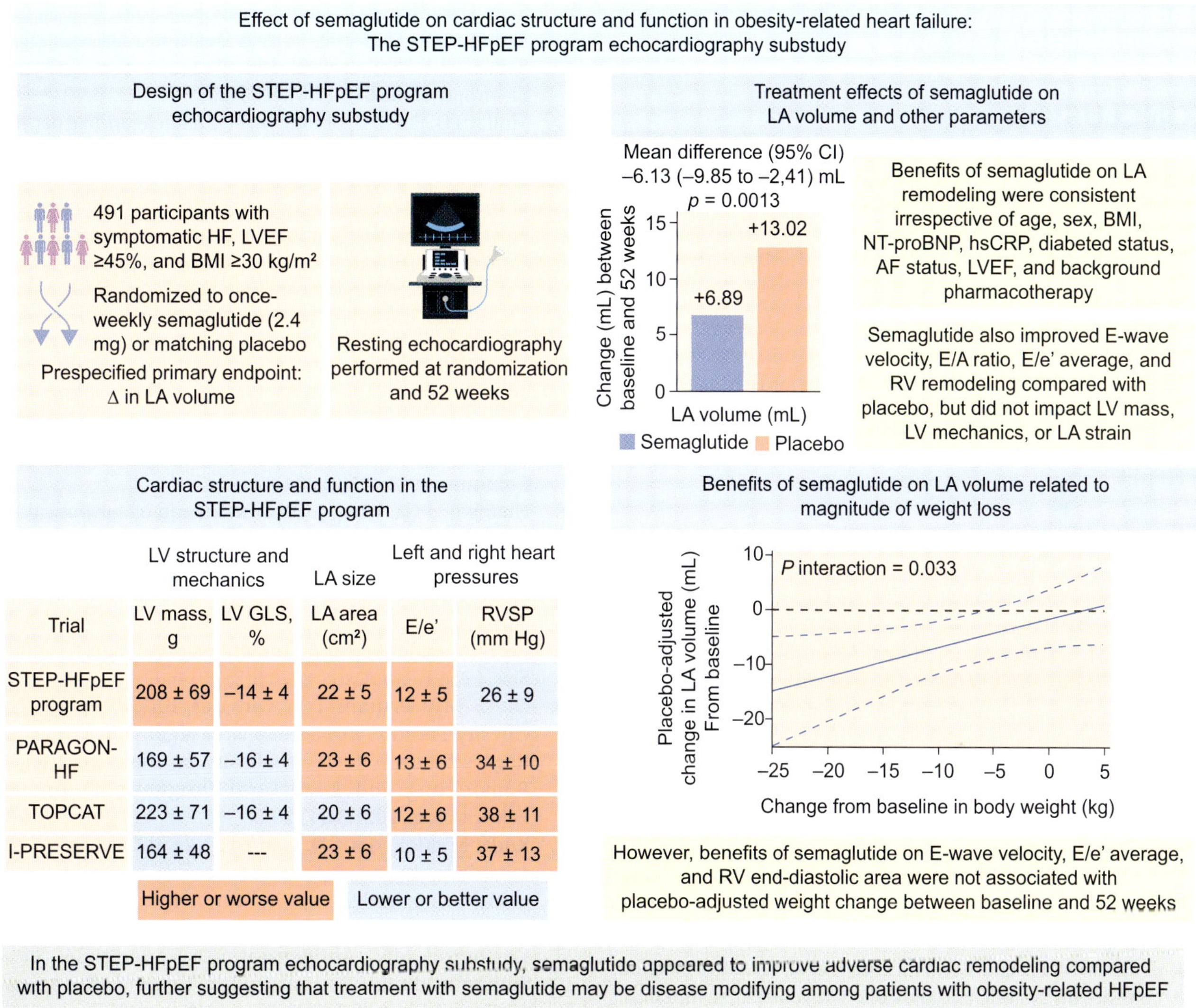

Fig. 3: *Central illustration*: Design and findings of the STEP-HFpEF Program Echocardiography Sub-study. (AF: atrial fibrillation; BMI: body mass index; E/A: ratio between early and late mitral inflow velocity; E/e': ratio between early mitral inflow velocity and early diastolic mitral annular velocity; GLS: global longitudinal strain; HF: heart failure; HFpEF: heart failure with preserved ejection fraction; hsCRP: high-sensitivity C-reactive protein; I-PRESERVE: Irbesartan in Heart Failure With Preserved Ejection Fraction; LA: left atrial; LV: left ventricular; LVEF: left ventricular ejection fraction; NT-proBNP: N-terminal pro-B-type natriuretic peptide; PARAGON-HF: Efficacy and Safety of LCZ696 compared to Valsartan, on Morbidity and Mortality in Heart Failure Patients With Preserved Ejection Fraction; RV: right ventricular; RVSP: right ventricular systolic pressure; STEP-HFpEF: Semaglutide Treatment Effect in People with Obesity and HFpEF; TOPCAT: Treatment of Preserved Cardiac Function Heart Failure With an Aldosterone Antagonist)
Source: Solomon SD, et al.[24]

and LA volume (WMD: –5.4 mL; 95% CI: –8.8 to –2.0; $p = 0.002$) compared with placebo.[27]

LIMITATIONS

Several limitations exist. First, the original trials were not specifically designed to study cardiac structure and function, which may have made the analysis underpowered. Second, obesity worsened echocardiographic image quality, causing some missing data and potential bias. Third, only resting echocardiography was performed; future work should examine the effect of semaglutide on exercise-related dysfunction. Participants also received other heart failure therapies, such as ARNI and SGLT2 inhibitors, which can affect cardiac remodeling. Finally, site expertise varied, particularly at sites without

CMR imaging specialists, potentially impacting image acquisition and interpretation.

CONCLUSION

Echocardiography is an extremely valuable noninvasive imaging technique in the assessment of cardiac modeling/reverse remodeling in obese subjects with HFpEF. In both the STEP-HFpEF program and the SUMMIT trial, treatment with semaglutide and tirzepatide was associated with favorable impact on cardiac remodeling compared with placebo. These findings provide important mechanistic insights into the benefits of GLP-1-based therapies in patients with obesity-related HFpEF, supporting their potential as disease-modifying agents in the pathobiology of HFpEF.

REFERENCES

1. Redfield MM, Borlaug BA. Heart failure with preserved ejection fraction: a review. JAMA. 2023;329(10):827-38.
2. Zile M, Gottdiener JS, Hetzel SJ, et al. Prevalence and significance of alterations in cardiac structure and function in patients with heart failure and a preserved ejection fraction. Circulation. 2011;124(23):2491-501.
3. Cimino G, Vaduganathan M, Lombardi CM, et al. Obesity, heart failure with preserved ejection fraction, and the role of glucagon-like peptide-1 receptor agonists. ESC Heart Fail. 2024;11(2):649-61.
4. Ferreira JP, Sharma A, Butler J, et al. Glucagon-like peptide-1 receptor agonists across the spectrum of heart failure. J Clin Endocrinol Metab. 2023;109(1):4-9.
5. Pascual M, Pascual DA, Vincente T, et al. Effects of isolated obesity on systolic and diastolic left ventricular function. Heart. 2003;89(10):1152-6.
6. Li L, Zhao Q, Kong W. Extracellular matrix remodeling and cardiac fibrosis. Matrix Biol. 2018;68-69:490-506.
7. Anthony SR, Guarnieri AR, Gozdiff A, et al. Mechanisms linking adipose tissue inflammation to cardiac hypertrophy and fibrosis. Clin Sci (Lond). 2019;133(23):2329-44.
8. Iacobellis G, Bianco AC. Epicardial adipose tissue: emerging physiological, pathophysiological and clinical features. Trends Endocrinol Metab. 2011;22(11):450-7.
9. Goldman SA, Requena-Ibanez JA, Devesa A, et al. Uncovering the role of epicardial adipose tissue in heart failure with preserved ejection fraction. JACC Adv. 2023;2(9):100657.
10. Koepp KE, Obokata M, Reddy YNV, et al. Hemodynamic and Functional Impact of Epicardial Adipose Tissue in Heart Failure with Preserved Ejection Fraction. JACC Heart Fail. 2020;8(8):657-66.
11. Cho JH. Sudden death and ventricular arrhythmias in heart failure with preserved ejection fraction. Korean Circ J. 2022;52(4):251-64.
12. Cho JH, Zhang R, Aynaszyan S, et al. Ventricular Arrhythmias Underlie Sudden Death in Rats with Heart Failure and Preserved Ejection Fraction. Circ Arrhythm Electrophysiol. 2018;11(8):e006452.
13. Muller TD, Finan B, Bloom SR, et al. Glucagon-like peptide 1 (GLP-1). Mol Metab. 2019;30:72-130.
14. Rowlands J, Heng J, Newsholme P, et al. Pleiotropic effects of GLP-1 and analogs on cell signaling, metabolism, and function. Front Endocrinol (Lausanne). 2018;9:672.
15. Dailey MJ, Moran TH. Glucagon-like peptide 1 and appetite. Trends Endocrinol Metab. 2013;24:85-91.
16. Chaudhuri A, Ghanim H, Vora M, et al. Exenatide exerts a potent anti-inflammatory effect. J Clin Endocrinol Metab. 2012;97:198-207.
17. Shiraishi D, Fujiwara Y, Komohara Y, et al. "Glucagon-Like Peptide-1 (GLP-1) Induces M2 Polarization of Human Macrophages via STAT3 Activation," Biochem Biophys Res Commun. 2012;425(2):304-8.
18. Huang J, Li Ga, Wang J, et al. Evaluation of subclinical left ventricular systolic dysfunction in obese patients by global myocardial work. Diabetol Metab Syndr. 2023;15:254.
19. Singh M, Sethi A, Mishra AK, et al. Echocardiographic Imaging Challenges in Obesity: Guideline Recommendations and Limitations of Adjusting to Body Size. J Am Heart Assoc. 2020;9(2):e014609.
20. Dietz MF, Prihadi EA, van der Bijl P, et al. The Obesity Paradox in Patients with Significant Tricuspid Regurgitation: Effects of Obesity on Right Ventricular Remodeling and Long-Term Prognosis. J Am Soc Echocardiogr. 2021;34(1):20-9.
21. Kodsi M, Makarious D, Gan GCH, et al Cardiac reverse remodeling by imaging parameters with recent changes to guideline medical therapy in heart failure. ESC Heart Fail. 2023;10(6):3258-75.
22. Kosiborod MN, Abildstrøm SZ, Borlaug BA, et al Semaglutide in Patients with Heart Failure with Preserved Ejection Fraction and Obesity. N Engl J Med. 2023;389(12):1069-84.
23. Kosiborod MN, Petrie MC, Borlaug BA, et al. Semaglutide in Patients with Obesity-Related Heart Failure and Type 2 Diabetes. N Engl J Med. 2024;390:1394-407.
24. Solomon SD, Ostrominski JW, Wang X, et al. Effect of Semaglutide on Cardiac Structure and Function in Patients with Obesity-Related Heart Failure. JACC. 2024;84(17):1587-602.
25. Packer M, Zile MR, Kramer CM, et al. Tirzepatide for Heart Failure with Preserved Ejection Fraction and Obesity. N Engl J Med. 2025;392(5):427-37.
26. Kramer CM, Borlaug BA, Zile MR, et al. Tirzepatide Reduces LV Mass and Paracardiac Adipose Tissue in Obesity-Related Heart Failure: SUMMIT CMR Sub-study. JACC. 2025;85(7):699-706.
27. Siddiqui HF, Waqas SA, Batool RM, et al. The effect of GLP-1 receptor agonists on cardiac remodeling in heart failure patients with preserved and reduced ejection fraction: a systematic review and meta-analysis. Heart Fail Rev. 2025;30(5):991-1004.

SECTION 16

Obesity and Intensive Care Unit

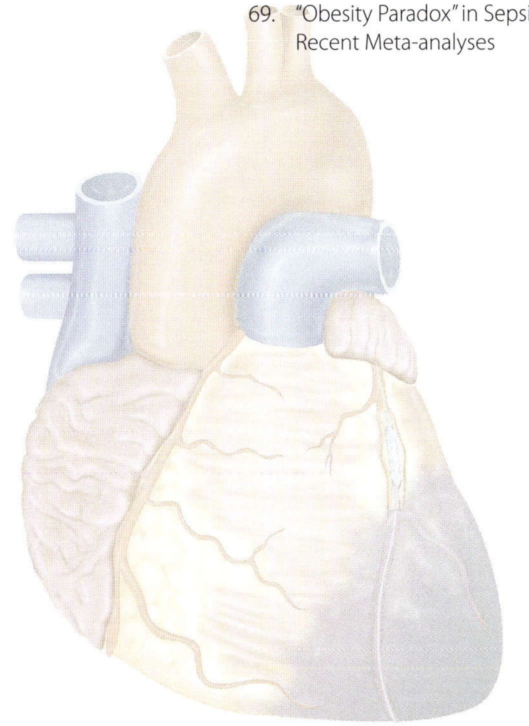

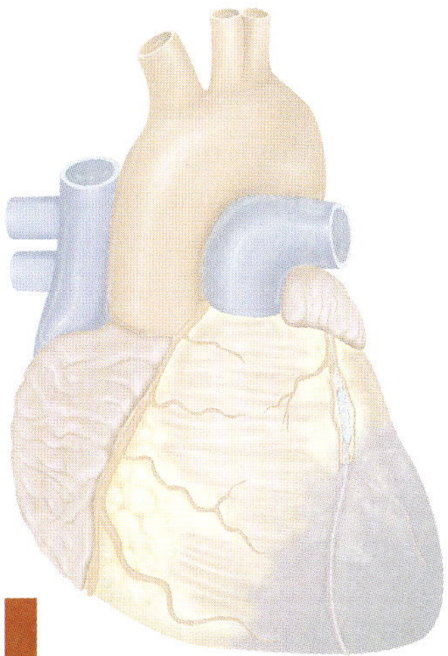

69

CHAPTER

"Obesity Paradox" in Sepsis: Multiple Recent Meta-analyses

HK Chopra, Md Inamul Haque, Abbas Ali Khatai, Rajesh Mishra

INTRODUCTION

Sepsis is a life-threatening condition characterized by acute organ dysfunction resulting from a dysregulated host response to infection.[1] Over the past several decades, the global prevalence of obesity has risen dramatically.[2] Although obesity is well established as a risk factor for numerous adverse health outcomes, including cardiovascular disease, a paradoxical survival advantage has been observed in certain clinical conditions, particularly among critically ill patients.[3-5] In recent years, this so-called obesity paradox has been increasingly reported in patients with sepsis.[6] Furthermore, multiple systematic reviews and meta-analyses indicate that patients with higher body mass index (BMI) experience improved survival following sepsis.[7]

OVERVIEW OF THE OBESITY PARADOX IN SEPSIS

The obesity paradox refers to the counterintuitive observation that overweight and obese patients sometimes exhibit better survival outcomes in acute and critical illnesses, including sepsis, compared with individuals of normal body weight. Although obesity is a well-established risk factor for chronic diseases, such as cardiovascular and metabolic disorders, numerous clinical studies have reported reduced mortality in septic patients with elevated BMI, challenging traditional paradigms regarding obesity and health outcomes.[8]

Despite supporting evidence, the existence and interpretation of the obesity paradox in sepsis remain subjects of debate. Critics emphasize that most supporting studies are observational and therefore vulnerable to confounding factors, including variations in illness severity, comorbidities, and treatment differences. Moreover, BMI itself is an imperfect surrogate for body composition and does not distinguish between lean muscle mass and fat distribution, which may have differential effects on outcomes. Consequently, it remains unclear whether the associations observed reflect true biological protection or are partly artifacts of study design and confounding.[9]

PATHOPHYSIOLOGICAL MECHANISMS EXPLAINING THE OBESITY PARADOX: CURRENT HYPOTHESES

The obesity paradox in critically ill patients has been the focus of prolonged scientific debate, with multiple hypotheses proposed to explain the observed survival advantage associated with obesity. Multiple pathophysiological mechanisms have been proposed to

TABLE 1: BMI categories for adult weight assessment.

BMI, kg/m²	<18.5	18.5–24.9	25–29.9	30–34.9	35–39.9	≥40
Classification	Underweight	Normal weight	Overweight	Class I (moderate)	Class II (severe)	Class III (very severe)

account for the obesity paradox observed in critically ill patients with sepsis.

First, obesity may provide greater metabolic reserves, which are beneficial during the highly catabolic state of acute illness. Second, adipose tissue can influence the inflammatory response by releasing anti-inflammatory mediators such as leptin[10,11] and soluble tumor necrosis factor receptor-2.[10] In addition, increased activation of the renin angiotensin system in obese patients may offer hemodynamic advantages during sepsis.[11]

Possible Pathophysiological Mechanisms of the Obesity Paradox

- Higher metabolic reserves in acute catabolic illnesses.
- Secretion of anti-inflammatory mediators by adipose tissue, e.g., leptin, soluble tumor necrosis factor-receptor-2.
- Hemodynamic benefits of renin-angiotensin system activation.
- High-density lipoproteins bind bacterial lipopolysaccharide.
- Obesity and resulting obstructive sleep apnea contribute to ischemic preconditioning.

Possible Biases in Studies Examining the Obesity Paradox (Fig. 1)

- Inadequate adjustment for confounding factors, e.g., smoking.
- Protective effect limited to certain subpopulations, e.g., older patients with comorbidities
- Relatively restrictive administration of medications in obese patients due to a nonweight-based principle.
- Misclassification of patients due to inaccurate BMI measurements.
- Decreased BMI may be due to sarcopenia.

Proposed biological mechanisms underlying the obesity paradox across diverse disease states, including cardiovascular disease, trauma, sepsis, burns, and pulmonary conditions. A consistent U-shaped association between BMI and clinical outcomes is observed across these settings.[12]

RECENT META-ANALYSES AND UPDATES (2025) ON THE OBESITY PARADOX IN SEPSIS

In recent years, a growing number of systematic reviews and meta-analyses have evaluated the association between BMI categories and outcomes in patients with sepsis, providing updated insights into the obesity paradox. Meta-analyses synthesizing observational data consistently suggest that overweight and obese patients with sepsis experience lower mortality compared with individuals of normal weight, while underweight status is associated with higher mortality. Morbid obesity did not show a consistent protective effect.

Observational Meta-analyses Supporting the Paradox (Fig. 2)[13,14]

A total of fifteen studies encompassing 105,159 patients were included in the pooled analysis. Overweight and obese BMI categories were associated with significantly reduced mortality (OR: 0.79, 95% CI: 0.70–0.88, and OR: 0.74, 95% CI: 0.67–0.82, respectively). However, these associations were not statistically significant among patients aged ≤50 years (OR: 0.89, 95% CI: 0.68–1.14 and OR: 0.77, 95% CI: 0.50–1.18, respectively). Furthermore, no significant association was observed between morbid obesity and mortality (OR: 0.91, 95% CI: 0.62–1.32).

Overweight and obese BMIs (25.0–39.9 kg/m^2) are associated with reduced mortality of patients with sepsis or septic shock, although such a survival advantage was not found in all crowds.

Individual and pooled results of the association of underweight, overweight, obese, and morbidly obese BMIs with mortality in patients with sepsis.[15]

Murine Sepsis Models Meta-analysis (2025) (Fig. 3)[16]

A systematic review/meta-analysis of mouse models found mixed effects of obesity on survival, with no significant pooled mortality benefit in the best-matched experiments. Heterogeneity drivers such as timing of high-fat diet, duration of obesity induction, and age at sepsis onset all affected outcomes in meta-regression analysis.

Overall, animal studies do not support a consistent biological survival advantage of obesity in sepsis, suggesting caution when interpreting human observational findings.

Comparison of the duration of individual periods (preresearch diet feeding, research diet feeding period, and observation period after sepsis induction) in the studies included in the meta-analysis.[17]

Confounding Effects of Comorbidities and Therapeutic Interventions[18-21]

After adjustment for underlying metabolic abnormalities, overweight status was no longer independently associated with improved 28-day survival. Importantly,

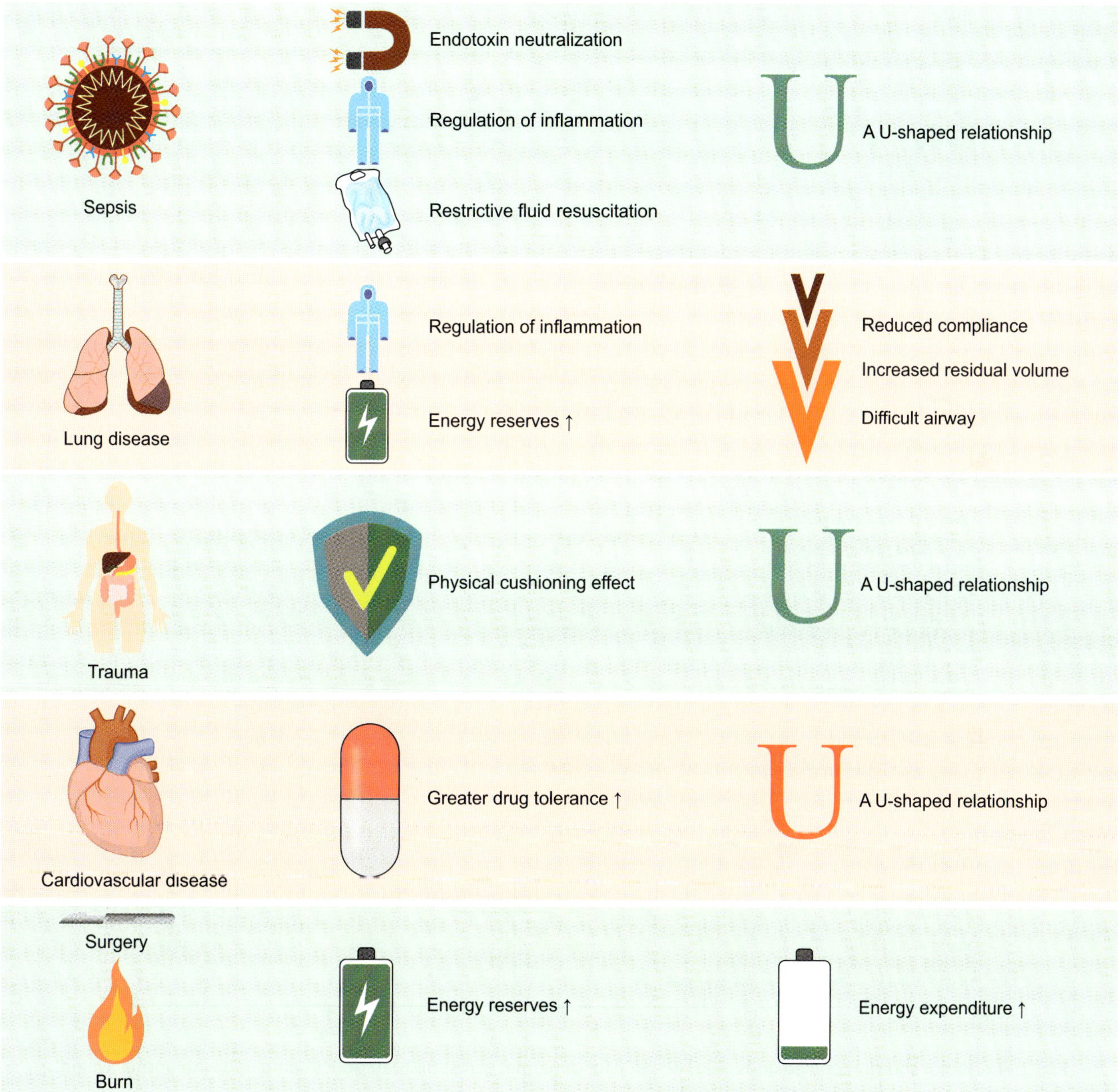

Fig. 1: Proposed relationships between body mass (or adiposity) and outcomes across critical illness and disease states

the previously observed survival advantage associated with metabolic abnormalities was largely attributable to the pharmacologic therapies used in their management, including biguanides, sulfonylureas, β-blockers, angiotensin converting enzyme inhibitors, angiotensin II receptor blockers, diuretics, and statins.

These findings call into question the traditional concept of the "obesity paradox" in sepsis and suggest that the apparent protective effect is primarily medication-driven rather than intrinsic to metabolic status itself. Optimizing evidence-based pharmacological strategies may therefore represent a critical avenue for improving outcomes in patients with sepsis.

LIMITATIONS AND CRITIQUES OF THE OBESITY PARADOX

Despite longstanding hypotheses of a survival advantage in obesity, emerging evidence suggests that the observed association is driven by a complex interplay

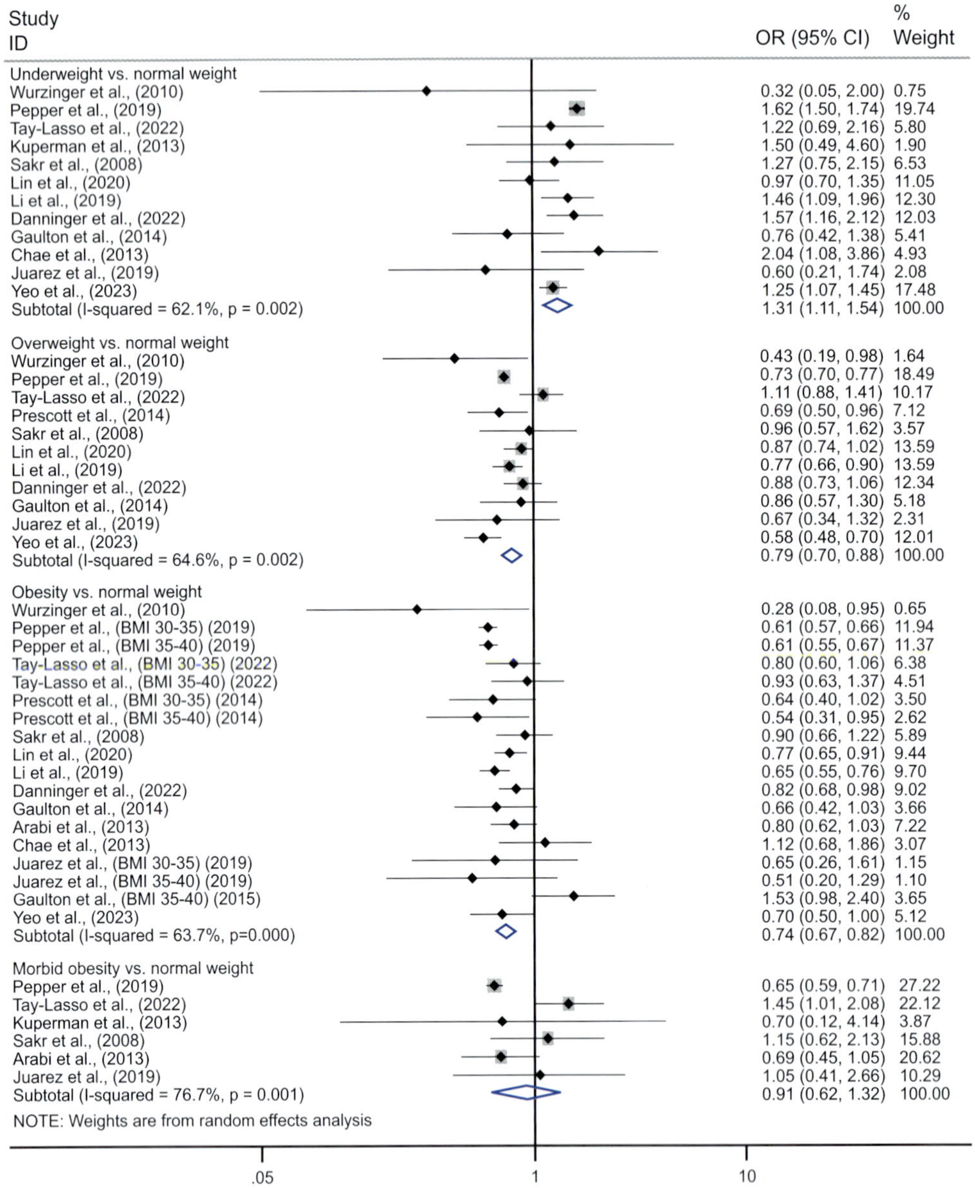

Fig. 2: Forest plot showing pooled odds ratios (95% CI) for outcomes across BMI categories compared with normal weight.

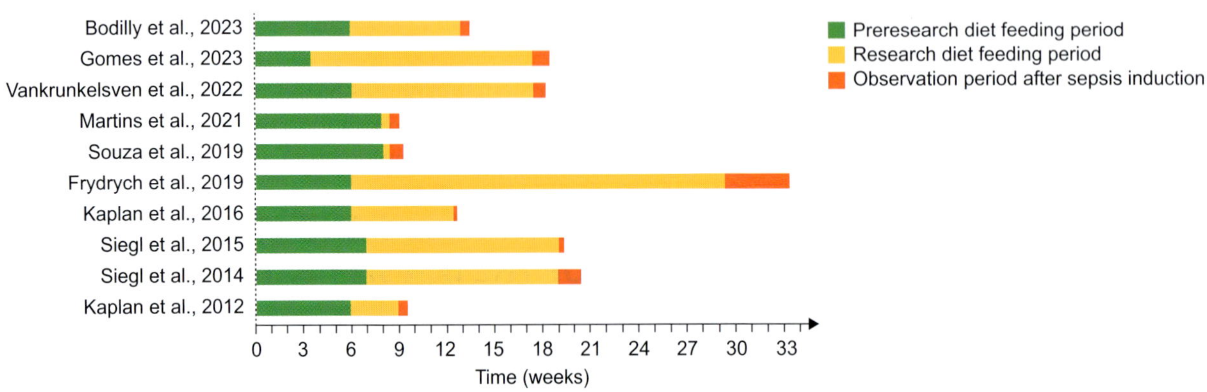

Fig. 3: Timeline of preresearch diet, research diet, and postsepsis observation periods across included experimental studies.

of methodological and biological factors, including confounding, imperfect adiposity measurement using BMI, chronic illness-related weight loss, heterogeneity of obesity phenotypes, and sampling bias.

Many of the observed links between BMI and mortality come from studies that have important limitations and cannot prove cause and effect. Illness-related weight loss before BMI is measured, and hidden medical conditions can distort results, making normal-weight patients appear at higher risk and obese patients seem protected.[22] In addition, most studies rely on only one weight measurement and do not account for weight changes over time. Therefore, without strong biological evidence, the obesity paradox may reflect a statistical artifact rather than a true protective effect.[23]

CONCLUSION

Recent meta-analyses up to 2025 consistently demonstrate that overweight and obese patients with sepsis experience lower mortality compared with normal weight patients, while underweight status remains a strong predictor of adverse outcomes. This survival advantage, widely termed by the obesity paradox, appears robust across multiple clinical settings and outcome measures, although substantial heterogeneity persists.

The observed association is likely multifactorial, involving metabolic reserves, immunomodulatory effects of adipose tissue, altered inflammatory responses, and differences in clinical management. Nevertheless, residual confounding and limitations of observational data preclude causal inference. Future prospective and mechanistic studies are required to better define the biological basis of this phenomenon and to inform risk stratified management strategies in septic patients.

REFERENCES

1. Singer M, Deutschman CS, Seymour CW, et al. The Third International Consensus Definitions for Sepsis and Septic Shock (Sepsis-3). JAMA. 2016;315(8):801-10.
2. Goda A, Masuyama T: Obesity and overweight in Asian people. Circ J. 2016;80(12):2425-6.
3. Karampela I, Chrysanthopoulou E, Christodoulatos GS, et al. Is there an obesity paradox in critical illness? Epidemiologic and metabolic considerations. Curr Obes Rep. 2020;9(3):231-44.
4. Cho WH, Oh JY, Yeo HJ, et al. Obesity survival paradox in pneumonia supported with extracorporeal membrane oxygenation: Analysis of the national registry. J Crit Care. 2018;48:453-7.
5. Schetz M, De Jong A, Deane AM, et al. Obesity in the critically ill: A narrative review. Intensive Care Med. 2019;45:757-69.
6. Jagan N, Morrow LE, Walters RW, et al. Sepsis and the obesity paradox: Size matters in more than one way. Crit Care Med. 2020;48:e776-82.
7. Trivedi V, Bavishi C, Jean R: Impact of obesity on sepsis mortality: A systematic review. J Crit Care. 2015;30(3):518-24.
8. Singer M, Deutschman CS, Seymour C, et al. The Third International Consensus Definitions for Sepsis and Septic Shock (Sepsis-3). JAMA. 2016;315:801-10.
9. Ni YN, Luo J, Yu H, et al. Can body mass index predict clinical outcomes for patients with acute lung injury/acute respiratory distress syndrome? A meta-analysis. Crit Care. 2017;21(1):36.
10. Ahima RS. Adipose tissue as an endocrine organ. Obesity (Silver Spring). 2006;14(Suppl 5):242S-9S.
11. Winkler G, Kiss S, Keszthelyi L, et al. Expression of tumor necrosis factor (TNF)-alpha protein in the subcutaneous and visceral adipose tissue in correlation with adipocyte cell volume, serum TNF-alpha, soluble serum TNF-receptor-2 concentrations and C-peptide level. Eur J Endocrinol. 2003;149(2):129-35.
12. Obesity Paradox in Critically Ill Patients: Do Patients with Critical Diseases Benefit from Obesity? Obes Facts 2025;1-12.
13. Kershaw EE, Flier JS. Adipose tissue as an endocrine organ. J Clin Endocrinol Metab. 2004;89(6):2548-5.
14. Singer M, Deutschman CS, Seymour CW, et al. The Third International Consensus Definitions for Sepsis and Septic Shock (Sepsis-3). JAMA. 2016;315(8):801-10.
15. Wang HE, Griffin R, Judd S, et al. Obesity and risk of sepsis: a population-based cohort study. Obesity (Silver Spring, Md). 2013;21(12):E762-9.
16. Bai L, Huang J, Wang D, et al. Association of body mass index with mortality of sepsis or septic shock: an updated meta-analysis. J Intensive Care. 2023;11:27.
17. Wasyluk W, Czop M, Wasyluk M, et al. The obesity paradox in murine sepsis models: a systematic review and meta-analysis. Anaesthesiol Intensive Ther. 2025;57(1):182-94.
18. Cecconi M, Evans L, Levy M, et al. Sepsis and septic shock Lancet. 2018;392(10141):75-87.
19. Rudd KE, Johnson SC, Agesa KM, et al. Global, regional, and national sepsis incidence and mortality, 1990-2017: analysis for the global burden of disease study. Lancet. 2020;395(10219):200-11.
20. Terblanche M, Almog Y, Rosenson RS, et al. Statins and sepsis: multiple modifications at multiple levels. Lancet Infect Dis. 2007;7(5):358-68.
21. Yeo HJ, Kim TH, Jang JH, et al. Obesity paradox and functional outcomes in sepsis: a multicenter prospective study. Crit Care Med. 2023;51(6):742-52.
22. Tobias DK. Addressing reverse causation bias in the obesity paradox is not "one size fits all". Diabetes Care. 2017;40(8):1000-1
23. Kalantar-Zadeh K, Rhee CM, Amin AN. To legitimize the contentious obesity paradox. Mayo Clin Proc. 2014;89(8):1033-5.

SECTION 17

Cardio-ophthalmology

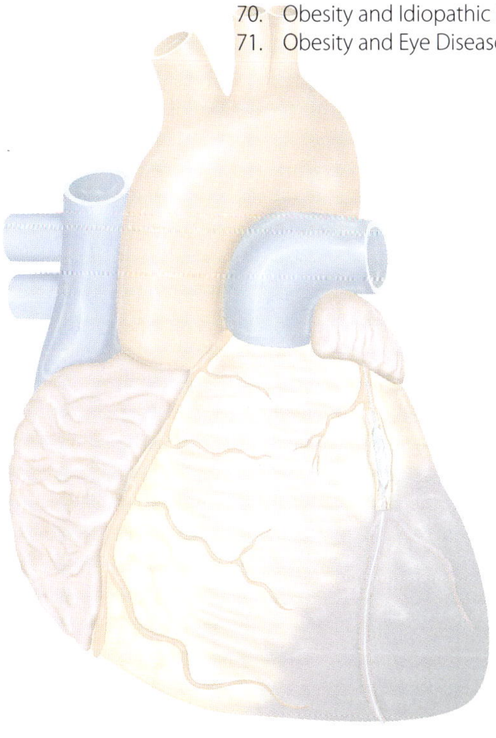

70

CHAPTER

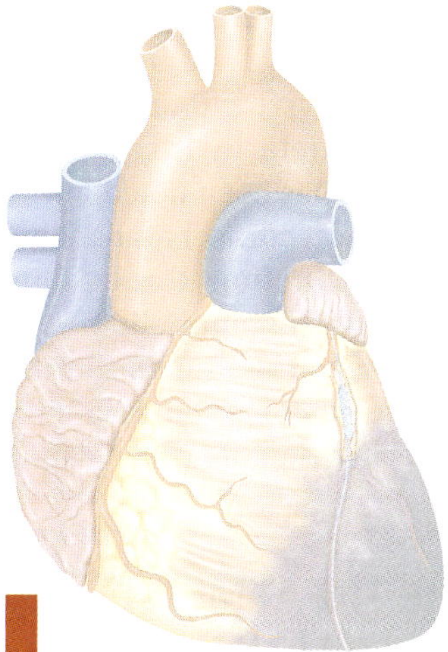

Obesity and Idiopathic Intracranial Hypertension

Krishna Vaitheeswaran, Preetinder Kaur, Monika Nadar

INTRODUCTION AND EPIDEMIOLOGY

Obesity is a global health problem affecting over half a billion individuals around the world. It is defined by the WHO as having a body mass index (BMI >30 kg/m^2). In the US, in 2018, over two-thirds of adults were overweight (BMI >25 kg/m^2), with one-third being obese (BMI >30 kg/m^2).

Obesity constitutes an important contributor to various comorbidities, including diabetes, cardiovascular diseases, cancer, hypertension, and premature death.

Obesity is associated with insulin resistance, dyslipidemia, an altered sexually dimorphic endocrine phenotype, increased proinflammatory cytokines, including IL-1β, leptin, and IL-6, as well as reduced levels of anti-inflammatory cytokines, such as adiponectin.[1]

Underlying this is a biochemical and hormonal alteration driven by adiposity and chronic low-level information. Given this biochemical phenotype, obesity affects all functioning of the human body, including the nervous system.

Idiopathic intracranial hypertension (IIH), in particular, has been known to be associated with an elevated BMI, with reduction in weight and obesity affording symptomatic and clinical relief. Over 70–80% of patients are obese, and over 90% are overweight.[2] The overall age-adjusted incidence of IIH is 11 per 100,000 population, but increases to 86 per 100,000 in the obese.

The risk of developing IIH increases with increasing BMI and percentage weight gain. The odds ratio increases from 19.5 with a BMI of 30–35 kg/m^2 to 26 with a BMI of >35 kg/m^3. With annual weight gain, the odds ratio increases from 3.6 with a 5–10% annual weight gain to 15.2 with a 11–15% annual weight gain.[4]

Nonobese patients (BMI <30 kg/m^2) are also at greater risk if they have a weight gain of 5% or more. A study of recurrent IIH also found a mean weight gain of 6% before the recurrence, mirroring the weight loss at which the disease resolves.[5]

The role of obesity in males is less clear for the development of IIH. Only 25% of men with IIH were overweight compared to 78% of women in the same cohort.[6] Other studies have shown that men with IIH were less obese but had more vision loss than women, including severe vision loss.[7,8] Another difference was that 24% of men had obstructive sleep apnea compared to only 4% of women.[9]

POSTULATED MECHANISMS AND PATHOPHYSIOLOGY OF OBESITY AND INTRACRANIAL HYPERTENSION

The mechanisms by which obesity contributes to the development of IIH is not fully understood. Several pathophysiological mechanisms have been proposed, but none account for all the features of the disease.

- *Enhanced CSF production*. Some authors have suggested and an increased CSF production from data obtained from ventricular infusion studies.[10] Other studies using velocity-sensitive magnetic resonance image mapping have shown no significant difference in CSF production in IIH patients and controls.[11]
- *Reduced absorption of CSF:*
  - *Thrombophilic conditions*. Occult microthrombosis has been stated to occur within the dural venous sinuses in the vicinity of the arachnoid granulations, reducing CSF absorption. A high

prevalence of prothrombotic abnormalities, including anti-phospholipid antibodies, abnormal protein S levels, factor 5 Leiden, and prothrombin 20, 210 mutations have been noted.[12] However, the studies show that the prothrombotic conditions were more common in nonobese individuals. Higher thrombophilic abnormalities have been noted in PCO syndrome with associated IIH.[13] 38% had homozygous methylenetetrahydrofolate mutations, and 29% had increased lipoprotein A levels in addition to fourteen percent having thrombophilic concentrations of factor VIII.

- *Elevated intra-abdominal pressure:* The increased intra-abdominal pressure increases the pleural and cardiac pressures, limiting venous return from the brain. Increased abdominal pressure also limits the expansion of CSF spaces and CSF homeostasis. However, IIH patients have been shown to have increased adiposity below the waist rather than above the waist.[14] Also, conditions with raised central venous pressure are not reported to have IIH.

- *Hormonal factors:* Adipocytes secret hormone leptin, which regulates appetite, food intake, and body weight. An absence of Leptin or a resistance to it can lead to uncontrolled eating and weight gain. Higher serum leptin levels have been found in IIH.[15] Elevated CSF pressure may impede the action of leptin, creating a relative leptin-resistant state. The hyperleptinemia may be a secondary effect, however, since leptin is found in higher levels in subcutaneous fat compared with visceral fat, and the distribution of obesity in IIH favors subcutaneous fat deposition. Ball et al.[16] found that IIH patients had higher CSF Leptin levels compared with controls after correction for age, gender, and BMI. It was suggested that obesity in IIH may result from hypothalamic Leptin resistance.
  In addition,
  - *Impaired sodium homeostasis:* Sodium homeostasis may also be impaired in IIH patients. A study demonstrated that 77% of patients with IIH had orthostatic oedema compared to none in the control group. Patients with IIH treated with diuretics lost weight and had less diurnal weight gain as compared to obesity matched controls.[17]
  - *Inflammation:* Obesity has been associated with chronic low-grade inflammation and an abnormal proinflammatory cytokine profile. However, in a study, profiles of inflammatory cytokines in IIH patients were not different from those of controls. Inflammatory markers correlate better with central obesity, and IIH have less marked central obesity than obese cohorts.[18]
  - *Cortisol dysregulation:* A dysregulation of the intracellular enzyme, 11 beta-hydroxysteroid dehydrogenase (11β-HSD1) has been noted in IIH patients, which mediates local cortisol availability. This may affect CSF production through its expression in choroidal plexus epithelium and arachnoid granulation tissue.[19] Reduction in the global 11β-HSD1 activity has been noted after a 3-month low-calorie diet in IIH patients, indicating a pathogenic mechanism.

WEIGHT LOSS IN THE TREATMENT OF IDIOPATHIC INTRACRANIAL HYPERTENSION

Several studies have demonstrated the beneficial effect of weight loss in the management of IIH further, further strengthening the association of the disease with obesity.

In 1974, Newborg[20] reported 9 IIH patients treated with Kempner's rice/reduction diet, comprising a daily allowance of 400–1,000 calories, 750–1,250 mL fluid, and less than 100 mg sodium. Within 3 months, the patients lost 13–38% of body weight and had resolution of papilledema.

Kupersmith et al.[21] reviewed the charts of 58 IIH patients treated with weight loss and diuretics. Papilledema was resolved in 74% of the 38 patients who lost weight compared with 40% of those who did not lose weight.

Sinclair reported that 20 patients, who lost an average of 15.7 kg after 3 months, had an improvement in headaches and papilledema and had an average reduction of CSF pressure of 8 cmH_2O.[22]

BARIATRIC SURGERY

Bariatric surgery is a proven weight loss method for morbidly obese individuals and is effective for long-term control of obesity. In a literature review of 62 reported cases of IIH treated with bariatric surgery, 92% had resolution of IIH symptoms, 97% had resolution of papilledema, and 92% had complete or nearly complete resolution of visual field deficits. The mean decrease in CSF opening pressure on lumbar puncture after surgery was 25 cmH_2O.[23]

Although bariatric surgery provides a mechanical alteration as to how food is processed post-prandially, the primary mode of weight loss is mediated through changes in gut-neuropeptides. This rebalancing of gut-neuropeptides alters feeding behavior and the metabolic metabolism, thus facilitating weight loss.

IDIOPATHIC INTRACRANIAL HYPERTENSION TRIAL

The idiopathic intracranial hypertension treatment trial (IIHTT)[24] was a randomized, double blind, placebo-controlled study of acetazolamide therapy in IIH. The study showed significantly more improvement at month 6 in the acetazolamide group compared with the control group. Patients treated with acetazolamide lost more weight over 6 months (mean loss 7.5 kg; 7.8%) than those given a placebo (mean loss 3.5 kg; 3.5%). Compared with the control group, the acetazolamide group also showed a greater decrease in mean BMI (3.3 vs. 1.3) and waist circumference (8.6 vs. 3.9 cm). Also, 28% of the control group gained weight compared with only 13% in the acetazolamide group. Acetazolamide-treated patients had a significant improvement in quality-of-life measures, which may have allowed them to pursue weight loss more diligently.

GLUCAGON-LIKE-PEPTIDE 1 RECEPTOR AGONISTS

Glucagon-like peptide-1 receptor agonists are widely used to treat obesity and diabetes. Its role in the management of IIH was evaluated by a systematic review. Nine clinical studies (one RCT, eight observational studies) with IIH patients receiving GLP-1 RAs were included. GLP-1 RA use was consistently associated with improvements in headache frequency, weight reduction, and reduced need for acetazolamide or surgical interventions. This may be further investigated in larger studies to further validate its use in the condition.

CONCLUSION

Obesity and weight gain is an important pathogenic mechanisms for the development of Idiopathic IIH mediated through various mechanisms. The use of measures to control obesity has been shown to be effective in managing the disease. The role of bariatric surgery and newer antiobesity drugs has been effective in clinical trials and may usher in a newer paradigm in the management of this vision-threatening condition.

REFERENCES

1. Mokdad AH, Ford ES, Bowman BA, et al. Prevalence of Obesity, Diabetes, and Obesity-Related Health Risk Factors, 2001. JAMA. 2003;289(1):76-9.
2. Markey KA, Mollan SP, Jensen RH, et al. Understanding idiopathic intracranial hypertension: mechanisms, management, and future directions. Lancet Neurol. 2016;15(1):78-91.
3. Raoof N, Sharrack B, Pepper IM, et al. The incidence and prevalence of idiopathic intracranial hypertension in Sheffield, UK. Eur J Neurol. 2011;18(10):1266-8.
4. Kesler A, Hadayer A, Goldhammer Y, et al. Idiopathic intracranial hypertension: risk of recurrences. Neurology. 2004;63(90):1737-9.
5. Ko MW, Chang SC, Ridha MA, et al. Weight gain and recurrence in idiopathic intracranial hypertension: a case-control study. Neurology. 2011;76(18):1564-7.
6. Kesler A, Goldhammer Y, Gadoth N. Do men with pseudomotor cerebri share the same characteristics as women? A retrospective review of 141 cases. J Neuroophthalmol. 2001;21(1):15-7.
7. Digre KB, Corbett JJ. Pseudotumor cerebri in men. Arch Neurol. 1988;45(8):866-72.
8. Bruce BB, Kedar S, Van Stavern GP, et al. Idiopathic intracranial hypertension in men. Neurology. 2009;72(4):304-9.
9. Fraser JA, Bruce BB, Rucker J, et al. Risk factors for idiopathic intracranial hypertension in men: a case-control study. J Neurol Sci. 2010;290(1-2):86-9.
10. Donaldson JO. Cerebrospinal fluid hypersecretion in pseudotumor cerebri. Trans Am Neurol Assoc. 1979;104: 196-8.
11. Gideon P, Sorensen PS, Thomsen C, et al. Assessment of CSF dynamics and venous flow in the superior sagittal sinus by MRI in idiopathic intracranial hypertension: a preliminary study. Neuroradiology. 1994;369(5):350-4.
12. Sussman J, Leach M, Greaves M, et al. Potentially prothrombotic abnormalities of coagulation in benign intracranial hypertension. J Neurol Neurosurg Psychiatry. 1997;62(3):229-33.
13. Glueck CJ, Aregawi D, Goldenberg N, et al. Idiopathic intracranial hypertension, polycystic-ovary syndrome, and thrombophilia. J Lab Clin Med. 2005;145(2):72-82.
14. Kesler A, Kliper E, Shenkerman G, et al. Idiopathic intracranial hypertension is associated with lower body adiposity. Ophthalmology. 2010;117(1):169-74.
15. Lampl Y, Eshel Y, Kessler A, et al. Serum leptin level in women with idiopathic intracranial hypertension. J Neurol Neurosurg Psychiatry. 2002;72(5):642-3.
16. Ball AK, Sinclair AJ, Curnow SJ, et al. Elevated cerebrospinal fluid (CSF) leptin in idiopathic intracranial hypertension (IIH): evidence for hypothalamic leptin resistance? Clin Endocrinol (Oxf). 2009;70(6):863-9.
17. Friedman DI, Streeten DH. Idiopathic intracranial hypertension and orthostatic edema may share a common pathogenesis. Neurology. 1998;50(4):1099-104.
18. Sinclair AJ, Ball AK, Burdon MA, et al. Exploring the pathogenesis of IIH: an inflammatory perspective. J Neuroimmunol. 2008;201-2:212-20.
19. Rauz S, Stewart PM. Expression and putative role of 11 beta-hydroxysteroid dehydrogenase isozymes within the human eye. Invest Ophthalmol Vis Sci. 2001;42(9):2037-42.

20. Newborg B. Pseudotumor cerebri treated by rice reduction diet. Arch Intern Med. 1974;133(5):802-7.
21. Kupersmith MJ, Gamell L, Turbin R, et al. Effects of weight loss on the course of idiopathic intracranial hypertension in women. Neurology. 1998;50(4):1094-8.
22. Sinclair AJ, Burdon MA, Nightingale PG, et al. Low energy diet and intracranial pressure in women with idiopathic intracranial hypertension: prospective cohort study. BMJ. 2010;341:c2701.
23. Fridley J, Foroozan R, Sherman V, et al. Bariatric surgery for the treatment of idiopathic intracranial hypertension. J Neurosurg. 2011;114(1):34-9.
24. Nordic Idiopathic Intracranial Hypertension Study Group Writing Committee; Wall M, McDermott MP, Kieburtz KD, et al. Effect of acetazolamide on visual function in patients with idiopathic intracranial hypertension and mild visual loss: the idiopathic intracranial hypertension treatment trial. JAMA. 2014;311(16):1641-51.

71

CHAPTER

Obesity and Eye Diseases

Monika Nadar, Preetinder Kaur, Krishna Vaitheeswaran

INTRODUCTION

Obesity is a chronic disease and is increasing worldwide. It is considered a global epidemic, which has a high impact on quality-of-life as well as increasing costs of healthcare in the community.

It has been reported that the prevalence of obesity worldwide has approximately tripled since 1980 in more than 70 countries and has increased steadily in most other countries, now exceeding two billion people worldwide.[1]

Worldwide, at least 2.8 billion people die each year due to obesity-related pathologies. It is estimated that 35.8 million (2.3%) of the global disability adjusted life years (DALYs) are caused by being overweight or due to obesity.

Obesity is also considered a significant risk factor for eye diseases. A multidisciplinary and a multidimensional approach to control and manage obesity will reflect in better ocular health. Eye diseases are serious worldwide health problems that negatively impact quality of life. The prevalence of age-related eye diseases is expected to increase worldwide as the aging population increases.[2] While 43.3 million people were estimated to be blind in 2020, it is estimated that this number will go up to 61 million by 2050.[3] In addition, the number of people with moderate severe visual employment is expected to increase worldwide from 216.6 million in 2015 to 587.6 million by 2050.

Although the negative effects of obesity on health have been well studied, the impact on the visual system is still being understood. Many eye conditions, known to be associated with obesity, are being studied, including cataracts, glaucoma, age-related macular degeneration (AMD), diabetic retinopathy, and dry eye syndrome.

The etiopathogenetic mechanisms behind the changes caused by obesity in the eye include inflammation, oxidative stress, and hormonal imbalances as also cardio-vascular effects of the metabolic syndrome on the eye. Adipose tissue is known to enhance proinflammatory cytokines, increasing tissue damage and contributing to disease.

In a systematic review of population based studies,[4] association between obesity and different anthropometric measures with four main age-related ocular diseases was reported—cataract, glaucoma, AMD, and diabetic retinopathy.

CATARACT

Cataracts are age-dependent ocular pathologies with some reports suggesting a significant association with obesity.

In 1995, Glynn et al. reported a strong correlation between BMI and incident cataracts, particularly posterior subcapsular cataract (PSC) and nuclear cataract. A two-unit increase in BMI value predicted a 12% major risk of cataract.[5]

In a study of 17,150 males, followed up 5 years, BMI and WHR were found to be independent risk factors for cataract.[6] Glynn et al. in 2009 reported that the type of cataract most strongly associated with high BMI is cortical cataract.[7]

There is evidence that, compared to obesity assessed by BMI, abdominal obesity is a better indicator for any type of incident cataract. In fact, waist circumference (WC), waist-to-hip circumference (WHR), and waist-to-height ratio (WHtR) are more reliable and specific indicators of intra-abdominal fat and visceral obesity than BMI.[8]

Elevated CRP levels, market of systemic inflammation, were found to be associated with an increased risk of cataracts.[9] Inflammation causes oxidative stress leading to oxidative damage to the lens. Obesity is correlated with a subclinical low-grade systemic inflammation and oxidative stress leading to the development of cataracts.

On the other hand, several studies have revealed that a higher level of physical activity is associated with reduced incidence of cataract. Cohorts engaged in physical activity such as walking or running had a lower risk of cataract.[10] This emphasizes the role of physical activity and obesity control measures as part of public health intervention for the control of cataract.

GLAUCOMA

Glaucoma is a multifactorial disease and a very important cause of irreversible blindness worldwide. Neurodegeneration, inflammation of retinal neurons as well as progressive loss of retinal ganglion cells are the most important aspects of glaucomatous optic neuropathy.

Glaucoma causes silent visual loss, which cannot be reversed. Early diagnosis requires recognition of high-risk factors enabling targeted intervention toward causative mechanisms aimed at preventing or stalling progression of the disease.

Elevated intraocular pressure is the most common and first called upon risk factor for open-angle glaucoma. Other significant risk factors for progression include higher baseline age, high baseline IOP, high BMI, high hematocrit levels, and various systemic diseases such as a dysthyroid state.[11]

Open-angle glaucoma, both hypertensive and normotensive, is associated with obstructive sleep apnea (OSA) syndrome. Glaucomatous damage in these patients may be induced by increased intraocular pressure due to sympathetic over stimulation or due to vascular insufficiency. Hypoxia at the peripapillary plexus and optic nerve head induces irreversible damage to axons, simulating glaucoma.[12]

Wish et al. in a prospective cohort study of African American women demonstrated that primary open and glaucoma was significantly associated with BMI, WC, waist-to-hip ratio, and smoking.[13]

In the mechanisms by which obesity may increase risk of primary open glaucoma, a greater level of oxidative stress due to an increase in androgen levels associated with obesity has been reported.[14] Oxidative damage at the trabeculae meshwork and directly to the optic nerve head results in the glaucomatous phenotype.

Systemic inflammation could lead to altered blood-retinal barrier, leading to ganglion cell death and neurodegeneration.[15]

AGE-RELATED MACULAR DEGENERATION

Age-related macular degeneration is a common cause of blindness all over the world. It is a complex disease for which multiple modifiable and nonmodifiable risk factors have been identified.[16]

The most proven consistent risk factor is smoking. Obesity has been associated with AMD but not its progression. A longitudinal study investigating the effect of weight loss on the incidence of AMD revealed that a 3% reduction in waist-to-hip ratio is associated with a decrease in the incidence of AMD.[17] A meta-analysis confirms that physical activity is protective against the development of both early and late AMD, emphasizing the importance of physical activity and weight control measures.[18]

In addition, a high intake of dietary fat is associated with a greater risk of AMD progression.[19] Specific nutrients such as antioxidant vitamins and omega-3 fatty acids are associated with a reduced progression of late AMD.[20]

Physical activity, control of obesity, and nutritional factors are important both in the development of AMD as well as its progression. This has many public health implications for preventing this blinding disease.

UVEITIS

Uveitis is an inflammatory process affecting the middle layers, uvea, of the eye. Obesity is a chronic disease characterized by an increase in adipose tissue with the corresponding increase in the production of inflammatory cytokines and overall systemic state of inflammation.

Behcet's disease is a chronic multisystem autoimmune vasculitis. Metabolic syndrome has been reported to be present in 25.52% of patients.[21] The risk of metabolic syndrome was noted to be 126% higher in the study group compared to controls.[22]

Considering that abdominal adiposity is a fundamental marker for metabolic syndrome, a link exists between obesity, particularly viscero-abdominal and uveitis.

DRY EYE SYNDROME

Dry eye syndrome is a very common eye disorder that often significantly affects quality of life and may be linked to systemic inflammatory diseases, localized eye diseases, or frequently used medications.

The main descriptive definition of dry eye (DEWS II, 2017) is a multifactorial disease of the ocular surface characterized by tear film dysfunction caused by tear production deficiency or excessive evaporation, accompanied by ocular symptoms such as ocular discomfort, pain, itching, light sensitivity, fatigue or strain, heavy or foreign body sensation, and discharge.[23]

Recent studies have reported a high incidence of dry eye with body fat composition and lipid metabolic changes. A positive correlation between fat percentage and symptoms of dry eye has been reported. Women with body fat values above 30% and men with values more than 20% were more likely to report symptoms of dry eye.[24]

Sedentary lifestyle and obesity induce a low-grade inflammation, which negatively impacts tear production and tear stability linking obesity with dry eye disease.

Lifestyle modification including a physical activity program combined with a Mediterranean diet characterized by 30-minute intense aerobic exercises three times revealed significant improvements in dry eye syndrome symptoms.[25]

In conclusion, an albeit moderate but positive correlation was found between body fat percentage and dry eye symptoms. There is also evidence that weight loss, caloric restriction, and an active lifestyle are associated with significant improvements in patients with dry eye syndrome.

OBSTRUCTIVE SLEEP APNEA AND EYE DISEASES

Obesity is a common finding and an important pathogenetic factor in OSAS, both in adults and children. It has been demonstrated that some ocular pathologies are frequently associated with OSAS both in adults and in children.[26] Ocular changes may even prompt investigation and diagnosis of sleep apnea syndrome.

A recent systematic review and meta-analysis revealed significant associations between OSAS and many ocular pathologies.[27] Those that seem to have the closest pathophysiological links are nonarteritic anterior ischemic optic neuropathy (NAION), proliferative diabetic retinopathy (RDP), central serous chorioretinopathy (CSCR), and floppy eyelid syndrome (FES). Other ocular pathologies, such as vascular occlusions, papilledema, and glaucoma, are also known to be associated with OSAS.

CONCLUSION

It has been long recognized that physical activity is a critical factor in preventing and controlling obesity as well as myopia in children and adolescents. The prevalence of comorbid obesity and myopia has been reported to have increased from 11.1% in 2019 to 17.9% in 2020. A favorable physical activity environment in school reduced the odds ratio and relative risk of comorbid obesity and myopia.[28] This underlines the need to emphasize physical activity and obesity control measures in children to prevent myopia progression.

REFERENCES

1. Global Burden of Disease Collaborative Network. Global Burden of Disease Study 2019 (GBD 2019) Covariates 1980–2019. Seattle, United States of America: Institute for Health Metrics and Evaluation (IHME), 2020.
2. Bourne RRA, Flaxman SR, Braithwaite T, et al. Magnitude, temporal trends, and projections of the global prevalence of blindness and distance and near vision impairment: a systematic review and meta-analysis. Lancet Glob Health. 2017;5:e888-e897.
3. Bourne R, Steinmetz JD, Flaxman S, et al. Trends in prevalence of blindness and distance and near vision impairment over 30 years: an analysis for the Global Burden of Disease Study. Lancet Glob Health. 2021;9: e130-e143.
4. Ng Yin Ling C, Lim SC, Jonas JB, et al. Obesity and risk of age-related eye diseases: a systematic review of prospective population-based studies. Int J Obes. 2021;45: 1863-85.
5. Glynn RJ. Body mass index: an independent predictor of cataract. Arch Ophthalmol. 1995;113:1131.
6. Schaumberg DA, Glynn RJ, Christen WG, et al. Relations of body fat distribution and height with cataract in men. Am J Clin Nutr. 2000;72:1495-502.
7. Glynn RJ, Rosner B, Christen WG. Evaluation of risk factors for cataract types in a competing risks framework. Ophthalmic Epidemiol. 2009;16:98-106.
8. Elffers TW, de Mutsert R, Lamb HJ, et al. Body fat distribution, in particular visceral fat, is associated with cardiometabolic risk factors in obese women. PLoS ONE. 2017;12:e0185403.
9. Schaumberg DA, Ridker PM, Glynn RJ, et al. High levels of plasma C-reactive protein and future risk of age-related cataract. Ann Epidemiol. 1999;9:166-171.
10. Zheng Selin J, Orsini N, Ejdervik Lindblad B, et al. Long-term physical activity and risk of age-related cataract. Ophthalmology. 2015;122:274-80.
11. Kim YK, Choi HJ, Jeoung JW, et al. Five-year incidence of primary open-angle glaucoma and rate of progression in health center-based Korean population: The Gangnam Eye Study. PLoS ONE. 2014;9:e114058.
12. Chuang L-H, Koh Y-Y, Chen HSL, et al. Normal tension glaucoma in obstructive sleep apnea syndrome: a structural and functional study. Medicine. 2020;99: e19468.
13. Wise LA, Rosenberg L, Radin RG, et al. A prospective study of diabetes, lifestyle factors, and glaucoma among African-American women. Ann Epidemiol. 2011;21: 430-9.

14. Zarei R, Anvari P, Eslami Y, et al. Retinal nerve fibre layer thickness is reduced in metabolic syndrome. Diabet Med. 2017;34:1061-6.
15. Pezzino S, Sofia M, Greco LP, et al. Microbiome dysbiosis: a pathological mechanism at the intersection of obesity and glaucoma. Int J Mol Sci. 2023;24:1166.
16. Wong WL, Su X, Li X, et al. Global prevalence of age-related macular degeneration and disease burden projection for 2020 and 2040: a systematic review and meta-analysis. Lancet Glob Health. 2014;2:e106-e116.
17. Peeters A. Changes in abdominal obesity and age-related macular degeneration: the atherosclerosis risk in communities study. Arch Ophthalmol. 2008;126:1554.
18. McGuinness MB, Le J, Mitchell P, et al. Physical activity and age-related macular degeneration: a systematic literature review and meta-analysis. Am J Ophthalmol. 2017;180:29-38.
19. Agrón E, Mares J, Clemons TE, et al. Dietary nutrient intake and progression to late age-related macular degeneration in the age-related eye disease studies 1 and 2. Ophthalmology. 2021;128:425-42.
20. Pameijer EM, Heus P, Damen JAA, et al. What did we learn in 35 years of research on nutrition and supplements for age-related macular degeneration: a systematic review. Acta Ophthalmol. 2022;100:e1541.
21. Yalçın B, Gür G, Artüz F, et al. Prevalence of metabolic syndrome in Behçet disease: a case-control study in Turkey. Am J Clin Dermatol. 2013;14:421-5.
22. Chen T, Shao X, Li H, et al. Association of Behçet's disease with the risk of metabolic syndrome and its components: a systematic review and meta-analysis. Clin Exp Med. 2023;23:2855-66.
23. Craig JP, Nichols KK, Akpek EK, et al. TFOS DEWS II definition and classification report. Ocul Surf. 2017;15:276-83.
24. Surmacz HU, Cotlinski AL, Gehlen ML, et al. Dry eye and percentage of body fat: a cross-sectional prospective study. Int Ophthalmol. 2021;41:1855-61.
25. Ismail AMA, El-Azeim ASA, Saif HFAEA. Effect of aerobic exercise alone or combined with Mediterranean diet on dry eye in obese hypertensive elderly. Ir J Med Sci. 2023;192(6):3151-61.
26. Pedrotti E, Demasi CL, Bruni E, et al. Prevalence and risk factors of eye diseases in adult patients with obstructive sleep apnoea: results from the SLE.E.P.Y cohort study. BMJ Open. 2017;7:e016142.
27. Bulloch G, Seth I, Zhu Z, et al. Ocular manifestations of obstructive sleep apnea: a systematic review and meta-analysis. Graefes Arch Clin Exp Ophthalmol. 2024;262:19-32.
28. Dang J, Cai S, Zhong P, et al. Associations of school physical activity environment with comorbid obesity and myopia in children and adolescents: Findings from a Chinese national follow-up study. Scand J Med Sci Sports. 2024;34(1):e14562.

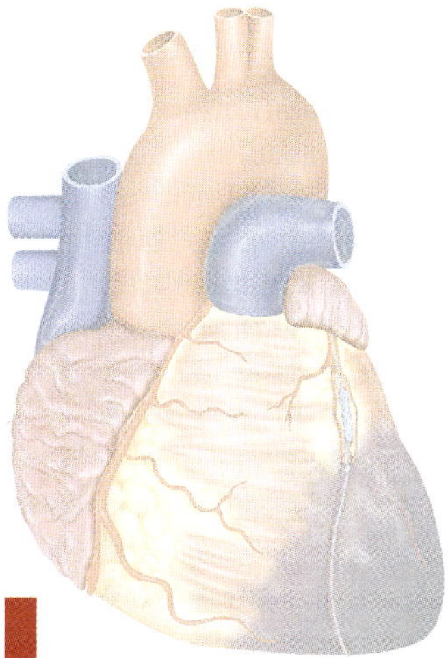

72

CHAPTER

Obesity and Retinopathy

Preetinder Kaur, Krishna Vaitheeswaran, Monika Nadar

INTRODUCTION

Diabetes mellitus is a pathological condition affecting a large number of individuals all over the world. The prevalence of diabetes in 2024 was 589 million adults (20–79 years) up from 200 million in 1990. It is expected to reach 853 million by 2050, impacting over 10% of adults worldwide. Diabetes is a disease driven by lifestyle changes, urbanization, and genetics.

It is classified as a metabolic disorder caused by chronic hyperglycemia and results in a number of microvascular complications such as retinopathy, nephropathy, ischemic heart disease, cerebrovascular disease, and peripheral vascular disease.[1]

The hyperglycemia in type 1 diabetes is a direct result of destruction of pancreatic beta cells while the hyperglycemia in diabetes type 2 is a result of insulin resistance and subsequent pancreatic beta cell dysfunction.[2]

The metabolic syndrome is a multifactorial condition of central obesity, hypertriglyceridemia, dyslipidemia, hypertension, fasting hyperglycemia, and insulin resistance. This in turn may lead to diabetes.

The review summarizes current literature on the link of obesity, metabolic syndrome, and retinopathy in diabetic and non-diabetic individuals.

THE METABOLIC SYNDROME OR THE PREDIABETIC STATE

Although guidelines for a clinical diagnosis of diabetes require a random blood sugar >200 mg/dL for a fasting blood sugar >125 mg/dL, current evidence suggests that the body undergoes significant metabolic alterations even before the development of frank diabetes.[3]

These changes include:

- Insulin resistance
- Hyperinsulinemia and hyperglycemia
- Vascular endothelial dysfunction
- Adiposity
- Inappropriate cytokine release from adipose tissue.

Clinically the metabolic syndrome has many definitions but is generally diagnosed in individuals presenting with three of the following clinical presentations.[4]

- Fasting glucose >6.1 mmol/L (110 mg/dL)
- HDL cholesterol
  - Male <1.0 mmol/L (40 mg/dL)
  - Female <1.3 mmol/L (50 mg/dL)
- Triglycerides >1.7 mmol/L (150 mg/dL)
- Abdominal obesity
  - Male waist circumference >102 cm
  - Female waist circumference >88 cm
- Blood pressure >130/85

The prevalence of the metabolic syndrome was reported to be 22% of adults in the United States with an age dependent increase in prevalence.[5] A recent study showed that the prevalence has increased to 34.5%.[6]

The metabolic syndrome increases the individual's risk of developing diabetes, cardiovascular disease, and all-cause mortality from cardiovascular disease.

OBESITY AND DIABETIC RETINOPATHY

Obesity and diabetes are positively correlated with the development of diabetic retinopathy, its progression as also the complications associated with the retinopathy.[7]

The global prevalence of diabetic retinopathy among people with diabetes was studied in a systematic literature review of 35 studies. 34.6% of diabetic patients were affected by any diabetic retinopathy, 6.81% by diabetic macular edema and 10% by vision threatening diabetic retinopathy.[8]

In a Chinese community based cross sectional study, 40% of diabetic patients were affected by diabetic retinopathy. Patients with diabetic retinopathy were both likely to be elderly ($p = 0.00003$), male ($p = 0.018$), hypertensive ($p < 0.0001$), have a high body mass index ($p < 0.0001$), metabolic abnormalities and a longer duration of diabetes ($p < 0.0001$).[9]

In a 2024 prospective cohort study, Chen et al. reported that visceral obesity, measured by the visceral adiposity index (VAI), lipid accumulation product (LAP), and Chinese VAI (CVAI), is independently associated with an increased risk of new-onset diabetic retinopathy in Chinese patients with type 2 diabetes.[10]

Studies indicate that visceral obesity as measured by visceral adiposity index is independently associated with an increased risk of new onset diabetic retinopathy in patients with diabetes.[10] The WHR is a more clinically relevant risk marker than BMI for individuals with type 2 diabetes.[11] In addition, data supports the protective effect of physical activity against diabetic retinopathy.[12]

INSULIN RESISTANCE AND THE METABOLIC SYNDROME

There are several mechanisms for the development of insulin resistance and metabolic syndrome.[13] These include:

- Genetic defects in proteins involved in the insulin action cascade
- Increased levels of visceral adiposity
- Increase levels of free fatty acids
- Indolent chronic inflammation

Insulin resistance reduces the free fatty acid uptake by fat cells and increases the free fatty acid release from fat cells.[13] This contributes to the chronic inflammatory state and vascular impairment seen in metabolic syndrome. Under the insulin resistance state there is an impaired glucose handling by skeletal muscle and adipose tissue. This leads to the hyperglycemia associated with the metabolic syndrome. Hyperglycemia in metabolic syndrome also contributes to the vascular endothelial damage seen in insulin resistant states.[14] In addition insulin is important for the release of nitric oxide which is responsible for vasodilatation, reduced vascular resistance and maintenance of blood pressure. Thus, there is a strong association between the presence of insulin resistance and hypertension due to increased vascular resistance in the metabolic syndrome. These changes in turn lead to microvascular and macrovascular alterations in the retina.

Hypertension causes retinal vascular endothelial damage similar to diabetic retinopathy. However, unlike diabetic retinopathy, the damage is induced by the altered mechanical blood flow rather than a metabolic damage seen in diabetes.[15] Poorly controlled systemic hypertension causes worsening of microvascular disease in the eye.[16]

DYSLIPIDEMIA AND DIABETIC RETINOPATHY

Diabetic dyslipidemia is characterized by high plasma triglycerides and low-density lipoprotein (LDL) and reduced levels of high-density lipoprotein cholesterol (HDL).

A recent meta-analysis revealed that triglycerides, total cholesterol, and LDL cholesterol were significantly elevated in patients with diabetic macular edema when compared to those without macular edema.[17]

In the Madrid Diabetes Study, higher LDL cholesterol level increased the 4-year risk for DR by eight-fold in type 2 diabetes.[18] In a follow-up analysis of the DCCT-EDIC trial from type-1 diabetic patients, the severity of retinopathy was positively associated with triglycerides (combined cohort) and negatively associated with HDL cholesterol in men from combined cohort.[19]

The impact of dyslipidemia in diabetic retinopathy initiated several studies examining the role of lipid lowering agents on diabetic retinopathy. Modjtahedi et al. in 2016, noted variable results in their review but the majority of these studies supported a protective role of lipid lowering agents such as fenofibrate in mitigating hard exudates in diabetic retinopathy.[20] Other studies have added evidence that lipid lowering agents such as fenofibrate significantly reduced diabetic progression in diabetic patients.[21] However, a multinational case control study showed that conventional serum lipid profiles are unlikely to show clear and dependent effects on the development of diabetic retinopathy.[22]

The published literature suggests an association between diabetic dyslipidemia and diabetic retinopathy. However, a more detailed and specific subtype of lipids or lipoproteins may have a more pathogenic role rather than a traditional lipid profile. The initial damage to the blood retinal barrier due to diabetes my facility leakage of lipids and its oxidized metabolite to exert local adverse effects that are not mirrored by alteration in serum lipid profile. The beneficial effects of lipid lowering agents are not fully attributed to correcting dyslipidemia and may be attributed to anti-inflammatory, antioxidants, and anti-apoptotic effects.

OBESITY AND RETINAL VASCULAR CHANGES

The retinal vascular system is a marker for microvascular disease and can predict cardiovascular events.

Retinal microvascular disease is associated with obesity and cardiovascular involvement. Individuals with high BMI and WHtR (waist to hip ratio) are associated with narrow retinal arteriolar caliber. Venular caliber shows a late association. These changes are also seen in children who are obese.[23] Obesity and adiposity, therefore, appear to exert a more negative effect on arteriolar retinal microcirculation which appears earlier than other changes.

Another study on young and adult obese subjects revealed a narrow arteriolar caliber and wider venular caliper independent of cardiovascular risk factors.[24]

Obesity is associated with active inflammatory and oxidative processes. The bioavailability of nitric oxide has been shown to decrease in individuals who are obese. Nitric oxide is a key endothelial relaxing and vasodilating agent that regulates perfusion. Low levels of nitric oxide may be a contributing factor to narrower arteriolar diameters.[25] Inflammation is associated with larger retinal venules.[26] Therefore sub-clinical inflammation may be the mechanism through which obesity alters retinal microcirculation.

The results of a cross-sectional study of 1,555 Chinese adults aged ≥50 years with no history of ocular disease showed that BMI and waist-to-hip ratio are positively associated with increased macular vessel density (VD) on optical coherence tomography angiography, both in the superficial capillary plexus and deep capillary plexus. Macular vessel alteration in obese individuals may contribute to disease onset and retinal changes.[27]

Obesity has also been associated with an increased risk of retinal vascular occlusions with all quartiles of BMI. Studies from the National Health and Nutrition Examination Survey, 1999–2006, show that a high BMI is related to an increased risk of developing both diabetes mellitus (DM) and retinal vein occlusion (RVO).[28] Several reviews have shown evidence supporting the association of hypercoagulability disorders with obesity and metabolic syndrome which may induce and contribute to the retinal vascular occlusive disease.[29]

Obesity is also linked with obstructive sleep apnea syndrome which causes severe dysfunction in the self-regulation of blood vessels leading to hypertensive retinopathy in the early phases and retinal vascular occlusions later on.[24]

The "Obesity Paradox"

A Korean population-based study showed that obesity has a different effect on the incidence of retinal vascular occlusion in the presence or absence of diabetes. In diabetics, higher BMI was associated with a lower risk of retinal vascular occlusion. This inverse association was related to the degree and duration of diabetes mellitus.

This obesity paradox is seen only in subjects with diabetes. A high BMI was associated with an increased risk of retinal vascular occlusions in normal individuals without diabetes. The main criticism to this finding arises from using BMI as the only indicator of obesity while it is known today that the distribution of fat is crucial to the development of vascular disease in obesity.

CONCLUSION

There is considerable evidence showing that central obesity, insulin resistance, and dyslipidemia are associated with retinopathy lesions in non-diabetic and diabetic patients. Patients with type 2 diabetes with dyslipidemia show higher tendency for DME and can benefit from cholesterol reducing agents such as fenofibrate in addition to antidiabetic agents.

The distribution of fat appears to be critical in the development of vascular lesions and retinopathy in obese individuals and needs to be assessed prior to intervention. In addition, public health programs must underline the need to institute dietary modifications and physical activity for reducing the burden of disease in the population.

REFERENCES

1. Hadi HA, Suwaidi JA. Endothelial dysfunction in diabetes mellitus. Vasc Health Risk Manag. 2007;3:853-76.
2. Olokoba AB, Obateru OA, Olokoba LB. Type 2 diabetes mellitus: a review of current trends. Oman Med J. 2012;27:269-273.
3. Kaur J. A comprehensive review on metabolic syndrome. Cardiol Res Pract. 2014;2014:943162.
4. Miranda PJ, DeFronzo RA, Califf RM, et al. Metabolic syndrome: definition, pathophysiology, and mechanisms. Am Heart J. 2005;149:33-45.
5. Ford ES, Giles WH, Mokdad AH. Increasing prevalence of the metabolic syndrome among U.S. Adults. Diabetes Care. 2004;27:2444-9.
6. Ford ES. Prevalence of the metabolic syndrome defined by the International Diabetes Federation among adults in the U.S. Diabetes Care. 2005;28:2745-49.
7. Gray N, Picone G, Sloan F, et al. Relation between BMI and diabetes mellitus and its complications among US older adults. South Med J. 2015;108:29-36.

8. Yau JWY, Rogers SL, Kawasaki R, et al. Global prevalence and major risk factors of diabetic retinopathy. Diabetes Care. 2012;35:556-64.
9. Yin L, Zhang D, Ren Q, et al. Prevalence and risk factors of diabetic retinopathy in diabetic patients: a community based cross-sectional study. Medicine (Baltimore) 2020;99:e19236.
10. Chen J, Li YT, Niu Z, et al. Association of visceral obesity indices with incident diabetic retinopathy in patients with diabetes: prospective cohort study. JMIR Public Health Surveill. 2024;10:e48120.
11. Man REK, Sabanayagam C, Chiang PP-C, et al. Differential association of generalized and abdominal obesity with diabetic retinopathy in Asian patients with type 2 diabetes. JAMA Ophthalmol. 2016;134:251.
12. AlQabandi Y, Nandula SA, Boddepalli CS, et al. Physical activity status and diabetic retinopathy: a review. Cureus. 2022.
13. Sutherland JP, McKinley B, Eckel RH. The metabolic syndrome and inflammation. Metab Syndr Relat Disord. 2004;2:82-104.
14. Muniyappa R, Sowers JR. Role of insulin resistance in endothelial dysfunction. Rev Endocr Metab Disord. 2013;14:5-12.
15. Garner A, Ashton N. Pathogenesis of hypertensive retinopathy: a review. J R Soc Med. 1979;72:362-5.
16. Chatterjee S, Chattopadhyay S, Hope-Ross M, et al. Hypertension and the eye: changing perspectives. J Hum Hypertens. 2002;16:667-75.
17. Das R, Kerr R, Chakravarthy U, et al. Dyslipidemia and Diabetic Macular Edema: A Systematic Review and Meta-Analysis. Ophthalmology. 2015;122:1820-27.
18. Salinero-Fort MÁ, San Andrés-Rebollo FJ, de Burgos-Lunar C, et al. Four-year incidence of diabetic retinopathy in a Spanish cohort: the MADIABETES study. PLoS One. 2013;8:e76417.
19. Lyons TJ, Jenkins AJ, Zheng D, et al. Diabetic retinopathy and serum lipoprotein subclasses in the DCCT/EDIC cohort. Invest Ophthalmol Vis Sci. 2004;45:910-8.
20. Modjtahedi BS, Bose N, Papakostas TD, et al. Lipids and Diabetic Retinopathy. Semin Ophthalmol. 2016;31:10-18.
21. Keech A, Simes RJ, Barter P, et al. Effects of long-term fenofibrate therapy on cardiovascular events in 9795 people with type 2 diabetes mellitus (the FIELD study): randomised controlled trial. Lancet. 2005;366:1849-61.
22. Sacks FM, Hermans MP, Fioretto P, et al. Association between plasma triglycerides and high-density lipoprotein cholesterol and microvascular kidney disease and retinopathy in type 2 diabetes mellitus: a global case-control study in 13 countries. Circulation. 2014;129:999-1008.
23. Liu M, Lycett K, Wong TY, et al. Do body mass index and waist-to-height ratio over the preceding decade predict retinal microvasculature in 11–12 year olds and midlife adults? Int J Obes. 2020;44:1712-22.
24. Boillot A, Zoungas S, Mitchell P, et al. Obesity and the microvasculature: a systematic review and meta-analysis. PLoS ONE. 2013;8:e52708.
25. Montero D, Walther G, Perez-Martin A, et al. Endothelial dysfunction, inflammation, and oxidative stress in obese children and adolescents: markers and effect of lifestyle intervention. Obes Rev. 2012;13:441-55.
26. Daien V, Carriere I, Kawasaki R, et al. Retinal vascular caliber is associated with cardiovascular biomarkers of oxidative stress and inflammation: The POLA Study. PLoS ONE. 2013;8:e71089.
27. Ding Q, Wu H, Wang W, et al. Association of body mass index and waist-to-hip ratio with retinal microvasculature in healthy Chinese adults: an optical coherence tomography angiography study. Am J Ophthalmol. 2023;246:96-106.
28. Nguyen NT, Nguyen X-MT, Lane J, et al. Relationship between obesity and diabetes in a US adult population: findings from the national health and nutrition examination survey, 1999–2006. Obes Surg. 2011;21:351-5.
29. Nieuwdorp M, Stroes ES, Meijers JC, et al. Hypercoagulability in the metabolic syndrome. Curr Opin Pharmacol. 2005;5:155-9.

SECTION 18

Obesity, HFpEF, Cardio-ENT, and Cardiopulmonary Disease

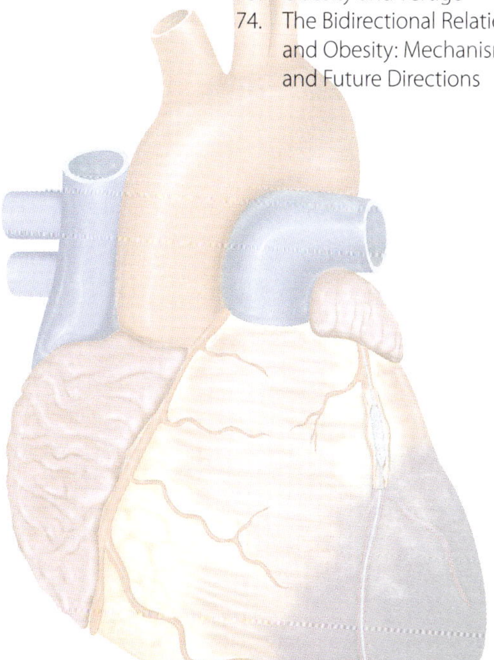

73

CHAPTER

Obesity and Vertigo

Poonam Singla

INTRODUCTION

Vertigo is a *hallucination or illusion of movement*. Most commonly felt as a *spinning (rotatory) sensation*. Results from a *mismatch or dysfunction* within the vestibular apparatus, vestibular pathways, or their central processing centers.

Obesity does not directly cause vertigo but contributes to *multiple systemic and vestibular pathophysiological mechanisms* that increase susceptibility to dizziness and vertigo.

VASCULAR MECHANISMS

Atherosclerosis and Microangiopathy[1]

Obesity is associated with:

- Hyperlipidemia
- Chronic inflammation
- Endothelial dysfunction

These changes lead to: These changes lead to the formation of atherosclerotic plaque, which leads to the narrowing of the lumen of arteries, as shown in **Figure 1** here:

- The labyrinthine artery 2 is an end artery, as shown in **Figure 2** and therefore even little vascular changes result in *reduced perfusion of the inner ear.*
- *Cochleovestibular ischemia*, producing vertigo, tinnitus, and imbalance.

Hypertension

Common in obesity due to:

- RAAS activation
- Sympathetic overactivity
- Insulin resistance

Blood pressure fluctuations can cause *vascular dysregulation and orthostatic hypotension. Orthostatic hypotension (OH) is relatively common among individuals with hypertension, affecting about 10% of hypertensive adults.*[2-4]

UNDERSTANDING ORTHOSTATIC HYPOTENSION AND VERTIGO

Normally, when standing, our bodies automatically constrict blood vessels and increase heart rate to maintain blood flow to the brain. In OH, this response is impaired, leading to a temporary reduction in blood flow to the brain, including areas involved in balance (the brainstem and cerebellum).

- *Symptoms:* The primary symptoms of OH are lightheadedness or dizziness immediately after standing up, which usually resolve quickly when sitting or lying down. Other symptoms can include:
    - Blurred vision
    - Weakness or fatigue
    - Nausea
    - Fainting (syncope) in severe cases
    - Confusion or difficulty concentrating

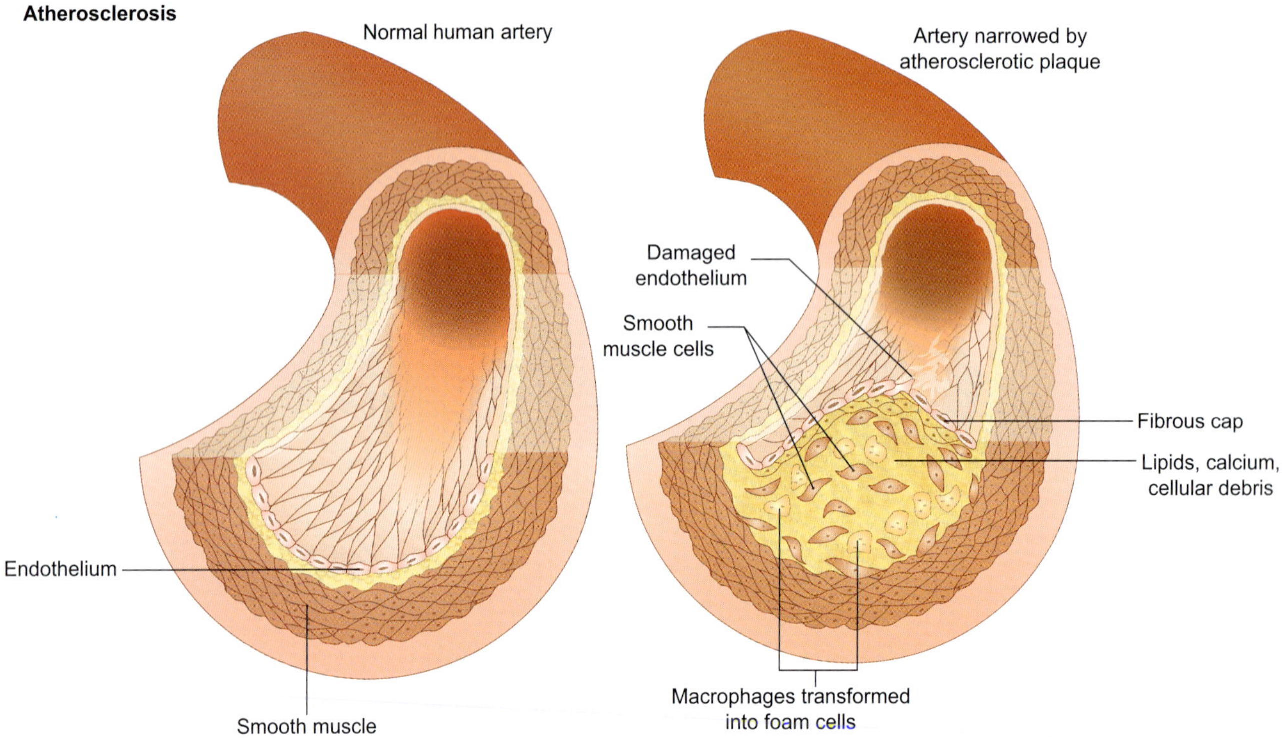

Fig. 1: Development of atherosclerosis in a human artery.

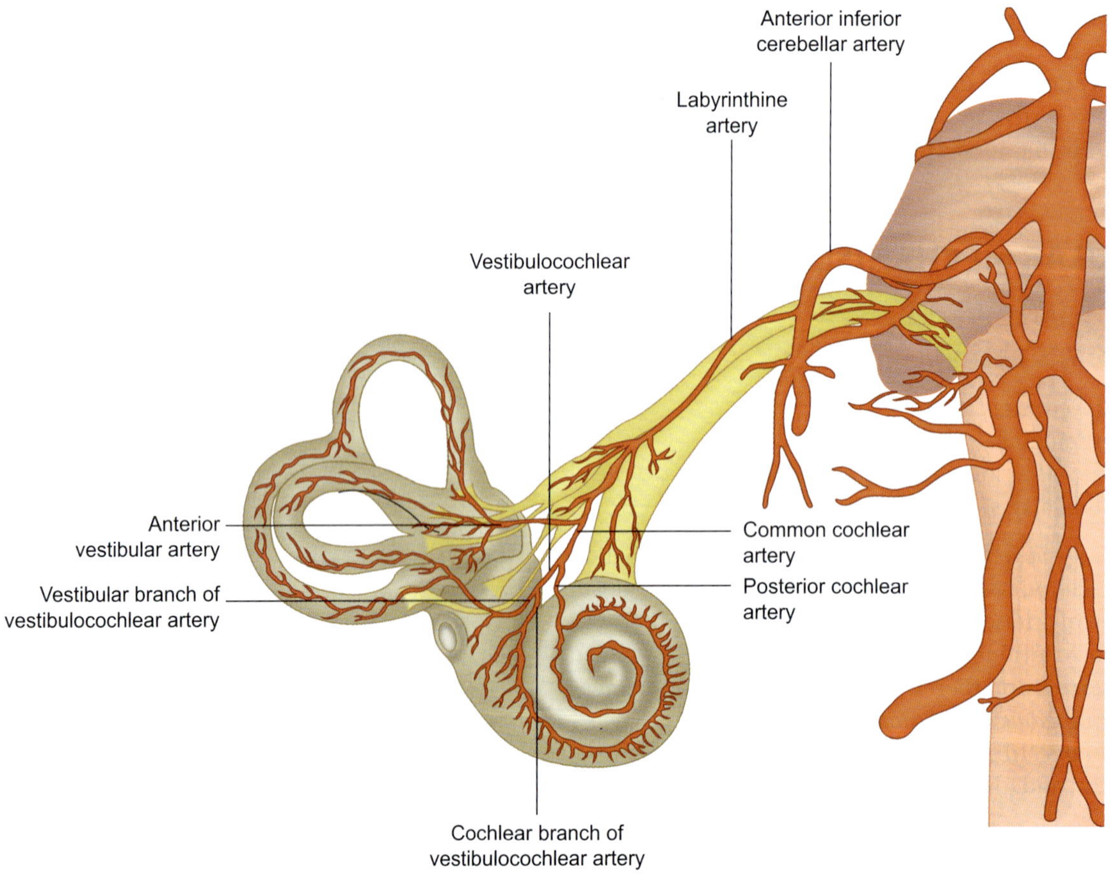

Fig. 2: Arterial supply of the inner ear (labyrinth).

- *Vertigo (spinning sensation):* While non-spinning dizziness is more common, studies show that a significant percentage (up to 39%) of patients with documented OH can experience rotatory vertigo during orthostatic challenges. This is thought to be caused by transient hypoperfusion (reduced blood flow) to the inner ear or cerebellum, which creates an imbalance in the vestibular system.

METABOLIC MECHANISMS (FLOWCHART 1)[5]

Obesity is linked with:

- Type 2 diabetes
- Dyslipidemia

Vertigo in metabolic disorders, especially DM,[6] arises because of:

Mechanism	*Explanation*
Microangiopathy	Damages vestibular structures → peripheral vertigo
Autonomic neuropathy	Orthostatic hypotension → dizziness/ vertigo
Hypoglycemia	Brainstem/cerebellar dysfunction → vertigo
Hyperglycemia	Osmotic disturbance of endolymph → vertigo
Peripheral neuropathy	Proprioceptive loss → imbalance (often mistaken for vertigo)
Infections	Otitis media/externa → acute vestibular dysfunction
Medications	Hypoglycemia or hypotension → vertigo

Dyslipidemia[7-8]

- Dyslipidemia → atherosclerosis of vertebrobasilar system → most important cause of vertigo.
- Labyrinthine artery is end-artery → highly susceptible to lipid-induced microvascular ischemia.
- Hypertriglyceridemia → hyperviscosity → reduced cochleovestibular perfusion.
- Metabolic syndrome increases risk of both peripheral and central vestibular dysfunction.
- Always evaluate vertigo patients for cardiovascular risk factors—including lipid profile.

INNER EAR/OTOLOGICAL ASSOCIATIONS

Benign Paroxysmal Positional Vertigo

Obesity is linked to a higher incidence of benign paroxysmal positional vertigo (BPPV) due to:

- Chronic inflammation
- Metabolic disturbances
- Sedentary lifestyle → decreased vestibular stimulation
- Vitamin D deficiency[9] (common in obesity) → otoconia degeneration

Ménière's Disease[10-11]

Obesity may contribute via:

- Sodium/water retention
- Metabolic syndrome-related microvascular dysfunction
- Hormonal changes affecting endolymph regulation

Leading to *endolymphatic hydrops* → episodic vertigo, tinnitus, aural fullness

Flowchart 1: Pathophysiological mechanisms linking metabolic disorders to vertigo.

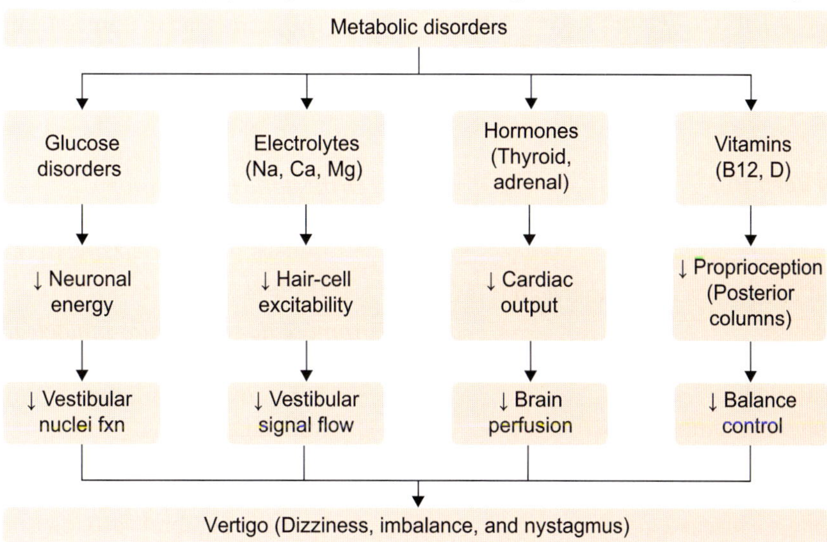

SLEEP-RELATED MECHANISMS

Obstructive Sleep Apnea[12]

Highly prevalent in obese individuals.

Consequences relevant to vertigo:

- Intermittent hypoxia → neuronal dysfunction
- Fluctuating intracranial pressure
- Autonomic instability
- Morning dizziness/vertigo
- Increased risk of *vestibular migraines*

Obstructive sleep apnea (OSA) also contributes to cardiovascular instability → compounding dizziness.

HORMONAL AND INFLAMMATORY FACTORS

Chronic Low-grade Inflammation

Obesity = adipose tissue releasing:

- TNF-α
- IL-6
- Leptin
- Adipokines

These affect:

- Vestibular nerve signaling
- Vascular tone
- Inner ear immune response

May worsen susceptibility to both peripheral and central vestibular disorders.

Thyroid Dysfunction[13-14]

Thyroid dysfunction—both hypothyroidism and hyperthyroidism—can contribute to vertigo, though the mechanisms are often indirect. Vertigo arises due to disruption in the vestibular system, cerebral perfusion, or neuromuscular control, all of which can be influenced by thyroid hormones.

Hypothyroidism and Vertigo

Vestibular system effects

- *Mucopolysaccharide Accumulation*
  - Hypothyroidism causes glycosaminoglycan (GAG) deposition in tissues.
  - This can occur in the inner ear, leading to:
    - Endolymphatic edema
    - Altered endolymph composition
    - Impaired hair cell function
  - This manifests as true vertigo, sometimes resembling Ménière's disease.

Eustachian Tube Dysfunction

Myxedematous changes in the nasopharyngeal mucosa → impaired eustachian tube ventilation → middle-ear pressure changes → imbalance or dizziness

Cardiovascular effects causing vertigo

- *Bradycardia and Reduced Cardiac Output*
  - *Thyroid hormone deficiency reduces*:
    - HR
    - Stroke volume
    - Cardiac output
  - → Reduced cerebral perfusion → lightheadedness or presyncopal dizziness, which patients may describe as "vertigo."

Diastolic Hypertension

Increased peripheral vascular resistance contributes to headaches and feeling of imbalance.

Neuromuscular and neurological effects

- *Peripheral Neuropathy*
  - *Chronic hypothyroidism may cause*:
    - Sensory neuropathy
    - Impaired proprioception
  - Loss of joint position sense → imbalance and "unsteady gait"

Cerebellar Ataxia (Rare)

Severe longstanding hypothyroidism can affect cerebellar pathways → ataxic gait, disequilibrium.

Hyperthyroidism and Vertigo

Cardiovascular effects

- *Tachyarrhythmias*
  - Hyperthyroidism increases β-adrenergic activity → tachycardia, atrial fibrillation.
  - These can lead to transient cerebral hypoperfusion, producing:
    - Dizziness
    - Presyncope
    - Feeling of spinning
- *Orthostatic Hypotension*
  - Due to vasodilation and relative volume depletion.
  - Causes postural dizziness, often misinterpreted as vertigo.

Neuromuscular and neuro-otological effects

- *Muscle weakness and tremors*
  - Thyrotoxic myopathy → poor postural control → imbalance
- *Anxiety and hyperventilation*
  - Common in hyperthyroidism
  - Leads to cerebral vasoconstriction → dizziness

- *Vestibular migraine triggering:*
    - Thyroid hormone fluctuations can trigger migraine pathways, and vestibular migraine presents with episodic vertigo.

Autoimmune Thyroid Disease and Vertigo

Hashimoto's thyroiditis:

- Strongly associated with autoimmune inner ear disease (AIED).
- Autoantibodies may attack vestibular epithelium → episodic vertigo, fluctuating sensorineural hearing loss (Ménière-like presentation).

Graves' disease: Autoimmune inflammation may indirectly affect microcirculation of the inner ear.

PHARMACOLOGICAL FACTORS

Obese patients are often on multiple medications:

- Antihypertensives (especially alpha/beta blockers) → orthostatic dizziness
- Hypoglycemics → risk of hypoglycemia-induced dizziness
- Diuretics (for BP or Ménière's) → electrolyte imbalance → vertigo
- Psychotropic drugs → vestibular suppression

Polypharmacy increases the risk of vertigo through:

- Sedation
- Hypotension
- Electrolyte disturbances

BIOMECHANICAL AND POSTURAL FACTORS[15-16]

Obesity affects balance through mechanical, neuromuscular, and sensory-perceptual mechanisms. Together, these changes increase the risk of postural instability, falls, and gait abnormalities.

Mechanical and Biomechanical Factors

Altered Centre of Gravity

- Excess adipose tissue—especially central/abdominal obesity—shifts the center of gravity anteriorly and superiorly.
- An altered center of gravity (COG) requires greater postural adjustments to maintain balance.
- This increases reliance on ankle and hip strategies, making balance correction slower and less efficient.

Increased Body Mass → Increased Joint Load

- Excess weight places greater stress on ankles, knees, hips, and the lumbar spine.
- *This leads to:*
    - Early joint fatigue
    - Osteoarthritis
    - Reduced range of motion
- These factors impair balance, especially during dynamic activities (walking and stair climbing).

Reduced Postural Stability

- Studies show obesity increases postural sway (antero-posterior and medio-lateral).
- Greater sway indicates poorer ability to maintain upright stance.

Neuromuscular Factors

Weakness of Postural Muscles

- *Obesity is associated with:*
    - Lower relative muscle strength (reduced strength-to-weight ratio)
    - Fat infiltration in muscle (myosteatosis)
- Weak trunk and lower-limb muscles impair postural responses and corrective reflexes.

Slower Reaction Time

- Increased body mass slows neuromuscular reaction to sudden perturbations (e.g., tripping), because:
    - More force is required to move the body.
    - Motor control becomes less efficient.

This leads to difficulty in regaining balance after minor disturbances.

Sensory and Proprioceptive Impairment

Reduced Proprioception

- Excess fat around joints (especially ankles and knees) may reduce proprioceptive feedback from:
    - Joint mechanoreceptors
    - Muscle spindles
- Impaired joint position sense makes balance maintenance more difficult.

Effect on Vestibular and Visual Systems

- Obesity does not directly damage these systems, but:
    - Reduced mobility → less sensory training → poor integration of vestibular cues
    - Comorbidities (diabetes and hypertension) may indirectly impair sensory systems.

Gait Abnormalities Associated with Obesity

Obese individuals commonly exhibit:

- Wider stance (compensatory)
- Shorter step length

- Slower walking speed
- Longer double-support phase

These are compensatory mechanisms to increase stability but indicate decreased balance confidence.

OBESITY AND VESTIBULAR MIGRAINE[17]

Vestibular migraine is a migraine disorder in which patients experience *recurrent vertigo, dizziness, imbalance,* often associated with migraine features (photophobia, phonophobia, and aura). Obesity does *not directly cause* vestibular migraine, but it is a *significant risk factor* and is associated with *more frequent and severe attacks.*

The relationship is mediated through *metabolic, vascular, hormonal,* and *inflammatory* pathways that influence migraine pathophysiology.

Obesity → Increased Migraine Susceptibility

Migraine, including vestibular migraine, is more common in individuals with obesity. Mechanisms include:

Chronic Low-grade inflammation

Adipose tissue secretes inflammatory mediators:

- TNF-α
- IL-6
- Calcitonin gene-related peptide (CGRP)—a key migraine mediator

These can lower the threshold for *trigeminovascular activation*, leading to more frequent migraine and vestibular symptoms.

Calcitonin Gene-related Peptide Overproduction

Calcitonin gene-related peptide is central to migraine and is also involved in vestibular processing.Excess CGRP release in obesity → increased susceptibility to:

- Headache
- Motion sensitivity
- Vertigo episodes

CONCLUSION

Obesity contributes to vertigo through vascular insufficiency, metabolic syndrome, diabetic and dyslipidemic complications, increased risk of BPPV and Ménière's disease, sleep apnea-related hypoxia, chronic inflammation, hormonal disturbances, and drug side effects.

REFERENCES

1. Haverich A, Boyle EC. Atherosklerose-Pathogenese und mikrovaskuläre Dysfunktion. Springer; 2023.
2. Fedorowski A, Burri P, Melander O. Orthostatic hypotension in genetically related hypertensive and normotensive individuals. J Hypertens. 2009;27:976-82.
3. Di Stefano C, Milazzo V, Totaro S, et al. Orthostatic hypotension in a cohort of hypertensive patients referring to a hypertension clinic. J Hum Hypertens. 2015;29:599-603.
4. Applegate WB, Davis BR, Black HR, et al. Prevalence of postural hypotension at baseline in the Systolic Hypertension in the Elderly Program (SHEP) cohort. J Am Geriatr Soc. 1991;39:1057-64.
5. Lehrer JF, Poole DC, Seaman M, et al. Identification and Treatment of Metabolic Abnormalities in Patients with Vertigo. Arch Intern Med. 1986;146(8):1497-1500.
6. Bittar RSM, Bottino MA, Simoceli L, et al. Vestibular impairment due to metabolic disorders of glucose: reality or myth? Braz J Otorhinolaryngol. 2004;70(6):800-5.
7. Saito T, Sato K, Saito H. An experimental study of auditory dysfunction associated with hyperlipoproteinemia. Arch Otorhinolaryngol. 1986;243(4):242-5.
8. Friedrich G, Pilger E. Lipoproteins in cochleovestibular disorders. Arch Otorhinolaryngol. 1981;232(2):101-5.
9. Sheikhzadeh M, Lotfi Y, Mousavi A, et al. Influence of supplemental vitamin D on intensity of benign paroxysmal positional vertigo: A longitudinal clinical study. Caspian J Intern Med. 2016;7(2):93-8.
10. Spencer JT Jr. Hyperlipoproteinemia, hyperinsulinism, and Meniere's disease. South Med J. 1981;74(10):1194-7.
11. Oğuz E, Cebeci A, Geçici CR. The relationship between nutrition and Ménière's disease. Auris Nasus Larynx. 2021;48(5):803-8.
12. Tsai MS, Lee LA, Tsai YT, et al. Sleep apnea and risk of vertigo: a nationwide population-based cohort study. Laryngoscope. 2018;128(3):763-8.
13. Brenner M, Hoistad DL, Hain TC. Prevalence of thyroid dysfunction in patients with Ménière's disease. Arch Otolaryngol Head Neck Surg. 2004;130(2):226-8.
14. Modugno GC, Pirodda A, Ferri GG, et al. A relationship between autoimmune thyroiditis and benign paroxysmal positional vertigo? Med Hypotheses. 2000;54(4):61-5.
15. Alice A, Yadav M, Verma R. Effect of obesity on balance: A literature review. Int J Health Sci. 2022;6(S4):3261-79.
16. Son SM. Influence of Obesity on Postural Stability in Young Adults. Osong Public Health Res Perspect. 2016;7(6):378-81.
17. Bond DS, Roth J, Nash JM, et al. Migraine and obesity: epidemiology, possible mechanisms and the potential role of weight loss treatment. Obes Rev. 2011;12(5):e362-71.

74

CHAPTER

The Bidirectional Relationship between Allergy and Obesity: Mechanisms, Clinical Implications, and Future Directions

Sarika Verma

INTRODUCTION

Allergic disorders including allergic rhinitis, asthma, urticaria, atopic dermatitis, and food allergies have risen dramatically in recent decades. Parallel to this, obesity has become a worldwide epidemic.[1,2] Although these conditions were once thought unrelated, extensive research now confirms a strong interconnection.[3,4]

In the past decades allergic diseases have become a household problem with almost 1 in 5 people suffering from some form of allergic disease, and the incidence in children is almost double. The usage of nebulizers in children has increased manifold with every fourth house in metropolitan cities having a nebulizer.

There are many reasons for this increase—sedentary lifestyles, eating processed foods, high calorie readymade "junk" foods and sweetened beverages, reduced outdoor activities, and air pollution have caused an increase in allergic disease. The same factors are responsible for the rising incidence of obesity. Add to that shrinking playgrounds and public spaces, increased screen time seems like an epidemic of allergy and obesity is set to hit the planet.

In my 23 years of clinical practice as an ENT surgeon and allergy specialist, I consistently observe that untreated allergies predispose individuals to weight gain, while excess weight significantly worsens allergic symptoms. This reciprocal relationship is supported by evidence involving inflammation, hormonal imbalance, immune changes, behavioral factors, and sleep disturbances.[5-10]

Understanding this two-way relationship is essential for meaningful prevention and treatment strategies.

HOW ALLERGY INCREASES OBESITY?

Systemic Inflammation and Metabolic Changes

Allergic diseases involve persistent inflammation driven by Th2 cytokines such as IL-4, IL-5, and IL-13, which interfere with insulin signaling and promote fat deposition.[5,8] Chronic allergic inflammation contributes to metabolic dysfunction and weight gain.[6]

Disrupted Sleep Cycle

Nasal obstruction from allergic rhinitis or sinusitis causes sleep fragmentation and mouth breathing.[9] Sleep deprivation increases ghrelin and decreases leptin, driving weight gain.[10] Patients wake up not feeling fresh and active, which lowers their activity levels throughout the day, including missing out on regular exercise.

Allergic patients often develop chronic fatigue, leading to reduced daytime activity.

Reduced Physical Activity

Exercise-induced bronchospasm and uncontrolled allergic asthma discourage physical activity.[2,11] Parents are afraid that activity might trigger coughing bouts or emergency visits and thus discourage allergic children from participating in sports or regular physical activity.

Children avoid outdoor play during pollen seasons or high pollution days, reducing energy expenditure. Schools have been advised to take online classes, postpone sports tournaments and cancel PE classes in view of poor air quality that North India faces for 3–4 months of the year.

During COVID lockdown and the 2 years post-COVID, we have seen the incidence of allergic disease go up exponentially. Most individuals, including young children, put on a lot of weight in this period. Screen time increased exponentially and many people have forgone their exercise and sports regimes.

Medication-related Weight Gain

Most oral antihistamines cause sedation, reducing energy and activity levels. Antihistamines used in children cause enough sedation to miss school and sports activities.

Long-term or repeated use of systemic corticosteroids in severe allergic rhinitis, chronic urticaria, and recurrent nasal polyps, and uncontrolled asthma increases appetite, central obesity, and insulin resistance,[12] further leading to gain in weight.

Psychological Stress and Emotional Eating

Chronic itching, nasal blockage, or wheezing leads to anxiety and emotional eating particularly in adolescents, contributing to increased body mass index (BMI).[12] Patients who are suffering from long-term mild illnesses turn to food for comfort and sometimes out of sheer boredom. High-calorie readymade foods are easily accessible in homes and online instamarts/instant home deliveries have made healthy eating even more challenging for young people. Chocolate and sweets release dopamine, and trigger binge eating worsening obesity.

HOW OBESITY AGGRAVATES ALLERGIC DISEASES?

Adipose Tissue as an Inflammatory Organ

Obesity is characterized by increased adipokines such as TNF-α, IL-6, and leptin, which amplify airway inflammation and worsen asthma and rhinitis.[6,11]

Children with obesity show more severe allergic airway inflammation than normal-weight peers.[13]

Mechanical Respiratory Effects

Increased abdominal fat reduces lung volumes, chest wall compliance, and diaphragmatic movement, worsening asthma severity.[7,14]

Obesity also increases obstructive sleep apnea, which aggravates rhinitis and asthma.[9]

Overweight people feel self-conscious and demotivated in active sports and outdoor activities. Obese children tend to be left behind in team sports activities. Bullying and social ostracism are real challenges for mental and physical health, more so for teens and younger children with obesity. Excess weight reduces agility and taking frequent breaks to catch their breath, make obese children vulnerable to jibes from their peers.

Impaired Immune Regulation

Obesity shifts the immune response toward Th17 dominance and reduces regulatory T-cell function.[5] This immune imbalance increases the severity of asthma, eczema, and urticaria.[15,16]

Allergic rhinitis, allergic bronchitis, hyper-reactive airway disease, atopy, and allergic asthma are mediated through Th2 (T-helper cells type 2) which cause characteristic inflammatory response by releasing cytokines such as IL-4, IL-5, and IL-13 that promote IgE production, mast cell activation, and eosinophil recruitment.

Gut Microbiome Dysbiosis

Both obesity and allergic diseases are associated with reduced microbial diversity.

Gut dysbiosis contributes to increased intestinal permeability and heightened allergic sensitization.[17] Earlier trends of avoiding allergenic foods in the first 1 year of life are now being replaced by early introduction of foods like egg, peanut, and cow's milk in the weaning phase of life to reduce food sensitizations and atopy.

CLINICAL IMPLICATIONS

Allergy Patients Require Weight Assessment

Body mass index, waist circumference, diet, and sleep quality should be assessed as part of routine allergy evaluation.[18] Patients must be counseled empathetically toward a healthier diet, regular exercise, and mood elevation mental interventions such as meditation and deep breathing exercises.

Weight Loss Improves Allergy Outcomes

Even a 5–10% reduction in body weight improves asthma control, nasal congestion, sleep quality, and overall inflammation.[14,19,20] Obstructive sleep apnea syndrome, snoring, nocturnal awakenings are directly worsened by weight gain. A healthier lifestyle, regular exercise and watchful eating causing weight loss improves sleep, mood, activity levels, and overall energy levels positively, improving allergy control of nasal symptom scores.

Multidisciplinary Management is Essential

Combining allergen avoidance, immunotherapy, breathing exercises, dietary changes, and increased physical activity offers the best long-term outcomes.[18]

Allergic patients need time and a patient ear. They need to be heard, and advice given should be practical and feasible, keeping their lifestyle in mind. Pharmacotherapy and inhaled steroids are safe, and their optimal use should be encouraged. Patients and families should be given a step-up/step-down plan regarding medication to avoid frequent doctor visits.

Mental wellness is a very important yet neglected part of patient counseling. Loneliness, fatigue, work, or study stress should be enquired about, discussed, and addressed. The importance of regular physical exercise should be highlighted in every patient visit.

Oral steroid usage should be judicious and clearly mentioned in the prescription to avoid refilling of prescriptions over-the-counter. Good symptomatic relief with pharmacotherapy is important for patients to believe that allergen avoidance and immunotherapy will relieve their long-term symptoms and their hopelessness regarding long-term suffering has to be addressed.

FUTURE DIRECTIONS

Further research is needed to understand:

- The role of microbiome restoration in reducing obesity-related allergy severity[17]
- Biomarkers for predicting obesity-driven allergic inflammation
- Personalized immunotherapy strategies for obese patients.[6,14]

CONCLUSION

Allergy and obesity are intricately linked in a vicious cycle of inflammation, immune disruption, lifestyle changes, and metabolic dysfunction. Recognizing and addressing this bidirectional relationship allows clinicians to provide more effective and holistic treatment. Treating allergies without addressing obesity and vice versa limits overall therapeutic success. An integrated, interdisciplinary, and empathetic approach is essential for long-term relief of symptoms and overall well-being of allergic patients.

REFERENCES

1. Beuther DA, Sutherland ER. Overweight, obesity, and incident asthma: a meta-analysis of prospective epidemiologic studies. Am J Respir Crit Care Med. 2007;175(7):661-6.
2. Fonseca-Junior SJ, Sá CGA, Rodrigues PA, et al. Obesity and asthma: the role of adipokines and physical activity. Can Respir J. 2014;21(6):376-81.
3. Zhang G, Spickett J, Rumchev K, et al. Obesity and respiratory diseases in children: the role of environmental factors. J Paediatr Child Health. 2009;45(11):646-50.
4. Boulet LP. Influence of obesity on the prevalence and clinical expression of asthma. Clin Invest Med. 2008;31(6):E386-90.
5. Scherzer R, Heyman MB, Lee D, et al. Altered immune balance in obesity: increased Th17 and reduced Treg cell frequencies. Int J Obes. 2011;35(4):623-9.
6. Peters U, Dixon AE, Forno E. Obesity and asthma. J Allergy Clin Immunol. 2018;141(4):1169-79.
7. Sharma S, Sherrill DL, Guerra S, et al. Airway hyperresponsiveness and obesity in children: the role of lung volumes. J Allergy Clin Immunol. 2009;123(4):825-30.
8. Hersoug LG, Linneberg A. The link between obesity and the development of allergic disease. Allergy. 2007;62(10):1205-13.
9. Khalili M, Sadr-Azodi O, Akerman M, et al. Sleep disturbances and allergic diseases: a bidirectional relationship. Chest. 2013;144(5):1466-73.
10. Van Leeuwen WM, Hublin C, Sallinen M, et al. Prolonged sleep restriction increases ghrelin and decreases leptin levels. Sleep. 2008;31(10):1351-9.
11. Farah CS, Salome CM. Asthma and obesity: a known association but unknown mechanism. Respirology. 2012;17(3):412-21.
12. Wright L, Aronne LJ. Causes of weight gain. Clin Cornerstone. 2012;12(3):19-25.
13. Santamaria F, Montella S, Greco L, et al. Obesity enhances allergic airway inflammation in children. Allergol Immunopathol. 2010;38(3):103-8.
14. Holguin F. Obesity as a risk factor for increased severity of asthma. Clin Chest Med. 2019;40(1):97-108.
15. Kim KW, Shin YH, Lee KE, et al. Relationship between adipokines and atopic dermatitis in children. Pediatr Allergy Immunol. 2010;21(4):530-8.
16. Novak N, Bieber T. The immune response in atopic dermatitis. J Allergy Clin Immunol. 2003;112(3):S128-39.
17. Pascoe CD, Tkaczyk ER, Kesavan A, et al. Obesity-related changes in the microbiome: implications for asthma and allergies. Curr Allergy Asthma Rep. 2020;20(12):77.
18. Bousquet J, Khaltaev N, Cruz AA, et al. Allergic Rhinitis and its Impact on Asthma (ARIA) update. Allergy. 2008;63(Suppl 86):8-160.
19. Gibson PG, McDonald VM, Marks GB. Asthma in older adults. Lancet. 2010;376(9743):803-13.
20. Hurbault H, Chan-Yeung M, Cheung J, et al. Impact of weight reduction on asthma control in obese patients. J Asthma. 2011;48(7):714-21.

SECTION 19

Obesity, HFpEF and Pediatrics

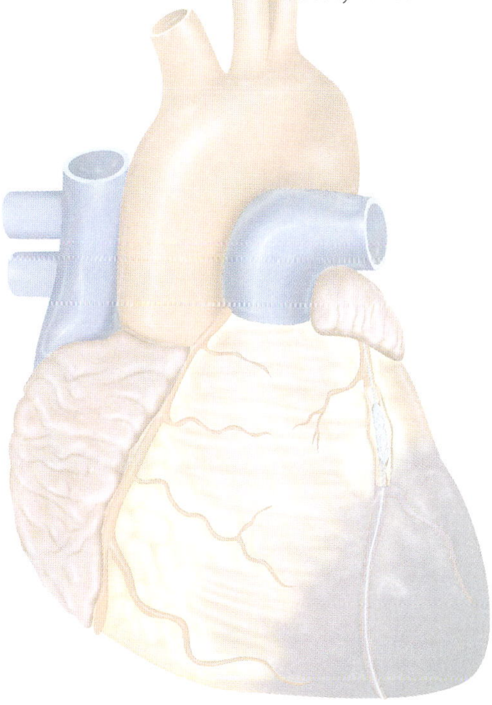

75

CHAPTER

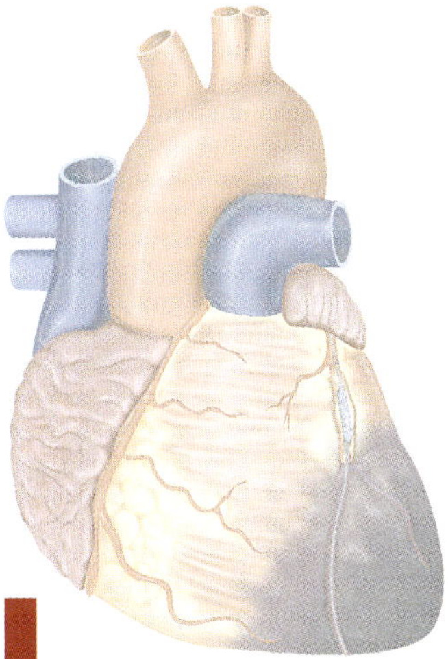

Obesity in Pediatrics

Hala Elmarsafawy, Shaimaa Zakariya

INTRODUCTION

The World Health Organization (WHO) defines obesity and overweight as excessive accumulation of body fat that can negatively impact an individual's health. Age must be considered when classifying overweight and obesity in children. According to a WHO study report published in June 2021, overweight in children under 5 years of age is defined as weight-for-height exceeding two standard deviations, while obesity is defined as weight-for-height exceeding three standard deviations from the WHO average child growth standard. Overweight and obesity in children aged 5–19 years are defined as a body mass index (BMI) exceeding one and two standard deviations, respectively, from the WHO average growth standard. The Centers for Disease Control and Prevention (CDC) classifies overweight as being at or above the 95th percentile for BMI,[1,2] while European researchers define overweight as being at or above the 85th percentile and obese as being at or above the 95th percentile for BMI.[3]

PREVALENCE

Childhood obesity rates are increasing globally in both developed and developing countries.[4,5] The prevalence of obesity nearly tripled between 1975 and 2016 worldwide. More than 60% of children who are overweight before puberty will be obese in adulthood.[6] Globally, 42 million children under the age of 5 years are overweight, including 35 million in developing countries, according to 2010 global data.[5] A 2020 WHO report showed that 39 million children under the age of 5 years and 340 million children aged 5–19 years were obese or overweight in 2016.[6]

FACTORS CONTRIBUTING TO CHILDHOOD OBESITY

Multiple factors contribute to childhood obesity. An energy imbalance between calories consumed and calories expended is the primary cause of overweight and obesity in children.

The world has witnessed an increase in the consumption of foods high in fat and sugar, coupled with a sedentary lifestyle. The causes of childhood obesity are numerous, and energy imbalance is one of them.[7] Sometimes, a discrepancy between energy intake and expenditure is observed in children, but excess fat accumulation occurs during their early years of growth when energy expenditure is less than calories consumed. Obesity is the product of a complex interaction between biological, developmental, behavioral, genetic, and environmental factors.[8]

Studies have revealed that agouti-related protein (AgRP), a signaling molecule in mammals involved in weight regulation, causes obesity in adulthood when overexpressed. It has been identified as a competitive antagonist of melanocortin receptors 3 and 4 (MC3R, MC4R), while MC4r is involved in the hypothalamic control of feeding behavior **(Fig. 1)**.[9]

Genetic Factors

A mother's prepregnancy BMI is an independent risk factor for childhood obesity.[10] When both parents are obese, the likelihood of the child developing obesity increases.[11]

Genetics is a major risk factor for childhood obesity.[12] Research indicates that BMI is 25–40% heritable.[13] However,

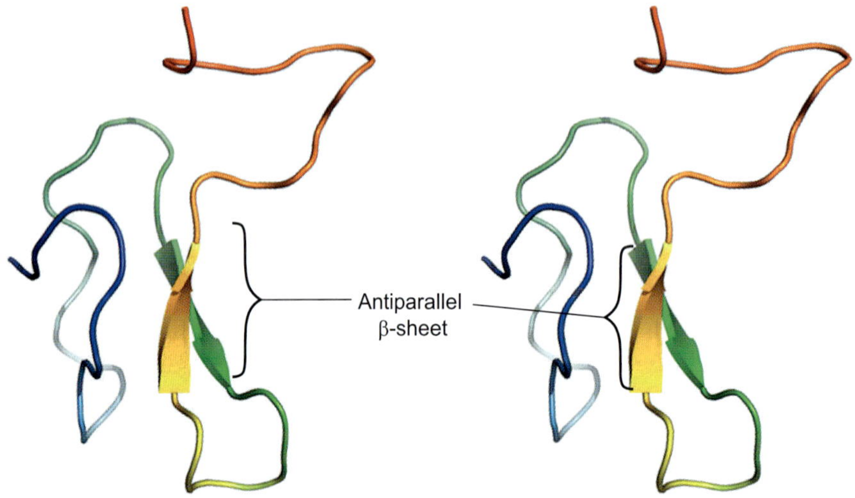

Fig. 1: 3D-stereo view representation of NMR structure of minimized agouti-related protein (AgRP) (87-132) [AC-AgRP(87-132)] PDB ID 1HYK.
Source: Bolin et al. (1999).

environmental and behavioral factors, in addition to genetic factors, influence weight. Genetic causes are divided into two types: Single-gene and multigene. Single-gene obesity is rare and results from mutations in genes of the leptin/melanocortin pathway in the hypothalamus, a region crucial for regulating food intake/satiety, body weight, and energy metabolism.[14]

The hormone leptin regulates eating behaviors, the onset of puberty, and T-cell immunity. Approximately 3% of overweight children have a mutation in the leptin gene and its receptor, exhibiting delayed puberty and immune system dysfunction.[15] Monogenic obesity and abnormal eating behaviors appear in children as young as 2 years old.[16]

Genetic syndromes associated with childhood obesity include Prader-Willi syndrome, Bardet-Biedl syndrome, and Alström syndrome.[17] Other syndromes include Beckwith-Wiedemann syndrome and Cohen syndrome. More than 25 syndromes of obesity have been identified, the most common being Prader-Willi syndrome.[18]

Polygenic obesity, a more common form of obesity, results from the interaction of genes with the environment.[19] Genetic variations in obese individuals influence their behaviors, such as their eating patterns, low physical activity, low metabolic rate, and increased predisposition to fat storage.[20,21] Recent studies reveal that epigenetic factors play a role in obesity.[22] Furthermore, maternal nutrition before birth or in the early postpartum period stimulates these epigenetic changes and increases the risk of developing chronic diseases, such as obesity.[23]

Endocrine Factors

Less than 1% of childhood obesity cases are due to hormonal factors.[24] Children with underlying hormonal disorders often experience mild-to-moderate obesity, short stature, and hypogonadism. Examples of hormonal conditions associated with obesity include growth hormone deficiency, hypothyroidism, pseudohypoparathyroidism, precocious puberty, leptin deficiency or resistance, prolactin-secreting tumors, polycystic ovary syndrome, and Cushing's syndrome.

Lifestyle and Dietary Practices

A child's eating habits develop during their early formative years, as they observe adults and their surrounding environment to shape their dietary patterns.[25] Due to the demands of daily life, parents often provide their children with processed, high-calorie ready-made foods, as illustrated in **Figure 2**. Studies have indicated that formula feeding instead of breastfeeding and the early introduction of protein into a child's diet are contributing factors to weight gain that may persist into adulthood.[26,27]

Furthermore, children are encouraged to finish their meals from large plates, a practice observed across various cultures.[28] In nurseries and schools, children are exposed to a wider variety of food options and enjoy greater independence in choosing different foods. The lack of physical activity in nurseries and schools is also a contributing factor to weight gain.[29]

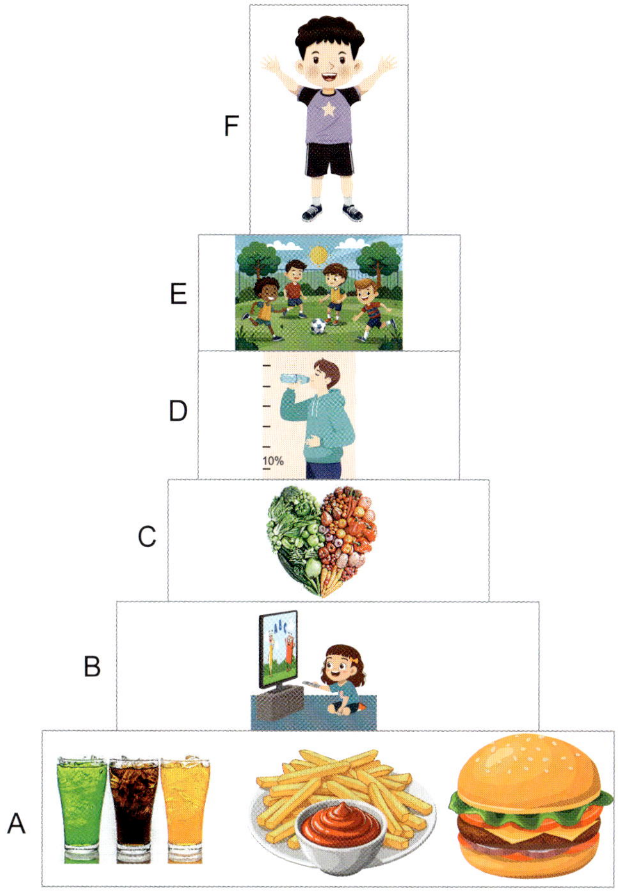

Fig. 2: Prevention of obesity in children. (A) No/less junk food; (B) less screen time; (C) eating more veggies/fruits; (D) plenty of fluids; (E) physical activities; and (F) healthy child.
Source: Pont et al. (2017).

Adolescents have gained greater autonomy regarding high-calorie foods. The affordability and easy availability of unhealthy foods, coupled with extensive brand advertising, encourage the consumption of high-calorie foods in public, a major contributor to obesity.[30] In the United States, the price of McDonald's and Coca-Cola decreased (by 5.44 and 34.89%, respectively) from 1990 to 2007, while the prices of fruits and vegetables increased by 17% between 1997 and 2003.[31]

Furthermore, playing video games and spending long periods in front of screens reduces physical activity and negatively impacts adolescents' mental health.[32] Adolescence is a stage in which teenagers become increasingly anxious about their appearance and weight, in addition to experiencing other psychological problems.[33] Therefore, a sedentary lifestyle, lack of physical activity, and unhealthy eating habits, such as drinking soda and sugary beverages and consuming large quantities of snacks, lead to increased energy expenditure and, consequently, higher rates of obesity.[34-36]

Sleep and Obesity

Sleep patterns affect a child's weight.[37] Studies indicate that 45% of children who get less sleep (<10.5 hours) at age 3 years are more likely to be obese at age 7 years compared to children who sleep >12 hours at the same age.[38,39] Technology disrupts children's sleep and eating patterns.[40] Using electronic devices during sleep reduces total sleep time, leading to decreased physical activity during the day and, consequently, weight gain.[41]

Psychological Factors

Childhood obesity leads to eating disorders. Severe body dissatisfaction and low self-esteem may contribute to both eating disorders and obesity.[42]

Early diagnosis of eating disorders, such as anorexia nervosa, bulimia nervosa, and binge eating disorder, can help prevent obesity or aid weight loss in adolescents with chronic obesity.[43]

Eating disorders may co-occur with obesity or develop after obesity treatment in children or adolescents.[44] Binge eating is associated with comorbid obesity, followed by bulimia nervosa, and approximately 30% of females with eating disorders are chronically obese.[45]

When emotional regulation is disrupted, it triggers binge eating episodes, which in turn lead to feelings of shame and guilt, creating a vicious cycle of loss of control over eating.[46]

Several socioeconomic factors are common risk factors for both eating disorders and obesity, such as frequent criticism, bullying, family/peer pressure, and social pressure.[47]

Furthermore, families experiencing overeating behaviors, parental separation, high parental demands, traumatic life events, and negative childhood experiences such as physical and sexual abuse are all risk factors for developing eating disorders and obesity.[48]

Medications and Toxins

Some medications can cause weight gain and obesity. Examples include antidepressants, glucocorticoids, progestins, propranolol, alpha-blockers (such as terazosin), and insulin.

Both bisphenol A and dichlorodiphenyltrichloroethane are endocrine-disrupting toxins, and these chemicals may contribute to obesity by disrupting estrogen receptors and metabolic programing.[49]

CONSEQUENCES OF OBESITY

Obesity significantly impacts children's physical health and their social and psychological well-being. Most children suffer from low self-esteem, poor academic performance, and a reduced quality of life. Chronic diseases: There are numerous chronic diseases that a child may develop as a result of obesity. A high BMI before the age of 5 years is a risk factor for obesity in adulthood, its associated diseases, and metabolic syndrome,[50,51] as illustrated in **Figure 3**.

Chronic health conditions associated with childhood obesity include cardiovascular diseases such as hypertension, dyslipidemia, and coronary artery disease; metabolic problems, e.g., prediabetes and type 2 diabetes; hormonal problems such as polycystic ovary syndrome; and other diseases such as fatty liver disease, precocious puberty, bone problems such as slipped femoral head, asthma, sleep apnea, poor balance,[52] and idiopathic intracranial hypertension.[53]

Diabetes

Childhood obesity quadruples the risk of developing glucose intolerance and type 2 diabetes. Approximately 85% of children diagnosed with noninsulin-dependent diabetes mellitus are overweight or obese.[54] Type 2 diabetes in children is characterized by severe symptoms and high rates of treatment failure. Children with diabetes may develop comorbidities and early complications, such as fatty liver disease, nephropathy, dyslipidemia, and polycystic ovary syndrome, especially in girls.[55,56] In clinics, obese children are routinely screened for type 2 diabetes.[57]

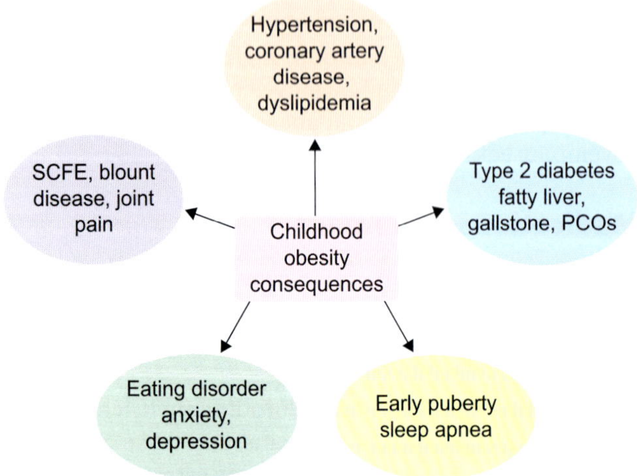

Fig. 3: Consequences of obesity.
Source: Whitaker et al. (1998); Jabakhanji et al. (2018).

Hypertension

Obesity is a major risk factor for hypertension in children. Approximately 25% of obese children develop hypertension. The mechanisms behind the development of hypertension in obese children are complex, but several factors have been identified, including activation of the renin-angiotensin-aldosterone system, activation of the sympathetic nervous system, disruption of blood sodium balance, oxidative stress, and impaired endothelial function. Leptin, resistin, and interleukin-6, all inflammatory adipocytes, stimulate the sympathetic nervous system, which in turn affects the renal blood vessels.[58] Furthermore, hyperinsulinemia leads to increased sodium retention in the kidneys, increased intracellular calcium, and stimulates the sympathetic nervous system,[59] resulting in hypertension.

Hepatic Steatosis

Nonalcoholic fatty liver disease (NAFLD) is a major cause of liver disease in obese children. Physicians should screen obese children for fatty liver using the alanine aminotransferase (ALT) test and ultrasound. NAFLD is associated with fat accumulation in the liver (steatohepatitis) and inflammation and damage to the liver (nonalcoholic steatohepatitis—NASH).[60] NAFLD is also associated with central obesity, insulin resistance, type 2 diabetes, dyslipidemia, and hypertension, all of which are factors associated with metabolic syndrome.[61] The progression of NAFLD to an advanced stage requiring liver transplantation is less well understood in children,[62] while some studies suggest that NAFLD is 14 times more common in children with the disease than in those without.

Gallstones

There are pigment gallstones associated with chronic hemolysis, cholesterol gallstones linked to environmental and genetic factors, and mixed gallstones. Cholesterol gallstones constitute 70% of all gallstones. Obese girls are more prone to gallstones than boys, and this condition becomes more common during periods of weight loss. Gallstone formation in obese adolescents is attributed to increased cholesterol production and bile saturation with cholesterol.[63] Pediatricians should consult a pediatric gastroenterologist if an obese child presents with unexplained abdominal pain or jaundice.

Sleep Disorders

Children and adolescents who are obese or overweight are more likely to develop obstructive sleep apnea.[64]

Neurocognitive disturbances, abnormal behaviors, and increased daytime sleepiness are common symptoms in children with obstructive sleep apnea.[65] Obstructive sleep apnea may cause systemic oxidative stress and inflammation in adolescents.[66] However, cardiovascular complications are less common in children with obstructive sleep apnea compared to adolescents and adults.[67,68]

Metabolic Syndrome

There is no clear-cut definition of metabolic syndrome in children; however, it is characterized by cardiovascular risk factors such as acanthosis nigricans, dyslipidemia, hypertension, prediabetes, and NASH which is caused by insulin resistance due to obesity.[69] Hyperinsulinism,[70] poor sleep behaviors, and low vitamin D levels increase the risk of metabolic syndrome. Regular screening and intervention of complications associated with metabolic syndrome in an obese child are vital to save the future of a child's health.

Asthma

Some studies indicate that asthma and its acute attacks are more common and severe in children who are obese or overweight. Asthma in obese children is slightly less responsive to inhaled corticosteroids compared to nonobese children. Asthma and obesity in children are mediated by abnormal systemic inflammation associated with obesity and oxidative stress, airway narrowing, reduced lung volume, restricted chest movement, obstructive sleep apnea, and gastroesophageal reflux disease.[71]

Growth and Puberty

Obesity can affect growth and puberty in children. Excessive weight gain accelerates the rate of linear growth in prepubertal children and accelerates bone aging.[72] Obese children may have abnormally high insulin levels, and leptin resistance may occur in children whose adipose tissue produces higher levels of leptin. Insulin, leptin, and sex hormones affect the maturation of growth plates, leading to premature bone aging.[72,73] Precocious puberty can begin in overweight children due to hormonal imbalances. They may exhibit signs of breast development, adrenal initiation, and precocious puberty.[74] Research indicates that precocious pubertal changes occur more frequently in girls, while obese boys show delayed puberty, and overweight boys may exhibit precocious puberty.[75] Precocious adrenal initiation in girls is a risk factor for developing polycystic ovary syndrome later in life.[76,77] Furthermore, rapid weight gain during infancy is a risk factor for childhood obesity and early puberty in girls.[78] Obese children tend to be taller and mature earlier than lean children, but their growth rate is relatively lower during adolescence compared to adolescents of normal weight.[79]

Social and Emotional Impacts

In addition to medical concerns, there are emotional and social impacts on children with obesity. Childhood obesity is one of the most socially stigmatized and least accepted conditions.[80] Children with obesity often experience discrimination and face challenges such as bullying, ridicule from peers, negative stereotypes, and social exclusion.[81,82]

They are frequently excluded from competitive physical activities because they tend to be slower than their peers. These negative experiences lead to low self-esteem, which affects their academic performance. Children with obesity experience problems at school and in their academic performance four times more often than their peers of normal weight, e.g., they are more likely to be absent from school.[80]

INITIAL ASSESSMENT

Epigenetics is believed to play a significant role in the dramatic rise in obesity rates over the past 30 years. Children are at increased risk of obesity if one parent is obese: The risk is 30% if one parent is obese, and 90% if both parents are obese. Childhood obesity is associated with a maternal prepregnancy BMI ≥30 kg/m^2, excessive weight gain during pregnancy, and gestational diabetes.[5,6,83]

Infants who are underweight for their gestational age due to tobacco use or insufficient maternal weight gain are also at risk of childhood obesity and metabolic disorders. Other factors that may lead to congenital changes that cause obesity include, but are not limited to, toxins, nutrition, medications, antibiotics, infections, and exogenous hormones.[11,84,85]

The weight of an obese child is assessed by considering both the child's age and the severity of the obesity. BMI is not measured in infants up to the age of 2 years. Instead, the infant's weight percentile is compared to their height percentile.

Body mass index charts are used for children aged 2–20 years. Developed by the CDC in 2000, these charts are color-coded according to BMI percentile: The 95th percentile is in red. The chart extends up to a BMI of 35 kg/m^2. An additional BMI chart has also been developed for children aged 2 to 20 years who are obese.[86]

Both BMI graphs show a J-shaped curve, where BMI in young children naturally declines between the ages of 2 and 6 years, then gradually rises between the ages of 6 and 20 years. This decline or fluctuation, followed by a rise in the BMI curve, is referred to as obesity rebound. If a child's BMI does not decline or rises prematurely between the ages of 2 and 6 years, the child is at risk of becoming obese or is already obese. This phenomenon is called early obesity rebound.[86]

Children, like adults, experience symptoms of obesity in most aspects of their physical and mental health. The term adipose tissue pathology is used to describe the hormonal and immune responses to increased adipose tissue, while the term fat-mass disease describes the physical response to increased adipose tissue.[7,87]

IMPORTANCE OF HISTORY TAKING FOR INITIAL ASSESSMENT

We need to obtain a detailed medical history that includes family history,[88-90] prenatal, intranatal, and postnatal care, as well as any childhood medical complications and medications used to treat coexisting conditions and obesity.[7,87] The social history includes not only dietary recall but also breastfeeding or formula feeding history, the timing of introducing complementary foods, and parenting style. Additionally, it is important to assess the child's activity level, including access to safe spaces for exercise and the availability of support for vigorous physical activity. Finally, the physician needs to evaluate the child's sedentary time and screen time for nonacademic purposes.[7,87]

APPROACH TO PHYSICAL EXAMINATION

Clinical examination is both important and precise in children with obesity.

Acanthosis nigricans is a skin condition associated with hyperinsulinemia, and parents or the child themselves often mistake it for dirt or eczema rather than melanin. Explaining the cause reassures the child and their parents and provides an opportunity to educate them about the physiology of glucose metabolism and the mechanism of insulin resistance.[20-22]

The physician should be aware of skeletal problems that may occur in children with obesity. Young children with Blount's disease are usually able to walk and may begin walking early without realizing there is a problem. Therefore, radiographic diagnosis is essential. Slipped femoral head may present with knee or hip pain, or it may be asymptomatic, which can lead to misdiagnosis. Therefore, immediate evaluation and referral to an orthopedic surgeon are crucial if the condition is diagnosed. Scoliosis is difficult to detect due to obesity, although it occurs in obese children at the same or higher rate than in children of normal weight **(Table 1)**.[20-22]

DIAGNOSTIC WORKUP: LABORATORIES AND STUDIES

From Cuda SE, Censani M, Scinta W, Joseph M, Green R, Pediatric Obesity Algorithm, 2016-17. www.pediatricobesityalgorithm.org

TABLE 1: Diagnostic workup: laboratories and studies.

Infancy (0–24 months)	*Toddler (ages 2–4 years)*	*Early childhood (ages 5–9 years)*	*Puberty (ages 10–14 years)*	*Adolescent (ages 15–18 years)*
Weight > length	BMI ≥95th percentile or ≥85th percentile with two or more risk factors (24–48 months)	BMI ≥95th percentile or ≥85th percentile with two or more risk factors	BMI ≥95th percentile or ≥85th percentile with two or more risk factors	BMI ≥95th percentile or ≥85th percentile with two or more risk factors
	• Fasting blood glucose and/or HbA1c • Fasting lipid panel/nonfasting if fasting not feasible • ALT, AST, consider GGT • Consider 25-OH vitamin D			
		• Consider sleep study • Consider liver ultrasound • Consider uric acid • Consider fasting serum insulin		
			• Consider urine microalbumin/creatinine ratio • Consider C-peptide, hs-CRP	

Source: From Cuda S, O'Hara V, Browne NT, et al. (2025). Pediatric Obesity Algorithm. 2016-2017. [online] Available from https://obesitymedicine.org/resources/obesity-algorithm/pediatric-obesity-algorithm/. [Last accessed January, 2026].

PREVENTIVE STRATEGIES AND MANAGEMENT OF CHILDHOOD OBESITY

World Health Organization recommendations: The WHO places great emphasis on preventive measures for childhood obesity by providing supportive environments and communities that are essential in shaping individual choices, such as choosing healthy foods and engaging in 60 minutes of daily physical activity, which is the easiest, most accessible, and most convenient option for children. The organization recommends increasing the consumption of fruits, vegetables, legumes, and nuts, and reducing energy intake from sugars and fats, as illustrated in **Figure 2**. The food industry can play a significant role in promoting healthy diets by reducing the sugar, salt, and fat content in processed foods; limiting the marketing of foods high in sugars, fats, and salt, especially those targeted at children and adolescents; and providing healthy food options in schools and workplaces.[91]

Motivational Interview

Motivational interviewing techniques are useful for encouraging positive behavior change in adolescents and children with obesity.[92] Research indicates that the language used by healthcare providers can sometimes reduce motivation to manage weight, potentially leading to avoidance of preventive care,[91] and even to overeating, decreased physical activity, social isolation, avoidance of healthcare facilities, and weight gain.[93] Effective communication between the caregiver and the patient is essential for encouraging positive behavior change.[94]

Anticipatory Guidance

Providing support to parents or guardians from healthcare providers to understand a child's expected growth and development is considered proactive guidance. This includes educating parents about healthy and unhealthy eating habits, the importance of physical activity, and the drawbacks of a sedentary lifestyle, such as excessive screen time. Children's lifestyles are significantly influenced by societal factors, including family habits.[95] Therefore, family based, multidisciplinary behavioral weight-loss therapy is considered the gold standard for managing childhood obesity, particularly in children aged 2–6 years.[96]

A structured weight management program: A multidisciplinary approach, involving physicians, dietitians, and psychologists, conducted once or twice weekly, is the next step in structured weight management for children and adolescents when lifestyle modifications fail,[97,98] but it is not effective in cases of severe obesity.

Pharmacological Treatment

Drug therapy for obesity management in children and adolescents is limited. However, the U.S. Food and Drug Administration (FDA) has approved two drugs for the treatment of obesity in children and adolescents: Orlistat and phentermine.[99]

Orlistat is FDA-approved for children over 12 years of age for long-term obesity management. Its use in adolescents was not approved until 2003.[100] The dosage is 120 mg three times daily with meals. Its mechanism of action is the inhibition of pancreatic and gastric lipase, which reduces fat absorption. Undesirable side effects limit its use, such as stomach upset, abdominal pain, fecal urgency and incontinence, and deficiencies in fat-soluble vitamins.[101]

Contraindications include malabsorption, pregnancy, and cholestasis.[102]

Phentermine is a short-term (12 weeks or less) treatment for obesity in individuals over 16 years of age. This drug is an amphetamine analog and is FDA-approved. The prescribed dosage is 15, 30, and 37.5 mg daily.[100] Phentermine works by enhancing the activity of catecholamines and serotonin in the central nervous system, leading to appetite suppression.[100] Common side effects include increased heart rate and blood pressure, gastrointestinal disturbances, tremors, headache, mood swings, and dry mouth.[103] A history of or uncontrolled cardiovascular disease, glaucoma, hyperthyroidism, and current use of monoamine oxidase inhibitors are contraindications for phentermine.[104]

Other medications for obesity, such as metformin, exenatide, topiramate, zonisamide, octreotide, and growth hormone, should not be used outside of this approved indication.

Phentermine should not be used outside of this approved indication. Growth hormone is used to treat syndromes of obesity, such as Prader–Willi syndrome.[105] It reduces fat mass and increases lean body mass. Octreotide (a somatostatin analog) is used to treat obesity caused by hypothalamic dysfunction, aiming to stabilize weight in adolescents.[106]

Dexamphetamine, used to treat attention deficit hyperactivity disorder (ADHD), is used to treat binge eating and obesity in adolescents.[107]

Metformin is used to treat children with insulin resistance and may have an effect on weight, but it is not FDA-approved for treating childhood obesity.

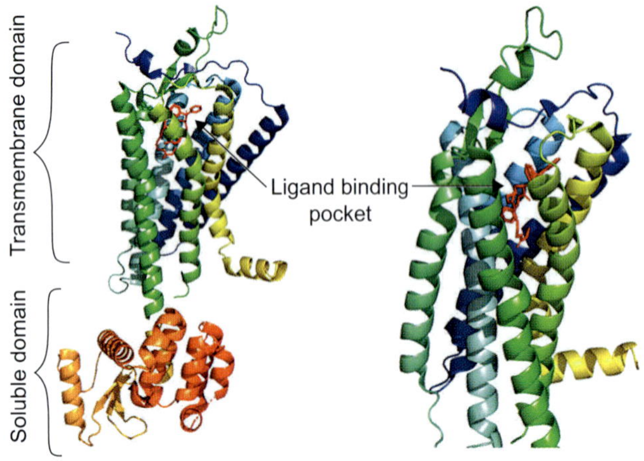

Fig. 4: The crystal structure of human neuropeptide Y Y1 receptor with BMS-193885. The receptor is shown in cartoon representation while the ligand is shown as the red stick.
Source: Park et al. (2022).

Neuropeptide Y (NPY) is abundant in the central nervous system. Its receptor belongs to the G protein receptor family and plays vital roles in eating, anxiety, and cancer biology. The NPY Y1R receptor is expressed in a variety of tissues and is involved in regulating several physiological functions associated with obesity and cancer[108] **(Fig. 4)**.

Bariatric Surgery

Weight loss surgery is considered necessary for individuals aged 14–18 with a BMI of 40 kg/m^2 or higher, or 35 kg/m^2 or higher with a serious comorbidity associated with obesity, such as type 2 diabetes. Before considering surgery, patients should participate in a structured weight loss program for at least 6 months under the supervision of a multidisciplinary team.[109] Roux-en-Y gastric bypass and laparoscopic sleeve gastrectomy (LASG) are currently approved for children under 18 years.

Gastric banding is not FDA-approved for adolescents. Research suggests that weight loss surgery has fewer severe side effects in adolescents compared to adults.[110] The long-term outcomes of surgery in adolescents are still unknown. Although data collected over 5 years on gastric bypass surgery are promising, the psychological and social effects after surgery remain uncertain in adolescents.[17]

CONCLUSION

Obesity rates are rising among children and adolescents globally, and it is well-known that it significantly impacts their physical and mental health, including their self-esteem and psychological well-being. Obesity in children results from several factors, including environmental factors, lifestyle, and cultural preferences, which play a pivotal role in its increasing global prevalence. Generally, overweight and obesity are believed to be caused by excessive consumption of calories and fats.

Lifestyle changes are crucial for preventing obesity, although their impact is limited in cases of severe childhood obesity. Parents need to adopt a healthy lifestyle, encouraging their children to eat more fruits and vegetables, reduce their consumption of fast food, limit screen time, and increase physical activity.

A combined intervention that includes dietary modification and physical activity, implemented in the community and integrated into schools, is more effective in preventing obesity or overweight in children, thus contributing to building a healthier society.

REFERENCES

1. Flegal KM, Wei R, Ogden C. Weight-for-stature compared with body mass index-for-age growth charts for the United States from the Centers for Disease Control and Prevention. Am J Clin Nutr. 2002;75(4):761-6.
2. Himes JH, Dietz WH. Guidelines for overweight in adolescent preventive services: recommendations from an expert committee. The Expert Committee on Clinical Guidelines for overweight in adolescent preventive services. Am J Clin Nutr. 1994;59(2):307-16.
3. Ghosh A. Explaining overweight and obesity in children and adolescents of Asian Indian origin: the Calcutta childhood obesity study. Indian J Public Health. 2014;58(2):125-8.
4. Popkin BM, Doak CM. The obesity epidemic is a worldwide phenomenon. Nutr Rev. 1998;56(4 Pt 1):106-14.
5. Sahoo K, Sahoo B, Choudhury AK, et al. Childhood obesity: causes and consequences. J Family Med Prim Care. 2015;4(2):187-92.
6. Nittari G, Scuri S, Petrelli F, et al. Fighting obesity in children from European World Health Organization member states. Epidemiological data, medical-social aspects, and prevention programs. Clin Ter. 2019;170(3):e223-e230.
7. Centers for Disease Control and Prevention (CDC). CDC grand rounds: childhood obesity in the United States. Morb Mortal Wkly Rep. 2011;60(2):42-6.
8. Qasim A, Turcotte M, J de Souza R, et al. On the origin of obesity: identifying the biological, environmental and cultural drivers of genetic risk among human populations. Obes Rev. 2018;19(2)121-49.
9. Bolin KA, Anderson DJ, Trulson JA, et al. NMR structure of a minimized human agouti related protein prepared by total chemical synthesis. FEBS Lett. 1999;451(2):125-31.
10. Catalano PM, Farrell K, Thomas A, et al. Perinatal risk factors for childhood obesity and metabolic dysregulation. Am J Clin Nutr. 2009;90(5):1303-13.
11. Sanyaolu A, Okorie C, Qi X, et al. Childhood and adolescent obesity in the United States: a public health concern. Glob Pediatr Health. 2019;6:2333794X19891305.

12. UNICEF. "Joint child malnutrition estimates," 2021 edition interactive dashboard. New York (NY): United Nations Children's Fund; report 2021. [online] Available from https://data.unicef.org/resources/joint-childmalnutrition-estimates-interactive-dashboard-2021.
13. Anderson PM, Butcher KE Childhood obesity: trends and potential causes. Future Child. 2006;16(1):19-45.
14. Ranadive SA, Vaisse C. Lessons from extreme human obesity: monogenic disorders. Endocrinol Metab Clin North Am. 2008;37(3):733-51.
15. Farooqi IS, Wangensteen T, Collins S, et al. Clinical and molecular genetic spectrum of congenital deficiency of the leptin receptor. N Engl J Med. 2007;356(3):237-47.
16. Huvenne H, Dubern B, Clement K, et al. Rare genetic forms of obesity: clinical approach and current treatments in 2016. Obes Facts. 2016;9(3):158-73.
17. Kansra AR, Lakkunarajah S, Jay MS. Childhood and adolescent obesity: a review. Front Pediatr. 2020;8:581461.
18. Geets E, Meuwissen MEC, Van Hul W. Clinical, molecular genetics and therapeutic aspects of syndromic obesity. Clin Genet. 2019;95(1):23-40.
19. Heianza Y, Qi L. Gene-diet interaction and precision nutrition in obesity. Int J Mol Sci. 2017;18(4):787.
20. Rask-Andersen M, Karlsson T, Ek WE, et al. Gene-environment interaction study for BMI reveals interactions between genetic factors and physical activity, alcohol consumption and socioeconomic status. PLoS Genet. 2017;13(9):e1006977.
21. Martinez JA. Body-weight regulation: causes of obesity. Proc Nutr Soc. 2000;59(3):337-45.
22. Sun X, Li P, Yang X, et al. From genetics and epigenetics to the future of precision treatment for obesity. Gastroenterol Rep (Oxf). 2017;5(4):266-70.
23. Li Y. Epigenetic mechanisms link maternal diets and gut microbiome to obesity in the offspring. Front Genet. 2018;9:342.
24. Reinehr T, Hinney A, de Sousa G, et al. Definable somatic disorders in overweight children and adolescents. J Pediatr. 2007;150(6):618-22, 622.e1-5.
25. Birch LL, Fisher JO. Development of eating behaviors among children and adolescents. Pediatrics. 1998;101 (3 Pt 2):539-49.
26. Indrio F, Martini S, Francavilla R, et al. Epigenetic matters: the link between early nutrition, microbiome, and long-term health development. Front Pediatr. 2017;5:178.
27. Koletzko B, Fishbein M, Lee WS, et al. Prevention of childhood obesity: a position paper of the Global Federation of International Societies of Paediatric Gastroenterology, Hepatology and Nutrition (FISPGHAN). J Pediatr Gastroenterol Nutr. 2020;70(5):702-10.
28. Nielsen SJ, Popkin BM. Patterns and trends in food portion sizes, 1977-1998. JAMA. 2003;289(4):450-3.
29. Institute of Medicine. Committee on food marketing and the diets of children and youth. In: McGinnis JM, Gootman JA, Kraak VI (Eds). Food Marketing to Children and Youth: Threat or Opportunity? Washington: National Academies Press; 2006. p. 516.
30. Benjamin R. Surgeon general's prevention priorities dovetail with health care reform law. JAMA. 2010;303(21):2123-4.
31. Friedlander SL, Larkin EK, Rosen CL, et al. Decreased quality of life associated with obesity in school-aged children. Arch Pediatr Adolesc Med. 2003;157(12):1206-11.
32. Liu M, Wu L, Yao S. Dose-response association of screen time-based sedentary behaviour in children and adolescents and depression: a meta-analysis of observational studies. Br J Sports Med. 2016;50(20):1252-8.
33. Lowe CJ, Morton JB, Reichelt AC. Adolescent obesity and dietary decision making—a brain-health perspective. Lancet Child Adolesc Health. 2020;4(5):388-96.
34. Schiffino FL, Siemian JN, Petrella M, et al. Activation of a lateral hypothalamic-ventral tegmental circuit gates motivation. PLoS One. 2019;14(7):e0219522.
35. Reilly JJ, Armstrong J, Dorosty AR, et al. Early life risk factors for obesity in childhood: cohort study. BMJ. 2005;330(7504):1357.
36. Di Cesare M, Sorić M, Bovet P, et al. The epidemiological burden of obesity in childhood: a worldwide epidemic requiring urgent action. BMC Med. 2019;17(1):212.
37. Lissak G. Adverse physiological and psychological effects of screen time on children and adolescents: literature review and case study. Environ Res. 2018;164:149-57.
38. Dev DA, McBride BA, Fiese BH, et al.; Behalf of the Strong Kids Research Team. Risk factors for overweight/obesity in preschool children: an ecological approach. Child Obes. 2013;9(5):399-408.
39. Vos MB, Welsh J. Childhood obesity: update on predisposing factors and prevention strategies. Curr Gastroenterol Rep. 2010;12(4):280-7.
40. Fuller C, Lehman E, Hicks S, et al. Bedtime use of technology and associated sleep problems in children. Glob Pediatr Health. 2017;4:2333794X17736972.
41. Chahal H, Fung C, Kuhle S, et al. Availability and night-time use of electronic entertainment and communication devices are associated with short sleep duration and obesity among Canadian children. Pediatr Obes. 2013;8(1):42-51.
42. Goldschmidt AB, Aspen VP, Sinton MM, et al. Disordered eating attitudes and behaviors in overweight youth. Obesity (Silver Spring). 2008;16(2):257-64.
43. Horsager C, Faerk E, Gearhardt AN, et al. Food addiction comorbid to mental disorders in adolescents: a nationwide survey and register-based study. Eat Weight Disord. 2022;27(3):945-59.
44. Stabouli S, Erdine S, Suurorg L, et al. Obesity and eating disorders in children and adolescents: the bidirectional link. Nutrients. 2021;13(12):4321.
45. Aguera Z, Lozano-Madrid M, Mallorqui-Bague N, et al. A review of binge eating disorder and obesity. Neuropsychiatr. 2021;35(2):57-67.
46. Puhl RM, Himmelstein MS, Pearl RL. Weight stigma as a psychosocial contributor to obesity. Am Psychol. 2020;75(2):274-89.
47. Libbey HP, Story MT, Neumark-Sztainer DR, et al. Teasing, disordered eating behaviors, and psychological

morbidities among overweight adolescents. Obesity (Silver Spring). 2008;16 Suppl 2:S24-9.
48. Striegel-Moore RH, Fairburn CG, Wilfley DE, et al. Toward an understanding of risk factors for binge-eating disorder in black and white women: a community-based case-control study. Psychol Med. 2005;35(6):907-17.
49. Warner M, Wesselink A, Harley KG, et al. Prenatal exposure to dichlorodiphenyltrichloroethane and obesity at 9 years of age in the CHAMACOS study cohort. Am J Epidemiol. 2014;179(11):1312-22.
50. Whitaker RC, Pepe MS, Wright JA, et al. Early adiposity rebound and the risk of adult obesity. Pediatrics. 1998;101(3):E5.
51. Jabakhanji SB, Boland F, Ward M, et al. Body mass index changes in early childhood. J Pediatr. 2018;(202):106-14.
52. Pulgaron ER. Childhood obesity: a review of increased risk for physical and psychological comorbidities. Clin Ther. 2013;35(1):A18-32.
53. Brara SM, Koebnick C, Porter AH, et al. Pediatric idiopathic intracranial hypertension and extreme childhood obesity. J Pediatr. 2012;161(4):602-7.
54. Silverstein J, Klingensmith G, Copeland K, et al. Care of children and adolescents with type 1 diabetes: a statement of the American Diabetes Association. Diabetes Care. 2005;28(1):186-212.
55. Dabelea D, Stafford JM, Mayer-Davis EJ, et al. Association of type 1 diabetes vs type 2 diabetes diagnosed during childhood and adolescence with complications during teenage years and young adulthood. JAMA. 2017;317(8):825-35.
56. Cioana M, Deng J, Nadarajah A, et al. Prevalence of polycystic ovary syndrome in patients with pediatric type 2 diabetes: a systematic review and meta-analysis. JAMA Netw Open. 2022;5(2):e2147454.
57. Zeitler P, Arslanian S, Fu J, et al. ISPAD Clinical Practice Consensus Guidelines 2018: type 2 diabetes mellitus in youth. Pediatr Diabetes. 2018;19 Suppl 27:28-46.
58. Brady TM. Obesity-related hypertension in children. Front Pediatr. 2017;5:197.
59. Bonner G. Hyperinsulinemia, insulin resistance, and hypertension. J Cardiovasc Pharmacol. 1994;24 Suppl 2:S39-49.
60. Anderson EL, Howe LD, Jones HE, et al. The prevalence of nonalcoholic fatty liver disease in children and adolescents: a systematic review and meta-analysis. PLoS One. 2015;10(10):e0140908.
61. Schwimmer JB, Pardee PE, Lavine JE, et al. Cardiovascular risk factors and the metabolic syndrome in pediatric nonalcoholic fatty liver disease. Circulation. 2008;118(3):277-83.
62. Feldstein AE, Charatcharoenwitthaya P, Treeprasertsuk S, et al. The natural history of non-alcoholic fatty liver disease in children: a follow-up study for up to 20 years. Gut. 2009;58(11):1538-44.
63. Koebnick C, Smith N, Black MH, et al. Pediatric obesity and gallstone disease. J Pediatr Gastroenterol Nutr. 2012;55(3):328-33.
64. Jehan S, Zizi F, Pandi-Perumal SR, et al. Obstructive sleep apnea and obesity: implications for public health. Sleep Med Disord. 2017;1(4):00019.
65. Narang I, Mathew JL. Childhood obesity and obstructive sleep apnea. J Nutr Metab. 2012;2012:134202.
66. Eisele HJ, Markart P, Schulz R. Obstructive sleep apnea, oxidative stress, and cardiovascular disease: evidence from human studies. Oxid Med Cell Longev. 2015;2015:608438.
67. Patinkin ZW, Feinn R, Santos M. Metabolic consequences of obstructive sleep apnea in adolescents with obesity: a systematic literature review and meta-analysis. Child Obes. 2017;13(2):102-10.
68. Kaditis A. From obstructive sleep apnea in childhood to cardiovascular disease in adulthood: what is the evidence? Sleep. 2010;33(10):1279-80.
69. Magge SN, Goodman E, Armstrong SC, et al. The metabolic syndrome in children and adolescents: shifting the focus to cardiometabolic risk factor clustering. Pediatrics. 2017;140(2):e20171603.
70. Weiss R, Dziura J, Burgert TS, et al. Obesity and the metabolic syndrome in children and adolescents. N Engl J Med. 2004;350(23):2362-74.
71. Lang JE. Obesity, nutrition, and asthma in children. Pediatr Allergy Immunol Pulmonol. 2012;25(2):64-75.
72. Chung S. Growth and puberty in obese children and implications of body composition. J Obes Metab Syndr. 2017;26(4):243-50.
73. Soliman AT, Yasin M, Kassem A. Leptin in pediatrics: a hormone from adipocyte that wheels several functions in children. Indian J Endocrinol Metab. 2012;16(Suppl 3): S577-87.
74. Burt Solorzano CM, McCartney CR. Obesity and the pubertal transition in girls and boys. Reproduction. 2010;140(3);399-410.
75. Lee JM, Wasserman R, Kaciroti N, et al. Timing of puberty in overweight versus obese boys. Pediatrics. 2016;137(2):e20150164.
76. Franks S. Polycystic ovary syndrome in adolescents. Int J Obes (Lond). 2008;32(7):1035-41.
77. Sadeeqa S, Mustafa T, Latif S. Polycystic ovarian syndrome-related depression in adolescent girls: a review. J Pharm Bioallied Sci. 2018;10(2):55-9.
78. Ong KK, Emmett P, Northstone K, et al. Infancy weight gain predicts childhood body fat and age at menarche in girls. J Clin Endocrinol Metab. 2009;94(5):1527-32.
79. Stovitz SD, Demerath EW, Hannan PJ, et al. Growing into obesity: patterns of height growth in those who become normal weight, overweight, or obese as young adults. Am J Hum Biol. 2011;23(5):635-41.
80. Schwimmer JB, Burwinkle TM, Varni JW. Health-related quality of life of severely obese children and adolescents. JAMA. 2003;289(14):1813-9.
81. Budd GM, Hayman LL. Addressing the childhood obesity crisis: a call to action. MCN Am J Matern Child Nurs. 2008;33(2):111-8, quiz 119-20.
82. Bacchini D, Licenziati MR, Garrasi A, et al., Bullying and victimization in overweight and obese outpatient children

and adolescents: an Italian multicentric study. PLoS One. 2015;10(11):e0142715.
83. Scuri S, Petrelli F, Tesauro M, et al. Energy drink consumption: a survey in high school students and associated psychological effects. J Prev Med Hyg. 2018;59(1):E75-9.
84. Ball GDC, Savu A, Kaul P. Changes in the prevalence of overweight, obesity, and severe obesity between 2010 and 2017 in preschoolers: a population-based study. Pediatr Obes. 2019;14(11):e12561.
85. Rao DP, Kropac E, Do MT, et al. Childhood overweight and obesity trends in Canada. Health Promot Chronic Dis Prev Can. 2016;36(9):194-8.
86. World Health Organization. (2016). The double burden of malnutrition: policy brief. [online] Available from https://apps.who.int/iris/handle/10665/255413. [Last accessed January, 2026].
87. Mazidi M, Banach M, Kengne AP, et al.; Lipid and Blood Pressure Meta-analysis Collaboration Group. Prevalence of childhood and adolescent overweight and obesity in Asian countries: a systematic review and meta-analysis. Arch Med Sci. 2018;14(6):1185-1203.
88. Niehoff V. Childhood obesity: a call to action. Bariatric Nursing Surgical Patient Care. 2009;4(1):17-23.
89. Rankin J, Matthews L, Cobley S, et al. Psychological consequences of childhood obesity: psychiatric comorbidity and prevention. Adolesc Health Med Ther. 2016;7:125-146.
90. Ruiz LD, Zuelch ML, Dimitratos SM, et al. Adolescent obesity: diet quality, psychosocial health, and cardiometabolic risk factors. Nutrients. 2019;12(1):43.
91. Pont SJ, Puhl R, Cook SR, et al.; Section on Obesity; Obesity Society. Stigma experienced by children and adolescents with obesity. Pediatrics. 2017;140(6):e20173034.
92. Simmonds M, Llewellyn A, Owen CG, et al. Predicting adult obesity from childhood obesity: a systematic review and meta-analysis. Obes Rev. 2016;17(2):95-107.
93. Puhl R, Suh Y. Health consequences of weight stigma: implications for obesity prevention and treatment. Curr Obes Rep. 2015;4(2):182-90.
94. Carcone AI, Jacques-Tiura AJ, Brogan Hartlieb KE, et al. Effective patient-provider communication in pediatric obesity. Pediatr Clin North Am. 2016;63(3):525-38.
95. Brown CL, Halvorson EE, Cohen GM, et al. Addressing childhood obesity: opportunities for prevention. Pediatr Clin North Am. 2015;62(5):1241-61.
96. Hayes JF, Fitzsimmons-Craft EE, Karam AM, et al. Disordered eating attitudes and behaviors in youth with overweight and obesity: implications for treatment. Curr Obes Rep. 2018;7(3):235-46.
97. Katzmarzyk PT, Barlow S, Bouchard C, et al. An evolving scientific basis for the prevention and treatment of pediatric obesity. Int J Obes (Lond). 2014;38(7):887-905.
98. Skjakodegard HF, Danielsen YS, Morken M, et al. Study protocol: a randomized controlled trial evaluating the effect of family-based behavioral treatment of childhood and adolescent obesity-The FABO-study. BMC Public Health. 2016;16(1):1106.
99. Singhal V, Sella AC, Malhotra S. Pharmacotherapy in pediatric obesity: current evidence and landscape. Curr Opin Endocrinol Diabetes Obes. 2021;28(1):55-63.
100. Woodard K, Louque L, Hsia DS. Medications for the treatment of obesity in adolescents. Ther Adv Endocrinol Metab. 2020;11:2042018820918789.
101. Maahs D, de Serna DG, Kolotkin RL, et al. Randomized, double-blind, placebo-controlled trial of orlistat for weight loss in adolescents. Endocr Pract. 2006;12(1):18-28.
102. Torgerson JS, Hauptman J, Boldrin MN, et al. XENical in the prevention of diabetes in obese subjects (XENDOS) study: a randomized study of orlistat as an adjunct to lifestyle changes for the prevention of type 2 diabetes in obese patients. Diabetes Care. 2004;27(1):155-61.
103. Ryder JR, Kaizer A, Rudser KD, et al. Effect of phentermine on weight reduction in a pediatric weight management clinic. Int J Obes (Lond). 2017;41(1):90-3.
104. Srivastava G, Apovian CM. Current pharmacotherapy for obesity. Nat Rev Endocrinol. 2018;14(1):12-24.
105. Wolfgram PM, Carrel AL, Allen DB. Long-term effects of recombinant human growth hormone therapy in children with Prader-Willi syndrome. Curr Opin Pediatr. 2013;25(4):509-14.
106. Lustig RH, Hinds PS, Ringwald-Smith K, et al. Octreotide therapy of pediatric hypothalamic obesity: a double-blind, placebo-controlled trial. J Clin Endocrinol Metab. 2003;88(6):2586-92.
107. Srivastava G, O'Hara V, Browne N. Use of lisdexamfetamine to treat obesity in an adolescent with severe obesity and binge eating. Children (Basel). 2019;6(2):22.
108. Park C, Kim J, Ko S-B, et al., Structural basis of neuropeptide Y signaling through Y1 receptor. Nat Commun. 2022;13(1):853.
109. Weiss AL, Mooney A, Gonzalvo JP. Bariatric surgery: the future of obesity management in adolescents. Adv Pediatr. 2017;64(1):269-83.
110. Lamoshi A, Chernoguz A, Harmon CM, et al. Complications of bariatric surgery in adolescents. Semin Pediatr Surg. 2020;29(1):150888.

SECTION 20

Obesity, HFpEF and Cardio-oncology

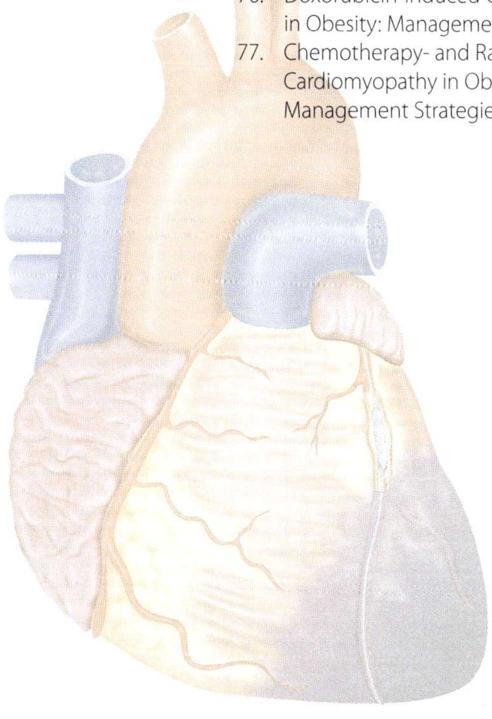

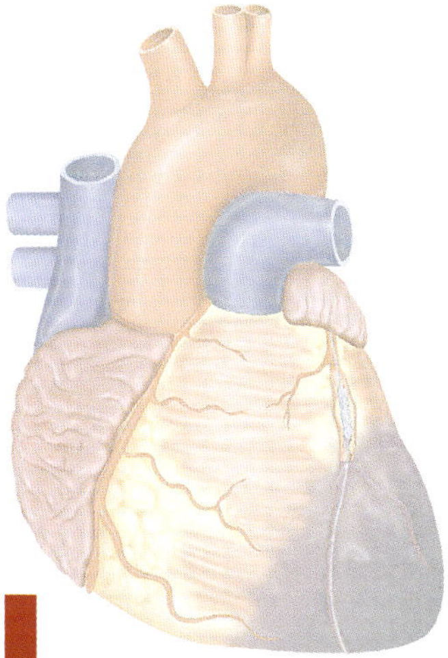

76

CHAPTER

Doxorubicin-induced Cardiotoxicity in Obesity: Management Strategies

Shipra Gupta, Indu Bansal Aggarwal, Harmesh Aggarwal

INTRODUCTION

The Clinical Problem of Doxorubicin Cardiotoxicity

Cancer patients and survivors have an increased risk of cardiovascular diseases (CVDs) as compared with the general population. Doxorubicin, an anthracycline, remains a cornerstone in cancer treatment due to its effectiveness against a range of tumors, including breast cancer, lymphomas, and sarcomas.[1] But it is also considered a major cause of the acute and chronic dose dependent cardiotoxicity, a feared side effect which can manifest immediately after cancer therapy or many years later.[2] The mechanism of doxorubicin-induced cytotoxicity is presented in **Flowchart 1**. The pathophysiology of cardiotoxicity involves injury to heart muscle cells, primarily through oxidative stress, mitochondrial damage, and activation of cell death pathways, which over time impair cardiac function and can lead to heart failure.[3]

The incidence of clinical heart failure varies, typically affecting about 3–5% of patients treated with standard doses (around 400–550 mg/m^2), but subclinical declines in cardiac function may reach 10–15%.[1] Early detection tools, such as blood biomarkers (troponin) and advanced imaging (strain echocardiography), enable clinicians to identify early myocardial injury.[4] When such injury is detected promptly, protective treatments—most notably ACE inhibitors and beta-blockers—can help preserve or recover cardiac function and prevent progression to symptomatic heart failure.[3] The current international guidelines emphasize vigilant heart monitoring before and during anthracycline therapy to mitigate long-term risks.[3]

The Global Burden of Obesity

Being overweight and obesity are complex health problems in a large number of people which increase the risk of cancer. Obesity has become the most rapidly increasing health challenge worldwide, with prevalence tripling since the mid-1970s.[5] Currently, >1 billion adults are classified as obese, which significantly increases the risk of hypertension, type 2 diabetes, and structural

Flowchart 1: Mechanism of doxorubicin-induced cytotoxicity.

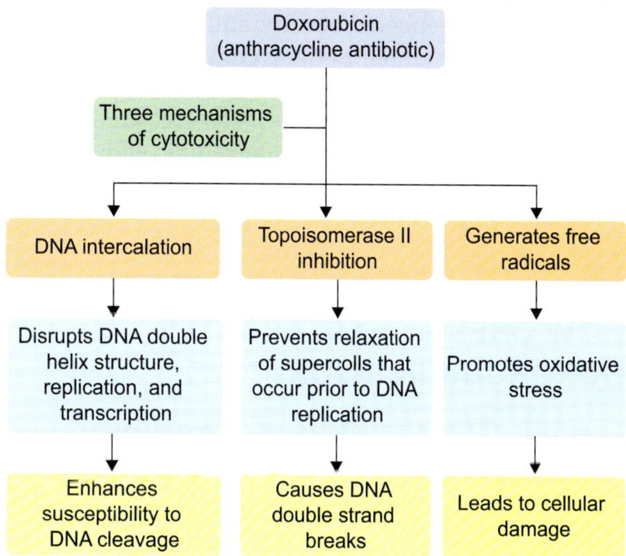

heart disease—each a risk factor for developing heart failure.[6] Each one-unit increase in BMI is associated with a 5–7% higher risk of heart failure, independent of other comorbidities or demographic factors.[7]

In cancer survivors, obesity not only elevates the baseline cardiovascular risk but also appears to worsen responses to cardiotoxic therapies like doxorubicin and other anthracyclines, potentially through metabolic and inflammatory pathways.[7] International guidelines have acknowledged obesity as a key comorbidity that amplifies vulnerability to chemotherapy-related cardiac injury, underscoring the importance of integrating weight management into cancer care protocols.[3] Usually, it is thought that excess adiposity is associated with reduced cancer survival but surprisingly few studies have emerged challenging this by saying that overweight and early obese states are associated with improved survival. This finding is termed the "obesity paradox" and needs further research.[8]

Flowchart 2: Pathophysiology of doxorubicin-induced cardiotoxicity.

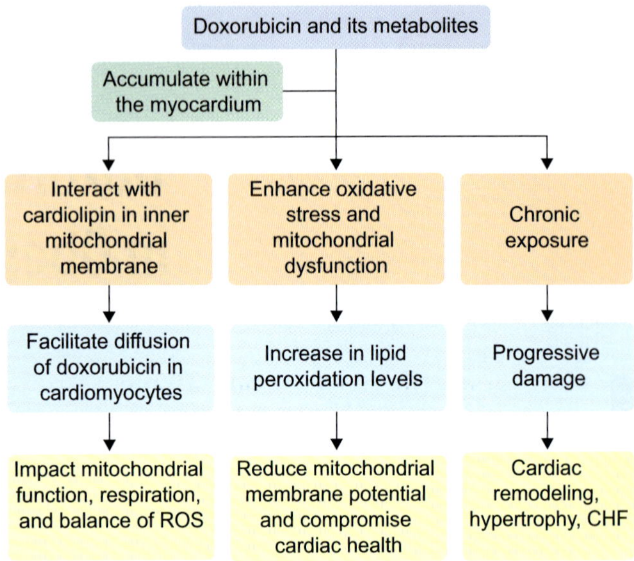

Confluence of Epidemics

With aging populations and rising obesity rates, the intersection of cancer and CVD (termed cardio-oncology) is a growing concern. Evidence suggests that obesity does not simply coexist with cancer; it actively worsens anthracycline-induced cardiac toxicity. The pathophysiology involves heightened oxidative stress, systemic inflammation, and hormonal disturbances—factors that intensify myocardial injury.[9] A meta-analysis encompassing nearly 9,000 women with breast cancer confirmed that overweight and obese patients had a 40% higher likelihood of developing cardiotoxicity compared to their lean counterparts.[7] In a meta-analysis, pooled odds ratio for cardiotoxicity was 1.38 for overweight or obesity (BMI >25), 1.47 for obesity, and 1.15 for overweight.[7]

This convergence of obesity and cancer creates a particularly vulnerable patient group. Understanding how excess weight amplifies the cardiotoxic effects of doxorubicin is crucial. It informs better risk stratification, preventive strategies, and early intervention efforts aimed at improving long-term cardiac outcomes for cancer survivors.

PATHOPHYSIOLOGICAL MECHANISMS: HOW OBESITY EXACERBATES DOXORUBICIN INJURY?

Canonical Mechanisms of Doxorubicin Cardiotoxicity

The risk of anthracycline-induced cardiotoxicity is dynamic and evolves during patients' journey. Doxorubicin causes type I cardiotoxicity which is irreversible. The mechanism of doxorubicin-induced cardiotoxicity is depicted in **Flowchart 2**. Doxorubicin-induced cardiac injury originates primarily from oxidative stress and mitochondrial dysfunction. The drug undergoes redox cycling within cardiac myocytes, generating reactive oxygen species (ROS) that damage DNA, proteins, and membrane lipids.[1] This oxidative burden impairs mitochondrial bioenergetics, leading to a decline in ATP production critical for cardiac contraction, and triggers cardiomyocyte apoptosis via both intrinsic and extrinsic pathways.[1,2] Additionally, doxorubicin intercalates DNA and forms complexes with topoisomerase II beta in cardiomyocytes, disrupting DNA repair and transcription, thereby exacerbating cellular injury.[3] These mechanisms collectively weaken cardiac structure and function over time.

Obesity-associated Metabolic Alterations

Obesity creates a systemic proinflammatory and pro-oxidative environment that synergizes with doxorubicin's toxic effects. Adipose tissue in obesity releases increased levels of inflammatory cytokines such as TNF-α, IL-6, and leptin, while adiponectin—an anti-inflammatory adipokine—is downregulated.[7] Chronic inflammation contributes to endothelial dysfunction and primes cardiac tissue for exaggerated injury when stressed by chemotherapeutics.[4] Furthermore, obesity induces insulin resistance and lipotoxicity, leading to abnormal myocardial fatty acid metabolism and accumulation of toxic lipid intermediates that worsen mitochondrial function.[3]

Synergistic Pathways of Injury

The convergence of doxorubicin toxicity and obesity-induced metabolic derangements potentiates cardiac dysfunction through multiple interactive pathways. ROS generated by doxorubicin is amplified in the context of obesity-related oxidative stress, overwhelming cardiomyocyte antioxidant defenses.[3] Altered adipokine profiles exacerbate inflammatory signaling cascades and further promote fibrosis and remodeling in cardiac tissue.[5] Insulin resistance and mitochondrial lipid overload also sensitize cardiomyocytes to apoptosis and necrosis. The mechanism of obesity and anthracyclines causing cardiotoxicity is depicted in **Flowchart 3**. Evidence from experimental models demonstrates that obese animals exhibit heightened susceptibility to anthracycline-induced reductions in left ventricular function compared to lean counterparts.[6]

Clinical Implications

Understanding these intersecting pathophysiological mechanisms reinforces the need for tailored cardiac monitoring and preventive strategies in obese cancer patients receiving doxorubicin. Biomarkers of oxidative stress and inflammation may identify high-risk individuals who would benefit from early cardioprotective interventions.[7] Lifestyle modifications including weight loss and pharmacologic approaches addressing metabolic dysfunction hold promise as adjunctive therapies to reduce anthracycline cardiotoxicity in obese populations.[7]

MANAGEMENT OF ANTHRACYCLINE-INDUCED CARDIOTOXICITY WITH CONSIDERATION OF OBESITY

Anthracycline-induced cardiotoxicity remains a significant clinical challenge, requiring tailored management approaches, especially in the vulnerable obese patient population. The goals include early detection, prevention, mitigation of progression, and treatment of established cardiac dysfunction.[9]

Prevention of Anthracycline-induced Cardiotoxicity

The European Society of Cardiology Guidelines on CVD[10] suggest to take primary as well as secondary measures to prevent the development of cardiotoxicity. The suggested preventive measures are to avoid risk factors such as obesity, cigarette smoking, and alcohol consumption; manage arterial hypertension; encourage physical activity; and encourage use of the liposomal doxorubicin, dexrazoxane, ACEi, ARB, beta-adrenergic receptor antagonists, and statins in high-risk patients. As a secondary preventive measure, left ventricular ejection fraction (LVEF) assessment before and within 12 months after the administration of anthracyclines should be done

Flowchart 3: Obesity and cardiotoxicity synergism.

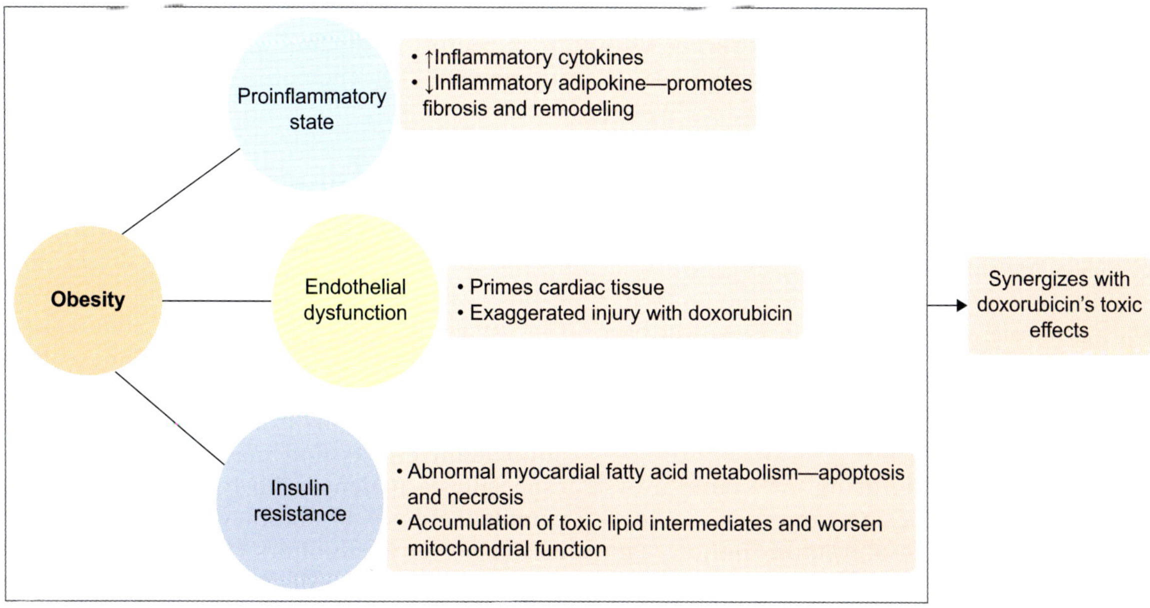

Flowchart 4: Management of cardiotoxicity.

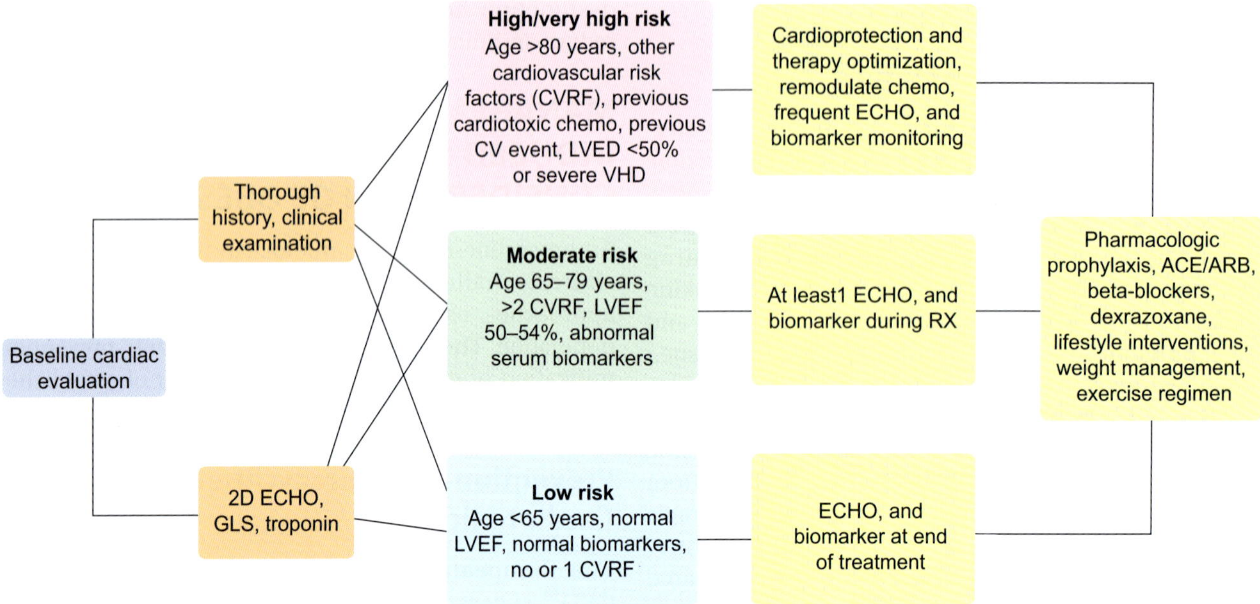

with additional assessments throughout the treatment for high-risk patients. The management algorithm for cardiotoxicity is given in **Flowchart 4**.

Early Detection and Risk Stratification

Baseline cardiovascular risk assessment is critical prior to anthracycline therapy. This involves clinical evaluation, imaging with echocardiographic parameters such as LVEF and global longitudinal strain (GLS), as well as biomarker measurements including high-sensitivity troponins and natriuretic peptides.[9,11] If the LVEF <53% and GLS is lower than normal and troponins are elevated, early cardiology consultation is advised.[12] Obesity may obscure clinical symptoms, highlighting the need for diligent imaging and biomarker surveillance to detect subclinical dysfunction.[9,11] Repeat echocardiography during treatment—every 3-6 months in high-risk patients—is advised.[9] High-risk patients are classified as patients with age >65 years, BMI >30 kg/m^2, obesity with cardiac abnormalities, preexisting cardiac disease, anthracycline dose >300 mg/m^2, elevated biomarkers, or those who have received prior chest radiation.[12]

Pharmacological Cardioprotection

Neurohormonal blockade using ACE inhibitors, angiotensin receptor blockers, and beta-blockers has shown mixed results in preventing anthracycline cardiotoxicity.[9,11] While some trials in low-to-moderate risk groups showed limited benefit, emerging evidence supports their use particularly in high-risk patients, including those with obesity or preexisting cardiovascular risk factors.[9,11] Specifically, carvedilol demonstrates antioxidant properties that may counteract mitochondrial damage, and nebivolol enhances endothelial function through nitric oxide pathways.[9] The approved cardioprotective agent dexrazoxane is recommended for patients receiving high cumulative anthracycline doses (>300 mg/m^2). It prevents DNA damage by inhibiting topoisomerase IIβ and chelates free iron to reduce oxidative injury, with demonstrated efficacy in reducing heart failure rates.[9,11] However, its use is currently limited by regulatory guidelines and concerns over potential interference with chemotherapy efficacy, which recent data refute.[9]

Lifestyle and Adjunctive Therapies

Weight management through diet and physical activity is foundational to reduce cardiometabolic stress and improve cardiac resilience against chemotherapy injury. Aerobic exercise programs improve cardiorespiratory fitness and potentially mitigate anthracycline cardiotoxicity, though larger randomized trials are ongoing.[9] Pharmacological agents such as statins exhibit anti-inflammatory and antioxidant effects and may offer cardioprotection, especially in patients with lymphoma receiving high cumulative doses of anthracyclines[9]. Sodium-glucose cotransporter 2 inhibitors (SGLT2i) and other novel metabolic modulators display promising preclinical data for cardioprotection.[9]

Advanced Therapeutic Interventions

For patients progressing to anthracycline-induced heart failure refractory to medical therapy, advanced therapies including implantable cardioverter-defibrillators, cardiac resynchronization therapy, left ventricular assist devices, and even heart transplantation represent viable options.[9] Despite the complexity added by cancer survivorship, outcomes with these therapies can approach those observed in nononcologic cardiomyopathy populations.[9]

Multidisciplinary and Patient-centered Care

Integration of cardio-oncology teams combining cardiology, oncology, pharmacology, nutrition, and rehabilitation expertise is essential to optimize outcomes. Patient education on lifestyle, medication adherence, and symptom awareness is imperative.[9,11] Emerging technologies such as artificial intelligence and machine learning hold promise to refine individualized risk prediction and management protocols.[9]

CONCLUSION

Despite advances in understanding the intersection between obesity and doxorubicin cardiotoxicity, several challenges inhibit optimal patient outcomes. Diagnostic tools for early cardiac injury often lack sensitivity or qualitative precision in obese populations due to altered biomarker kinetics and imaging limitations.[1,2] There remain gaps in predicting individual susceptibility based on genomic or metabolomic profiles, limiting tailored preventive strategies.[3]

Moreover, pharmacologic cardioprotective agents such as ACE inhibitors and beta-blockers, while beneficial, do not fully eliminate myocardial damage in at-risk obese patients, highlighting the need for novel therapeutic targets.[4,7] Investigational therapies aiming to modulate mitochondrial function, reduce oxidative stress more effectively, or counteract inflammation are promising but require rigorous clinical validation.[3]

Lifestyle changes, although foundational, can be challenging to implement and sustain in the cancer survivorship setting, necessitating integrated multidisciplinary programs that combine cardiology, oncology, nutrition, and behavioral psychology expertise.[3]

Future research priorities include:

- Developing sensitive and specific biomarkers for early detection in obese cancer patients
- Elucidating molecular mechanisms underpinning obesity's amplification of doxorubicin toxicity
- Clinical trials testing emerging cardioprotective agents in high-risk populations
- Designing comprehensive survivorship care models incorporating individualized metabolic and cardiac monitoring
- Leveraging machine learning to integrate clinical, imaging, and -omics data for precision cardio-oncology

Addressing these challenges promises to improve long-term cardiovascular health and quality of life for the growing population of obese cancer survivors receiving anthracyclines.

REFERENCES

1. Cardinale D, Lacopo F, Cipolla CM. Cardiotoxicity of anthracyclines. Front Cardiovasc Med. 2020;7:26.
2. Ferrera A, Fiorentini V, Reale S, et al. Anthracyclines-induced cardiac dysfunction: what every clinician should know? Rev Cardiovasc Med. 2023;24(5):148.
3. Armenian SH, Lacchetti C, Barac A, et al. Prevention and monitoring of cardiac dysfunction in survivors of adult cancers: ASCO Clinical Practice Guideline. J Clin Oncol. 2017;35(8):893-911.
4. Gilchrist SC, Barac A, Ades PA, et al. Cardio-oncology rehabilitation to manage cardiovascular outcomes in cancer patients and survivors: a scientific statement from the American Heart Association. Circulation. 2019;139(21):3997-e1012.
5. World Health Organization. (2025). Obesity and overweight. [online] Available from https://www.who.int/news-room/fact-sheets/detail/obesity-and-overweight. [Last accessed January, 2026].
6. Kenchaiah S, Evans JC, Levy D, et al. Obesity and the risk of heart failure. N Engl J Med. 2002;347(5):305-13.
7. Guenancia C, Lefebvre A, Cardinale D, et al. Obesity as a risk factor for anthracyclines and trastuzumab cardiotoxicity in breast cancer: a systematic review and meta-analysis. J Clin Oncol. 2016;34(26):3157-65.
8. Lennon H, Sperrin M, Badrick E, et al. The obesity paradox in cancer: a review. Curr Oncol Rep. 2016;18:56.
9. Camilli M, Cipolla CM, Dent S, et al. Anthracycline cardiotoxicity and management in adult cancer patients. JACC CardioOncol. 2024;6(5):655-77.
10. Lyon AR, López-Fernández T, Couch LS, et al. 2022 ESC guidelines on cardio-oncology developed in collaboration with the European Hematology Association (EHA), the European Society for Therapeutic Radiology and Oncology (ESTRO) and the International Cardio-oncology Society (IC-OS). Eur Heart J. 2022;43(41):4229-361.
11. Salvatorelli E, Menna P, Minotti G. Managing anthracycline-induced cardiotoxicity beginning with the end in mind. Future Cardiol. 2015;11(4):363-6.
12. Plana JC, Galderisi M, Barac A, et al. Expert consensus for multimodality imaging of adult patients during and after cancer therapy: a report from the American Society of Echocardiography and the European Association of Cardiovascular Imaging. Eur Heart J. 2014;15:1063-93.

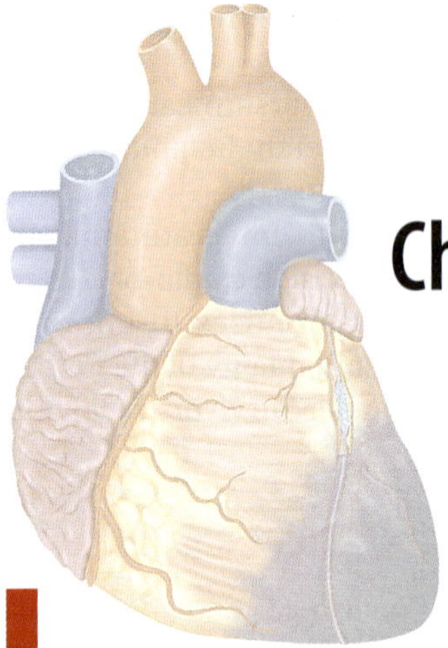

77

CHAPTER

Chemotherapy- and Radiotherapy-induced Cardiomyopathy in Obese Individuals: Management Strategies

Kanika Sood Sharma, Jhanja Mohapatra

INTRODUCTION

Chemotherapy and radiotherapy are an integral part of treatment of many cancers and significantly improve overall survival in those patients. But certain subgroup of chemotherapeutic agents and radiotherapy for thoracic malignancies, such as lung cancer, breast cancer, and lymphomas, also involves some inevitable cardiac complications leading to chemoradiation-induced cardiac diseases.[1] Chemoradiation-induced cardiac dysfunction comprises a spectrum of disease, including cardiomyopathy, pericarditis, coronary artery disease, valvular heart diseases, and conduction abnormalities. Risk of development of cardiac diseases is further increased in obese individuals. Obesity is independently associated with higher rates and greater severity of chemotherapy-induced cardiotoxicity, notably for anthracyclines and trastuzumab.[2] With the advancement of newer techniques of radiotherapy, intense monitoring, early interventions, dose modifications, and other preventive measures, chemoradiation-induced cardiac disease can be reduced.[3] Also, with screening recommendations and timely follow-up, it can be diagnosed early and managed accordingly.

DESCRIPTION

Radiotherapy has improved 5-year survival rate of 80% in Hodgkin's lymphoma and 90% in breast cancer patients.[4] However, radiotherapy also induces cardiac dysfunction as late toxicity in patients who have undergone mediastinal or breast radiotherapy. Patients who underwent chest radiotherapy have a 2% higher risk of cardiac morbidity and death at 5 years, and 23% increased absolute risk after 20 years.[5] Chemoradiation-induced cardiac diseases comprise a spectrum of heart disease, including pericarditis, cardiomyopathy, coronary artery disease, valvular heart disease, and cardiac conduction abnormality.[6] The incidence of each kind of heart disease varies greatly among breast cancer patients, ranging from 0.5 to 37%.[7] In lymphoma patients, the incidence of radiation-induced heart disease (RIHD) is higher than that of breast cancer patients, reaching 49.5–54.6%, and the incidence of various heart diseases ranges from 11 to 31%.[8]

Risk Factors for Development of Radiation-induced Heart Diseases[9]

- Anterior or left chest irradiation
- High cumulative dose of radiation (>30 Gy)
- Younger age (<50 years) at the time of radiation therapy
- High dose of radiation fractions (>2 Gy/day)
- Proximity of tumor to the heart
- Concomitant chemotherapy (e.g., anthracyclines)
- Cardiovascular risk factors such as smoking, diabetes, hypertension, obesity, and dyslipidemia
- Preexisting cardiovascular disease

Pathophysiology

Cardiomyopathy due to chemoradiation therapy is mainly due to myocardial fibrosis due to multiple complex pathways.[10] Radiation-induced oxidative stress and inflammation, endoplasmic reticulum, and mitochondrial damage are the main reasons for cardiac toxicity.[11] Many researchers also believe that miRNAs regulate the production of various cytokines, which in turn play an important role in the development of late cardiac injury related to radiation.[12] Chest radiotherapy may cause both systolic and diastolic dysfunction, and dilated as well as restrictive cardiomyopathy.[13] Higher dose of radiotherapy causes more systolic dysfunction in patients undergoing thoracic radiotherapy. Chemotherapy-induced cardiomyopathy (CIC) is a serious concern for obese individuals receiving cancer treatment. Obesity compounds risk due to increased systemic inflammation, altered pharmacokinetics, and a higher prevalence of metabolic comorbidities. The most implicated drugs include anthracyclines, HER2-targeted agents, alkylating agents, antimetabolites, taxanes, and tyrosine kinase inhibitors, each with unique mechanisms and risk profiles.[14-18]

Obesity is a proinflammatory state; adipose tissue secretes adipokines (e.g., leptin, adiponectin) and proinflammatory cytokines (TNF-α, IL-6) that can impair endothelial function and worsen oxidative stress. Obesity causes left ventricular (LV) hypertrophy, increased mass, and diastolic dysfunction, even in absence of overt cardiomyopathy, increasing the risk of cardiac diseases in postradiation therapy patients.[19] Also, obese patients have higher baseline cardiac output and volume load, which could stress myocardium **(Table 1)**.

Clinical presentation: Radiation-induced cardiomyopathy is mainly asymptomatic, so the diagnostic rate is as low as 10%.[20] Later, it may develop regional wall motion abnormality, mild LV hypertrophy, and diastolic dysfunction, which can present as severe congestive cardiac insufficiency (dyspnea, chest pain).[21]

Diagnosis: [Adapted from the European Association of Cardiovascular Imaging and the American Society of Echocardiography][9]

- *Echocardiography:* Cardiomyopathy is characterized by increased stiffness of the myocardium and a small LV with an increased left atrial (LA) size. This causes an early rapid rise in LV pressure during LV filling. Systolic function assessed by traditional echocardiographic techniques is usually normal.
- *Color Doppler:* Doppler measurements of the transmitral flow reveal a typical pattern consisting of a short mitral E deceleration duration and a low A wave velocity resulting in a high E/A ratio. The E0-wave by tissue Doppler imaging is usually decreased. The corresponding finding during invasive catheterization is the dip-plateau pattern of early diastolic pressure traces. A combined occurrence of constrictive pericarditis and restrictive cardiomyopathy may lead to a more difficult interpretation of the transmitral LV filling pattern.

  A constellation of findings, consisting of decreased mean LV mass, end-diastolic dimension, and end-diastolic wall thickness, together with self-reported dyspnea, is also suggestive of restrictive cardiomyopathy in this population.
- *Cardiac MRI:* Restrictive cardiomyopathy occurs because of diffuse myocardial fibrosis. T1 mapping can be used to quantify the concentration of gadolinium-based extracellular contrast agents in the myocardium and in the blood pool.
- *Cardiac CT scan:* Cardiac CT in the diagnosis of restrictive cardiomyopathy after radiotherapy has little value. Dilation of both atria in the presence of a small LV chamber in a patient with chest radiation therapy, symptoms of heart failure, and without any history of atrial fibrillation might raise the suspicion of restrictive cardiomyopathy. The disease must be confirmed or ruled out by echocardiography or cardiac magnetic resonance (CMR).
- *Nuclear scan:* There is no proven value of nuclear cardiology in the detection of restrictive cardiomyopathy after radiation exposure.

TABLE 1: Cardiotoxic chemotherapy drugs: Key agents and mechanisms.

Drug class	*Examples*	*Cardiac effects*	*Mechanism of cardiotoxicity*
Anthracyclines	Doxorubicin, daunorubicin, mitoxantrone	Irreversible heart failure, reduced LVEF	Free radical/ROS production, mitochondrial injury
HER2-targeted	Trastuzumab, lapatinib	Reversible LV dysfunction	Inhibition of neuregulin pathway in myocytes
Alkylating agents	Cyclophosphamide, ifosfamide	Acute myocarditis, HF	Endothelial injury, direct cytotoxicity
Antimetabolites	5-FU, capecitabine	Vasospasm, arrhythmias, rare HF	Coronary vasospasm/ischemia
Taxanes	Paclitaxel, docetaxel	Arrhythmias, heart block	Microtubule disruption altering conduction
VEGF/PDGF inhibitors	Bevacizumab, sunitinib, imatinib, dasatinib	Hypertension, HF, thrombosis	Vascular/endothelial dysfunction

- *Predictive biomarkers: Troponin, NT-proBNP,* and *galectin-3* help in early detection of subclinical myocardial injury.

MANAGEMENT STRATEGIES

Baseline cardiac assessment should be done in high-risk and obese patients before undergoing chemoradiation therapy. Patient should be counseled for risk of late cardiac toxicity, lifestyle modifications, and management of high-risk factors such as hypertension, dyslipidemia. CIC is more complex in obese individuals due to both increased baseline cardiac risk and altered drug pharmacokinetics. Each regimen requires individualized surveillance and intervention based on the patient's risk profile, with obese patients warranting enhanced vigilance and preventive strategies. Effective management involves multifactorial approaches with early identification, careful cardiac and metabolic assessment, judicious drug selection, and tailored interventions.[22-25]

Patient should be on regular follow-up and screening for cardiac functions for early detection and management of chemoradiation-induced cardiac diseases. Collaboration between oncologists, cardiologists, and nutritionists is required for tailored therapy and risk reduction.

Screening Recommendations [Adapted from the European Association of Cardiovascular Imaging and the American Society of Echocardiography][9]

- *Before chemoradiotherapy:* Baseline transthoracic echocardiography to detect cardiac anomalies
- *Annual follow-up:* Cardiovascular history and examination; transthoracic echocardiography if murmur detected; careful investigation of symptoms
- *5-year follow-up:* Transthoracic echocardiography for high-risk asymptomatic patients; noninvasive coronary artery disease assessment with stress echocardiography or stress CMR imaging; repeat transthoracic echocardiography at 5-year intervals
- *10-year follow-up:* Transthoracic echocardiography for asymptomatic nonhigh-risk patients; repeat transthoracic echocardiography every 5 years thereafter.

Drug Therapy

- *Statins:* In addition to lowering cholesterol, statins activate adenosine 5′-monophosphate-activated protein kinase (AMPK) to achieve anti-inflammatory effects. *Atorvastatin* can protect the heart by inhibiting inflammatory reactions and oxidative stress.[26]

TABLE 2: Summary of cardiotoxic chemotherapeutic agents and management.

Drug/class	*Prevention/management*
Anthracyclines	Dexrazoxane, ACEI, β-blocker
HER2 agents	Discontinue/rechallenge, monitor
Alkylators	Surveillance, supportive care
Antimetabolites	Antianginals, monitor
Taxanes	Monitor, antiarrhythmic therapy
VEGF/PDGF TKIs	BP control, anticoagulation

Lovastatin can inhibit the activation of transcription factor NF-κB and the expression of inflammatory cell adhesion molecules, thereby inhibiting the acute inflammatory response. It also inhibits the mRNA expression of fibrotropic factor CTGF, which is induced by radiation, thus preventing tissue fibrosis.[27] *Pravastatin* reduces the expression of transforming growth factor (TGF)-β_1, CTGF, RhoA, and cyclin D1, thereby reducing tissue fibrosis. *Pravastatin* could also protect against tissue damage caused by radiation by reducing DNA double-strand breakage in normal tissue cells.[28]

- *ACE inhibitors (ACEI):* ACEI drugs can reduce myocardial perivascular fibrosis and myocardial cell apoptosis through anti-inflammation and reducing oxygen-free radicals after radiation exposure of heart and lungs, thereby inhibiting myocardial fibrosis and decreasing cardiac diastolic function.[29] These also increase the production of nitric oxide to protect vascular cells by reducing the negative effects on the bradykinin system, and inhibit production of reactive oxygen species to reduce myocardial injury.[30]
- *Anti-inflammatory and antioxidant compounds:* Antioxidants such as *pentoxifylline, α-tocopherol, melatonin, amifostine, L-carnitine, caffeic acid phenethyl ester* (*CAPE*) have antioxidative stress and antiapoptotic properties, thereby reducing vasculitis and cardiac fibrosis.[31]
- Recombinant *human neuregulin-1* (*rhNRG-1*β) reduces myocardial damage and protects cardiac function.[32]

Heart transplant may be considered as a treatment option for end-stage heart failure in selected patients **(Table 2)**.

PREVENTION OF RADIATION-INDUCED CARDIAC DISEASE

Reducing the Radiation Dose

The risk of major cardiac disease increases linearly by ~7.4% per Gray increase in mean heart dose.[33]

Recommended Dose Constraints[34]

- Mean heart dose <5 Gy
- V25 (volume receiving ≥25 Gy) <10%
- LAD mean dose <10 Gy, and maximum point dose <20 Gy

Reducing the Radiation Field and Volume

Computed tomography-based planning with multiple static fields to shape the dose around the target volume and cardiac sparing by optimizing beam angles and applying customized blocks for heart reduces the risk of cardiac toxicity.

Dose-volume histogram (DVH) analysis must be routinely performed for the heart and substructures.

Documentation of heart and LAD doses is mandatory in all thoracic and breast cancer radiotherapy plans.

Adoption of the *QUANTEC* (Quantitative Analyses of Normal Tissue Effects in the Clinic) guidelines improves consistency in dose constraints.[35]

Reduction of radiation field from extended field, such as mantle field, to the involved node and involved site radiotherapy fields can decrease mean heart dose. A study in patients with early Hodgkin's lymphoma found a mean heart dose of 27.5 Gy with mantle field therapy compared with 7.7 Gy with involved-node therapy. This decrease in mean heart dose was associated with a reduction in the 25-year absolute excess cardiac risk from 9.1 to 1.4% and a reduction in cardiac mortality from 2.1 to 1%.[36]

Newer Technique for Radiation Planning and Delivery

Newer techniques such as IMRT and VMAT offer better dose conformity and reduce mean heart dose, thereby reducing risk of radiation-induced cardiomyopathy.

Deep inspiratory breath-hold (DIBH) technique: During deep inspiration, the heart moves posteriorly and inferiorly, increasing the distance between heart and chest wall, thus reducing exposure in left-sided breast irradiation.[37]

Respiratory gating and real-time tracking: Radiation is delivered only during specific respiratory phases, minimizing motion-induced cardiac exposure.

Image-guided radiotherapy (IGRT): Incorporates daily imaging (CBCT or kV imaging) to verify tumor position and cardiac proximity and enables adaptive planning if cardiac position shifts significantly over treatment course.[38]

Adaptive radiotherapy: Periodic replanning based on anatomical or physiological changes over the period of treatment (e.g., tumor shrinkage, weight loss). It helps in reduction of unintended cardiac dose escalation during long-treatment courses.

Proton beam therapy: Proton therapy deposits maximum dose at a finite depth with minimal exit dose (Bragg peak effect), thus sparing normal tissue beyond the target. It is particularly valuable in mediastinal tumors and left-sided breast cancer in young or high-risk patients.[39] Proton therapy reduces mean heart dose by 50–70% compared with photon-based techniques.

SUMMARY

As discussed earlier, obese patients undergoing chemoradiation therapy for thoracic tumors have higher risk of development of cardiomyopathy, but it can be minimized and well managed with the following measures:

Pretreatment measures: Assess cardiovascular risks, including obesity, optimize comorbidities, plan radiation and chemotherapy with cardioprotective measures, and counsel on weight control and lifestyle modification.

During treatment: Monitor cardiac functions with imaging and biomarkers, adjust therapy if early signs of toxicity develop, manage hypertension, diabetes, etc. aggressively, and implement exercise/diet modification.

Post-treatment measures: Long-term surveillance, especially in high-risk patients, early diagnosis and treatment of cardiomyopathy per guidelines, ongoing weight management, and multidisciplinary follow-up

CONCLUSION

Obesity significantly increases the risk of chemotherapy- and radiotherapy-induced cardiomyopathy. Early detection, prevention through both oncologic and cardiovascular means, and prompt management are required to reduce morbidity and improve both cardiac and cancer-related outcomes. As cancer survivorship is increasing day by day with newer techniques of radiotherapy, integrating modern cancer therapy with obesity management may be beneficial in reducing as well as managing chemoradiation-induced cardiomyopathy.

REFERENCES

1. Vejpongsa P, Yeh ET. Prevention of anthracycline-induced cardiotoxicity: challenges and opportunities. J Am Coll Cardiol. 2014;64(9):938-45.
2. Yeh ET, Tong AT, Lenihan DJ, et al. Cardiovascular complications of cancer therapy: diagnosis, pathogenesis, and management. Circulation. 2004;109(25):3122-31.

3. Lee Chuy K, Groarke JD, Avila M, et al. Association of body mass index and cardiotoxicity related to anthracyclines and trastuzumab. Breast Cancer Res Treat. 2019;179(2):307-15.
4. Jemal A, Siegel R, Ward E, et al. Cancer statistics, 2009. CA Cancer J Clin. 2009;59(4):225-49.
5. Galper SL, Yu JB, Mauch PM, et al. Clinically significant cardiac disease in patients with Hodgkin lymphoma treated with mediastinal irradiation. Blood. 2011;117(2):412-8.
6. Donnellan E, Phelan D, McCarthy CP, et al. Radiation-induced heart disease: a practical guide to diagnosis and management. Cleve Clin J Med. 2016;83(12):914-22.
7. Hooning MJ, Botma A, Aleman BM, et al. Long-term risk of cardiovascular disease in 10-year survivors of breast cancer. J Natl Cancer Inst. 2007;99(5):365-75.
8. Van Nimwegen FA, Schaapveld M, Janus CP, et al. Cardiovascular disease after Hodgkin lymphoma treatment: 40-year disease risk. JAMA Intern Med. 2015;175(6):1007-17.
9. Lancellotti P, Nkomo VT, Badano LP, et al.; European Society of Cardiology Working Groups on Nuclear Cardiology and Cardiac Computed Tomography and Cardiovascular Magnetic Resonance, American Society of Nuclear Cardiology, Society for Cardiovascular Magnetic Resonance, Society of Cardiovascular Computed Tomography. Expert consensus for multi-modality imaging evaluation of cardiovascular complications of radiotherapy in adults: a report from the European Association of Cardiovascular Imaging and the American Society of Echocardiography. Eur Heart J Cardiovasc Imaging. 2013;14(8):721-40.
10. Tapio S. Pathology and biology of radiation-induced cardiac disease. J Radiat Res. 2016;57(5):439-48.
11. Slezak J, Kura B, Babal P, et al. Potential markers and metabolic processes involved in the mechanism of radiation-induced heart injury. Can J Physiol Pharmacol. 2017;95(10):1190-203.
12. Kura B, Babal P, Slezak J. Implication of microRNAs in the development and potential treatment of radiation-induced heart disease. Can J Physiol Pharmacol. 2017;95(10):1236-44.
13. Heidenreich PA, Hancock SL, Vagelos RH, et al. Diastolic dysfunction after mediastinal irradiation. Am Heart J. 2005;150(5):977-82.
14. Barish R, Lynce F, Unger K, et al. Trastuzumab-induced cardiomyopathy: incidence and risk factors in a large multicenter cohort. J Cancer Res Clin Oncol. 2019;145(5):1435-43.
15. Volkova M, Russell R 3rd. Anthracycline cardiotoxicity: prevalence, pathogenesis and treatment. Curr Cardiol Rev. 2011;7(4):214-20.
16. Zamorano JL, Lancellotti P, Rodriguez Muñoz D, et al. 2016 ESC position paper on cancer treatments and cardiovascular toxicity developed under the auspices of the ESC Committee for Practice Guidelines. Eur Heart J. 2016;37(36):2768-801.
17. Ewer MS, Ewer SM. Cardiotoxicity of anticancer treatments: what the cardiologist needs to know. Nat Rev Cardiol. 2010;7(10):564-75.
18. Moslehi JJ. Cardiovascular toxicity of targeted cancer therapies. N Engl J Med. 2016;375(15):1457-67.
19. Tavora F, Zhang Y, Zhang M, et al. Cardiomegaly is a common arrhythmogenic substrate in adult sudden cardiac deaths and is associated with obesity. Pathology. 2012;44(3):187-91.
20. Chang HM, Moudgil R, Scarabelli T, et al. Cardiovascular complications of cancer therapy: best practices in diagnosis, prevention, and management: part 1. J Am Coll Cardiol. 2017;70(20):2536-51.
21. Filopei J, Frishman W. Radiation-induced heart disease. Cardiol Rev. 2012;20(4):184-8.
22. Rahman AM, Yusuf SW, Ewer MS, et al. Chemotherapy-related cardiomyopathy: pathogenesis, diagnosis and management. J Natl Cancer Inst. 2012;104(17):1287-96.
23. Goetz MP, Reeves JH, Jain S, et al. Appropriate systemic therapy dosing for obese adult patients with cancer. J Clin Oncol. 2012;20:4836-49.
24. de Boer RA, van der Meer P, van Veldhuisen DJ. Mechanisms and biomarkers to detect chemotherapy-induced cardiomyopathy. Clin Cancer Investig J. 2017;6(5):207-13.
25. Wang X, Wang X, Zhang S, et al. Cardiac toxicity of cancer therapies: mechanisms, surveillance and clinical implications. Int J Cardiovasc Acad. 2025;2(1):12-18.
26. Mahmoudi M, Gorenne I, Mercer J, et al. Statins use a novel Nijmegen breakage syndrome-1-dependent pathway to accelerate DNA repair in vascular smooth muscle cells. Circ Res. 2008;103(7):717-25.
27. Ostrau C, Hülsenbeck J, Herzog M, et al. Lovastatin attenuates ionizing radiation-induced normal tissue damage in vivo. Radiother Oncol. 2009;92(3):492-9.
28. Matsumoto S, Odawara S, Shikata T, et al. Pravastatin reduces radiation-induced damage in normal tissues. Exp Ther Med. 2017;13(5):1765-72.
29. Ghosh SN, Zhang R, Fish BL, et al. Renin-Angiotensin system suppression mitigates experimental radiation pneumonitis. Int J Radiat Oncol Biol Phys. 2009;75(5):1528-36.
30. Bertrand ME, Ferrari R, Remme WJ. Provision of cardiovascular protection by ACE inhibitors: a review of recent trials. Curr Med Res Opin. 2004;20(10):1559-69.
31. Gürses İ, Özeren M, Serin M, et al. Histopathological evaluation of melatonin as a protective agent in heart injury induced by radiation in a rat model. Pathol Res Pract. 2014;210(12):863-71.
32. Hu Y, Xia W, Hou M. Macrophage migration inhibitory factor serves a pivotal role in the regulation of radiation-induced cardiac senescence through rebalancing the microRNA-34a/sirtuin 1 signaling pathway. Int J Mol Med. 2018;42(5):2849-58.
33. Schneider U, Ernst M, Hartmann M. The dose-response relationship for cardiovascular disease is not necessarily linear. Radiat Oncol. 2017;12(1):74.

34. Darby SC, Ewertz M, McGale P, et al. Risk of ischemic heart disease in women after radiotherapy for breast cancer. N Engl J Med. 2013;368(11):987-98.
35. Gagliardi G, Constine LS, Moiseenko V, et al. Radiation dose-volume effects in the heart. Int J Radiat Oncol Biol Phys. 2010;76(3):S77-85.
36. Maraldo MV, Brodin NP, Vogelius IR, et al. Risk of developing cardiovascular disease after involved node radiotherapy versus mantle field for Hodgkin lymphoma. Int J Radiat Oncol Biol Phys. 2012;83(4):1232-7.
37. Aznar MC, Corradini S, Mast M, et al. ESTRO-ACROP guideline: recommendations on implementation of breath-hold techniques in radiotherapy. Radiother Oncol. 2023;185:109734.
38. Lemanski C, Thariat J, Ampil FL, et al. Image-guided radiotherapy for cardiac sparing in patients with left-sided breast cancer. Front Oncol. 2014;4:257.
39. Nangia S, Burela N, Noufal MP, et al. Proton therapy for reducing heart and cardiac substructure doses in Indian breast cancer patients. Radiat Oncol J. 2023;41(2):69.

78

CHAPTER

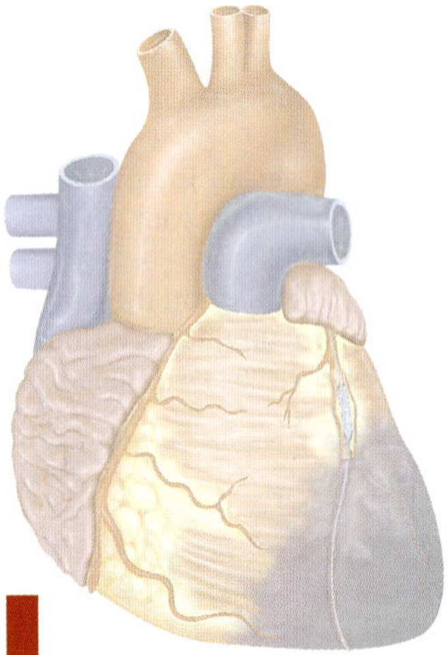

Obesity and Thyroid Carcinoma (Medullary Thyroid Carcinoma and Differentiated Thyroid Carcinoma)

Akriti Rastogi, Bhawani Pathak

INTRODUCTION

Images related to MTC are given in **Figure 1**.

Obesity has *no clearly established association* with the development of medullary thyroid carcinoma.[1-3] While obesity significantly increases the risk of papillary thyroid carcinoma (PTC), no such correlation exists for MTC, largely due to differences in cellular origin. MTC arises from *parafollicular (C) cells*, which are not regulated by obesity-associated pathways such as hyperinsulinemia, IGF-1, leptin signaling, and adipokine-driven inflammation.[4-9]

In hereditary MTC (MEN2A/2B), *germline RET mutations fully determine tumorigenesis,* with no metabolic influence.

PATHOPHYSIOLOGY AND C-CELL BIOLOGY

C-cells express *low levels of leptin receptors* and demonstrate *minimal responsiveness* to IGF-1, insulin, or inflammatory cytokines.[10,11] Unlike follicular cells, C-cells do not proliferate in response to TSH or adipokine-mediated pathways. Thus, the *mechanistic basis for an obesity-MTC link is weak,* consistent with epidemiologic findings.

DIAGNOSTIC CHALLENGES INTRODUCED BY OBESITY

Ultrasonography in Obesity

Obesity substantially *reduces ultrasound sensitivity* for detecting small thyroid lesions and central compartment lymph nodes.[12,13] Neck adiposity impairs visualization of Level VI/VII and deep lateral nodal basins.

For MTC patients, where preoperative nodal mapping is essential, CT or MRI is frequently required.

Biochemical Markers

Serum *calcitonin and CEA* remain reliable regardless of BMI. Calcitonin doubling time is *not affected by obesity.*[14]

SURGICAL IMPLICATIONS IN OBESITY

Airway and Anesthetic Concerns

Obesity increases:

- Difficult mask ventilation
- Difficult intubation (large neck circumference)
- Higher OSA prevalence
- Need for postoperative airway monitoring[15,16]

Central Compartment Dissection

Obesity leads to:

- Thickened pretracheal fat obscuring RLN
- Difficulty identifying parathyroids
- Longer operative times
- Increased blood loss
- Higher wound complication rates[15,16]

Given that MTC requires *routine central ± lateral lymphadenectomy*, obesity complicates operative exposure but does not contraindicate adequate dissection in experienced hands.

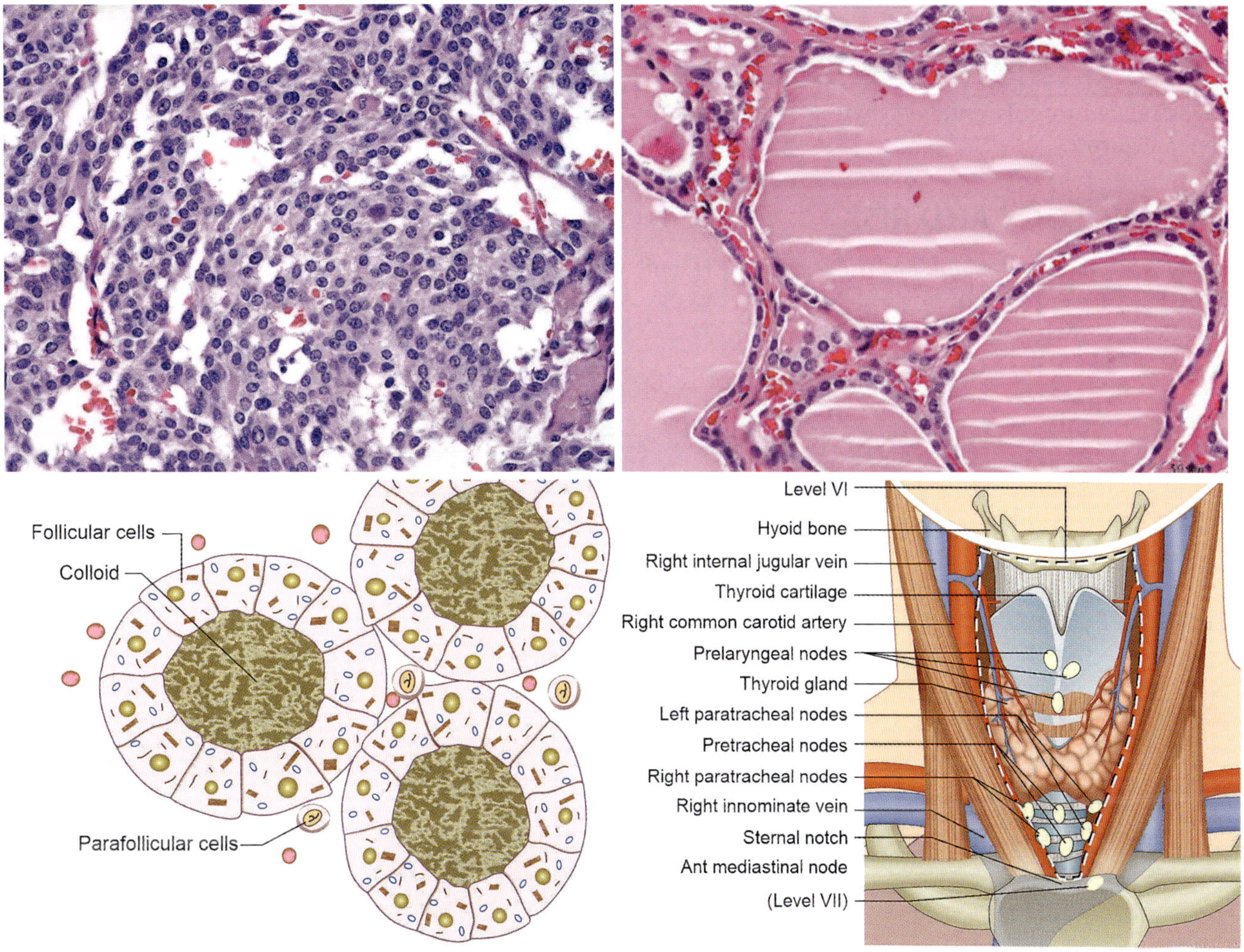

Fig. 1: Overview images related to MTC (histology, C-cells, central compartment dissection, and limitations of ultrasound in obesity).

SYSTEMIC THERAPY CONSIDERATIONS

RET inhibitors (selpercatinib, pralsetinib) improve outcomes, but obesity influences their toxicity profiles:[17,18]

- *Hypertension* worsened by obesity
- *Hepatic steatosis* increases risk of TKI hepatotoxicity
- *QT prolongation* more likely in metabolic syndrome

Obese MTC patients require enhanced cardiovascular and hepatic monitoring.

OBESITY MANAGEMENT IN MTC

Lifestyle Therapy

High-protein, moderate-calorie diets are preferred, especially in patients with metastasis or TKI-associated anorexia/diarrhea.

Pharmacotherapy

Contraindicated:

- GLP-1 agonists (semaglutide, liraglutide, tirzepatide) due to FDA black-box warnings for C-cell tumors.[19-21]

Permitted:

- Orlistat
- Phentermine–topiramate
- Bupropion–naltrexone
- Metformin

Bariatric Surgery

Suitable after biochemical stability.

Sleeve gastrectomy preferred over bypass due to predictable drug absorption and fewer diarrheal issues.[22]

DIFFERENTIATED THYROID CARCINOMA

Images related to differentiated thyroid carcinoma are given in **Figure 2**.

EPIDEMIOLOGY AND RISK

Obesity is a *strong, well-established risk factor* for PTC and likely FTC.[4-6] Risk rises with:

- BMI
- Central (visceral) adiposity
- Insulin resistance
- Metabolic syndrome

PHYSIOLOGICAL EFFECTS

Metabolic–Hormonal Effects

- *Hyperinsulinemia* activates IGF-1 pathways → follicular-cell proliferation.[8]

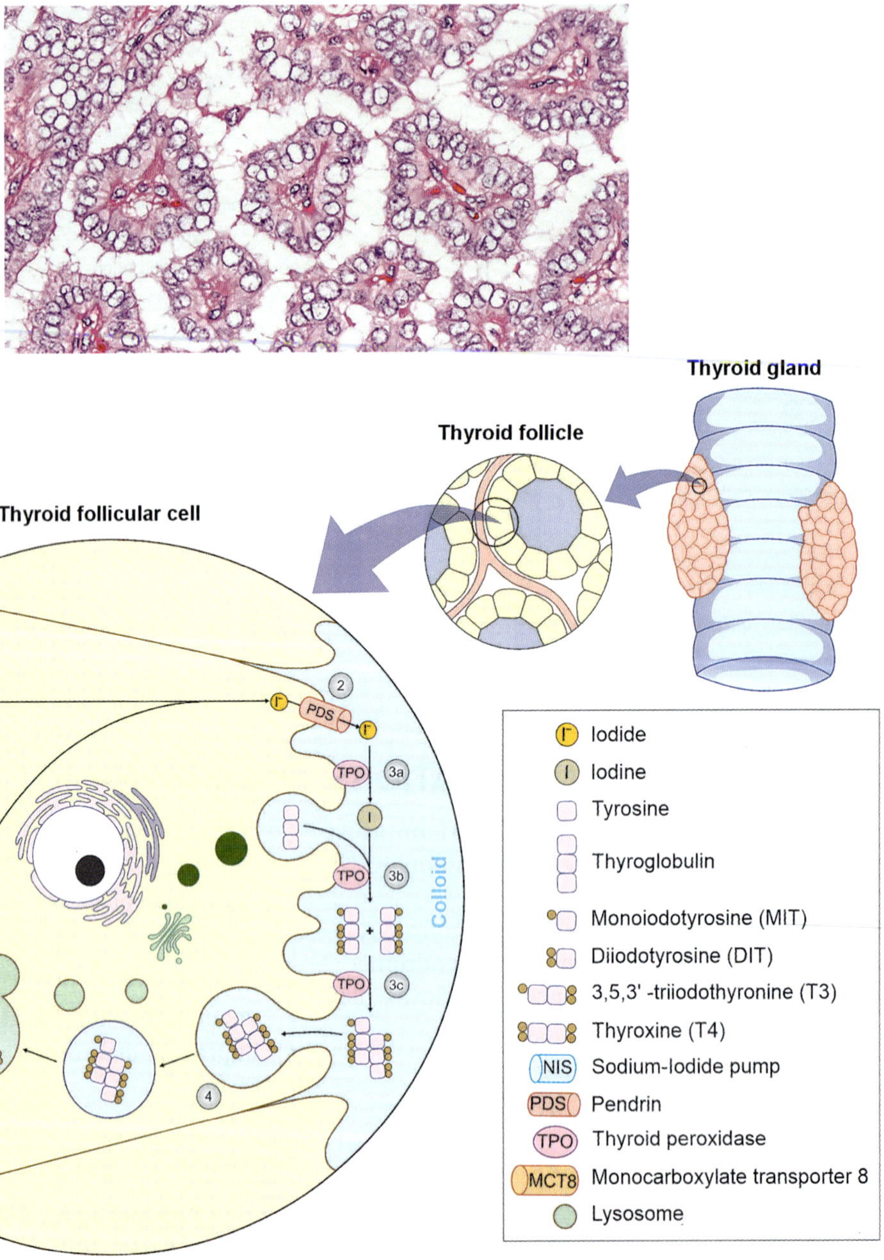

Fig. 2: Differentiated thyroid carcinoma.

- *Leptin elevation* stimulates PI3K/Akt and MAPK pathways → tumor growth.[7]
- *Increased estrogen* from adipose aromatase enhances mitogenic signaling.

Chronic Inflammation

Obese adipose tissue secretes TNF-α, IL-6, and MCP-1 → increases oxidative stress and DNA damage.[9]

Thyroid Axis Alterations

Subtle TSH elevations frequently occur in obesity, promoting *follicular epithelial hyperplasia.*

TUMOR PRESENTATION AND DISEASE BIOLOGY IN OBESITY

Obese patients more frequently present with:
- Larger tumors
- Multifocal disease
- Extrathyroidal extension
- Higher nodal metastases[23,24]
- More aggressive tumor phenotypes (selected cohorts)

These features contribute to higher recurrence risk.[25,26]

DIAGNOSTIC CONSIDERATIONS

Ultrasound sensitivity is reduced in obese patients:[12,13]
- Difficulty detecting small nodules
- Poor visualization of central nodes
- Lower accuracy in postoperative surveillance

FNAC adequacy decreases in deep nodules, requiring adjunct CT/MRI.

SURGICAL CONSIDERATIONS

Obesity increases:
- Flap thickness and exposure difficulty
- Operative duration
- Blood loss
- Hematoma and wound infection rates
- RLN neuropraxia risk
- Airway challenges[27,28]

Despite this, surgical *extent is unchanged* and follows oncologic guidelines **(Fig. 3)**.

RADIOACTIVE IODINE THERAPY

Obesity modifies RAI kinetics:
- Larger distribution volume
- Lower radiation dose per gram
- Altered clearance[29,30]

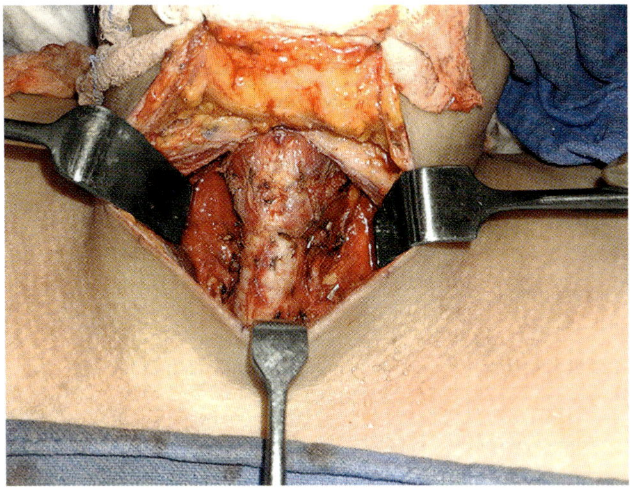

Fig. 3: Surgery image.

Individualized dosimetry may be beneficial in selected obese patients.

TSH SUPPRESSION THERAPY

Aggressive suppression increases risks of:
- Atrial fibrillation
- Hypertension
- Coronary artery disease[31,32]

High-risk DTC requires strong suppression; low/intermediate-risk disease should receive *moderate suppression* to avoid cardiovascular morbidity.

OBESITY TREATMENT IN DTC

GLP-1 Receptor Agonists (Safe)

GLP-1 agonists *are safe in DTC* and show no association with PTC/FTC incidence.[33,34]

Other Agents

All antiobesity medications (orlistat, phentermine-topiramate, bupropion-naltrexone, metformin) are safe.

Levothyroxine Dose Adjustment

Weight loss decreases levothyroxine requirements. TSH monitoring every *6–8 weeks* is recommended.

BARIATRIC SURGERY

Suitable after:
- Completion of RAI (if required)
- Stable TSH suppression
- No evidence of persistent/recurrent disease[35]

TABLE 1: Comparison of obesity's impact: MTC vs. DTC.

Feature	*MTC*	*DTC*
Obesity as risk factor	No association	Strong association
Cell origin	C-cells	Follicular cells
Obesity → tumor biology	Minimal	Strong (IGF-1, leptin, TSH)
Ultrasound accuracy	↓	↓↓
Calcitonin/Tg impact	Calcitonin unaffected	Tg unaffected
Surgery difficulty	↑	↑↑
RAI considerations	Not used	Altered kinetics
GLP-1 agonists	Contraindicated	Safe
Bariatric surgery	Allowed (sleeve preferred)	Allowed (sleeve preferred)

Sleeve gastrectomy is preferred for predictable LT4 absorption.[25,36]

PROGNOSIS

Obese DTC patients show:

- Higher recurrence[26]
- More aggressive tumor features[37]
- Reduced surveillance sensitivity

Despite this, overall survival remains high due to excellent DTC biology.

Comparison of obesity impact between MTC and DTC is given in **Table 1**.

CONCLUSION

Management of Obesity in MTC Patients

Assess MTC status → Calcitonin, CEA, imaging, *exclude advanced disease with diarrhea/cachexia, lifestyle therapy* → high-protein diet, *avoid GLP-1 agonists, use alternative pharmacotherapy (if needed), consider sleeve gastrectomy only after biochemical stability.*

Management of Obesity in DTC Patients

Confirm DTC status → Tg, imaging, establish TSH suppression target, start lifestyle therapy, *GLP-1 agonists permitted,* adjust LT4 dose during weight loss, bariatric surgery (sleeve) if indicated, Continue long-term surveillance

REFERENCES

1. Kitahara CM, Platz EA, Freeman LE, et al. Body fatness and risk of thyroid cancer in the NIH-AARP cohort. Int J Cancer. 2012;131(11):E1004-14.
2. Schmid D, Ricci C, Behrens G, et al. Associations of overweight and obesity with thyroid cancer risk by histology: a meta-analysis. Obes Rev. 2015;16(12):1042-54.
3. Durante C, Costante G, Lucisano G, et al. The natural history of benign thyroid nodules. JAMA. 2015;313(9): 926-35. (Includes BMI-MTC epidemiologic data from large Italian cohorts.)
4. Kitahara CM, Pfeiffer RM, Sosa JA, et al. Impact of obesity on papillary thyroid cancer incidence trends. Cancer Epidemiol Biomarkers Prev. 2020;29(6):1307-15.
5. Schmid D, Behrens G, Jochem C, et al. Physical activity, diabetes, and thyroid cancer risk: a systematic review. Eur J Epidemiol. 2013;28(6):403-13.
6. Yeh MW, Bauer AJ, Bernet VA, et al. The epidemiology of thyroid carcinoma. Endocrinol Metab Clin North Am. 2019;48(1):1-23.
7. Arihara Z, Takano T, Tagami T, et al. Leptin augments proliferation of papillary thyroid carcinoma cells via PI3K/Akt. J Clin Endocrinol Metab. 2001;86(12):5982-5.
8. Rezzonico J, Rezzonico M, Pusiol E, et al. Insulin resistance is a key factor in rising rates of thyroid cancer. Endocr Relat Cancer. 2008;15(4):1063-71.
9. Alyusuf RH. Obesity, inflammation, and thyroid cancer. Cytokine. 2020;125:154814.
10. Kameda M, Ito M, Nishimura K. Leptin and endocrine regulation: implications for thyroid cancer. J Endocrinol. 2012;214(1):1-3.
11. Melvin A. C-cell physiology and calcitonin regulation. Endocr Rev. (classic reference; year varies by edition).
12. Moon HJ, Kwak JY, Kim MJ, et al. Ultrasound limitations in obese individuals: thyroid interpretation study. AJR Am J Roentgenol. 2010;195(4):e89-94.
13. Kim ES, Kim TY, Lee HS, et al. Impact of BMI on thyroid ultrasound diagnostic performance. Thyroid. 2013;23(5):585-91.
14. Barbet J, Campion L, Kraeber-Bodéré F, et al. Prognostic value of calcitonin and calcitonin doubling-time in medullary thyroid carcinoma. J Clin Endocrinol Metab. 2005;90(11):6077-84.
15. Sanders G, Royle GT. The impact of obesity on thyroid surgery. Surgery. 2014;155(1):43-50.
16. Kim J, Park S, Jeong JS, et al. Influence of body mass index on surgical outcomes in thyroidectomy. Ann Surg Oncol. 2016;23(2):403-10.
17. Wirth LJ, Sherman E, Robinson B, et al. Selpercatinib in RET-altered thyroid cancer. N Engl J Med. 2020;383(9): 825-35.
18. Subbiah V, Hu MI, Wirth LJ, et al. Pralsetinib for RET-mutant and RET-fusion thyroid cancers. Lancet Diabetes Endocrinol. 2021;9(8):491-501.
19. Roman SA. Medullary thyroid cancer: management and outcomes. Ann Surg Oncol. 2006;13(9):1171-9.

20. Food and Drug Administration (FDA). Liraglutide/semaglutide drug safety communication regarding thyroid C-cell tumors. Silver Spring (MD): FDA; 2011.
21. Marso SP, Daniels GH, Brown-Frandsen K, et al. Liraglutide and cardiovascular outcomes in type 2 diabetes. N Engl J Med. 2016;375(4):311-22.
22. Mechanick JI, Apovian C, Brethauer S, et al. Clinical practice guidelines for the perioperative nutrition, metabolic, and nonsurgical support of bariatric surgery patients—2020 update. Surg Obes Relat Dis. 2020;16(2):175-247.
23. Makay Ö, Icoz G, Yilmaz M, et al. The effect of obesity on thyroid carcinoma aggressiveness. Ann Surg Oncol. 2013;20(7):2286-92.
24. Pappa T, Alevizaki M. Obesity as a prognostic factor in thyroid cancer. Thyroid. 2015;25(2):145-6.
25. Mechanick JI, Youdim A, Jones DB, et al. Guidelines for bariatric surgery nutritional management. Surg Obes Relat Dis. 2020;16(2):175-247.
26. Park S, Lee YM, Lee YH, et al. Body mass index and recurrence risk in papillary thyroid carcinoma. Thyroid. 2018;28(4):439-46.
27. Carter YM, Mazeh H, Sippel RS, et al. Influence of BMI on thyroidectomy outcomes. Surgery. 2014;156(5):1142-6.
28. Sosa JA, Bowman HM, Tielsch JM, et al. Surgeon volume and outcomes in thyroidectomy. Ann Surg. 1998;228(3):320-30.
29. Thomas D. Biodistribution of radioactive iodine differs by body weight. Eur J Nucl Med Mol Imaging. 2013;40(5):799-807.
30. Verburg FA. Body mass influences effective half-life of I-131. Thyroid. 2014;24(4):621-7.
31. Biondi B, Cooper DS. Benefits and risks of thyroid hormone suppression therapy. J Clin Endocrinol Metab. 2010;95(1):186-93.
32. Tuttle RM, Haugen BR, Perrier ND. 2015 ATA Guidelines for management of thyroid nodules and DTC. Thyroid. 2015;25(1):1-133.
33. Davies MJ, Bergenstal RM, Bode BW, et al. Efficacy and safety of semaglutide for weight management. Diabetes Care. 2015;38(12):2241-9.
34. Azoulay L, Filion KB, Platt RW, et al. Incretin drugs and thyroid cancer: population-based cohort. BMJ. 2016;352:i581.
35. Sjöström L. Long-term outcomes after bariatric surgery. N Engl J Med. 2013;369(14):1307-14.
36. Snyder ML. Levothyroxine malabsorption following Roux-en-Y gastric bypass. Obes Surg. 2016;26(3):538-42.
37. Trésallet C, Seman M, Tissier F, et al. Obesity correlates with aggressive behavior in PTC. Surgery. 2014;156(5):1144-52.

SECTION 21

Obesity and Therapeutics

79

CHAPTER

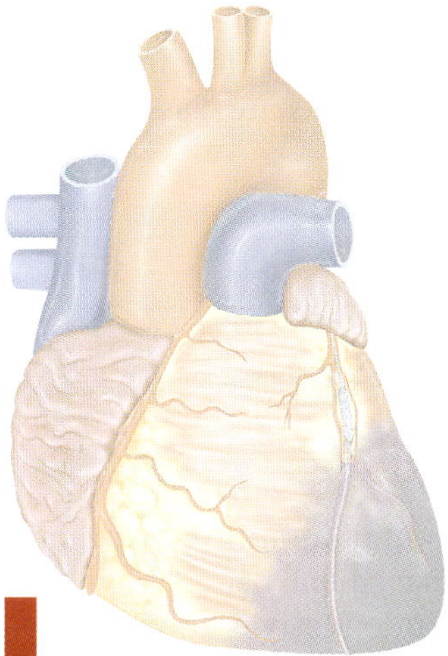

Advances in Obesity and Lipid Management in Cardiovascular Disease

Manotosh Panja, Prakas Chandra Mondal

INTRODUCTION

Traditionally, central abdominal obesity was acknowledged as one of the modifiable minor risk factors and OBESITY PARADOX[1] was once thought to be protective after acute myocardial infarction, heart failure especially with preserved ejection fraction. Prevalence of obesity has increased dramatically over the last few decades and is linked to reduced life expectancy.[2]

In 2021, European Commission acknowledged obesity as a definite pathological entity with a chronic, relapsing, and noncommunicable disease state.[3,4]

CONTROL OF ENERGY MILIEU SYSTEM AND ITS REGULATORS

Human internal milieu regulates the amount of adipose tissue over time by balancing caloric consumption and food intake to maintain energy reserve through multiple systems: The homeostatic system, referred to as the metabolic brain, the hedonic system, referred to as the "emotional brain" and the cognitive system.[4]

The primary homeostatic energy system allows the bidirectional communication between the brain, mainly the hypothalamus and the peripheral organs through neuronal, hormonal, or food-derived chemical signals. These neural circuits can be orexigenic which stimulate hunger or anorexigenic which lead to satiety.[4] Leptin, a protein produced primarily by adipose tissue, is a key circulating mediator of neural circuits. Serum leptin levels are positively associated with fat mass.

Leptin levels increase after meals suppressing the feeling of hunger and promote satiety and decrease during fasting.[5]

Following food intake, chemicals with satiety-promoting effects are released by the duodenum, small intestine, and pancreas. In contrast, during fasting, the hunger-stimulating gastrointestinal hormone, ghrelin, is released from the stomach and activates the orexigenic pathway.

The hedonic system in the mesocorticolimbic area governs the reward control system through the neurotransmitters serotonin and dopamine. These reward-related brain regions respond to visual cues of desirable foods and reinforce cravings independent of hunger. Increased serotonergic signaling typically results in reduced food intake and weight loss, while an increased dopaminergic signaling is associated with food overconsumption and weight gain.

The cognitive system situated in the prefrontal cortex modulates voluntary control including social and impulse control which influence food choices and eating frequency.[6]

DISRUPTION OF HOMEOSTASIS CAUSING OBESITY

In general, obesity occurs when a genetically predisposed individual is exposed to an obesogenic environment. Obesity is influenced by variety of factors including genetic and epigenetic, metabolic, vascular, behavioral, or pharmacological factors. Genetic mutations affecting key proteins in energy homeostasis and genes can predispose individuals to develop obesity.[7] Mutations leading to alteration in leptin structure or leptin receptor (LEPR), leading to the inability of leptin to bind to its receptor and contributing to obesity.

Genetics cannot completely explain the significant global surge of obesity in the last few decades. Environmental and behavioral factors such as nutrition and lifestyle may have positive influences on gene expression without affecting DNA sequence, a phenomenon known as epigenetics.[7] Some clinical conditions or pharmacological agents such as some beta-blockers (metoprolol) and some antidiabetic agents (insulin or sulfonylurea) may trigger excess adipose tissue accumulation.[8]

An excess in visceral adipose tissue triggers a pathological process mediated by an increased cytokine secretion, variations in immune system activity, fat hypertrophy, increased fibrosis, and alterations in vascular function and structures. Obesity is clinically associated with cardiovascular diseases (CVDs), type 2 diabetes mellitus, atrial fibrillation, heart failure, particularly with preserved ejection fraction, metabolic dysfunction associated with steatotic liver disease and related chronic liver disease, polycystic ovary disease (PCOD) in females, and low serum testosterone with erectile dysfunction in males. These conditions are called sick fat disease or adiposopathy by the Obesity Medicine Association.

Fat mass disease includes the biomechanical complications of obesity such as obstructive sleep apnea and joint stress and damage.

RECENT STATUS OF DIAGNOSING OBESITY

Body measurements such as body mass index (BMI), waist circumference (WC), and waist-hip ratio (WHR) with their gender and ethnic adjustments are good correlates of obesity. These parameters are insufficient in obesity evaluation because of inability to distinguish body composition, the location of adipose tissue, and impact of excess adiposity.

Body composition analyzing technologies such as bioelectrical impedance analysis (BIA), dual-energy X-ray absorptiometry (DEXA), and air displacement plethysmography can improve obesity characterization. CT and MRI are considered the gold standard, but DEXA is also accurate in obesity characterization.

EDMONTON OBESITY STAGING SYSTEM[9]

The Edmonton Obesity Staging System (EOSS) is a frequently used classification tool to evaluate the presence of weight-related risk factors or comorbidities, physical symptoms, psychological symptoms, and functional limitations.[9] Based on EOSS, patients are classified into "five" stages, as follows:

- *Stage 0:* No risk factor
- *Stage 1:* Subclinical risk factors
- *Stage 2:* Established disease
- *Stage 3:* Severe disease
- *Stage 4:* End-stage disease

Management of Obesity

Obesity is multifactorial, and a multidisciplinary approach is needed for management. Three modalities of obesity management include lifestyle interventions, pharmacotherapy to reduce body weight and combat associated metabolic risk, and metabolic bariatric interventions and surgeries.

The foundation of obesity management is lifestyle intervention, even when pharmacological therapy or surgery is indicated. A structured meal plan with an aim to limit caloric intake can be evidence-based Mediterranean diet or a ketogenic diet, like very low-calorie ketogenic (VLCK) diet, may be implemented based on preferences and need. Increased physical activity aiming for >150 minutes per week of moderate exercise divided into "three" to "five" sessions per week. Patients should be encouraged to self-monitor weight, food intake, and physical activities.

For drug treatment, a decision is needed whether to treat obesity first or concomitant treatment of comorbidities is also needed.[10] The Obesity Management Association has suggested treating obesity first in those without any acute adiposopathic metabolic consequences of obesity (i.e., severely elevated blood glucose, blood pressure, CVD, thrombosis, or cancer) to avoid risk of hypoglycemia or hypotension during initiation of anti-obesity measures. A potential exception should be dyslipidemia with elevated LDL cholesterol, where statins can be initiated if the ASCVD risk is high.

Several pharmacologic therapies have been approved for long-term management of obesity. Pharmacologic agents with incretin mimetic effects such as liraglutide (3 mg), semaglutide (2.4 mg), and tirzepetide (5, 10, and 15 mg) have demonstrated significant weight reduction in clinical trials.

In STEP program, semaglutide 2.4 mg resulted in greater body weight loss targets than lifestyle intervention alone in patients with BMI >27 kg/m^2 with at least one weight-related complication or BMI >30 kg/m^2 with or without weight related complication.[11]

Recently FDA has approved tirzepatide, a novel, first-in-class, glucose-dependent insulinotropic polypeptide

(GIP), and glucagon-like peptide-1 (GLP-1) receptor agonist. In the SURMOUNT-1 trial, tirzepetide was associated with a decrease in body weight of 15, 19.5, and 20.9% at a dose of 5, 10, and 15 mg, respectively.[12]

Setmelanotide has also been approved for the treatment of obesity and hunger due to genetic disorders such as Bardet–Biedl syndrome, proopiomelanocortin (POMC) loss of function, including proprotein convertase subtilisin/kexin-type-1 (PCSK1), and LEPR deficiency.[13]

Metabolic bariatric surgery can be a highly effective treatment including improvements of metabolic and mechanical complications of obesity with improved quality of life.[14]

OBESITY MANAGEMENT: AN INTEGRAL COMPONENT OF ADVANCED CARDIOMETABOLIC CARE

Improvement in CVD risk factors and adverse CV events is an integral outcome of body weight reduction. The LOOK AHEAD Trial highlighted the role of lifestyle intervention.[15] In the SELECT double-blind trial against placebo, semaglutide led to a 20% reduction in death from cardiovascular causes, nonfatal MI or nonfatal stroke, and an 8.15% reduction in body weight. The STEP HFpEF study demonstrated that semaglutide improved Kansas City Cardiomyopathy Questionnaire clinical summary score (KCCQ-CSS) by 7.8 points, increased 6-minute walk distance by 20.3 m, and reduced body weight by 10.7%, compared to placebo.[16]

CONCLUSION

New horizons in the management of adiposity and CV risk should see the emergence of combination of therapies including pharmacotherapy, surgery, and lifestyle interventions delivered either face-to-face or via electronic media. Comprehensive structured programs would be beneficial involving expertise from multidisciplinary team including psychologists, dietitians, general/family physicians, cardiologists, obesity medicine specialists, and bariatric surgeons.

REFERENCES

1. Curtis JP, Selter JG, Wang Y, et al. The obesity paradox: body mass index and outcomes in patients with heart failure. Arch Intern Med. 2005;165(1):55-61.
2. Bucholz EM, Beckman AL, Krumholz HA, et al. Excess weight and life expectancy after acute myocardial infarction: the obesity paradox reexamined. Am Heart J. 2016;172:173-81.
3. Burki T. European Commission classifies obesity as a chronic disease. Lancet Diabetes Endocrinol. 2021;9(7): 418.
4. Lazarus E, Ortiz-Pujols S. Increasing clinical awareness of obesity as a serious, chronic, relapsing, and treatable disease. Am J Manag Care. 2022;28(15):S271-8.
5. Gjermeni E, Kirstein AS, Kolbig F, et al. Obesity—an update on the basic pathophysiology and review of recent therapeutic advances. Biomolecules. 2021;11(10):1426.
6. Majeed M, Majeed S, Nagabhushanam K, et al. Lesse investigated natural ingredients for the management of obesity. Nutrients. 2021;13(2):510.
7. Mahmoud AM. An overview of epigenetics in obesity: the role of lifestyle and therapeutic interventions. Int J Mol Sci. 2022;23(3):1341.
8. Lopez-Jimenez F, Almahmeed W, Bays H, et al. Obesity and cardiovascular disease: mechanistic insights of management strategies. A joint position paper by the World Heart Federation and World Obesity Federation. Eur J Prev Cardiol. 2022;29(17):2218-37.
9. Busetto L, Dicker D, Fruhbeck G, et al. A new framework for the diagnosis, staging and management of obesity in adults. Nat Med. 2024;30(9):2395-9.
10. Bays HE, Bindlish S, Clayton TL. Obesity diabetes mellitus, and cardiometabolic risk: an Obesity Medicine Association (OMA) Clinical Practice Statement (CPS) 2023. Obes Pillars. 2023;5:100056.
11. Wilding JPH, Batterham RL, Calanna S, et al. Once weekly semaglutide in adults with overweight or obesity. N Engl J Med. 2021;384(11):989-1002.
12. Jastreboff AM, Aronne LJ, Ahmed NN, et al. Tirzepatide once weekly for the treatment of obesity. N Engl J Med. 2022;387(3):205-16.
13. European Medicines Agency. (2024) Imcivree: setmelanotide. [online] Available from http://ema.europa.eu/en/medicines/human/EPAR/imcivree. [Last accessed January, 2026].
14. Eisenberg D, Shikora SA, Aarts E, et al. 2022 American Society for Metabolic and Bariatric Surgery (ASMBS) and International Federation for the Surgery of Obesity and Metabolic Disorders (IFSO): indications for metabolic and bariatric surgery. Surg Obes Relat Dis. 2022; 18(12):1345-56.
15. Look AHEAD Research Group, Wing RR, Bolin P, et al. Cardiovascular effects of intensive lifestyle intervention in type 2 diabetes. N Engl J Med. 2013;369(2):145-54.
16. Lincoff AM, Brown-Frandsen K, Colhoun HM, et al. Semaglutide and cardiovascular outcomes in obesity without diabetes. N Engl J Med. 2023;389(24):2221-32.

80

CHAPTER

Top 10 Take-home Messages from the ACC/AHA and HESA/HFSA on Empagliflozin in HFpEF with Obesity (Including EMPEROR-Preserved)

Tarun Kumar, Ashima Gosai

INTRODUCTION

Obesity is a major and independent risk factor for developing *heart failure with preserved ejection fraction (HFpEF)*, and obesity-related HFpEF is recognized as a distinct clinical phenotype of the disease.[1,2] The excess fat causes unique pathological changes that complicate diagnosis and require specific treatment strategies.[1]

PATHOPHYSIOLOGY

Obesity contributes to HFpEF through multiple interconnected mechanisms **(Fig. 1)**:[1]

- *Systemic inflammation:* Excess visceral and epicardial fat are metabolically active and release proinflammatory cytokines, which lead to chronic and low-grade systemic inflammation.[1] This inflammation causes microvascular damage and fibrosis (stiffening) in the heart muscle and blood vessels, impairing the heart's ability to relax and fill properly.[1]
- *Hemodynamic changes:* Increased body mass requires a higher cardiac output and expanded total blood volume.[1,2] A stiffened heart cannot accommodate this extra volume, leading to elevated left ventricular (LV) filling pressures and congestion.[1] The mechanical restraint from increased epicardial fat also contributes to these elevated pressures.[1]
- *Neurohormonal activation:* Obesity triggers the activation of the sympathetic nervous system and the renin-angiotensin-aldosterone system, promoting sodium retention, high blood pressure, and further cardiac remodeling.[1]
- *Metabolic alterations:* Insulin resistance and abnormal fatty acid metabolism in obese individuals can lead to the accumulation of fat within heart muscle cells (cardiac lipotoxicity), further impairing heart function.[1]

Heart failure with preserved ejection fraction is a heterogeneous syndrome in which obesity is a frequent and prognostically important comorbidity. Sodium-glucose cotransporter-2 inhibitors (SGLT2i)—notably empagliflozin—have emerged as the first pharmacologic therapy to demonstrate a consistent reduction in composite heart failure (HF) events in HFpEF in large randomized trials, most importantly the EMPEROR-Preserved trial.[3] Recent guideline documents from ACC/AHA (with input from HF societies) have incorporated SGLT2i into management pathways for HFpEF, usually with cautious class/level recommendations reflecting the evolving evidence base.[4]

Top 10 Take-home Messages

Below are the top 10 practical messages combining the EMPEROR-Preserved evidence, guideline guidance (ACC/AHA and HF society documents), and obesity-specific data.

1. Empagliflozin reduces the primary composite of CV death or HF hospitalization in HFpEF.
   EMPEROR-Preserved (empagliflozin 10 mg daily) showed a statistically significant reduction (~21%) in time to CV death or HF hospitalization versus placebo in patients with LVEF >40%. Benefit was seen in patients with and without diabetes.[3,5]

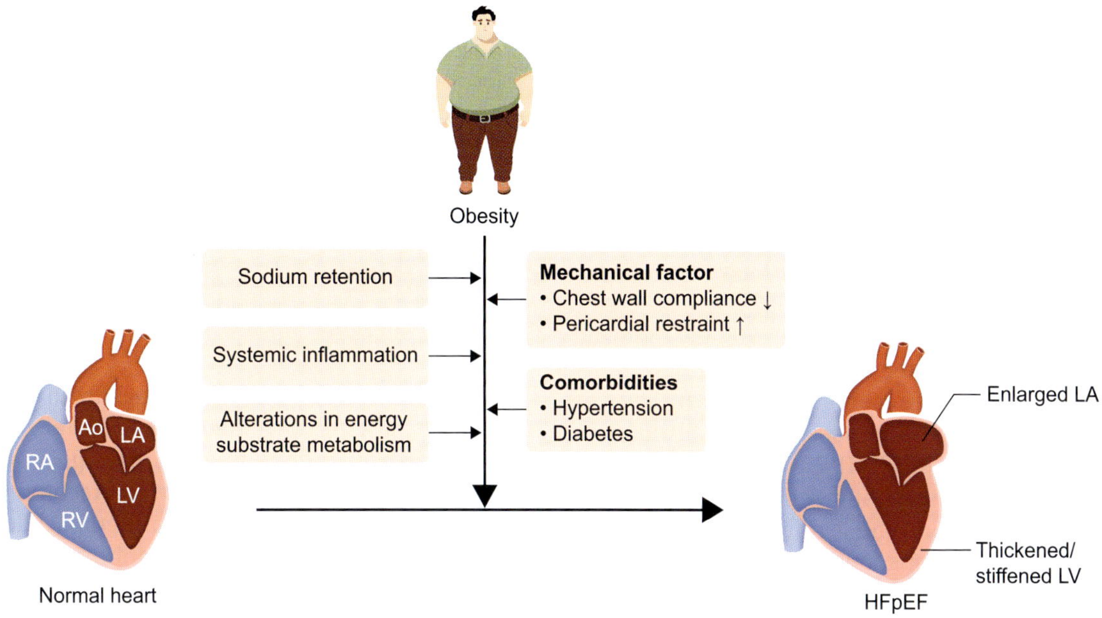

Fig. 1: Pathophysiological links between obesity and heart failure with preserved ejection fraction (HFpEF).

2. Benefit extends across BMI categories—obesity does not negate effect.
   Prespecified and post-hoc analyses indicate that empagliflozin lowers HF events and improves outcomes across BMI strata; treated patients who were overweight/obese also experienced greater absolute weight loss versus placebo, but the event-reduction effect was preserved across BMI ranges. Thus, obesity is not a contraindication and may bring metabolic advantages.[6,7]
3. Dosing and practical initiation: 10 mg once daily.
   EMPEROR-preserved used empagliflozin 10 mg once daily; this is the commonly recommended HF dose for trials in HFpEF and HFrEF unless specific local labeling differs. Check renal function and volume status prior to initiation.[3]
4. Safety profile in HFpEF is acceptable—monitor renal function, BP, and genital infections.
   Empagliflozin showed good tolerability; expect modest initial eGFR dip, small BP lowering, and a known small increase in genital mycotic infections. Serious events were not increased in EMPEROR-Preserved compared with placebo. Monitor electrolytes and renal function, especially when combined with diuretics.[6,8]
5. Empagliflozin's diuretic-like effects do not mandate stopping background diuretics but may reduce diuretic needs.
   Analyses found empagliflozin-reduced HF events independent of background diuretic use and in some patients allowed diuretic dose reduction; carefully monitor for symptomatic hypotension or volume depletion when starting or uptitrating other diuretics.[8]
6. Empagliflozin benefits are independent of diabetes status—treat HFpEF patients regardless of glycemia if they meet HF criteria.
   The EMPEROR-preserved trial included patients with and without type 2 diabetes; primary benefits were seen irrespective of diabetes. Guidelines therefore recommend consideration of SGLT2i for HFpEF independent of diabetes.[4,9]
7. Empagliflozin preserves renal function slope in HFpEF.
   One of EMPEROR-Preserved's secondary findings was slower decline in eGFR with empagliflozin versus placebo—an important organ-protective effect, especially relevant in obese patients who often have CKD risk.[9,10]
8. Combine SGLT2i with guideline-directed therapies but individualize in obesity phenotype.
   ACC/AHA guidance places SGLT2i as a recommended therapy for HFpEF (class IIa/IIb depending on EF band and evidence updates). In obese HFpEF patients, consider multidisciplinary care including weight-management strategies (lifestyle, antiobesity pharmacotherapy where indicated) alongside empagliflozin to target symptoms and cardiometabolic risk.[4]

9. Expect modest weight loss and symptomatic benefit but do not use empagliflozin as a primary weight-loss agent.
   Empagliflozin produces small but consistent weight loss; however, trials of GLP-1 receptor agonists (GLP-1RA) (e.g., semaglutide) show larger weight and symptomatic HFpEF improvements in obese patients. Empagliflozin should be seen as HF therapy with metabolic benefits, not a primary antiobesity drug.[7]
10. Limitations exist—heterogeneity in HFpEF and need for individualized care.
    Heart failure with preserved ejection fraction is heterogeneous (age, sex, obesity, atrial fibrillation, and renal disease). EMPEROR-preserved was positive overall but subgroup signals require cautious interpretation; combine evidence with clinical judgment for obese patients with HFpEF. Ongoing trials and meta-analyses further refine indications.[4,10]

See **Flowchart 1** for Initiation and monitoring of empagliflozin in HFpEF.

LIMITATIONS

- *Heterogeneity of HFpEF:* EMPEROR-Preserved enrolled a broad HFpEF population (EF >40%); effect size varies by EF bands and phenotypes. Post-hoc subgroup analyses are hypothesis-generating.[3]
- *Obesity-specific data limited:* While analyses show consistent benefit across BMI ranges and modest weight loss, trials were not designed specifically for obesity-targeted HFpEF care; trials of targeted weight-loss agents (e.g., semaglutide) show potentially larger effects on symptoms.[6]
- *Long-term outcomes/real-world adoption:* Longer follow-up and registry data will better define safety in diverse populations.

Flowchart 1: Initiation and monitoring of empagliflozin in HFpEF.

Patient with suspected HFpEF (symptoms ± signs) → Confirm HF with EF ≥40–50% + objective evidence (NT-proBNP, echo, structural markers

↓

Assess contraindications (type 1 diabetes, pregnancy, active genitourinary infection, and hypersensitivity)

↓

Check laboratories: eGFR, electrolytes, BP, and volume status

↓

If suitable → start empagliflozin 10 mg once daily

↓

Follow-up 1–2 weeks: Check BP, symptoms, renal function; adjust diuretics if volume depletion

↓

Long term: Monitor eGFR periodically, counsel re: genital hygiene, assess weight, symptoms, and HF events

Source: Based on EMPEROR-preserved and ACC/AHA guidance.[4,9]

GUIDELINES

Guideline synoptic points (ACC/AHA + HF society synthesis):

- Use SGLT2i (empagliflozin/dapagliflozin) in suitable HFpEF patients to reduce HF hospitalization and combined CV endpoints—ACC/AHA gives a class IIa (or IIb depending on EF and update) recommendation for SGLT2i in HFpEF. Start at 10 mg empagliflozin daily after baseline laboratories.[4] Monitor renal function and volume.

Summary algorithm:

1. Confirm HFpEF diagnosis (EF and natriuretic peptides/imaging)
2. Screen for contraindications
3. Baseline laboratories (eGFR, electrolytes, and glucose if diabetic), BP, and volume status.
4. Start empagliflozin 10 mg daily
5. Early follow-up for volume status and renal laboratories; adjust diuretics as needed
6. Combine with obesity management as appropriate (diet, exercise, and consider GLP-1RA if indicated).[3,10]

CONCLUSION

Empagliflozin represents a meaningful advance in the care of HFpEF—including patients with obesity—reducing the risk of HF hospitalization and the composite of cardiovascular death or HF hospitalization in EMPEROR-preserved. Benefits are observed regardless of diabetes status and across BMI categories, with modest associated weight loss and renal preservation. Current ACC/AHA/HF Society guidance incorporates SGLT2 inhibitors into HFpEF management pathways; clinicians should individualize decisions, monitor safety (renal function and volume status), and combine pharmacotherapy with obesity-targeted strategies where indicated.[3,4,6]

REFERENCES

1. Jung MH, Shin MS. Obesity-related heart failure with preserved ejection fraction: diagnostic and therapeutic challenges. Korean J Intern Med. 2023;38(2):157-66.

2. Li C, Qin D, Hu J, et al. Inflamed adipose tissue: A culprit underlying obesity and heart failure with preserved ejection fraction. Front Immunol. 2022;13:947147.
3. Anker SD, Butler J, Filippatos Get al. Empagliflozin in heart failure with a preserved ejection fraction. N Engl J Med. 2021;385(16):1451-61.
4. Heidenreich PA, Bozkurt B, Aguilar D, et al. 2022 AHA/ACC/HFSA Guideline for the Management of Heart Failure: A Report of the American College of Cardiology/American Heart Association Joint Committee on Clinical Practice Guidelines. Circulation. 2022;145(18):e895-e1032. Erratum in: Circulation. 2022;145(18):e1033. Erratum in: Circulation. 2022;146(13):e185. Erratum in: Circulation. 2023;147(14):e674.
5. Bhatt DL, Verma S, Pitt B. EMPEROR-preserved: A promise fulfilled. Cell Metab. 2021;33(11):2099-103.
6. Nicholls S, Hansen JE, Vlahopoulos J, et al. Impact of baseline body mass index on key primary outcome in the EMPEROR-preserved trial. Heart Lung Circ. 2022;31: S85-S86.
7. Sattar N, Butler J, Lee MMY, et al. Body mass index and cardiorenal outcomes in the EMPEROR-preserved trial: Principal findings and meta-analysis with the DELIVER trial. Eur J Heart Fail. 2024;26(4):900-9.
8. Butler J, Usman MS, Filippatos G, et al. Safety and efficacy of empagliflozin and diuretic use in patients with heart failure and preserved ejection fraction: A post-hoc analysis of the EMPEROR-preserved trial. JAMA Cardiol. 2023;8(7):640-9.
9. Solomon SD, McMurray JJV, Claggett B, et al. Dapagliflozin in heart failure with mildly reduced or preserved ejection fraction. N Engl J Med. 2022;387(12): 1089-98.
10. Kosiborod MN, Verma S, Borlaug BA, et al.; STEP-HFpEF Trial Committees and Investigators. Effects of semaglutide on symptoms, function, and quality of life in patients with heart failure with preserved ejection fraction and obesity: a prespecified analysis of the STEP-HFpEF trial. Circulation. 2024;149(3):204-16.

81

CHAPTER

Impact of Empagliflozin on Metabolic Syndrome Components in Heart Failure

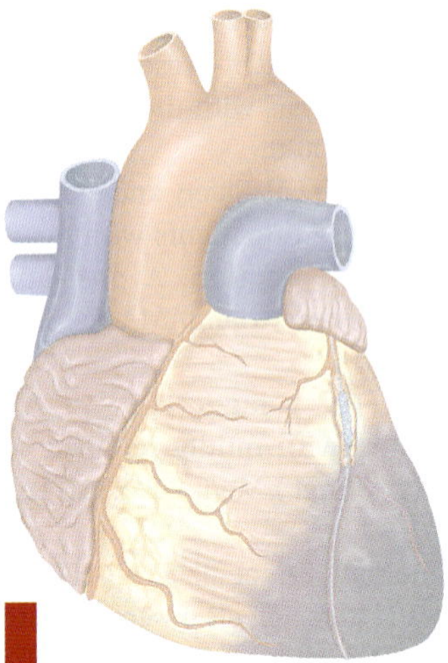

Rahul Mehrotra, Mayank Butola

INTRODUCTION

Metabolic syndrome is a cluster of interrelated metabolic risk factors that promote the development of atherosclerotic cardiovascular disease (ASCVD). It includes diabetes, abdominal obesity, atherogenic dyslipidemia, and hypertension. According to the International Diabetes Federation (IDF) worldwide consensus,[1] about 20–25% of the world's adult population have metabolic syndrome and are thrice as likely to develop and twice as likely to die from ASCVD or stroke, when compared to the people without the syndrome. People with metabolic syndrome also have a fivefold greater risk of developing type 2 diabetes mellitus (T2DM).[2] Pooled estimates suggest that one-third of the Indian population suffers from metabolic syndrome. In India, prevalence of metabolic syndrome is 13% for the age group of 18–29 years and rises steeply to 50% in the 50–59 years age group.

Overall, both men and women are equally affected, but men seem to be affected more in younger age groups, while women are mostly affected in the postmenopausal period. In the Indian population, women have a higher prevalence than men.[3] The cardiovascular complications of diabetes, which is also a leading cause of blindness, amputation and kidney failure, account for much of the social and financial burden of the disease.[4]

With the metabolic syndrome driving the twin global epidemics of type 2 diabetes and CVD, there is an overwhelming moral, medical, and economic imperative to identify those individuals with metabolic syndrome early, so that lifestyle interventions and treatment may prevent the development of diabetes and/or cardiovascular disease.

Empagliflozin is a sodium-glucose cotransporter-2 (SGLT-2) inhibitor that was initially approved by the FDA for the management of diabetes in 2014. It acts by inhibiting the SGLT-2 found in proximal renal tubules, thus reducing absorption of glucose and increasing urinary excretion of glucose **(Fig. 1)**. It also reduces sodium and volume load, causing intravascular contraction through its diuretic and natriuretic properties attributing to its role in reducing cardiovascular mortality in heart failure and renal protection.[5] Further studies reveal that empagliflozin also assists weight loss and loss of visceral adipose tissue as a consequence of increased glucagon secretion, which in turn stimulates fatty acid oxidation.[6] Beyond its direct renal and cardiovascular effects, empagliflozin also provides systemic metabolic benefits. Its anti-inflammatory and antifibrotic properties, influenced by alterations in arachidonic acid and n-3 PUFA metabolism, contribute to overall metabolic health. Thus, it addresses multiple avenues associated with the pathogenesis of metabolic syndrome. These combined effects establish empagliflozin as an important therapeutic agent for enhancing metabolic health in patients suffering from metabolic syndrome.

PATHOGENESIS

The pathogenesis of metabolic syndrome and each of its components is complex and not well understood; however, central obesity and insulin resistance are acknowledged as the most important causative factors.

Central obesity can be easily established by measuring waist circumference; however, if BMI is >30 kg/m^2, central obesity can be assumed, and waist circumference does not

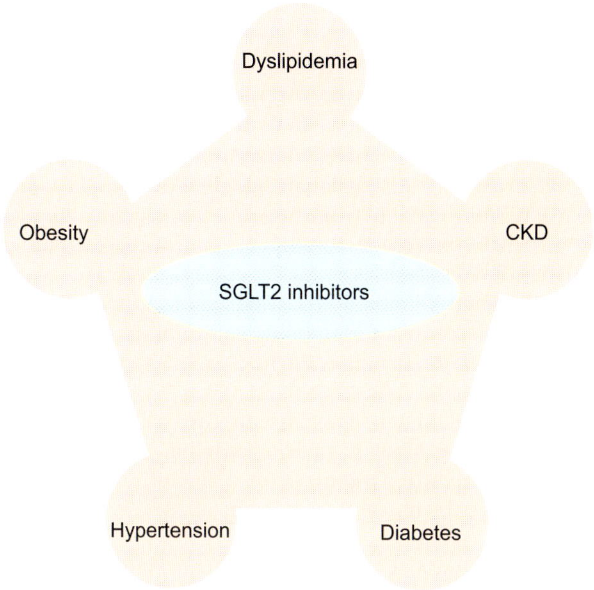

Fig. 1: Role of sodium-glucose cotransporter-2 (SGLT2) inhibitors in managing key components of metabolic syndrome and cardiovascular risk factors, including obesity, dyslipidemia, chronic kidney disease (CKD), hypertension, and diabetes.

need to be measured. Obesity contributes to hypertension, high serum cholesterol, low HDL-C, and hyperglycemia, and is independently associated with higher CVD risk.

Insulin resistance occurs when cells in the body (liver, skeletal muscle, and adipose/fat tissue) become less sensitive and eventually resistant to insulin, the hormone which is produced by the beta cells in the pancreas to facilitate glucose absorption. Glucose can no longer be absorbed by the cells but remains in the blood, triggering the need for more and more insulin (hyperinsulinemia) to be produced in an attempt to process the glucose. The production of ever-increasing amounts of insulin weakens and may eventually wear out the beta cells. Once the pancreas is no longer able to produce enough insulin, then a person becomes hyperglycemic and is then diagnosed with diabetes mellitus. Insulin resistance is difficult to measure in day-to-day clinical practice and is thus not an essential requirement but can be measured by assessing fasting insulin/proinsulin levels, HOMA-IR levels wherever possible.

Atherogenic dyslipidemia describes the combination of raised triglycerides (TG) and low concentrations of HDL-C together with elevated apolipoprotein B (ApoB), small dense LDL, and small HDL particles, all of which are independently atherogenic.[7] The adipose tissue of obesity exhibits abnormalities in the production of several adipokines that may separately affect insulin resistance and/or modify risk for ASCVD. These include increased production of inflammatory cytokines,[8] plasminogen activator inhibitor-1,[9] and other bioactive products;[10,11] at the same time the potentially protective adipokine, adiponectin, is reduced.[12] All of these changes have been implicated as causes of the metabolic risk factors.

Other associated conditions can be physical inactivity,[13] aging,[14] prothrombotic states,[15] and hormonal imbalance.[16] An atherogenic diet (e.g., a diet rich in saturated fat and cholesterol) can enhance risk for developing cardiovascular disease in people with the syndrome, although this diet is not listed specifically as an underlying risk factor for the condition.[17]

WORLDWIDE DEFINITION FOR USE IN CLINICAL PRACTICE

The IDF definition[1] for metabolic syndrome states that for a person to be defined as having the metabolic syndrome, they must have central obesity plus any *two* of the following *four* risk factors:

1. *Raised TG*: TG ≥150 mg/dL or specific treatment for this lipid abnormality
2. *Reduce HDL cholesterol*: HDL <40 mg/ dL in males, and <50 mg/dL in females or specific treatment for this lipid abnormality
3. *Raised blood pressure (BP)*: Systolic BP ≥130 mm Hg or diastolic BP ≥85 mm Hg or treatment of previously diagnosed hypertension
4. *Raised fasting plasma glucose (FPG)*: FPG ≥100 mg/dL or previously diagnosed T2DM

EMPAGLIFLOZIN AS A CORNERSTONE THERAPY IN MANAGEMENT OF METABOLIC SYNDROME

Experts regard empagliflozin as a game changer due to its extensive benefits across multiple health conditions. Initially prescribed by diabetologists, its role has expanded as cardiologists and nephrologists recognize its cardiovascular and renal protection advantages. The shift from a glucose-focused approach to a broader cardiorenal-metabolic profile was emphasized. Most experts agreed that the key reasons for initiating therapy include glycemic control, cardiovascular, and renal protection, and weight loss, all of which constitute important pathways to the development of metabolic syndrome.

Empagliflozin is commonly initiated at a 10 mg once-daily dose for the treatment of T2DM. If additional glycemic control is needed and well tolerated, the dosage may be increased to 25 mg once daily.[18] Research from trials such as EMPA-REG OUTCOME and EMPA-Kidney has demonstrated that the standard 10 mg dose effectively supports cardiovascular and renal health.[19,20] It is now a key pillar in the management of heart failure across all ejection fraction spectrums and is a class 1A recommendation as evidenced by the ESC heart failure guidelines.[21]

How empagliflozin helps with metabolic syndrome?

- *Improved glycemic control and insulin sensitivity*: Increased urinary glucose excretion, lowers plasma glucose and HbA1c levels, reducing glucotoxicity, and improving overall insulin sensitivity in peripheral tissues
- *Weight and adipose tissue reduction*: The excretion of excess glucose represents a loss of calories (240–400 kcal/day), which leads to modest but clinically significant weight loss. The caloric loss leads to significant body weight reduction, primarily through loss of fat mass, including visceral adipose tissue.
- *Blood pressure lowering*: The osmotic diuresis and natriuresis (sodium excretion) effects reduce sodium and volume load, which consistently lowers both systolic and diastolic BP, normalizing circadian BP rhythms in hypertensive models.
- *Favorable lipid profile changes*: Empagliflozin has been shown to increase HDL-cholesterol and potentially decrease TG, though effects on LDL can be variable.
- *Cardiorenal protection*: Beyond metabolic effects, it reduces intraglomerular pressure, has anti-inflammatory, and antioxidative stress properties, and enhances mitochondrial function in cardiomyocytes, which are central to its established cardiovascular benefits.

LIMITATIONS

Research data for the role of empagliflozin in management of metabolic syndrome currently remains limited to animal models, while only one post-hoc analysis of patients from EMPA-REG OUTCOME trial aimed to assess role of empagliflozin in patients with metabolic syndrome. Thus although results seem promising adjudicating a positive role of empagliflozin in the management of metabolic syndrome, data remains lacking.

CONCLUSION

Empagliflozin's ability to address the multifactorial nature of metabolic syndrome—targeting hyperglycemia, hypertension, obesity, and dyslipidemia simultaneously, while providing robust cardiorenal protection—positions it as an ideal candidate for a cornerstone therapy. The drug has not yet been approved by the FDA for the management of metabolic syndrome, but ongoing clinical trials continue to gather more data on nondiabetic populations. The official therapeutic role of empagliflozin is likely to expand, moving it closer to becoming an established foundational treatment for this complex condition.

REFERENCES

1. International Diabetes Federation. Clinical Guidelines Task Force. (2012). Global Guideline or Type 2 Diabetes. [online] Available from https://idf.org/media/uploads/2023/05/attachments-49.pdf [Last accessed January, 2026].
2. Obeidat AA, Ahmad MN, Ghabashi MA, et al. Developmental Trends of Metabolic Syndrome in the Past Two Decades: A Narrative Review. J Clin Med. 2025;14(7):2402.
3. Bhalwar R. Metabolic syndrome: The Indian public health perspective. Med J Armed Forces India. 2020;76(1):8-16.
4. World Health Organization. Prevention of diabetes mellitus. Technical Report Series no. 844. WHO: Geneva; 1994.
5. Heise T, Jordan J, Wanner C, et al. Acute Pharmacodynamic Effects of Empagliflozin With and Without Diuretic Agents in Patients With Type 2 Diabetes Mellitus. Clin Ther. 2016;38(10):2248-64.e5.
6. Ozcelik S, Celik M, Vural A, et al. The effect of low and high dose empagliflozin on HbA1c and lipid profile in type 2 diabetes mellitus: a real-world data. North Clin Istanb. 2020;7(2):167-73.
7. Brunzell JD, Ayyobi AF. Dyslipidemia in the metabolic syndrome and type 2 diabetes mellitus. Am J Med. 2003;115 Suppl 8A:24S-28S.
8. You T, Yang R, Lyles MF, et al. Abdominal adipose tissue cytokine gene expression: relationship to obesity and metabolic risk factors. Am J Physiol Endocrinol Metab. 2005;288:E741-E747.
9. Juhan-Vague I, Alessi MC, Mavri A, et al. Plasminogen activator inhibitor-1, inflammation, obesity, insulin resistance and vascular risk. J Thromb Haemost. 2003;1:1575-9.
10. Morton NM, Paterson JM, Masuzaki H, et al. Novel adipose tissue-mediated resistance to diet-induced visceral obesity in 11 beta-hydroxysteroid dehydrogenase type 1-deficient mice. Diabetes. 2004;53:931-8.
11. Ruan H, Lodish HF. Regulation of insulin sensitivity by adipose tissue-derived hormones and inflammatory cytokines. Curr Opin Lipidol. 2004;15:297-302.
12. Hara T, Fujiwara H, Shoji T, et al. Decreased plasma adiponectin levels in young obese males. J Atheroscler Thromb. 2003;10:234-8.
13. Gustat J, Srinivasan SR, Elkasabany A, et al. Relation of self-rated measures of physical activity to multiple risk factors of insulin resistance syndrome in young adults: the Bogalusa Heart Study. J Clin Epidemiol. 2002;55:997-1006.
14. Ford ES, Giles WH, Dietz WH. Prevalence of the metabolic syndrome among US adults: findings from the Third National Health and Nutrition Examination Survey. JAMA. 2002;287:356-9.

15. Pearson TA, Blair SN, Daniels SR, et al. AHA Guidelines for Primary Prevention of Cardiovascular Disease and Stroke: 2002 Update: Consensus Panel Guide to Comprehensive Risk Reduction for Adult Patients Without Coronary or Other Atherosclerotic Vascular Diseases. American Heart Association Science Advisory and Coordinating Committee. Circulation. 2002;106:388-91.
16. Apridonidze T, Essah PA, Iuorno MJ, et al. Prevalence and characteristics of the metabolic syndrome in women with polycystic ovary syndrome. J Clin Endocrinol Metab. 2004;90:1929-35.
17. National Cholesterol Education Program (NCEP) Expert Panel on Detection, Evaluation, and Treatment of High Blood Cholesterol in Adults (Adult Treatment Panel III). Third Report of the National Cholesterol Education Program (NCEP) Expert Panel on Detection, Evaluation, and Treatment of High Blood Cholesterol in Adults (Adult Treatment Panel III) final report. Circulation. 2002;106:3143-421.
18. Ridgefield, CT: Boehringer Ingelheim Pharmaceuticals, Inc. (2023). Jardiance. [online] Available from https://www.ema.europa.eu/en/documents/product-information/jardiance-epar-product-information_en.pdf
19. Zinman B, Wanner C, Lachin JM, et al.; EMPA-REG OUTCOME Investigators. Empagliflozin, cardiovascular outcomes, and mortality in type 2 diabetes. N Engl J Med. 2015;373(22):2117-28.
20. The EMPA-KIDNEY Collaborative Group. Empagliflozin in patients with chronic kidney disease. N Engl J Med. 2023;388(2):117-27.
21. McDonagh TA, Metra M, Adamo M, et al. 2021 ESC Guidelines for the diagnosis and treatment of acute and chronic heart failure: Developed by the Task Force for the diagnosis and treatment of acute and chronic heart failure of the European Society of Cardiology (ESC). With the special contribution of the Heart Failure Association (HFA) of the ESC. Eur J Heart Fail. 2022;24(1):4-131.

82

CHAPTER

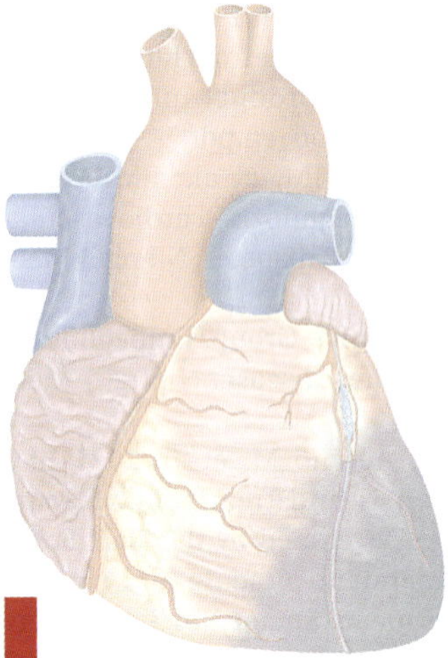

Comparison of Empagliflozin versus Dapagliflozin in Obesity Management in Heart Failure

Mohan Bhargava, Prasun Sagar

INTRODUCTION

Empagliflozin and dapagliflozin are SGLT2 inhibitors that have been recommended for heart failure management, and emerging data continue to clarify nuanced differences in obesity management effectiveness, safety, and patient-centric outcomes in heart failure populations. Empagliflozin and dapagliflozin share a common mechanism as SGLT2 inhibitors, lowering glucose reabsorption in the renal proximal convoluted tubule by an effect that also facilitates osmotic diuresis, natriuresis, weight loss, blood pressure reduction, and beneficial cardiac remodeling in patients with heart failure, irrespective of diabetic status.[1]

Recent studies highlight additional beneficial metabolic effects: Reduction in epicardial adipose tissue, mitigation of insulin resistance, and attenuation of obesity-driven inflammatory mediators.

Empagliflozin has demonstrated consistent improvement in composite outcomes including all-cause mortality and heart failure hospitalizations.[2] Dapagliflozin is equally recommended for heart failure, with large trials confirming reductions in cardiovascular events and hospitalizations, including both preserved and reduced ejection fraction and across the BMI spectrum.[3]

Major multicenter cohort analyses suggest that empagliflozin may offer incremental advantages in reducing all-cause mortality or hospitalization when compared directly to dapagliflozin in some cohorts, though these differences may reflect baseline population heterogeneity or trial design. Comprehensive network meta-analyses show dapagliflozin may modestly decrease all-cause mortality over empagliflozin, while both offer comparable reductions in heart failure hospitalizations.[4]

WEIGHT LOSS AND OBESITY MANAGEMENT

Both SGLT2 inhibitors lead to meaningful reductions in weight and BMI, and the magnitude may be more pronounced in patients with obesity:[5]

- Empagliflozin promotes marked weight loss, with 17.4% of patients achieving >5% reduction over a 1-year period in HFrEF cohorts.
- Dapagliflozin also causes weight loss, with some studies noting a greater percentage reduction in BMI and epicardial adipose tissue, especially in obese heart failure patients. Dapagliflozin's effect on weight and symptoms is also more pronounced in those with higher BMI.

SYMPTOM BURDEN AND QUALITY OF LIFE

- Dapagliflozin produces greater improvement in symptoms in obese heart failure patients, measured by Kansas City Cardiomyopathy Questionnaire scores, compared to lower BMI patients.
- Empagliflozin has demonstrated robust improvements in quality of life across the heart failure spectrum, independent of baseline BMI.[6]

SAFETY PROFILES

Both drugs appear safe in obese heart failure populations with low rates of hypoglycemia and no significant increase in adverse events. Variations in renal effects, blood pressure lowering, and weight reduction exist, but neither

TABLE 1: Comparison of empagliflozin and dapagliflozin across clinical outcomes in heart failure.

Parameter	*Empagliflozin*	*Dapagliflozin*
HF hospitalization	Significant reduction	Significant reduction
All-cause mortality	Potential incremental benefit	May modestly outperform empagliflozin in meta-analysis
Weight/BMI reduction	17% experience >5% loss at 1 year	Greater weight reduction in higher BMI
Symptom improvement	Significant QoL gains	Greater effect in obesity
Safety in obesity	Safe, low hypoglycemia	Safe, low hypoglycemia
Cost-effectiveness	Equivalent or less cost-effective	Shown more cost-effective

agent markedly increases risk in obese cohorts. Both drugs can modestly improve lipids and blood pressure, but side effect differences are minimal.[7]

PRACTICAL CONSIDERATIONS

Selection between empagliflozin and dapagliflozin for heart failure patients with obesity should factor in patient comorbidities, cost, formulary constraints, and possible incremental differences in symptomatic benefit or mortality reduction **(Table 1)**. Dapagliflozin may be more cost-effective in some healthcare systems and lead to slightly greater symptom improvement in those with high BMI, while empagliflozin may provide greater reductions in mortality in select cohorts.[8]

CONCLUSION

Both agents are effective and safe for heart failure with obesity. Patient-specific factors and nuanced data may guide choice, but both remain central to evidence-based management. Ongoing head-to-head and subgroup analyses will further clarify distinctions.

For obesity management in heart failure, dapagliflozin may offer slightly greater benefit in symptomatic improvement and weight reduction, particularly for patients with class II/III obesity, while empagliflozin may have a mortality benefit in select settings. Final selection should integrate clinical goals and individual patient context.

REFERENCES

1. Modzelewski KL, Pipilas A, Bosch NA. Comparative outcomes of empagliflozin to dapagliflozin in patients with heart failure. JAMA Netw Open. 2024;7(5):e249305.
2. Anker SD, Khan MS, Butler J, et al. Weight change and clinical outcomes in heart failure with reduced ejection fraction: insights from EMPEROR-Reduced. Eur J Heart Fail. 2023;25(1):117-27.
3. Adamson C, Kondo T, Jhund PS, et al. Dapagliflozin for heart failure according to body mass index: the DELIVER trial. Eur Heart J. 2022;43(41):4406-17.
4. Shi Z, Gao F, Liu W, et al. Comparative efficacy of dapagliflozin and empagliflozin of a fixed dose in heart failure: a network meta-analysis. Front Cardiovasc Med. 2022;9:869272.
5. Reddy YNV, Melenovsky V, Asokan AK, et al. Dapagliflozin, peptide YY, and weight loss in heart failure with preserved ejection fraction. Eur Heart J. 2024;45(37):3889-91.
6. Voors AA, Angermann CE, Teerlink JR, et al. The SGLT2 inhibitor empagliflozin in patients hospitalized for acute heart failure: a multinational randomized trial. Nat Med. 2022;28(3):568-74.
7. Khan RH, Qureshi H, Ahmed Z, et al. Dapagliflozin's role in heart failure: an overview of clinical trial evidence. Cureus. 2024;16(10):e70727.
8. Rane A, Nechi RN, Imam M, et al. Comparative value of dapagliflozin vs empagliflozin in patients with heart failure and preserved ejection fraction: a cost-effectiveness analysis. J Manag Care Spec Pharm. 2023;29(9):1045-53.

83

CHAPTER

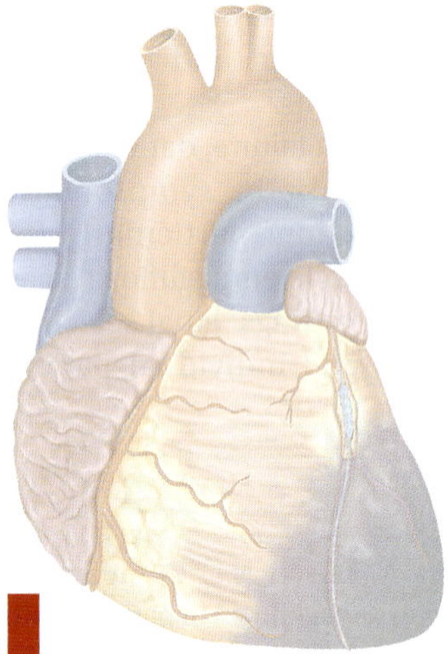

Clinical Evidence of Empagliflozin-induced Weight Loss in Obese Patients

Rakesh Varma, Shekhar Kunal

INTRODUCTION

Obesity is a major driver of cardiometabolic disease, contributing significantly to the global burden of type 2 diabetes mellitus (T2DM), coronary artery disease, heart failure, hypertension, atrial fibrillation, and non-alcoholic fatty liver disease (NAFLD). The strong association between excess adiposity—particularly central and visceral fat—and cardiovascular morbidity underscores the importance of effective weight management strategies for cardiologists. However, despite lifestyle modification being the primary approach to weight loss, long-term success remains challenging, and pharmacologic options have often been limited by modest efficacy or undesirable side effects.

In recent years, sodium-glucose cotransporter-2 (SGLT2) inhibitors have emerged as an important therapeutic class with benefits extending beyond glycemic control. Among them, empagliflozin is distinguished by robust cardiovascular outcome data, renal protection, and consistent evidence of weight loss. Although originally developed as a glucose-lowering agent, empagliflozin exhibits a unique metabolic profile that facilitates sustained reductions in body weight, visceral fat mass, and ectopic adipose depots such as epicardial adipose tissue (EAT). These effects are clinically meaningful for cardiologists, given the established links between obesity, diastolic dysfunction, HFpEF, and systemic inflammation. This chapter provides a comprehensive narrative review of the mechanisms, clinical trials, real-world evidence, and practical implications of empagliflozin-induced weight loss in obese individuals.

PHYSIOLOGICAL BASIS OF OBESITY AND CARDIOMETABOLIC DYSFUNCTION

Obesity is characterized by an imbalance between energy intake and expenditure, leading to adipocyte hypertrophy, ectopic fat deposition, and metabolic dysregulation.

Visceral adiposity is particularly harmful because visceral fat is metabolically active and releases pro-inflammatory cytokines, including TNF-α, IL-6, resistin, and leptin, while reducing protective adipokines such as adiponectin. These changes contribute to insulin resistance, endothelial dysfunction, hypertension, and accelerated atherosclerosis.

Excess epicardial adipose tissue exerts local inflammatory effects on the myocardium and coronary arteries. Increased EAT thickness correlates with impaired diastolic function, left atrial enlargement, atrial fibrillation, and HFpEF. Hepatic fat accumulation plays a central role in NAFLD and contributes to systemic insulin resistance. Therefore, therapies that target visceral and ectopic fat—not merely total body weight—offer substantial cardiometabolic benefits.

PHARMACOLOGY OF EMPAGLIFLOZIN

Empagliflozin is a highly selective SGLT2 inhibitor with approximately 2500-fold selectivity over SGLT1 **(Fig. 1)**.

Key pharmacokinetics:

- *Oral bioavailability:* 78%
- *Peak plasma concentration:* 1.5 hours

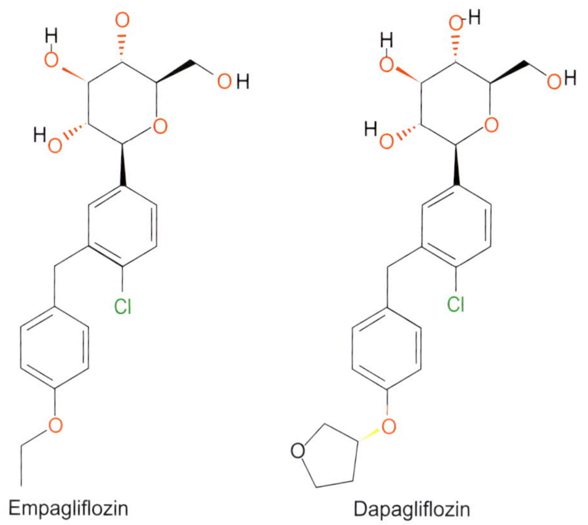

Fig. 1: Comparative molecular structures of empagliflozin and dapagliflozin.

- *Elimination half-life:* 12 hours
- *Renal excretion:* Major route
- *Dosing:* 10 mg and 25 mg once daily

No titration is typically needed, and efficacy is consistent across BMI ranges.

Side-by-side 2D chemical structures of empagliflozin (left) and dapagliflozin (right), highlighting key structural differences between the two SGLT2 inhibitors. Both molecules share a conserved β-D-glucopyranoside core (atoms shown in red for oxygen and light blue for hydrogen) and an aryl–C-glycosidic linkage. Empagliflozin features an *ethoxy substituent* on the terminal phenyl ring, whereas dapagliflozin contains a *tetrahydrofuran (THF) ring* attached through an ether linkage (highlighted in contrasting color). The shared para-chloro-phenyl ring is labelled in green to emphasize conserved pharmacophoric elements. The figure visually contrasts the molecular extensions contributing to differences in potency, selectivity, and pharmacokinetic behavior.

MECHANISMS OF EMPAGLIFLOZIN-INDUCED WEIGHT LOSS (TABLE 1)

Although glycosuria is the primary mechanism associated with weight loss, the effects of empagliflozin are multifactorial and extend to deep metabolic pathways.

Glucosuria and Caloric Deficit

Empagliflozin blocks SGLT2 receptors in the proximal renal tubule, preventing reabsorption of 60–80 g of filtered glucose per day. This results in a caloric deficit of approximately 240–320 kcal/day. While compensatory hyperphagia may occur, sustained negative energy balance is maintained, leading to gradual weight loss.

TABLE 1: Mechanisms of empagliflozin-induced weight loss.

Mechanism	Description
Glucosuria-induced caloric loss	Promotes urinary glucose excretion of 60–80 g/day, creating a caloric deficit of ~240–320 kcal/day
Reduction in visceral fat	Decreases hepatic, epicardial, and visceral adipose tissue; preferential fat-mass reduction
Improved insulin sensitivity	Lowers fasting insulin, enhances lipolysis, reduces adipocyte hypertrophy
Shift toward ketone metabolism	Increases β-hydroxybutyrate levels, improves metabolic efficiency, enhances fat oxidation
Natriuresis and osmotic diuresis	Causes initial extracellular volume reduction, followed by sustained fat-mass loss

Reduction in Visceral Adiposity

Imaging studies using MRI and CT consistently show preferential reduction of visceral adipose tissue. This includes reductions in hepatic fat, abdominal visceral fat, and importantly, epicardial adipose tissue, which is strongly implicated in HFpEF pathophysiology. Visceral fat reduction is more clinically relevant than changes in total body weight, making empagliflozin particularly valuable to cardiologists.

Improvement in Insulin Sensitivity

Empagliflozin decreases glucotoxicity, lowers fasting insulin levels, and enhances insulin sensitivity in skeletal muscle and liver. This promotes lipolysis, reduces adipocyte hypertrophy, and improves adipose tissue metabolic flexibility.

Shift Toward Ketone Metabolism

By promoting mild ketosis (increased β-hydroxybutyrate levels), empagliflozin induces a fasting-mimicking metabolic state. Enhanced mitochondrial efficiency and fat oxidation contribute further to reductions in fat mass.

Natriuresis and Osmotic Diuresis

Initially, empagliflozin produces small reductions in extracellular fluid volume due to natriuresis. However, long-term weight reductions primarily reflect true fat-mass loss rather than water loss.

TABLE 2: Major clinical trials demonstrating weight loss.

Trial	Population	Key weight-related findings
EMPA-REG Outcome	T2DM with established CVD	Sustained weight loss of 2–3 kg, maintained over 3.1 years
EMPA-REG Metabolic	Subgroup imaging analysis	10% reduction in visceral fat area; reduced epicardial fat
EMPA-REG BP	Hypertensive T2DM patients	2.0–2.6 kg weight loss within 12 weeks
EASE Trials	Patients with type 1 diabetes	1.8–3.4 kg reduction; independent of insulin sensitivity
EMPEROR Trials	HFpEF/HFrEF patients	1.2–1.8 kg weight loss; reduced epicardial fat in sub-studies
NAFLD Studies	Obese, non-diabetic adults	2.5–4.0 kg loss with 10–20% reduction in liver fat

CLINICAL TRIALS DEMONSTRATING EMPAGLIFLOZIN-INDUCED WEIGHT LOSS (TABLE 2)

EMPA-REG OUTCOME

This landmark cardiovascular outcomes trial was a paradigm shift, confirming not only cardiovascular safety but superiority. EMPA-REG OUTCOME trial enrolled 7020 T2DM patients with established cardiovascular disease. Over a median follow-up of 3.1 years, empagliflozin consistently reduced body weight by 2–3 kg. Importantly, this reduction was sustained and attributed largely to loss of fat mass, including visceral adiposity. This trial demonstrated that the weight-reducing effect is durable over the long term in a high-risk population.

EMPA-REG METABOLIC Sub-study

This analysis provided detailed body composition data. Empagliflozin reduced:

- Visceral fat area by ~10%
- Subcutaneous fat by ~7%
- Epicardial fat in MRI sub-studies

These reductions correlated with improved insulin sensitivity and metabolic markers.

EMPA-REG BP

In hypertensive patients with T2DM, empagliflozin demonstrated 2.0–2.6 kg weight loss within 12 weeks. This early reduction highlights the combined effect of caloric loss and improved metabolic efficiency.

EASE Trials (Type 1 Diabetes)

In type 1 diabetes patients, empagliflozin reduced weight by 1.8–3.4 kg, demonstrating that its weight-loss effect is independent of insulin resistance and driven largely by glucosuria and fat oxidation.

EMPEROR-Reduced and EMPEROR-Preserved

Among heart failure patients, empagliflozin led to modest reductions of 1.2–1.8 kg, along with significant improvements in symptoms and functional capacity. Sub-studies confirmed reductions in epicardial fat, a key contributor to HFpEF.

NAFLD and Non-diabetic Obesity Studies

Emerging trials in obese adults without diabetes show:

- 2.5–4.0 kg weight reduction
- 10–20% reduction in hepatic fat
- Improvements in ALT, AST, and liver stiffness

Given the tight link between NAFLD and cardiovascular disease, this represents a major metabolic advantage.

COMPARATIVE EFFICACY WITH OTHER SGLT2 INHIBITORS

While the SGLT2 inhibitor class as a whole is associated with weight loss, direct and indirect comparisons provide insights into the relative efficacy of individual agents, particularly empagliflozin, within the class.

HEAD-TO-HEAD CLINICAL TRIALS

Few direct head-to-head trials are powered for weight loss as a primary endpoint, but available data suggest a high degree of similarity.

- *Empagliflozin vs. dapagliflozin:* A 2017 randomized, open-label study directly compared empagliflozin 25 mg and dapagliflozin 10 mg in patients with T2D. After 24 weeks, the reduction in body weight was nearly identical: -2.39 kg with dapagliflozin versus -2.36 kg with empagliflozin, confirming no significant clinical difference in overall weight loss effect.
- *Empagliflozin vs. canagliflozin:* Similarly, a meta-analysis comparing various SGLT2 inhibitors found that the weight reduction between empagliflozin and canagliflozin at standard doses (100 mg) was comparable, typically falling within the -2.0 to -3.0 kg range.

Meta-analyses and Pooled Data

Large-scale systematic reviews and network meta-analyses provide the broadest view of class effects.

- *Class-wide effect:* As noted in the query, meta-analyses consistently report a class-wide placebo-corrected weight loss of *1.8–3.0 kg* over 24–26 weeks. This effect is dose-dependent for some agents (e.g., canagliflozin 300 mg leads to greater weight loss than 100 mg).
- *Position of empagliflozin:* Within this range, empagliflozin, particularly at the 25 mg dose, is often found on the *higher end of the spectrum (~2.5–3.0 kg)*. This can be attributed to its high selectivity and potent SGLT2 inhibition, leading to a slightly greater daily glucose excretion compared to some other agents in the class at their standard doses.

BODY COMPOSITION ACROSS THE CLASS

The critical question is not just total weight loss, but its composition. Evidence suggests that the favorable fat-mass-to-lean-mass ratio observed with empagliflozin is a class effect, though some subtle differences may exist.

- *Dapagliflozin:* Studies using DEXA scans show that dapagliflozin also leads to a significant reduction in fat mass, with a preservation of lean mass similar to empagliflozin.
- *Canagliflozin:* Data from the CANVAS program and dedicated body composition studies confirm that the majority of weight loss with canagliflozin is also from fat mass, including visceral and subcutaneous adipose tissue.
- *Ertugliflozin:* As a newer agent, data is more limited but follows the same pattern, with significant reductions in body weight and a composition favoring fat loss.

COMPARISON WITH OTHER WEIGHT-LOSS MEDICATIONS (TABLE 3)

Modern obesity treatments include GLP-1 receptor agonists, dual agonists like tirzepatide, and older agents such as orlistat. While empagliflozin produces more modest total weight loss (2–4 kg), its visceral fat reduction, cardio-renal benefits, and excellent tolerability make it uniquely valuable. Studies comparing empagliflozin with other glucose-lowering agents further highlight its weight benefit.

- *Versus sulfonylureas/insulin*: Empagliflozin consistently shows superior weight loss, as these older agents are associated with weight gain.
- *Versus DPP-4 inhibitors*: Empagliflozin leads to significantly greater weight reduction.

TABLE 3: Comparative evidence with other weight-loss pharmacotherapies.

Agent	*Expected weight loss*	*Notes*
Empagliflozin	2–4 kg	Cardioprotective profile; improves HF outcomes
GLP-1 RA (semaglutide)	10–15% body weight	Superior weight loss; injectable
Tirzepatide	Up to 20%	Currently gold standard
Orlistat	2–3 kg	Poor tolerability
Metformin	1–2 kg	Minimal effect in established obesity

- *Versus GLP-1 receptor agonists:* While GLP-1 RAs generally produce greater weight loss (10–20% body weight), empagliflozin offers a favorable weight profile, especially for patients who may not tolerate GLP-1 RA side effects. Empagliflozin additionally complements these agents and is often used in combination therapy—particularly in cardiometabolic disease.

EFFECT ON VISCERAL AND EPICARDIAL ADIPOSE TISSUE

Among all adipose depots, reductions in visceral fat, hepatic fat, and epicardial adipose tissue (EAT) are most relevant to clinicians. EAT reduction may improve diastolic function, reduce inflammation, and decrease atrial arrhythmia burden. Visceral fat reduction improves blood pressure, lipid profile, and systemic inflammation.

COMPOSITION OF WEIGHT LOSS: FAT MASS VS. LEAN MASS

A concern with any weight-loss intervention is the potential loss of lean body mass (muscle). The evidence for empagliflozin is reassuring.

- *DEXA scan studies:* Several studies using Dual-Energy X-ray Absorptiometry (DEXA) have analyzed body composition. They consistently show that approximately two-thirds to three-quarters of the weight lost with empagliflozin is fat mass, particularly visceral adipose tissue, which is metabolically detrimental.
- *Proportion of loss:* The remaining fraction is a combination of fluid and a small amount of lean tissue. This ratio is considered favorable compared to weight loss from diet alone and is similar to or better than that seen with other pharmacotherapies. The mild diuretic effect also contributes to a reduction in extracellular water volume.

REAL-WORLD EVIDENCE SUPPORTING WEIGHT LOSS

Large observational studies such as CVD-REAL confirm consistent weight loss and improved cardiovascular outcomes with empagliflozin in routine clinical practice. Asian and Indian real-world cohorts show even greater reductions in visceral fat due to ethnicity-specific adiposity patterns.

SAFETY, TOLERABILITY, AND PRACTICAL USE

Empagliflozin is generally well tolerated. The most common effects are genital mycotic infections and transient diuresis. Euglycemic ketoacidosis is rare and typically occurs in type 1 diabetes or ketogenic diets. Renal function should be monitored, though empagliflozin remains effective down to eGFR 20 mL/min/1.73 m^2.

For obese patients with T2DM, heart failure, metabolic syndrome, or NAFLD, empagliflozin represents an excellent choice. It can be started at 10 mg once daily, increasing to 25 mg if needed.

CONCLUSION

Empagliflozin induces consistent, modest, and sustained weight loss in obese patients, with or without T2D. The average loss of 2–3 kg is clinically significant, as a 3–5% reduction in body weight is associated with improvements in cardiovascular risk factors. The composition of this loss is favorable, being predominantly fat mass. This effect, combined with its proven cardiorenal benefits, positions empagliflozin as a valuable therapeutic agent, especially for the large patient population with overlapping T2D, obesity, and cardiovascular disease.

Future research directions include:
- Investigating empagliflozin in combination with GLP-1 receptor agonists for synergistic weight loss.
- Conducting larger, long-term trials specifically in non-diabetic obese populations.
- Exploring its effects on specific body composition parameters, including ectopic fat (liver, pancreas) in obese individuals.

BIBLIOGRAPHY

1. Anker SD, Butler J, Filippatos G, et al. Empagliflozin in heart failure with preserved ejection fraction. N Engl J Med. 2021;385(16):1451-61.
2. Bonora BM, Avogaro A, Fadini GP. Effects of SGLT2 inhibitors on body weight: metabolic mechanisms and clinical results. Nutrients. 2020;12(5):1338.
3. Cho YK, Kang YM, Lee SE, et al. Effects of SGLT2 inhibitors on NAFLD: a meta-analysis. Diabetes Metab J. 2022;46(3):362-75.
4. Lee PCH, Ganguly S, Goh SY. Weight loss associated with empagliflozin in Asian populations: a meta-analysis. J Diabetes Investig. 2019;10(2):464-72.
5. Neeland IJ, McGuire DK, Chilton R, et al. Empagliflozin reduces body weight and adiposity in type 2 diabetes: EMPA-REG METABOLIC study. Diabetes Care. 2016;39(12):e213-4.
6. Packer M, Anker SD, Butler J, et al. Cardiovascular and renal outcomes with empagliflozin in heart failure. N Engl J Med. 2020;383(15):1413-24.
7. Sattar N, Fitchett D, Hantel S, George JT, Zinman B. Empagliflozin is associated with modest weight loss and improved cardiometabolic profile. Diabetologia. 2019;62(2):358-64.
8. Scheen AJ. SGLT2 inhibitors and body weight loss: pathophysiologic mechanisms and clinical evidence. Diabetes Metab. 2020;46(3):220-9
9. Shimizu M, Suzuki K, Kato K, et al. Evaluation of dapagliflozin on epicardial fat volume in type 2 diabetes using cardiac CT. Circ J. 2019;83(5):1098-104.
10. Zinman B, Wanner C, Lachin JM, et al. Empagliflozin, cardiovascular outcomes, and mortality in type 2 diabetes. N Engl J Med. 2015;373(22):2117-28.

84

CHAPTER

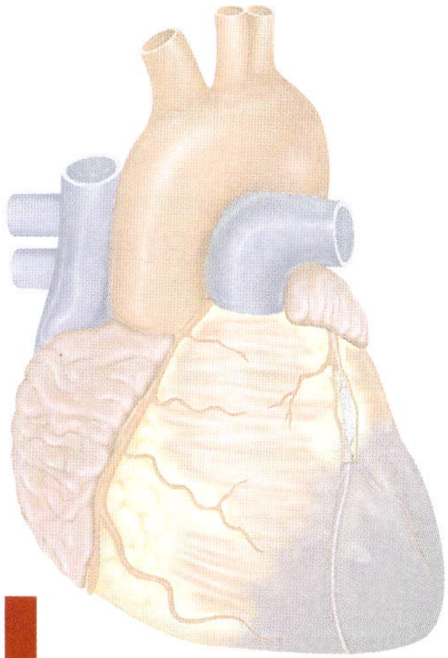

Effects of SGLT2i and GLP-1 RA on Epicardial Fat

Naveen Garg, Rekha Mishra

INTRODUCTION

Obesity is considered as a major risk factor for cardiovascular events. Adipose tissues are considered to be metabolically active tissues and are proinflammatory. Thus, the anthropometric indices like BMI index and waist-to-hip ratios were designed to screen the population for cardiovascular risks. But, further studies have indicated that it is not the subcutaneous fat but the visceral fat which is more vicious.[1-4] This emphasizes that many lean persons with high visceral fat content are more prone to cardiovascular events than of otherwise obese people. For almost the last decade, the effects of fat around the heart on cardiovasculature have become the center of research. The association between coronary artery disease (CAD) and the fat around the coronary arteries (also known as epicardial fat) is now being established.[4-7] This association has led to the addition of a new risk factor. The thickness of epicardial fat, which is often measured by noninvasive techniques such as CT scan, MRI, or echocardiography, is the novel predictor for development of CAD.

The fat around the heart is divided into two compartments, viz., pericardial fat and epicardial fat. This division is well depicted in **Figure 1 and Table 1**.

The fat around the myocardium is of major interest as the main coronary arteries are embedded in these areas. The coronaries have their own vasculature, i.e., vasa vasorum, which are in direct contact with the fat around them.[8-10] This fat is metabolically active fat, and it affects the pathophysiology of coronary vessels. In normal circumstances, this epicardial fat contributes to increase in vasa vasorum, coronary relaxation via nitric oxide (NO), production of antioxidants and anti-inflammatory substances, and thermoregulation. However, the phenotypic shift of this fat leads to vasoconstriction, release of proatherogenic, proinflammatory, and pro-oxidative substances **(Table 2)**. This behavioral change from friend to foe of epicardial fat is still a matter of research but the increase in its thickness (or volume) and some systemic inflammatory insult is thought to trigger this change. The concept that atherosclerosis occurs because of insult to vascular endothelium that later produces stenosis is also challenged as the phenotypic change in epicardial fat may also induce stenosis of coronaries without endothelial injury. Thus, atheroma are formed not only from "inside to outside" of the vessel but can also propagate from "outside to inside" the coronaries.[10-17]

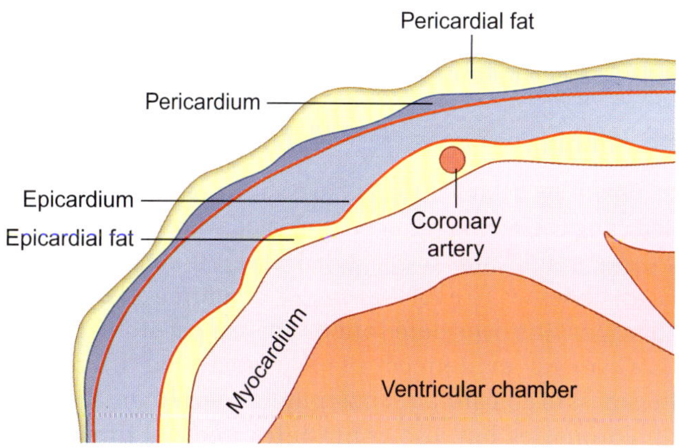

Fig. 1: Depicting diagrammatic location of epicardial fat and pericardial fat.

TABLE 1: Comparison of epicardial fat and pericardial fat.

Variable	Epicardial fat	Pericardial fat
Location	Between the myocardial surface and the visceral pericardium	Outside the visceral pericardium, between the visceral and parietal pericardium and on the external surface of the parietal pericardium
Embryologic origin	Splanchnopleuric mesoderm	Primitive thoracic mesenchyme
Blood supply	Branches from the coronary arteries	Noncoronary sources (branches from the internal mammary artery)
Amount	20% of total heart weight	20–50% of cardiac mass
Metabolic	Active	Less active
Relation to myocardium	No fascia, contiguity with adventitia and myocardium	No compact relation to myocardium
Adipocytes	Generally smaller, more preadipocytes, high-energy consuming metabolism	Mature adipocyte
Morphology	Brown	More white

TABLE 2: Vasoactive and inflammatory mediators secreted by epicardial adipose tissue: protective ("friendly") and deleterious ("adversary") substances.

Friendly substances	Adversary substances
Adiponectin and adrenomedullin	Leptin
ADRF	Omentin
PAME	Visfatin
NO	Resistin
PGI2	TNF

(ADRF: adventitium-derived relaxing factors; NO: nitric oxide; PAME: palmitic acid methyl ester; PGI2: prostacyclin; TNF: tumor necrosis factor)

Many systematic studies have shown that sensitivity of detecting CAD (which can be evaluated with measuring the volume or thickness of epicardial fat) is 70–90%. Epicardial fat thicknesses (EFTs) >5 mm, or a volume >125 mL or 68 mL/m^2, are considered abnormal in most of studies.[17-26]

Growing evidences also suggest that increased thickness of epicardial fat not only has decremental effects on coronaries but also contributes to atrial fibrillation (AF), heart failure (HF), microvascular dysfunction, sudden cardiac death, and cardiomyopathies, as well as predicting major adverse cardiovascular events (MACE).[26-30] These observations led to the interventions to reduce the thickness of epicardial fat. These include regular exercise, diet therapies, and drug therapies.

METHODS TO MEASURE EPICARDIAL FAT THICKNESS

Epicardial fat thickness can be measured by various methods such as CT scan, MRI, or echocardiography. The merits and demerits of these diagnostic modalities are tabulated in **Table 3**.

Echocardiography is considered as most economically, rapid, portable, and easily assessable screening tool for measuring epicardial fat for evaluation of risk analysis.[31-35] The EFT is measured in PLAX or short axis view (SAX view), as depicted in **Figures 2A and B**.

The echocardiography measures the thickness not volume of epicardial fat, which is also well correlated with the results of other expensive modalities.[36-39] Echocardiography measurements are operator dependent; they need expertise and demand a good acoustic window for analysis.

SEVERITY GRADING

Though there is no consensus on normal value of epicardial thickness or its volume, due to many ethnic and geographic variations, the exact measurements may vary. Many studies have indicated that EFT value above 7 mm has definitely correlated with cardiovascular disease and also carries prognostic value. However, the EFT <3 mm may be considered as safe limit.[17]

THERAPY

Sodium–glucose Cotransporter-2 Inhibitors aka Gliflozins

It is no wonder that this era of medicine is dedicated to sodium–glucose cotransporter-2 inhibitors (SGLT2i) or rather to say that treatment of cardiac elements is through kidneys. Three SGLT2i drugs, viz., empagliflozin, dapagliflozin, and canagliflozin (also known as gliflozins) were first to get approved for clinical use and were extensively studied.[17,40-44]

Gliflozins were antidiabetic glycosuric drugs that were found to have advantageous effects on heart. Studies such as EMPA-REG OUTCOME, CANVAS, DECLARE-TIMI, SOLOIST-WHT, CREDENCE, DAPA-HF, and EMPA-VISION showed that MACE and rehospitalization were markedly lower in patients with heart diseases (CAD, HF, etc.) who

TABLE 3: Methods to measure epicardial fat thickness.

	MRI	*CT scan*	*Echocardiography*
Resolution	Best	Better	Good
Measurements	Volume and thickness	Volume and thickness	Thickness only
Reproducibility	High	High	Good
Cost	High	High	Low
Hazards	None	Radiation exposure	None
Time taken to study	Excess	Excess	Low
Accessibility	Low	Low	High
Portability	None	None	Portable
Advantages	Gold standard	Coronaries can be accessed simultaneously	Good screening tool

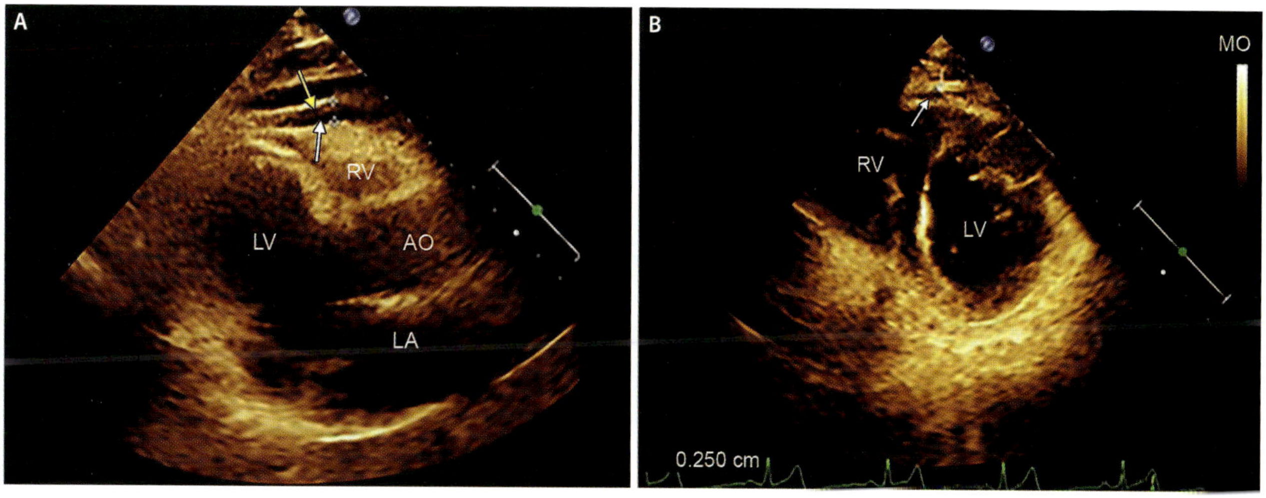

Figs. 2A and B: (A) PLAX view in transthoracic echocardiographic, depicting white arrow as epicardial fat tissue; an echo-lucent space between epicardial surface and parietal pericardium; anterior to the right ventricular free wall. Yellow arrow depicts pericardial fat. (B) Showing epicardial fat as white arrow in SAX view in transthoracic echocardiography. (AO: aorta; LA: left atrium; LV: left ventricle; RV: right ventricle)

were treated with gliflozins irrespective of their diabetic status. These studies confirm their beneficial role in heart diseases even in nondiabetic patients, which postulates that these effects are due to their anti-inflammatory properties. These molecular effects of gliflozins were elucidated in many experimental studies. These studies also confirmed to have not only anti-inflammatory but also antiobesity, anti-insulin resistant, as well as antiendothelial dysfunction properties of gliflozins. Their effects to reduce EFT as well as reduction in cardiac risk profile are well studied[45-49] **(Figs. 3A and B)**.

The effect on EFT is more if the duration of therapy is lengthened. Thus, the beneficial effects of gliflozins can be summarized in **Flowchart 1**.

It is emphasized that the role of gliflozins in reduction of epicardial fat is studied in diabetic patients only. However, as the drug authorities of many countries have approved the use of gliflozins in nondiabetic patients with HF (both HFrEF and HFpEF), it is possible that futuristic studies may be able to prove that this promising molecule is advantageous to nondiabetic patients too. Following are the studies and meta-analysis of gliflozins use in reducing EFT[49-53] **(Tables 4 and 5)**.

Glucagon-like Peptide-1 Receptor Agonists

Glucagon-like peptide-1 receptor agonists (GLP-1 RA) (also known as "Glutides") were originally used for treatment of diabetes but later these were being widely recognized for treatment of obesity, metabolic syndrome, as well as cardiovascular protection in nondiabetics. The popular GLP-1 RA are exenatide, liraglutide, semaglutide,

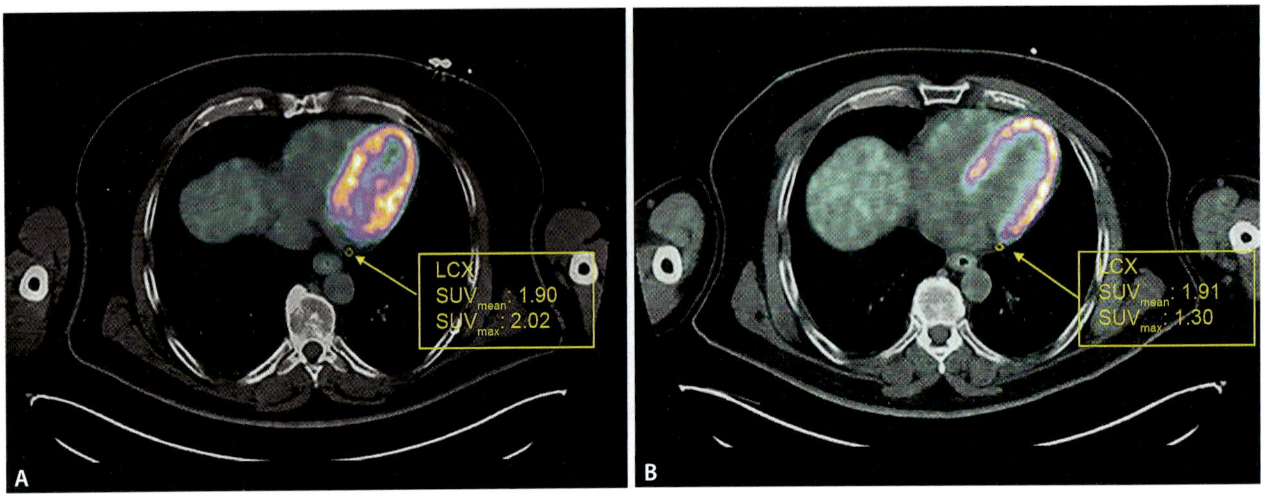

Figs. 3A and B: Epicardial adipose tissue reduction clearly seen after 4 weeks of dapagliflozin therapy by FDG-PET/CT scan. (A) Baseline, (B) after therapy. (LCX: left circumflex artery; SUV: standardized uptake value)
Source: Adapted from Cinti et al. (2023).

Flowchart 1: Depicting the pathways by which gliflozins decrease the epicardial fat thickness (or volume).

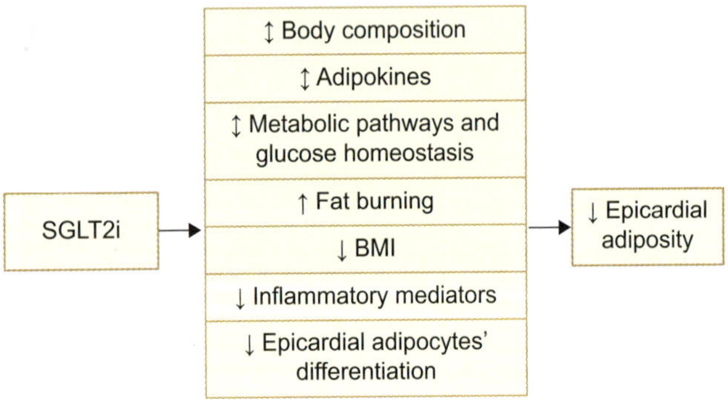

Source: Adapted from Yaribeygi et al. (2023).

and dulaglutide. These agents reduce visceral adiposity and so led to similar observations in epicardial fat. The effect on epicardial fat is found to be 20–35% reduction and improvement in lipid metabolism. These have demonstrated reduced risk of MACE including heart attack, stroke, and cardiovascular death both in diabetics as well as in nondiabetics. Though the studies indicating the effects of GLP-1 RA on epicardial fat among nondiabetics are few, these studies indicate that this is futuristic molecule to reduce the cardiovascular events in population at large.[53-57]

The meta-analysis of various studies in diabetic patients has shown their beneficial effects, as summarized in **Table 6**.

It is also observed through molecular studies that increased expressions of GLP-1 receptors in EAT indicate transformation of fat from white to brown, decreased inflammation, or fibrosis. The therapeutic role of GLP-1 RA to reduce epicardial fat though not yet recommended but there is promising possibility of the same in the near future.

CONCLUSION[58-61]

Epicardial fat is a new risk predictor for cardiovascular event. It is recommended to analyze EFT in risk profiling CAD patients. Echocardiography is the most rapid, cheap, and hazard-free tool to estimate EAT. MRI remains gold standard for EAT. Gliflozins and glutides are futuristic molecules for decreasing cardiovascular risks or MACE, irrespective of diabetic status of patient. Larger RCTs with longer follow-up to see the sustainability of EAT reduction and whether this translates to cardiovascular outcome improvements (e.g., reduced coronary disease progression and HF). More data in nondiabetic populations, or in populations with less obesity, to see how generalizable the effects are Standardization of measurement techniques, so comparisons across studies are more reliable.

TABLE 4: Various gliflozins used to study epicardial fat.

Study/author	*Drug*	*Duration*	*Method*	*Key findings*
Yagi et al. (2017) PMID: 29034006	Canagliflozin	6 months	Ultrasound (EFT)	↓ EFT thickness from 9.3 to 7.3 mm
Fukuda et al. (2017) PMID: 28253918	Luseogliflozin	12 weeks	MRI (EFV)	↓ EFV (117 → 111 cm^3)
Iacobellis et al. (2017) PMID: 28616806	Ipragliflozin	12 weeks	MRI (EFV)	↓ EFV (102 → 89 cm^3)
Sato et al. (2018) PMID: 29301516	Dapagliflozin	6 months	CT (EFV)	↓ EFV (–16.4 cm^3 vs. +4.7 cm^3)
Bosch et al. (2020) PMID: 32352644	Dapagliflozin + Metformin	24 weeks	Ultrasound (EFT)	↓ EAT thickness by ~20%
Aoyama et al. (2021) J-STAGE	Dapagliflozin	6 months	CT (EFV) + ECG	↓ EFV and ↓ P-wave dispersion
JAR Ibáñezetal (2021) PMID: 34325888	Empagliflozin	6 months	CMR	↓ EFV by 10%
B Gaborit et al. (2021) PMID: 33648515	Empagliflozin	12 weeks	CMR	↓ EFV (10^8–10^6 mL)
El Mahdiui et al. (2024) PMID: 38115004	Dapagliflozin	4 weeks	PET/CT (EFT)	↓ EAT thickness (~19%)

TABLE 5: Meta-analysis of epicardial fat.

Study/author	*Studies/size*	*Key findings*
Wang et al. (2024) PMID: 39819408	11 studies	↓ EFT volume (–6.57 mL), ↓ EF thickness (–1.55 mm); significant versus control
Yang et al. (2021) PMID: 34440918	3 RCTs	↓ EFT with SGLT2-i versus control (SMD = –0.82); HbA1c ↓ more consistent than BMI changes
Guo et al. (2023) PMID: 36721184	Multidrug comparison	SGLT2-i significantly ↓ EFT; GLP-1 RA may show stronger effect in some comparisons
Mori et al. (2024) PMID: 39639835	16 trials, $n = 867$	SGLT2-i > GLP-1 RA > placebo for EFT reduction; consistent across imaging methods

TABLE 6: Glucagon-like peptide-1 receptor agonists.

Study/meta-analysis	*GLP-1 RA*	*Measurement and methods*	*Key findings*
Exenatide versus "reference treatment"	Exenatide	MRI/MR spectroscopy	Exenatide reduced EAT by ~8.8% versus ~1.2%
Liraglutide 6-months RCT (metformin + liraglutide vs. metformin alone)	Liraglutide	Ultrasound	EAT reduced by ~29% at 3 months and ~36% at 6 months in liraglutide group; no change in metformin-only group
Liraglutide in T2D with abdominal obesity	Liraglutide	Cardiac MRI	EAT thickness dropped from ~5–7 to ~3.95 mm
Semaglutide versus dulaglutide	Semaglutide or dulaglutide	Ultrasound	~20% reduction in EAT thickness in both GLP-1 RA groups

REFERENCES

1. Iozzo P. Myocardial, perivascular, and epicardial fat. Diabetes Care. 2011;34(Suppl. 2):S371-9.
2. Wu Y, Zhang A, Hamilton DJ, et al. Epicardial fat in the maintenance of cardiovascular health. Methodist Debakey Cardiovasc J. 2017;13(1):20-4.
3. Fitzgibbons TP, Czech MP. Epicardial and perivascular adipose tissues and their influence on cardiovascular disease: basic mechanisms and clinical associations. J Am Heart Assoc. 2014;3:e000582.
4. Lobeek M, Rienstra M, Gorter TM. Epicardial adipose tissue and cardiac dysfunction: progress in knowledge but questions remain. Eur J Heart Failure. 2023;25: 1944-6.
5. Pruthvi G, Naidu OA, Praveen N, et al. Correlation of epicardial adipose tissue thickness by echocardiography with waist circumference, lipid profile, and severity of lesion by coronary angiography in patients with acute coronary syndrome. J Pract Cardiovasc Sci. 2020;6: 61-7.
6. Mancio J, Barros AS, Conceicão G, et al. Influence of EPICardial adipose tissue in HEART diseases (EPICHEART) study: protocol for a translational study in coronary atherosclerosis. Rev Port Cardiol (Engl Ed). 2020;39(11):625-33.
7. Mahmoud I, Dykun I, Kärner L, et al. Epicardial adipose tissue differentiates in patients with and without coronary microvascular dysfunction. Int J Obes (Lond). 2021;45(9):2058-63.
8. Duyuler S, Duyuler PT. Epicardial adipose tissue in coronary microvascular dysfunction. Int J Obes (Lond). 2022;46(8):1564.
9. Iacobellis G. Epicardial adipose tissue in contemporary cardiology. Nat Rev Cardiol. 2022;19(9):593-606.
10. Cerit L. The tip of the iceberg: non-calcified coronary plague and epicardial adipose tissue. Arq Bras Cardiol. 2017;108(4):383-5.
11. Nagy E, Jermendy AL, Merkely B, et al. Clinical importance of epicardial adipose tissue. Arch Med Sci. 2017;13(4):864-74.
12. Talman AH, Psaltis PJ, Cameron JD, et al. Epicardial adipose tissue: far more than a fat depot. Cardiovasc Diagn Ther. 2014;4(6):416-29.
13. Wang Q, Chi J, Wang C, et al. Epicardial adipose tissue in patients with coronary artery disease: a meta-analysis. J Cardiovasc Dev Dis. 2022;9(8):253.
14. Leone A. Morphology of coronary arteries in relation to ischemic heart disease. J Cardiol Curr Res. 2021;14(2): 27-32.
15. Conceição G, Martins D, Miranda IM, et al. Unraveling the role of epicardial adipose tissue in coronary artery disease: partners in crime? Int J Mol Sci. 2020;21:8866.
16. Nelson MR, Mookadam F, Thota V, et al. Epicardial fat: an additional measurement for subclinical athero-sclerosis and cardiovascular risk stratification? J Am Soc Echocardiogr. 2011;24:339-45.
17. Iacobellis G, Willens HJ. Echocardiographic epicardial fat: a review of research and clinical applications. J Am Soc Echocardiogr. 2009;22:1311-9.
18. Petersen JW, Pepine CJ. Microvascular coronary dysfunction and ischemic heart disease—where are we in 2014? Trends Cardiovasc Med. 2015;25(2):98-103.
19. Braescu L, Sturza A, Aburel OM, et al. Assessing the relationship between indexed epicardial adipose tissue thickness, oxidative stress in adipocytes, and coronary artery disease complexity in open-heart surgery patients. Medicina. 2024;60:177.
20. Pompei G, Ganzorig N, Kotanidis CP, et al. Novel diagnostic approaches and management of coronary microvascular dysfunction. Am J Prev Cardiol. 2024;19:100712.
21. Sena CM. Epicardial adipose tissue: an important therapeutic target. Rev Port Cardiol (Engl Ed). 2019;38(6):425-6.
22. Dey D, Nakazato R, Li D, et al. Epicardial and thoracic fat—noninvasive measurement and clinical implications of epicardial fat. Cardiovasc Diagn Ther. 2012;2(2):85-93.
23. Tran T, Small G, Cocker M, et al. A single slice measure of epicardial adipose tissue can serve as an indirect measure of total epicardial adipose tissue burden and is associated with obstructive coronary artery disease. Eur Heart J Cardiovasc Imaging. 2014;15(4):423-30.
24. Afrăsânie I, Matei IT, Leancă SA, et al. Ischemia with nonobstructive coronary artery disease and atrial cardiomyopathy—two sides of the same story? Life (Basel). 2023;13:443.
25. Sinha SK, Thakur R, Jha MJ, et al. Epicardial adipose tissue thickness and its association with the presence and severity of coronary artery disease in clinical setting: a cross-sectional observational study. J Clin Med Res. 2016;8(5):410-9.
26. Zhao E, Giamberardino SN, Pagidipati NJ, et al. Branched-chain amino acids in computed tomography-defined adipose depots and coronary artery disease: a PROMISE trial biomarker substudy. J Am Heart Assoc. 2023;12:e028410.
27. Wong CX, Mahajan R, Pathak R, et al. The role of pericardial and epicardial fat in atrial fibrillation pathophysiology and ablation outcomes. J Atr Fibrillation. 2013;5(5):790.
28. Ansari MA, Mohebati M, Poursadegh F, et al. Is echocardiographic epicardial fat thickness increased in patients with coronary artery disease? A systematic review and meta-analysis. Electron Physician. 2018;10(9): 7249-58.
29. Rossi VA, Nebunu D, Haider T, et al. Diverging role of epicardial adipose tissue across the entire heart failure spectrum. ESC Heart Fail. 2023;10:3419-29.
30. Filtz A, Lorenzatti D, Scotti A, et al. Relationship between epicardial adipose tissue and coronary atherosclerosis by CCTA in young adults (18–45). Am J Prev Cardiol. 2024;19:100711.
31. Eroğlu S. How do we measure epicardial adipose tissue thickness by transthoracic echocardiography? Anatol J Cardiol. 2015;15:416-9.

32. Hong H, Aksenov S, Guan X, et al. Remodeling of small intramyocardial coronary arteries distal to a severe epicardial coronary artery stenosis. Arterioscler Thromb Vasc Biol. 2002;22:2059-65.
33. Hirata Y, Yamada H, Kusunose K, et al. Clinical utility of measuring epicardial adipose tissue thickness with echocardiography using a high-frequency linear probe in patients with coronary artery disease. J Am Soc Echocardiogr. 2015;28:1240-6.e1.
34. Iacobellis G, Assael F, Ribaudo MC, et al. Epicardial fat from echocardiography: a new method for visceral adipose tissue prediction. Obes Res. 2003;11(2):304-10.
35. Rostamzadeh A, Khademvatani K, Mohammadzadeh MHS, et al. Association of epicardial fat thickness assessed by echocardiography with the severity of coronary artery disease. J Cardiovasc Thorac Res. 2020;12(2):114-9.
36. Nerlekar N, Baey Y-W, Brown AJ, et al. Poor correlation, reproducibility, and agreement between volumetric versus linear epicardial adipose tissue measurement: a 3D computed tomography versus 2D echocardiography comparison. JACC Cardiovasc Imaging. 2018;11(7):1035-6.
37. Trimarchi G, Carerj ML, Zito C, et al. Epicardial adipose tissue: a multimodal imaging diagnostic perspective. Medicina (Kaunas). 2025;61:961.
38. Chong B, Jayabaskaran J, Ruban J, et al; Epicardial adipose tissue assessed by computed tomography and echocardiography are associated with adverse cardiovascular outcomes: a systematic review and meta-analysis. Circ Cardiovasc Imaging. 2023;16:e015159.
39. Panda S, Vimala LR, Livingstone R, et al. Can epicardial and pericardial adipose tissue volume predict the presence and severity of coronary artery disease? Pol J Radiol. 2022;87:e348-53.
40. Santulli G, Varzideh F, Forzano I, et al. Functional and clinical importance of SGLT2 inhibitors in frailty: from the kidney to the heart. Hypertension. 2023;80:1800-9.
41. Checa Ros A, Okojie O-J, D'Marco L. SGLT2 inhibitors: multifaceted therapeutic agents in cardio metabolic and renal diseases. Metabolites. 2025;15:536.
42. Fulvio C, Ciro M, Valentina C, et al. Cardiometabolic crossroads: obesity, sleep-disordered breathing, and epicardial adipose tissue in heart failure with preserved ejection fraction—a mini-review. Heart Mind. 2025;9:147-56.
43. Yaribeygi H, Maleki M, Butler AE, et al. Sodium-glucose co-transporter-2 inhibitors and epicardial adiposity. Eur J Pharm Sci. 2023;180:106322.
44. Cinti F, Leccisotti L, Sorice GP, et al. Dapagliflozin treatment is associated with a reduction of epicardial adipose tissue thickness and epicardial glucose uptake in human type 2 diabetes. Cardiovasc Diabetol. 2023;22(1):349.
45. Bao Y, Hu Y, Shi M, et al. SGLT2 inhibitors reduce epicardial adipose tissue more than GLP-1 agonists or exercise interventions in patients with type 2 diabetes mellitus and/or obesity: a systematic review and network meta-analysis. Diabetes Obes Metab. 2025;27(3):1096-112.
46. Mullens W, Martens P. Empagliflozin-induced changes in epicardial fat: the centerpiece for myocardial protection? JACC Heart Fail. 2021;9(8):590-3.
47. Sato T, Aizawa Y, Yuasa S, et al. The effect of dapagliflozin treatment on epicardial adipose tissue volume and P-wave indices: an ad-hoc analysis of the previous randomized clinical trial. J Atheroscler Thromb. 2020;27(12):1348-58.
48. Ionică LN, Lința AV, Bătrîn AD, et al. The off-target cardio protective mechanisms of sodium-glucose cotransporter 2 inhibitors: an overview. Int J Mol Sci. 2024;25(14):7711.
49. Masson W, Lavalle-Cobo A, Nogueira JP. Effect of SGLT2 Inhibitors on epicardial adipose tissue: a meta-analysis. Cells. 2021;10(8):2150.
50. Iacobellis G, Gra-Menendez S. Effects of dapagliflozin on epicardial fat thickness in patients with type 2 diabetes and obesity. Obesity. 2020;28:1068-74.
51. Santosgallego CG, Requena-Ibanez JA, Botija MBP, et al. Abstract 15407: Benefits of the Sglt2 inhibitor empagliflozin on epicardial adipose tissue in non-diabetic Hfref. Circulation. 2022;146:15407.
52. Cinti F, Laborante R, Cappannoli L, et al. The effects of SGLT2i on cardiac metabolism in patients with HFpEF: fact or fiction? Cardiovasc Diabetol. 2025;24:208.
53. Banerjee M. Epicardial fat paradox and differential effects of GLP-1 receptor agonists across heart failure phenotypes. Circulation: Heart Fail. 2023;16(12):010966.
54. Yaribeygi H, Maleki M, Nasimi F, et al. Benefits of GLP-1 mimetics on epicardial adiposity. Curr Med Chem. 2023;30(37):4256-65.
55. Berg G, Barchuk M, Lobo M, et al. Effect of glucagon-like peptide-1 (GLP-1) analogues on epicardial adipose tissue: a meta-analysis. Diabetes Metab Syndr Clin Res Rev. 2022;16(7):102562.
56. Iacobellis G, Malavazos AE. How semaglutide effects on epicardial fat inflammation can be good for the heart. J Am Coll Cardiol. 2025;85(1):e7.
57. Dozio E, Vianello E, Malavazos AE, et al. Epicardial adipose tissue GLP-1 receptor is associated with genes involved in fatty acid oxidation and white-to-brown fat differentiation: a target to modulate cardiovascular risk? Int J Cardiol. 2019:292:218-24.
58. Schwartz RS, Burke A, Farb A, et al. Microemboli and microvascular obstruction in acute coronary thrombosis and sudden coronary death: relation to epicardial plaque histopathology. J Am Coll Cardiol. 2009;54(23):2167-73.
59. Benčević M, Galić I, Habijan M, et al. Recent progress in epicardial and pericardial adipose tissue segmentation and quantification based on deep learning: a systematic review. Appl Sci. 2022;12:5217.
60. Fred HL. Pericardial fat necrosis: a review and update. Tex Heart Inst J. 2010;37(1):82-4.
61. Couto J, dos Santos LP, Mendes EM, et al. Epicardial fat necrosis: a rare and benign cause of chest pain. Revista Portuguesa de Cardiologia. 2020;39:113-4.

85

CHAPTER

Empagliflozin versus Dapagliflozin in Diabetic Kidney Disease

Muthu Jayaraman, Rajeevalochana Parthasarathy,
Guhan Senthilkumaran, Veenaa Manjari S

INTRODUCTION

Chronic kidney disease (CKD) is fast becoming one of the world's most prevalent chronic noncommunicable diseases. The World Health Organization (WHO) projects CKD to become the fifth most common chronic disease by 2040.[1] This CKD pandemic is driven primarily by an aging global population and the rampant rise of metabolic risk factors such as diabetes, hypertension, and obesity. These stark realities underscore the urgent need for effective therapeutic interventions for CKD.

Diabetic Kidney Disease—The Principal Catalyst of the Chronic Kidney Disease Surge

Diabetic kidney disease (DKD) stands out as the major etiology of CKD and end-stage kidney disease (ESKD) worldwide. Almost 30% of diabetics can have kidney disease and the presence of kidney disease amplifies cardiovascular morbidity and mortality.[2] The clinical spectrum of DKD is remarkably heterogeneous, ranging from modest albuminuria with preserved estimated glomerular filtration rate (eGFR) to rapidly progressive disease. In India, it is estimated that over 100 million adults are living with diabetes, with an additional 130 million at risk of developing the disease.[3,4]

EVOLVING THERAPEUTIC STRATEGIES FOR DIABETIC KIDNEY DISEASE

While the statistics surrounding diabetes and DKD have been alarming, we have thankfully witnessed a significant evolution in the therapeutic armamentarium for DKD. While initial care generally focused on glycemic and blood-pressure control and on delaying the progression to end-stage renal disease, well-evidenced interventions have contributed significantly to sustained improvement in patient outcomes over the last two decades. Contemporary reviews and clinical guidelines now recommend a "four-pillar" strategy for comprehensive kidney protection in DKD. This strategy encompasses (1) renin–angiotensin–aldosterone system (RAAS) blockade, (2) sodium–glucose cotransporter 2 inhibitors (SGLT2i), (3) GLP-1 agonists, and (4) nonsteroidal mineralocorticoid receptor antagonists.[5]

DISCOVERY OF SODIUM–GLUCOSE COTRANSPORTER 2 INHIBITORS—A STORY OF SWEET SERENDIPITY

Sodium-glucose cotransporter 2 inhibition has emerged as a truly paradigm-shifting therapeutic approach. The story of the discovery of SGLT2i, quite remarkably, begins from the bark of an apple tree. In 1835, Belgian chemists Laurent-Guillaume de Koninck and Jean Servais Stas isolated natural glycoside "phlorizin" from the tree and proposed that it may be utilized for its anti-inflammatory properties similar to prior bark extracts.[6] Later in the 19th and 20th centuries, von Mering made interesting observations as to the blood–glucose lowering effects of the drug by increasing urinary sugar levels. The sodium–glucose cotransport with SGLT-1 and SGLT-2 receptors was later enlightened by Dr Robert Kellogg Crane, whose team also proved that phlorizin was a potent inhibitor of both. The breakthrough came with the design of C-glucoside scaffolds by along with other structural refinements that produced potent, orally bioavailable, SGLT2-selective agents with better pharmacokinetic stability and clinical profiles.[7] The first clinically available gliflozin was dapagliflozin which received the U.S. Food and Drug Administration (FDA) approval in 2014. Empagliflozin and Canagliflozin soon followed as added agents to this class of drugs.

THE SODIUM–GLUCOSE COTRANSPORTER 2 INHIBITORS MECHANISM: A RISING TIDE FOR THE NEPHRONS

To understand the relative parity of dapagliflozin and empagliflozin, it is crucial to appreciate their shared mechanism of action. These agents block the SGLT2 protein in the kidney's proximal tubules, which is responsible for reabsorbing about 90% of filtered glucose and induce glycosuria and natriuresis.[8] **Figure 1 and Table 1** elucidate the mechanism of action of SGLT2i and differences between the types of SGLT receptors. The resulting benefits, beyond glucose control, include:

- *Reduced intraglomerular pressure:* The increased sodium delivery to the macula densa restores the tubuloglomerular feedback mechanism, which constricts the afferent arteriole and reduces intraglomerular pressure.
- *Mitigation of inflammation and fibrosis:* SGLT2i have demonstrated anti-inflammatory and antifibrotic effects, which help combat the underlying pathological processes that drive DKD progression.
- *Lowered blood pressure and weight:* The osmotic diuresis and reduced systemic volume load lead to modest but clinically significant decreases in blood pressure and body weight, which further reduce kidney damage.

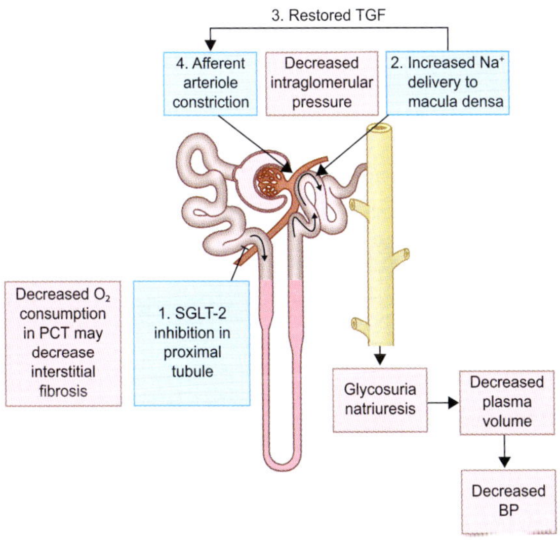

Fig. 1: Mechanism of action of SGLT2 inhibitors. SGLT2 inhibition in the proximal convoluted tubule prevents sodium and glucose reabsorption. Increased sodium delivery to distal tubules is sensed by the macula densa. Macula densa signals the afferent arteriole to constrict via tubuloglomerular feedback, reducing blood flow to the glomerulus and lowering the GFR. (TGF: tubuloglomerular feedback)

Pharmacokinetic and Pharmacodynamic Differences Between Dapagliflozin and Empagliflozin

It is important to understand the differences in the molecular characteristics of empagliflozin and dapagliflozin. **Table 2** shows the differences in characteristics of the two molecules. Empagliflozin is more water soluble with higher affinity to SGLT2 while dapagliflozin is more lipophilic with better tissue penetration.[9]

Trials of Empagliflozin and Dapagliflozin in Kidney Disease

Multiple large randomized controlled trials have established the benefits of both empagliflozin and dapagliflozin in CKD, significantly reducing the risk of

TABLE 1: Comparison of SGLT1 and SGLT2 receptors.

Characteristic	*SGLT1*	*SGLT2*
Primary location	Small intestine; late proximal convoluted tubule (segment 3)	Early proximal convoluted tubule (segments 1 and 2)
Transport capacity	Low	High
Affinity for glucose	High	Low
Contribution to renal glucose reabsorption	~10%	~90%
Genetic/functional defect	Glucose–galactose malabsorption	Familial renal glycosuria
Clinical manifestations of defect	Severe diarrhea in infancy	Benign course
Natural course (if untreated)/inhibitors	Fatal without lactose/galactose-free diet	Currently available SGLT2 inhibitors

TABLE 2: Differences in the pharmacokinetic and pharmacodynamic profile of dapagliflozin and empagliflozin.

Property	Dapagliflozin	Empagliflozin	Significance
Chemical formula	$C_{21}H_{25}ClO_6$	$C_{23}H_{27}ClO_7$	Empagliflozin is slightly bulkier and more hydroxylated, contributing to subtle differences in solubility and affinity
Molecular weight	408.88 g/mol	450.91 g/mol	
Aryl substituent	4-chloro-3-(4-ethoxybenzyl) phenyl group	4-chloro-3-(4-(3-hydroxy-tetrahydrofuran-3-yl)oxy-benzyl)phenyl group	Empagliflozin has a more polar, oxygen-rich side chain, enhancing hydrogen bonding with SGLT2 residues
Hydroxyl groups	Fewer hydroxyl moieties	Additional hydroxyl group on the side chain	Empagliflozin shows higher water solubility and selectivity for SGLT2 over SGLT1
SGLT2:SGLT1 selectivity	1,200:1	2,500:1	
Lipophilicity (logP)	1.8	1.4	Dapagliflozin is more lipophilic-increased nonspecific binding, broader tissue penetration

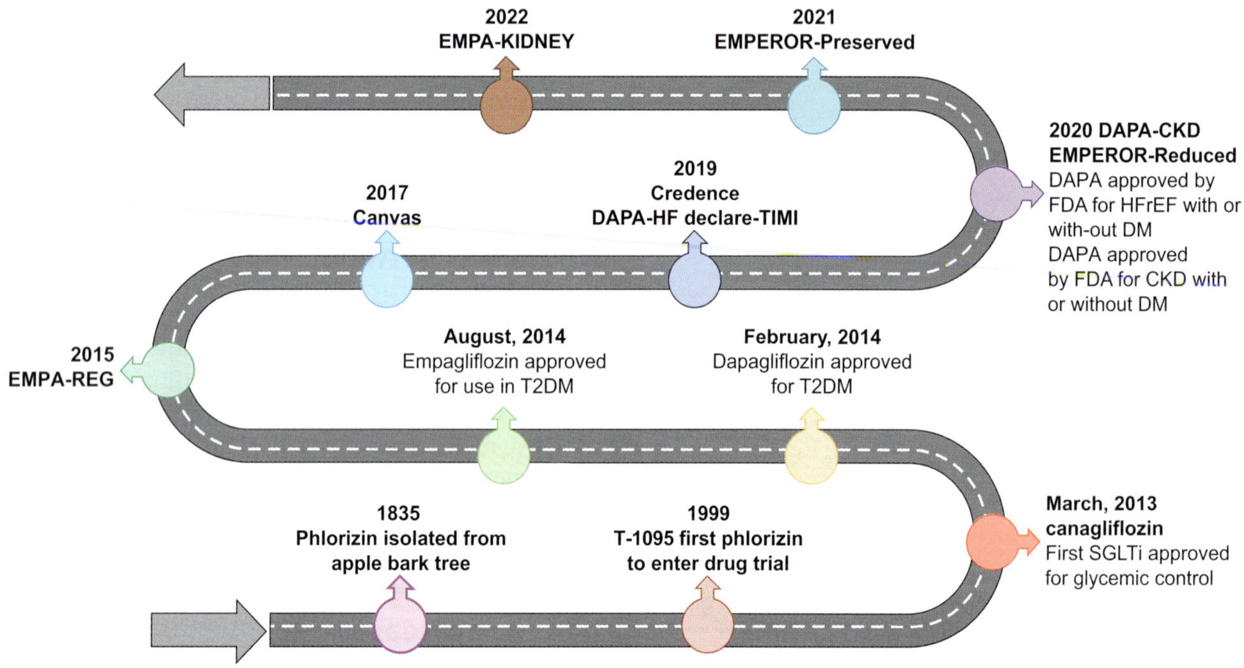

Fig. 2: Roadmap of SGLT2i and the major trials. Timeline summarizing development and approval of SGLT2i with important trials. SGLT2i: sodium–glucose cotransporter-2 inhibitors; HFrEF: heart failure with reduced ejection fraction.

kidney disease progression, cardiovascular events, and mortality in both diabetic and nondiabetic populations. The initial trials EMPA-REG,[10] CANVAS,[11] and DECLARE-TIMI 58[12] were cardiovascular trials, primarily designed to satisfy the FDA guidance on proving cardiovascular safety, which serendipitously revealed not just safety but reduced adverse cardiovascular and kidney outcomes with these drugs. CREDENCE was the first study to focus on patients at high risk of kidney outcomes and promote those outcomes to the primary end point. After CREDENCE,[13] SGLT2i were firmly entrenched as the standard of care in the treatment of DKD.

The EMPA-KIDNEY[14] and DAPA-CKD trials[15] are landmark studies evaluating SGLT2i for CKD. Both trials demonstrated significant benefit in reducing kidney disease progression and cardiovascular events, but there are differences in design, populations, and outcome magnitude. **Figure 2** illustrates the roadmap of the trials and discovery of the various SGLT2i.

Empagliflozin in Kidney Disease

- The *EMPA-KIDNEY* trial[14] was a large, randomized, controlled study enrolling 6,609 patients with CKD, irrespective of diabetes status. Participants received empagliflozin 10 mg or placebo. Over a median of 2 years, empagliflozin reduced the composite risk of kidney disease progression (including ESKD, sustained large drop in eGFR, or death from cardiovascular causes) with a hazard ratio (HR) of 0.72 (95% CI: 0.64–0.82; $p < 0.001$). Benefits were consistent across both diabetic and nondiabetic groups.[16] The trial also found fewer hospitalizations for any cause in the empagliflozin group, while adverse events were similar between groups. Secondary analyses confirmed renoprotective effects across a spectrum of primary kidney diseases like IgA nephropathy and DKD.[17]

Dapagliflozin in Kidney Disease

- The *DAPA-CKD* trial,[15] a randomized double-blind placebo-controlled multicenter study, enrolled 4,304 patients with CKD (eGFR 25–75 mL/min/1.73 m^2, urinary ACR 200–5,000 mg/g), randomizing them to dapagliflozin 10 mg or placebo. The trial was stopped early for the profound efficacy it demonstrated. Over a median of 2.4 years, dapagliflozin reduced the primary outcome risk (sustained ≥50% eGFR decline, kidney failure, or renal/cardiovascular death) with an HR of 0.61 (95% CI: 0.51–0.72; $p < 0.001$). Mortality was reduced (HR for death: 0.69, 95% CI: 0.53–0.88). Benefits were observed in both those with and without diabetes. Longer term modeling of trial data predicted that dapagliflozin could delay time to kidney failure by more than 6 years for patients at risk.[18,19] The DAPA-CKD trial served as a powerful illustration of dapagliflozin's broad renoprotective effects.

Both the trials provide a powerful illustration of the independence of SGLT2i-related kidney benefits from its glucose-lowering effects. Both agents provided a consistent benefit across the trial population, proving that the reno- and cardioprotective mechanisms of SGLT2 inhibition are not strictly tied to the presence of diabetes. This was a watershed moment, solidifying SGLT2i place as a cornerstone therapy for CKD, extending its use far beyond its initial indication for type 2 diabetes.[20]

Key Safety Signals for Empagliflozin Versus Dapagliflozin in Chronic Kidney Disease

Empagliflozin and dapagliflozin have comparable and favorable safety profiles in CKD patients, with key adverse events overall infrequent and consistent between agents according to head-to-head analyses and major trials.[21]

Safety Profiles of Empagliflozin and Dapagliflozin

- *Genital infections:* Slightly increased risk of genital mycotic infections for both, but mostly mild and manageable
- *Volume depletion/hypotension:* Both agents may cause low blood pressure or dehydration, especially in frail or elderly patients with concomitant diuretic use; monitoring is advised. Patients should be counseled regarding the importance of hydration and "Sick day" rules.[22]
- *Acute kidney injury:* The risk is not higher than placebo and may even be lower due to protective effects, despite transient eGFR dip after initiation.[23]
- *Diabetic ketoacidosis:* Rare, more frequent in type 1 diabetes or insulin-dependent patients, but caution and patient selection are important.
- *No increase in hyperkalemia or hypoglycemia:* Not significantly increased over placebo in large-scale studies
- Both drugs have been confirmed safe in CKD patients down to eGFR 20–25 mL/min/1.73 m^2, and safety is maintained even in high-risk comorbid populations when proper precautions are taken.
- Specific exclusion of patients with type 1 diabetes, recent serious infection, or pregnancy applies equally to both agents.

Comparative Findings (Empagliflozin vs. Dapagliflozin)

- Direct comparisons and post hoc analyses suggest no substantial difference in major adverse events between empagliflozin and dapagliflozin in CKD.[21]
- The rates of discontinuation due to adverse events are similar.
- Some analyses show dapagliflozin prevention value is higher for cardiovascular disease, while empagliflozin may show slightly better results for preventing CKD progression, but these are efficacy signals rather than distinct adverse event profiles.
- Both agents appear safe and well tolerated, with similar rates of infections, hypovolemia, acute illness-associated temporary eGFR fall, or serious adverse events.

Cost Implications

- In the Indian context, a head-to-head cost comparison of the innovator molecules for empagliflozin (Jardiance™) and dapagliflozin (Forxiga™) is almost similar at around 520–550 INR. In addition, with the expiry of the patent period, multiple generic brands that are quite effective have been made available at far more affordable rates for both molecules. Hence, cost considerations alone do not warrant preferential selection of one molecule over the other.

CONCLUSION

To summarize, when comparing dapagliflozin and empagliflozin in the context of DKD, the practical illustration is one of functional equivalence for the vast majority of patients. The choice between them, therefore, often boils down to subtle differences in cost, availability, or nuanced secondary outcomes that emerged from trial analyses. While one study may hint at a slightly different effect on blood pressure or specific cardiovascular endpoints, these differences are not consistently observed in head-to-head comparisons for diabetic patients and do not indicate a significant clinical superiority of one drug over the other for DKD.

In essence, dapagliflozin and empagliflozin are two artists working with the same palette of therapeutic tools. Their landmark trials, DAPA-CKD and EMPA-KIDNEY, are distinct masterpieces that, when viewed together, illustrate the same powerful truth: SGLT2i offer a new and indispensable standard of care for patients with DKD, providing a strong armamentarium against the forces of renal decline and cardiovascular risk.[24] For most clinicians and patients, the focus can be placed on adopting this therapeutic class, as the choice between these equally effective agents is of secondary importance.

Table 3 demonstrates the main differences between EMPA-KIDNEY and DAPA-KIDNEY trials.

TABLE 3: Main differences between EMPA-KIDNEY and DAPA-KIDNEY trials.

	EMPA-KIDNEY	*DAPA-CKD*
Drug/dose	Empagliflozin 10 mg daily	Dapagliflozin 10 mg daily
Sample size	6,609	4,304
Median follow-up (years)	2.0	2.4
Population	CKD with and without diabetes (54% diabetes)	CKD with and without diabetes (67% diabetes)
Inclusion–eGFR/uACR	• 20–<45 mL/min/1.73 m^2 or 45–<90 with uACR ≥ 200 mg/g • ≥200 mg/g if eGFR ≥ 45; no minimum if <45	• 25–75 mL/min/1.73 m^2 • 200–5000 mg/g (required)
Background therapy	RAAS blockade encouraged (not mandatory)	Mandatory maximally tolerated ACEi/ARB (unless contraindicated)
Primary composite outcome	Kidney disease progression (≥40% eGFR decline, ESKD, renal, or CV death)	Sustained ≥50% eGFR decline, ESKD, renal, or CV death
Primary outcome event rate	Empa 13.1% versus placebo 16.9%	Dapa 9.2% versus placebo 14.5%
Primary outcome HR (95% CI)	0.72 (0.64–0.82), $p < 0.001$	0.61 (0.51–0.72), $p < 0.001$
Relative risk reduction (RRR) (%)	28	39
Absolute risk reduction (ARR) (%)	3.8	5.3
All-cause mortality HR	0.84 (0.73–0.96)	0.69 (0.53–0.88)
Kidney-specific outcome HR	0.71 (0.62–0.81)	0.56 (0.45–0.68)
Effect in nondiabetic CKD	HR 0.78 (0.66–0.91)	HR 0.50 (0.35–0.72)
Effect in diabetic CKD	HR 0.68 (0.57–0.81)	HR 0.64 (0.52–0.79)
Effect by baseline eGFR	Benefit consistent down to eGFR <30	Benefit consistent down to eGFR 25
Hospitalization (any cause)	HR 0.86 (0.78–0.95)	HR 0.79 (0.71–0.89)
Safety	Genital infections ↑; no increase in AKI or DKA	Genital infections ↑; no excess AKI; rare DKA
Distinctive feature	Broader CKD population, including low albuminuria and advanced CKD	Required albuminuria; stronger signal in proteinuric CKD
Clinical implication	Extends SGLT2i benefit to broader CKD phenotypes	Confirms renal and mortality benefit in albuminuric CKD

Note: DAPA-CKD showed stronger absolute benefit in a higher-risk, albuminuric cohort. EMPA-KIDNEY expanded generalizability to patients with lower albuminuria and more advanced CKD, including nondiabetic etiologies.

REFERENCES

1. Borg R, Carlson N, Søndergaard J, et al. The growing challenge of chronic kidney disease: an overview of current knowledge. Int J Nephrol. 2023;2023:9609266.
2. Hoogeveen EK. The epidemiology of diabetic kidney disease. Kidney Dial. 2022;2:433-42.
3. Anjana RM, Unnikrishnan R, Deepa M, et al. Metabolic non-communicable disease health report of India: the ICMR-INDIAB national cross-sectional study (ICMR-INDIAB-17). Lancet Diabetes Endocrinol. 2023; 11(7):474-89.
4. Afkarian M, Sachs MC, Kestenbaum B, et al. Kidney disease and increased mortality risk in type 2 diabetes. J Am Soc Nephrol. 2013;24:302-8.
5. Naaman SC, Bakris GL. Diabetic nephropathy: update on pillars of therapy slowing progression. Diabetes Care. 2023;46(9):1574-86.
6. Ehrenkranz JRL, Lewis NG, Kahn CR, et al. Phlorizin: a review. Diabetes Metab Res Rev. 2005;21(1):31-8.
7. Panchapakesan U, Pegg K, Gross S, et al. Effects of SGLT2 inhibition in human kidney proximal tubular cells—renoprotection in diabetic nephropathy? PLoS One. 2013;8(2);e54442.
8. Fonseca-Correa JI, Correa-Rotter R. Sodium-glucose cotransporter 2 inhibitors mechanisms of action: a review. Front Med (Lausanne). 2021;8:777861.
9. Ramani J, Shah H, Vyas VK, et al. A review on the medicinal chemistry of sodium-glucose co-transporter 2 (SGLT2) inhibitors (SGLT2-I): update from 2010 to present. Eur J Med Chem Rep. 2022;6:100074.
10. Zinman B, Wanner C, Lachin JM, et al.; EMPA-REG OUTCOME Investigators. Empagliflozin, cardiovascular outcomes, and mortality in type 2 diabetes. N Engl J Med. 2015;373(22):2117-28.
11. Neal B, Perkovic V, Mahaffey KW, et al.; CANVAS Program Collaborative Group. Canagliflozin and cardiovascular and renal events in type 2 diabetes. N Engl J Med. 2017;377(7):644-57.
12. Wiviott SD, Raz I, Bonaca MP, et al.; DECLARE–TIMI 58 Investigators. Dapagliflozin and cardiovascular outcomes in type 2 diabetes. N Engl J Med. 2019;380(4):347-57.
13. Perkovic V, Jardine MJ, Neal B, et al.; CREDENCE Trial Investigators. Canagliflozin and renal outcomes in type 2 diabetes and nephropathy. N Engl J Med. 2019;380(24):2295-306.
14. The EMPA-KIDNEY Collaborative Group; Herrington WG, Staplin N, et al. Empagliflozin in patients with chronic kidney disease. N Engl J Med. 2023;388(2):117-27.
15. Heerspink HJL, Stefánsson BV, Correa-Rotter R, et al.; DAPA-CKD Trial Committees and Investigators. Dapagliflozin in patients with chronic kidney disease. N Engl J Med. 2020;383(15):1436-46.
16. EMPA-KIDNEY Collaborative Group. Impact of primary kidney disease on the effects of empagliflozin in patients with chronic kidney disease: secondary analyses of the EMPA-KIDNEY trial. Lancet Diabetes Endocrinol. 2024;12(1):51-60.
17. EMPA-KIDNEY Collaborative Group. Effects of empagliflozin on progression of chronic kidney disease: a prespecified secondary analysis from the empa-kidney trial. Lancet Diabetes Endocrinol. 2024;12(1):39-50.
18. McEwan P, Gabb PD, Davis JA, et al. The long-term effects of dapagliflozin in chronic kidney disease: a time-to-event analysis. Randomized Controlled Trial. 2024;39(12):2040-7.
19. Chertow GM, Correa-Rotter R, Vart P, et al.; DAPA-CKD Trial Committees and Investigators. Effects of dapagliflozin in chronic kidney disease, with and without other cardiovascular medications: DAPA-CKD Trial. J Am Heart Assoc. 2023;12(9):e028739.
20. Krishnan A, Shankar M, Lerma EV, et al.; GlomCon Editorial Team. Sodium glucose cotransporter 2 (SGLT2) inhibitors and CKD: Are You a #Flozinator? Kidney Med. 2023;5(4):100608.
21. Alnsasra H, Tsaban G, Solomon A, et al. Dapagliflozin versus empagliflozin in patients with chronic kidney disease. Front Pharmacol. 2023;14:1227199.
22. Lam D, Shaikh A. Real-life prescribing of SGLT2 inhibitors: how to handle the other medications, including glucose-lowering drugs and diuretics. Kidney360. 2021;2(4):742-6.
23. Menne J, Dumann E, Haller H, et al. Acute kidney injury and adverse renal events in patients receiving SGLT2-inhibitors: a systematic review and meta-analysis. PLoS Med. 2019;16(12):e1002983.
24. Qiu M, Ding LL, Zhang M, et al. Safety of four SGLT2 inhibitors in three chronic diseases: a meta-analysis of large randomized trials of SGLT2 inhibitors. Diab Vasc Dis Res. 2021;18(2):14791641211011016.

CHAPTER 86

Future Directions: Empagliflozin in Obesity Prevention and Treatment Paradigms

Ajay K Sinha

INTRODUCTION

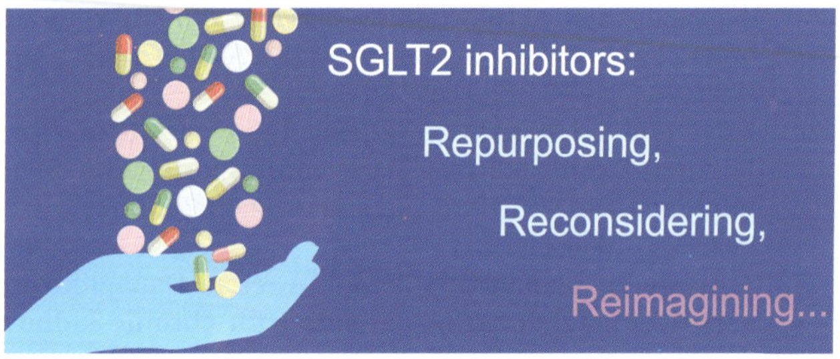

Empagliflozin represents a paradigm shift from simple weight reduction to holistic metabolic restoration. By targeting insulin resistance, ectopic fat deposition and cardiometabolic risk rather than only BMI reduction, empagliflozin is expected to play an increasingly significant role in future obesity management frameworks—possibly forming the backbone of next-generation precision-metabolic therapy.

Obesity is a chronic, multifactorial, and morbid disease. It represents a growing public health challenge in India, with prevalence rates rising rapidly due to urbanization, dietary shifts, and sedentary lifestyles. Recent data indicate high burdens, particularly abdominal obesity, linked to noncommunicable diseases (NCDs) such as diabetes and cardiovascular issues. Economic costs are projected to escalate dramatically by 2030.[1]

National surveys show obesity affecting a significant portion of adults aged 18–54 years, with overweight and obesity more than doubling since 1980. India ranks third globally in obese population percentage, using a BMI threshold above 27.5 tailored to Asian populations. Projections estimate India among the top three countries for obesity by 2050, especially among women.[2]

EPIDEMIOLOGY AND PATHOPHYSIOLOGY OF OBESITY

Obesity is a global health crisis, contributing to increased morbidity and mortality through its association with type 2 diabetes, cardiovascular disease, chronic kidney disease, and heart failure. The pathophysiology of obesity is multifactorial, involving dysregulation of energy homeostasis, adipokine secretion, chronic inflammation, and ectopic fat deposition.[3,4]

Visceral adiposity, in particular, is a key driver of metabolic complications, with epicardial and hepatic fat depots implicated in the pathogenesis of heart failure with preserved ejection fraction (HFpEF) and nonalcoholic fatty liver disease.[5]

EMPAGLIFLOZIN IN OBESITY

Empagliflozin, a sodium-glucose cotransporter-2 (SGLT2) inhibitor, has emerged as a promising agent in the evolving landscape of obesity prevention and treatment. While its primary indication remains glycemic control in type 2 diabetes, accumulating evidence suggests that empagliflozin exerts pleiotropic effects on adipose tissue biology, metabolic homeostasis, and organ protection, positioning it as a candidate for future obesity management strategies.

MECHANISMS OF EMPAGLIFLOZIN IN ADIPOSE TISSUE AND METABOLIC REGULATION

Sodium-glucose cotransporter-2 inhibitors increase urinary glucose excretion (UGE), thereby reducing hyperglycemia and weight with apparent pleiotropic effects. When large amounts of glucose are forced into urinary excretion processes, whole-body metabolism undergoes adaptive changes involving glucose fluxes, hormonal responses, and fuel selection. Recent clinical studies have shown that the treatment of type 2 diabetes with SGLT2 inhibitors paradoxically increases endogenous glucose production (EGP) despite an overall reduction in fasting hyperglycemia. Moreover, the chronic administration of empagliflozin drives a fuel shift in which tissue glucose disposal decreases, and lipid use increases, although the mechanisms underlying these effects have yet to be determined.

Sodium-glucose cotransporter-2 inhibition by empagliflozin increases glucosuria, thereby reducing hyperglycemia and weight with pleiotropic effects in obesity: (1) Empagliflozin promotes fat utilization by activating AMPK in skeletal muscle. (2) Empagliflozin increases fibroblast growth factor (FGF) 21 levels in blood and promotes browning of adipose tissue, thereby increasing thermogenesis and energy expenditure. (3) Empagliflozin reduces M1-polarised macrophage accumulation while inducing the anti-inflammatory M2 phenotype of macrophages within fat and liver, attenuating obesity-induced inflammation and insulin resistance.

The primary and secondary mechanisms contributing to empagliflozin's anti-obesity effects include:

- *Caloric loss via glucosuria:* By blocking SGLT2, empagliflozin prevents approximately 90% of glucose reabsorption back into the bloodstream from the kidney's proximal tubules. This excess glucose (and its associated calories) is excreted in the urine (glucosuria), creating a negative energy balance that leads to weight loss.
- *Increased energy expenditure:* Preclinical studies suggest that empagliflozin increases whole-body energy expenditure and heat production (thermogenesis). This is partly achieved by promoting the "browning" of white adipose tissue (WAT) into brown-like adipocytes, which are more metabolically active and burn energy instead of storing it as fat.
- *Enhanced fat utilization:* The body compensates for the loss of glucose-derived energy by shifting its metabolism towards increased fat utilization and oxidation. This involves:
  - Activation of AMP-activated protein kinase (AMPK) in skeletal muscle, which promotes the breakdown of fatty acids.
  - Increased levels of fibroblast growth factor 21 (FGF21), a hormone that helps regulate energy metabolism and fat oxidation.

Reduction of adiposity and inflammation: Empagliflozin leads to a reduction in both subcutaneous and visceral fat depots, with particular efficacy in reducing visceral adipose tissue (VAT), which is highly associated with metabolic risk. It also attenuates obesity-induced chronic inflammation by reducing pro-inflammatory M1 macrophages and promoting anti-inflammatory M2 macrophages in fat and liver tissues.

Improved insulin sensitivity: The reduction in body weight, fat mass, and inflammation helps improve overall insulin sensitivity, thereby breaking the cycle of hyperglycemia and hyperinsulinemia commonly associated with type 2 diabetes and obesity.[6]

CLINICAL EVIDENCE: EMPAGLIFLOZIN IN OBESITY AND METABOLIC DISEASE

Short-term RCTs consistently demonstrate benefits, with greater effects observed at higher doses and in specific subgroups **(Tables 1 and 2)**.

ONGOING AND EMERGING EVIDENCE

Trials such as NCT05042973 assess metabolic effects in non-T2D obesity, while NCT06762314 evaluates empagliflozin versus tirzepatide in overweight T1D, targeting 5–10% reductions. Long-term data from EMPRISE (real-world) show sustained 2–4 kg loss over 2 years with CV/renal protection. Gaps remain in primary obesity prevention of RCTs without diabetes comorbidity.

Clinical studies have demonstrated that empagliflozin reduces body mass index, body fat, and visceral fat in patients with obesity and type 2 diabetes, with additional benefits on leptin resistance and renal function. The EmDia trial identified significant alterations in plasma lipid classes, notably lysophosphatidylcholines (LPCs), after empagliflozin treatment, correlating with improvements in estimated glomerular filtration rate, uric acid, and blood pressure. These findings suggest that empagliflozin-induced lipidome remodeling may contribute to its metabolic and organ-protective effects.[3,7]

The Empire Prevent trial program is currently evaluating empagliflozin in elderly and obese patients without diabetes or established heart failure, focusing on its impact on physical capacity, cardiac structure,

TABLE 1: Overview of included studies, study populations, intervention characteristics, and reported weight-related outcomes.

Trial/study	Population (n)	Duration	Intervention	Weight change (kg)	Other outcomes	Citation
2025 RCT (Nature) nature	T2D/prediabetes with obesity (n = NR)	12 weeks	Empagliflozin 10 mg QD	–6.3 (max); dose-dependent	↓BMI, ↓HbA1c, ↓waist; greater in males, GFR >90	nature
EMPA-REG OUTCOME substudy pmc.ncbi.nlm.nih	T2D (n = NR)	24 weeks	Empagliflozin 10/25 mg	–2.0 to –3.0 vs. placebo	↓Adipose inflammation, ↓visceral fat	pmc.ncbi.nlm.nih
NCT01131676 (Phase III) clinicaltrials	T2D (n = 986)	24 weeks	Empagliflozin 10/25 mg	–2.2 to –2.96 vs. placebo	↓Body weight indices	clinicaltrials
NCT01210001 (Phase III) clinicaltrials	T2D (n = NR)	24 weeks	Empagliflozin mono	–2.5 avg	↓BMI, safety profile	clinicaltrials

TABLE 2: Overview of analytical approaches, study populations, and reported weight reduction outcomes.

Analysis	Studies/population	Key findings	Weight reduction	Citation
SGLT2i dosage meta (2023) onlinelibrary.wiley	25 RCTs, T2D (n >10 k)	Dose-response: higher dose > weight loss	1–3 kg (10–25 mg)	onlinelibrary.wiley
SGLT2i weight loss review onlinelibrary.wiley	Multiple RCTs	Mechanisms: glucosuria, fat utilization	1.5–2.5 kg sustained	onlinelibrary.wiley
Emerging SGLT2 role pmc.ncbi.nlm.nih	T2D/obesity reviews	Beyond glucose: cardiometabolic benefits	Consistent 2–4% body weight	pmc.ncbi.nlm.nih

epicardial adipose tissue, and volume homeostasis. This investigator-initiated, double-blind, randomized clinical trial represents a critical step toward elucidating the preventive potential of SGLT2 inhibition in high-risk populations.[8] Mechanistic endpoints, such as changes in epicardial adipose tissue and extracellular volume, will provide insights into the role of empagliflozin in modulating cardiac-adipose tissue interactions and preventing heart failure **(Flowchart 1)**.[8]

RENAL PROTECTION AND INFLAMMATION MODULATION

Obesity-related kidney disease is an emerging concern, with chronic inflammation and oxidative stress driving renal injury. Empagliflozin has demonstrated renoprotective effects in obese mice, alleviating lipid deposition, glomerular and tubular injury, and regulating metabolites involved in phospholipid, purine, and biliverdin metabolism. These metabolic changes are associated with improved oxidative stress and inflammation balance, supporting the potential of empagliflozin to delay the progression of obesity-related kidney disease.[7,9]

While empagliflozin's weight reduction is modest compared to incretin analogues, its unique effects on visceral adiposity, adipokine modulation, and organ protection distinguish it from other agents. Ongoing trials, including those evaluating dapagliflozin, will further clarify the role of SGLT2 inhibitors in obesity management.[4,5]

FUTURE RESEARCH DIRECTIONS

The future of empagliflozin in obesity prevention and treatment will be shaped by ongoing and future clinical trials, mechanistic studies, and real-world evidence. Key research priorities include (1) Elucidating the long-term effects of empagliflozin on weight maintenance, visceral adiposity, and metabolic health in non-diabetic populations;[8,9] (2) Defining the optimal patient populations for empagliflozin therapy, including those with high cardiometabolic risk, established organ dysfunction, or leptin resistance;[7-9] (3) Investigating the molecular mechanisms underlying empagliflozin's effects on adipose tissue biology, adipokine secretion, and lipid metabolism;[7,5] (4) Assessing the impact of empagliflozin on obesity-related complications, including heart failure, chronic kidney disease, and non-alcoholic fatty liver disease;[4,7-9] and (5) Evaluating cost-effectiveness, accessibility, and long-term safety in diverse and underrepresented populations.[4]

Flowchart 1: Overview of the Empire Prevent trial program illustrating the proposed cardiac and metabolic effects of empagliflozin.

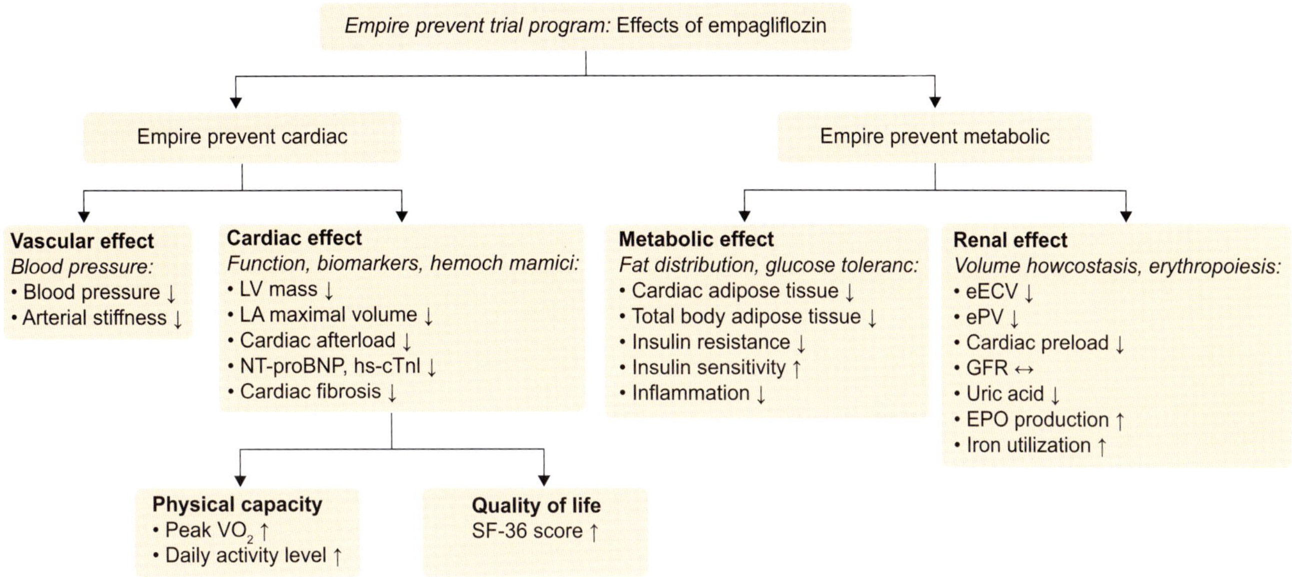

Large-scale RCTs are needed to evaluate empagliflozin monotherapy or combinations (e.g., with GLP-1 agonists) for primary obesity prevention in high-risk groups such as prediabetes or metabolic syndrome. Long-term studies should assess cardiovascular, renal, and NAFLD outcomes in non-diabetic obese populations, building on mouse models showing aortic protection via fatty acid metabolism improvements. Precision dosing based on GFR, sex, and ethnicity, plus biomarkers for responders, warrants investigation.[10,11]

CONCLUSION

Empagliflozin represents a novel and multifaceted approach to obesity prevention and treatment, with mechanistic, translational, and clinical evidence supporting its role in modulating adipose tissue biology, metabolic homeostasis, and organ protection. While its weight loss effects are modest, the disproportionate reduction in visceral adiposity, favorable adipokine profile, and organ-protective properties position empagliflozin as a candidate for future obesity management paradigms. Ongoing clinical trials and mechanistic studies will further define their place in the therapeutic armamentarium, with the potential to address the unmet needs of patients with obesity and related cardiometabolic complications.

Empagliflozin represents a pivotal therapeutic evolution from weight-loss orientation to *comprehensive metabolic restoration*. By influencing insulin resistance, adipose distribution, hepatic steatosis, and cardiovascular risk—rather than focusing solely on BMI—it holds the potential to redefine obesity management. Future obesity paradigms are likely to integrate empagliflozin into *combination regimens, early prevention strategies and precision-based metabolic phenotyping*. With ongoing trials in non-diabetic obesity and NAFLD, empagliflozin may soon become a cornerstone of next-generation obesity therapeutics that link metabolic health, cardiovascular protection, and weight control.

REFERENCES

1. Gupta RD, Tamanna N, Siddika N, et al. Obesity and Abdominal Obesity in the Indian Population: Findings from a Nationally Representative Study of 698,286 Participants. Epidemiologia. 2023;4(2):163-72.
2. Kalra S, Kapoor N, Verma M, et al. Defining and Diagnosing Obesity in India: A Call for Advocacy and Action. J Obes. 2023;2023:4178121.
3. Szekeres Z, Sandor B, Bognar Z, et al. Clinical Study of Metabolic Parameters, Leptin and the SGLT2 Inhibitor Empagliflozin Among Patients with Obesity and Type 2 Diabetes. Int J Mol Sci. 2023;24(5):4405.
4. Kokkorakis M, Chakhtoura M, Rhayem C, et al. Emerging Pharmacotherapies for Obesity: A Systematic Review. Pharmacol Rev. 2025;77(1):100002.
5. Packer M. The Adipokine Hypothesis of Heart Failure with a Preserved Ejection Fraction: A Novel Framework to Explain Pathogenesis and Guide Treatment. J Am Coll Cardiol. 2025;86(16):1269-73.
6. Xu L, Nagata N, Nagashimada M, et al. SGLT2 Inhibition by Empagliflozin Promotes Fat Utilization and Browning

and Attenuates Inflammation and Insulin Resistance by Polarizing M2 Macrophages in Diet-induced Obese Mice. EBioMedicine. 2017;20:137-49.

7. Izzo C, Carrizzo A. Empagliflozin-Induced Lipidome Remodeling in Type 2 Diabetes: Mechanistic Insights and Translational Perspectives. Cardiovasc Diabetol. 2025;24(1):421.
8. Andersen CF, Larsen JH, Jensen J, et al. Empagliflozin to Elderly and Obese Patients With Increased Risk of Developing Heart Failure: Study Protocol for the Empire Prevent Trial Program. Am Heart J. 2024;271:84-96.
9. Chen X, Chen S, Ren Q, et al. A Metabonomics-Based Renoprotective Mechanism Analysis of Empagliflozin in Obese Mice. Biochem Biophys Res Commun. 2022; 621:122-9.
10. Cai X, Yang W, Gao X, et al. The Association Between the Dosage of SGLT2 Inhibitor and Weight Reduction in Type 2 Diabetes Patients: A Meta-Analysis. Obesity (Silver Spring). 2018;26(1):70-80
11. Hasan I, Rashid T, Jaikaransingh V, et al. SGLT2 inhibitors: Beyond glycemic control. J Clin Transl Endocrinol. 2024; 35:100335.

87

CHAPTER

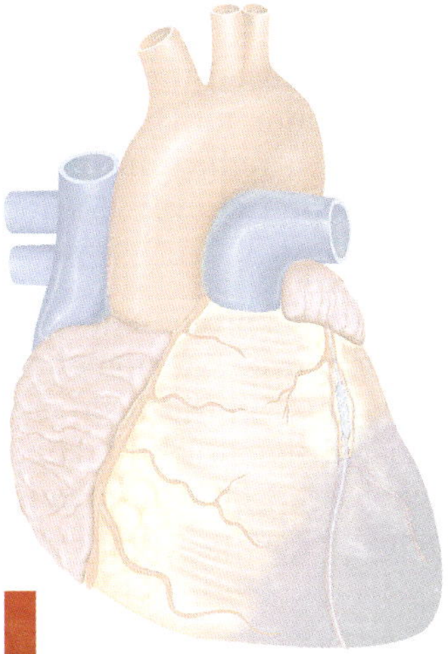

ESC Recommendation: Empagliflozin in Type 2 Diabetes Mellitus with Obesity and Obesity-related HFpEF

Prayaag Kini, Reeta Varyani

INTRODUCTION

Empagliflozin, a sodium–glucose cotransporter 2 (SGLT2) inhibitor, has evolved from a glucose-lowering agent to a cornerstone therapy with robust cardiovascular (CV) and heart failure (HF) benefits across a range of phenotypes. This chapter synthesizes ESC-relevant recommendations and the latest evidence for empagliflozin in two clinically challenging settings: (1) Type 2 diabetes mellitus (T2DM) with obesity and (2) obesity with heart failure with preserved ejection fraction (HFpEF). It also integrates insights from the EMPA-REG OUTCOME program, the SEESAW trial, and contemporary real-world cohort data. The ESC and other authoritative guidelines are continuously updated, and the most current data is presented here.

WHY EMPAGLIFLOZIN IS CLINICALLY IMPORTANT IN OBESITY?

Obesity amplifies CV risk in T2DM and contributes to HFpEF pathophysiology through dysmetabolism, inflammation, and increased preload/afterload. SGLT2 inhibitors, including empagliflozin, offer benefits beyond glycemic control: Diuresis/natriuresis, modest weight reduction, blood pressure effects, renal protection, and favorable effects on HF outcomes. The ESC framework increasingly endorses SGLT2 inhibitors for cardio-renal-metabolic risk reduction across T2DM, obesity, and HF phenotypes, with particular emphasis on HFpEF where traditional neurohormonal therapies yield limited mortality benefits.[1]

Empagliflozin in Type 2 Diabetes Mellitus with Obesity: Evidence and ESC Implications—Key Evidence

EMPA-REG OUTCOME (empagliflozin 10 and 25 mg) studied T2DM with established CV disease (high CV risk; obesity common in this population). Key findings included significant reductions in major adverse cardiovascular events (MACE), CV death, and hospitalization for heart failure (HFH). Weight loss was modest but clinically relevant given the obesity comorbidity. The investigators postulated that mechanisms beyond glucose lowering such as empagliflozin providing diuretic effects, reductions in blood pressure, improvements in energy/metabolic substrate utilization, and potential renal protection were also contributing to the beneficial effect.[2,3]

Key Findings

Primary outcome: The primary composite endpoint of this study was the first occurrence of CV death, nonfatal myocardial infarction, or nonfatal stroke. Empagliflozin treatment resulted in a statistically significant reduction of this outcome. *CV death*: A significant reduction in CV death was observed, with one analysis reporting a 38% decrease in CV mortality. *HF*: Empagliflozin reduced the risk of hospitalization for HF. *Composite endpoint*: The study showed a reduction in the composite endpoint of CV death or hospitalization for HF.[4]

Consistent effects: The benefits of empagliflozin were consistent across various subgroups of patients, including those with or without a history of HF at baseline.

Further T2DM trials/cohorts (e.g., REWIND and real-world cohorts) also consistently show CV risk reduction with empagliflozin in diverse T2DM populations, including those with obesity, and with modest weight loss.[5]

Relevant Recommendations from the ESC

- For patients with T2DM and obesity who have established ASCVD or high ASCVD risk, empagliflozin should be considered to reduce CV events and HF hospitalization, with added weight and metabolic benefits.
- In obesity coexisting with T2DM and high CV risk, empagliflozin is a reasonable first-line SGLT2 inhibitor option, particularly when HF risk mitigation is a priority.

Practical Considerations

Dosing should ideally start with 10 mg once daily; this may be escalated to 25 mg daily if tolerated when additional CV/metabolic benefit is desired. Benefits include CV risk reduction, HF risk reduction, weight reduction (modest), BP lowering, and potential renal protection.

Safety has been a concern from various studies, including the occurrence of volume depletion, increased incidence of genital mycotic infections, rare cases of diabetic ketoacidosis (particularly in specific contexts), especially requiring monitoring in renal impairment.

EMPAGLIFLOZIN IN OBESITY + HFpEF: WHY THIS SUBGROUP MATTERS?

Heart failure with preserved ejection fraction is prevalent in obesity and metabolic syndrome. Treatments with clear mortality benefits in HFrEF have historically underperformed in HFpEF; thus, therapies addressing metabolic dysfunction are of high interest. SGLT2 inhibitors have demonstrated HF hospitalization risk reductions across EF ranges, including HFpEF in broader HF populations (e.g., EMPEROR-Preserved program and related analyses).

HFpEF-focused Data with SGLT2 Inhibitors—Key Evidence Landscape

Trials such as EMPEROR-Preserved indicate reductions in HF hospitalizations among HFpEF patients, with favorable effects that extend to those with metabolic comorbidity, obesity, and diabetes. Mechanistically, SGLT2 inhibition lowers preload/afterload, improves myocardial energetics, and reduces systemic inflammation and edema.

Key Findings from the EMPEROR-Preserved Trial

Primary outcome: Empagliflozin reduced the primary endpoint of CV death or hospitalization for HF by 21%. The most significant benefit was a reduction in HF hospitalizations, with a risk reduction of over 25% for recurrent hospitalizations.

Cardiovascular death: Nominal, nonsignificant reduction in the risk of CV death. The drug improved symptoms and health-related quality of life for patients. Empagliflozin also led to a slower decline in estimated glomerular filtration rate (eGFR) and a reduced risk of severe hospitalizations, including those requiring intensive care or vasopressor drugs.

Impact on subgroups: The benefits of empagliflozin were consistent across all subgroups, including those with and without diabetes, and across different age groups.

The SEESAW trial (empagliflozin and obesity-related HF phenotypes), in its early-phase data exploring empagliflozin in obesity-associated HFpEF or metabolic-risk-heavy phenotypes, reported signals include improvements in exercise capacity, diastolic function, and body composition. The SEESAW trial (SGLT2 Inhibitor Empagliflozin Effects on Appetite and Weight Regulation) was a 24 weeks, randomized, double-blind, placebo-controlled study that investigated why the observed weight loss with empagliflozin in patients with type 2 diabetes is less than the predicted energy deficit from increased urinary glucose excretion. The main goal was to determine if compensatory changes in appetite-regulating hormones or increased energy intake explained the weight loss discrepancy. The trial had four arms for male and postmenopausal female participants with type 2 diabetes and a BMI of 25 kg/m^2 or higher:

1. Placebo only
2. Placebo plus an energy-restricted diet (~360 kcal/day deficit)
3. Empagliflozin 25 mg daily only
4. Empagliflozin 25 mg daily plus an energy-restricted diet

Researchers measured various outcomes, including appetite-regulating gut peptides (e.g., total PYY, GLP-1, and acylated ghrelin), body weight and composition (using DEXA scans), energy expenditure and physical activity, and glycemic control (HbA1c, glucose, and insulin).

Key Findings

Published in Diabetes, Obesity and Metabolism in 2022, key results of the SEESAW trial showed that empagliflozin did not produce significant differences in the levels of appetite-regulating peptides (PYY, GLP-1, or ghrelin) compared to the placebo group. However, significant weight loss occurred across all intervention groups. The empagliflozin-plus-diet group achieved the greatest weight loss, followed by the empagliflozin-only and placebo-plus-diet groups. The study did not find significant changes in daily energy intake or self-reported physical activity across the groups, suggesting the weight loss discrepancy might involve other complex energy balance adaptations not fully captured by the measured parameters. Empagliflozin-treated groups showed significant improvements in HbA1c and glucose levels compared to placebo.

The SEESAW trial concluded that the effect of empagliflozin on appetite regulation remains inconclusive and does not appear to significantly impact the measured appetite-regulating hormones over 24 weeks. The observed weight loss with empagliflozin may be due to other mechanisms or long-term energy balance adaptations that require further investigation.

How ESC Views this Space? Relevant Recommendations from the ESC

- ESC guidelines increasingly advocate SGLT2 inhibitors for HF across EF spectrums, including HFpEF, especially in patients with diabetes or metabolic risk factors.
- In obesity-associated HFpEF, empagliflozin is a rational therapeutic option to reduce HF-related events and potentially improve functional status, while also addressing metabolic derangements.

Practical Considerations

- *Initiation*: Consider empagliflozin in obesity-related HFpEF where there are no contraindications to SGLT2 inhibitors. Monitoring with regular assessment of renal function (eGFR), volume status, blood pressure, and signs of genital infections or ketoacidosis risk is the key to using this class of drugs safely in this cohort. Though initial dosing of 10 mg daily is standard, higher doses of 25 mg daily can be considered for augmented CV/ metabolic benefit if tolerated.
- *Safety*: As with T2DM, monitor for volume depletion, euglycemic ketoacidosis (especially in catabolic states or low insulin reserves), and genital infections must be monitored for.

Real-World and Cohort Data: Practical Insights

Across diverse populations, real-world cohorts show consistent reductions in HF hospitalizations with empagliflozin, including patients with obesity and metabolic syndrome. There is also a modest but meaningful weight loss benefit, contributing to improved metabolic profiles. Safety profiles that align with RCTs, with ongoing vigilance for rare adverse events, support generalizable CV and HF benefits in everyday clinical practice, reinforcing ESC guidance to consider empagliflozin for cardiometabolic risk reduction in eligible patients.

Practical Guidance for Clinicians—How to Use These Drugs?

- *Patient selection:* In patients with T2DM and obesity who have high CV risk or established ASCVD, empagliflozin is a strong therapeutic option for CV risk reduction and metabolic benefits. Especially in the cohort of obesity with HFpEF, empagliflozin can be considered to reduce HF events and potentially improve symptoms, in line with broader HFpEF management and metabolic risk reduction.
- *Start/up-titration:* Begin at 10 mg daily, consider 25 mg daily if additional CV or weight/metabolic benefit is desired and well tolerated.
- *Monitoring:* eGFR and renal function at baseline and periodically must be done. A note of volume status, blood pressure, and hydration, along with regular screening for genital infections, must be carried out. We must educate patients and their families about signs/symptoms of ketoacidosis (particularly in at-risk individuals or during catabolic states).

Drug Interactions and Concomitant Therapy

Generally, this class of drugs is compatible with metformin and many other antidiabetic agents; monitor interactions with diuretics and antihypertensives due to additive volume depletion risk.

Lifestyle management and integration play an extremely vital role in reaching their action to fruition—hence, it is essential to combine with structured weight management programs, physical activity, and dietary optimization to maximize obesity-related benefits.

CONCLUSION

SEESAW and similar obesity/HFpEF-focused studies are crucial for refining patient selection and understanding long-term outcomes in obesity-linked HFpEF. Ongoing and future real-world analyses will clarify the durability of benefits across diverse populations and help identify subgroups most likely to benefit from empagliflozin in obesity-related HFpEF. As guidelines evolve, explicit ESC recommendations may increasingly emphasize SGLT2 inhibitors as disease-modifying agents in metabolic dysfunction-driven HFpEF and obesity-related CV risk.

REFERENCES

1. Zinman B, Wanner C, Lachin JM, et al. Empagliflozin, cardiovascular outcomes, and mortality in type 2 diabetes. N Engl J Med. 2015;373:2117-28.
2. Anker SD, Butler J, Filippatos G, et al.; EMPEROR-Preserved Trial Investigators. Empagliflozin in heart failure with a preserved ejection fraction. N Engl J Med. 2021;385:1451-61.
3. Sargeant JA, King JA, Yates T, et al. The effects of empagliflozin, dietary energy restriction, or both on appetite-regulatory gut peptides in individuals with type 2 diabetes and overweight or obesity: The SEESAW randomized, double-blind, placebo-controlled trial. Diabetes Obes Metab. 2022;24(8):1509-21.
4. ESC Guidelines: Integrate SGLT2 inhibitors for CV risk reduction in T2DM with high CV risk and endorse HFpEF benefits with SGLT2 inhibitors in appropriate patients.
5. Real-World Cohort Studies: Observational analyses supporting CV/HF benefits and weight-related outcomes with empagliflozin in obesity/metabolic syndrome contexts.

88

CHAPTER

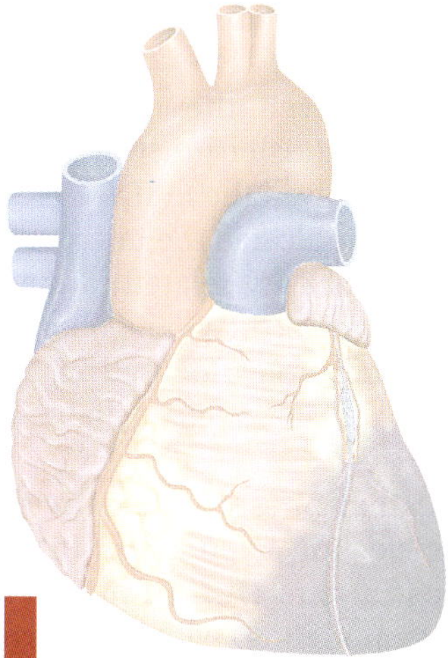

Dapagliflozin in the Management of Obesity-associated all Spectrum of Heart Failure

Zakia A Khan, Shakil Shaikh

INTRODUCTION

Obesity has reached worldwide epidemic proportions, adversely impacting health on a global scale. Overweight and abdominal obesity adversely impact cardiac structure and function. Obesity is an abnormal change caused by multiple factors, including genetics, environment, and behavior. The increased risk of cardiovascular disease in obese patients makes obesity an independent risk factor for heart failure, coronary heart disease, and other cardiovascular diseases.

Dapagliflozin (Dapa) is considered one of the most important pillars of heart failure across the spectrum of LV dysfunction and has shown significant morbidity and mortality benefits. However, there are currently no available studies or trials in humans to study the specific benefits of this agent in obesity-related heart failure. There are studies done in mice, which we will discuss subsequently.[1-5]

PATHOGENESIS AND PROPOSED MECHANISMS OF HEART FAILURE IN OBESITY

Ferroptosis is a type of cell death discovered by Dixon et al. in 2012 and is characterized by abnormal intracellular iron metabolism, glutathione (GSH)-dependent antioxidant system dysfunction, and a large accumulation of lipid hydroperoxides.[6] Studies have found that ferroptosis may be involved in the pathogenic process of various cardiovascular diseases, including myocardial ischemia-reperfusion injury,[7] cardiomyopathy,[8] inflammatory response after heart transplantation,[9] and atherosclerosis.[10] However, studies on whether ferroptosis is involved in the pathological process of obesity cardiomyopathy are rare. Recently, it has been found that Dapa can reduce excessive activation of the hypoxia-inducible factor-1α/heme oxygenase-1 axis (HIF-1α/HO-1), which serves a renal protective role in the progression of diabetic nephropathy by inhibiting ferroptosis.[11]

It is well-known that increased BMI is closely related to the incidence of early cardiovascular disease or cardiometabolic syndrome.[12] Obesity can cause hypertension and abnormal glucose and lipid metabolism, which are associated with each other and aggravate the damage to myocardial structure and function. BMI is the obesity classification standard used internationally; however, some studies have demonstrated that some obese patients may not have metabolic syndrome and thus shorten the expected survival time and may even produce "benefits" in some cases, which researchers call "obesity paradox."[13] In addition, studies have found that obesity itself, especially severe obesity and persistent obesity, can also cause extensive changes in myocardial structure and function, leading to obesity cardiomyopathy[14] ultrastructural changes in the heart tissue caused by obesity, including collagen deposition, muscle fiber breakage, and mitochondrial swelling. These abnormalities in the myocardium will further cause cardiac structural remodeling and heart failure.

Some researchers have hypothesized that hemodynamic abnormalities caused by excessive weight gain can increase cardiac load and reduce cardiac compliance, and systolic and diastolic functions, thus finally leading to myocardial fibrosis, massive deposition of interstitial collagen, and accelerated cardiac remodeling.[15]

Others have found that obesity can induce abnormal regulatory function of adipose tissue, leading to imbalance of secretion of anti-inflammatory fat factor and proinflammatory fat factor, which causes inflammatory reaction and metabolic disorder, and then promotes oxidative stress damage of myocardial cells and mitochondrial dysfunction.[16] Cardiomyocyte death is a key process of cardiomyopathy. Autophagy, apoptosis, and other related pathways all participate in the pathogenesis of obesity-related cardiomyopathy.

Therefore, how to reverse myocardial apoptosis is important for the treatment of obesity cardiomyopathy. Zhang et al. found that urolithin A could reverse the PTEN-induced kinase 1/Parkin-dependent mitophagy in high-fat-induced metabolic cardiomyopathy by alleviating the mitochondrial defects.[17] In recent years, ferroptosis, as a novel type of cell death, has been confirmed to be involved in numerous cardiovascular diseases, and it has gradually attracted the attention of scholars. Du et al. found that the contents of total iron and Fe^{2+}, and the expression levels of TFR1 and FPN1 were markedly increased in rats with diabetic cardiomyopathy, while the GSH and FPN levels were reduced.[18] It has been confirmed that ferroptosis is involved in metabolic cardiomyopathy. Although ferroptosis has been demonstrated to be involved in ischemic cardiomyopathy[19] and diabetic cardiomyopathy,[20] to the best of our knowledge, whether it is also involved in the development of obesity cardiomyopathy remains unknown.

PROPOSED MECHANISM OF BENEFIT WITH DAPA IN OBESITY-RELATED HEART FAILURE

The KEGG analysis demonstrated that the ferroptosis pathway was involved in the process of obesity-induced myocardial injury, and GO enrichment analysis identified ferroptosis-related genes. Therefore, ferroptosis is involved in the pathogenesis of obesity cardiomyopathy. SGLT2 inhibitors (SGLT2is) are emerging hypoglycemic drugs and have been confirmed to be effective in treating hyperglycemia in patients with type 2 diabetes. Numerous studies have demonstrated that they not only have a hypoglycemic effect but can also improve cardiovascular disease-related risk factors and reduce the risk of worsening heart failure and in-hospital death in patients with type 2 diabetes.[21] In addition, some studies have found that SGLT2is still have a significant role in improving heart failure after excluding major influencing factors such as blood pressure, blood lipids, and blood sugar, making the role of SGLT2is in myocardial protection more prominent.[22]

Dapagliflozin not only improved the metabolic parameters, including body weight, islet function, and TC and LDL-C levels, but also improved the LVIDs, LVFS, LVEF, E/A, and E/E′ levels, which indicated the improved systolic and diastolic function of obesity-related cardiac dysfunction. There are few studies on SGLT2is and obesity cardiomyopathy, and previous studies have focused on the mechanism of metabolic heart disease, such as diabetic cardiomyopathy.

Some researchers found that obese patients with heart failure with preserved ejection fraction exhibited increased epicardial adipose tissue (EAT) thickness and concentric ventricular remodeling, which in turn were associated with parameters of greater pericardial restraint and ventricular diastolic dysfunction compared with the nonobese counterparts,[23] whereas SGLT2is could markedly reduce the EAT mass and fibrosis and inflammatory biomarkers.[24,25]

Sun et al. also demonstrated that empagliflozin reduced HFD-induced fat mass and insulin levels, and markedly improved diastolic function, which manifested as an enhanced E/A ratio.[26] Using histological analysis, it was found that Dapa alleviated structural remodeling, such as mitochondrial structural abnormalities caused by high lipids, indicating that Dapa could alleviate cardiac dysfunction by improving mitochondrial function. A study by Jhuo et al. examined myocardial mitochondrial function in HFD-induced metabolic disorders and obesity, and the authors found that empagliflozin-treated rats exhibited improved cardiomyocyte mitochondrial biogenesis function.[27] In a study on SGLT2is and ischemia–reperfusion injury, Dapa was demonstrated to improve myocardial injury and cardiac function in rats by inhibiting ferroptosis through inhibition of ACSL4 and upregulation of the SLC7A11/GPX4 axis and FTH.[28] Many studies have confirmed that SGLT2i can regulate ferroptosis. Min et al.[28] found that trastuzumab can overtly promote adverse myocardial remodeling, oxidative stress, lipid peroxidation, mitochondrial ultrastructural damage, DNA damage, and ferroptosis in C57BL/6 mice. Empagliflozin intervention can significantly improve cardiac injury and oxidative stress by inhibiting ferroptosis.[28]

Chen et al. found that Dapa significantly ameliorated myocardial injury, reperfusion arrhythmia, and cardiac function via reducing ferroptosis and the MAPK signaling pathway.[29] Huang et al. showed the inhibitory effects and potential mechanism of Dapa against diabetes-related ferroptosis in the HFD and STZ mice model.[30] It is noteworthy that some researchers have hypothesized that an excess of iron,[31,32] whether from supplementation or due to iron-overload disorders, could potentially lead to cardiac damage when using SGLT2is. Given the association between myocardial iron overload and ferroptosis, it is reasonable to infer that SGLT2is may, at least in part, offer protection against iron-overload-mediated cardiomyocyte injury. Therefore, we hypothesized that these key factors regulating ferroptosis may also be involved in the development of obesity-related cardiomyopathy and aimed to investigate whether Dapa was involved in the regulation of these key factors, thereby ameliorating obesity-related heart failure.

As one of the important trace elements in organisms, iron participates in the regulation of various physiological processes in the body. Intracellular iron homeostasis is mainly regulated by TFR1, FPN1 on the cell membrane surface, and intracellular ferritin.[33] When the cellular iron homeostasis is out of balance, it can cause intracellular iron overload and damage mitochondria, proteins, and nucleic acids, resulting in cell damage.[34] Accumulating evidence has indicated that ferroptosis serves an important role in cardiovascular disease.[35] Studies have demonstrated that iron deficiency can damage the energy regulation function of mitochondria and produce harmful substances of active oxygen, reduce the contractility of cardiomyocytes, and damage cardiac function and structure, while excessive free iron in cardiomyocytes can inhibit the influx of calcium ions, affecting cardiomyocyte excitation–contraction coupling, leading to heart failure and cardiomyopathy.[36] Huang et al. found that Dapa could reduce the ubiquitination of FPN1 in a rat model of diabetic nephropathy, thereby inhibiting ferroptosis.[30] This result was consistent with experimental results, indicating that Dapa may reduce the iron ion concentration in cardiomyocytes mainly by affecting FPN1 expression. GPX4, as a core regulator of ferroptosis, can convert intracellular toxic lipid hydroperoxide into nontoxic lipid alcohols to remove harmful substances and block the occurrence of chain lipid peroxidation, and its upstream cystine/glutamate antiporter can transport cystine into the cell to ensure the synthesis of GSH, which is a cofactor of GPX4 and also serves an important role in ferroptosis and oxidative stress.

ACSL4 is another specific biomarker of ferroptosis and also an important regulator of lipid metabolism. It can catalyze polyunsaturated fatty acids such as arachidonic acid and epinephrine, enhance the process of lipid peroxidation, and accelerate the progress of ferroptosis.[37] Dixon et al. found that the level of lipid peroxidation can be inhibited via downregulation of the ACSL4 and lysophosphatidylcholine acyltransferase-3 genes, and thus, inhibiting ferroptosis key factors could effectively improve the antioxidant capacity.[38] This study first detected the contents of GSH and MDA and revealed that Dapa reversed the changes of GSH and MDA caused by OHF, indicating that Dapa could inhibit high-fat-induced oxidative stress and lipid peroxidation. Subsequently, the present study analyzed the expression levels of GPX4, SLC7A11, and ACSL4. At present, there are no relatively accurate means for precise and hierarchical classification of obesity. Therefore, how to determine the harmful effect of obesity on cardiovascular disease early and how to prevent and control the adverse effects of obesity are problems that need to be solved urgently. Although the present study confirmed that Dapa could ameliorate obesity cardiomyopathy by inhibiting ferroptosis, how it regulates them and the related signaling pathway will be further explored in our in vitro study in the future.

CONCLUSION

Dapagliflozin is a novel hypoglycemic agent with multiple cardiovascular protective effects, and it is widely used in the treatment of heart failure patients. Dapa could improve the myocardial structure and function of obesity cardiomyopathy rats by inhibiting ferroptosis and may serve an important role in the prevention and treatment of obesity-related heart failure. Although there is no trial that has studied specific subgroup analysis of obese patients with heart failure where Dapa has specifically benefited these individuals, current knowledge is derived from studies done in mice.

REFERENCES

1. Mu L, Liu J, Zhou G, et al. Obesity prevalence and risks among Chinese adults: findings from the China PEACE Million Persons Project, 2014-2018. Circ Cardiovasc Qual Outcomes. 2021;14:e007292.
2. Smith U. Dietary fibre, diabetes and obesity. Int J Obes (Lond). 1987;11:27-31.
3. Wong C, Marwick TH. Obesity cardiomyopathy: pathogenesis and pathophysiology. Nat Clin Pract Cardiovasc Med. 2007;4:436-43.
4. Velliou M, Polyzogopoulou E, Ventoulis I, et al. Clinical pharmacology of SGLT-2 inhibitors in heart failure. Expert Rev Clin Pharmacol. 2023;16:149-60.
5. Chen HB, Yang YL, Meng RS, et al. Indirect comparison of SGLT2 inhibitors in patients with established heart failure: evidence based on Bayesian methods. ESC Heart Fail. 2023;10:1231-41.
6. Dixon SJ, Lemberg KM, Lamprecht MR, et al. Ferroptosis: an iron-dependent form of nonapoptotic cell death. Cell. 2012;149:1060-72.
7. Ma L, Liu X, Zhang M, et al. Paeoniflorin alleviates ischemia/reperfusion induced acute kidney injury by inhibiting Slc7a11-mediated ferroptosis. Int Immunopharmacol. 2023;116:109754.

8. Zhou YJ, Duan DQ, Lu LQ, et al. The SPATA2/CYLD pathway contributes to doxorubicin-induced cardiomyocyte ferroptosis via enhancing ferritinophagy. Chem Biol Interact. 2022;368:110205.
9. Li W, Feng G, Gauthier JM, et al. Ferroptotic cell death and TLR4/Trif signaling initiate neutrophil recruitment after heart transplantation. J Clin Invest. 2019;129:2293-304.
10. Bai T, Li M, Liu Y, et al. Inhibition of ferroptosis alleviates atherosclerosis through attenuating lipid peroxidation and endothelial dysfunction in mouse aortic endothelial cell. Free Radic Biol Med. 2020;160:92-102.
11. Wang Y-H, Chang D-Y, Zhao M-H, et al. Dapagliflozin alleviates diabetic kidney disease via HIF1α/HO1 mediated ferroptosis. Antioxid Redox Signal. 2024;40(7-9):492-509.
12. Świątkiewicz I, Wróblewski M, Nuszkiewicz J, et al. The role of oxidative stress enhanced by adiposity in cardiometabolic diseases. Int J Mol Sci. 2023;24:6382.
13. Kim SA, Lim K, Lee JK, et al. Metabolically healthy obesity and the risk of all-cause and cardiovascular disease mortality in a Korean population: a prospective cohort study. BMJ Open. 2021;11:e049063.
14. Aune D, Sen A, Norat T, et al. Body mass index, abdominal fatness, and heart failure incidence and mortality: a systematic review and dose-response meta-analysis of prospective studies. Circulation. 2016;133:639-49.
15. Ren J, Wu NN, Wang S, et al. Obesity cardiomyopathy: evidence, mechanisms, and therapeutic implications. Physiol Rev. 2021;101:1745-807.
16. Achari AE, Jain SK. Adiponectin, a therapeutic target for obesity, diabetes, and endothelial dysfunction. Int J Mol Sci. 2017;18:1321.
17. Zhang W, Wang X, Tang Y, et al. Melatonin alleviates doxorubicin-induced cardiotoxicity via inhibiting oxidative stress, pyroptosis and apoptosis by activating Sirt1/Nrf2 pathway. Biomed Pharmacother. 2023;162:114591.
18. Du S, Shi H, Xiong L, et al. Canagliflozin mitigates ferroptosis and improves myocardial oxidative stress in mice with diabetic cardiomyopathy. Front Endocrinol (Lausanne). 2022;13:1011669.
19. Liu C, Li Z, Li B, et al. Relationship between ferroptosis and mitophagy in cardiac ischemia reperfusion injury: a mini-review. PeerJ. 2023;11:e14952.
20. Zhao Y, Pan B, Lv X, et al. Ferroptosis: roles and molecular mechanisms in diabetic cardiomyopathy. Front Endocrinol (Lausanne). 2023;14:1140644.
21. Chrysant SG, Chrysant GS. Beneficial cardiovascular and remodeling effects of SGLT 2 inhibitors. Expert Rev Cardiovasc Ther. 2022;20:223-32.
22. Garg V, Verma S, Connelly K. Mechanistic insights regarding the role of SGLT2 inhibitors and GLP1 agonist drugs on cardiovascular disease in diabetes. Prog Cardiovasc Dis. 2019;62:349-57.
23. Obokata M, Reddy YNV, Pislaru SV, et al. Evidence supporting the existence of a distinct obese phenotype of heart failure with preserved ejection fraction. Circulation. 2017;136:6-19.
24. van Tassell BW, Arena R, Biondi-Zoccai G, et al. Effects of interleukin-1 blockade with anakinra on aerobic exercise capacity in patients with heart failure and preserved ejection fraction (from the D-HART pilot study). Am J Cardiol. 2014;113:321-7.
25. Everett BM, Cornel JH, Lainscak M, et al. Anti-inflammatory therapy with canakinumab for the prevention of hospitalization for heart failure. Circulation. 2019;139:1289-99.
26. Sun X, Han F, Lu Q, et al. Empagliflozin ameliorates obesity-related cardiac dysfunction by regulating Sestrin2-mediated AMPK-mTOR signaling and redox homeostasis in high-fat diet-induced obese mice. Diabetes. 2020;69:1292-305.
27. Jhuo SJ, Lin YH, Liu IH, et al. Sodium glucose cotransporter 2 (SGLT2) inhibitor ameliorate metabolic disorder and obesity induced cardiomyocyte injury and mitochondrial remodeling. Int J Mol Sci. 2023;24:6842.
28. Min J, Lin W, Liu Y, et al. Empagliflozin attenuates trastuzumab-induced cardiotoxicity through suppression of DNA damage and ferroptosis. Life Sci. 2023;312:121207.
29. Chen W, Zhang Y, Wang Z, et al. Dapagliflozin alleviates myocardial ischemia/reperfusion injury by reducing ferropotosis via MAPK signaling inhibition. Front Pharmacol. 2023;20:1078205.
30. Huang B, Wen W, Ye S. Dapagliflozin ameliorates renal tubular ferroptosis in diabetes via SLC40A1 stabilization. Oxid Med Cell Longev. 2022;2022:9735555.
31. Cirovic A, Cirovic A. Iron status screening in individuals with heart failure before initiating sodium-glucose cotransporter 2 inhibitor therapy: is it necessary? Cardiovasc Drugs Ther. 2024;38:859-60.
32. Packer M. Potential interactions when prescribing SGLT2 inhibitors and intravenous iron in combination in heart failure. JACC Heart Fail. 2023;11:106-14.
33. Nemeth E, Ganz T. Hepcidin-ferroportin interaction controls systemic iron homeostasis. Int J Mol Sci. 2021;22:6493.
34. Hoes MF, Grote Beverborg N, Kijlstra JD, et al. Iron deficiency impairs contractility of human cardiomyocytes through decreased mitochondrial function. Eur J Heart Fail. 2018;20:910-9.
35. Park TJ, Park JH, Lee GS, et al. Quantitative proteomic analyses reveal that GPX4 downregulation during myocardial infarction contributes to ferroptosis in cardiomyocytes. Cell Death Dis. 2019;10:835.
36. Sugishita K, Asakawa M, Usui S, et al. A case of iron overload cardiomyopathy: beneficial effects of iron chelating agent and calcium channel blocker on left ventricular dysfunction. Int Heart J. 2009;50:829-38.
37. Yang Y, Zhu T, Wang X, et al. ACSL3 and ACSL4, distinct roles in ferroptosis and cancers. Cancers (Basel). 2022;14:5896.
38. Dixon SJ, Winter GE, Musavi LS, et al. Human haploid cell genetics reveals roles for lipid metabolism genes in nonapoptotic cell death. ACS Chem Biol. 2015;10:1604-9.

CHAPTER 89

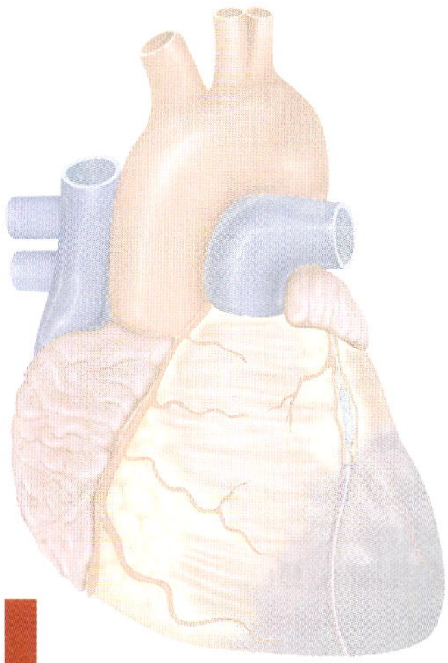

Renoprotection with SGLT2 Inhibitors in Nondiabetic CKD: A Paradigm Shift

Shreyasee Borah, Sunil Prakash

INTRODUCTION

Chronic kidney disease (CKD) is a leading global health problem with substantial morbidity, mortality, and health-system costs. Recent guideline estimates place the global prevalence of CKD at approximately 9.1% (95% CI 8.5–9.8%), highlighting its widespread public-health impact. Progressive loss of kidney function culminates in end-stage kidney disease (ESKD), imposing profound consequences on survival and quality of life and creating a significant societal burden. Historically, disease-modifying treatments for CKD have focused on blood-pressure control, blockade of the renin–angiotensin system (RAS) and, in diabetics, glycemic control; despite these measures, a large residual risk of progression to ESKD and of cardiovascular events persists across CKD etiologies.[1,2]

Sodium–glucose cotransporter-2 inhibitors (SGLT2i) were introduced as oral antihyperglycemic agents for type 2 diabetes mellitus (T2DM), acting principally by inhibiting SGLT2-mediated glucose and sodium reabsorption in the proximal renal tubule, thereby promoting glucosuria and natriuresis.[3] Unexpectedly, large cardiovascular outcome trials in people with T2DM demonstrated consistent renal and cardiac benefits that were disproportionate to the modest glucose-lowering effect, prompting mechanistic and clinical investigation into nonglycemic mechanisms and broader indications.[4,5] Subsequent dedicated CKD outcome trials have demonstrated that SGLT2 inhibitors slow kidney function decline and reduce risk of ESKD and cardiovascular events in patients with CKD irrespective of diabetes status, thereby reframing SGLT2i as renoprotective agents rather than solely antihyperglycemic drugs.[6,7] This chapter reviews the pathophysiological rationale, summarizes the clinical evidence base, details safety and monitoring considerations, discusses guideline recommendations and practical implementation, and highlights future research directions in nondiabetic CKD.

PATHOPHYSIOLOGICAL BASIS FOR SGLT2 INHIBITOR BENEFIT IN NONDIABETIC CKD

Sodium–glucose cotransporter-2 inhibitors confer renoprotection through multifactorial pathways that are relevant regardless of glycemic state. These include hemodynamic modulation [restoration of tubulo-glomerular feedback (TGF)], anti-inflammatory and anti-fibrotic effects, systemic metabolic changes, and favorable cardiorenal interactions. Together, these mechanisms attenuate the maladaptive processes that drive CKD progression.

Restoration of Tubuloglomerular Feedback and Hemodynamic Reset

A central driver of CKD progression is glomerular hyperfiltration and elevated intraglomerular pressure. Under normal physiology, the macula densa senses distal sodium chloride delivery and modulates afferent arteriolar tone via TGF. Enhanced proximal tubular reabsorption of sodium (and glucose) reduces distal sodium delivery, blunts TGF, and sustains afferent arteriolar dilation and intraglomerular hypertension; over time, this promotes podocyte stress, mesangial expansion, and glomerulosclerosis.[8,9]

Sodium-glucose cotransporter-2 inhibition reduces proximal sodium and glucose reabsorption, increasing sodium chloride delivery to the macula densa and restoring TGF. The resulting afferent vasoconstriction lowers intraglomerular pressure, diminishing hyperfiltration injury. Importantly, this hemodynamic mechanism is glycemia-independent, explaining why SGLT2i benefit is observed in nondiabetic CKD.[10]

Anti-inflammatory and Antifibrotic Effects

Chronic kidney disease progression is also mediated by chronic inflammation, oxidative stress, and fibrogenesis. Preclinical and translational studies indicate that SGLT2i reduce renal cortical hypoxia (by lowering proximal tubular oxygen consumption), attenuate mitochondrial oxidative stress, and downregulate proinflammatory cytokines and chemokines (e.g., TNF-α, IL-6, and MCP-1).[11-13] Inhibition of profibrotic pathways, including TGF-β signaling, and reduction in extracellular matrix deposition have been demonstrated, together with preservation of podocyte structure and function. These actions limit tubulointerstitial fibrosis and glomerulosclerosis—key determinants of long-term renal outcome—independently of glucose lowering.[14]

Metabolic and Hemodynamic Modulation

Sodium-glucose cotransporter-2 inhibitors produce several systemic metabolic effects that enhance organ resilience: They induce modest, physiologic ketosis that provides the myocardium and kidney with a more energy-efficient substrate, promote uricosuria and lower serum uric acid, produce sustained natriuresis and mild osmotic diuresis (leading to modest reductions in blood pressure and extracellular volume), and contribute to weight loss.[15-17] These combined effects reduce cardiac preload and afterload and mitigate factors that accelerate renal injury, such as hypertension and volume overload.

Cardiovascular-renal Cross-talk

Cardiovascular disease is the major cause of mortality in CKD. Heart failure and reduced cardiac output exacerbate renal hypoperfusion and venous congestion, accelerating kidney dysfunction. SGLT2i reduces hospitalizations for heart failure across the spectrum of ejection fraction and in patients without diabetes, improving cardiac function and hemodynamics; these cardiac benefits feedback to preserve kidney function by improving perfusion and reducing venous congestion.[18,19] Thus, SGLT2i act on both sides of the cardiorenal axis.

EVIDENCE FROM CLINICAL TRIALS

Many randomized clinical trials and meta-analyses have established the efficacy of SGLT2 inhibitors for renal protection in both diabetic and nondiabetic CKD.

Early Diabetes Cardiovascular Outcome Trials

Renoprotective signals first emerged in cardiovascular outcome trials of SGLT2i in people with T2DM. EMPA-REG OUTCOME showed marked reductions in cardiovascular mortality and benefits on renal endpoints with empagliflozin.[4] CANVAS and DECLARE-TIMI 58 further supported class effects for cardiovascular and renal outcomes and shaped the hypothesis that SGLT2i protect kidneys via nonglycemic mechanisms.[5,20]

DAPA-CKD

DAPA-CKD was a pivotal trial that enrolled 4,304 patients with CKD (eGFR 25–75 mL/min/1.73 m^2 and UACR 200–5,000 mg/g); notably, 32% of participants did not have diabetes.[6] Participants randomized to dapagliflozin 10 mg daily experienced a 39% reduction in the primary composite endpoint of sustained ≥50% eGFR decline, onset of ESKD, or renal/cardiovascular death (HR 0.61; 95% CI 0.51–0.72; $p < 0.001$). The benefit was consistent in the nondiabetic subgroup (HR ≈ 0.50). DAPA-CKD also demonstrated reductions in all-cause mortality and heart-failure hospitalizations, firmly establishing dapagliflozin as renoprotective in nondiabetic CKD.

EMPA-KIDNEY

EMPA-KIDNEY enrolled 6,609 participants with a wide range of eGFR (20–90 mL/min/1.73 m^2) and UACR thresholds, of whom 54% were nondiabetic.[7] Empagliflozin 10 mg daily reduced the primary composite of kidney disease progression or cardiovascular death by 28% (HR 0.72; 95% CI 0.64–0.82). Benefits were observed across etiologies, albuminuria strata, and eGFR levels—extending even to patients with lower albuminuria and advanced CKD—thereby broadening the applicability of SGLT2i in CKD care.

DIAMOND and Other Mechanistic/Short-term Studies

DIAMOND, a small randomized crossover study in proteinuric nondiabetic CKD, did not show short-term antiproteinuric effects of dapagliflozin; however, the trial's size and brief duration limit interpretation, and longer trials demonstrate structural and outcome benefits that rely on sustained therapy.[21] Mechanistic studies and biomarker analyses from large trials support effects on tubular injury markers and inflammatory mediators.

TABLE 1: Major SGLT2i trials—renal outcomes summary.

Trial	*Year*	*Population (key features)*	*Primary renal outcome*
DAPA-CKD (dapagliflozin)	2020	CKD (*n* = 4,304); 32% nondiabetic	0.61 (0.51–0.72)
EMPA-KIDNEY (empagliflozin)	2023	CKD (*n* = 6,609); 54% nondiabetic	0.72 (0.64–0.82)
CREDENCE (canagliflozin)	2019	T2DM with CKD (*n* = 4,401)	0.70 (0.59–0.82)
DECLARE-TIMI 58 (dapagliflozin)	2019	T2DM (*n* = 17,160); cardiorenal secondary outcome	0.76 (0.67–0.87)—cardiorenal composite
EMPA-REG OUTCOME (empagliflozin)	2015	T2DM with CV disease (*n* = 7,020)	Approximately 0.61—worsening nephropathy reduction (~39%)
DIAMOND (dapagliflozin)	2020	Proteinuric nondiabetic CKD (*n* = 53)	NS (short-term)

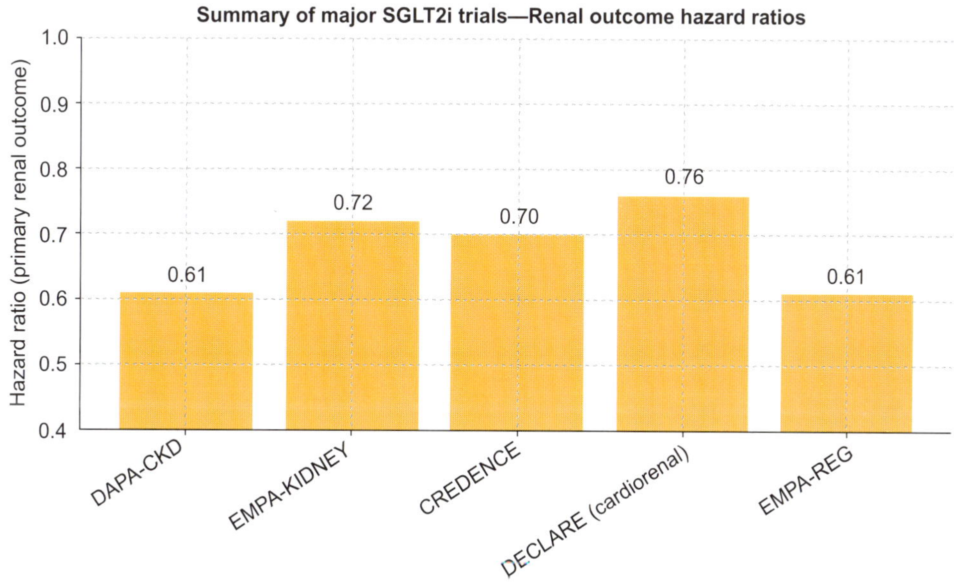

Fig. 1: Major SGLT2 inhibitor trials demonstrating consistent renoprotective benefits across diabetic and nondiabetic CKD populations, confirming a class-wide reduction in primary renal outcomes.

Meta-analyses and Real-world Data

Meta-analyses of major trials and pooled individual patient data show consistent relative risk reductions in kidney failure and composite renal endpoints in the range of ~30–40%, with similar relative effect sizes for diabetic and nondiabetic participants **(Table 1)**.[22,23] Observational registry data corroborate trial results in more heterogeneous, real-world populations, supporting safety and generalizability **(Fig. 1)**.

SAFETY AND TOLERABILITY IN NONDIABETIC CHRONIC KIDNEY DISEASE

Sodium-glucose cotransporter-2 inhibitors are generally well tolerated in CKD and in patients without diabetes; overall safety profiles in pivotal trials were comparable to placebo.

Transient eGFR Dip

An early, modest decline in eGFR (commonly 2–5 mL/min/1.73 m^2) often occurs after initiation, reflecting the hemodynamic reduction in intraglomerular pressure. This "dip" stabilizes within weeks and is predictive of long-term renal benefit rather than nephrotoxicity; continuation is recommended unless the eGFR falls by >30% or other concerning signs appear.[24]

Volume Depletion and Blood Pressure Effects

Osmotic diuresis and natriuresis may cause mild reductions in blood pressure and occasional volume-depletion symptoms, particularly in elderly or diuretic-treated patients. Initial assessment of volume status and adjustment of loop/thiazide diuretics when necessary minimize this risk.

Genital and Urinary Tract Infections

Genital mycotic infections are the most frequent adverse events (more common in women); these are typically mild and respond to standard antifungal therapy and preventive hygiene counseling. Rates of serious urinary tract infections have not been consistently increased in trials.[25]

Euglycemic Ketoacidosis and Metabolic Effects

Euglycemic diabetic ketoacidosis is rare and primarily a concern in type 1 diabetes; it is exceptionally uncommon in nondiabetic CKD. Nevertheless, temporary discontinuation during acute illness, fasting, or perioperative periods (sick-day rules) is prudent. SGLT2i are metabolically neutral with respect to hypoglycemia in nondiabetic patients and reduce serum uric acid—an ancillary benefit.[26]

Acute Kidney Injury and Electrolytes

Contrary to early theoretical concerns, SGLT2i have not increased AKI risk in large trials; pooled analyses suggest reduced AKI hospitalizations. No consistent increases in clinically significant hyperkalemia have been observed; mild changes in magnesium and phosphate are reported but are typically asymptomatic.[27]

GUIDELINE RECOMMENDATIONS AND PRACTICAL IMPLEMENTATION

Major international guidelines now recommend SGLT2 inhibitors for eligible adults with CKD irrespective of diabetes status, reflecting the robust evidence from DAPA-CKD, EMPA-KIDNEY, and supporting trials.

Indications and Thresholds

KDIGO 2024 and other bodies endorse SGLT2i for adults with CKD when eGFR is ≥20 mL/min/1.73 m^2 (for initiation) and with albuminuria thresholds often cited as UACR ≥200 mg/g in trials, though the benefit extends across albuminuria strata.[1,6,7] Clinical judgment guides initiation in cases with lower albuminuria or other specific circumstances.

Initiation and Monitoring

Standard dosing (dapagliflozin 10 mg or empagliflozin 10 mg daily) is used without glycemic titration. Before initiation, evaluate baseline eGFR, electrolytes, blood pressure, and volume status; recheck eGFR and electrolytes within 1 month. Anticipate and counsel about the transient eGFR dip and genital infection risk. Hold SGLT2i during acute severe illness, major surgery, or significant dehydration.

Concomitant Therapies

Sodium-glucose cotransporter-2 inhibitors are additive to RAS blockade and complement other renoprotective agents, including nonsteroidal mineralocorticoid receptor antagonists; close monitoring for hyperkalemia is recommended when combining these agents. Diuretic doses may need adjustment to avoid volume depletion.

Special Populations and Implementation Barriers

Evidence supports safety and benefit down to eGFR 20 mL/min/1.73 m^2; data for dialysis and transplant populations are limited and under active investigation. Implementation challenges—cost, access, clinician awareness—are pronounced in low- and middle-income settings and require policy, education, and system-level interventions to ensure equitable uptake.

FUTURE DIRECTIONS

Research will prioritize on expansion to specific CKD etiologies, combination regimens, identification of biomarkers for precision therapy, and strategies to increase global access.

COMBINATION THERAPIES

Combinations of SGLT2i with agents targeting inflammation and fibrosis (e.g., nonsteroidal MRAs such as finerenone), GLP-1 receptor agonists, or endothelin receptor antagonists are under investigation and may yield additive benefits for renal and cardiovascular outcomes.[28-30]

DISEASE-SPECIFIC TRIALS

Subgroup signals in IgA nephropathy and other glomerulonephritis suggest meaningful benefit; dedicated trials (e.g., disease-specific SGLT2i studies) are underway. Trials in polycystic kidney disease and kidney transplant recipients are exploring safety and efficacy in these special populations.

MECHANISTIC AND BIOMARKER RESEARCH

Deeper understanding of SGLT2i effects on mitochondrial bioenergetics, immune cell phenotypes, endothelial glycocalyx, and renal repair pathways will refine indications and guide combinatorial approaches. Biomarker development—urinary KIM-1, NGAL, metabolomic signatures—may identify responders and permit precision nephrology.[31]

GLOBAL IMPLEMENTATION

Translating trial evidence into population health gains requires overcoming cost and access barriers, integrating SGLT2i into CKD care bundles, and training multidisciplinary teams—particularly in resource-limited settings.

CONCLUSION

Sodium-glucose cotransporter-2 inhibitors represent a seminal therapeutic advance in nephrology. Robust trial evidence demonstrates that they slow CKD progression, reduce the risk of ESRD, and lower cardiovascular events in patients with and without diabetes. These benefits arise from pleiotropic mechanisms—hemodynamic reset via TGF restoration, anti-inflammatory and antifibrotic effects, metabolic modulation, and cardiorenal interactions—that are independent of glycemia. Contemporary guidelines endorse SGLT2i as foundational therapy for eligible CKD patients, and ongoing research will define combination strategies, expand indications, and facilitate precise use. Adoption of SGLT2i in global CKD practice promises to reduce the burden of kidney failure and cardiovascular disease worldwide.

REFERENCES

1. Kidney Disease: Improving Global Outcomes (KDIGO) CKD Work Group. KDIGO 2024 clinical practice guideline for the evaluation and management of chronic kidney disease. Kidney Int. 2024;105(4S):S117-314.
2. Jha V, Garcia-Garcia G, Iseki K, et al. Chronic kidney disease: global dimension and perspectives. Lancet. 2013;382(9888):260-72.
3. Vallon V, Thomson SC. Targeting renal glucose reabsorption to treat hyperglycaemia: the pleiotropic effects of SGLT2 inhibition. Diabetologia. 2017;60:215-25.
4. Zinman B, Wanner C, Lachin JM, et al. Empagliflozin, cardiovascular outcomes, and mortality in type 2 diabetes. N Engl J Med. 2015;373:2117-28.
5. Neal B, Perkovic V, Mahaffey KW, et al. Canagliflozin and cardiovascular and renal events in type 2 diabetes. N Engl J Med. 2017;377:644-57.
6. Heerspink HJL, Stefánsson BV, Correa-Rotter R, et al. Dapagliflozin in patients with chronic kidney disease. N Engl J Med. 2020;383:1436-46.
7. Herrington WG, Staplin N, Wanner C, et al. Empagliflozin in patients with chronic kidney disease. N Engl J Med. 2023;389:1855-66.
8. Hostetter TH. Hyperfiltration and glomerulosclerosis. Semin Nephrol. 2003;23(2):194-9.
9. Vallon V, Thomson SC. The tubular hypothesis of nephron filtration and diabetic hyperfiltration. Nat Rev Nephrol. 2020;16(6):317-36.
10. Heerspink HJL, de Zeeuw D. The kidney protective effects of SGLT2 inhibitors in diabetes mellitus. Nat Rev Nephrol. 2011;7(6):295-302.
11. O'Neill J, Fasching A, Pihl L, et al. Acute SGLT inhibition normalizes O_2 tension in the renal cortex but causes medullary hypoxia in rats. Acta Physiol (Oxf). 2015;213(4):803-15.
12. Li C, Zhang J, Xue M, et al. SGLT2 inhibition attenuates renal oxidative stress and fibrosis via the AGE-RAGE-Nox4 pathway in diabetic mice. J Cell Mol Med. 2018;22(12):5734-45.
13. Dekkers CCJ, Petrykiv S, Laverman GD, et al. Effects of the SGLT2 inhibitor dapagliflozin on glomerular and tubular injury markers. Diabetes Obes Metab. 2018;20(8):1988-93.
14. Zhao Y, Xu L, Tian D, et al. Empagliflozin attenuates renal fibrosis and inflammation in adenine-induced CKD rats. Eur J Pharmacol. 2021;905:174185.
15. Ferrannini E, Mark M, Mayoux E. CV protection in the EMPA-REG OUTCOME trial: a "thrifty substrate" hypothesis. Diabetes Care. 2016;39(7):1108-14.
16. Chino Y, Samukawa Y, Sakai S, et al. SGLT2 inhibitor lowers serum uric acid via altered renal urate transport. Biopharm Drug Dispos. 2014;35(7):391-404.
17. Lambers Heerspink HJ, de Zeeuw D, Wie L, et al. Dapagliflozin reduces albuminuria in patients with diabetes and hypertension receiving RAS blockade: a randomized, double-blind, placebo-controlled trial. Lancet Diabetes Endocrinol. 2014;2(9):737-46.
18. McMurray JJV, Solomon SD, Inzucchi SE, et al. Dapagliflozin in patients with heart failure and reduced ejection fraction. N Engl J Med. 2019;381:1995-2008.
19. Anker SD, Butler J, Filippatos G, et al. Empagliflozin in heart failure with preserved ejection fraction. N Engl J Med. 2021;385:1451-61.
20. Wiviott SD, Raz I, Bonaca MP, et al. Dapagliflozin and cardiovascular outcomes in type 2 diabetes. N Engl J Med. 2019;380:347-57.
21. Cherney DZI, Dekkers CCJ, Barbour SJ, et al. Effects of the SGLT2 inhibitor dapagliflozin on proteinuria in non-diabetic patients with CKD (DIAMOND trial). Kidney Int. 2020;97(6):1130-9.

22. Wheeler DC, Stefánsson BV, Jongs N, et al. Effects of dapagliflozin on major adverse kidney and cardiovascular events in patients with CKD. Lancet Diabetes Endocrinol. 2021;9(1):22-31.
23. Staplin N, Herrington WG, Judge PK, et al. Empagliflozin and dapagliflozin for CKD: a meta-analysis of major trials. Kidney Int. 2024;106(2):205-18.
24. Heerspink HJL, de Zeeuw D. Initial eGFR decline after SGLT2i: a sign of renal protection. Kidney Int. 2018; 94(5):1046-9.
25. Johnsson KM, Ptaszynska A, Schmitz B, et al. Vulvovaginitis and balanitis in SGLT2 inhibitor trials. Diabetes Ther. 2013;4(2):409-25.
26. Ueda P, Svanström H, Melbye M, et al. SGLT2 inhibitors and risk of ketoacidosis in routine practice. N Engl J Med. 2018;379:2300-2.
27. Neuen BL, Ohkuma T, Neal B, et al. SGLT2 inhibitors and risk of acute kidney injury: a systematic review and meta-analysis. Lancet Diabetes Endocrinol. 2019;7(11): 938-48.
28. Agarwal R, Kolkhof P, Bakris GL, et al. Combination therapy with finerenone and SGLT2 inhibitors in CKD: a path forward. Kidney Int. 2023;104(5):883-95.
29. Gerstein HC, Colhoun HM, Dagenais GR, et al. Dulaglutide and renal outcomes in type 2 diabetes. Lancet Diabetes Endocrinol. 2019;7(11):845-54.
30. Mann JFE, Birkelo BC, de Zeeuw D, et al. Endothelin antagonists and SGLT2 inhibitors: complementary kidney protection. Clin J Am Soc Nephrol. 2022;17(3):451-60.
31. Dekkers CCJ, Petrykiv S, Laverman GD, et al. Biomarkers of response to SGLT2 inhibitors in CKD. Diabetes Obes Metab. 2023;25(5):1322-32.

CHAPTER 90

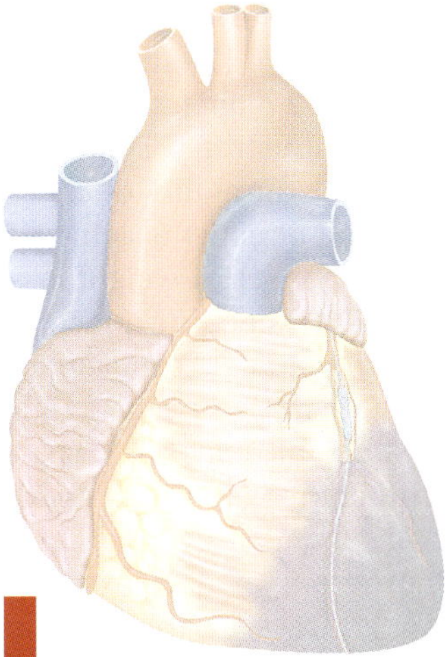

Top 6 CVOT Trials of Semaglutide in Cardiology: Evidence from Landmark Clinical Trials and Practical Protocol

HK Chopra, Anu Grover, Viveka Kumar, CK Ponde, Tiny Nair

INTRODUCTION

Obesity and cardiometabolic disease have evolved into dominant drivers of global cardiovascular morbidity and mortality. The relationship between excess adiposity and cardiovascular disease extends far beyond mechanical loading or hemodynamic stress. It encompasses a complex interplay of systemic inflammation, neurohormonal dysregulation, endothelial dysfunction, autonomic imbalance, renal impairment, lipotoxicity, and progressive myocardial, as well as vascular remodeling.[1,2] Within this biological landscape, the advent of glucagon-like peptide-1 receptor agonists (GLP-1 RAs) represents one of the most transformative therapeutic milestones in contemporary cardiometabolic medicine.

Semaglutide is currently the most comprehensively evaluated GLP-1 RA, supported by an extensive clinical trial portfolio spanning obesity management, type 2 diabetes, cardiovascular prevention, heart failure with preserved ejection fraction (HFpEF), CKD, and metabolic liver disease. Importantly, its clinical trajectory follows a coherent scientific progression: Initial cardiovascular safety validation in diabetes (SUSTAIN-6); demonstration of profound and durable weight loss through STEP; translation of biological benefit into functional cardiac improvement including HFpEF; confirmation of major adverse cardiovascular event (MACE) reduction in a strictly nondiabetic population (SELECT, complemented conceptually by real-world STEER and SCORE); validation of efficacy and cardiovascular protection in an oral formulation (SOUL); and reinforcement of effectiveness in routine clinical practice through real-world evidence.

This chapter synthesizes evidence from the landmark programs STEP, STEER, SCORE, SELECT (conceptually supportive), SOUL, and SUSTAIN to illustrate how semaglutide has transitioned from a metabolic agent to a therapy with direct cardiovascular importance. Collectively, these trials demonstrate that semaglutide modifies cardiovascular risk, improves symptomatic cardiovascular syndromes associated with obesity, and contributes significantly to secondary prevention strategies. For modern cardiology, this evidence redefines obesity management as a cardiovascular imperative and expands the therapeutic relevance of GLP-1-based treatment.

PHARMACOLOGICAL AND MECHANISTIC RATIONALE

Semaglutide is a potent, long-acting GLP-1 RA with a plasma half-life of approximately 7 days, enabling once-weekly subcutaneous administration or daily oral dosing with a bioavailability-optimized formulation.[3] Although developed originally for glucose regulation in type 2 diabetes, semaglutide engages multiple biological pathways directly relevant to cardiovascular health.

At the central nervous system level, semaglutide modulates hypothalamic appetite-regulatory systems and corticolimbic reward networks, decreasing hunger, enhancing satiety, and suppressing hedonic feeding behavior.[4] These effects facilitate sustained caloric reduction, durable weight loss, and recalibration of distorted appetite signaling characteristic of chronic obesity.

Peripherally, semaglutide improves insulin sensitivity, decreases hepatic glucose production, corrects atherogenic dyslipidemia, and preferentially reduces visceral and ectopic fat depots including hepatic steatosis and epicardial adipose tissue, pathological fat reservoirs closely linked to cardiometabolic injury.[5,6]

Additionally, semaglutide demonstrates anti-inflammatory, endothelial protective, autonomic stabilizing, and hemodynamic benefits, including reductions in C-reactive protein and inflammatory cytokines, improved endothelial function, lowered blood pressure, improved myocardial energetics, and favorable impact on cardiac filling pressures.[7] These mechanisms align precisely with biological pathways underlying atherosclerosis, plaque vulnerability, HFpEF pathophysiology, renal deterioration, and CKM disease progression.

Importantly, mediation analyses from major trials indicate that semaglutide's cardiovascular benefits cannot be explained solely by weight loss or glycemic improvement. A substantial proportion of benefit appears weight independent, reinforcing semaglutide's classification as a cardiovascularly active therapeutic rather than merely a metabolic adjunct.

STEP PROGRAM: ESTABLISHING WEIGHT LOSS AS A CARDIOVASCULAR THERAPEUTIC STRATEGY

The STEP (Semaglutide Treatment Effect in People with Obesity) clinical program forms the cornerstone of semaglutide's evidence base in obesity and cardiometabolic management. Across STEP 1–8 and the STEP TEENS trial, once-weekly subcutaneous semaglutide 2.4 mg has been consistently shown to induce large, sustained reductions in body weight across a wide spectrum of patients, including those with and without diabetes, adolescents, ethnically diverse populations, and individuals with established cardiovascular disease phenotypes.

The pivotal trials collectively evaluated semaglutide in individuals with obesity (BMI ≥30 kg/m^2) or overweight (BMI ≥27 kg/m^2 with at least one weight-related comorbidity), with STEP 1, 3, 4, 5, and 7[8-12] primarily enrolling nondiabetic populations, while STEP 2 specifically included individuals with type 2 diabetes. Other studies extended the evidence to East Asian populations (STEP 6 and 7)[12,13] and directly compared semaglutide with liraglutide (STEP 8).[14] The STEP TEENS trial[15] further established efficacy in adolescents aged 12–<18 years with severe obesity, highlighting the potential for early cardiometabolic risk modification.

Across these trials, semaglutide consistently produced clinically meaningful weight loss, with mean reductions typically ranging from approximately 13–16% at 68 weeks in nondiabetic adults (STEP 1, 3, 4, 6, 7, and 8) and around 10% in individuals with type 2 diabetes (STEP 2). Long-term data from STEP 5 demonstrated sustained benefit over 2 years, reinforcing the durability of effect. Importantly, a very high proportion of patients achieved key clinical thresholds of ≥5, ≥10, and ≥15% weight loss, with response rates dramatically exceeding placebo. STEP 4 demonstrated that discontinuation of semaglutide following initial weight loss results in significant weight regain underscoring obesity as a chronic relapsing disease requiring sustained pharmacotherapy rather than short-term intervention.

Importantly, the STEP program evolved beyond weight-centric outcomes to address cardiovascular syndromes directly linked to obesity. The STEP-HFpEF[16] and STEP-HFpEF DM[17] trials evaluated semaglutide in patients with obesity-related HFpEF, with and without diabetes. In these studies, semaglutide significantly improved patient-reported symptoms, functional capacity, and quality of life as assessed by the Kansas City Cardiomyopathy Questionnaire, alongside substantial weight reduction and favorable congestion biomarkers. These trials represent a major advance, positioning semaglutide as a therapy capable of modifying a high-burden cardiovascular phenotype for which effective treatments have historically been limited.

The STEP-UP trial[18] further explored dose-response relationships, demonstrating that higher weekly doses of semaglutide achieved even greater weight reduction, approaching magnitudes previously seen only with metabolic surgery. These findings inform future therapeutic optimization and underscore the central role of adiposity reduction in cardiometabolic disease modulation.

Across the STEP program, weight reduction was accompanied by consistent improvements in cardiovascular risk markers, including reductions in waist circumference, blood pressure, atherogenic lipids, glycemic indices, and inflammatory markers such as C-reactive protein. Preferential reduction in visceral and ectopic adipose tissue further supports mechanistic pathways linking weight loss to cardiovascular benefit.

Safety outcomes across the STEP program were consistent. Gastrointestinal adverse events, primarily nausea, vomiting, and diarrhea, were the most frequently reported, generally dose-related and transient. Cholelithiasis occurred infrequently and was largely associated with rapid weight reduction, while pancreatitis remained rare. Overall, serious adverse events were comparable to placebo, supporting a favorable long-term safety profile.

Collectively, the STEP program, summarized in **Table 1**, unequivocally establishes semaglutide 2.4 mg as a highly effective, durable, and broadly applicable pharmacologic

TABLE 1: Summary of STEP program trials evaluating semaglutide.

Trial	*Population*	*Duration (weeks)*	*Intervention*	*Primary endpoint*	*Key outcomes*	*Cardiovascular relevance*
STEP-1	Obesity/overweight without diabetes	68	Semaglutide 2.4 mg weekly versus placebo	% change in body weight	–14.9 versus –2.4%; 86% achieved ≥5% WL	Marked reduction in adiposity, BP, CRP
STEP-2	T2DM with overweight/obesity	68	Semaglutide 2.4 mg versus 1.0 mg versus placebo	% change in body weight	–9.6 versus –3.4%	Glycemic + cardiometabolic risk reduction
STEP-3	Obesity with intensive behavioral therapy	68	Semaglutide 2.4 mg versus placebo	% change in body weight	–16.0 versus –5.7%	Synergistic lifestyle + pharmacotherapy effect
STEP-4	Obesity after 20-week semaglutide run-in	48 (post run-in)	Continue semaglutide versus withdrawal	Weight change maintenance	–7.9 versus +6.9% regain	Demonstrates need for chronic therapy
STEP-5	Obesity without diabetes	104	Semaglutide 2.4 mg versus placebo	Long-term weight loss	–15.2 versus –2.6%	Confirms the durability of cardiometabolic benefit
STEP-6	East Asian obesity ± T2DM	68	Semaglutide 2.4 mg or 1.7 mg versus placebo	% change in body weight	–13.2 versus –2.1%	Ethnic generalizability
STEP-7	East Asian overweight/obesity ± T2DM	44	Semaglutide 2.4 mg versus placebo	% change in body weight	–12.1 versus –3.6%	Confirms consistency across populations
STEP-8	Obesity/overweight (no diabetes)	68	Semaglutide 2.4 mg versus liraglutide 3.0 mg	% weight change	–15.8 versus –6.4%	Superior efficacy versus liraglutide
STEP-TEENS	Adolescents (12–<18 years) with obesity	68	Semaglutide 2.4 mg versus placebo	% change in BMI	–16.1 versus +0.6%	Early cardiometabolic risk modification
STEP-HFpEF	HFpEF + obesity (no diabetes)	52	Semaglutide 2.4 mg versus placebo	KCCQ-CSS, % weight change	↑ KCCQ, ↑ exercise capacity, ↓ weight	Direct HFpEF symptom and functional benefit
STEP-HFpEF DM	HFpEF + obesity with T2DM	52	Semaglutide 2.4 mg versus placebo	KCCQ-CSS, % weight change	Similar improvements as non-DM cohort	Extends HFpEF benefit to diabetics
STEP-UP	Obesity without diabetes	72	Semaglutide 7.2 mg versus 2.4 mg versus placebo	% weight change	–18.7 (7.2 mg) versus –15.6% (2.4 mg)	Dose–response, future therapeutic optimization

therapy for obesity. Beyond pure weight reduction, the STEP trials laid the scientific foundation for semaglutide's cardiovascular relevance, providing biological plausibility for subsequent demonstration of cardiovascular benefit in outcome-driven studies.

SELECT: DEFINITIVE CARDIOVASCULAR RISK REDUCTION IN NONDIABETIC ASCVD

The SELECT trial[19] represents a landmark in cardiometabolic therapeutics, providing the first definitive evidence that pharmacologic treatment of overweight and obesity can reduce cardiovascular events independent of diabetes. SELECT was a large, randomized, double-blind, placebo-controlled cardiovascular outcomes trial that enrolled 17,604 adults aged ≥45 years with established atherosclerotic cardiovascular disease and BMI ≥27 kg/m^2, explicitly excluding individuals with diabetes. Participants were randomized to semaglutide 2.4 mg once weekly or placebo and followed for a mean duration of 39.8 months. The primary endpoint was time to first three-point MACE, comprising cardiovascular death, nonfatal myocardial infarction, or nonfatal stroke.

Semaglutide significantly reduced the incidence of MACE by 20% compared with placebo (6.5 vs. 8.0%; HR 0.80; 95% CI 0.72–0.90), establishing clear cardiovascular benefit in a nondiabetic secondary prevention population. Importantly, treatment effects were consistent across age groups, sex, geographic regions, baseline BMI categories, and cardiovascular disease subtypes, confirming broad applicability. Although adverse-event-related discontinuation was higher with semaglutide, driven primarily by gastrointestinal events, the overall safety profile was consistent with the established GLP-1 RA class and without excess serious adverse events.

A prespecified adiposity-trajectory analysis provided critical mechanistic insight.[20] The reduction in cardiovascular events was observed across all baseline adiposity levels and was not dependent on early or magnitude of weight loss. Approximately one third of the cardiovascular benefit was mediated by reductions in waist circumference, indicating that a substantial proportion of benefit arose from weight-independent mechanisms, likely including reductions in systemic inflammation, improvements in endothelial function, vascular biology, and myocardial-metabolic efficiency. Notably, no increase in serious adverse events was seen with greater weight or waist reduction, while unintentional weight loss in the placebo group was associated with higher mortality, underscoring the distinction between therapeutic and disease-related weight change.

SELECT therefore marks a paradigm shift in cardiovascular prevention, demonstrating that semaglutide provides direct cardiovascular protection beyond glycemic control and beyond weight loss alone. The trial firmly establishes semaglutide as a disease-modifying therapy in patients with obesity-related ASCVD and positions it alongside established cardioprotective agents within contemporary secondary prevention strategies.

STEER AND SCORE: REAL-WORLD CARDIOVASCULAR REINFORCEMENT

The translation of randomized clinical trial evidence into routine clinical practice is a critical step in validating therapeutic relevance. Two pivotal real-world datasets, the SCORE[21] and STEER[22] studies provide compelling confirmation that the cardiovascular benefits of semaglutide observed in SELECT extend to heterogeneous, everyday patient populations.

SCORE evaluated >9,300 adults with overweight or obesity and established ASCVD treated with semaglutide 2.4 mg, matched against 18,600 nonusers. Across clinically meaningful cardiovascular endpoints, semaglutide therapy was associated with substantial event reduction, including:

- ≈57% lower risk of MACE-3 (myocardial infarction, stroke, and all-cause mortality)
- ≈45% lower risk of MACE-5 (MACE-3 plus heart failure hospitalization and coronary revascularization)

These outcomes indicate not only cardiovascular protection but also a reduction in heart-failure-related morbidity of particular relevance in obesity-associated cardiovascular disease.

The STEER study examined 21,250 individuals with overweight/obesity and established ASCVD without diabetes, highlighting the cardioprotective value of semaglutide in a truly nondiabetic secondary-prevention setting. Compared with tirzepatide, semaglutide was associated with:

- 57% reduction in revised MACE-3, hazard ratio: 0.43 (95% CI 0.24–0.78)
- Lower absolute event rates (4.4 vs. 10.3 events per 1,000 patient-years)

This finding is particularly striking because it reinforces semaglutide's benefit beyond glycemic modulation and suggests meaningful cardiovascular superiority in comparable real-world cohorts.

Viewed collectively, the SCORE and STEER datasets deliver an integrated and compelling interpretation. They demonstrate that the cardiovascular risk reductions associated with semaglutide are robust, consistent, and clinically meaningful, reinforcing the therapeutic signal observed in randomized trials. Importantly, these benefits extend beyond controlled research environments into routine clinical practice, encompassing diverse patient populations with real-world variation in comorbid burden, adherence, and clinical management. In doing so, these studies significantly strengthen the external validity of semaglutide's cardioprotective effect. Equally noteworthy, SCORE and STEER consolidate semaglutide's position as a legitimate secondary prevention therapy in patients with overweight or obesity and established ASCVD, including those without diabetes, a critical expansion of therapeutic relevance. Across both datasets, no new safety concerns emerged, further increasing clinician confidence regarding its broad clinical application.

From a safety standpoint, real-world findings remain highly concordant with randomized evidence. Gastrointestinal adverse events are the most frequently encountered effects, typically dose dependent, predictable, and self-limiting in nature. A modest increase in cholelithiasis has been observed, primarily attributable to rapid weight loss rather than intrinsic drug toxicity. Retinopathy progression, when reported, appears related to abrupt glycemic improvement in individuals with long-standing diabetes, echoing earlier observations from SUSTAIN-6 and supporting the need for ophthalmological surveillance in high-risk patients. Importantly, serious adverse events are not generally increased; in several programs, including HFpEF and cardiovascular outcome trials, serious event rates were numerically lower than placebo.

Taken together, these real-world data provide decisive validation that semaglutide not only reduces cardiovascular events but does so with a consistent and reassuring safety profile. SCORE and STEER therefore reinforce semaglutide's evolving role as a cornerstone therapy within modern secondary cardiovascular prevention and the broader cardiometabolic care paradigm.

SOUL: VALIDATING ORAL SEMAGLUTIDE FOR CARDIOVASCULAR OUTCOMES

The SOUL trial was a large, multinational, double-blind cardiovascular outcomes study designed to evaluate whether oral semaglutide confers cardiovascular protection in high-risk individuals with type 2 diabetes.[23] The trial enrolled 9,650 participants aged ≥50 years with established atherosclerotic cardiovascular disease and/or chronic kidney disease, HbA1c between 6.5 and 10%, and followed them for a mean duration of approximately 47.5 months across 33 countries. Participants were randomized to oral semaglutide titrated up to 14 mg daily or placebo, with the primary endpoint being time to first MACE, defined as cardiovascular death, nonfatal myocardial infarction, or nonfatal stroke.

SOUL demonstrated a 14% relative risk reduction in MACE with oral semaglutide compared with placebo (HR 0.86; 95% CI 0.77–0.96). Importantly, the cardiovascular benefit was consistent irrespective of concurrent SGLT2 inhibitor therapy, highlighting its additive therapeutic value within contemporary cardioprotective treatment regimens. Safety outcomes were reassuring, with serious adverse events comparable to placebo, no increase in severe hypoglycemia or diabetic ketoacidosis, and gastrointestinal adverse effects remaining the most common class-related events.

Overall, SOUL confirms that oral semaglutide provides clinically meaningful cardiovascular risk reduction in high-risk T2DM populations, broadens therapeutic accessibility for patients unwilling or unsuitable for injectable therapy, and reinforces that cardiovascular protection with semaglutide represents a formulation-independent clinical effect.

SUSTAIN-6: FROM SAFETY CONFIRMATION TO A DEFINITIVE CARDIOVASCULAR SIGNAL

SUSTAIN-6 was a pivotal, double-blind, randomized cardiovascular outcomes trial conducted across 20 countries to evaluate the cardiovascular safety of injectable semaglutide in individuals with type 2 diabetes at elevated cardiovascular risk. The trial enrolled 3,297 adults, including those aged ≥50 years with established cardiovascular disease, chronic kidney disease, or heart failure, or ≥60 years with at least one additional cardiovascular risk factor, all with HbA1c ≥7%. Participants were assigned to once-weekly semaglutide 0.5 or 1.0 mg versus placebo and followed for 104 weeks with an additional 5-week observation period.

The primary endpoint was time to first occurrence of three-point MACEs, comprising cardiovascular death, nonfatal myocardial infarction, or nonfatal stroke. Semaglutide significantly reduced MACE to 6.6 versus 8.9% with placebo, corresponding to a 26% relative risk reduction (HR 0.74; 95% CI 0.58–0.95), thereby meeting both noninferiority and superiority criteria (p = 0.02). Component analyses demonstrated marked reductions in nonfatal stroke (HR 0.61) and nonfatal myocardial infarction (HR 0.74). Additionally, semaglutide was associated with a reduced risk of new or worsening nephropathy (HR 0.64) and overall lower rates of serious adverse events compared with placebo.

The safety profile was consistent with the GLP-1 RA class, with gastrointestinal adverse effects being most frequent. A higher incidence of diabetic retinopathy complications was observed (HR 1.76), largely attributed to rapid glucose lowering in individuals with preexisting advanced retinopathy, emphasizing the importance of ophthalmologic surveillance in such patients. Rates of pancreatitis, malignancy, and other major safety outcomes were comparable to placebo, with only a mild increase in heart rate noted.

SUSTAIN-6 therefore not only confirmed cardiovascular safety but provided one of the earliest and strongest indications that semaglutide confers meaningful cardiovascular protection, setting the stage for subsequent definitive outcome trials, and reshaping its role from a glucose-lowering therapy to a cardiometabolic agent of major clinical relevance.

Semaglutide's role in cardiology is anchored by six landmark clinical programs that collectively define its cardiovascular efficacy, safety, and translational relevance. A summary of these pivotal trials is presented in **Figures 1A to F**.

PRACTICAL SEMAGLUTIDE PROTOCOL FOR USE IN CARDIOLOGY PRACTICE

With the expansion of evidence supporting semaglutide's cardiovascular benefit, a structured and pragmatic approach is essential for its safe and effective integration

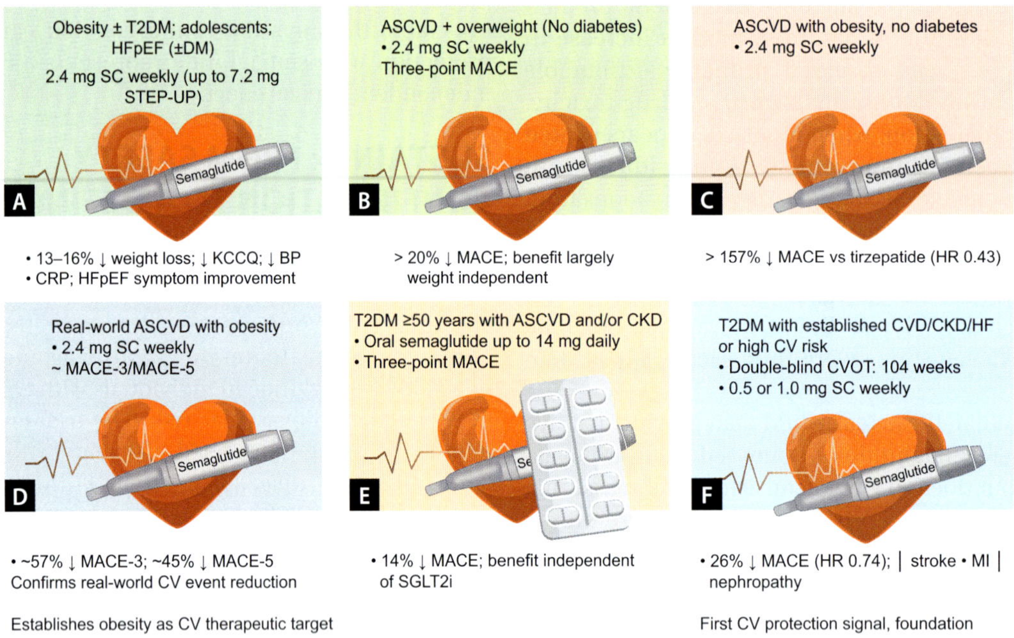

Figs. 1A to F: Summary of six pivotal trials evaluating cardiovascular outcomes with semaglutide. (A) STEP program; (B) SELECT; (C) STEER; (D) SCORE; (E) SOUL; (F) SUSTAIN-6.

TABLE 2: Comprehensive clinical protocol for semaglutide use in cardiology practice.

Domain	Key points
Indications	• Obesity/adiposity: Waist circumference >90 cm (men), >80 cm (women); BMI ≥30 kg/m² or ≥27 kg/m² with comorbidities • Type 2 diabetes mellitus • Cardiovascular disease: ASCVD, heart failure (especially obesity-related HFpEF), CKM multimorbidity • Age: ≥12 years
Contraindications/caution	• Absolute: Personal or family history of medullary thyroid carcinoma, MEN-2, pregnancy or lactation, known hypersensitivity to semaglutide • Use with caution: History of pancreatitis, significant GI disease (gastroparesis, severe IBD), advanced age/frailty, sarcopenic obesity, marasmic state, multiorgan failure

Contd...

Contd...

Domain	*Key points*
Baseline clinical evaluation	• Anthropometry: Weight, BMI, waist circumference • Metabolic profile: Fasting glucose, HbA1c, lipid profile, CRP • Renal and hepatic: Serum creatinine, eGFR, AST, ALT • Thyroid: TSH, T3, T4 • Cardiac: BP, HR, ECG, echocardiography • Abdominal ultrasound (fatty liver, gallbladder) • Retinal examination (baseline; repeat ~6 months in diabetes) • Pregnancy test where applicable; history of pancreatitis, gallbladder disease, thyroid cancer
Patient counseling	• Reduced appetite and early satiety • Sustained weight loss • Improved glycemic control and HbA1c reduction • Reduction in ASCVD and HF burden • Common AEs: nausea, vomiting, diarrhea, constipation • Rare AEs: Pancreatitis, gallstones, transient retinopathy worsening • Emphasize gradual dose escalation and long-term therapy
Dose escalation protocol (SC)	• Weeks 1–4: 0.25 mg weekly • Weeks 5–8: 0.5 mg weekly • Weeks 9–12: 1.0 mg weekly • Weeks 13–16: 1.7 mg weekly • ≥Week 17: 2.4 mg weekly (target dose) *Delay escalation by 4 weeks if intolerance occurs*
Maintenance dose	• Preferred: 2.4 mg weekly • If not tolerated: 1.7 mg weekly
Monitoring during therapy	• Every 2–4 weeks/monthly: GI tolerance, adherence, weight, waist circumference, BP, HR, fasting glucose, HbA1c, renal function • Every 6 months: HbA1c, LFTs, lipid profile, retinal evaluation (diabetes)
Concomitant drug adjustment	• Reduce insulin or sulfonylurea doses to prevent hypoglycemia • Avoid DPP-4 inhibitors • Safe to combine with SGLT2 inhibitors, metformin, statins, ACEi/ARB/ARNI, beta-blockers
When to discontinue	• Persistent or severe GI intolerance • Symptoms suggestive of pancreatitis • New or worsening visual symptoms • Detection of thyroid nodules or suspected malignancy
Follow-up and lifestyle reinforcement	• Nutritional optimization with adequate protein intake • Regular physical activity (aerobic + resistance training) • Adequate sleep • Behavioral modification support • Reinforce dosing schedule and adherence
Longitudinal checklist/ trajectory	• Waist circumference and weight • BP and HR • Fasting glucose and HbA1c • LFTs, KFTs, lipid profile • Retinal status • In HF: Echocardiography and NT-proBNP/BNP trends • Sarcopenia surveillance • CRP ± adipokines (optional/research)

into routine cardiology practice. **Table 2** summarizes the key clinical considerations, including indications, contraindications, baseline evaluation, dosing, monitoring, and follow-up, to guide cardiologists in the evidence-based use of semaglutide across diverse cardiometabolic scenarios.

CONCLUSION

Semaglutide's evolution from a glucose-lowering therapy to a cornerstone cardiometabolic treatment represents a defining paradigm shift in contemporary cardiovascular medicine. Cumulative evidence from the STEP, SELECT,

STEER, SCORE, SOUL, and SUSTAIN programs demonstrates not only durable and clinically meaningful durable weight reduction, but also robust reduction in cardiovascular events, improvements in symptom burden and quality of life in obesity-related cardiac syndromes, and consistent benefit across both randomized trials and real-world clinical practice.

Importantly, the incorporation of a structured, evidence-based clinical protocol enables translation of these findings into routine cardiology care. Semaglutide now holds a justified and actionable role across cardiovascular spectrum, HFpEF management, CKM intervention, and obesity-driven cardiovascular disease modulation, marking a decisive transition toward upstream cardiometabolic therapeutic strategy in modern cardiology, thereby enhancing CVD morbidity and mortality benefits.

REFERENCES

1. Bray GA, Kim KK, Wilding JPH. Obesity: a chronic relapsing progressive disease process. A position statement of the World Obesity Federation. Obes Rev. 2017;18(7):715-23.
2. Kyle TK, Dhurandhar EJ, Allison DB. Regarding obesity as a disease: evolving policies and their implications. Endocrinol Metab Clin North Am. 2016;45(3):511.
3. Kommu S, Whitfield P. Semaglutide. Pharma-Kritik. 2024;40(8):29-31.
4. Park JS, Kim KS, Choi HJ. Glucagon-like peptide-1 and hypothalamic regulation of satiation: cognitive and neural insights from human and animal studies. Diabetes Metab J. 2025;49(3):333.
5. Jensterle M, Ferjan S, Ležaič L, et al. Semaglutide delays 4-hour gastric emptying in women with polycystic ovary syndrome and obesity. Diabetes Obes Metab. 2023;25(4):975-84.
6. Sokary S, Bawadi H. Exploring beyond numeric weight loss: the metabolic effects of semaglutide. Clin Nutr ESPEN. 2025;67:435-40.
7. Mosenzon O, Capehorn MS, De Remigis A, et al. Impact of semaglutide on high-sensitivity C-reactive protein: exploratory patient-level analyses of SUSTAIN and PIONEER randomized clinical trials. Cardiovasc Diabetol. 2022;21(1):172.
8. Rubino D, Abrahamsson N, Davies M, et al. Effect of continued weekly subcutaneous semaglutide vs placebo on weight loss maintenance in adults with overweight or obesity: the STEP 4 randomized clinical trial. JAMA. 2021;325(14):1414-25.
9. Wadden TA, Bailey TS, Billings LK, et al. Effect of subcutaneous semaglutide vs placebo as an adjunct to intensive behavioral therapy on body weight in adults with overweight or obesity: the STEP 3 randomized clinical trial. JAMA. 2021;325(14):1403-13.
10. Wilding JPH, Batterham RL, Calanna S, et al. Once-weekly semaglutide in adults with overweight or obesity. N Engl J Med. 2021;384(11):989-1002.
11. Garvey WT, Batterham RL, Bhatta M, et al. Two-year effects of semaglutide in adults with overweight or obesity: the STEP 5 trial. Nat Med. 2022;28(10):2083-91.
12. Mu Y, Bao X, Eliaschewitz FG, et al. Efficacy and safety of once weekly semaglutide 2.4 mg for weight management in a predominantly East Asian population with overweight or obesity (STEP 7): a double-blind, multicentre, randomised controlled trial. Lancet Diabetes Endocrinol. 2024;12(3):184-95.
13. Kadowaki T, Isendahl J, Khalid U, et al. Semaglutide once a week in adults with overweight or obesity, with or without type 2 diabetes in an East Asian population (STEP 6): a randomised, double-blind, double-dummy, placebo-controlled, phase 3a trial. Lancet Diabetes Endocrinol. 2022;10(3):193-206.
14. Rubino DM, Greenway FL, Khalid U, et al. Effect of weekly subcutaneous semaglutide vs daily liraglutide on body weight in adults with overweight or obesity without diabetes: the STEP 8 randomized clinical trial. JAMA. 2022;327(2):138-50.
15. Weghuber D, Barrett T, Barrientos-Pérez M, et al. Once-weekly semaglutide in adolescents with obesity. N Engl J Med. 2022;387(24):2245-57.
16. Kosiborod MN, Abildstrøm SZ, Borlaug BA, et al. Semaglutide in patients with heart failure with preserved ejection fraction and obesity. N Engl J Med. 2023;389(12):1069-84.
17. Kosiborod MN, Petrie MC, Borlaug BA, et al. Semaglutide in patients with obesity-related heart failure and type 2 diabetes. N Engl J Med. 2024;390(15):1394-407.
18. Wharton S, Freitas P, Hjelmesæth J, et al. Once-weekly semaglutide 7.2 mg in adults with obesity (STEP UP): a randomised, controlled, phase 3b trial. Lancet Diabetes Endocrinol. 2025;13(11):949-63.
19. Lincoff AM, Brown-Frandsen K, Colhoun HM, et al. Semaglutide and cardiovascular outcomes in obesity without diabetes. N Engl J Med. 2023;389(24):2221-32.
20. Deanfield J, Lincoff AM, Kahn SE, et al. Semaglutide and cardiovascular outcomes by baseline and changes in adiposity measurements: a prespecified analysis of the SELECT trial. Lancet. 2025;406(10516):2257-68.
21. Zhao Z, Song J, Faurby M, et al. Lower risk of mace and all-cause death in patients initiated on semaglutide 2.4 mg in routine clinical care: results from the SCORE study (semaglutide effects on cardiovascular outcomes in people with overweight or obesity in the real world). J Am Coll Cardiol. 2025;85(12):380.
22. Reuters. (2025). Novo Nordisk's Wegovy cuts heart risk by 57% versus rival Lilly weight-loss drug in study. [online] Available from https://www.reuters.com/business/healthcare-pharmaceuticals/novo-nordisks-wegovy-cuts-heart-risk-by-57-versus-rival-lilly-weight-loss-drug-2025-08-31/. [Last accessed January, 2026].
23. Marx N, Deanfield JE, Mann JFE, et al. Oral semaglutide and cardiovascular outcomes in people with type 2 diabetes, according to SGLT2i use: prespecified analyses of the SOUL randomized trial. Circulation. 2025;151(23):1639-50.

91

CHAPTER

Cardiovascular Benefits of Weight Loss: The Position of Glucagon-like Peptide-1 Receptor Agonists

Tiny Nair

INTRODUCTION

Glucagon-like peptide-1 receptor agonists (GLP-1 RAs) have rapidly emerged as one of the most important therapeutic classes in modern metabolic and cardiovascular medicine. Originally designed to address the diminished incretin effect in type 2 diabetes mellitus (T2DM), these agents are now recognized as potent weight-loss medications, cardioprotective agents, modulators of systemic inflammation, and key components of long-term risk reduction strategies.[1,2] Their capacity to influence multiple physiological pathways has positioned them at the center of contemporary discussions on obesity, diabetes, cardiovascular disease prevention, and metabolic health. This expanded review examines their mechanisms, clinical trial evidence, cardiometabolic benefits, renal outcomes, safety, and future directions, integrating insights from landmark trials and mechanistic studies.

PHYSIOLOGICAL OVERVIEW AND MECHANISTIC FOUNDATIONS

Glucagon-like peptide-1 is an incretin hormone secreted by L-cells in the distal small intestine in response to nutrient intake. It enhances glucose-dependent insulin secretion, suppresses inappropriate glucagon release, delays gastric emptying, and promotes satiety.[3] Pharmacological GLP-1 RAs replicate and amplify these effects, with extended half-lives enabling daily or weekly dosing.

CENTRAL MECHANISMS OF APPETITE AND WEIGHT REGULATION

Glucagon-like peptide-1 receptors in the hypothalamic arcuate nucleus modulate satiety by activating proopiomelanocortin (POMC) neurons and inhibiting neuropeptide-Y/agouti-related peptide (NPY/AgRP) neurons.[3] These neural circuits are critical for regulating hunger and caloric intake. GLP-1 RAs also influence mesolimbic dopaminergic pathways, reducing hedonic eating and the reward value of high-calorie foods. This dual action—homeostatic and hedonic—explains the robust and sustained weight loss observed in clinical trials.

Peripheral Metabolic Effects

Peripherally, GLP-1 RAs slow gastric emptying, reduce postprandial glucose excursions, and promote insulin secretion during hyperglycemia while minimizing hypoglycemia.[3] They also reduce hepatic steatosis, modulate adipokine secretion, improve endothelial function, and reduce visceral fat. These effects collectively translate into broad improvements in metabolic health.

Weight Loss Efficacy: Lessons from STEP and SURMOUNT

One of the most transformative findings in obesity pharmacotherapy has been the magnitude of weight loss achieved with GLP-1 RAs. Semaglutide 2.4 mg (STEP Program): STEP-1 demonstrated a mean weight reduction of 14.9% among nondiabetic individuals with overweight or obesity, with nearly one third losing ≥20% of baseline weight.[4] STEP-2 and STEP-3 extended these findings to individuals with diabetes and those undergoing intensive lifestyle intervention, consistently showing reductions far superior to earlier pharmacotherapies.

Tirzepatide (SURMOUNT-1)

Tirzepatide, a dual GIP/GLP-1 RA, achieved weight loss up to 21% in SURMOUNT-1.[5] Importantly, MRI substudies revealed dramatic reductions in visceral adipose tissue, liver fat, and inflammatory biomarkers. These findings carry major implications for cardiometabolic risk, as visceral fat—rather than total fat mass—drives insulin resistance and adverse cardiovascular outcomes.

Cardiovascular Benefits: Evidence from Major Trials

Cardiovascular outcome trials (CVOTs) represent a cornerstone in understanding GLP-1 RA benefits beyond glycemic control.

LEADER

LEADER enrolled 9,340 individuals with T2DM at high cardiovascular risk and demonstrated a 13% reduction in major adverse cardiovascular events (MACE), with a particularly notable 22% reduction in cardiovascular death.[6] Liraglutide also reduced renal endpoints and hospitalizations for heart failure.

SUSTAIN-6

SUSTAIN-6, examining semaglutide, demonstrated a 26% reduction in MACE, primarily driven by stroke reduction.[7] These benefits emerged early and were consistent across subgroups.

REWIND

Unique among CVOTs, REWIND enrolled a majority of patients without prior cardiovascular disease. Dulaglutide reduced MACE by 12%, highlighting the potential for primary prevention.[8]

HARMONY

HARMONY showed a 22% MACE reduction with albiglutide.[9] Though the drug was later withdrawn for commercial reasons, the trial strengthened the evidence that GLP-1 RAs provide class-wide cardiovascular benefit.

Mechanistic Basis for Cardiovascular Protection

Several mechanisms explaining the cardioprotective effects of GLP-1 RAs have been postulated. They include the following:

- *Reduction in blood pressure:* GLP-1 receptor agonists consistently lower systolic blood pressure by 3–6 mm Hg.[10] While part of this decline is due to weight loss, GLP-1-mediated natriuresis and vasodilation also contribute directly.
- *Improved lipid profile:* Modest reductions in triglycerides and LDL cholesterol, along with increases in HDL cholesterol, have been documented.[11] Improvements in postprandial lipemia may help slow atherosclerotic plaque growth.
- *Anti-inflammatory and antiatherosclerotic effects:* GLP-1 receptor agonists decrease inflammatory cytokines, including C-reactive protein and interleukin-6.[11] They enhance endothelial nitric oxide availability, reduce oxidative stress, and lower markers of endothelial dysfunction.
- *Reduction in epicardial and visceral fat:* Excess epicardial fat is linked to coronary inflammation and diastolic dysfunction. GLP-1 receptor agonists decrease epicardial adipose thickness, which correlates with better diastolic function.[11] This is especially relevant in India, where visceral adiposity is a major driver of cardiovascular disease.
- *Renal protection:* Complementary to SGLT2 inhibitors: Although SGLT2 inhibitors remain the primary treatment for diabetic kidney disease, GLP-1 receptor agonists provide additional renal benefits.

Mann et al. showed reduced progression to macroalbuminuria and slower eGFR decline with liraglutide.[12] Likely contributing factors include decreased renal inflammation, better metabolic control, and weight loss. These findings support combined therapies for patients with obesity-related cardiovascular and renal risks.

Benefits in Nondiabetic Individuals

A significant paradigm shift recognizes that GLP-1 receptor agonists benefit people without diabetes. In STEP-1, metabolic syndrome parameters improved regardless of initial blood sugar levels.[4] Similar results appeared in SURMOUNT-1,[5] showing benefits such as:

- Reduction in liver fat
- Less severe sleep apnea
- Decreased systemic inflammation
- Enhanced fitness and mobility
- Improved quality of life[13]

This indicates that GLP-1 receptor agonists are effective metabolic treatments independent of their glucose-lowering effects.[14]

SAFETY AND TOLERABILITY

Glucagon-like peptide-1 receptor agonists are generally safe. Gastrointestinal symptoms such as nausea, vomiting, and constipation affect up to 30–40% of users, but usually lessen with dose titration.[15] Rare issues include gallbladder disease and pancreatitis. There is no strong evidence linking them to increased thyroid cancer risk in humans, though rodent studies suggest caution for those with MEN2 or medullary thyroid carcinoma.

Long-term safety data are favorable, supported by over 10 years of postmarketing experience.

FUTURE DIRECTIONS: THE ERA OF MULTIAGONISTS

Next-generation incretin therapies—triple agonists targeting GLP-1, GIP, and glucagon receptors—have shown weight loss exceeding 24% in early trials.[16] These drugs improve metabolic rate, reduce liver fat, and boost insulin sensitivity. They may narrow the gap between drugs and bariatric surgery. Other emerging areas include:

- Oral GLP-1 receptor agonists with greater potency
- Combination therapy with SGLT2 inhibitors
- Personalized obesity medicine based on genetic and metabolic profiling
- Investigating GLP-1 benefits in neurodegenerative diseases.

CONCLUSION

Glucagon-like peptide-1 receptor agonists represent a groundbreaking step forward in the treatment of metabolic and cardiovascular conditions. With strong evidence of significant weight loss, cardiovascular risk reduction, kidney protection, and improvements in metabolic health—even in nondiabetic people—they are now key in managing obesity and cardiometabolic diseases. As new incretin therapies develop, the treatment landscape will grow, offering new opportunities to improve population health.

REFERENCES

1. Nauck MA, Meier JJ. Incretin hormones: their role in health and disease. Diabetes Obes Metab. 2018;20:5-21.
2. Drucker DJ. Mechanisms of action of GLP-1-based therapies. Cell Metab. 2018;27:740-56.
3. Holst JJ. The physiology of glucagon-like peptide-1. Physiol Rev. 2007;87:1409-39.
4. Wilding JPH, Batterham RL, Calanna S, et al. Once-weekly semaglutide in adults with overweight or obesity. N Engl J Med. 2021;384:989-1002.
5. Jastreboff AM, Aronne LJ, Ahmad NN, et al. Tirzepatide once weekly for the treatment of obesity. N Engl J Med. 2022;387:205-16.
6. Marso SP, Daniels GH, Brown-Frandsen K, et al. Liraglutide and cardiovascular outcomes in type 2 diabetes. N Engl J Med. 2016;375:311-22.
7. Marso SP, Bain SC, Consoli A, et al. Semaglutide and cardiovascular outcomes in patients with type 2 diabetes. N Engl J Med. 2016;375:1834-44.
8. Gerstein HC, Colhoun HM, Dagenais GR, et al. Dulaglutide and cardiovascular outcomes in type 2 diabetes (REWIND): a double-blind, randomised placebo-controlled trial. Lancet. 2019;394:121-30.
9. Hernandez AF, Green JB, Janmohamed S, et al. Albiglutide and cardiovascular outcomes in patients with type 2 diabetes and cardiovascular disease (Harmony Outcomes): a double-blind, randomised placebo-controlled trial. Lancet. 2018;392:1519-29.
10. Teslaa T, et al. Circulation. 2019;140:1801-11.
11. Lee M, et al. Diabetes Care. 2020;43:2830-8.
12. Mann JFE, et al. Lancet Diabetes Endocrinol. 2017;5:605-17.
13. Davies M, Færch L, Jeppesen OK, et al. Semaglutide 2.4 mg once a week in adults with overweight or obesity, and type 2 diabetes (STEP 2): a randomised, double-blind, double-dummy, placebo-controlled, phase 3 trial. Lancet. 2021;397:971-84.
15. Bethel MA, Patel RA, Merrill P, et al. Cardiovascular outcomes with glucagon-like peptide-1 receptor agonists in patients with type 2 diabetes: a meta-analysis. Lancet Diabetes Endocrinol. 2018;6:105-13.
16. Coskun T, et al. Cell Metab. 2022;34:843-56.

92

CHAPTER

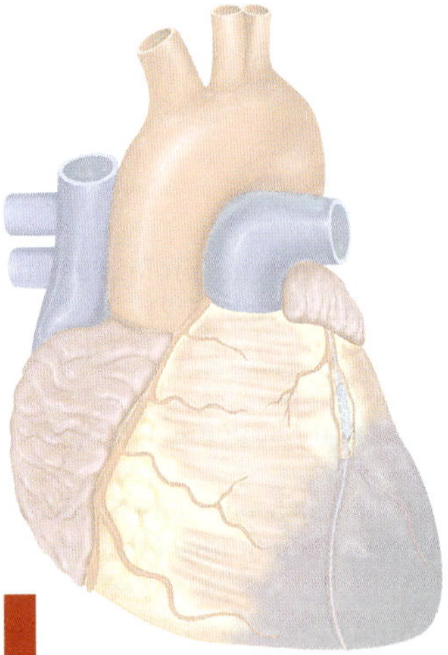

Semaglutide for Managing Obesity and Diabetes: What do the Guidelines Recommend?

Ranjit Unnikrishnan, V Mohan

INTRODUCTION

The glucagon-like peptide 1 receptor agonists (GLP-1 RAs) are novel therapeutic agents, originally launched as glucose-lowering drugs for use in individuals with type 2 diabetes (T2D). Clinical experience right from the time of introduction of these agents has revealed that they possess pleiotropic benefits over and beyond their glucose-lowering effects. While there exists evidence for these benefits with most of the newer GLP-1 RAs, semaglutide stands out as the agent with the most robust clinical trial evidence base not only for benefits in glucose-lowering, but with respect to other metabolic parameters such as body weight, cardiovascular risk, and renal dysfunction. Semaglutide also has the advantage of being the only GLP-1 RA currently available in an oral formulation.

Clinical practice guidelines have recognized the mounting evidence for benefits of semaglutide by amending their recommendations and expanding the indications for use of this agent in individuals with and without T2D. However, even the most regularly updated practice guidelines have struggled to keep up with the explosion of evidence on this drug. In this chapter, we discuss the current status of semaglutide in popularly quoted clinical practice guidelines, review the evidence base for the various indications of this drug, and provide a crystal ball for the likely expansion of the recommended indications in the near future.

AMERICAN DIABETES ASSOCIATION GUIDELINES

The 2025 edition of the American Diabetes Association (ADA)'s Standards of Care in Diabetes recommends the use of GLP-1 RAs with proven benefits in reducing cardiorenal adverse outcomes, as initial antihyperglycemic therapy in individuals with atherosclerotic cardiovascular disease (ASCVD), heart failure (HF), and diabetic kidney disease, along with lifestyle modification. These therapies are to be prescribed without reference to the prevailing HbA1c levels.[1]

It should be noted that these guidelines do not explicitly mention semaglutide; however, as current evidence supports the use of both oral and injectable semaglutide in reducing major adverse cardiovascular events, and that of injectable semaglutide in improving outcomes in HF and diabetic kidney disease, these guidelines can be construed as an endorsement of the use of semaglutide for these indications.

The ADA guidelines also state that GLP-1 RAs with proven benefits are preferred glucose-lowering agents in individuals with T2D and metabolic dysfunction-associated steatotic liver disease (MASLD). Here again, semaglutide is the only GLP-1 RA for which there exists Phase 3 clinical trial evidence of benefit in MASLD (albeit in an interim analysis).[2]

AMERICAN COLLEGE OF CARDIOLOGY/AMERICAN HEART ASSOCIATION GUIDELINES

The 2025 American College of Cardiology/American Heart Association (ACC/AHA) guidelines on management of obesity in HF,[3] while recognizing that semaglutide improves functional capacity and symptoms in individuals with obesity and heart failure with preserved ejection fraction (HFpEF), stop short of recommending it for this indication, as trials have not shown robust evidence of reduction in HF events and hospitalizations in this population.

SUMMARY OF EVIDENCE

There is now a large body of evidence on the benefits of both oral and injectable semaglutide in reducing glycemia in individuals with T2D. There is also considerable evidence on its benefits for weight reduction and improvement of adverse cardiorenal outcomes, in individuals with and without T2D.

Semaglutide as a Glucose-lowering Agent

The SUSTAIN trial program investigated the effects of injectable semaglutide in >8,000 individuals with T2D.[4] These trials have clearly shown that semaglutide (both at 0.5 and 1 mg doses) is associated with statistically superior reductions in HbA1c compared to placebo and active comparators (basal insulin, sitagliptin, exenatide, and dulaglutide) in a range of patient populations with T2D **(Table 1)**.

Similarly, the PIONEER program evaluated the effects of oral semaglutide in individuals with T2D.[5] Overall, oral semaglutide was found to be superior to placebo, sitagliptin, and empagliflozin and noninferior to liraglutide in bringing about reductions in HbA1c **(Table 2)**.

As glucose-lowering drugs, semaglutide and other GLP-1 RAs have the major advantage that they do not cause hypoglycemia when used as monotherapy or in combination with other glucose-lowering agents (except insulin and sulfonylureas). This, along with the pleiotropic benefits noted elsewhere in this article, has led to it being promoted in the hierarchy of glucose-lowering

TABLE 1: Summary of trials of injectable semaglutide on HbA1c reduction.

Trial	*N; Duration*	*Comparator*	*HbA1c reduction (%)*			
SUSTAIN 1 Monotherapy in drug-naive	388; 30 weeks	Placebo	**Sema 0.5 mg**	**Sema 1.0 mg**	Placebo	
			–1.5*	–1.6*	<–0.1	
SUSTAIN 2 Add on to metformin, TZD, or metformin/TZD	1,231; 56 weeks	Sitagliptin	**Sema 0.5 mg**	**Sema 1.0 mg**	Placebo	
			–1.3*	–1.6*	–0.5	
SUSTAIN 3 Add on to 1 or 2 OADs	813; 56 weeks	Exenatide ER	**Sema 1.0 mg**		Exe 2.0 mg	
			–1.5*		–0.9	
SUSTAIN 4 Add on to metformin ± SU	1,089; 30 weeks	Insulin glargine	**Sema 0.5 mg**	**Sema 1.0 mg**	Glargine	
			–1.2*	–1.6*	–0.8	
SUSTAIN 5 Add on to basal insulin	397; 30 weeks	Placebo	**Sema 0.5 mg**	**Sema 1.0 mg**	Placebo	
			–1.4*	–1.8*	–0.1	
SUSTAIN 6 CVOT	3,297; 104 weeks	Placebo	**Sema 0.5 mg**	**Sema 1.0 mg**	Placebo 0.5 mg	Placebo 1.0 mg
			–1.1*	–1.4*	–0.4	–0.4
SUSTAIN 7 Add on to metformin	1,201; 40 weeks	Dulaglutide	**Sema 0.5 mg**	**Dula 0.75 mg**	**Sema 1.0 mg**	Dula 1.5 mg
			–1.5*	–1.1	–1.8*	–1.4

Source: Aroda et al.[4]

**p* < 0.05 for estimated treatment difference between injectable semaglutide and placebo/active comparator.

(CVOT: cardiovascular outcome trial; OAD: oral antidiabetic agent; SU: sulfonylurea; TZD: thiazolidinedione)

TABLE 2: Summary of trials of oral semaglutide on HbA1c reduction.

Trial	*N; Duration*	*Comparator*	*HbA1c reduction (%)*				
PIONEER 1 Monotherapy in drug-naive	703; 26 weeks	Placebo	**Sema 3 mg**	**Sema 7 mg**	**Sema 14 mg**	Placebo	
			−0.9*	−1.2*	−1.4*	−0.3	
PIONEER 2 Add on to metformin	822; 52 weeks	Empagliflozin	**Sema 14 mg**			Empa 25 mg	
			−1.3*			−0.9	
PIONEER 3 Add on to metformin ± SU	1,864; 78 weeks	Sitagliptin	**Sema 3 mg**	**Sema 7 mg**	**Sema 14 mg**	Sita 100 mg	
			−0.6	−0.8	−1.1*	−0.7	
PIONEER 4 Add on to metformin ± SGLT2i	711; 52 weeks	Liraglutide Placebo	**Sema 14 mg**	Lira 1.8 mg		Placebo	
			−1.2*	−0.9		−0.2	
PIONEER 5 Moderate renal impairment Add on to metformin ± SU or basal insulin ± metformin	324; 26 weeks	Placebo	**Sema 14 mg**			Placebo	
			−1.0*			−0.2	
PIONEER 6 CVOT	3,183; Event-driven	Placebo	**Sema 14 mg**			Placebo	
			−1.0			−0.3	
PIONEER 7 Add on to 1–2 OADs	504; 52 weeks	Sitagliptin	**Sema 14 mg**			Sita 100 mg	
			−1.3*			−0.8	
PIONEER 8 Add on to insulin ± metformin	731; 52 weeks	Placebo	**Sema 3 mg**	**Sema 7 mg**	**Sema 14 mg**	Placebo	
			−0.6*	−0.8*	−1.2*	−0.2	
PIONEER 9 Drug-naive or on stable dose of 1 OAD	243; 52 weeks	Liraglutide Placebo	**Sema 3 mg**	**Sema 7 mg**	**Sema 14 mg**	Lira 0.9 mg	Placebo
			−0.9*	−1.4*	−1.5*	−1.2	−0.1
PIONEER 10 Stable dose of 1 OAD	458; 52 weeks	Dulaglutide	Sema 3 mg	Sema 7 mg	Sema 14 mg	Dula 0.75 mg	
			−0.9	−1.4	−1.7*	−1.4	

Source: Thethi et al.[5]
*$p < 0.05$ for estimated treatment difference between oral semaglutide and placebo/active comparator.
(CVOT: cardiovascular outcome trial; OAD: oral antidiabetic agent; SGLT2i: sodium glucose cotransporter 2 inhibitor; SU: sulfonylurea)

agents (even to the first-line agent in some situations) in individuals with certain compelling indications.

Semaglutide and Obesity

The double-blind STEP-1 trial randomized 1,961 adults with BMI of ≥30 (≥27 in persons with ≥1 weight-related comorbidity) but without diabetes, to once-weekly subcutaneous semaglutide (at a dose of 2.4 mg) or placebo, plus lifestyle intervention for a period of 68 weeks.[6] Individuals randomized to semaglutide demonstrated a mean change in body weight of −14.9% as compared with −2.4% with placebo [estimated treatment difference of −12.4 percentage points; 95% confidence interval (CI): −13.4 to −11.5; $p < 0.001$]. Individuals randomized to semaglutide also had greater improvement in cardiometabolic risk factors and participant-reported physical functioning compared to placebo.

In the SUSTAIN trial program in individuals with T2D, use of semaglutide was consistently associated with weight loss compared to the placebo or active comparator.[4] The magnitude of the weight loss was lower than that noted in STEP-1, but it should be noted that SUSTAIN used a maximum semaglutide dose of 1 mg, compared to 2.4 mg in STEP. However, it should be noted that trials of other GLP-1 RAs have consistently shown lower magnitudes of weight loss in individuals with T2D compared to those without, even when comparable doses were used.

In the PIONEER trial program, oral semaglutide at a dose of up to 14 mg was associated with greater weight loss than placebo, sitagliptin, or injectable liraglutide, but similar to empagliflozin.[5] The magnitude of achieved weight loss was lower than that noted for injectable semaglutide. This has led to the investigation of higher doses of oral semaglutide for promoting greater magnitudes of weight loss. In the OASIS study, oral semaglutide at a dose of

25 mg/day was associated with a mean weight loss of 13.9%,[7] while 50 mg/day produced a mean weight loss of 15.1% (comparable to the weight loss obtained with injectable semaglutide).[8] These doses, however, are not licensed for clinical use at present.

Semaglutide and Cardiovascular Outcomes

Since 2008, the US Food and Drug Administration (USFDA) has mandated the demonstration of cardiovascular safety prior to approval of any new glucose-lowering agent. Accordingly, the SUSTAIN-6 trial randomly assigned 3,297 patients with T2D to receive once-weekly semaglutide (0.5 or 1.0 mg) or placebo,[9] in addition to standard care, for 104 weeks. While rates of cardiovascular death, nonfatal myocardial infarction, or nonfatal stroke were significantly lower among patients receiving semaglutide than among those receiving placebo, the trial could only conclude noninferiority as it was designed as part of regulatory protocol and not for demonstrating superiority. Subsequently, the SELECT trial in overweight and obese individuals without diabetes has shown that injectable semaglutide at a weekly dose of 2.4 mg is superior to placebo with respect to risk of cardiovascular death, nonfatal stroke, and nonfatal myocardial infarction.[10]

In the STEP-HFpEF trial, 529 patients who had HFpEF and BMI of ≥30 kg/m² were randomized to receive once-weekly semaglutide (2.4 mg) or placebo for 52 weeks.[11] Use of semaglutide was associated with larger reductions in symptoms and physical limitations, improvements in exercise function, and more weight loss compared to placebo. These findings are important as HFpEF has long been considered an unsolved riddle in cardiology, with few approved effective treatments. The findings of STEP-HFpEF therefore represent a major advance in management of this relatively common condition.

Cardiovascular benefits have been reported for oral semaglutide as well. In the SOUL conducted in 9,650 individuals with T2D and ASCVD, chronic kidney disease, or both, use of oral semaglutide was associated with a significantly lower risk of major adverse cardiovascular events compared to placebo.[12]

Semaglutide and Kidney

Post hoc analyses of cardiovascular outcome trials of liraglutide and dulaglutide suggested that these agents might have a beneficial role in preventing adverse outcomes in individuals with diabetic kidney disease. To further explore this hypothesis, the FLOW trial randomly assigned 3,530 individuals with T2D and chronic kidney disease to receive subcutaneous semaglutide at a dose of 1 mg/week or placebo.[13] The trial was prematurely terminated (due to benefit) at a median follow-up of 3.4 years, at which time individuals randomized to semaglutide had a significantly lower risk of kidney-specific adverse outcomes as well as death from cardiovascular causes compared to placebo.

Semaglutide and Metabolic Dysfunction-associated Steatotic Liver Disease

ESSENCE is a Phase 3, multicenter, randomized, double-blind, placebo-controlled trial of injectable semaglutide in individuals with MASLD.[2] The interim results of ESSENCE were reported recently. Use of semaglutide was associated with significantly greater likelihood of resolution of steatohepatitis without worsening of fibrosis and reduction in liver fibrosis without worsening of steatohepatitis.

Semaglutide and Peripheral Arterial Disease

There are a few therapeutic options that improve outcomes in clinically significant peripheral arterial disease (PAD). In the STRIDE trial, 792 individuals with T2D and PAD with intermittent claudication were randomly assigned to receive injectable semaglutide (1 mg/week) or placebo for 52 weeks.[14] Use of semaglutide was associated with significantly greater improvements in maximum walking distance compared to placebo.

ISSUES AND CONCERNS

As with any other GLP-1 RA, use of semaglutide has been associated with gastrointestinal adverse effects, which can occasionally be severe and necessitate discontinuation of the drug. Cases of acute pancreatitis have also been reported, although causality has not been proven. Another side effect reported in animal studies is the development of medullary thyroid carcinoma (MTC). Although no human cases have been reported, this finding has led to the recommendation that GLP-1 RAs be avoided in individuals with a personal or family history of MTC, or of multiple endocrine neoplasia (MEN) syndromes.

Recently, there has been concern over certain ophthalmologic side effects of semaglutide. In the SUSTAIN-6 trial, use of semaglutide was associated with worsening of diabetic retinopathy, but subsequent trials did not replicate this finding, in part due to the exclusion of individuals with significant diabetic retinopathy from participation.[15] An ongoing trial (FOCUS) aims to evaluate the risk of diabetic retinopathy with semaglutide use, and is expected to report in 2028. Till such time, it would be wise to avoid use of semaglutide in individuals with any grade of retinopathy higher than mild nonproliferative retinopathy. A more worrying concern relates to recent reports of nonarteritic ischemic optic neuropathy (NAION) with semaglutide use, although this correlation has not been consistently shown. In view of the above, it is advisable to obtain ophthalmologic opinion prior to initiating semaglutide, especially in individuals with T2D.[16]

When semaglutide is used for the primary indication of weight loss, the benefits last only as long as the drug is used. Most, if not all, the weight lost is regained once the drug is discontinued. This raises concerns of safety and cost if the drug needs to be taken long-term (even lifelong).

LIKELY EXPANSION OF THE ROLE OF SEMAGLUTIDE IN GUIDELINES

In view of the above evidence, there is likely to be a significant expansion in the indications for semaglutide in subsequent iterations of clinical practice guidelines promulgated by various organizations. Recognizing the central role of obesity in the development of metabolic dysfunction, the ADA has decided to publish Standards of Medical Care for obesity (separate from those for diabetes), and the process of preparing these guidelines is underway.[17] Central to this decision is the availability of medical therapies such as semaglutide that have the potential to bring about magnitudes of weight loss comparable to surgical interventions. It is also likely that semaglutide will be recommended as the first-line glucose-lowering agent in a larger proportion of individuals with T2D than is currently the case. Potential additional indications for choosing semaglutide as a first-line agent include comorbidities such as osteoarthritis, obstructive sleep apnea, PAD, and polycystic ovarian disease, for some of which clinical trial evidence is already available.[18]

With respect to cardiovascular indications, the ACC/AHA guidelines are likely to expand indications of semaglutide from HFpEF with obesity to a broader category of ASCVD with obesity as clinical trials have shown outcome benefits in this population, irrespective of the coexistence of T2D. With injectable semaglutide cementing its place as one of the pillars of management of diabetic kidney disease, renal society guidelines, such as KDIGO, are also likely to support its use for this indication.

CONCLUSION

From their initial introduction as glucose-lowering agents, GLP-1 RAs have now evolved to form a major class of metabolic medications. Among these, semaglutide stands apart as a true "broad-spectrum antidysmetabolic drug," with proven benefits on hyperglycemia, obesity, ASCVD, HF, kidney disease, and PAD, favorably modifying almost all components of the newly described cardiovascular-kidney-metabolic (CKM) syndrome.[19] It is therefore not surprising that indications for this agent are rapidly expanding and that clinical practice guidelines across the world are embracing it as a major tool in the fight against noncommunicable disease. There is an enormous number of ongoing clinical trials exploring the wider effects of semaglutide on different aspects of metabolic health. Information from these trials will help us further define the role of this molecule in metabolic care, and will also clear the air on its long-term safety and tolerability.

REFERENCES

1. American Diabetes Association Professional Practice Committee. 9. Pharmacologic approaches to glycemic treatment: standards of care in diabetes—2025. Diabetes Care. 2025;48(Suppl. 1):S181-206.
2. Sanyal AJ, Newsome PN, Kliers I, et al.; ESSENCE Study Group. Phase 3 trial of semaglutide in metabolic dysfunction-associated steatohepatitis. N Engl J Med. 2025;392:2089-99.
3. Kittleson MM, Benjamin EJ, Blumer V, et al. 2025 ACC scientific statement on the management of obesity in adults with heart failure: a report of the American College of Cardiology. J Am Coll Cardiol. 2025;86:1953-75.
4. Aroda VR, Ahmann A, Cariou B, et al. Comparative efficacy, safety, and cardiovascular outcomes with once-weekly subcutaneous semaglutide in the treatment of type 2 diabetes: insights from the SUSTAIN 1-7 trials. Diabetes Metab. 2019;45:409-18.
5. Thethi TK, Pratley R, Meier JJ. Efficacy, safety and cardiovascular outcomes of once-daily oral semaglutide in patients with type 2 diabetes: the PIONEER programme. Diabetes Obes Metab. 2020;22:1263-77.
6. Wilding JPH, Batterham RL, Calanna S, et al.; STEP 1 Study Group. Once-weekly semaglutide in adults with overweight or obesity. N Engl J Med. 2021;384:989-1002.
7. Wharton S, Lingvay I, Bogdanski P, et al.; OASIS 4 Study Group. Oral semaglutide at a dose of 25 mg in adults with overweight or obesity. N Engl J Med. 2025;393:1077-87.
8. Knop FK, Aroda VR, do Vale RD, et al.; OASIS 1 Investigators. Oral semaglutide 50 mg taken once per day in adults with overweight or obesity (OASIS 1): a randomised, double-blind, placebo-controlled, phase 3 trial. Lancet. 2023;402:705-19.
9. Marso SP, Bain SC, Consoli A, et al.; SUSTAIN-6 Investigators. Semaglutide and cardiovascular outcomes in patients with type 2 diabetes. N Engl J Med. 2016;375:1834-44.
10. Lincoff AM, Brown-Frandsen K, Colhoun HM, et al.; SELECT Trial Investigators. Semaglutide and cardio-vascular outcomes in obesity without diabetes. N Engl J Med. 2023;389:2221-32.

11. Kosiborod MN, Abildstrøm SZ, Borlaug BA, et al.; STEP-HFpEF Trial Committees and Investigators. Semaglutide in patients with heart failure with preserved ejection fraction and obesity. N Engl J Med. 2023;389:1069-84.
12. McGuire DK, Marx N, Mulvagh SL, et al.; SOUL Study Group. Oral semaglutide and cardiovascular outcomes in high-risk type 2 diabetes. N Engl J Med. 2025;392: 2001-12.
13. Perkovic V, Tuttle KR, Rossing P, et al.; FLOW Trial Committees and Investigators. Effects of semaglutide on chronic kidney disease in patients with type 2 diabetes. N Engl J Med. 2024;391:109-21.
14. Bonaca MP, Catarig AM, Houlind K, et al.; STRIDE Trial Investigators. Semaglutide and walking capacity in people with symptomatic peripheral artery disease and type 2 diabetes (STRIDE): a phase 3b, double-blind, randomised, placebo-controlled trial. Lancet. 2025;405:1580-93.
15. Bloomgarden ZT. Semaglutide and the retina. J Diabetes. 2025;17:e70085.
16. Natividade GR, Spiazzi BF, Baumgarten MW, et al. Ocular adverse events with semaglutide: a systematic review and meta-analysis. JAMA Ophthalmol. 2025;143:759-68.
17. Bannuru RR; ADA Professional Practice Committee (PPC). Introduction and methodology: standards of care in overweight and obesity-2025. BMJ Open Diabetes Res Care. 2025;13(Suppl. 1):e004928.
18. Bliddal H, Bays H, Czernichow S, et al.; STEP 9 Study Group. Once-weekly semaglutide in persons with obesity and knee osteoarthritis. N Engl J Med. 2024;391:1573-83.
19. Ndumele CE, Neeland IJ, Tuttle KR, et al.; American Heart Association. A synopsis of the evidence for the science and clinical management of cardiovascular-kidney-metabolic (CKM) syndrome: a scientific statement from the American Heart Association. Circulation. 2023;148:1636-64.

93

CHAPTER

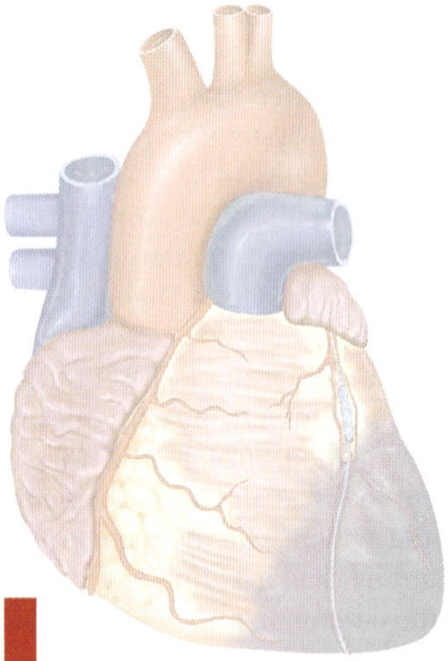

Obesity, Diabetes Management, and Cardiovascular Risk Reduction Strategies: Semaglutide and Tirzepatide Major Trials Update

JPS Sawhney, Nitin Saini, KM Vivek

INTRODUCTION

Obesity is a major global health challenge which is strongly associated with major cardiovascular disease (CVD), type 2 diabetes mellitus (T2DM), and heart failure with preserved ejection fraction (HFpEF). Two modern drugs—semaglutide and tirzepatide—have shown impressive results in weight reduction and cardiometabolic risk improvement. Semaglutide is a glucagon-like peptide-1 receptor agonist (GLP-1 RA), and tirzepatide is a newer drug that acts on both glucose-dependent insulinotropic polypeptide (GIP) and GLP-1 receptor. Both drugs lead to major weight loss and improve cardiovascular and metabolic health. They are especially useful for people who are overweight, diabetic, and have heart-related problems such as HFpEF.[1] Their superior efficacy in weight reduction and cardiometabolic risk reduction makes them important novel treatments for obesity and cardiovascular risk reduction, marking a shift in therapy especially for high-risk groups such as patients with HFpEF.[2,3]

SEMAGLUTIDE: CLINICAL TRIALS OVERVIEW

Subcutaneous semaglutide as 2.4 mg once weekly has been extensively studied through STEP trials and consistently showed significant weight loss and HbA1c reduction. The STEP trial studied once-weekly semaglutide 2.4 mg injections: Semaglutide 2.4 mg subcutaneous once weekly, as studied in STEP-1, caused 14.9% mean weight reduction versus 2.4% with placebo over 68 weeks ($p < 0.001$),[4] in 1,961 adults with obesity having BMI ≥30 or ≥27 kg/m^2 with comorbidities (excluding diabetes). Similarly, in 1,210 patients with type 2 diabetes enrolled in STEP-2, semaglutide led to 9.6 versus 3.4% weight loss as compared to placebo with concurrent HbA1c reduction of –1.6%.[5] Semaglutide as demonstrated in STEP-3 caused a more robust weight loss when combined with intensive behavioral therapy (IBT) in comparison to placebo plus IBT(16.0 vs. 5.7%).[6] Long-term treatment with semaglutide as studied in STEP-4, causes additional weight loss but discontinuation leads to weight regain.[7] STEP-5 showed long-term effects in about 3,043 overweight/obese adults with CVD, confirmed 15.2% weight loss maintained over 104 weeks.[8]

The PIONEER program evaluated the effect of different doses of oral semaglutide formulation in people with type 2 diabetes. It looked at how well this new, noninjectable form of a GLP-1 medicine works through a series of randomized controlled trials of oral semaglutide. The studies showed that oral semaglutide lowers blood sugar effectively and also helps with weight loss. This makes it a convenient alternative to the injectable versions of the same type of medication. In total, 703 adults whose diabetes was not well controlled with diet and exercise took oral semaglutide 14 mg daily in the PIONEER 1 study. After 26 weeks, their HbA1c dropped by 1.3% and they lost about 4.5 kg compared with people taking a placebo.[9] Oral semaglutide was compared to injectable liraglutide in PIONEER 4 and was found noninferior to liraglutide for HbA1c reduction and superior in terms of weight loss. In total, 711 patients taking metformin (with or without a sulfonylurea) were given either oral semaglutide 14 mg, injectable liraglutide 1.8 mg, or a placebo. Oral semaglutide lowered HbA1c just as well as liraglutide and led to greater weight loss.[10] Subsequent trials such as PIONEER 7 and PIONEER 10 confirmed these benefits in wider groups of patients, including those taking different diabetes medications and older adults, showing consistent effectiveness and safety profiles.[11,12]

TIRZEPATIDE: CLINICAL TRIALS OVERVIEW

The clinical data for safety and efficacy of tirzepatide is also substantial and evolving. The SURPASS trial series evaluated the efficacy of tirzepatide in people with type 2 diabetes. These studies found that higher doses led to greater weight loss and more significant drop in HbA1c compared with medicines such as semaglutide and insulin analogs. In SURPASS-2, tirzepatide led to dose-dependent weight loss up to 11.2 kg with 15 mg, 9.3 kg with 10 mg, and 7.6 kg with 5 mg as compared to 5.5 kg with semaglutide 1 mg, and also superior HbA1c reductions (–2.3 vs. –1.9%) over 40 weeks in 1,879 patients with T2DM inadequately controlled on metformin.[13]

Efficacy of tirzepatide in patients with inadequately controlled diabetes on metformin ± sulfonylureas was evaluated and compared to insulin in the large clinical trial SURPASS-3. Tirzepatide proved to be superior to insulin degludec leading to more robust HbA1c reduction and weight loss with a lesser risk of hypoglycemia in 1999 patients over 52 weeks.[14] Tirzepatide was also found to be safe and efficacious in T2DM patients with high cardiovascular risk as evaluated in SURPASS-4.[15]

The SURMOUNT trials series established the efficacy of tirzepatide in obese patients. In SURMOUNT-1 study tirzepatide 5, 10, or 15 mg once weekly versus placebo, over 72 weeks with lifestyle intervention in 2,539 adults with obesity or overweight with at least one weight-related comorbidity, excluding diabetes led to dose-dependent mean weight loss of 15.0, 19.5, and 20.9%, respectively, versus 3.1% with placebo in addition to significant improvements in waist circumference and cardiometabolic parameters.[16]

Similarly, in SURMOUNT-2, 938 adults with type 2 diabetes and obesity/overweight who received tirzepatide had dose-dependent weight loss up to 17.9% at 15 mg over 72 weeks and also reported greater HbA1c reductions and improvement in cardiometabolic parameters as compared to placebo.[17] SURMOUNT-3 demonstrated efficacy of tirzepatide in patients who had previous unsuccessful weight management attempts or lost some weight using different methods. In total, 806 adults who already tried and had ≥5% weight loss with some other modalities when treated with tirzepatide achieved up to 18.4% of additional weight loss over 72 weeks.[18]

HEAD-TO-HEAD COMPARISON: SURMOUNT-5 AND SURPASS-2

The efficacy and safety of semaglutide and tirzepatide have been evaluated through multiple dedicated large clinical trials such as SURPASS-2 and SURMOUNT-5. In SURPASS-2, tirzepatide led to dose-dependent weight loss up to 11.2 kg with 15 mg, 9.3 kg with 10 mg, and 7.6 kg with 5 mg as compared to 5.5 kg with semaglutide 1 mg, and also superior HbA1c reductions (–2.3 vs. –1.9%) over 40 weeks in 1,879 patients with T2DM inadequately controlled on metformin.[13]

In the SURMOUNT-5 trial, tirzepatide (10 or 15 mg) produced greater weight loss than semaglutide (1.7 or 2.4 mg), with an average 21.6% reduction versus 15.4% over 72 weeks in 750 adults with obesity or overweight. More people taking tirzepatide reached ≥25% weight loss (32 vs. 19%).[19] Both drugs had similar rates of gastrointestinal side effects and treatment discontinuation (around 7–8%), though tirzepatide caused slightly more injection-site reactions.

Cardiovascular Benefits and Safety

Semaglutide has shown important cardiovascular and clinical benefits across multiple trials. A larger cardiovascular study (PIONEER-6 trial) of 3,183 high-risk patients showed that oral semaglutide (14 mg once daily) was safe for the heart. It did not increase major cardiovascular events [major adverse cardiovascular events (MACE): CV death, nonfatal MI, or stroke] compared with placebo (3.8 vs. 4.8%) and showed HR 0.79 (p <0.001) for noninferiority, proving it met the standard for cardiovascular noninferiority over 15.9 months.[20]

In the SUSTAIN-6 trial of 3,297 high-risk patients with type 2 diabetes, it reduced major adverse cardiovascular events (MACE) by 26%.[21] In another trial (SOUL trial), 9,650 patients with type 2 diabetes and high CV risk, oral semaglutide lowered three-point MACE (CV death, nonfatal heart attack, or nonfatal stroke) by 14% compared with placebo (12.0 vs. 13.8%; HR 0.86; p = 0.006) over 4 years.[22] The STEP-HFpEF trial (529 obese patients with HFpEF) showed that semaglutide improved symptoms (KCCQ-CSS improvement of 7.8 points), increased exercise capacity (+20.3 m in the 6-minute walk), and significantly reduced CRP and weight (–13.3 vs. –2.6% placebo). It also lowered serious adverse events.[2]

Alternatively, the SURPASS-CVOT trial aims to demonstrate the cardiovascular safety of tirzepatide versus dulaglutide in 13,029 high-risk T2DM patients ≥40 years with established ASCVD showed a 8% lower MACE incidence as compared to liraglutide meeting the criteria for noninferiority. Tirzepatide demonstrated significant benefits in reducing all-cause mortality and improving kidney function and HbA1c compared to dulaglutide.[23] The SUMMIT trial (731 HFpEF obese patients) revealed a 38% reduction in cardiovascular death or worsening heart failure events, showed improved KCCQ-CSS (+6.9 points), and better functional capacity (+18.3 m walk).[3] SURMOUNT-1 and SURMOUNT-2 trials also showed that tirzepatide, in addition to weight loss and HbA1c reduction, led to improvement in other cardiometabolic parameters such as reductions in blood pressure and improvement in dyslipidemia. The observed benefits are likely mediated through favorable effects on inflammation, myocardial remodeling, and vascular function.

Adverse Effects and Limitations

The most common adverse effect (AE) seen with both semaglutide and tirzepatide are related to gastrointestinal system and are comparable for both drugs. These are mostly mild to moderate, more pronounced at the starting of therapy and dose dependent for tirzepatide. Gastrointestinal AEs were primarily mild-moderate; nausea occurred in 17–22% (tirzepatide) versus 18% (semaglutide), vomiting in 6–10 versus 8%, and diarrhea in 13–16 versus 12%. Serious AEs noted were 5–7% in tirzepatide versus 3% in semaglutide; and discontinuations due to AEs occurred in 4–10% (tirzepatide) versus 2% (semaglutide) as reported in SURPASS-2.[13] Similarly data from SURMOUNT-5 reported serious AEs 4.8% (tirzepatide) versus 3.5% (semaglutide); discontinuations due to AEs 7.1 versus 8.0% (GI-related: 2.7 vs. 5.6%). Tirzepatide had more injection site reactions (8.6 vs. 0.3%), and semaglutide had more vomiting (21.3 vs. 15.0%).[19] Rare side effects of semaglutide may include pancreatitis, increased risk of nonarteritic anterior ischemic optic neuropathy (NAION) and increased risk of developing neovascular age-related macular degeneration (AMD).[24,25] There is also a theoretical risk of developing thyroid carcinoma as observed in rodent studies but no such risk has been observed in various human trials.

Both drugs need to be administered chronically for sustained effects and discontinuation of therapy leads to weight regain. STEP-4 was designed to be a 68-week randomized withdrawal trial in 803 adults with obesity/overweight (excluding T2D) who achieved ≥5% weight loss on semaglutide 2.4 mg. One group who continued semaglutide maintained weight loss (–7.9% from randomization) while those who were randomized to receive placebo regained +6.9% from randomization. In total, 86.6% patients on semaglutide were able to achieve ≥5% weight loss as compared to 16.6% on placebo.[7]

Similarly for tirzepatide, in the SURMOUNT-4 trial, participants who received 36 weeks of tirzepatide (10/15 mg MTD) achieved a mean weight loss of 20.9%, and those randomized to placebo regained 14.0% of body weight over 52 weeks (resulting in a net –9.9% change from baseline), whereas those who continued tirzepatide experienced an additional 5.5% reduction (net –25.3%). Notably, 89.5% patients who continued on tirzepatide maintained ≥80% of lead-in weight loss versus 16.6% on placebo, confirming chronic therapy.[26]

CURRENT GUIDELINES AND RECOMMENDATIONS

The US Food and Drug Administration (FDA) approved semaglutide 2.4 mg once weekly under the brand name Wegovy in June 2021 for chronic weight management. The drug is indicated for adults with obesity (BMI ≥30 kg/m^2) or overweight (BMI ≥27 kg/m^2) with at least one weight-related comorbidity such as hypertension, type 2 diabetes, or dyslipidemia, to be used as an adjunct to a reduced-calorie diet and increased physical activity. FDA approval of subcutaneous semaglutide for the treatment of type 2 diabetes was granted earlier (December 2017) for improving glycemic control as an adjunct to diet and exercise. In September 2019, FDA approved oral semaglutide tablets (3, 7, and 14 mg daily dosing) for improving glycemic control in adults with type 2 diabetes.

Subcutaneous tirzepatide (Mounjaro) was approved by the FDA in May 2022 for the treatment of T2DM as an adjunct to diet and exercise. It is available in once-weekly subcutaneous doses of 5, 10, and 15 mg. Tirzepatide received FDA approval for chronic weight management in adults with obesity or overweight with comorbidities in May 2023, based on data from the SURMOUNT trials, allowing its use as an adjunct to lifestyle modifications. Based on recent cardiovascular outcomes evidence (SURPASS-CVOT), the FDA updated tirzepatide's label in 2025 to include a reduction in risk of MACE in adults with type 2 diabetes and established CVD or multiple risk factors.

CONCLUSION

Semaglutide and tirzepatide represent significant advancements in the pharmacological management of obesity and type 2 diabetes along with substantial benefits on cardiovascular health. Tirzepatide achieves greater reductions in body weight, glucose, and cardiometabolic risk than semaglutide. Both drugs improve cardiovascular outcomes, but semaglutide has longer follow-up supporting its established safety. The durability of treatment effects requires continuous therapy, as discontinuation leads to weight regain. Their safety profiles are generally favorable, with primarily mild-to-moderate gastrointestinal side effects. These therapies mark a paradigm shift, providing integrated metabolic and cardiovascular benefits beyond traditional glucose-lowering and weight-loss strategies but treatment selection should be tailored to individual patient needs and tolerability.

REFERENCES

1. NCD Risk Factor Collaboration (NCD-RisC). Worldwide trends in underweight and obesity from 1990 to 2022: a pooled analysis of 3663 population representative studies with 222 million children, adolescents, and adults. Lancet. 2024;403:1027-50.
2. Kosiborod MN, Abildstrøm SZ, Borlaug BA, et al. Semaglutide in patients with heart failure with preserved ejection fraction and obesity. N Engl J Med. 2023;389:1069-84.
3. Packer M, Zile MR, Kramer CM, et al. Tirzepatide for heart failure with preserved ejection fraction and obesity. N Engl J Med. 2025;392:427-37.
4. Wilding JPH, Batterham RL, Calanna S, et al. Once-weekly semaglutide in adults with overweight or obesity. N Engl J Med. 2021;384(11):989-1002.
5. Davies MJ, Bergenstal R, Bode B. et al. Once-weekly semaglutide in adults with overweight or obesity, and type 2 diabetes. Lancet. 2021;397(10278):971-84.
6. Wadden TA, Bailey TS, Billings LK, et al. Effect of subcutaneous semaglutide vs placebo as adjunct to intensive behavioral therapy on body weight in adults with overweight or obesity: the STEP 3 randomized clinical trial. JAMA. 2021;325(14):1403-13.
7. Rubino D, Abrahamsson N, Davies M, et al. Effect of continued weekly subcutaneous semaglutide vs placebo on weight loss maintenance in adults with overweight or obesity: the STEP 4 randomized clinical trial. JAMA. 2021;325(14):1414-25.
8. Koh Y, Rubino D, Wang C. et al. Long-term efficacy and safety of once-weekly subcutaneous semaglutide 2.4 mg in adults with overweight or obesity (STEP 5): a randomised, double-blind, placebo-controlled, phase 3 trial. Lancet. 2023;401(10383):878-89.
9. Aroda VR, Rosenstock J, Terauchi Y, et al. PIONEER 1: randomized clinical trial of the efficacy and safety of oral semaglutide monotherapy in comparison with placebo in patients with type 2 diabetes. Diabetes Care. 2019;42(9):1724-32.
10. Pratley RE, Aroda VR, Lingvay I, et al. Oral semaglutide versus subcutaneous liraglutide and placebo in type 2 diabetes (PIONEER 4): a randomised, double-blind, multi-centre, phase 3a trial. Lancet. 2019;394(10215):1395-1404.
11. Meneghini L, Avilés-Santa ML, Buse JB. et al. Once-daily oral semaglutide with flexible dose adjustment versus sitagliptin in type 2 diabetes (PIONEER 7): a multicentre, open-label, randomised, parallel-group, phase 3b trial. Lancet Diabetes Endocrinol. 2020;8(4):297-308.
12. Pratley RE, Aroda VR, Lingvay I. et al. Efficacy and safety of oral semaglutide in older adults with type 2 diabetes: PIONEER 10. Diabetes Obes Metab. 2020;22(3):465-74.
13. Frías JP, Davies MJ, Rosenstock J, et al. Tirzepatide versus semaglutide once weekly in patients with type 2 diabetes. N Engl J Med. 2021;385(6):503-15.
14. Ludvik B, Giorgino F, Jódar E, et al. Once-weekly tirzepatide versus once-daily insulin degludec as add-on to metformin with or without SGLT2 inhibitors in patients with type 2 diabetes (SURPASS-3): a randomised, open-label, parallel-group, phase 3 trial. Lancet. 2021;398(10300):583-98.
15. Del Prato S, Andersen KR, Zacho M, et al. Efficacy and safety of tirzepatide vs insulin glargine in type 2 diabetes and increased cardiovascular risk (SURPASS-4): a randomized, open-label, parallel-group, phase 3 trial. Lancet Diabetes Endocrinol. 2021;9(6):401-13.
16. Jastreboff AM, Aronne LJ, Ahmad NN, et al. Tirzepatide once weekly for the treatment of obesity. N Engl J Med. 2022;387(3):205-16.
17. Garvey WT, Frias JP, Jastreboff AM, et al. Tirzepatide once weekly for the treatment of obesity in people with type 2 diabetes (SURMOUNT-2): a double-blind, randomised, multicentre, placebo-controlled, phase 3 trial. Lancet. 2023;402(10402):613-26.
18. Wadden TA, Chao AM, Machineni S, et al. Tirzepatide after intensive lifestyle intervention in adults with overweight or obesity: the SURMOUNT-3 phase 3 trial. Nat Med. 2023;29(11):2909-18.
19. Aronne LJ, Horn DB, le Roux CW, et al. Tirzepatide as compared with semaglutide for the treatment of obesity. N Engl J Med. 2025;393(1):26-36.
20. Husain M, Birkenfeld AL, Donsmark M, et al. Oral semaglutide and cardiovascular outcomes in patients with type 2 diabetes. N Engl J Med. 2019;381(9):841-51.
21. Marso SP, Bain SC, Consoli A, et al. Semaglutide and cardiovascular outcomes in patients with type 2 diabetes. N Engl J Med. 2016;375(19):1834-44.
22. McGuire DK, Busui RP, Deanfield J, et al. Effects of oral semaglutide on cardiovascular outcomes in individuals with type 2 diabetes and established atherosclerotic cardiovascular disease and/or chronic kidney disease: design and baseline characteristics of SOUL, a randomized trial. Diabetes Obes Metab. 2023;25(7):1932-41.
23. Nicholls SJ, Bhatt DL, Buse JB, et al. Comparison of tirzepatide and dulaglutide on major adverse cardiovascular events in participants with type 2 diabetes and atherosclerotic cardiovascular disease: SURPASS-CVOT design and baseline characteristics. Am Heart J. 2024;267:1-11.
24. Hathaway JT, Shah MP, Hathaway DB, et al. Risk of nonarteritic anterior ischemic optic neuropathy in patients prescribed semaglutide. JAMA Ophthalmol. 2024;142(8):732-9.
25. Shor R, Mihalache A, Noori A, et al. Glucagon-like peptide-1 receptor agonists and risk of neovascular age-related macular degeneration. JAMA Ophthalmol. 2025;143(7):587-94.
26. Aronne LJ, Sattar N, Horn DB, et al. Continued treatment with tirzepatide for maintenance of weight reduction in adults with obesity: the SURMOUNT-4 randomized clinical trial. JAMA. 2024;331(1):38-48.

94

CHAPTER

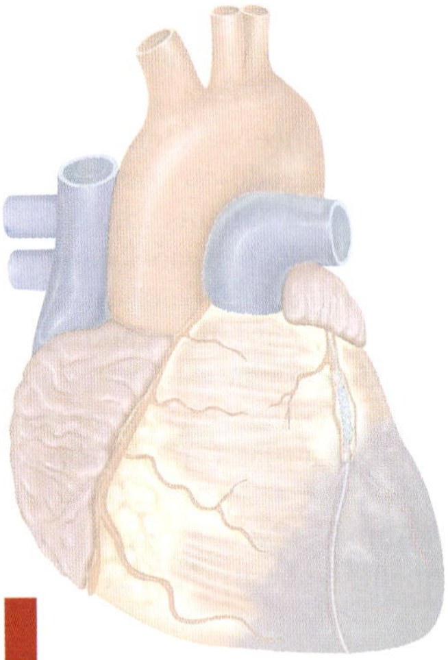

Role of Semaglutide in Patients with Obesity, Heart Failure, and High Atherosclerotic Cardiovascular Disease Risk

Himanshu Garg, Abhishek Garg, Akash Batta, Gurpreet Singh Wander

INTRODUCTION

Obesity, heart failure (HF), and atherosclerotic cardiovascular disease (ASCVD) represent interlinked conditions that contribute substantially to the global burden of morbidity and mortality. The prevalence of obesity has risen to pandemic levels, with over 650 million adults worldwide classified as obese, and this trajectory is mirrored in India and other developing nations, where rapid urbanization and lifestyle changes drive escalating rates of cardiometabolic disease.[1] Obesity serves as a pivotal risk factor not only for type 2 diabetes mellitus (T2DM) but also for hypertension, dyslipidemia, and ultimately the development of HF and ASCVD.[2]

The pathophysiological overlap between obesity, HF, and ASCVD reflects their shared underpinnings in the cardiometabolic continuum. Excess adiposity promotes systemic inflammation, insulin resistance, endothelial dysfunction, and neurohormonal activation, thereby accelerating atherosclerosis, adverse cardiac remodeling, and progression to HF—particularly heart failure with preserved ejection fraction (HFpEF)[3] **(Flowchart 1)**. Importantly, patients with obesity and metabolic syndrome often present with multiple comorbidities that amplify cardiovascular risk and complicate long-term management.[4]

Despite the availability of established therapies for diabetes, dyslipidemia, and HF, the residual risk of ASCVD events and the limited efficacy of lifestyle modification alone show the unmet need for novel therapeutic strategies. Conventional pharmacologic agents for weight management have often been associated with modest efficacy or unfavorable safety profiles, while the management of obesity-related HF and ASCVD remains challenging.[5] Thus, interventions that target both metabolic derangements and cardiovascular outcomes are highly desirable.

Flowchart 1: Pathophysiological mechanisms linking obesity with heart failure and ASCVD.

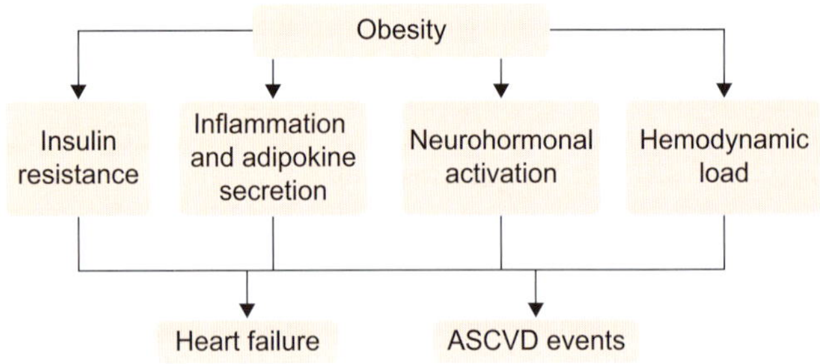

Glucagon-like peptide-1 (GLP-1) receptor agonists have emerged as a transformative class of agents bridging the gap between metabolic and cardiovascular medicine. Among these, semaglutide has shown robust efficacy in producing sustained weight loss, improving glycemic control, and reducing cardiovascular events. Evidence from large outcome trials has expanded its role beyond diabetes management to obesity treatment, ASCVD risk reduction, and symptomatic improvement in HFpEF.[6] Consequently, semaglutide represents a paradigm shift, offering a single therapeutic option that addresses the interrelated triad of obesity, HF, and atherosclerotic disease.

This chapter examines the evolving role of semaglutide in the treatment of ASCVD, HF, and obesity, highlighting its clinical evidence and foundation in cardiometabolic care.

SEMAGLUTIDE: MECHANISM OF ACTION

Semaglutide is a long-acting GLP-1 receptor agonist with a half-life of approximately 7 days, allowing for once-weekly subcutaneous administration or once-daily oral dosing.[7] It is a modified human GLP-1 analog with 94% sequence homology, engineered with structural substitutions and fatty acid side-chain attachment to enhance binding to albumin and resist degradation by dipeptidyl peptidase-4, thereby prolonging its duration of action.[8]

The primary mechanism of semaglutide involves activation of the GLP-1 receptor, a G-protein–coupled receptor expressed in pancreatic islets, the gastrointestinal tract, the cardiovascular system, and the central nervous system.[9] Its effects can be broadly classified into metabolic, cardiovascular, and cardiac actions, as shown in **Box 1**. Through this multisystem profile, semaglutide addresses not only hyperglycemia and obesity but also directly and indirectly improves cardiovascular and HF outcomes.

SEMAGLUTIDE IN OBESITY

Obesity is recognized as a chronic, relapsing, and multifactorial disease that significantly increases the risk of T2DM, hypertension, dyslipidemia, and ASCVD.[10] While lifestyle modification remains the cornerstone of weight management, long-term adherence and efficacy are often limited, and traditional pharmacotherapies have shown modest outcomes with concerns about tolerability and safety.[11] This has created a strong demand for more effective and durable medical therapies for obesity.

Semaglutide has emerged as a highly effective option for weight reduction through its action on central appetite regulation and peripheral metabolic pathways.[12] The pivotal Semaglutide Treatment Effect in People with Obesity (STEP) trials demonstrated unprecedented efficacy in nondiabetic individuals with overweight or obesity, as shown in **Table 1**. In STEP 1, once-weekly semaglutide (2.4 mg) achieved a mean weight reduction of nearly 15% from baseline over 68 weeks compared with 2.4% with placebo, alongside improvements in cardiometabolic parameters.[13] The STEP 3 study demonstrated that semaglutide, combined with intensive behavioral therapy, resulted in even greater weight loss.[15] Importantly, STEP 4 highlighted the importance of treatment continuation, as withdrawal of semaglutide led to weight regain.[16]

In populations with T2DM, STEP 2 confirmed significant weight loss, slightly less than in nondiabetic participants, with additional benefits in glycemic control and cardiovascular risk markers.[14] Furthermore, semaglutide demonstrated improvement in obesity-related health-related quality of life and physical functioning, which is of particular importance in patients with comorbid conditions such as HFpEF.[17]

Real-world and extension studies suggest that semaglutide's benefits are sustained with continued therapy and extend beyond weight loss, including reductions in waist circumference, blood pressure, and C-reactive protein levels, thereby addressing obesity-related cardiometabolic risk.[18]

Reflecting this robust evidence, the 2025 American College of Cardiology (ACC) Society recommends semaglutide as a first-line pharmacologic option for adults with obesity (BMI ≥30 kg/m^2) or overweight (BMI ≥27 kg/m^2) with comorbidities who do not achieve adequate weight loss through lifestyle modification alone.[19] The guidelines emphasize semaglutide as part of a comprehensive, long-term management strategy for obesity, given its chronic, relapsing course.

Similarly, the 2024 European Society of Cardiology (ESC) guidelines on cardiovascular disease prevention endorse semaglutide as an effective treatment for obesity with proven cardiometabolic benefits, while advising

BOX 1: Cardiometabolic effects of semaglutide.

Metabolic regulation:
- Enhances glucose-dependent insulin secretion and suppresses inappropriate glucagon release, improving glycemic control
- Delays gastric emptying and promotes satiety through hypothalamic appetite centers, leading to reduced caloric intake and significant weight loss

Cardiovascular effects:
- Reduces blood pressure, likely through weight loss, natriuresis, and improved endothelial function
- Improves lipid metabolism, with reductions in triglycerides and non-HDL cholesterol
- Exerts anti-inflammatory and antiatherosclerotic effects by attenuating oxidative stress and vascular inflammation

Cardiac effects:
- Modulates myocardial metabolism by promoting a shift from fatty acid to glucose utilization, thereby improving cardiac efficiency
- Reduces epicardial and visceral adiposity, reduces adverse ventricular remodeling in obesity-related HF
- Improves exercise capacity and health-related quality of life in patients with HFpEF and obesity

TABLE 1: Key step trials of semaglutide in obesity.

Trial	Population	Intervention/comparator	Duration	Primary outcome	Main results
STEP 1[13]	Adults with overweight/ obesity without diabetes	Semaglutide 2.4 mg weekly versus placebo + lifestyle	68 weeks	Percentage change in body weight	−14.9% with semaglutide versus −2.4% with placebo
STEP 2[14]	Adults with overweight/ obesity with T2DM (HbA1c 7–10%)	Semaglutide 2.4 mg versus semaglutide 1.0 mg versus placebo + lifestyle	68 weeks	Percentage change in body weight	−9.6% with semaglutide versus −3.4% placebo
STEP 3[15]	Adults with overweight/ obesity without diabetes all received IBT	Semaglutide 2.4 mg versus placebo + low-calorie diet + IBT	68 weeks	Percentage change in body weight	−16.0% with semaglutide versus −5.7% placebo
STEP 4[16]	Adults with overweight/ obesity without diabetes all received a 20-week semaglutide run-in (16 weeks of dose escalation; 4 weeks of maintenance dose)	Continued semaglutide versus switched to placebo	48 weeks (after 20-week run-in)	Percentage change in body weight after randomization	−7.9% additional loss with continued semaglutide versus +6.9% regain with placebo: Highlights need for continued therapy

(IBT: intensive behavioral therapy; STEP: Semaglutide Treatment Effect in People with Obesity; T2DM: type 2 diabetes mellitus)

individualized use in older adults where the "obesity paradox" may alter risk–benefit considerations.[20]

SEMAGLUTIDE IN HEART FAILURE

Heart failure, particularly HFpEF, is frequently associated with obesity, metabolic syndrome, and T2DM, which exacerbate myocardial remodeling, diastolic dysfunction, and systemic inflammation.[21] Traditional HF therapies primarily target neurohormonal pathways and symptomatic relief, but residual risk remains high in patients with obesity-related HF.[21]

Semaglutide, through its weight-reducing, metabolic, and anti-inflammatory properties, has emerged as a promising adjunct therapy in HF management. Mechanistically, GLP-1 receptor activation improves myocardial energy utilization by shifting substrate preference from fatty acids to glucose, reduces epicardial and visceral adiposity, and reduces systemic inflammation, all of which can attenuate the progression of HFpEF.[22]

The STEP-HFpEF trial investigated the effects of semaglutide 2.4 mg weekly in obese patients with HFpEF. Over 52 weeks, participants experienced significant reductions in body weight, waist circumference, and systolic blood pressure, alongside improvements in exercise capacity, symptom burden (assessed by the Kansas City Cardiomyopathy Questionnaire), and health-related quality of life.[17] Importantly, these benefits were achieved without adverse impact on left ventricular ejection fraction or renal function, showing the safety of semaglutide in this population.[17]

Building on this, the STEP-HFpEF DM trial extended the findings to individuals with both HFpEF and T2DM—a population with even higher cardiometabolic risk. Semaglutide not only improved HF symptoms and exercise tolerance but also enhanced glycemic control and reduced body weight, demonstrating consistent benefits across metabolic and cardiovascular domains,[23] as shown in **Table 2**.

Current guidelines have begun to reflect these emerging data. While the 2023 ACC expert consensus management of HFpEF does not yet formally recommend semaglutide as a primary HF therapy, concerns persist that GLP-1 receptor agonists may reduce not only adipose tissue but also lean muscle mass, which could worsen sarcopenia in HF patients.[24] Current expert consensus recommends that patients with BMI ≥35 kg/m^2 and HFpEF be considered for referral to a multidisciplinary obesity management team—including medical, surgical, and nutritional specialists—where available, to improve symptoms and address obesity-related comorbidities.[24]

Collectively, semaglutide offers a dual benefit in HF management: Substantial weight loss and improvement in cardiometabolic parameters, which may translate into symptomatic and functional improvements in patients with obesity-related HFpEF.

SEMAGLUTIDE IN ATHEROSCLEROTIC CARDIOVASCULAR DISEASE

Atherosclerotic cardiovascular disease remains the leading cause of morbidity and mortality globally, with

TABLE 2: KEY trials of semaglutide in heart failure.

Trial	Population	Intervention/ comparator	Duration (weeks)	Primary outcome	Main results
STEP-HFpEF[17]	529 patients with obesity and HFpEF (LVEF ≥ 45%)	Semaglutide 2.4 mg weekly versus placebo	52	Change in KCCQ-CSS—greater improvement with semaglutide (+16.6 vs. +8.7)	Weight loss −13.3% versus −2.6%, improved 6MWD +21.5 m versus 1.2 m, reduced NT-proBNP. Reduced CRP
STEP-HFpEF DM[23]	616 patients with obesity, HFpEF (LVEF ≥45%), and T2DM	Semaglutide 2.4 mg weekly versus placebo	52	Change in KCCQ-CSS—greater improvement with semaglutide (+13.7 vs. +6.4)	Weight loss −9.8% versus −3.4%, improved 6MWD +14.3 m versus 1.58 m, reduced NT-proBNP. Reduced CRP

(6MWD: 6-minute walk distance; CRP: C-reactive protein; KCCQ-CSS: Kansas City Cardiomyopathy Questionnaire–Clinical Summary Score; NT-proBNP: N-terminal pro-B-type natriuretic peptide; T2DM: type 2 diabetes mellitus)

obesity, T2DM, and other cardiometabolic risk factors driving accelerated atherosclerosis.[25] Traditional strategies focusing on lipid-lowering, antihypertensives, and lifestyle modification have improved outcomes, but residual cardiovascular risk persists, particularly in patients with obesity and diabetes.[26]

Glucagon-like peptide-1 receptor agonists, including semaglutide, have demonstrated favorable effects on major adverse cardiovascular events (MACE) in patients with T2DM and high cardiovascular risk. The SUSTAIN-6 trial established that once-weekly semaglutide significantly reduced the composite outcome of cardiovascular death, nonfatal myocardial infarction, and nonfatal stroke compared with placebo in patients with T2DM, highlighting its potential beyond glycemic control.[6] Importantly, the cardiovascular benefits appeared to be largely independent of its glucose-lowering effect, suggesting direct vascular and antiatherosclerotic mechanisms, including improved endothelial function, reduced inflammation, and favorable lipid profile modulation.[9]

Extending the evidence to nondiabetic populations, the SELECT trial evaluated semaglutide 2.4 mg weekly in overweight or obese individuals with established ASCVD but without diabetes. Semaglutide significantly reduced the risk of MACE, alongside robust weight reduction and improvements in blood pressure, waist circumference, and inflammatory markers.[27] These findings position semaglutide as a dual-purpose therapy, targeting both weight management and cardiovascular risk mitigation.

Reflecting these trial data, major guidelines now incorporate semaglutide in ASCVD prevention strategies. The 2025 ACC Expert Consensus Statement recognizes GLP-1 receptor agonists as a therapeutic consideration in patients with established ASCVD, particularly those with concomitant obesity or T2DM, to reduce MACE risk.[19]

Collectively, semaglutide represents a paradigm shift in ASCVD management by addressing both traditional cardiometabolic risk factors and body weight, offering a pharmacological strategy that complements lifestyle and standard cardiovascular therapies.

PLEOTROPIC BENEFITS OF SEMAGLUTIDE

Beyond its established efficacy in weight reduction, HF symptom improvement, and ASCVD risk mitigation, semaglutide demonstrates a spectrum of additional benefits that extend across organ systems including positive effects on renal and hepatic outcomes. Significant reductions in albuminuria and preservation of estimated glomerular filtration rate (eGFR) indicate potential renoprotective properties that complement its cardiovascular benefits. Semaglutide has also been associated with improvements in nonalcoholic steatohepatitis (NASH), with histologic data showing reductions in hepatic fat content and inflammatory markers—an important finding given the close metabolic link between obesity, liver disease, and cardiovascular risk. Furthermore, semaglutide contributes to blood pressure reduction with an average 4–6 mm Hg systolic decrease across studies, and anti-inflammatory effects, as evidenced by consistent reductions in high-sensitivity C-reactive protein levels across trials. Preliminary evidence also points toward improvements in sleep apnea severity, mobility, and osteoarthritis-related pain, driven by both weight loss and anti-inflammatory mechanisms. Taken together, these pleiotropic benefits reinforce semaglutide's role as not merely an antidiabetic or antiobesity agent, but as a comprehensive metabolic modulator capable of improving multiorgan health and long-term outcomes.

TABLE 3: Overview of trials of semaglutide in ASCVD patients.

Trial	Population	Intervention/ comparator	Duration (weeks)	Primary outcome	Main results
SUSTAIN-6[6]	3,297 patients with Type 2 diabetes and high ASCVD risk	Semaglutide 0.5 mg or 1.0 mg weekly versus placebo	104	Composite of CV death, nonfatal MI, or nonfatal stroke (MACE)	Significant reduction in MACE with semaglutide—confirmed noninferiority of semaglutide
SELECT[27]	17,604 patients with overweight/obesity and established ASCVD, without diabetes	Semaglutide 2.4 mg weekly versus placebo	40	Composite of CV death, nonfatal MI, or nonfatal stroke (MACE)	MACE—6.5% versus 8.0%—confirmed superiority of semaglutide

(ASCVD: atherosclerotic cardiovascular disease; CV: cardiovascular; MACE: major adverse cardiovascular events; MI: myocardial infarction; SELECT: Semaglutide Effects on Cardiovascular Outcomes in People with Overweight or Obesity; SUSTAIN: Evaluate Cardiovascular and Other Long-term Outcomes with Semaglutide in Subjects with Type 2 Diabetes)

SAFETY AND ADVERSE EFFECTS OF SEMAGLUTIDE

While semaglutide has demonstrated robust efficacy in obesity, ASCVD, and HF, its safety profile is an important consideration for clinical use. Overall, semaglutide is well-tolerated, with most adverse events being mild to moderate and transient.[19]

The most frequently reported side effects are gastrointestinal in nature, including nausea, vomiting, diarrhea, and constipation. Across the STEP trials, nausea was reported in approximately 44–47% of participants receiving semaglutide 2.4 mg weekly compared with 16% in placebo groups, while vomiting and diarrhea occurred in about 25 and 30%, respectively. Permanent discontinuation due to GI side effects occurred in 4–7% of participants, compared with <1% in placebo arms. These events are generally dose-dependent and often diminish over time with continued therapy.[19] Initiation with gradual dose escalation is recommended to minimize gastrointestinal intolerance. Rare but clinically significant adverse effects include acute pancreatitis and gallbladder-related complications, such as cholelithiasis. Meta-analyses of the STEP and SUSTAIN trials suggest that the absolute risk is low, but vigilance is warranted, particularly in patients with a prior history of pancreatitis or biliary disease.[19]

Concerns regarding thyroid C-cell tumors originate from rodent studies; however, human data to date have not demonstrated an increased risk of medullary thyroid carcinoma, and semaglutide remains contraindicated in patients with a personal or family history of this malignancy.[19]

CONCLUSION

Semaglutide represents a breakthrough in the management of obesity and related cardiometabolic disorders, providing substantial, sustained weight loss, and improvements in glycemic control, blood pressure, and lipid profiles. Evidence from STEP, SUSTAIN-6, and SELECT trials demonstrates meaningful reductions in cardiovascular risk and symptomatic benefits in HFpEF. Major guidelines now support its use as part of individualized, long-term therapy **(Table 3)**. With a generally favorable safety profile, semaglutide bridges metabolic and cardiovascular care, offering a comprehensive strategy to improve patient outcomes.

Obesity initiates multiple maladaptive processes—including insulin resistance, chronic inflammation with altered adipokine secretion, neurohormonal activation, and increased hemodynamic load that converge to promote both heart failure (predominantly HFpEF) and ASCVD events. These interrelated pathways highlight obesity as a central upstream driver of cardiometabolic disease.

REFERENCES

1. World Health Organization. (2025). Obesity and overweight. [online] Available from https://www.who.int/news-room/fact-sheets/obesity-and-overweight. [Last accessed January, 2026].
2. Eckel RH, Grundy SM, Zimmet PZ. The metabolic syndrome. Lancet. 2005;365(9468):1415-28.
3. Abel ED, Litwin SE, Sweeney G. Cardiac remodeling in obesity. Physiol Rev. 2008;88(2):389-419.
4. Packer M. Epicardial adipose tissue, inflammation, and cardiovascular disease. J Am Coll Cardiol. 2018;71(20):2360-72.
5. Garvey WT, Mechanick JI, Brett EM, et al. American Association of Clinical Endocrinologists and American College of Endocrinology comprehensive clinical practice guidelines for medical care of patients with obesity. Endocr Pract. 2016;22(Suppl 3):1-203.
6. Marso SP, Bain SC, Consoli A, et al. Semaglutide and cardiovascular outcomes in patients with type 2 diabetes. N Engl J Med. 2016;375(19):1834-44.

7. Lau J, Bloch P, Schaffer L, et al. Discovery of the once-weekly glucagon-like peptide-1 (GLP-1) analogue semaglutide. J Med Chem. 2015;58(18):7370-80.
8. Buckley ST, Baekdal TA, Vegge A, et al. Transcellular stomach absorption of a derivatized GLP-1 analogue enables oral administration of semaglutide in humans. Sci Transl Med. 2018;10(467):eaar7047.
9. Drucker DJ. Mechanisms of action and therapeutic application of glucagon-like peptide-1. Cell Metab. 2018;27(4):740-56.
10. Gadde KM, Martin CK, Berthoud HR, et al. Obesity: pathophysiology and management. J Am Coll Cardiol. 2018;71(1):69-84.
11. Bray GA, Heisel WE, Afshin A, et al. The science of obesity management: an Endocrine Society scientific statement. Endocr Rev. 2018;39(2):79-132.
12. Nauck MA, Quast DR, Wefers J, et al. GLP-1 receptor agonists in the treatment of type 2 diabetes—state of the art. Mol Metab. 2021;46:101102.
13. Wilding JPH, Batterham RL, Calanna S, et al. Once-weekly semaglutide in adults with overweight or obesity. N Engl J Med. 2021;384(11):989-1002.
14. Davies M, Færch L, Jeppesen OK, et al. Semaglutide 2.4 mg once a week in adults with overweight or obesity, and type 2 diabetes (STEP 2): a randomized, double-blind, double-dummy, placebo-controlled, phase 3 trial. Lancet. 2021;397(10278):971-84.
15. Wadden TA, Bailey TS, Billings LK, et al. Effect of subcutaneous semaglutide vs placebo as an adjunct to intensive behavioral therapy on body weight in adults with overweight or obesity: the STEP 3 randomized clinical trial. JAMA. 2021;325(14):1403-13.
16. Wilding JPH, Batterham RL, Davies M, et al. Weight regain and cardiometabolic effects after withdrawal of semaglutide: the STEP 4 trial. Diabetes Obes Metab. 2022;24(8):1553-64.
17. Kosiborod MN, Abildstrøm SZ, Borlaug BA, et al. Semaglutide in patients with heart failure with preserved ejection fraction and obesity. N Engl J Med. 2023;389(12):1069-84.
18. Kushner RF, Calanna S, Davies M, et al. Semaglutide 2.4 mg for the treatment of obesity: key lessons from the STEP program. Nat Rev Endocrinol. 2022;18(9): 555-69.
19. Gilbert O, Gulati M, Gluckman TJ, et al. 2025 Concise clinical guidance: an ACC expert consensus statement on medical weight management for optimization of cardiovascular health. J Am Coll Cardiol. 2025;85(24): e215-37.
20. Visseren FL, Mach F, Smulders YM, et al. 2021 ESC guidelines on cardiovascular disease prevention in clinical practice. Eur Heart J. 2021;42(34):3227-337.
21. Pfeffer MA, Shah AM, Borlaug BA. Heart failure with preserved ejection fraction in perspective. Circ Res. 2019; 124(11):1598-617.
22. Ussher JR, Drucker DJ. Cardiovascular actions of incretin-based therapies. Circ Res. 2014;114(11):1788-803.
23. Kosiborod MN, Petrie MC, Borlaug BA, et al. Semaglutide in patients with obesity-related heart failure and type 2 diabetes. N Engl J Med. 2024;390(15):1394-407.
24. Kittleson MM, Panjrath GS, Amancherla K, et al. 2023 ACC expert consensus decision pathway on management of heart failure with preserved ejection fraction. J Am Coll Cardiol. 2023;81(18):1835-78.
25. Roth GA, Mensah GA, Johnson CO, et al. Global burden of cardiovascular diseases and risk factors, 1990–2020: update from the GBD 2020 study. J Am Coll Cardiol. 2020; 76(25):2982-3021.
26. Vijayaraghavan K, Baum S, Desai NR, et al. Intermediate and long-term residual cardiovascular risk in patients with established cardiovascular disease treated with statins. Front Cardiovasc Med. 2024;10:1308173.
27. Wilding JPH, Batterham RL, Calanna S, et al. Cardiovascular outcomes in non-diabetic patients with overweight or obesity: the SELECT trial. N Engl J Med. 2023; 389(8):773-84.

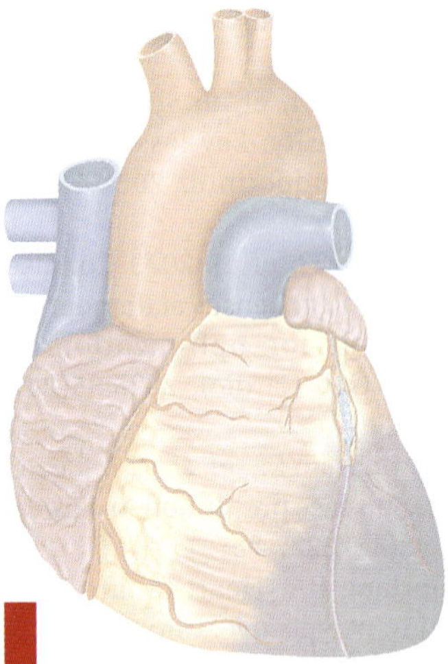

95

CHAPTER

Semaglutide and Cardiovascular Outcomes in Obesity with and without Diabetes

Mohan Bhargava, Sneha Garg

INTRODUCTION

Cardiovascular disease (CVD) remains the leading cause of mortality worldwide and is strongly linked to metabolic dysfunction. Both obesity and type 2 diabetes mellitus (T2DM) amplify atherosclerotic risk through shared mechanisms such as endothelial dysfunction, inflammation, and dyslipidemia. Until recently, pharmacologic weight-loss interventions lacked robust CV outcome data, and most cardioprotective evidence came from glucose-lowering agents tested in diabetic cohorts.

Glucagon-like peptide receptor agonists (GLP-1RAs) emerged as a promising class capable of addressing weight, glycemia, and vascular risk simultaneously. Semaglutide, a long-acting GLP-1 analog with weekly subcutaneous administration, demonstrated significant reductions in cardiovascular events in the SUSTAIN-6 trial among diabetic patients. The subsequent SELECT trial broadened this paradigm, showing CV benefit in obese individuals without diabetes, establishing obesity as an independent and treatable cardiovascular risk state.

SEMAGLUTIDE IN TYPE 2 DIABETES: THE SUSTAIN-6 TRIAL

The SUSTAIN-6 trial, a randomized, double-blind, placebo-controlled study involving 3,297 adults with T2DM and high CV risk, was designed to meet regulatory safety requirements for new antidiabetic agents. Participants received semaglutide 0.5 or 1.0 mg weekly versus placebo for 104 weeks. The primary endpoint was a composite of CV death, nonfatal myocardial infarction (MI), or nonfatal stroke.

Key results: Primary MACE occurred in 6.6% of the semaglutide group versus 8.9% with placebo (HR 0.74; 95% CI 0.58–0.95; $p = 0.02$ for superiority). Nonfatal stroke was significantly reduced (HR 0.61), and nephropathy declined by 36%. Retinopathy complications were higher (HR 1.76). Body weight decreased by 3.6–4.9 kg, HbA1c by 1.1–1.4%, and systolic blood pressure (BP) by up to 5 mm Hg. Adverse events were mainly gastrointestinal (GI). SUSTAIN-6 demonstrated both CV safety and potential cardioprotection in T2DM.

SEMAGLUTIDE IN OBESITY WITHOUT DIABETES: THE SELECT TRIAL

The SELECT trial ($n = 17,604$) enrolled adults ≥45 years with established CVD and BMI ≥27 kg/m^2 but without diabetes (HbA1c <6.5%). Participants were randomized to semaglutide 2.4 mg weekly or placebo for ~40 months. The primary endpoint was a composite of CV death, nonfatal MI, or nonfatal stroke.

Key findings: MACE occurred in 6.5% of semaglutide versus 8.0% of placebo participants (HR 0.80; 95% CI 0.72–0.90; $p < 0.001$). All-cause mortality fell by 19%, MI by 28%, and heart failure composite by 18%. Mean weight loss was –9.4% versus –0.9%, systolic BP fell by 3.8 mm Hg, and hs-CRP by 38%. Discontinuation (16.6%) was due to GI intolerance. SELECT proved that obesity treatment alone can confer CV benefit, independent of diabetes or glucose lowering.

COMPARATIVE INSIGHTS: SUSTAIN-6 VERSUS SELECT

Both trials show consistent CV protection across metabolic states. In T2DM (SUSTAIN-6), MACE fell by 26%; in nondiabetic obesity (SELECT), it fell by 20%. Benefits in both stem from improved weight, BP, inflammation, and endothelial function. Effects appear early, suggesting mechanisms beyond glycemia. Semaglutide thus bridges the diabetes–obesity continuum, offering CV benefit across metabolic risk profiles.

Mechanisms of Cardiovascular Benefit

Semaglutide exerts cardioprotection through multiple pathways:

- Appetite suppression reduces adiposity and cardiac load.
- BP and lipid improvement lower vascular risk.
- Anti-inflammatory effects (↓CRP, cytokines) stabilize plaques.
- Enhanced endothelial function improves nitric oxide bioavailability.
- Renal protection reduces albuminuria and oxidative stress.
- Decreased ectopic fat improves metabolic flexibility.

The early divergence of event curves indicates possible direct vascular or anti-inflammatory effects.

Safety Considerations

Adverse events were primarily GI—nausea, vomiting, diarrhea—manageable with slow dose titration. Gallbladder events were slightly more frequent. No increase in pancreatitis or malignancy was noted. Retinopathy complications in SUSTAIN-6 likely relate to rapid glucose reduction; they were absent in SELECT. Overall, semaglutide demonstrated favorable tolerability and safety.

Clinical Implications

Semaglutide's evidence base redefines obesity as a target for cardiovascular prevention. SELECT validates obesity treatment as cardiovascular risk reduction. GLP-1RAs now extend from diabetic to nondiabetic populations. In secondary prevention, semaglutide complements statins, ACE inhibitors, and antiplatelets by addressing residual cardiometabolic risk. With obesity prevalence rising globally, its public health implications are transformative.

LIMITATIONS AND FUTURE DIRECTIONS

Despite strong outcomes, both trials included primarily secondary prevention populations, limiting generalizability to primary prevention. The cohorts were mostly White and male. GI intolerance led to discontinuation in up to 17%. Long-term (>4 years) outcomes are still under investigation. Future research should explore combination therapy (GLP-1RA + SGLT2i), primary prevention efficacy, and cost-effectiveness in diverse populations.

CONCLUSION

The continuum of evidence from SUSTAIN-6 and SELECT confirms semaglutide's capacity to lower major cardiovascular events across diabetic and nondiabetic obesity. With 20–26% MACE reduction and improvements in weight, inflammation, and BP, semaglutide redefines metabolic and cardiovascular prevention. Integrating GLP-1RA therapy into cardiology heralds a new era in holistic risk reduction.

BIBLIOGRAPHY

1. Drucker DJ. The cardiovascular biology of glucagon-like peptide-1. Cell Metab. 2016;24(1):15-30.
2. Gorgojo-Martínez JJ, Feher M, Strem M, et al. Real-world safety and effectiveness of semaglutide in type 2 diabetes management. J Clin Med. 2022;12(1):145.
3. He L, Petersen KS, Hron B, et al. Association between glucagon-like peptide-1 receptor agonists and risk of mortality and major cardiovascular events: a systematic review and meta-analysis. JAMA Intern Med. 2022;182(5):513-19.
4. Heymsfield SB, Wadden TA. Mechanisms, pathophysiology, and management of obesity. N Engl J Med. 2017;376(3):254-66.
5. Iacobellis G. Epicardial adipose tissue in contemporary cardiology. Nat Rev Cardiol. 2022;19(10):593-606.
6. Lincoff AM, Omar M, Wang T, et al. Semaglutide and cardiovascular outcomes in obesity without diabetes. N Engl J Med. 2023;389(24):2221-32.
7. Magkos F, Fraterrigo G, Yoshino J, et al. Effects of moderate and severe weight loss on metabolic function and adipose tissue biology. Cell Metab. 2016;23(4):591-601.
8. Marso SP, Bain SC, Consoli A, et al. Semaglutide and cardiovascular outcomes in patients with type 2 diabetes. N Engl J Med. 2016;375(19):1834-44.
9. Ryan DH, Lingvay I, Colhoun HM, et al. Semaglutide in cardiometabolic medicine: clinical evidence and practical considerations. Am Heart J. 2020;229:61-9.
10. Sattar N, Lee MMY, Kristensen SL, et al. Cardiovascular effects of glucagon-like peptide-1 receptor agonists: a review of data from large clinical trials. Lancet Diabetes Endocrinol. 2021;9(10):653-62.

96

CHAPTER

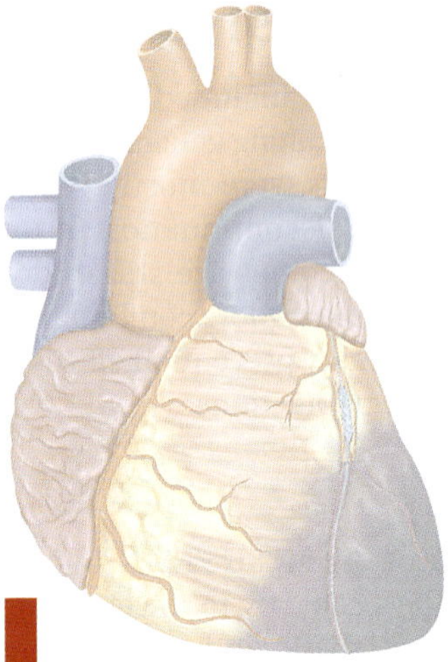

Glucagon-like Peptide-1 Receptor Agonists and Cardiovascular Health

Srikanta Sharma, Rajesh Ranjan Behera, Sudhir Kumar Satpathy, HK Chopra

INTRODUCTION

Glucagon-like peptide-1 receptor agonists (GLP-1RAs) represent one of the most transformative pharmacological advances in the management of type 2 diabetes mellitus (T2DM) and cardiometabolic disease. Initially developed as glucose-lowering agents, GLP-1RAs have demonstrated significant cardiovascular (CV) benefits independent of glycemic control. The CV protective role of these agents is now well-established, particularly in patients with established atherosclerotic cardiovascular disease (ASCVD) or those at high risk. The mechanisms of benefit extend beyond glucose regulation, encompassing weight loss, blood pressure reduction, improved endothelial function, and anti-inflammatory properties.[1]

CONTENTS AND DESCRIPTION

Physiology of Glucagon-like Peptide-1 and Receptor Activation

Glucagon-like peptide-1 is an incretin hormone secreted by intestinal L-cells in response to food intake. It stimulates insulin secretion, suppresses glucagon release, delays gastric emptying and promotes satiety. Pharmacologic GLP-1RAs mimic these effects while resisting degradation by dipeptidyl peptidase-4 (DPP-4). Major GLP-1RAs include liraglutide, semaglutide, dulaglutide, exenatide, and lixisenatide. Tirzepatide is a dual GLP-1 and GIP receptor agonist. Retatrutide is a triple GLP-1, GIP, and glucagon agonist **(Table 2)**.[2-8]

Mechanisms of Cardiovascular Protection

The cardioprotective effects of GLP-1RAs are multifactorial:

- *Direct cardiac effects:* In myocardium, GLP-1 receptors in cardiomyocytes enhance glucose uptake and efficiency of ATP generation during ischemia. It also increases nitric oxide (NO), reduces oxidative stress and apoptosis, so there is ischemia-reperfusion protection. Left ventricular function improves diastolic function and myocardial contractility in some studies.
- *Endothelial function: Increases endothelial nitric oxide synthase (eNOS) activity leading to vasodilation and improved endothelial function.* Reduction of oxidative stress leading to reduced NADPH oxidase activity and ROS generation.
- *Anti-inflammatory actions:* Downregulation of NF-κB pathway and reduction of inflammatory cytokines. It reduces TNF-α, IL-6, and MCP-1; and inhibits adhesion molecule expression (VCAM-1 and ICAM-1). Improved adiponectin levels leading to anti-inflammatory and anti-atherogenic effects.
- *Atherogenesis deceleration:* Less foam-cell formation and plaque stabilization. Decreased macrophage infiltration and plaque stabilization.
- *Weight and blood pressure reduction:* Average weight loss of 3–5 kg and systolic BP reduction of 2–5 mm Hg.
- *Myocardial effects:* Enhanced myocardial glucose uptake and improved left ventricular function.
- *Hemodynamic and renal mechanisms:* Promote natriuresis by inhibiting NHE3 (Na^+/H^+ exchanger) in the renal tubule. Reduce preload and afterload

TABLE 1: Major cardiovascular outcome trials.

Trial	Drug	Population	Primary CV outcome	Result
LEADER	Liraglutide	T2DM + CVD	3-point MACE	13% RRR
SUSTAIN-6	Semaglutide	T2DM + High risk	3-point MACE	26% RRR
REWIND	Dulaglutide	T2DM (mixed risk)	3-point MACE	12% RRR
EXSCEL	Exenatide ER	Broad population	3-point MACE	Neutral trend
HARMONY	Albiglutide	Established CVD	3-point MACE	22% RRR
ELIXA	Lixisenatide	Post-ACS	3-point MACE	Neutral

[RRR: relative risk reduction; MACE: major adverse cardiovascular event (CV death, myocardial infarction, and stroke)].

leading to improved cardiac efficiency. Indirect renal protection means less cardiorenal stress and improved volume homeostasis.

Major Cardiovascular Outcome Trials

Major cardiovascular outcome trials (CVOTs) are given in **Table 1**.

These trials demonstrated consistent cardiovascular benefit, especially with human-based GLP-1RAs such as liraglutide, semaglutide, and dulaglutide.[2-4]

Beyond Cardiovascular Outcomes

Glucagon-like peptide-1 receptor agonists also impact heart failure (HF), renal function, and metabolic syndrome components:

- *Heart failure:* Modest reduction in hospitalization, particularly in HFpEF patients.
- *Renal protection:* Reduction in albuminuria and slowing of eGFR decline.
- *Metabolic profile:* Weight reduction, improved lipid profile, and reduced visceral adiposity.

Comparative Benefits Across Glucagon-like Peptide-1 Receptor Agonists

Once-weekly agents (semaglutide and dulaglutide) show superior adherence and glycemic efficacy compared to daily formulations. Semaglutide (both injectable and oral) has shown the most significant weight loss and CV benefit in the STEP and SELECT trials.[3,4,9,10]

LIMITATIONS

- *Cost:* GLP-1RAs remain expensive compared to conventional therapies.
- *Gastrointestinal side effects:* Nausea, vomiting, and diarrhea are common.

TABLE 2: Generational classification of glucagon-like peptide-1 receptor agonists (GLP-1RAs) with representative agents and routes of administration.

Generation	Examples	Route
First generation	Exenatide and lixisenatide	Injectable (short-acting)
Second generation	Liraglutide, dulaglutide, and semaglutide	Injectable (daily or weekly)
Third generation/ dual/oral	Tirzepatide and retatrutide	Injectable or oral (multiagonist and next generation)

- *Limited long-term safety data:* Especially for oral formulations.
- *Access and adherence:* Injectable route and cost may limit widespread use.
- *Limited data in advanced HF:* Benefit less robust compared to SGLT2 inhibitors.

GUIDELINES/ALGORITHM/SUMMARY

Guideline Highlights

- *ADA/EASD 2024:* Recommends GLP-1RAs for patients with T2DM and ASCVD or high CV risk, irrespective of baseline HbA1c.[11]
- *ESC 2023:* Endorses GLP-1RAs as first-line add-on in diabetic patients with CVD.[12]
- *AHA 2023:* Supports use in obesity-related cardiometabolic risk reduction.[1]

Algorithm: GLP-1RA Use in Cardiovascular Risk Management

1. *Assess CV risk:* Established ASCVD or high risk (age > 55 + risk factors).
2. *Initiate GLP-1RA:* Prefer liraglutide, semaglutide, or dulaglutide.[2-4]

3. *Evaluate response:* Monitor weight, HbA1c, BP, and renal profile at 3–6 months.
4. *Combine with SGLT2i:* For additional HF and renal benefit.
5. *Review tolerability:* Manage GI side effects and adherence.

Summary Points

- GLP-1RAs confer robust CV protection independent of glycemic control
- *Dual benefit:* Weight loss and ASCVD risk reduction.
- Best outcomes with human-based long-acting GLP-1RAs.[13]

Illustration

Case Example

A 58-year-old male with T2DM, BMI 32 kg/m^2, and prior MI is started on liraglutide 1.8 mg daily. After 12 months, his HbA1c drops from 8.5% to 6.7%, weight decreases by 4.8 kg, and BP reduces by 6 mm Hg. Follow-up echocardiography shows improved LV diastolic function. The patient reports better exercise tolerance. This case exemplifies the cardiometabolic synergy of GLP-1RA therapy.[1,2]

CONCLUSION

Glucagon-like peptide-1 receptor agonists represent a paradigm shift in CV prevention among patients with diabetes and obesity. Their benefits extend beyond glycemic control to encompass reduction in atherosclerotic events, improvement in endothelial and myocardial function, and favorable effects on weight and blood pressure. Integration of GLP-1RAs into cardiometabolic management aligns with current guidelines emphasizing organ protection and outcome-driven care. Future directions include combination therapy with SGLT2 inhibitors and exploration of cardiovascular benefits in nondiabetic populations.[1]

REFERENCES

1. Sharma A, Verma S, McGuire DK, et al. Cardiometabolic effects of GLP-1 receptor agonists. J Am Coll Cardiol. 2020;75:1426-40.
2. Marso SP, Daniels GH, Brown-Frandsen K, et al. Liraglutide and cardiovascular outcomes in type 2 diabetes. N Engl J Med. 2016;375:311-22.
3. Marso SP, Bain SC, Consoli A, et al. Semaglutide and cardiovascular outcomes in type 2 diabetes. N Engl J Med. 2016;375:1834-44.
4. Gerstein HC, Colhoun HM, Dagenais GR, et al. Dulaglutide and cardiovascular outcomes in type 2 diabetes (REWIND). Lancet. 2019;394:121-30.
5. Pfeffer MA, Claggett B, Diaz R, et al. Lixisenatide in patients with type 2 diabetes and acute coronary syndrome (ELIXA). N Engl J Med. 2015;373:2247-57.
6. Holman RR, Bethel MA, Mentz RJ, et al. Exenatide once weekly and cardiovascular outcomes (EXSCEL). N Engl J Med. 2017;377:1228-39.
7. Drucker DJ, Nauck MA, Bailey CJ, et al. The incretin system: physiology and pharmacology. Diabetes Care. 2020;43:S223-S229.
8. Jastreboff AM, Aronne LJ, Ahmad NN, et al. Tirzepatide once weekly for obesity. N Engl J Med. 2022;387:205-16.
9. Wilding JPH, Batterham RL, Calanna S, et al. Once-weekly semaglutide in adults with overweight or obesity (STEP). N Engl J Med. 2021;384:989-1002.
10. Rubino DM, Cohen RV, Mingrone G, et al. Effect of semaglutide on cardiovascular events in obesity without diabetes (SELECT). N Engl J Med. 2023;389:2225-37.
11. Davies MJ, Aroda VR, Collins BS, et al. Management of hyperglycemia in type 2 diabetes: ADA/EASD Consensus 2024. Diabetologia. 2024;67:1-32.
12. Cosentino F, Grant PJ, Aboyans V, et al. ESC guidelines on diabetes and cardiovascular diseases. Eur Heart J. 2023;44:1231-319.
13. Pratley RE, Nauck MA, Bailey CJ, et al. Long-acting GLP-1 RAs and CV outcomes. Diabetes Obes Metab. 2020;22:2144-55.

97

CHAPTER

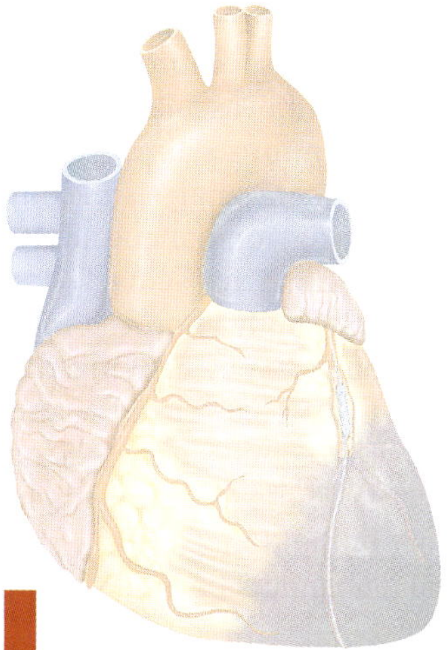

Role of Semaglutide in Managing Cardiometabolic Syndrome in Cardiovascular Disease

Sarita Bajaj

INTRODUCTION

Cardiometabolic syndrome refers to a group of metabolic abnormalities, including central obesity, insulin resistance, dyslipidemia, and hypertension, which collectively lead to a significantly increased risk of cardiovascular disease (CVD). The coexistence of these risk factors not only accelerates atherosclerosis but also worsens outcomes in patients with established CVD. 1.95 million CVD deaths were attributed to obesity and obesity-related complications in 2021.[1] While CV mortality has decreased over the past two decades, overweight- and obesity-related CV deaths have increased threefold.[2] The growing global prevalence of obesity and type 2 diabetes has increased the burden of cardiometabolic disease, with India witnessing a rapid increase in incidence due to urbanization, dietary transitions, and sedentary lifestyles.

Among newer therapeutic agents, glucagon-like peptide-1 receptor agonists (GLP-1RAs) have emerged as a cornerstone in managing multiple components of cardiometabolic disease. Semaglutide, a long-acting GLP-1RA, has demonstrated substantial benefits extending beyond glycemic control, including weight reduction, improvement in lipid profile and blood pressure, and significant reductions in major adverse cardiovascular events (MACE). Its multifactorial mechanisms make it a key therapeutic option in addressing the complex interplay between metabolic dysfunction and cardiovascular risk.

PATHOPHYSIOLOGY OF CARDIOMETABOLIC SYNDROME AND CARDIOVASCULAR DISEASE

Cardiometabolic syndrome develops because of a complex interplay between excess adiposity, insulin resistance, and chronic low-grade inflammation. In obesity, particularly with increased visceral fat, adipocyte hypertrophy, and hypoxia lead to macrophage infiltration and the release of proinflammatory cytokines such as TNF-α, IL-6, and IL-1β. These mediators activate the NF-κB and JNK pathways, impairing insulin signaling through phosphorylation of IRS-1. The resulting systemic insulin resistance promotes dyslipidemia, endothelial dysfunction, and oxidative stress all of which leads to increased cardiometabolic risk. Given this pathophysiology, agents that improve insulin sensitivity, reduce adipose inflammation, and protect the endothelium can meaningfully decrease both metabolic and cardiovascular risk.[3]

SEMAGLUTIDE PHYSIOLOGY AND MECHANISM OF ACTION

Glucagon-like peptide-1 is an incretin hormone secreted by intestinal L-cells in response to nutrient intake. It enhances glucose-dependent insulin secretion, suppresses glucagon release, delays gastric emptying, and promotes satiety through central hypothalamic pathways. GLP-1 also exerts direct cardiovascular effects, enhancing endothelial nitric oxide (NO) bioavailability, reducing oxidative stress, and improving myocardial glucose utilization. Semaglutide, a potent and long-acting GLP-1RA with 94% sequence homology to native GLP-1, resists degradation by dipeptidyl peptidase-4 (DPP-4) and binds strongly to albumin, permitting once-weekly subcutaneous or once-daily oral dosing. Through these mechanisms, semaglutide acts on multiple targets to improve glycemia, promote weight loss, and reduce cardiovascular risk.

Semaglutide is available in two formulations: A once-weekly subcutaneous injection and a once-daily oral tablet coformulated with the absorption enhancer SNAC. The subcutaneous formulation is initiated at 0.25 mg once weekly, titrated gradually to 0.5 mg, 1.0 mg, and up to 2.4 mg weekly depending on the therapeutic indication, up to 1.0 mg for type 2 diabetes and 2.4 mg for obesity and cardiometabolic risk reduction. The oral formulation, evaluated in the PIONEER program, is administered once daily on an empty stomach with no more than 4 ounces of water, at doses of 3 mg, 7 mg, or 14 mg daily for glycemic control in type 2 diabetes. The SUSTAIN trials evaluated the efficacy and cardiovascular safety of once-weekly subcutaneous semaglutide, while the PIONEER trials investigated similar outcomes with the oral formulation of semaglutide in patients with type 2 diabetes. Both trials showed consistent glycemic and weight-loss efficacy of semaglutide across diverse populations with diabetes.

CARDIOMETABOLIC EFFECTS OF SEMAGLUTIDE

Semaglutide significantly lowers HbA1c (by 1.0–1.8%) and fasting plasma glucose in patients with through glucose-dependent enhancement of insulin secretion and suppression of glucagon. Improvement in HOMA-IR and other indices of insulin sensitivity has been consistently demonstrated across the SUSTAIN-1 to SUSTAIN-10 trials for subcutaneous semaglutide and PIONEER trials for oral semaglutide. These glycemic benefits occur without an increased risk of hypoglycemia, attributable to its glucose-dependent mechanism of action.[4]

Semaglutide causes substantial and sustained weight loss through appetite suppression, delayed gastric emptying, and hypothalamic satiety signaling. The STEP trials reported mean body weight reductions of 10–15% at doses of 2.4 mg weekly, far exceeding previous pharmacotherapies.[5] Importantly, semaglutide preferentially reduces visceral and hepatic fat, thereby mitigating the metabolic and inflammatory drivers of CVD. Weight loss has a beneficial impact on multiple cardiovascular risk factors. Reductions in body weight can lower blood pressure, improve lipid profiles, decrease blood glucose levels, reduce insulin resistance, and diminish systemic inflammation. These improvements collectively contribute to lowering cardiovascular risk.

Semaglutide has also shown to improve lipid profile in patients with obesity. A recent meta-analysis of four randomized controlled trials involving nondiabetic adults with overweight or obesity demonstrated that semaglutide 2.4 mg weekly over ≥68 weeks significantly improved lipid parameters. It reduced total cholesterol by 6.39 mg/dL, LDL-C by 6.01 mg/dL, VLDL-C by 10.67 mg/dL, and triglycerides by 14.75 mg/dL, while modestly increasing HDL-C by 1.82 mg/dL (all $p < 0.01$). These results highlight semaglutide's favorable impact on lipid metabolism and cardiovascular risk, extending its benefits beyond weight loss and glycemic control.[6]

Semaglutide also has a positive impact on blood pressure. An individual patient data meta-analysis of three randomized controlled trials found that semaglutide 2.4 mg weekly reduced systolic blood pressure (SBP) by approximately 4.95 mm Hg (95% CI, –5.86 to –4.05) compared with placebo over 68 weeks. The reduction was consistent across hypertensive subgroups and largely mediated by weight loss, with a concurrent decrease in antihypertensive medication intensity (–0.51; 95% CI, –0.71 to –0.32).[7] A pooled post-hoc analysis of the STEP trials evaluated the impact of semaglutide 2.4 mg on the need for antihypertensive and lipid-lowering therapy in adults with overweight or obesity, with or without type 2 diabetes. The study found that participants receiving semaglutide were more likely to reduce or discontinue these medications and less likely to require treatment intensification compared with placebo. These benefits were accompanied by greater weight reduction, suggesting that semaglutide improves cardiometabolic health sufficiently to lower dependence on adjunctive cardiovascular medications.[8]

CARDIOVASCULAR OUTCOME EVIDENCE

Semaglutide has emerged as a pivotal agent in the management of type 2 diabetes and obesity, offering not only glycemic and weight-lowering effects but also clinically proven cardiovascular benefits. Among currently available antiobesity medications, semaglutide is the only therapy supported by dedicated Cardiovascular Outcomes Trials (CVOTs) demonstrating significant reduction in MACE including cardiovascular death, nonfatal heart attack, and nonfatal stroke. The evidence from the SUSTAIN, PIONEER, and SELECT trials collectively establish semaglutide's role as a disease-modifying agent that goes beyond glucose control to provide comprehensive cardiometabolic protection. These trials highlight its

TABLE 1: Major cardiovascular outcomes trials of semaglutide.

Trial	*Population*	*Semaglutide dose and route*	*Comparator*	*Primary outcome (MACE)*	*Key findings*	*Comments/significance*
SUSTAIN-6[10]	3,297 adults with type 2 diabetes and high cardiovascular risk	0.5 mg and 1.0 mg subcutaneous weekly	Placebo	Composite of CV death, nonfatal MI, or nonfatal stroke	26% reduction in MACE (HR 0.74; 95% CI 0.58–0.95)	Demonstrated clear CV risk reduction and established CV safety of semaglutide
PIONEER-6[11]	3,183 adults with type 2 diabetes and high CV risk	14 mg oral daily	Placebo	Composite of CV death, nonfatal MI, or nonfatal stroke	Noninferior for MACE; trend toward lower all-cause and CV mortality	Confirmed CV safety for oral formulation and suggested class-wide cardioprotection
SELECT[12]	17,604 adults with overweight/obesity (BMI ≥27 kg/m^2) and established CVD, without diabetes	2.4 mg subcutaneous weekly	Placebo	Composite of CV death, nonfatal MI, or nonfatal stroke	20% reduction in MACE (HR 0.80; 95% CI 0.72–0.90)	First antiobesity drug to demonstrate CV benefit independent of glycemic control

efficacy across both diabetic and nondiabetic populations, showing its potential as a cornerstone therapy in reducing cardiovascular morbidity and mortality. **Table 1** highlights the details of the relevant cardiovascular outcome trials of semaglutide.

MECHANISTIC PATHWAYS UNDERLYING CARDIOVASCULAR BENEFIT OF SEMAGLUTIDE

The cardioprotective effects of semaglutide extend beyond its effects on body weight, reflecting a combination of metabolic, vascular, and anti-inflammatory mechanisms. In a subanalysis of the SELECT trial, semaglutide 2.4 mg weekly significantly reduced MACE consistently across all baseline weight and waist circumference categories, with an average 4% lower MACE risk per 5 kg lower body weight (HR 0.96; 95% CI 0.94–0.99) and per 5 cm smaller waist circumference (HR 0.96; 95% CI 0.93–0.99). Importantly, only 33% of the overall cardiovascular benefit was mediated through reductions in waist circumference, indicating that mechanisms beyond adiposity reduction contribute substantially to vascular protection.[9]

Semaglutide improves endothelial function and reduces arterial stiffness through enhanced no bioavailability and suppression of oxidative stress. It attenuates vascular inflammation by downregulating NF-κB–mediated cytokine release (IL-6 and TNF-α) and by reducing macrophage infiltration within vascular tissue. Additionally, semaglutide improves lipid metabolism, lowering total cholesterol, LDL-C, VLDL-C, and triglycerides, and promotes mild blood pressure reduction via natriuresis and suppression of RAAS. Central GLP-1 receptor activation further reduces sympathetic drive and systemic inflammation leading to decrease in proinflammatory markers. Collectively, these effects establish semaglutide as a cardiometabolic agent, exerting protective that are partly independent of weight loss and glycemic control.[6,7]

CONCLUSION

Semaglutide represents a paradigm shift in the management of cardiometabolic disease. Beyond its potent glucose-lowering and weight-reducing effects, it improves lipid metabolism, blood pressure, and vascular function, resulting in substantial cardiovascular risk reduction. Robust evidence from SUSTAIN, PIONEER, and SELECT trials confirms semaglutide's efficacy across diabetic and nondiabetic populations. Its multifaceted mechanisms, addressing adiposity, inflammation, insulin resistance, and vascular dysfunction, make semaglutide a cornerstone therapy in reducing obesity-related cardiometabolic risk.

REFERENCES

1. Vaduganathan M, Mensah GA, Turco JV, et al. The Global Burden of Cardiovascular Diseases and Risk. J Am Coll Cardiol. 2022;80(25):2361-71.

2. Raisi-Estabragh Z, Kobo O, Mieres JH, et al. Racial Disparities in Obesity-related Cardiovascular Mortality in the United States: Temporal Trends From 1999 to 2020. J Am Heart Assoc. 2023;12(18):e028409.
3. Kawai T, Autieri M V, Scalia R. Adipose tissue inflammation and metabolic dysfunction in obesity. Am J Physiol Cell Physiol. 2021;320(3):C375-91.
4. Cherney DZI, Hadjadj S, Lawson J, et al. Hemoglobin A1c reduction with the GLP-1 receptor agonist semaglutide is independent of baseline eGFR: post-hoc analysis of the SUSTAIN and PIONEER programs. Kidney Int Rep. 2022;7(11):2345-55.
5. Bergmann NC, Davies MJ, Lingvay I, et al. Semaglutide for the treatment of overweight and obesity: A review. Diabetes Obes Metab. 2023;25(1):18-35.
6. Miranda S, Choudhari J, Chauhan N, et al. Impact of semaglutide on lipid profiles in overweight and obese non-diabetic adults: A systematic review and meta-analysis of randomized controlled trials. Eur J Pharmacol. 2025;1003:177953.
7. Kennedy C, Hayes P, Cicero AFG, et al. Semaglutide and blood pressure: an individual patient data meta-analysis. Eur Heart J. 2024;45(38):4124-34.
8. Tchang BG, Knight MG, Adelborg K, et al. Effect of semaglutide 2.4 mg on use of antihypertensive and lipid-lowering treatment in five randomized controlled STEP trials. Obesity. 2025;33(2):267-77.
9. Deanfield J, Lincoff AM, Kahn SE, et al. Semaglutide and cardiovascular outcomes by baseline and changes in adiposity measurements: a prespecified analysis of the SELECT trial. Lancet. 2025;406(10516):2257-68.
10. Marso SP, Bain SC, Consoli A, et al. Semaglutide and cardiovascular outcomes in patients with type 2 diabetes. New Engl J Med. 2016;375(19):1834-44.
11. Husain M, Birkenfeld AL, Donsmark M, et al. Oral semaglutide and cardiovascular outcomes in patients with type 2 diabetes. New Engl J Med. 2019;381(9):841-51.
12. Lincoff AM, Brown-Frandsen K, Colhoun HM, et al. Semaglutide and cardiovascular outcomes in obesity without diabetes. New Engl J Med. 2023;389(24):2221-32.

98

CHAPTER

Indications, Contraindications, Uniqueness, Cardiovascular Outcome Trials, and Adverse Effects of Semaglutide in Obesity

HK Chopra, Manvika Tiwari, CK Ponde, Viveka Kumar

INTRODUCTION

Obesity has emerged as one of the most formidable public health challenges of the 21st century. Global obesity rates have surged dramatically since 1990, becoming a major pandemic, with over a billion adults affected, especially in Asia and Africa, necessitating urgent public health action.[1] India is no longer immune to this epidemic; rapid urbanization, sedentary lifestyles, and nutritional transitions have led to a steady rise in obesity across both urban and rural populations. Importantly, Asian Indians develop obesity-related complications at lower body mass index (BMI) thresholds, amplifying cardiometabolic risk even at modest weight gain.[2]

Far from being a cosmetic concern, obesity is now recognized as a chronic, progressive, relapsing, multifactorial, neurobehavioral disease that results from an increase in body fat.[3] Excess body fat leads to dysfunction in adipose tissue that causes adverse metabolic (adiposopathy), biomechanical (fat mass disease), and psychosocial effects. Obesity is a central driver of type 2 diabetes mellitus (T2DM), hypertension, dyslipidemia, nonalcoholic fatty liver disease, chronic kidney disease, and atherosclerotic cardiovascular disease (ASCVD). Consequently, effective obesity management is fundamental to reducing long-term morbidity, mortality, and healthcare burden.

Lifestyle modification—comprising dietary intervention, physical activity, and behavioral therapy—remains the cornerstone of obesity management. However, real-world evidence consistently demonstrates that lifestyle measures alone are often insufficient to achieve and sustain clinically meaningful weight loss, particularly in individuals with long-standing obesity or multiple metabolic comorbidities.[4] Biological adaptations such as increased appetite, reduced energy expenditure, and hormonal counter-regulation frequently undermine long-term success, underscoring the need for adjunctive pharmacotherapy.

In this context, glucagon-like peptide-1 receptor agonists (GLP-1RAs) have transformed the therapeutic landscape of obesity. By targeting central appetite regulation, gastric emptying, and glucose homeostasis, GLP-1 RAs address key pathophysiological mechanisms underlying obesity, positioning them as disease-modifying agents rather than mere weight-loss drugs.

Semaglutide, a long-acting GLP-1 receptor agonist, represents a major advance in this class. Initially developed for the treatment of T2DM, semaglutide has since gained approval for chronic weight management in individuals with obesity or overweight with comorbidities. Beyond robust and sustained weight reduction, semaglutide has demonstrated significant cardiovascular risk reduction in high-risk populations, reinforcing its role at the intersection of obesity, diabetes, and cardiovascular disease.[5] As evidence continues to evolve, semaglutide exemplifies a paradigm shift toward integrated cardiometabolic care in obesity management.

INDICATIONS FOR SEMAGLUTIDE

Semaglutide is approved for chronic weight management as an adjunct to diet and physical activity in adults with obesity or overweight who are at increased risk of cardiometabolic disease. Regulatory approval is supported by robust clinical evidence demonstrating clinically meaningful and sustained weight reduction, along with improvement in obesity-related comorbid conditions.

Approved indications include:
- BMI ≥30 kg/m² (obesity), or
- BMI ≥27 kg/m² (overweight) in the presence of at least one weight-related comorbidity

Weight-related comorbidities include:
- *T2DM:* Semaglutide improves glycemic control, reflected by reductions in glycated hemoglobin, while concurrently facilitating weight loss.
- *Hypertension:* Weight reduction contributes to blood pressure lowering, with downstream benefits on vascular function and left ventricular workload.
- *Dyslipidemia:* Weight loss is associated with favorable changes in lipid parameters, particularly triglycerides and non-HDL cholesterol.
- *Obstructive sleep apnea (OSA):* Pharmacological intervention may support patients unable to achieve sustained weight loss through lifestyle measures alone.
- *ASCVD or high cardiovascular risk:* Including coronary artery disease, cerebrovascular disease, and other manifestations of established or high-risk CVD.

Special populations in whom semaglutide has particular clinical relevance include:
- *Obesity with heart failure:* Weight reduction may improve functional capacity, metabolic efficiency, and symptom burden, especially in patients with heart failure with preserved ejection fraction.
- *Prediabetes:* Semaglutide has been shown to delay progression to overt diabetes, underscoring its disease-modifying potential.

In patients with overweight or obesity and established cardiovascular disease, semaglutide offers the advantage of dual therapeutic action—sustained weight reduction and improvement in cardiovascular risk profile, reinforcing the concept of obesity as a central driver of cardiometabolic disease rather than an isolated risk factor.

CONTRAINDICATIONS AND CAUTIONS

Appropriate use of semaglutide requires careful patient selection, with a clear distinction between absolute contraindications and conditions warranting caution.

Absolute contraindications:
- Personal or family history of medullary thyroid carcinoma
- Multiple endocrine neoplasia syndrome type 2 (MEN 2)
- Pregnancy and lactation, due to the absence of safety data and the nontherapeutic intent of weight reduction during these periods
- Known severe hypersensitivity to semaglutide or any constituent in the formulation

Relative contraindications and cautions:
- *History of pancreatitis:* Although a causal relationship has not been definitively established, semaglutide should be prescribed cautiously, with appropriate monitoring.
- *Severe gastroparesis or significant gastrointestinal motility disorders:* The drug's effect on gastric emptying may exacerbate preexisting symptoms.
- *Advanced chronic kidney disease:* Gastrointestinal adverse effects with resultant dehydration may precipitate renal dysfunction, necessitating close surveillance.
- *Rapid weight reduction:* Accelerated weight loss may increase the risk of gallstone formation, particularly in susceptible individuals.

Overall, semaglutide demonstrates a favorable safety profile when used judiciously.

UNIQUENESS OF SEMAGLUTIDE

Semaglutide distinguishes itself within the class of GLP-1 receptor agonists through a combination of pharmacokinetic advantages, receptor potency, and clinical efficacy, translating mechanistic strengths into superior real-world outcomes.

Key attributes include:
- *High GLP-1 receptor affinity*, resulting in potent and sustained receptor activation
- *Prolonged half-life (~1 week)*, enabling convenient *once-weekly dosing*
- *Central appetite suppression*
- *Slowing of gastric emptying*, contributing to early satiety and reduced caloric intake

Mechanism-to-outcome Linkage

The sustained receptor activation achieved with semaglutide translates into durable appetite suppression and clinically meaningful weight loss, even in individuals with prior failure of lifestyle-based interventions.

When compared with other agents:
- *Liraglutide*, an earlier GLP-1 receptor agonist, requires daily administration and is associated with more modest weight loss.
- *Tirzepatide*, a dual GIP/GLP-1 receptor agonist, has shown promising weight-loss efficacy in emerging

trials; however, long-term cardiovascular outcome data in obesity populations are still evolving.

Semaglutide's balance of efficacy, dosing convenience, and outcome data positions it as a benchmark therapy within contemporary pharmacological obesity management.

CARDIOVASCULAR OUTCOME TRIAL EVIDENCE

Why Cardiovascular Outcome Trials Matter in Obesity Pharmacotherapy?

Historically, several antiobesity drugs have failed due to cardiovascular safety concerns, underscoring the necessity for rigorous cardiovascular outcome trials (CVOTs). Given that obesity is intrinsically linked to cardiovascular morbidity and mortality, any pharmacotherapy intended for long-term use must demonstrate not only weight loss efficacy but also cardiovascular safety.

Key Trials Informing Clinical Practice

SUSTAIN-6 (Type 2 Diabetes Mellitus Population)

This landmark trial evaluated semaglutide in patients with T2DM at high cardiovascular risk. Semaglutide demonstrated a significant reduction in major adverse cardiovascular events (MACE) (26% reduction) in high cardiovascular risk patients with T2DM using semaglutide, providing early reassurance regarding cardiovascular safety and suggesting benefit beyond glycemic control **(Fig. 1)**.[6]

Importantly, CV risk reduction occurred alongside meaningful weight loss, reinforcing the interconnected nature of metabolic and cardiovascular pathways **(Fig. 2)**.

SELECT Trial (Obesity without Diabetes)

The SELECT trial represents a paradigm shift by specifically evaluating cardiovascular outcomes in patients with *overweight or obesity without diabetes*, a population previously lacking outcome-driven evidence. Semaglutide significantly reduced MACE, establishing, for the first time, that targeted pharmacological treatment of obesity can directly translate into cardiovascular benefit independent of glucose lowering.[7]

Key Clinical Insights from Cardiovascular Outcome Trials

- Reduction in MACE, including cardiovascular death, nonfatal myocardial infarction, and nonfatal stroke
- Glycemic control, reinforcing obesity as a modifiable cardiovascular risk factor in its own right
- A consistent relationship between weight reduction and improved cardiovascular outcomes
- Reassuring safety profile, with no signs of excess cardiovascular harm.

ADVERSE EFFECTS

The adverse-effect profile of semaglutide is generally predictable, dose dependent, and manageable with appropriate counseling and titration.

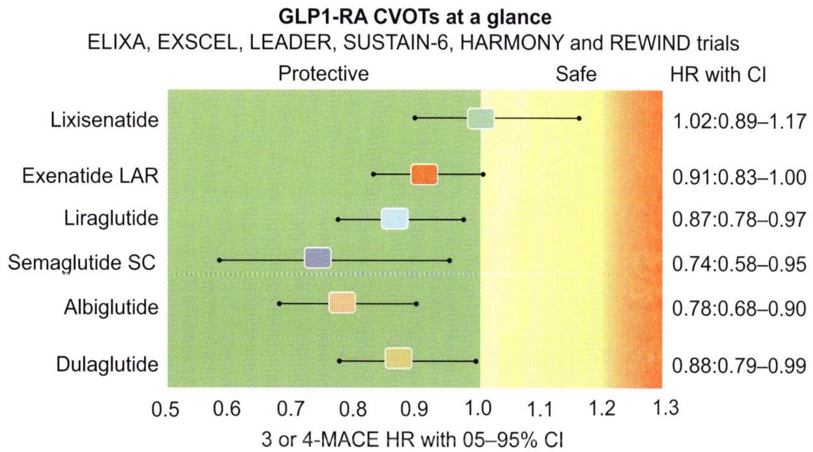

Fig. 1: Summary of the primary endpoint results of the six GLP1-RA studied in six CVOTs. Lixisenatide and exenatide (exendin-4 derivatives) like DPP-4i demonstrated noninferiority or safety. GLP1 analogs (liraglutide, semaglutide, albiglutide, and dulaglutide) demonstrated superiority or efficacy. Oral semaglutide (PIONEER 6 trial) is not included since its definitive CVOT (SOUL trial) is ongoing. (CI: confidence interval; CVOTs: cardiovascular outcomes trials; HR: hazard ratio; MACE: major adverse cardiovascular events)

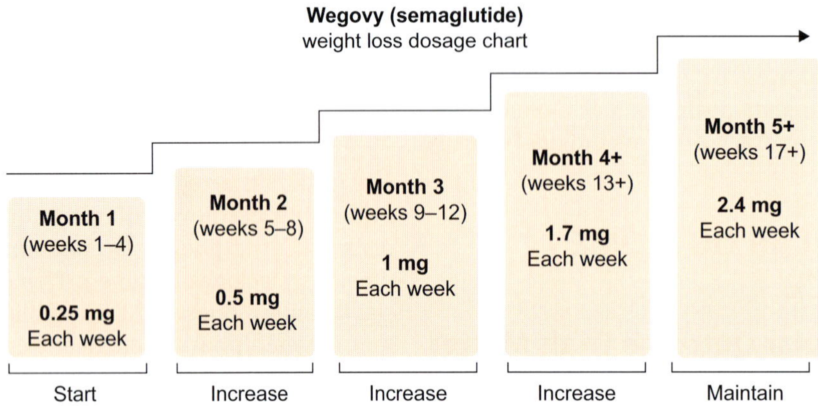

Fig. 2: Semaglutide weight-loss dose escalation schedule for chronic weight management.
Source: Adapted from NiceRx Editorial Team. (2025). Semaglutide weight loss dosage chart. [online] Available from https://www.nicerx.com/blog/semaglutide-weight-loss-dosage-chart/ [Last accessed January, 2026].

Common Adverse Effects

Common adverse effects include:
- Nausea
- Vomiting
- Diarrhea
- Constipation

These gastrointestinal symptoms are most prominent during dose escalation and tend to diminish with continued therapy.

Less Common Adverse Effects

- *Gallbladder disease*, particularly cholelithiasis, associated with rapid weight loss
- *Injection-site reactions*, usually mild and self-limiting

Rare but clinically important considerations:
- *Pancreatitis:* An association has been reported, though causality remains unproven; clinicians should remain vigilant for suggestive symptoms.
- *Thyroid C-cell tumors:* Observed in rodent models but not demonstrated in human trials; nonetheless, this underpins existing contraindications.

Suggestions to minimize adverse effects:
- Gradual dose escalation is essential to minimize gastrointestinal intolerance.
- Patient counseling should emphasize:
  - Eating smaller meals
  - Avoiding high-fat foods during initiation
  - Recognizing early satiety as an expected effect rather than an adverse one
- Temporary dose de-escalation may help manage persistent symptoms.

As per SELECT trial, in the semaglutide group, 12.0% of patients achieved normal weight status at week 104 (from 0% at baseline), compared with 1.2% (from 0% at baseline) for placebo. BMI classes: Healthy (BMI $<25\,kg\,m^{-2}$), overweight (25 to $<30\,kg\,m^{-2}$), class I obesity (30 to $<35\,kg\,m^{-2}$), class II obesity (35 to $<40\,kg\,m^{-2}$), and class III obesity (BMI $\geq 40\,kg\,m^{-2}$) **(Fig. 3)**.[8]

LIMITATIONS

Despite its robust efficacy and favorable cardiovascular profile, semaglutide has several practical limitations that must be acknowledged in routine clinical practice. Cost and access remain significant barriers, particularly in low- and middle-income countries such as India, where long-term affordability and limited insurance coverage may restrict sustained use. This economic constraint may affect real-world uptake despite strong clinical evidence.

The injectable route of administration can be a deterrent for some patients, especially those with needle aversion or limited familiarity with self-injection techniques. As obesity is a chronic disease, long-term adherence is paramount.

Another important limitation is weight regain after treatment discontinuation. 1 year after withdrawal of once-weekly subcutaneous semaglutide 2.4 mg and lifestyle intervention, participants regained two-thirds of their prior weight loss, with similar changes in cardiometabolic variables. Findings confirm the chronicity of obesity, and suggest ongoing treatment is required to maintain improvements in weight and health.[9]

Finally, although global evidence is robust, there is limited real-world data from Indian populations,

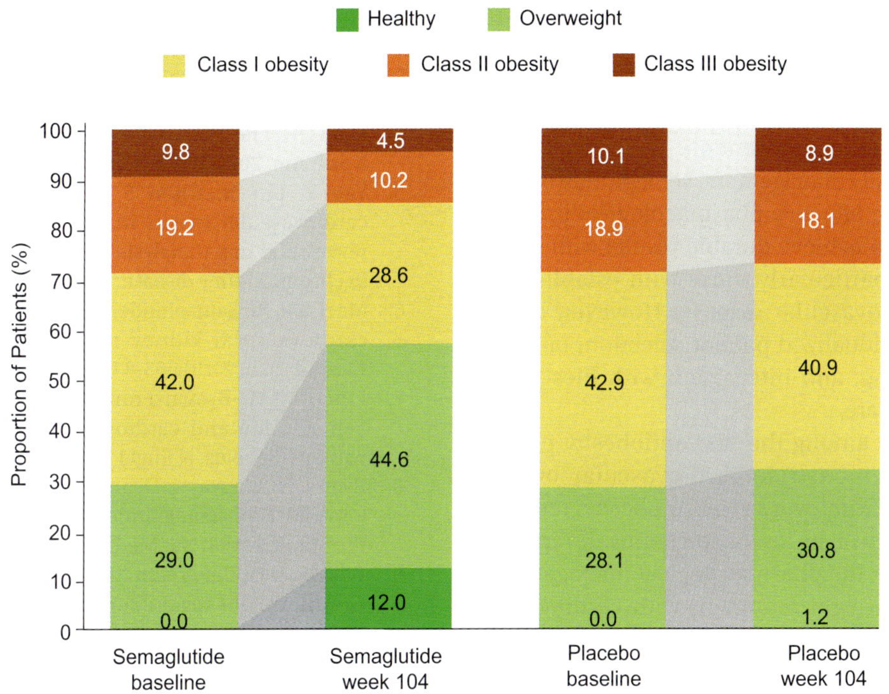

Fig. 3: Change in BMI category (healthy, overweight, class I obesity, class II obesity, and class III obesity) at baseline and week 104 for in-trial patients.[8]

particularly regarding long-term cardiovascular outcomes, cost-effectiveness, and implementation across diverse healthcare systems. Generation of region-specific evidence will be essential to optimize patient selection and guide policy-level decisions.

GUIDELINE/ALGORITHM/SUMMARY ILLUSTRATIONS

Semaglutide is increasingly positioned as a core pharmacological therapy within modern obesity management frameworks, particularly for individuals with established or high risk of cardiometabolic disease. Contemporary guidelines emphasize that obesity requires structured, stepwise, and long-term treatment, analogous to other chronic noncommunicable diseases.

A stepwise clinical algorithm is recommended:

1. *Lifestyle intervention* for all patients:
   - Nutritional therapy
   - Physical activity
   - Behavioral modification
2. *Pharmacotherapy:*
   - Initiated in patients with BMI ≥30 kg/m^2, or ≥27 kg/m^2 with comorbidities, who fail to achieve adequate weight loss with lifestyle therapy alone.
   - GLP-1 receptor agonists such as semaglutide are preferred in patients with T2DM, ASCVD, or high cardiovascular risk.
3. *Metabolic/bariatric surgery:* Reserved for selected patients with severe obesity or refractory disease, after failure of nonsurgical approaches.

Guideline Alignment

- The *American Diabetes Association (ADA)* recommends GLP-1 receptor agonists for individuals with overweight or obesity, particularly when cardiovascular risk reduction is a therapeutic priority.[10]
- The *European Society of Cardiology (ESC)* recognizes obesity as a major modifiable cardiovascular risk factor and supports therapies that demonstrate both cardiovascular safety and outcome benefit.[11]

CONCLUSION

Semaglutide has redefined the therapeutic approach to obesity by targeting the underlying neurohormonal mechanisms that drive weight gain and metabolic dysfunction. Rather than functioning solely as a weight-loss agent, it represents a disease-modifying therapy with the capacity to favorably influence the broader cardiometabolic continuum. Evidence from large CVOTs has established the dual benefit of sustained weight reduction and cardiovascular risk lowering, extending its relevance beyond glycemic control and into primary and secondary cardiovascular prevention.

In modern obesity management, semaglutide occupies a pivotal role as an effective pharmacological option for patients who fail to achieve durable results with lifestyle measures alone, particularly those with established or high risk of cardiovascular disease. However, optimal use requires individualized patient selection, long-term treatment planning, and integration with lifestyle and multidisciplinary care.

Semaglutide is among the first antiobesity pharmacotherapies to demonstrate cardiovascular outcome benefit in patients with overweight or obesity, redefining expectations from weight-loss medications. It represents a paradigm shift in the pharmacological management of obesity, aligning weight reduction with cardiovascular risk reduction.

REFERENCES

1. Ahmed SK, Mohammed RA. Obesity: Prevalence, causes, consequences, management, preventive strategies and future research directions. Metabol Open. 2025;27: 100375.
2. Wolf RM, Nagpal M, Magge SN. Diabetes and cardiometabolic risk in South Asian youth: a review. Pediatr Diabetes. 2021;22(1):52-66.
3. Fitch AK, Bays HE. Obesity definition, diagnosis, bias, standard operating procedures (SOPs), and telehealth: An Obesity Medicine Association (OMA) Clinical Practice Statement (CPS) 2022. Obese Pillars. 2022;1:100004.
4. Ryan DH. Lifestyle-Based Obesity Care. Gastroenterol Clin North Am. 2023;52(4):645-60.
5. Yao Y, Liu N, Chen S, et al. Semaglutide reduces cardiovascular events in type 2 diabetes: a systematic review and meta-analysis highlighting enhanced benefits in chronic kidney disease. Eur J Med Res. 2025;30(1):1059.
6. MacIsaac RJ. Semaglutide: a key medication for managing cardiovascular-kidney-metabolic syndrome. Future Cardiol. 2025;21(9):663-83.
7. Lincoff AM, Brown-Frandsen K, Colhoun HM, et al. Semaglutide and cardiovascular outcomes in obesity without diabetes. N Engl J Med. 2023;389:2221-32.
8. Ryan DH, Lingvay I, Deanfield J, et al. Long-term weight loss effects of semaglutide in obesity without diabetes in the SELECT trial. Nat Med. 2024;30:2049-57.
9. Wilding JPH, Batterham RL, Davies M, et al.; STEP 1 Study Group. Weight regain and cardiometabolic effects after withdrawal of semaglutide: The STEP 1 trial extension. Diabetes Obes Metab. 2022;24(8):1553-64.
10. Turkistani Y. Glucagon-like peptide-1 receptor agonists: a review from a cardiovascular perspective. Front Cardiovasc Med. 2025;12:1535134.
11. Vrints C, Andreotti F, Koskinas KC, et al. 2024 ESC Guidelines for the management of chronic coronary syndromes. Developed by the Task Force for the management of chronic coronary syndromes of the European Society of Cardiology (ESC), endorsed by the European Association for Cardio-Thoracic Surgery (EACTS). Eur Heart J. 2024;45(36):3415-537.

CHAPTER 99

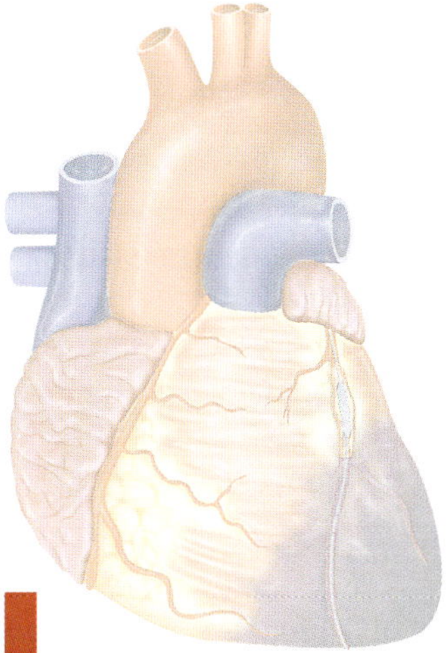

Practical Considerations of Using Semaglutide in Obese Patients with CVD Outcome Data

Saumitra Ray, Sujoy Majumdar

INTRODUCTION

GLP 1 receptor agonists (GLP-1RAs) are medications that mimic the action of the human GLP-1 hormone, normally released from the L cells of the intestine. GLP-1RAs particularly those with a human GLP-1 background chain (liraglutide, dulaglutide, and semaglutide) have been shown to have positive cardiovascular (CV) outcome data in randomized controlled trials (RCT).[1-4]

In addition, they have been shown to have independent action in suppression of the appetite by acting on the homeostatic pathway concerned with the regulation of appetite. Homeostatic feeding maintains energy balance by modulating food intake in response to the metabolic needs of the body. In contrast, nonhomeostatic feeding (hedonic feeding) is driven by the pleasure of food.[5] This can override this homeostatic mechanism and lead to overeating, thereby contributing to the obesity.

GLP 1 RECEPTOR AGONIST: MODE OF ACTION

GLP 1 receptor agonists bind to the GLP-1 receptors on the nucleus of tractus solitarius and area postrema in the brainstem, enhancing the activity of serotonergic neurons and thereby promoting satiety.[6] In addition, this also activates the dopaminergic pathway, that reduces the reward of food intake. The nucleus tractus solitarius and area postrema further convey these signals to the arcuate nucleus of the hypothalamus.[7] Anorexigenic neurons in the hypothalamus, in response to the GLP-1 stimulus, release anorexigenic (appetite suppressing) peptides [proopiomelanocortin (POMC)] and inhibit release of orexigenic (appetite stimulating) peptides [neuropeptide Y (NPY) and agouti-related peptide (AgRP)]. This leads to appetite suppression, resulting in reduced food intake and increased energy expenditure.[8]

Peripherally GLP-1RA stimulates the action of gut hormones such as peptide YY and cholecystokinin. Peptide YY, produced from the intestine and colon, acts as a peripheral hormone, reducing the gastric emptying and thereby contributing to satiety.[8] Cholecystokinin, produced from small intestine, promotes digestion and brings about a feeling of satiety.[9] GLP-1RA also inhibits the release of appetite stimulating hormone ghrelin, thereby contributing to the reduced appetite.[10]

To summarize GLP-1RAs act through central and peripheral ways to promote satiety, reduce food intake and thereby contribute to the reduction of obesity.

GLP-1 RECEPTOR AGONIST AND CARDIOVASCULAR OUTCOME BENEFITS

The vast majority of CV outcome studies conducted with liraglutide, dulaglutide, and semaglutide has been done on patients with type 2 diabetes mellitus (T2DM), where they have shown significant CV outcome benefits, manifested by relative risk reduction (RRR) as outlined in **Table 1**. A subsequent meta-analysis by Sattar et al.[11] of eight trials involving 60,080 patients showed that on the whole, GLP-1RA in patients with T2DM reduced 3P MACE by 14% [HR: 0·86 (95% CI: 0·80–0·93); p <0·0001], all-cause

TABLE 1: Select CV outcome trials in patients of T2DM with GLP-1RA.[1-4]

Name of the trial and GLP-1RA	3P MACE RRR	CV death RRR	Nonfatal MI RRR	Nonfatal stroke RRR
LEADER (liraglutide)	13% (95% CI: 0.78–0.97); $p = 0.01$ for superiority	22% (95% CI: 0.66–0.93); $p = 0.007$	12% (95% CI: 0.75–1.03); $p = 0.11$*	11% (95% CI: 95% CI: 0.72–1.11); $p = 0.30$*
REWIND (dulaglutide)	12% (95% CI: 0·79–0·99); $p = 0.026$	9% (95% CI: 0.78–1.06); $p = 0.21$*	4% (95% CI: 0.79–1.16); $p = 0.65$*	24% (95% CI: 0.61–0.95); $p = 0.017$
SUSTAIN 6 (injectable semaglutide)	26% (95% CI: 0.58–0.95); $p = 0.02$ for superiority	2% (95% CI 0.65–1.48); $p = 0.92$*	26% (95% CI: 0.51–1.08); $p = 0.12$*	39% (95% CI: 0.38–0.99); $p = 0.04$
SOUL (oral semaglutide)	14% (95% CI: 0.77–0.96); $p = 0.006$ for superiority	7% (95% CI: 0.80–1.09)*	26% (95% CI: 0.61–0.89)	12% (95% CI: 0.70–1.11)*

(*: statistically not significant; RRR: relative risk reduction)

mortality by 12% [HR: 0·88 (95% CI: 0·82–0·94); $p = 0{\cdot}0001$], hospitalization for heart failure by 11% [HR: 0·89 (95% CI: 0·82–0·98); $p = 0{\cdot}013$], and the composite kidney outcome by 21% [HR: 0·79 (95% CI: 0·73–0·87); $p < 0{\cdot}0001$]. The greatest RRR was on fatal or nonfatal stroke, followed by CV death, and lastly, fatal and nonfatal myocardial infarction. There was no significant heterogeneity across GLP-1RA structural homology or eight other examined subgroups (all p interaction ≥0.14), though there were signals that human backbone-based GLP-1RA performed better than exendin-4-based GLP-1RA.[12] The overall number needed to treat (NNT) to prevent one MACE outcome was 65 for 3 years. The meta-analysis did not demonstrate any increased risk of pancreatitis or pancreatic carcinoma, worsening of retinopathy (this was a concern raised in SUSTAIN 6 trial)[3] or severe hypoglycemia.

However as most of these trials demonstrated a significant weight reduction and judging by the mechanism of action of GLP-1RA, it was hypothesized that even in nondiabetic obese patients, this class of molecules would demonstrate CV outcome benefits, because glucose lowering effect of these drugs was not deemed to play a major role in CV outcomes.

SEMAGLUTIDE AND CV OUTCOME BENEFITS IN OBESE NONDIABETIC PATIENTS

Injectable semaglutide (Wegovy) 2.4 mg has shown considerable benefits of weight reduction in obese nondiabetic patients in the STEP trials 1-4.[13-16] However, these studies were not powered to look into CV outcome benefits as a primary endpoint. A meta-analysis of all the STEP trials (except STEP 7)[17] however did highlight the fact that majority of the patients had at least one comorbidity and >25% had three comorbidities. Hypertension, dyslipidemia, and obstructive sleep apnea were the most common comorbidities, all of which are recognized risk factors for poor outcome in CV disease including myocardial infarction and stroke. Injectable semaglutide 2.4 mg was, on the whole, seen to produce an average of 12.1% weight loss in comparison with placebo in these studies and at least 1/3 had 20% weight loss. Earlier studies had shown that a modest weight loss of 5–10% is associated with improvements in cardiovascular risk factors.[18] It was therefore expected that injection semaglutide 2.4 mg would demonstrate a significant CV outcome benefit in a dedicated CV outcome trial.

SELECT Trial (Semaglutide and Cardiovascular Outcomes in Obesity without Diabetes)[19] was the first placebo compared RCT that tried to answer the question as to whether semaglutide can bring about a positive CV outcome benefit in obese patients without diabetes. Cardiovascular disease was defined as either previous myocardial infarction, with or without heart failure, previous stroke, or symptomatic peripheral arterial disease.

17,604 patients were enrolled of whom 8,803 were in the semaglutide arm while 8,801 received placebo. The mean duration of exposure to semaglutide or placebo was 34.2 ± 13.7 months, and the mean duration of follow-up was 39.8 ± 9.4 months. Mean BMI was 33.3 ± 5 in the semaglutide arm versus 33.4 ± 5 in the placebo arm. Mean HbA1c was 5.78 ± 0.34 in semaglutide arm versus 5.78 ± 0.33 in the placebo arm. Cardiovascular comorbidity was equally distributed among the two arms [myocardial infarction only: 67.7% (semaglutide arm) vs. 67.5% (placebo arm); stroke only: 17.9% (semaglutide arm) vs. 17.7% (placebo arm); Peripheral arterial disease only 4.3% (semaglutide arm) vs. 4.6% (placebo arm); more than two comorbidities in 8.2% patients in both the arms]. Majority of the patients were Caucasians but there was a sizeable proportion of other ethnicities in both the groups.

Semaglutide was shown to produce a 20% RRR of 3P MACE (95% CI: 0.72–0.9, $p < 0.01$ for superiority),

18% RRR of composite heart failure endpoint (95% CI: 0.71–0.96), 19% RRR of all-cause mortality (95% CI: 0.71–0.93). Nonfatal myocardial infarction showed a RRR of 28% (95% CI: 0.61–0.85). There was no statistically significant reduction of CV death, nonfatal stroke, coronary revascularization or hospitalization for heart failure. Apart from gastrointestinal side effects, there were few causes of treatment discontinuation. Treatment discontinuation occurred in 16.6% of semaglutide patients as against 8.2% of patients in the placebo arm.

The interesting fact remains that 3P MACE benefits of semaglutide occurred early after the initiation of treatment, (within first 4 weeks) when no significant weight loss is expected. This was directionally similar across cardiovascular endpoints among prespecified patient subgroups. Obviously only weight loss could not explain the CV outcome benefit. Semaglutide also demonstrated changes in multiple biomarkers such as blood pressure, lipid levels, CRP, glycemic control, and nephropathy, thereby providing the mechanistic explanation for the 3P MACE benefit. However, a major limitation of this trial was the fact that patients having multiple risk factors but without documented atherosclerotic CV disease were not included. Hence, the CV outcome of intervention of semaglutide in nondiabetic obese patients without documented atherosclerotic CV disease remains unknown till date.

STEP-HFpEF (Semaglutide in Patients with Heart Failure with Preserved Ejection Fraction and Obesity) study was done on 529 patients with obesity and heart failure with preserved ejection fraction (HFpEF).[20] Patients received injection semaglutide 2.4 mg or placebo for 52 weeks. Dual primary endpoints were the change in the body weight from baseline and change in the Kansas City Cardiomyopathy Questionnaire Clinical Summary Score (KCCQ-CSS; scores 0–100, with higher scores indicating a better state). Confirmatory secondary endpoints included the change in the 6-minute walk distance; a hierarchical composite endpoint that included death, heart failure events, and differences in the change in the KCCQ-CSS and 6-minute walk distance. Changes in the CRP level were also noted.

At the end of 52 weeks, change in KCCQ-CSS from baseline to week 52 was 16.6 (semaglutide) versus 8.7 (placebo) (95% CI: 4.8–10.9, p <0.001) and body weight reduction was 13.3% (semaglutide) versus 2.6% (placebo) [95% CI: -11.9 to -9.4, p <0.001]. Of the secondary endpoints, 6-minute walk distance was 21.5 m (semaglutide) versus 1.2 m (placebo) (95% CI: 8.6–32.1, p <0.001). CRP levels were reduced by 43.5% (semaglutide) versus 7.3% (placebo) (95% CI: 0.51–0.72, p <0.001). This study validated the role of reduction of obesity in improving the outcome of HFpEF, as visceral adiposity is associated with the worsening of inflammatory markers, systolic and diastolic dysfunction, along with skeletal muscle, arterial and physical dysfunction.

A predefined SOUL trial post-hoc analysis was presented in the annual conference of the European Society of Cardiology 2025 at Madrid evaluated the effect of oral semaglutide on the HF events (composite outcome or HF hospitalization, urgent HF visit, and CV death) in the participants with or without HF at baseline. The patients had T2DM with ASCVD and/or CKD. There was a significant benefit with semaglutide in those with HF at baseline, especially with HFpEF. There was no safety signal in any subgroup. There was high rate of SGLT2I and MRA use at baseline, which neither reduced the benefit nor increased the side effects.

Another study presented in the same conference (JAMA 31st August 2025, DOI 10/1001/jama 2025.14092) looked into semaglutide versus tirzepatide in cardiometabolic HFpEF. There was a >40% reduction of composite of HHF and all-cause mortality compared to placebo. There was no difference between the two molecules.

USE OF SEMAGLUTIDE IN OBESITY AND COEXISTENT CV DISEASE

Injection semaglutide can be used in patients with obesity (BMI >27 kg/m^2) with associated CV disease like atherosclerotic CV disease with or without HFpEF. Starting dose is 0.25 mg once weekly SC injection. Every 4 weeks the dose has to be increased to 0.5 mg—1.0 mg—1.7 mg—2.4 mg, the maximum dose being attained by 16 weeks. Gastrointestinal side effects such as nausea, vomiting, and diarrhea are common, which are of particular concern at higher dosage. In case a patient develops GI symptoms at a particular dosage, it would be prudent to revert back to the previously followed dose. Pancreatitis is a relatively rare side effect of semaglutide. Nonetheless, if the patient develops any acute abdomen, it would be worthwhile to withhold the treatment and evaluate for pancreatitis. Also, like other GLP-1RA, semaglutide is also associated with an increased risk of cholelithiasis. Semaglutide, while causing loss of visceral adiposity, also causes sarcopenia. It is, therefore, recommended that patients on semaglutide should indulge in isotonic and resistance exercise under supervision, and high-protein diet, provided there is no contraindication.[21]

In SUSTAIN 6 study,[3] semaglutide was shown to worsen diabetic retinopathy, and as a consequence, patients with established retinopathy were excluded from the SOUL study.[4] A more dreaded complication is non-arteritic ischemic optic neuropathy (NAION) which can lead to complete unilateral visual loss. Though the incidence is rare (affecting 1 in 10,000 patients using semaglutide for 1 year), both the WHO and EMA have issued this as a potential warning for all users of semaglutide.[22] Semaglutide should therefore be stopped immediately if the patient complains of any visual problem and an urgent ophthalmologic review is imperative. Also, semaglutide is contraindicated in patients with a personal or family history of medullary carcinoma of thyroid or MEN syndrome 2. Appearance of depressive symptoms should also call for discontinuation of the medicine. An increase in the heart rate up to 20 beats/min has been observed in some studies, but this is hardly a concern in real life.

CONCLUSION

Semaglutide is a useful medication in improving the CV outcome in obesity. But one has to be careful about the side effects when using the medicine in order to get the desirable effects.

REFERENCES

1. Marso SP, Daniels GH, Brown-Frandsen K, et al. Liraglutide and Cardiovascular Outcomes in Type 2 Diabetes. N Engl J Med. 2016;375(4):311-22.
2. Gerstein HC, Colhoun HM, Dagenais GR, et al. Dulaglutide and cardiovascular outcomes in type 2 diabetes (REWIND): a double-blind, randomised placebo-controlled trial. Lancet. 2019;394(10193):121-30.
3. Marso SP, Bain SC, Consoli A, et al. Semaglutide and Cardiovascular Outcomes in Patients with Type 2 Diabetes. N Engl J Med. 2016;375(19):1834-44.
4. McGuire DK, Marx N, Mulvagh SL, et al. Oral Semaglutide and Cardiovascular Outcomes in High-Risk Type 2 Diabetes. N Engl J Med. 2025;392(20):2001-12.
5. Lutter M, Nestler EJ. Homeostatic and hedonic signals interact in the regulation of food intake. J Nutr. 2009;139(3):629-32.
6. Wang GJ, Volkow ND, Thanos PK, et al. Similarity between obesity and drug addiction as assessed by neurofunctional imaging: a concept review. J Addict Dis. 2004;23(3):39-53.
7. Alhadeff AL, Rupprecht LE, Hayes MR. GLP-1 neurons in the nucleus of the solitary tract project directly to the ventral tegmental area and nucleus accumbens to control for food intake. Endocrinology. 2012;153(2):647-58.
8. Geloneze B, de Lima-Júnior JC, Velloso LA. Glucagon-Like Peptide-1 Receptor Agonists (GLP-1RAs) in the Brain-Adipocyte Axis. Drugs. 2017;77(5):493-503. Erratum in: Drugs. 2017;77(10):1141.
9. Alhabeeb H, AlFaiz A, Kutbi E, et al. Gut hormones in health and obesity: the upcoming role of short chain fatty acids. Nutrients. 2021;13(2):481.
10. Ronveaux CC, Tomé D, Raybould HE. Glucagon-like peptide 1 interacts with ghrelin and leptin to regulate glucose metabolism and food intake through vagal afferent neuron signaling. J Nutr. 2015;145(4):672-80.
11. Sattar N, Lee MMY, Kristensen SL, et al. Cardiovascular, mortality, and kidney outcomes with GLP-1 receptor agonists in patients with type 2 diabetes: a systematic review and meta-analysis of randomised trials. Lancet Diabetes Endocrinol. 2021;9:653-62.
12. Longato E, Di Camillo B, Sparacino G, et al. Cardiovascular effectiveness of human-based *vs* exendin-based glucagon like peptide-1 receptor agonists: a retrospective study in patients with type 2 diabetes. Eur J Prev Cardiol. 2021;28:22-9.
13. Wilding JPH, Batterham RL, Calanna S, et al. Once-weekly semaglutide in adults with overweight or obesity. N Engl J Med. 2021;384(11):989-1002.
14. Davies M, Færch L, Jeppesen OK, et al. Semaglutide 2·4 mg once a week in adults with overweight or obesity, and type 2 diabetes (STEP 2): a randomised, double-blind, double-dummy, placebo-controlled, phase 3 trial. Lancet. 2021;397(10278):971-84.
15. Wadden TA, Bailey TS, Billings LK, et al. Effect of subcutaneous semaglutide vs placebo as an adjunct to intensive behavioral therapy on body weight in adults with overweight or obesity: The STEP 3 Randomized Clinical Trial. JAMA. 2021;325(14):1403-13.
16. Rubino D, Abrahamsson N, Davies M, et al. Effect of continued weekly subcutaneous semaglutide vs placebo on weight loss maintenance in adults with overweight or obesity: The STEP 4 randomized clinical trial. JAMA. 2021;325(14):1414-25.
17. Moiz A, Levett JY, Filion KB, et al. Long-term efficacy and safety of once-weekly semaglutide for weight loss in patients without diabetes: a systematic review and meta-analysis of randomized controlled trials. Am J Cardiol. 2024;222:121-30.
18. Ryan DH, Yockey SR. Weight loss and improvement in comorbidity: differences at 5%, 10%, 15%, and over. Curr Obes Rep. 2017;6(2):187-94.
19. Lincoff AM, Brown-Frandsen K, Colhoun HM, et al. Semaglutide and cardiovascular outcomes in obesity without diabetes. N Engl J Med. 2023;389(24):2221-32.
20. Kosiborod MN, Abildstrøm SZ, Borlaug BA, et al. Semaglutide in patients with heart failure with preserved ejection fraction and obesity. N Engl J Med. 2023;389(12):1069-84.
21. Wegovy. (2025). Semaglutide tablets 25 mg and Semaglutide injection 2.4 mg. [online] Available from https://www.novo-pi.com/wegovy.pdf [Last accessed January, 2026].
22. EMA. (2025). PRAC concludes eye condition NAION is a very rare side effect of semaglutide medicines Ozempic, Rybelsus and Wegovy. [online] Available from https://www.ema.europa.eu/en/news/prac-concludes-eye-condition-naion-very-rare-side-effect-semaglutide-medicines-ozempic-rybelsus-wegovy [Last accessed January, 2026].

100

CHAPTER

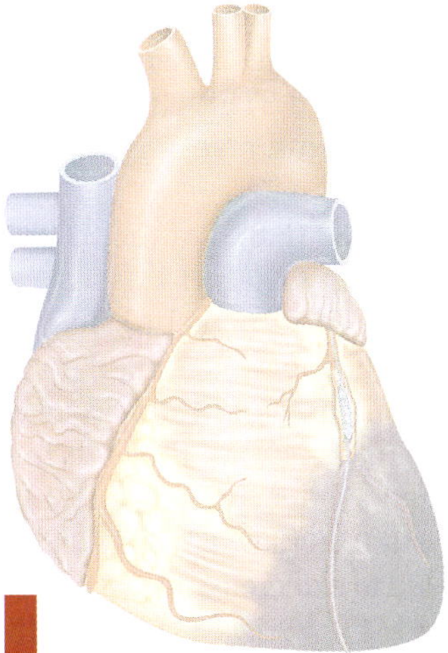

Semaglutide in Obesity with Heart Failure: Emerging Outcome Data and Clinical Implications

Satyendra Tewari, B Hilbert Sahoo

INTRODUCTION

Heart failure with preserved ejection fraction (HFpEF) constitutes more than one half of all heart failure cases and is on the rise in prevalence.[1] In India, the incidence of HFpEF is around 19–25%, which is considerably lower compared to Western populations.[2] It is likely that many instances remain undiagnosed in developing nations such as India.[2] A significant number of individuals with this condition are either overweight or obese, and increasing evidence indicates that obesity and excess fat are not merely coincidental but could contribute to the onset and worsening of HFpEF.[3-5] Since 1980, obesity rates have increased significantly. In the USA, the current prevalence has surpassed 40%, a dramatic rise from 15% in the 1970s, with projections suggesting that one in two adults in the USA will be obese by 2030.[3,6,7] Patients with obesity and HFpEF experience more negative hemodynamic and clinical characteristics, a heavier symptom burden, diminished functional capacity, and a more significantly impacted quality of life compared to those with HFpEF without obesity.[8-10] The presence of visceral fat is linked to heightened inflammation, left ventricular hypertrophy, insulin resistance, and both diastolic and systolic left ventricular dysfunction, as well as dysfunction in arterial, skeletal muscle, and physical capacities.[11] For patients already diagnosed with HFpEF, those exhibiting the obesity phenotype show unique clinical and hemodynamic traits, such as increased plasma and stressed blood volume, reduced venous capacitance, higher exercise pulmonary wedge pressures, poor hemodynamic reactions to diuresis, elevated inflammatory markers, and more severe hypertension, along with heightened symptoms and limited exercise tolerance.[8-12] Moreover, obesity results in a deficiency of natriuretic peptides due to decreased production and heightened clearance, which reduces the ability for vasodilation and natriuresis.[13,14] Agonists of the glucagon-like peptide-1 (GLP-1) receptor are utilized for managing type 2 diabetes and addressing overweight or obesity, and they have also been noted to diminish the risk of major adverse cardiovascular events among high-risk patients with type 2 diabetes.[15] Semaglutide, a long-acting GLP-1 analog administered at 2.4 mg subcutaneously once a week for 104 weeks, was shown to achieve a mean weight loss of 15.2% in patients who are overweight or obese and do not have diabetes.[16]

EMERGING DATA

Recent studies, including the STEP-HFpEF trial, have transformed the treatment approach for individuals with HFpEF and obesity.[1]

STEP-HFpEF Trial

In the STEP-HFpEF trial, the objective was to evaluate the safety and effectiveness of semaglutide in patients suffering from HFpEF and obesity. A total of 529 patients with a left ventricular ejection fraction (LVEF) of 45% or more, a body mass index (BMI) of 30 kg/m^2 or greater, and symptoms classified as New York Heart Association (NYHA) functional class II, III, or IV were randomly assigned in a 1:1 ratio to receive either once-weekly subcutaneous semaglutide ($n = 263$) or a matching placebo ($n = 266$). Treatment with semaglutide at a dose of 0.25 mg once weekly for the first month was increased every month until a maintenance dose of 2.4 mg was achieved by week 16.

- The median follow-up duration was 52 weeks.
- The median age of participants was 69 years.
- The percentage of female participants was 56.1%.
- Patients with a history of diabetes were not included in the study.

The coprimary endpoints comparing semaglutide to placebo from baseline to week 52 were:

- *Change in KCCQ-CSS:* 16.6 for semaglutide versus 8.7 for placebo ($p < 0.001$)
- *Percentage change in body weight:* –13.3% for semaglutide versus –2.6% for placebo ($p < 0.001$)

Key secondary outcomes for semaglutide in comparison to placebo included:

- Change in the 6-minute walk distance from baseline to week 52: 21.5 m for semaglutide versus 1.2 m for placebo ($p < 0.001$)
- Percentage reduction in NT-proBNP from baseline to week 52: –20.9% for semaglutide versus –5.3% for placebo ($p < 0.05$)
- Number of hospitalizations or urgent visits for heart failure: 1 for semaglutide compared to 12 for placebo ($p < 0.05$)
- The occurrence of adverse events was similar between the groups.

Although the trial lacked sufficient power to evaluate clinical events, a reduction in heart failure occurrences was documented.

SELECT Trial

- A total of 17,604 participants were randomly allocated in a 1:1 ratio to receive a weekly subcutaneous dose of 2.4 mg semaglutide or a placebo.
- The primary cardiovascular endpoint was defined as a composite of cardiovascular death, nonfatal myocardial infarction, or nonfatal stroke, analyzed for the time until the first event.
- For those with preexisting cardiovascular disease who were overweight or obese but did not have diabetes, weekly subcutaneous semaglutide at a 2.4 mg dose was found to be more effective than placebo in lowering the incidence of cardiovascular deaths, nonfatal myocardial infarction, or nonfatal stroke over a mean follow-up period of 39.8 months.
- The heart failure composite endpoint hazard ratio (HR) 0.82 (95% CI, 0.71–0.96)

A post hoc pooled participant-level analysis of four randomized, placebo-controlled trials (SELECT, FLOW, STEP-HFpEF, and STEP-HFpEF DM) aimed to investigate the effects of the once-weekly subcutaneous semaglutide (2.4 mg in SELECT, STEP-HFpEF, and STEP-HFpEF DM; 1.0 mg in FLOW) on heart failure events, revealing clinical benefits.

Across these four studies, 3,743 (16.8%) of the 22,282 participants had a history of HFpEF (1,914 assigned to semaglutide and 1,829 assigned to placebo). In the subgroup with HFpEF, semaglutide was linked to a reduced risk of the composite outcome of cardiovascular death or heart failure events [103 (5.4%) of those in the semaglutide group experienced events compared to 138 (7.5%) in the placebo group; HR 0.69 (95% CI, 0.53–0.89); $p = 0.0045$]. Semaglutide also led to a decrease in the risk of worsening heart failure events [54 (2.8%) vs 86 (4.7%); HR 0.59 (95% CI, 0.41–0.82); $p = 0.0019$]. No significant effect was detected for cardiovascular death alone [59 (3.1%) vs. 67 (3.7%); HR 0.82 (95% CI, 0.57–1.16); $p = 0.25$]. The rate of serious adverse events was lower in the semaglutide group compared to the placebo group [572 (29.9%) vs. 708 (38.7%)].

CONCLUSION

Semaglutide, classified as a GLP-1 receptor agonist, emerges as a promising therapeutic alternative for individuals with obesity and HFpEF, regardless of whether they have diabetes. Recent clinical studies have indicated that semaglutide significantly enhances symptoms, exercise performance, and quality of life while facilitating weight loss. Long-term data on clinical advantages, however, remain limited.

REFERENCES

1. Kosiborod MN, Abildstrøm SZ, Borlaug BA, et al. Semaglutide in patients with heart failure with preserved ejection fraction and obesity. N Engl J Med. 2023;389:1069-84.
2. Harikrishnan S, Oomman A, Jadhav UM, et al. Heart failure with preserved ejection fraction: management guidelines (from Heart Failure Association of India, endorsed by Association of Physicians of India). J Assoc Physicians India. 2022;70:71-3.
3. Borlaug BA, Kitzman DW, Redfield MM, et al. Obesity and heart failure with preserved ejection fraction: new insights and pathophysiological targets. Cardiovasc Res. 2023;118:3434-50.
4. Haass M, Obokata M, Reddy YNV, et al. Body mass index and adverse cardiovascular outcomes in heart failure patients with preserved ejection fraction: results from the Irbesartan in Heart Failure with Preserved Ejection Fraction (I-PRESERVE) trial. Circ Heart Fail. 2011;4:324-31.

5. Newman AB, Lee JS, Visser M, et al. Weight change and the conservation of lean mass in old age: The Health, Aging and Body Composition Study. Am J Clin Nutr. 2005;82: 872-8.
6. Ng ACT, Delgado V, Borlaug BA, et al. Diabesity: the combined burden of obesity and diabetes on heart disease and the role of imaging. Nat Rev Cardiol. 2021;18: 291-304.
7. Ward ZJ, Bleich SN, Cradock AL, et al. Projected U.S. state-level prevalence of adult obesity and severe obesity. N Engl J Med. 2019;381:2440-50.
8. Obokata M, Reddy YNV, Pislaru SV, et al. Evidence supporting the existence of a distinct obese phenotype of heart failure with preserved ejection fraction. Circulation. 2017;136:6-19.
9. Sorimachi H, Obokata M, Reddy YNV, et al. Obesity, venous capacitance, and venous compliance in heart failure with preserved ejection fraction. Eur J Heart Fail. 2021;23:1648-58.
10. Reddy YNV, Obokata M, Chung BB, et al. Characterization of the obese phenotype of heart failure with preserved ejection fraction: a RELAX trial ancillary study. Mayo Clin Proc. 2019;94:1199-209.
11. Kitzman DW, Nicklas BJ. Pivotal role of excess intra-abdominal adipose in the pathogenesis of metabolic/obese HFpEF. JACC Heart Fail. 2018;6:1008-10.
12. Obokata M, Reddy YNV, Pislaru SV, et al. Role of diastolic stress testing in the evaluation for heart failure with preserved ejection fraction: a simultaneous invasive-echocardiographic study. Circulation. 2017;135:825-38.
13. Shah SJ. BNP: biomarker not perfect in heart failure with preserved ejection fraction. Eur Heart J. 2022;43:1952-54.
14. Wang TJ. The natriuretic peptides and fat metabolism. N Engl J Med. 2012;367:377-8.
15. Sattar N, Lee MMY, Kristensen SL, et al. Cardiovascular, mortality, and kidney outcomes with GLP-1 receptor agonists in patients with type 2 diabetes: a systematic review and meta-analysis of randomised trials. Lancet Diabetes Endocrinol. 2021;9:653-62.
16. Garvey WT, Birkenfeld AL, Dicker D, et al. Two-year effects of semaglutide in adults with overweight or obesity: the STEP 5 trial. Nat Med. 2022;28:2083-91.

101

CHAPTER

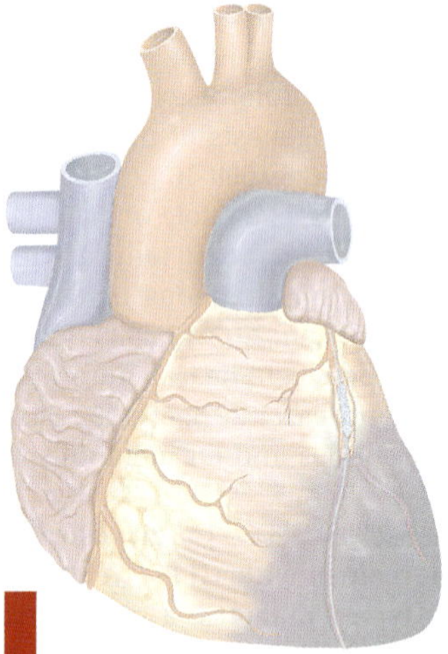

Impact of Semaglutide on Body Composition and Fat Distribution

Archit Dahiya, Isha Nandal, Harsh Wardhan

INTRODUCTION

Obesity and its sequelae, such as type 2 diabetes mellitus (T2DM) and atherosclerotic cardiovascular disease (ASCVD),[1-6] are escalating public health threats worldwide.[2,3] With the tripling of global obesity rates since the 1970s comes an urgent need for pharmacotherapeutics that target not just body weight but also body composition and fat distribution, given the particular risks associated with excess visceral adipose tissue (VAT) in our body.[7-9] Semaglutide's approval for chronic weight management is underpinned by compelling evidence of its ability to drive sustained, clinically meaningful weight loss, with impacts that extend into significant improvements in regional fat distribution and cardiometabolic risk.[3,7-9]

MECHANISM OF ACTION

Refer to **Figure 1**.

Metabolic Pathways Targeted by GLP-1 Receptor Agonism

The therapeutic actions of semaglutide flow from its agonism of the GLP-1 receptor, resulting in several complementary metabolic events. It acts by enhancing glucose-dependent insulin secretion, thereby lowering postprandial glucose excursions with a low risk of hypoglycemia in monotherapy settings.[2,3]

It suppresses glucagon secretion and decelerates gastric emptying, which results in blunting the postprandial

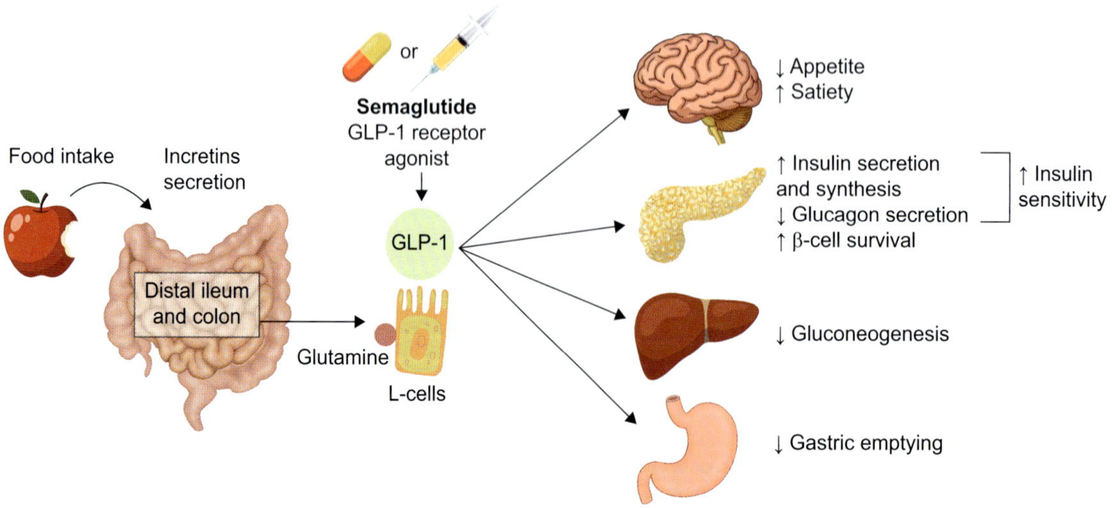

Fig. 1: Mechanism of action of semaglutide.

glycemic surges and increasing early satiety, leading to reduced caloric intake and, ultimately, energy deficit.[3,4,6]

It also modulates the hypothalamic and mesolimbic circuits through both central and vagal mechanisms, thereby attenuating hunger and spontaneously reducing reward-driven food-seeking behavior.[4-7]

Collectively, these mechanisms converge to produce a persistent negative energy balance that underlies semaglutide's effects on total body weight, fat reduction, and favorable redistribution of adiposity.[7]

MAJOR TRIALS ON SEMAGLUTIDE

The STEP and SUSTAIN trials, and corroborative real-world observational studies, have consistently shown that semaglutide leads to durable weight loss that is disproportionately attributable to reductions in VAT, which is established as the most pathogenic form of adiposity.[8-11]

Unlike nonspecific weight loss modalities, semaglutide is associated with preferential retention of lean (fat-free) mass as a percentage of total body weight, a quality especially relevant to the management of metabolic disease and physical function in at-risk populations.[8-10]

Also, semaglutide therapy is associated with substantial improvements in glycemic control (HbA1c reduction), reductions in liver transaminases, and favorable modulation of lipid profiles—with notably larger reductions in LDL cholesterol and total cholesterol than have been observed with other agents in the GLP-1 RA class.[11-14]

However, like with other weight reduction modalities, weight regain is a common issue when semaglutide is discontinued, underscoring the need for ongoing therapy or comprehensive maintenance approaches.[8,15]

METABOLIC EFFECTS ON BODY COMPOSITION AND FAT DISTRIBUTION

Total and Regional Fat Loss

A pivotal exploratory analysis from STEP 1 trial demonstrated that subjects randomized to 68 weeks of semaglutide experienced mean reductions in total fat mass of −19.3% and, more impressively, a −27.4% reduction in visceral fat mass. Taken together, these changes corresponded to absolute declines of −3.5 and −2.0% points in total and visceral fat, respectively, as proportions of overall body mass.[8]

Despite an absolute decrease in lean mass of 9.7%, the relative proportion of lean mass to total body weight actually increased by 3.0% points, indicating favorable repartitioning of lost weight toward more metabolically active tissue preservation. This profile contrasts with many hypocaloric weight-loss diets, which often result in proportionally greater losses of lean mass.[8,9]

Global Validation

Data from a Chinese cohort receiving semaglutide alongside lifestyle interventions for 6 months reinforce these findings: Participants lost on average 9.9 ± 3.9 kg, including substantial decreases in fat mass (−5.6 ± 3.7 kg) and visceral fat area (−24.4 ± 17.7 cm^2); meanwhile, skeletal muscle mass fell only slightly (−1.4 ± 1.3 kg) with the skeletal muscle index nearly unchanged (from 8.1 to 7.9 kg/m^2).[9]

Evidence from Type 2 Diabetes Mellitus Patients in Trials

Japanese patients with T2DM demonstrated a reduction in fat mass of −2.8 kg after 24 weeks of oral semaglutide, but only a minimal impact on muscle mass (−0.5 kg), supporting the agent's safety for preserving functional lean tissue in at-risk diabetic populations.[10]

Thus, multiple studies converge to demonstrate that semaglutide preferentially reduces VAT and total adiposity while either maintaining or even improving the proportion of body mass accounted for by lean tissue.[8-10] These changes are central to improvements in insulin sensitivity, reductions in hepatic steatosis, and long-term cardiovascular risk abatement.

Effects on Resting Metabolic Rate

The evidence about the direct effects of semaglutide on resting metabolic rate (RMR) is limited. However, in a randomized, double-blind, placebo-controlled clinical trial investigating RMR specifically, semaglutide produced significant decreases in energy intake and body weight versus placebo, but no meaningful differences in RMR when values were normalized to lean body mass.[16] This suggests that weight loss is achieved primarily by reducing caloric intake and that semaglutide does not inherently suppress or stimulate basal metabolic rate.

Glycemic Outcomes

Semaglutide's impacts on glycemic control are significant across populations with varying baseline glycemia. Trials demonstrate that weekly dosing at 0.5 or 1.0 mg leads to HbA1c reductions of 1.2–1.8% from an initial baseline of 8.1–8.7%—effects potentiated by concurrent reductions in hepatic and visceral fat and improved insulin action.[10,15] These improvements are strongly correlated with both the degree of total weight loss and the partitioning of fat loss toward high-risk depots (notably, the abdomen and liver).

EFFECTS ON LIPID PROFILE AND CARDIOVASCULAR RISK

SUSTAIN Trials

Comprehensive data from the SUSTAIN 1–7 trials demonstrate that semaglutide consistently lowers atherogenic lipid fractions: The 0.5 mg dose reduced total cholesterol [estimated treatment ratio (ETR) 0.95–0.97] and LDL-C (ETR 0.94–0.96); the 1.0 mg dose achieved even greater reductions in total cholesterol (ETR 0.92–0.96), triglycerides (ETR 0.87–0.94), and LDL-C (ETR 0.92–0.93), with modest improvements in HDL-C (ETR 1.02–1.04).[15]

Network Meta-analysis

A comprehensive 2024 network meta-analysis covering 76 trials found that semaglutide is the only GLP-1 RA with statistically significant reductions in LDL-C (–0.16 mmol/L) and total cholesterol (–0.48 mmol/L).[11] This distinction may reflect unique molecular and mechanistic properties of semaglutide within the GLP-1 RA class.[12,13]

Semaglutide may improve cholesterol homeostasis by upregulating ABCA1-dependent cholesterol efflux (via downregulation of microRNA-19b) and through statin-like inhibition of HMG-CoA reductase and downstream SREBP-1c signaling.[12-14] These mechanisms are likely additive to weight loss and may contribute specifically to the pronounced impact of semaglutide on atherogenic lipids.

Therapeutic Durability and Treatment Continuation

Despite its efficacy, discontinuation of semaglutide typically results in rapid weight regain—often approaching the initial baseline, as shown in follow-up cohorts—reinforcing the importance of continued pharmacotherapy or structured transition for durable long-term benefits.[8,15]

There is also no evidence to support adjunctive use of semaglutide to minimize weight regain or stimulate renewed weight loss after plateau or suboptimal outcomes following bariatric surgery **(Table 1)**.[10,15]

CLINICAL IMPLICATIONS

Targeting Visceral Adipose Tissue and Ectopic Fat

Given the clear link between visceral/ectopic fat and cardiometabolic disease, clinical strategies should prioritize reductions in VAT and hepatic fat. These changes directly improve insulin sensitivity, lower triglycerides, normalize liver function tests, and mitigate hypertension risk.[9,11,15]

Preservation of Lean Mass

Clinicians should combine semaglutide with interventions to maximize skeletal muscle preservation, including resistance exercise and high-protein dietary patterns—especially important for frail or older adults vulnerable to sarcopenia.[8-10]

Lipid Management Synergy

Semaglutide produces LDL and total cholesterol improvements that may be synergistic with statins and can meaningfully lower overall cardiovascular risk in high-risk patients.[11,12,14] Longitudinal follow-up is required to establish the full scope of risk reduction in primary and secondary prevention settings.

Maintenance and Relapse Prevention

Guidance for patients should emphasize sustained therapy or structured transitions, including behavioral supports, consistent physical activity, and regular monitoring to prevent recurrence of weight and cardiometabolic risk factors.[8,15]

The long-term dynamics of VAT and hepatic fat, particularly beyond 2 years of continuous treatment or

TABLE 1: Metabolic and cardiovascular effects of semaglutide.

Parameter	*Reported effect*	*Key study/trial*	*Statistical significance*	*Notes*
HbA1c (%, reduction)	–1.2 to –1.8%	SUSTAIN 1–7[15]	Yes	Dose-dependent, 0.5 mg/1.0 mg
LDL-C (mmol/L, reduction)	–0.16	Meta-analysis[11]	Yes	Significant versus other GLP-1 RAs
Total cholesterol (mmol/L, reduction)	–0.48	Meta-analysis[11]	Yes	Significant versus other GLP-1 RAs
Triglycerides (mmol/L, reduction)	0.87–0.94 ETR	SUSTAIN 1–7[15]	Yes	Greater effect at higher dose

(ETR: estimated treatment ratio)

postdiscontinuation, are still not known completely. More research is needed on standardized reporting of body composition across ages, sex, and phenotypes.[8,9]

Optimal resistance training regimens and protein distribution protocols need further clarification for lean mass retention when using GLP-1 RAs. Future trials need to also examine impacts on bone health, reproductive function, and the identification of biomarkers for responders versus nonresponders.

CONCLUSION

Semaglutide is a multidimensional therapy that addresses the root drivers of metabolic disease by promoting weight loss that selectively depletes VAT and ectopic fat, while substantially preserving lean mass proportion. The resultant shifts in body composition, alongside superior glycemic and lipid outcomes, help in achieving significant cardiometabolic risk reductions. These benefits are best sustained with ongoing therapy and a program integrated with resistance training, high-protein diets, and behavioral support. Future research will refine these approaches, optimize protocols for specific populations, and further clarify long-term efficacy and safety.

REFERENCES

1. Roder ME. Clinical potential of treatment with semaglutide in type 2 diabetes patients. Drugs Context. 2019;8:212585.
2. Meier JJ. GLP-1 receptor agonists for individualized treatment of type 2 diabetes mellitus. Nat Rev Endocrinol. 2012;8(12):728-42.
3. Al-Massadi O, Fernø J, Diéguez C, et al. Glucagon control on food intake and energy balance. Int J Mol Sci. 2019;20(16):3905.
4. Drucker DJ. Mechanisms of action and therapeutic application of GLP-1. Cell Metab. 2018;27(4):740-56.
5. Knudsen LB, Lau J. Discovery and development of liraglutide and semaglutide. Front Endocrinol. 2019;10:155.
6. Seufert J, Gallwitz B. Extra-pancreatic effects of GLP-1 RAs. Diabetes Obes Metab. 2014;16(8):673-88.
7. Christou GA, Katsiki N, Blundell J, et al. Semaglutide as a promising antiobesity drug. Obes Rev. 2019;20(6):805-15.
8. Wilding JPH, Batterham RL, Calanna S, et al. Impact of semaglutide on body composition: STEP 1 exploratory analysis. J Endocr Soc. 2021;5(Suppl_1):A16-7.
9. Xiang J, Ding X-Y, Zhang W, et al. Clinical effectiveness of semaglutide on weight loss, body composition, and muscle strength in Chinese adults. Eur Rev Med Pharmacol Sci. 2023;27(20):9908-15.
10. Uchiyama S, Sada Y, Mihara S, et al. Oral semaglutide induces loss of body fat mass without affecting muscle mass in patients with type 2 diabetes. J Clin Med Res. 2023;15(7):377-83.
11. Yao H, Zhang A, Li D, et al. Comparative effectiveness of GLP-1 receptor agonists on glycaemic control, body weight, and lipid profile for type 2 diabetes: systematic review and network meta-analysis. BMJ. 2024;384:e076410.
12. Yao Y, Li Q, Wang W, et al. Glucagon-like peptide-1 modulates cholesterol homeostasis by suppressing the miR-19b-induced downregulation of ABCA1. Cell Physiol Biochem. 2018;50(2):679-93.
13. Patel V, Joharapurkar A, Kshirsagar S, et al. Coagonist of GLP-1 and glucagon decreases liver inflammation and atherosclerosis in dyslipidemic condition. Chem Biol Interact. 2018;282:13-21.
14. Hasegawa Y, Hori M, Nakagami T, et al. Glucagon-like peptide-1 receptor agonists reduced the low-density lipoprotein cholesterol in Japanese patients with type 2 diabetes mellitus treated with statins. J Clin Lipidol. 2018;12(1):62-9.
15. Aroda VR, Ahmann A, Cariou B et al. Comparative efficacy, safety, and cardiovascular outcomes with once weekly subcutaneous semaglutide in the treatment of type 2 diabetes: insights from the SUSTAIN 1 7 trials. Diabetes Metab. 2019;45(5):409-18.
16. Blundell J, Finlayson G, Axelsen M, et al. Effects of once-weekly semaglutide on appetite, energy intake, control of eating, food preference and body weight in subjects with obesity. Diabetes Obes Metab. 2017;19(9):1242-51.

102

CHAPTER

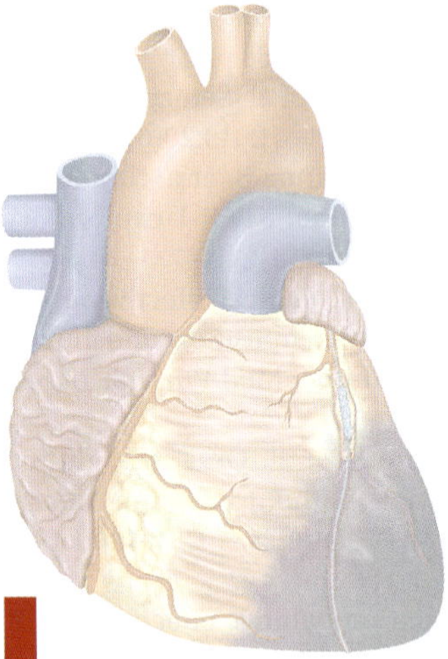

Comparative Effectiveness of Semaglutide in Different Obesity Phenotypes with Cardiovascular Disease

Ameet G Sattur

INTRODUCTION

Obesity is now firmly believed to be a biologically complex, chronic, progressive, and relapsing heterogeneous disease that requires individualized, phenotype- and complication-driven therapeutic strategies.[1] The nature of clinical improvement depends not only on weight reduction but also on the specific mechanism of action of the treatment and the underlying phenotype.

The introduction of newer pharmacotherapies, including glucagon-like peptide-1 receptor agonists (GLP-1 RA), dual glucose-dependent insulinotropic polypeptide/glucagon-like peptide-1 (GIP/GLP-1) agonists, has made a shift from weight-centric goals to precision-based phenotype-based obesity care.

OBESITY PHENOTYPES

The journey of obesity has evolved from body mass index (BMI) to obesity paradox to visceral obesity and different phenotypes.

Obesity is categorized across four groups with different metabolic profiles as shown in **Table 1**.

Obesity phenotypes and cardiovascular (CV) risk are shown in **Table 2**.

THERAPEUTIC STRATEGIES IN MANAGEMENT OF OBESITY PHENOTYPES

It is known that the different obesity phenotypes have different responses to obesity management interventions such as diet for weight loss, medications, devices, and surgery.[2]

In the modern pharmacological treatment of obesity, GLP1-RA has shown promising results independent of diabetes. The beneficial effects of GLP1-RA semaglutide are shown in **Figure 1**.

Semaglutide is effective in promoting significant weight loss and improving cardiometabolic risk factors in *both*

TABLE 1: Obesity categorized across four groups with different metabolic profiles.

	MUNW	*MHNW*	*MHO*	*MUO*	*SO*
Waist circumference	N/↑	N	N	↑	↑WC and/or BMI >25
BMI	18.5–24.9	18.5–24.9	>25	>25	>25
Visceral adipose tissue	↑	↓	↓	↑	↑
Lean mass	—	—	↑	—	↓
Metabolic abnormalities	Present	Absent	Absent	Present	Present

(MHNW: metabolically healthy normal weight; MHO: metabolically healthy obesity; MUNW: metabolically unhealthy normal weight; MUO: metabolically unhealthy obese; SO: sarcopenic obese)

TABLE 2: Obesity phenotypes and cardiovascular risk.

MUHN	*MHO*	*MUO*	*SO*
Higher risk of: • Dysmetabolism • LVH • HF • CV mortality • Stroke • Metabolic cardiomyopathy	*Higher risk of:* • MI, ischemic stroke, or CV death than MUO • HF • AF	*Higher risk of:* • Dysmetabolism • LVH • HFrEF • CV mortality • Stroke • Metabolic cardiomyopathy • HF • MI • Arrythmias	*Higher risk of:* • CV diseases and HF than MNHW • STEMI-mortality

(CV: cardiovascular; HFrEF: heart failure with reduced ejection fraction; LVH: left ventricular hypertrophy; MI: myocardial infarction; MHO: metabolically healthy obesity; MUHN: metabolically unhealthy normal weight; MUO: metabolically unhealthy obesity; SO: sarcopenic obesity; STEMI: ST-segment Elevation Myocardial Infarction)

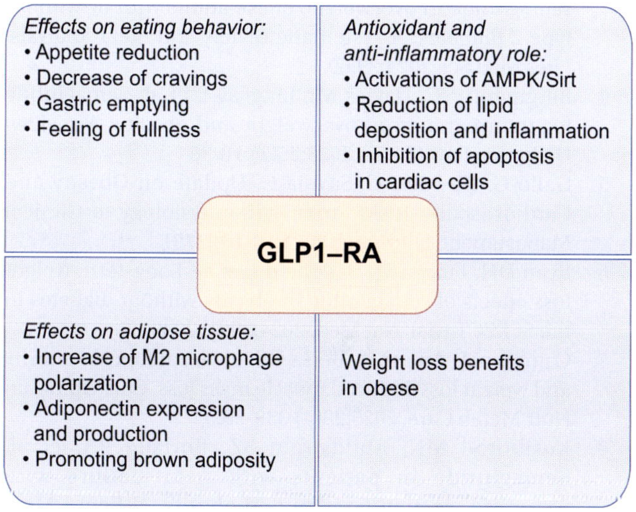

Fig. 1: Beneficial effects of GLP1-RA semaglutide.
(AMPK: adenosine monophosphate-activated protein kinase; GLP1-RA: glucagon-like peptide-1 receptor agonist)

metabolically unhealthy obese (MUO) and metabolically healthy obesity (MHO) individuals.

Its use in normal-weight individuals, whether metabolically healthy or unhealthy, is generally considered off-label and lacks extensive clinical trial data.

Metabolically unhealthy obese: Semaglutide is highly effective in this subset with substantial improvements.

- *Significant weight loss*: STEP program studies have consistently shown significant weight reduction (mean loss of 9.6–17.4% over 68–104 weeks, depending on the dosage and the trial) in obese individuals.[3,4]
- *Metabolic benefits*: Improves multiple cardiometabolic risk factors—improves glycemic control, reduces blood pressure, reduces low-density lipoprotein (LDL)/total cholesterol/triglycerides while increasing high-density lipoprotein (HDL).
- *Reduces CV risk*: SELECT trial showed a 20% reduction in major adverse CV events regardless of diabetic status.[5]

Metabolically healthy obese: Semaglutide is effective in this subset as well.

- *Weight loss and body composition*: Significant weight loss and reductions in waist circumference and overall fatness.
- *Improved health markers*: While MHO individuals do not have inherent metabolic issues, semaglutide treatment helps them move further from the risk threshold.
- Preventing progression of MHO to MUO.[6]

As mentioned earlier, the use of semaglutide in the Management of Unhealthy Nutrition and Weight (MUNW) and Medical/Management of Healthy Nutrition and Weight (MHNW) literature is limited and not advised.

Sarcopenic obese: Studies have shown that semaglutide effectively reduces fat mass, particularly visceral fat, while preserving lean muscle mass, which is beneficial for body composition. This suggests semaglutide may have favorable benefits, but dedicated studies on this phenotype are necessary.[7,8]

Benefits of semaglutide in cardiorenal-metabolic complications:

- *Atherosclerotic cardiovascular disease (ASCVD) and HF*: The SELECT trial used semaglutide 2.4 mg once weekly and reduced MACE by 20%, and all-cause mortality by 19% in patients with obesity and established ASCVD without diabetes.[6]

The STEP-HF trial: Trial enrolled 529 nondiabetic patients with Heart failure with preserved ejection fraction (HFpEF) and obesity who were randomly assigned to once-weekly semaglutide (2.4 mg) or placebo for 52 weeks. A statistically significant improvement in the quality of life score and in weight loss was observed. Statistically significant improvements were also seen in the 6 min walk distance, levels of C-reactive protein, and N-terminal pro-B-type natriuretic peptide levels.

Thus semaglutide should be used and preferred in patients with obesity and ASCVD or HFpEF, even without diabetes mellitus.

Chronic kidney disease (CKD): SELECT trial reduced the composite renal end points by 22% than placebo. It reduced the eGFR decline, onset of macroalbuminuria, and need for renal replacement therapy.

Thus, semaglutide should be used and preferred in patients with obesity and CKD.

- *Prediabetes and diabetes*: Semaglutide should be preferred in patients with diabetes and obesity, as both weight loss and glycemic control are desired based on the STEP 2 trial, which showed a 9.6% reduction in mean weight and glycated hemoglobin (HBA1c) reductions of 1.6% with improved insulin sensitivity.[9] The SUSTAIN 6 trial showed benefit in patients with secondary prevention of ASCVD.[10]
- *Metabolic dysfunction associated with steatotic liver disease*: Studies also suggest that Semaglutide can also be used with obesity associated with MASLD.[11]
- *Osteoarthritis*: STEP 9 trial involving adults with obesity and knee osteoarthritis, semaglutide resulted in significantly greater weight loss (–13.7% vs. –3.2%) and improvement in physical function (SF-36 + 12.0 vs. +6.5 points) compared to placebo (all $p < 0.001$) at 68 weeks.[12]

  Hence, semaglutide should be used with obesity and knee OA who meet criteria for pharmacologic weight management, particularly when pain and function impair quality of life.

CONCLUSION

- Semaglutide, a glucagon-like peptide-1 receptor agonist (GLP-1 RA), has shown promise in multiple comorbidities, offering potential benefits in obesity phenotypes based on clinical trials, including SUSTAIN 6 (Semaglutide Unabated Sustainability in Treatment of Type 2 Diabetes 6), PIONEER 6 (Peptide InnOvatioN for Early diabEtes tReatment 6), STEP HFpEF (Semaglutide Treatment Effect in People with Obesity-related Heart Failure with Preserved Ejection Fraction), and STEP HFpEF DM.
- Semaglutide is more beneficial in MUO and MHO obesity phenotypes as well as obesity-related HFpEF.

REFERENCES

1. Bray GA, Kim KK, Wilding JPH, World Obesity Federation. Obesity: a chronic, relapsing progressive disease process. A position statement of the world obesity federation. Obes Rev. 2017;18(7):715-23.
2. Heymsfield SB, Wadden TA. Mechanisms, pathophysiology, and management of obesity. N Engl J Med. 2017;376(3):254-66.
3. Yang L, Duan X, Hua P, et al. Effectiveness and safety of semaglutide in overweight/obese adults with or without type 2 diabetes: A systematic review and meta-analysis. J Res Med Sci. 2024;29:60.
4. Bergmann NC, Davies MJ, Lingvay I, et al. Semaglutide for the treatment of overweight and obesity: A review. Diabetes Obes Metab. 2023;25(1):18-35.
5. Gallo G, Desideri G, Savoia C. Update on Obesity and Cardiovascular Risk: From Pathophysiology to Clinical Management. Nutrients. 2024;16(16):2781.
6. Ryan DH, Lingvay I, Deanfield J, et al. Long-term weight loss effects of semaglutide in obesity without diabetes in the SELECT trial. Nat Med. 2024;30(7):2049-57.
7. Caturano A, Amaro A, Berra CC, et al. Sarcopenic obesity and weight loss-induced muscle mass loss. Curr Opin Clin Nutr Metab Care. 2025;28(4):339-50.
8. Kosiborod MN, Abildstrøm SZ, Borlaug BA, et al. Semaglutide in patients with heart failure with preserved ejection fraction and obesity. N Engl J Med. 2023;389(12):1069-84.
9. Davies M, Færch L, Jeppesen OK, et al. Semaglutide 2.4 mg once a week in adults with overweight or obesity, and type 2 diabetes (STEP 2): a randomised, double-blind, double-dummy, placebo-controlled, phase 3 trial. Lancet. 2021;397(10278):971-84.
10. Marso SP, Bain SC, Consoli A, et al. Semaglutide and cardiovascular outcomes in patients with type 2 diabetes. N Engl J Med. 2016;375(19):1834-44.
11. Sanyal AJ, Newsome PN, Kliers I, et al. Phase 3 trial of semaglutide in metabolic dysfunction-associated steatohepatitis. N Engl J Med. 2025;392(21):2089-99.
12. Bliddal H, Bays H, Czernichow S, et al. Once-weekly semaglutide in persons with obesity and knee osteoarthritis. N Engl J Med. 2024;391(17):1573-83.

103
CHAPTER

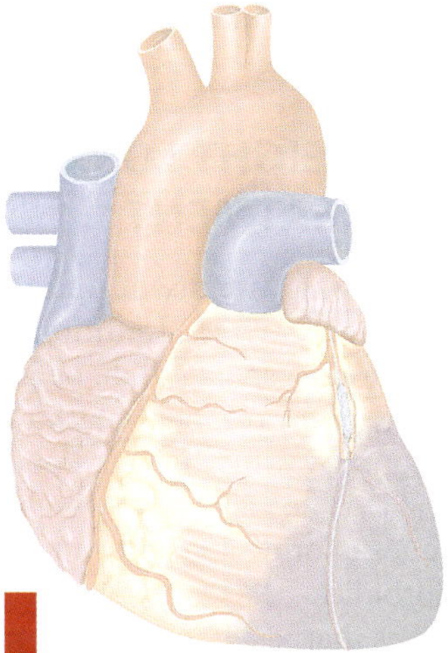

Long-term Safety and Sustainability of Weight Loss with Semaglutide

Pradeep Jain, Himanshu Jain, SN Pathak

INTRODUCTION

The global obesity epidemic is well established, with increase in obesity prevalence for most countries since the 1980s. Obesity contributes directly to incidence of cardiovascular risk factors, including dyslipidemia, type 2 diabetes, hypertension, and sleep disorders. Obesity also leads to the development of cardiovascular disease and cardiovascular disease mortality independent of other cardiovascular risk factors. More recent data highlight abdominal obesity, as determined by waist circumference, as a cardiovascular disease risk marker that is independent of body mass index. Obesity is a significant health concern worldwide, resulting in several diseases and increased mortality. Lifestyle changes and traditional weight loss methods such as diet, exercise, and behavioral therapy have shown results. However, the magnitude of weight loss achieved through these interventions is difficult to maintain in the long run. This has necessitated the need and growing demand for pharmacological options that can help reduce weight without any adverse effects.

Obesity is a multifactorial disease with a complex pathogenesis related to biological,[1] psychosocial,[2] socioeconomic,[3] and environmental[4,5] factors and heterogeneity in the pathways and mechanisms by which it leads to adverse health outcomes.[6-8]

Glucagon-like peptide-1 receptor agonists (GLP-1 RAs) such as semaglutide have shown encouraging outcomes. Semaglutide demonstrates robust efficacy in achieving significant weight loss and improving metabolic parameters in patients with and without diabetes.

Semaglutide has emerged as an anti-obesity medication for long-term weight management. It is effective for weight loss in obese patients, leading to its approval as chronic weight management treatment. A number of clinical trials have proved the efficacy of semaglutide in treating obesity. The STEP, i.e., semaglutide treatment effects in people with obesity, is the most notable program that has been instrumental in determining the long-term efficacy of semaglutide for weight loss.

LONG-TERM SAFETY PROFILE OF SEMAGLUTIDE TREATMENT

Significant data has been found to support the fact that semaglutide is a safe and effective treatment for chronic weight management. You may experience mild to moderate side effects such as nausea, vomiting, diarrhea, and constipation. These side effects are short-term and will go away once your body adapts to the medication.

Cardiovascular Safety

The SUSTAIN-6 trial, which was conducted on participants with type 2 diabetes, proved that semaglutide is effective in minimizing the risk of major adverse cardiovascular events by 26% compared to placebo.[9]

Additionally, in patients with heart failure with preserved ejection fraction (HFpEF) and obesity, semaglutide produced large improvements in HFpEF-related symptoms.[10] Semaglutide treatment is also found to decrease myocardial diastolic stiffness and improve actin–myosin and muscle contraction pathways.[11] Semaglutide therapy also reduced the incidence of any stroke when compared to a placebo through significant reductions in risk of small-vessel occlusion in a post hoc analysis of the SUSTAIN-6 and PIONEER 6 trials.[12]

Renal Function

The FLOW clinical trial investigated whether semaglutide can slow the progression of CKD in people with T2DM. They had demonstrated benefits for kidney-specific outcomes, cardiovascular death, and other secondary outcomes, including a slower decline in kidney function.[13]

Pancreases Concerns

Although GLP-1 receptor agonists, including semaglutide, have raised concerns about the increased risk of pancreatitis and gallbladder diseases, the risk is relatively low.

Thyroid Health

Glucagon-like peptide-1 receptor agonists have been associated with the increased risk of medullary thyroid carcinoma, but it has not been scientifically proven. However, if you have a past medical history of MTC, you must avoid using semaglutide. Semaglutide is also contraindicated for those with multiple endocrine neoplasia type 2 (MEN 2) syndrome, a rare genetic condition that increases the risk of MTC.

Bone Health

Long-term weight loss is often considered a reason for reduced bone density and increased fractures. Some studies reveal that minor changes in bone density are bound to occur, but the risk of fractures is quite low.

Metabolic Benefits

One of the best and most significant benefits of semaglutide is the ability to lose weight and sustain it for a longer period. Patients who use semaglutide treatment in continuity experience improved metabolic health. This sustained weight loss minimizes the risk of health complications caused due to obesity, including type 2 diabetes, hypertension, and cardiovascular diseases.

Diabetic Retinopathy

In SUSTAIN-6 trial, semaglutide therapy was associated with a significantly higher rate of diabetic retinopathy complications when compared to the placebo group.[14]

Quality of Life

Participants in clinical trials have witnessed improvement in their quality of life due to semaglutide, including increased physical health, better social interactions, improved psychological well-being, and sustainable lifestyle changes.

ACHIEVE LONG-TERM WEIGHT LOSS WITH SEMAGLUTIDE TREATMENT

Semaglutide is a promising and safe treatment option for long-term weight management. Where traditional methods fail to deliver desired results, semaglutide helps reduce weight, control glucose, and promote healthier eating habits. This led to its approval by the U.S. Food and Drug Administration (FDA) for chronic weight management in adults with obesity or overweight with at least one weight-related comorbidity.

Unlike diet plans or exercises that result in short-term weight loss, semaglutide has proved its ability to achieve improved and sustained weight loss outcomes. However, you can gain maximum benefits by combining it with healthier lifestyle choices such as a healthy diet, regular physical activity, and behavioral therapy.

GUIDELINES FOR SAFE USE AND MONITORING

The medication is typically administered as a once-weekly subcutaneous injection, on the same day each week, at any time of day, with or without meals. The injection site should be rotated among the abdomen, thigh, or upper arm.

When semaglutide is used with other medications that lower blood sugar, such as insulin or sulfonylureas, there is an increased risk of hypoglycemia. In such cases, the dosage of insulin or sulfonylureas may need to be adjusted to reduce this risk. If a dose is missed, it should be administered as soon as possible within 5 days of the missed dose. If >5 days have passed, the missed dose should be skipped, and the regular dosing schedule resumed.

PREGNANCY

Due to sporadic cases of atrial septal defect, the manufacturer advised stopping this semaglutide treatment 2 months prior to conception of the fetus.[15]

CONCLUSION

In conclusion, semaglutide represents a significant advancement in the pharmacological management of T2DM, offering improvements in glycemic control, cardiovascular outcomes, and obesity. Its multifaceted mechanism of action, targeting both central and peripheral pathways involved in glucose and energy homeostasis, positions it as a promising agent in the evolving landscape of metabolic and neurodegenerative disease management.

REFERENCES

1. Loos RJ. Genetic determinants of common obesity and their value in prediction. Best Pract Res Clin Endocrinol Metab. 2012;26:211-26.
2. Gebreab SZ, Vandeleur CL, Rudaz D, et al. Psychosocial stress over the lifespan, psychological factors, and cardiometabolic risk in the community. Psychosom Med. 2018;80:628-39.
3. Sommer I, Griebler U, Mahlknecht P, et al. Socioeconomic inequalities in non-communicable diseases and their risk factors: an overview of systematic reviews. BMC Public Health. 2015;15:914.
4. Sallis JF, Glanz K. Physical activity and food environments: solutions to the obesity epidemic. Milbank Q. 2009; 87:123-54.
5. Franks PW, McCarthy MI. Exposing the exposures responsible for type 2 diabetes and obesity. Science. 2016;354:69-73.
6. Jastreboff AM, Kotz CM, Kahan S, et al. Obesity as a disease: the Obesity Society 2018 position statement. Obesity (Silver Spring). 2019;27:7-9.
7. Jensen MD, Ryan DH, Apovian CM, et al. 2013 AHA/ACC/TOS guideline for the management of overweight and obesity in adults: a report of the American College of Cardiology/American Heart Association Task Force on Practice Guidelines and The Obesity Society. Circulation. 2014;129(suppl 2):S102-38.
8. Gordon-Larsen P, Heymsfield SB. Obesity as a disease, not a behavior. Circulation. 2018;137:1543-5.
9. Marso SP, Bain SC, Consoli A, et al. Semaglutide and cardiovascular outcomes in patients with type 2 diabetes. N Engl J Med. 2016;375:1834-44.
10. Kosiborod MN, Verma S, Borlaug BA, et al. Effects of semaglutide on symptoms, function, and quality of life in patients with heart failure with preserved ejection fraction and obesity: a prespecified analysis of the STEP-HFpEF trial. Circulation. 2024;149:204-16.
11. Withaar C, Meems LMG, Nollet EE, et al. The cardioprotective effects of semaglutide exceed those of dietary weight loss in mice with HFpEF. JACC Basic Transl Sci. 2023;8:1298-314.
12. Strain WD, Frenkel O, James MA, et al. Effects of semaglutide on stroke subtypes in type 2 diabetes: post hoc analysis of the randomized SUSTAIN 6 and PIONEER 6. Stroke. 2022;53:2749-57.
13. Perkovic V, Tuttle KR, Rossing P, et al. Effects of semaglutide on chronic kidney disease in patients with type 2 diabetes. N Engl J Med. 2024;391:109-21.
14. Wang F, Mao Y, Wang H, et al. Semaglutide and diabetic retinopathy risk in patients with type 2 diabetes mellitus: a meta-analysis of randomized controlled trials. Clin Drug Investig. 2022;42:17-28.
15. Dogan SE, Kuskonmaz SM, Koc G, et al. Case series: exposure to glucagon-like peptide-1 receptor agonist in the first trimester of pregnancy in two siblings. Endocr Metab Immune Disord Drug Targets. 2024;24:1237-9.

104

CHAPTER

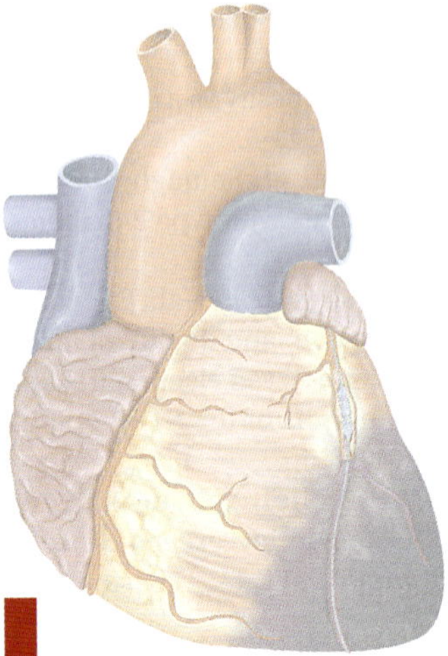

Mechanistic Insights: Semaglutide and Gut Microbiota Modulation

Urvashi Gupta

INTRODUCTION

Obesity and T2DM represent global health burdens, characterized by insulin resistance, chronic inflammation, and metabolic dysregulation.[1] GLP-1 receptor agonists (GLP-1 RAs) such as semaglutide (popularly marketed as Ozempic[2]/Rybelsus/Wegovy) have transformed treatment paradigms, demonstrating robust reductions in body weight, glycemia, and cardiovascular risk.

Beyond central and peripheral mechanisms, emerging evidence implicates gut microbiota modulation as a key mediator of semaglutide's therapeutic effects. Gut microbes influence host metabolism, immunity, appetite regulation, and even cognitive function via the gut–brain axis. Dysbiosis is often characterized by an increased Firmicutes/Bacteroidota ratio, and loss of beneficial taxa such as *Akkermansia muciniphila* is a hallmark of obesity and metabolic disease.[3]

Exploring how semaglutide reshapes the gut microbial ecosystem offers mechanistic insight and potential translational benefits.[4] The data is reviewed across obesity, NAFLD, T2DM, PCOS, and cognitive impairment models, focusing on microbiota diversity, specific taxa shifts, microbial metabolites (e.g., SCFAs, acetate), fecal microbiota transplantation (FMT)-mediated transfer, and barrier integrity. We have highlighted the interplay between altered microbiota and host metabolic pathways—central appetite regulation via hypothalamic circuits, lipid metabolism gene regulation, inflammatory markers, and the potential for human translation.

BACKGROUND ON SEMAGLUTIDE AND GUT MICROBIOTA

Semaglutide, a long-acting GLP-1 RA with a ~1 week half-life, mimics endogenous GLP-1, potentiating insulin secretion, inhibiting glucagon, delaying gastric emptying, and reducing appetite via hypothalamic GLP-1 receptor activation. Its metabolic benefits extend to improved insulin sensitivity, lipid metabolism, and weight loss.

Simultaneously, gut microbiota comprising trillions of micro-organisms play a pivotal role in nutrient harvesting, immune modulation, gut barrier integrity, and metabolite production (e.g., SCFAs). In obesity and T2DM, dysbiosis is marked by decreased *Akkermansia* and increased proinflammatory taxa such as *Romboutsia* and *Dubosiella*.

Recent preclinical evidence positions semaglutide as a modulator of gut ecology, reversing HFD-induced dysbiosis and promoting barrier function. The hormonal and metabolic effects may thus be partially mediated via these microbial shifts, motivating a deeper mechanistic exploration.

PRECLINICAL MECHANISTIC INSIGHTS

Cognitive Function and Inflammation via Microbiota

In obese mice, semaglutide significantly altered gut microbiota compared to HFD alone, restoring levels of *Akkermansia*, *Muribaculaceae*, *Coriobacteriaceae*

UCG-002, and *Clostridia UCG-014* while reducing *Romboutsia*, *Dubosiella*, and *Enterorhabdus*.

These changes coincided with improved cognitive performance (e.g., Morris water maze) and lowered serum proinflammatory cytokines (IL-6, IL-1β). Correlation analysis revealed positive associations between cognitive metrics and *Muribaculaceae/Clostridia UCG-014*, and negative associations with *Romboutsia* and *Dubosiella*; the latter positively correlated with inflammatory markers.

HFD-induced dysbiosis[3] increasing Firmicutes and Desulfobacterota reducing Verrucomicrobiota and Proteobacteria—reversed by semaglutide, which restored phyla balance.

The rapid 166-fold increase in *A. muciniphila* stood out, noted for improving mucosal integrity, glycemic control, and cognition. Its functions include promoting GLP-1 secretion via secreted protein P9, anti-inflammatory effects, and mucin degradation toward SCFA production **(Table 1)**.

Energy Balance, Hypothalamic Pathways, and SCFAs

Semaglutide also modulates appetite via gut–brain axis pathways. It enriches acetate-producing bacteria such as *Bacteroides acidifaciens* and *Blautia coccoides*, increasing hypothalamic acetate levels. These activate GPR43+/POMC+ neurons via PI3K-Akt, suppressing FoxO1 to reduce food intake.

Additionally, semaglutide countered gut inflammation—reducing TLR4/NF-κB/TNF-α/IL-1β and LPS levels while enhancing tight-junction proteins such as occludin, thereby restoring gut barrier integrity and reducing systemic inflammation.

Metabolism, Lipid Handling, and Fecal Microbiota Transplantation

Through metabolomics studies and FMT, semaglutide's microbial modulation was shown to be transferable. In HFD mice, semaglutide reduced weight, fat mass, fasting glucose, and insulin; it regulated hepatic/adipose lipid-metabolism genes (*PPAR-α*, *PPAR-γ*, *CPT-1a*, and *PGC-1α*) and hypothalamic appetite genes (*Leptin*, *AgRP*, *NPY*, and *POMC*).

Importantly, FMT from semaglutide-treated mice to pseudogerm-free mice transmitted these metabolic benefits reducing adiposity and improving insulin sensitivity and metabolic gene expression, demonstrating a direct role of the altered gut microbiota.

Semaglutide also influenced metabolomic pathways: Phenylalanine/tyrosine/tryptophan biosynthesis, arginine/proline metabolism, and more-linking microbiota shifts to host metabolite profiles.

Other Disease Models: NAFLD, T2DM, and PCOS

- *NAFLD/db/db mice:* Semaglutide improved lipid and glucose parameters, reduced hepatic steatosis, restored gut barrier integrity, and modulated gut microbiota—particularly increasing *Alloprevotella*, *Alistipes*, *Ligilactobacillus*, and *Lactobacillus*.
- *T2DM and β-cell function:* In diabetic mice, semaglutide improved islet morphology, boosted METTL14/PDX-1 expression (via m6A RNA modification), and modulated gut microbiota by increasing *Bacteroides* and *Muribaculaceae*, while reducing *Firmicutes*, *Actinobacteriota*, and *Lactobacillus*. SCFA production was also enhanced.
- *PCOS model:* In DHEA-induced PCOS mice, semaglutide altered gut microbiota composition differently from liraglutide-enriching phylum *Campylobacterota*, family *Helicobacteraceae*, genus *Helicobacter*, and species *Alistipes muris* **(Table 2)**.

Flowchart 1 shows how *semaglutide modulates gut microbiota* and downstream metabolic pathways such as SCFAs, LPS, and bile acids, leading to improved clinical outcomes.

TABLE 1: Effects of semaglutide on gut microbiota composition in preclinical models.

Taxonomic group	*Change after semaglutide*	*Implications*	*Study reference*
Akkermansia muciniphila	↑ (166-fold)	Improves mucosal integrity, reduces inflammation	Feng et al.[1]
Muribaculaceae	↑	Associated with improved cognition	Feng et al.[1]
Romboutsia	↓	Linked to inflammation and dysbiosis	Feng et al.[1]
Blautia coccoides	↑	Produces acetate, supports satiety	Hu et al. (2024)[5]
Bacteroides acidifaciens	↑	SCFA producer; enhances gut–brain signaling	Hu et al. (2024)[5]
Dubosiella	↓	Associated with metabolic dysfunction	Feng et al.[1]
Enterorhabdus	↓	Correlated with proinflammatory state	Feng et al.[1]

TABLE 2: Comparative effects of semaglutide on gut microbiota in disease models.

Model	Microbiota changes	Metabolic outcomes
HFD-induced obesity	↑ *Akkermansia*, ↓ *Romboutsia*, ↑ *Muribaculaceae*	↓ Weight, ↑ cognition
db/db diabetic mice	↑ *Bacteroides*, ↑ SCFAs	↑ β-cell function, ↓ glucose
NAFLD	↑ *Alistipes*, ↑ *Lactobacillus*	↓ Hepatic steatosis

Flowchart 1: Mechanistic insights: Semaglutide and gut microbiota.

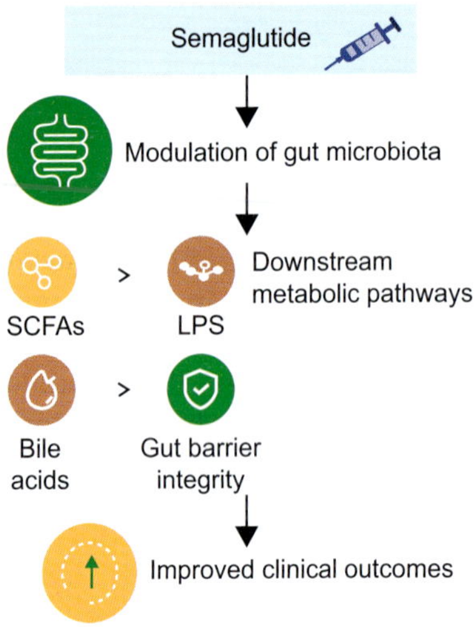

INTESTINAL BARRIER AND HUMAN IMPLICATIONS

While animal studies illustrate semaglutide's microbiota-mediated benefits, human data remain preliminary. GLP-1 RAs have shown improved gut barrier integrity and reduced colonic inflammation in animal colitis models, but direct human evidence on intestinal permeability is lacking.

Semaglutide similarly restores human gut integrity, attenuates systemic inflammation, and conveys metabolic gains via microbiota alterations. Clinical studies incorporating microbiome profiling, intestinal permeability assays, and inflammatory biomarker evaluation during semaglutide therapy will be vital for translation.

DISCUSSION AND FUTURE DIRECTIONS

The mechanistic evidence underscores a compelling narrative: Semaglutide's metabolic benefits are mediated in part by orchestrating gut microbiota shifts—restoring beneficial taxa, reducing proinflammatory bacteria, enhancing SCFA production, and improving intestinal and hypothalamic signaling.

Key mechanistic axes include:

- *Anti-inflammatory and cognitive effects* via *Akkermansia*, *Muribaculaceae*, and *Clostridia UCG-014* restoration.
- *Anorexigenic appetite suppression* through acetate production and GPR43/POMC neuronal activation.
- *Metabolic regulation* occurs via gene expression (PPAR pathways), lipid oxidation, and via metabolome shifts.
- *Translatability via FMT* proves causality of microbiota in metabolic improvement.

Knowledge gaps and future research:

- Can human microbiome data mirror these findings—taxa changes, SCFA shifts, microbiota as biomarker?
- Could combining semaglutide with prebiotics, probiotics, or targeted microbiota therapies amplify outcomes?
- Does gut barrier function improve in humans on semaglutide, and how does it correlate with metabolic/inflammatory parameters?
- Clinical trials with microbiome, metabolome, immune, and barrier markers should confirm and extend preclinical observations.

CONCLUSION

Semaglutide's metabolic efficacy extends beyond GLP-1 receptor activation to encompass profound modulation of gut microbiota. Preclinical studies reveal that altering the gut ecosystem contributes to decreased inflammation, improved cognition, suppressed appetite, better glucose and lipid metabolism, and possibly restored gut barrier integrity. The translational potential is promising, but validation in human studies is essential. Integrating microbiota-targeted strategies with semaglutide therapy could herald a new frontier in treating obesity and metabolic disease.

REFERENCES

1. Feng J, Teng Z, Yang Y, et al. Effects of semaglutide on gut microbiota, cognitive function and inflammation in obese mice. Peer J. 2024;12:e17891.

2. Wilding JPH, Batterham RL, Calanna S, et al.; STEP 1 Study Group. Once-weekly semaglutide in adults with overweight or obesity. N Engl J Med. 2021;384(11):989-1002.
3. Breton J, Galmiche M, Déchelotte P. Dysbiotic gut bacteria in obesity: an overview of the metabolic mechanisms and therapeutic perspectives of next-generation probiotics. Microorganisms. 2022;10(2):452.
4. He X, Zimo Z, Sun Y. Unraveling the safety profile of GLP-1 receptor agonists: mechanistic insights with a focus on semaglutide. Eur J Med Chem. 2025;300:118163.
5. Hu T, Mao T, Liu Q, et al. Semaglutide alters gut microbiota and improves NAFLD in db/db mice. Biochemical and Biophysical Research Communications. 2024;710: 149882.

105

CHAPTER

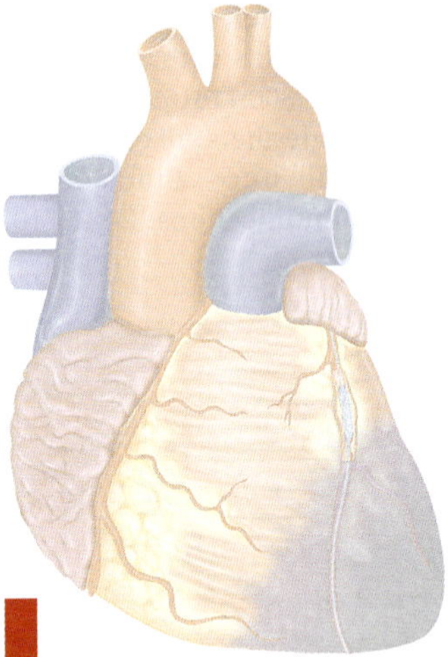

Future Directions: Combination Therapies Involving Semaglutide in Obesity and Cardiovascular Disease

Namrata Gaur, Dushyant Singh Gaur, Anu Gaur

INTRODUCTION

Obesity has been on the rise and is almost an epidemic. Similarly, cardiovascular diseases (CVDs) and diabetes are also rising at an alarming rate and now even developing countries are getting an epidemic like situation with even young adults getting affected.

Heart failure with reduced ejection fraction and heart failure with preserved ejection fraction have many clinical features in common but their cause and response to treatment are different, with the benefits of traditional treatments for heart failure with reduced ejection fraction less clear than in patients with preserved ejection fraction. SGLT2 inhibitors have been shown to improve outcomes in both, heart failure with preserved ejection fraction as well as reduced ejection fraction. In patients with or without diabetes, there is a considerable unmet clinical need, especially in patients with obesity.

Semaglutide, a glucagon-like peptide-1 (GLP-1) receptor agonist (RA), first introduced to manage dysglycemia, results in both weight loss and reduction in major adverse cardiac events (MACE) in patients with diabetes.

HISTORY OF GLUCAGON-LIKE PEPTIDE-1 AGONISTS

Semaglutide is an incretin hormone produced in the upper gastrointestinal tract. The term incretin hormone was coined by Labarre in 1932, describing endogenous factors produced by the intestine to influence pancreatic secretions.[1] In the later part of the 20th century, Nauck et al.[2] described GLP-1 and its biology in humans. GLP-1 is a 30-peptide-residue hormone that is secreted by L-cells in the ileum and colon in response to overall nutrient intake, primarily carbohydrates and amino acids.

Glucagon-like peptide-1 is quickly metabolized by dipeptidyl peptidase-4 (DPP-4) limiting its half-life to 2 minutes. In addition to pancreas and hypothalamus, GLP-1 receptors are also found on vascular endothelium and cardiac myocytes at lower concentrations.[3,4] The physiologic effects of GLP-1 are well studied. Their primary biologic impact on the pancreas is to secrete insulin and glucagon and induce early satiety by delaying gastric emptying and acting on hypothalamic receptors. On the other hand, GLP-1 effects on vascular endothelium resulting in vasodilation and modulation of atherosclerosis via anti-inflammatory pathways.[5,6] Since cardiovascular complications are the most common cause of morbidity and mortality in diabetes, it is essential to study the impact of GLP-1 agonists on CV outcomes in these patients.

Exenatide, a synthetic GLP-1 analog, was the first GLP-1 analog approved by the FDA in 2005 for clinical use in diabetes, as once-daily subcutaneous injection.[7,8]

Since then, there have been gradual but significant improvements in our understanding and availability of pharmacological alternatives that primarily work by stimulating GLP-1 receptors with a longer duration of action of up to 7 days following a single dose.

Liraglutide, dulaglutide, and semaglutide are three GLP-1 approved for once-a-week doses. Semaglutide is the most studied with proven outcomes in patients with or without diabetes, obesity, and CVD.[9-11]

Role of Semaglutide in Obesity and Cardiovascular Disease

SELECT was a multicenter, randomized, double-blind, parallel-group, placebo-controlled, event-driven trial evaluating the effect of once-weekly subcutaneous semaglutide 2.4 mg (vs. placebo) on MACE and other cardiovascular endpoints in individuals with ASCVD and overweight or obesity but without diabetes.

Subsequently, effect of semaglutide on patients post-CABG, with obesity, was studied by other groups,[12] and it was found that in addition to its known antiatherosclerotic effects, semaglutide may affect graft patency which could contribute to the reduction in nonfatal MI and is an important driver of long-term prognosis in these patients.

The observation that semaglutide reduces the incidence of new-onset biochemical diabetes, a risk factor for graft occlusion, may also contribute to its benefits. In CABG patients, despite weight loss being less, there was a consistent reduction in risk and semaglutide offered cardiovascular protection.

Most of the studies have shown a significant benefit of semaglutide in patients with diabetes with obesity, and semaglutide seems like a wonder drug causing both control of diabetes as well as weight loss.

However, its effect on patients with obesity and CVD but without diabetes was less studied. A multicenter study, which was double-blind, randomized, placebo-controlled, event-driven superiority trial[11] where patients above 45 years with preexisting CVD and body mass index of 27 or greater, but no history of diabetes, has shown that weekly dose of 2.4 mg of subcutaneous semaglutide reduced the incidence of death from cardiovascular causes, nonfatal MI, or nonfatal stroke at a mean follow-up of 39.8 months.

Mechanism of cardiovascular risk reduction with semaglutide may include those related to physiological benefits from the reduction of excess abnormal body fat and actions of semaglutide other than weight loss. Perivascular and epicardial adipose tissue impose direct adverse effects on the vascular endothelium and myocardium.[13] In addition, reductions in excess abnormal body fat ameliorate the systemic proinflammatory and prothrombotic milieu associated with obesity.[14]

Thus, semaglutide not only helps control of blood sugar but also reduces weight and abnormal fat which further helps in better glycemic control. Its effects on vasculature are remarkable, and consistent reduction in atherothrombotic events (MI and stroke) in CVOTs strongly points to the vasculature as primary site of action for GLP-1 RAs.

Atherosclerosis is a complex pathology driven by endothelial dysfunction, chronic inflammation, and lipid deposition within the arterial wall. Studies have revealed that GLP-1 RAs mount a coordinated, multipronged attack on these core processes, intervening at multiple steps to halt or reverse the disease. This multitarget engagement likely explains the robustness of the MACE reduction seen in clinical trials, distinguishing these agents from the therapies that target only a single pathway. In addition, effect of GLP-1 RAs on endothelium and NO bioavailability enhances cardiac protective effect.

Emerging evidence also suggests that they prevent the formation of new plaque, but more importantly, stabilize existing plaques, making them less vulnerable to rupture.

Semaglutide treatment increases the secretion of antithrombotic protein gelsolin while decreasing levels of the proinflammatory adipokine mechanism, whereby the drug alters the immediate paracrine environment of the coronary arteries to be less thrombotic and inflammatory.

Heart failure with preserved ejection fraction remained a challenge for decades with no effective pharmacotherapies. This syndrome is characterized by obesity, metabolic dysfunction, and a state of chronic low-grade systemic inflammation. The landmark STEP-HFpEF and STEP-HFpEF DM trials represented major therapeutic breakthrough. In these studies, treatment with semaglutide led to dramatic improvements in the primary end points.

There was substantial weight loss in obese patients with HFpEF with or without DM. This is due to semaglutide's ability to target the core pathophysiological drivers of the obesity-related HFpEF phenotype. The mechanism of benefit is multifaceted and synergistic.

Recent large-scale trials suggest potential benefits regardless of ejection fraction. In the FLOW trial, semaglutide response for heart failure indicates no harm and suggests possible benefits even in failure with reduced ejection fraction. The success of GLP-1 RAs in HFpEF validates the concept of the phenotype-specific therapy, where treatments are rationally selected to target the dominant underlying pathophysiology of a specific disease subtype **(Tables 1 and 2)**.

SIDE EFFECTS AND SAFETY

Ever since semaglutide received marketing approval in 2017, it has become popular and is being prescribed for obesity, diabetes, and atherosclerotic CVD.

The main side effects of this drug are gastrointestinal effects. Patients should be explained about these before prescribing. It may also affect absorption of some medications as it delays gastric emptying. Therefore, patients on warfarin must keep monitoring INR to know warfarin levels, although no dose adjustment of

TABLE 1: Impact of GLP-1 analogs and semaglutide on outcomes in patients with heart failure.

Trial	*HF subtype*	*Diabetic patients*	*Nondiabetic patients*	*BMI >30*	*BMI <30*	*Outcome in diabetic patients*	*Outcome in nondiabetic patients*	*Outcome in patients with BMI >30*	*Outcome in patients with BMI <30*
STEP-HFpEF	HFpEF	Yes	Yes	Yes (median BMI ~37)	Not explicitly analyzed	Improvement in symptoms and exercise capacity	Improvement in exercise capacity and weight loss	Significant weight loss and functional improvement	Not analyzed separately
SUSTAIN-6	Mixed (not heart failure specific)	Yes	No	Mixed	Mixed	Reduced CV events, including heart failure hospitalizations	Not applicable (only diabetic population studied)	Not clearly reported	Not analyzed separately
FIGHT	HFrEF	Yes	Yes	Not reported	Not reported	No significant improvement in outcomes or LV function	No significant improvement in outcomes	Not reported	Not reported
LIVE	HFrEF	Yes	Yes	Not reported	Not reported	No significant improvement in outcomes or LV function	No significant improvement in outcomes	Not reported	Not reported

TABLE 2: Impact of semaglutide on ischemic cardiovascular outcomes.

	Primary endpoint: Composite cardiovascular death			*Secondary endpoint: Nonfatal myocardial infarction*		
	Semaglutide (%)	*Placebo (%)*	*Hazard ratio (95 % CI)*	*Semaglutide (%)*	*Placebo (%)*	*Hazard ratio (95% CI)*
SUSTAIN-6	6.6	8.9	0.74	2.9	3.9	0.74*
SELECT	6.5	8.0	0.80	2.7	3.7	0.72

Note: Primary cardiovascular endpoint is defined as a composite of death from cardiovascular causes, nonfatal myocardial infarction, or nonfatal stroke.

*Hazard ratio (0.51–1.08); all other hazard ratios did not cross 1.0, indicating a protective mechanism.

semaglutide is required. Delayed gastric emptying can cause risk of aspiration, and therefore, it is suspended in perioperative phase, during general anesthesia, Cath Lab Procedures, and CABG. If it is being given once weekly, the dose may be given a few days prior to surgery or dose resumed 2–3 days after surgery.

The effect on pancreas and thyroid (pancreatic cancer, thyroid cancer, and pancreatitis) is not fully understood and is still being evaluated.

The safety profile of semaglutide is like that of other GLP-1 RAs.[15] Official blackbox warnings have been issued in the United States regarding thyroid C-cell cancer and also against compounding medications (mixing two or more drugs to create a customized drug), as these drugs are still being studied and evaluated.[16,17]

Semaglutide is contraindicated in patients with family history of medullary thyroid cancer or endocrine neoplasia.[18]

No dose adjustment is required for mild renal or hepatic impairment, but in patients above 70 years and with delayed clearance with moderate dysfunction, it is recommended to adjust the dose. In severe dysfunction, semaglutide should not be prescribed.

CONCLUSION

Semaglutide emerged as a wonder drug and its effect on *diabetes* and *obesity* was well documented. But what caught everyone's attention was its positive effect on patients with CVD and obesity. It received FDA approval in 2023 for managing type 2 DM and chronic weight management.[19,20] Subsequently, in 2024, it also received approval for adults with CVD and obesity, for prevention of adverse effects, and also in patients with diabetes and heart disease.

In conclusion, what was considered as antidiabetic medication has emerged as beneficial in patients of CVD with obesity, even without diabetes. It has shown a promising role in prevention of MACE including primary prevention. Their effect is more pronounced in obese patients than in nonobese patients.

Affordability is a barrier to universal use. It also remains to be seen whether patient will develop tolerance and whether a patient needs lifelong administration for continued benefits. Availability too is a factor in compliance, when drug needs frequent doses.

SURPASS-2 trial showed that tirzepatide has synergistic action with GLP-1 and glucagon insulinotropic polypeptide (GIP) is more effective in managing diabetes, weight loss, and lipid control. SUMMIT trial also showed similar benefits in preventing adverse cardiac events, preventing exacerbation of heart failure, and improving functional capacity in patients.[21,22]

Further studies are needed to study long-term effects (>2-year follow-up) and dosage, and safety profiles; to understand the mechanistic process behind its cardiovascular benefits; and to assess a more diverse patient pool before it can be added to the guidelines for the management of CVDs.

REFERENCES

1. Labarre J. (1932). Sur les possibilities d'un traitement du diabete par l'incretinine. [online] Available from https://www.semanticscholar.org/paper/Sur-les-possibilites-d%27un-traitement-du-diabete-par-Labarre/b4ea8ec486db924054d70827aed214da2b85c33f. [Last accessed January, 2026].
2. Nauck M, Stöckmann F, Ebert R, et al. Reduced incretin effect in type II (non-insulin-dependent) diabetes. Diabetologia. 1986;29:46-52.
3. Kreymann B, Williams G, Ghatei MA, et al. Glucagon-like peptide-1 7-36: a physiological incretin in man. Lancet. 1987; 330:1300-4.
4. Gasbjerg LS, Bergmann NC, Stensen S, et al. Evaluation of the incretin effect in humans using GIP and GLP-1 receptor antagonists. Peptides. 2020;125:170183.
5. Jorsal A, Kistorp C, Holmager P, et al. Effect of liraglutide, a glucagon-like peptide-1 analogue, on left ventricular function in stable chronic heart failure patients with and without diabetes (LIVE)—a multicentre, double-blind, randomised, placebo-controlled trial. Eur J Heart Fail. 2017;19:69-77.
6. Pandey A, LaMonte M, Klein L, et al. Relationship between physical activity, body mass index, and risk of heart failure. J Am Coll Cardiol. 2017;69:1129-42.
7. Parkes DG, Mace KF, Trautmann ME. Discovery and development of exenatide: the first antidiabetic agent to leverage the multiple benefits of the incretin hormone, GLP-1. Expert Opin Drug Discov. 2013;8: 219-44.
8. Nauck MA, Quast DR, Wefers J, et al. GLP-1 receptor agonists in the treatment of type 2 diabetes—state-of-the-art. Mol Metab. 2021;46:101102.
9. Marso SP, Bain SC, Consoli A, et al. Semaglutide and cardiovascular outcomes in patients with type 2 diabetes. N Engl J Med. 2016;375:1834-44.
10. Nauck MA, Quast DR. Cardiovascular safety and benefits of semaglutide in patients with type 2 diabetes: findings from SUSTAIN 6 and PIONEER 6. Front Endocrinol (Lausanne). 2021;12:645566.
11. Lincoff AM, Brown-Frandsen K, Colhoun HM, et al. Semaglutide and cardiovascular outcomes in obesity without diabetes. N Engl J Med. 2023;389: 2221-32.
12. Verma S, Emerson S, Plutzky J, et al. Semaglutide improves cardiovascular outcomes in patients with history of coronary artery bypass graft and obesity. J Am Coll Cardiol. 2025;85: 541-5.
13. Lacobellis G. Epicardial adipose tissue in contemporary cardiology. Nat Rev Cardiol. 2022;19:593-606.
14. Magkos F, Fraterrigo G, Yoshino J, et al. Effects of moderate and subsequent progressive weight loss on metabolic function and adipose tissue biology in humans with obesity. Cell Metab. 2016;23:591-601.
15. Elashoff M, Matveyenko AV, Gier B, et al. Pancreatitis, pancreatic and thyroid cancer with glucagon-like peptide-1-based therapies. Gastroenterology. 2011;141:150-6.
16. Dmour I. Content analysis of US FDA warning letters issued to compounding pharmacies regarding violations of current good manufacturing practices between 2017 and 2022. J Pharm Innov; 2022. pp. 1-15.
17. Spitery A, Elder MJ, Farhat N, et al. Legal, safety, and practical considerations of compounded injectable semaglutide. J Am Coll Clin Pharm. 2024;7:941-6.
18. Chao AM, Tronieri JS, Amaro A, et al. Clinical insight on semaglutide for chronic weight management in adults: patient selection and special considerations. Drug Des Devel Ther. 2022;16:4449-61.
19. Gourgari E, Wilhelm EE, Hassanzadeh H, et al. A comprehensive review of the FDA-approved labels of diabetes drugs: indications, safety, and emerging cardiovascular safety data. J Diabetes Complicat. 2017;31:1719-27.
20. Singh G, Krauthamer M, Bjalme-Evans M. Wegovy (semaglutide): a new weight loss drug for chronic weight management. J Investig Med. 2022;70:5-13.
21. Frías JP, Davies MJ, Rosenstock J, et al. Tirzepatide versus semaglutide once weekly in patients with type 2 diabetes. N Engl J Med. 2021;385:503-15.
22. Packer M, Zile MR, Kramer CM, et al. Tirzepatide for heart failure with preserved ejection fraction and obesity. N Engl J Med. 2025;392:427-37.

106

CHAPTER

Semaglutide in the Management of Obesity-related Comorbidities

SN Pathak

INTRODUCTION

Obesity is a mounting global health challenge, and recent advancements in pharmacologic interventions have brought new hope to this complex issue. Obesity, a chronic and complex disease, is linked to various comorbidities, including type 2 diabetes, hypertension, dyslipidemia, stroke, coronary heart disease, and cancers, resulting in a substantial economic burden. Worldwide obesity prevalence is 13%.[1]

Effective weight management is crucial to reduce morbidity and mortality. Lifestyle modification is the guideline-recommended foundation of treatment for individuals with overweight or obesity,[2-5] but typically achieves only modest weight loss that is often regained.[6-8] Furthermore, this loss is challenging to maintain because of metabolic adaptation that promotes gradual weight regain.[4] Pharmacological treatments for obesity provide a valuable adjunct to lifestyle interventions, but until recently, the available agents only offered moderate weight loss over that achieved with lifestyle intervention.[9] Semaglutide, initially developed as a GLP-1 receptor agonist for treating type 2 diabetes, is now being explored for its potential in addressing obesity. Its utilization is expanding to chronic weight management as it mimics the effects of GLP-1, regulating blood sugar levels and appetite. The FDA approved the use of a 2.4 mg injection of semaglutide once weekly for chronic weight management. The approval of oral semaglutide for obesity is based on results from the OASIS 4 phase 3 clinical trial.[10] Semaglutide proves efficacy for weight loss in obesity, endorsed by STEP trial findings and real-world data, with safety akin to GLP-1 receptor agonists (RAs) class, promoting long-term adherence. Its notable effects on albuminuria, HbA1c, heart failure, and quality of life herald a transformative paradigm in obesity and associated comorbidity management.

In the SELECT cardiovascular outcomes trial, semaglutide showed a 20% reduction in major adverse cardiovascular events in 17,604 adults with preexisting cardiovascular disease, overweight or obesity, without diabetes. GLP-1 RAs are recommended for diabetics and, increasingly, for nondiabetics with stable coronary artery disease and overweight/obesity, with semaglutide specifically indicated for weight and cardiovascular events reduction (class IIb, level of evidence B).[11,12]

PLEIOTROPIC EFFECT OF SEMAGLUTIDE (FIG. 1)

In people with overweight/obesity without diabetes, semaglutide achieved 10.8–14.8% and tirzepatide 17.4–20.8% greater weight loss than placebo. These agents' pleiotropic effects have translated into clinical trials showing improvement in cardiovascular outcomes, improved quality of life, and/or heart failure events in heart failure with preserved ejection fraction (HFpEF), resolution of steatohepatitis and improvement in liver fibrosis, prevention and treatment of type 2 diabetes, and improvement in renal function in chronic kidney disease. Semaglutide has additionally been shown to

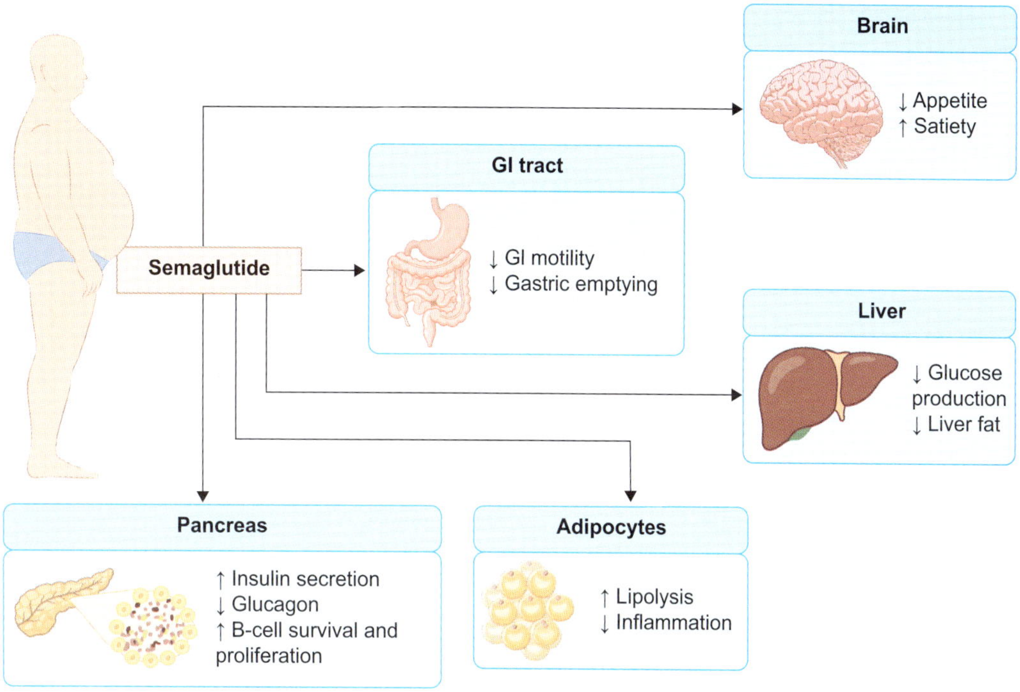

Fig. 1: Pleiotropic effect of semaglutide.

improve osteoarthritis symptoms and tirzepatide reduces obstructive sleep apnea severity.

An overall reduction in body weight was observed with semaglutide regardless of age, sex, race, ethnicity, baseline BMI, or renal function in the STEP trials. Secondary outcomes also showed semaglutide improved cardiometabolic risk factors in adolescents and adults, including waist circumference, blood pressure (BP), lipids, while also improving quality of life **(Flowchart 1)**.

The SUSTAIN-6 trial, which was conducted on participants with type 2 diabetes, proved that semaglutide is effective in minimizing the risk of major adverse cardiovascular events by 26% compared to placebo.[13]

Additionally, patients with HFpEF and obesity, semaglutide produced large improvements in HFpEF-related symptoms.[14] Semaglutide treatment is also found to decrease myocardial diastolic stiffness and improve actin–myosin and muscle contraction pathways.[15] Semaglutide therapy also reduced the incidence of any stroke when compared to a placebo through significant reductions in risk of small-vessel occlusion in a post hoc analysis of the SUSTAIN-6 and PIONEER 6 trials.[16]

The FLOW clinical trial investigated whether semaglutide can slow the progression of CKD in people with T2DM. They had demonstrated benefits for kidney-specific outcomes, cardiovascular death, and other secondary outcomes, including a slower decline in kidney function.[17]

CONCLUSION

Semaglutide, in its subcutaneous (Ozempic) and oral (Rybelsus) formulations, has been shown to be significantly effective in the treatment of DM2. In addition to improving glycemic control, semaglutide promotes significant reductions in body weight, with additional benefits on cardiovascular health and the prevention of metabolic complications. Promising results in weight loss with semaglutide in individuals with DM2 have led to the expansion of indications for the treatment of obesity or overweight associated with comorbidities. Clinical studies confirm the superiority of semaglutide over most other treatments in the same class of GLP-1 RAs, highlighting its ability to induce weight loss safely and effectively, even in populations with comorbidities. In summary, the STEP studies were important to confirm the efficacy of semaglutide in weight loss in individuals with obesity or overweight associated with comorbidities, leading to the approval of the indication of semaglutide 2.4 mg (Wegovy) for weight loss in this subpopulation.

Flowchart 1: Efficacy of semaglutide and tirzepatide in obesity and weight-related comorbidities.

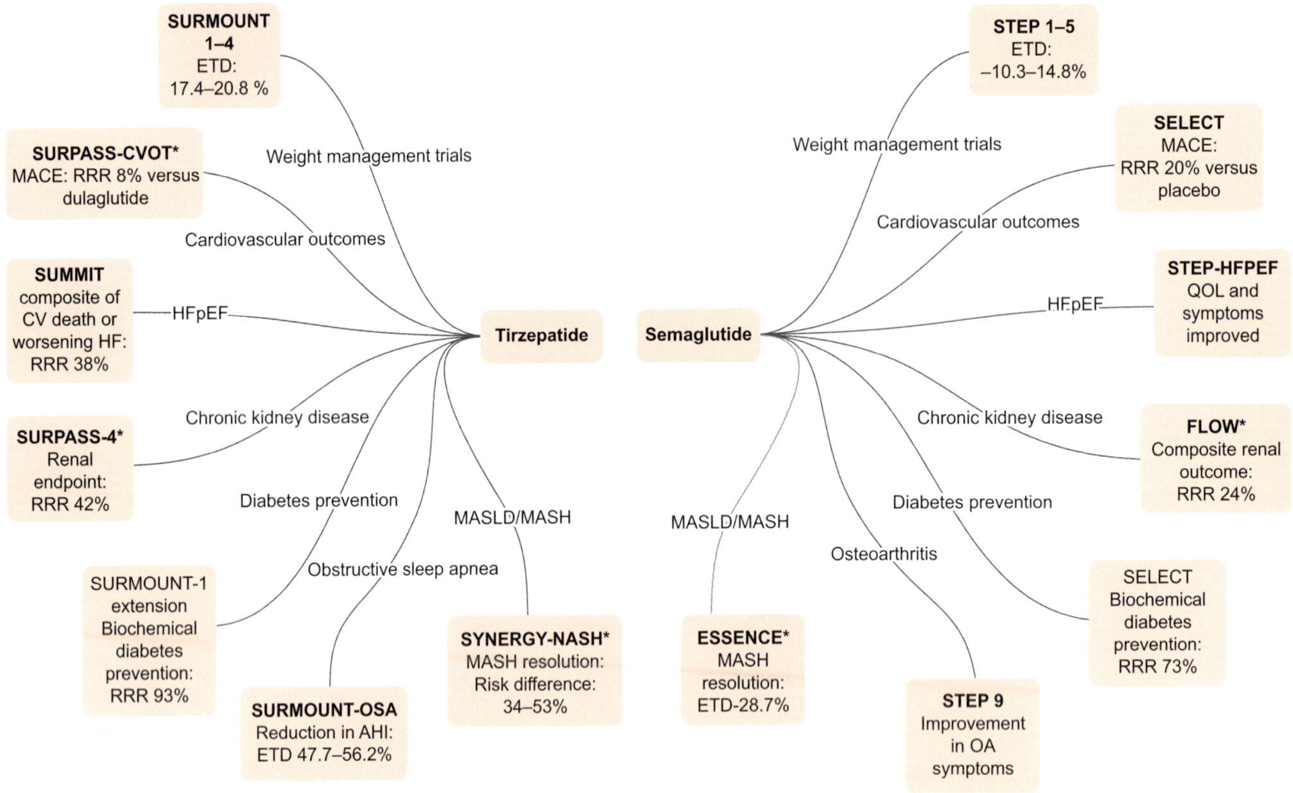

Note: Bolded conditions and trial names indicate outcomes that were the primary endpoint of the randomized controlled trial (RCT). Unbolded conditions and trial names indicate outcomes from RCTs that were either prespecified analyses or pooled analyses but not the primary outcome.

*Indicates an RCT not specifically conducted in a population with overweight or obesity.

[AHI: apnea–hypopnea index; CV: cardiovascular; ETD: estimated treatment difference; HFpEF: heart failure with preserved ejection fraction; MACE: major adverse cardiovascular events; MASLD: metabolic-associated steatotic liver disease; MASH: metabolic-associated steatohepatitis; OA: osteoarthritis; QOL: quality of life; RRR: relative risk reduction (1–hazard ratio)]

REFERENCES

1. World Health Organization. (2025). Obesity and overweight. [online] Available from https://www.who.int/news-room/fact-sheets/detail/obesity-and-overweight. [Last accessed January, 2026].
2. Garvey WT, Mechanick JI, Brett EM, et al. American Association of Clinical Endocrinologists and American College of Endocrinology comprehensive clinical practice guidelines for medical care of patients with obesity. Endocr Pract. 2016;22(Suppl 3):1-203.
3. Durrer Schutz D, Busetto L, Dicker D, et al. European practical and patient-centred guidelines for adult obesity management in primary care. Obes Facts. 2019;12(1):40-66.
4. Jensen MD, Ryan DH, Apovian CM, et al. AHA/ACC/TOS guideline for the management of overweight and obesity in adults: a report of the American College of Cardiology/American Heart Association Task Force on Practice Guidelines and The Obesity Society. J Am Coll Cardiol. 2014;63(25 Pt B):2985-3023.
5. Yumuk V, Tsigos C, Fried M, et al. European guidelines for obesity management in adults. Obes Facts. 2015;8(6):402-24.
6. Wadden TA, Tronieri JS, Butryn ML. Lifestyle modification approaches for the treatment of obesity in adults. Am Psychol. 2020;75(2):235-51.
7. Kushner RF, Calanna S, Davies M, et al. Semaglutide 2.4 mg for the treatment of obesity: key elements of the STEP trials 1 to 5. Obesity (Silver Spring). 2020;28(6):1050-61.
8. Sumithran P, Prendergast LA, Delbridge E, et al. Long-term persistence of hormonal adaptations to weight loss. N Engl J Med. 2011;365(17):1597-1604.
9. Singh AK, Singh R. Pharmacotherapy in obesity: a systematic review and meta-analysis of randomized

controlled trials of anti-obesity drugs. Expert Rev Clin Pharmacol. 2020;13(1):53-64.

10. Wharton S, Lingvay I, Bogdanski P, et al. Oral semaglutide at a dose of 25 mg in adults with overweight or obesity. N Engl J Med. 2025;393:1077-87.
11. Vrints C, Andreotti F, Koskinas KC, et al. 2024 ESC guidelines for the management of chronic coronary syndromes. Eur Heart J. 2024;45:3415-537.
12. Virani SS, Newby LK, Arnold SV, et al. 2023 AHA/ACC/ACCP/ASPC/NLA/PCNA guideline for the management of patients with chronic coronary disease: a report of the American Heart Association/American College of Cardiology Joint Committee on Clinical Practice Guidelines. J Am Coll Cardiol. 2023;82:833-955.
13. Marso SP, Bain SC, Consoli A, et al. Semaglutide and cardiovascular outcomes in patients with type 2 diabetes. N Engl J Med. 2016;375:1834-44.
14. Kosiborod MN, Verma S, Borlaug BA, et al. Effects of semaglutide on symptoms, function, and quality of life in patients with heart failure with preserved ejection fraction and obesity: a prespecified analysis of the STEP-HFpEF trial. Circulation. 2024;149:204-16.
15. Withaar C, Meems LMG, Nollet EE, et al. The cardioprotective effects of semaglutide exceed those of dietary weight loss in mice with HFpEF. JACC Basic Transl Sci. 2023;8:1298-314.
16. Strain WD, Frenkel O, James MA, et al. Effects of semaglutide on stroke subtypes in type 2 diabetes: post hoc analysis of the randomized SUSTAIN 6 and PIONEER 6. Stroke. 2022;53:2749-57.
17. Perkovic V, Tuttle KR, Rossing P, et al. Effects of semaglutide on chronic kidney disease in patients with type 2 diabetes. N Engl J Med. 2024;391:109-21.

107

CHAPTER

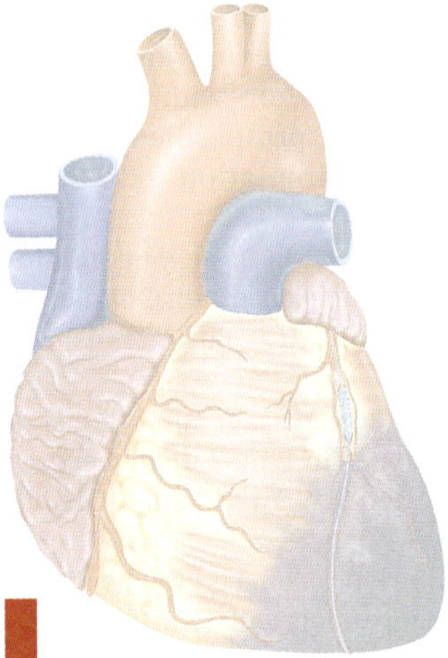

Pharmacokinetics and Pharmacodynamics of Semaglutide with Cardiovascular Outcomes

Anil Pareek, Shweta Sharma, Rupesh Salve

INTRODUCTION

Glucagon-like peptide-1 (GLP-1RA) receptor agonists are one of the important class of antidiabetic agents for the management of type 2 diabetes mellitus (T2DM) and obesity. GLP-1RAs act on multiple pathophysiologies of T2DM, resulting in significant reductions in HbA1c levels, weight loss due to decreased energy intake and delayed stomach emptying, cardiovascular (CV) benefits, and carry a low risk of hypoglycemia. Some of the GLP-1RAs are exenatide, liraglutide, dulaglutide, and semaglutide.[1]

HISTORICAL ASPECT OF GLUCAGON-LIKE PEPTIDE-1 THERAPY DEVELOPMENT

- *1930s:* The concept of incretin hormones emerged. Gut extracts were found to lower blood glucose in animals.
- *Late 1970s:* Discovery of the proglucagon gene, which encodes glucagon and related peptides.
- *Early 1980s:* Identification of GLP-1 as a product of the proglucagon gene. In 1984, synthetic GLP-1 was shown to stimulate insulin secretion and lower blood glucose in T2DM patients, confirming its therapeutic potential.
- *Early 1990s:* Recognition that native GLP-1 has a very short $T_{1/2}$ (<1 minute) due to rapid degradation by the DPP-4 enzyme.
- *1991:* Isolation of exendin-4 from Gila monster venom, a peptide similar to GLP-1 but more stable.
- *2005:* Exenatide (Exena) became the first GLP-1RA to be approved for T2DM treatment.
- *2006:* Approval of sitagliptin, the first dipeptidyl peptidase-4 inhibitor (DPP-4i), offering an oral incretin-based therapy.
- *2010:* Approval of subcutaneous (SC) liraglutide, a once-daily GLP-1RA with improved glycemic and weight benefits.
- *2014 and 2017:* Development of dulaglutide and semaglutide, long-acting once-weekly (QW) GLP-1 analogues with enhanced efficacy.
- *2019:* The first oral GLP-1RA to receive FDA approval was semaglutide, and the PIONEER 6 trial was the first cardiovascular outcomes trial (CVOT) for an oral GLP-1 RA **(Fig. 1)**. Highlight the key milestones in GLP-1RA research and development.

GLUCAGON-LIKE PEPTIDE-1 RECEPTOR AGONISTS AND DIPEPTIDYL PEPTIDASE-4 INHIBITOR

Incretin-based treatments for T2DM include GLP-1RAs and DPP-4i. Both enhance glycemic control with minimal hypoglycemia risk; however, their mechanism of actions and outcomes are different. DPP-4 is modestly enhanced endogenous GLP-1 levels by two to three times. While GLP-1RAs provide supraphysiological GLP-1 stimulation, which contributes to high glycemic efficacy, significant weight loss, and improved CV benefits. Guidelines recommend GLP-1RAs over DPP-4is for overweight, at rate of CVD, and T2DM patients.[3]

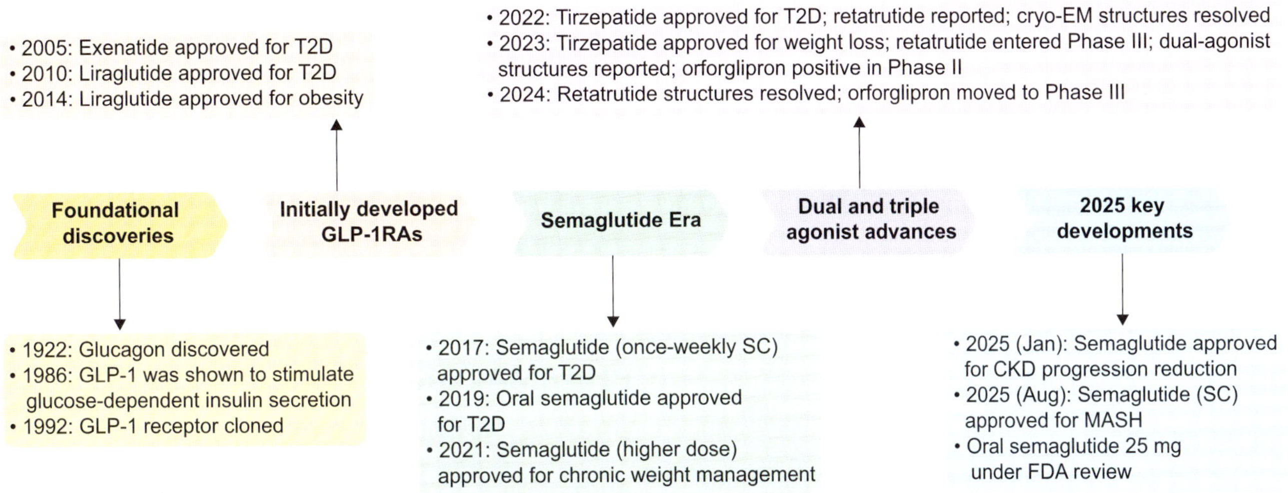

Fig. 1: Milestones of GLP-1RA research and recent drug development.[2]

Role of Visceral Adipose Tissue and Low-grade Inflammation in Pathophysiology of DM and Associated CVD

Visceral adipose tissue (VAT) is one of the most important determinants of insulin resistance (IR). It triggers chronic low-grade inflammation, enhances lipolysis, and elevates free fatty acids (FFAs), which exacerbates IR in peripheral tissues and prolongs metabolic dysfunction.[4] Framingham Heart Study links VAT to elevated inflammatory and oxidative stress markers, underscoring its pivotal role in vascular dysfunction and cardiometabolic risk. Diabetes, often associated with obesity, contributes to the development of atherosclerosis leading to high risk of myocardial infarction (MI), stroke, and mortality.[5,6]

This book chapter will cover semaglutide, which is a long-acting GLP-1RA and its clinical relevance in the treatment of T2DM and weight loss.[1]

SEMAGLUTIDE

Semaglutide demonstrates greater efficacy in improving glycemia and other cardiometabolic risk factors in T2DM patients. Considering clinical evidence, it appears to be at least as potent and possibly more effective than previous GLP-1RAs in reducing HbA1c levels, body weight, and body mass index.[7]

Semaglutide is available in both SC and oral formulations **(Table 1)**.

Subcutaneous Formulation

- Approved by USFDA, 2017 for T2DM patients and 2021 for obesity management/weight reduction
- Approved by DCGI, India: October 2025 for T2DM

TABLE 1: Subcutaneous and oral formulations of semaglutide, including available strengths and routes of administration.

Formulations	*Available strengths*	*Route of administration*
Injection	Prefilled, single-dose pen that delivers doses of 0.25 mg, 0.5 mg, 1 mg, 1.7 mg, 2 mg, and 2.4 mg[8,9]	SC
Tablet	3 mg, 7 mg, and 14 mg[10]	Oral

Oral Formulation

- Approved by USFDA, September 2019 for T2DM patients
- Approved by DCGI, India: November 2025 for T2DM patients

Approved Indications

For SC: Lower dose semaglutide indicated as an adjunct:

- To diet and exercise to improve glycemic control in adults with T2DM.
- To reduce the risk of major adverse CV events in adults with T2DM and established CV disease.
- To reduce the risk of sustained eGFR decline, end-stage kidney disease, and CV death in adults with T2DM and chronic kidney disease (CKD).[8]

Higher dose semaglutide indicated as an adjunct:

- To reduce the risk of major adverse CV events (CV death, nonfatal MI, or nonfatal stroke) in adults with established CV disease and either obesity or overweight.
- To reduce excess body weight and maintain weight reduction long-term in:

    - Adults and pediatric patients aged 12 years and older with obesity.
    - Adults with overweight in the presence of at least one weight-related comorbid condition.
- For the treatment of noncirrhotic metabolic dysfunction-associated steatohepatitis (MASH), formerly known as nonalcoholic steatohepatitis (NASH), with moderate to advanced liver fibrosis in adults.[9]

For oral: As an adjunct to diet and exercise to improve glycemic control in adults with T2DM.

Dosage and Administration

Subcutaneous

- *For T2DM:* Administer once-weekly semaglutide as an adjunct to diet and physical activity, on the same day each week, with or without food. Inject SC into the abdomen, thigh, or upper arm. Start at 0.25 mg once weekly for 4 weeks, then titrate every 4 weeks to 0.5 mg and 1 mg subsequently.[8,9]
- *For MASH:* The maintenance dosage is 2.4 mg once weekly. If patients do not tolerate 2.4 mg once weekly, the dosage can be decreased to 1.7 mg once weekly.[9]

Oral

- *For T2DM:* Oral semaglutide should be taken once daily (OD) on an empty stomach in the morning with up to 120 mL of water only, at least 30 minutes before eating, drinking, or taking other oral medications. Start with 3 mg OD for the first 30 days, then increase to 7 mg OD for the next 30 days. If needed, further increase to 14 mg OD thereafter. Swallow tablets whole. Do not split, crush, or chew tablets.[10]

MOLECULAR STRUCTURE OF SEMAGLUTIDE

As shown in **Figure 2**, semaglutide is a 31-amino acid peptide sharing 94% homology with native GLP-1, minimizing immunogenicity.[11] The alanine at position 8 is replaced with Aib (2-aminoisobutyric acid) to resist DPP-4 degradation. Additionally, the lysine at position 26 is acylated, enabling albumin binding, prolonged half-life, and reduced renal clearance.

PHARMACOKINETICS

Pharmacokinetics of Semaglutide

Absorption

After SC administration: Semaglutide is slowly absorbed and reaches maximum plasma concentration (T_{max}) approximately 1 to 3 days post-dose. The absolute bioavailability is 89%.[13] Semaglutide exposure remains consistent regardless of the injection site.[13] Thus, it has a predictable absorption profile.[14]

After oral administration: Semaglutide is coformulated with salcaprozate sodium (SNAC), an absorption enhancer which facilitates the absorption of semaglutide after oral administration. After oral administration, it is primarily absorbed in the stomach, with an absolute bioavailability of ~0.4–1% for 3, 7, and 14 mg, and ~1–2% for 1.5, 4, and 9 mg doses.[15] The maximum concentration is reached about 1-hour post-dose. Absorption is affected by water volume and post-dose fasting; higher exposure occurs with smaller water volume (50 mL vs. 240 mL) and longer fasting periods after dosing.[9,10]

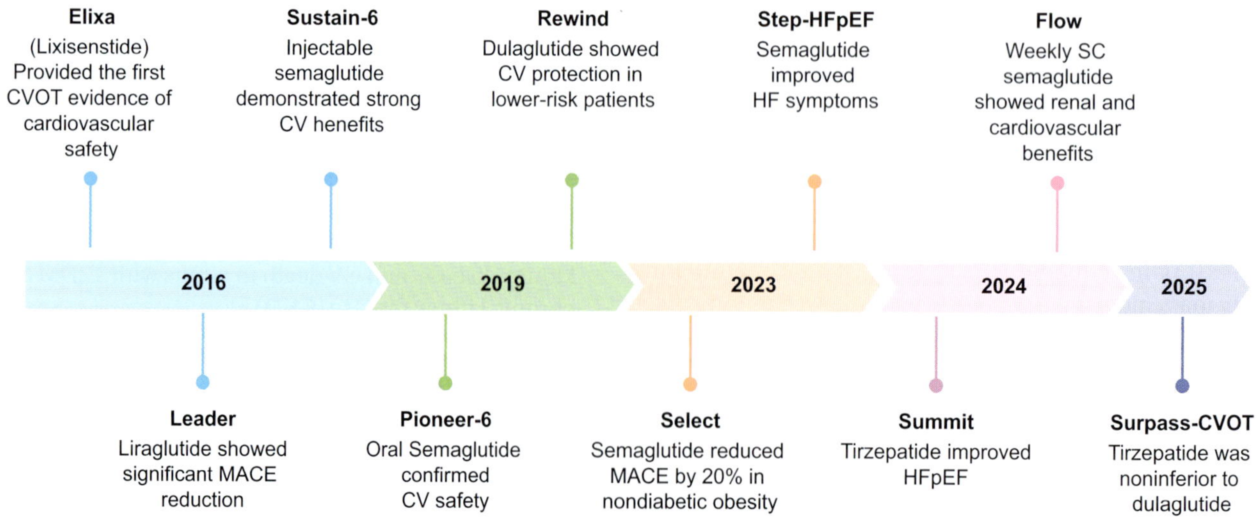

Fig. 2: Timeline of major CVOTs.

Distribution

After SC administration: The mean volume of distribution (V_d) of semaglutide following SC administration in patients with T2DM and obesity or overweight is approximately 12.5 L. It is extensively bound to plasma albumin (>99%), which results in decreased renal clearance and protection from degradation.[8,9] Steady state is achieved in 4–5 weeks with consistent dosing.

After oral administration: V_d is approximately (approximately) 8 L. Semaglutide is >99% bound to plasma albumin.[10]

Metabolism

After SC and oral administration: Semaglutide is not metabolized by a single organ but is degraded across tissues through proteolytic cleavage of the peptide backbone and sequential β-oxidation of its fatty acid side chain, which together represent its primary elimination pathway.[8-10]

Elimination

After SC and oral administration: The primary excretion routes of semaglutide-related material are via the urine and feces. Approximately 3% of the dose is excreted in the urine as intact semaglutide.[8,9] Elimination half-life is 1 week, and the drug remains in circulation for about 5 weeks after the last dose.[10]

Special Populations and Drug Interactions

Semaglutide shows a consistent PK profile across populations. Renal or hepatic impairment (of any severity) does not significantly affect its exposure, and dose adjustment is not required. Moreover, oral semaglutide does not interact with major CYP450 isoforms, indicating a low potential for drug–drug interactions.[1]

Both SC and oral formulations of semaglutide delay gastric emptying, which may influence the absorption of concomitantly administered oral medications. Use caution when coadministering drugs with a narrow therapeutic index or those requiring close clinical or laboratory monitoring. Regular monitoring and appropriate dose adjustments of the affected medications are recommended. Semaglutide is not established for pediatric use in T2DM but is approved for long-term weight management in adolescents aged ≥12 years with obesity, with a safety profile largely comparable to adults, although certain adverse events are more frequent. In older adults, including those aged ≥75 years, clinical trials demonstrate comparable efficacy and safety to younger patients; however, greater sensitivity and an increased risk of adverse events in very elderly individuals cannot be excluded.[8-10]

Safety Considerations: Pregnancy, Lactation, and Reproductive Potential

Use of semaglutide during pregnancy may cause fetal harm; discontinue treatment as soon as pregnancy is recognized. For individuals planning pregnancy, semaglutide should be stopped at least 2 months beforehand due to its long half-life and prolonged washout period. Use during pregnancy for conditions such as MASH should be considered only when the potential benefit outweighs the potential risk to the fetus. Breastfeeding is not recommended while taking semaglutide.[8-10]

PHARMACODYNAMICS

Semaglutide is a GLP-1RA, mimicking the action of the endogenous incretin hormone GLP-1. Refer to **Figure 3** for the effects of GLP-1 on various target organs.

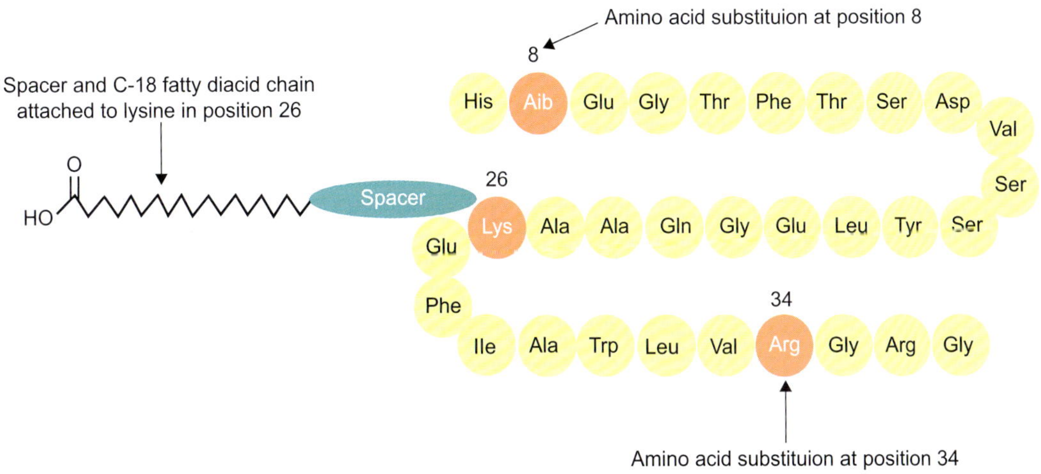

Fig. 3: Structure of semaglutide.[12]

Role of Semaglutide in Glycemic Control and Weight Loss

Semaglutide stimulates insulin secretion and reduces glucagon secretion in a glucose-dependent manner. It enhances glucose uptake in muscle and fat by promoting glucose transporter type 4 (GLUT4) activity and improving insulin sensitivity. These effects can lead to a reduction of blood glucose.

For weight loss, it reduces appetite by activating satiety pathways Pro-opiomelanocortin/Cocaine- and Amphetamine-Regulated Transcript (POMC/CART) and inhibiting hunger signals Neuropeptide Y/Agouti-Related Peptide (NPY/AgRP) in the hypothalamus, thereby decreasing caloric intake, slowing gastric emptying, and possibly improving leptin sensitivity. Overall, it acts centrally and peripherally to regulate glucose, reduce energy intake, and enhance metabolic efficiency.[16]

The PIONEER trial clinical program evaluated the efficacy and safety of oral semaglutide. PIONEER trials 1–5 demonstrated significant HbA1c and body weight reductions compared to placebo and several active comparators, including PIONEER 2 trial (Empagliflozin) and PIONEER 3 trial (Sitagliptin), while showing noninferiority to PIONEER 4 trial (Liraglutide). In patients with moderate renal impairment, PIONEER 5 trial Semaglutide maintained glycemic efficacy with a comparable safety profile to those with normal renal function. Overall, the PIONEER trial program established oral semaglutide as an effective, safe, and convenient OD oral alternative to injectable GLP-1RA for the management of T2DM.[12] Additionally, it showed increased insulin sensitivity, which is probably due to a general decrease in body weight **(Fig. 4)**.[1]

In studies with obesity and overweight patients, mean weight reduction ranged from 6.0% to 13.8%, and in the STEP 1 trial, once-weekly 2.4 mg SC semaglutide achieved a –14.9% body weight change versus –2.4% with placebo **(Table 2)**.[17]

Cardiovascular Outcomes and Semaglutide

Semaglutide has been extensively evaluated in CV outcomes trials, demonstrating a significant reduction in CV risk. Beyond glycemic control, GLP-1RAs modulate key cardiometabolic pathways, including lipid metabolism, endothelial function, and inflammatory processes, through mechanisms involving LDL receptor regulation, reduced lipid oxidation, inhibition of macrophage activation and foam cell formation, and decreased extracellular lipid deposition **(Fig. 5)**.[22] Across major trials such as SUSTAIN-6, SELECT, and PIONEER-6, semaglutide reduced MACE, including CV death, MI, and stroke, by approximately 18–20% in patients with T2DM and in individuals with obesity and established CV disease. These cardioprotective effects are driven by improvements in body weight, blood pressure, lipid profile, and systemic inflammation and are consistent across high-risk subgroups, including patients with CKD and heart failure.[23] For a summary of the clinical trials assessing semaglutide's CVOTs, see **Table 3**.

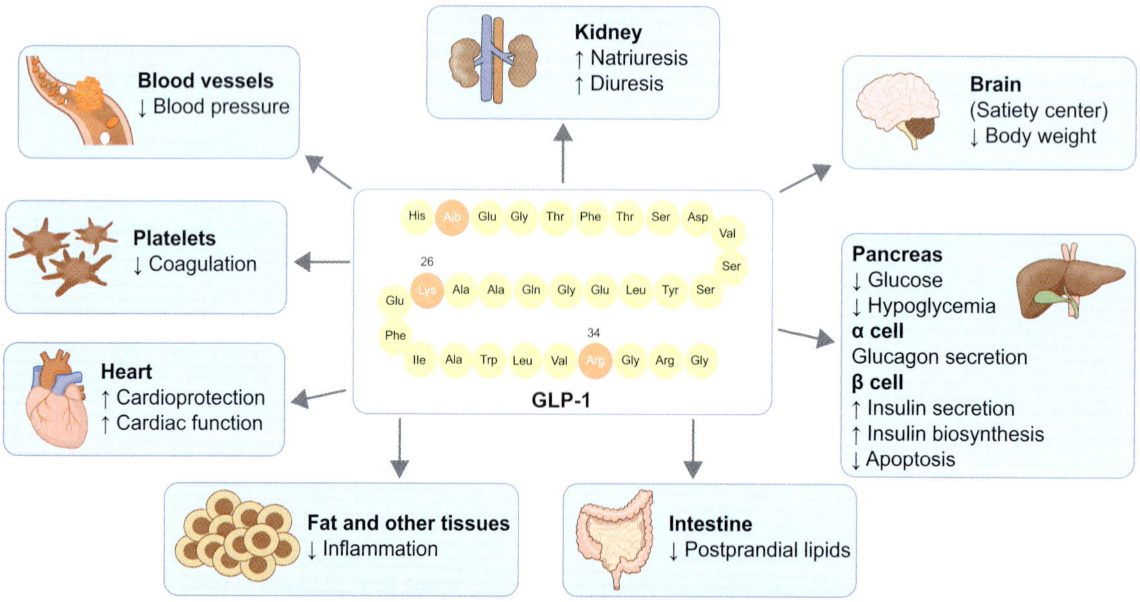

Fig. 4: Summary of the effect of GLP-1 on target organs.[16]

TABLE 2: Landmark trials of semaglutide in obesity.

Trial (Year)	*Population (n)*	*Primary outcome*	*Conclusion*	*Key points*
STEP-1 trial (2021)[18]	Obesity without diabetes $N = 1{,}961$	% body weight change once-weekly SC, C_{max} ~1–3 days	−14.9% with semaglutide vs. −2.4% with placebo $p < 0.001$	• Landmark weight loss efficacy • Appetite suppression, ↑ satiety
STEP-2 trial (2021)[19]	Obesity + T2DM $N = 1{,}210$	% body weight change	−9.6% vs. −3.4% (placebo) $p < 0.0001$	• Less weight reduction than STEP-1 due to diabetes • Similar PK profile
STEP-3 trial (2021)[20]	Obesity + intensive behavioral therapy $N = 611$	% body weight change	−16% vs. −5.7% $p < 0.0001$	• Additive benefit with lifestyle modification
STEP-4 trial (2021)[21]	Obesity; withdrawal trial $N = 902$	% body weight regain vs. continuation	Continued Semaglutide: sustained −15% loss; withdrawal: regain. $p < 0.001$	• Demonstrated need for ongoing therapy • Long-term maintenance critical

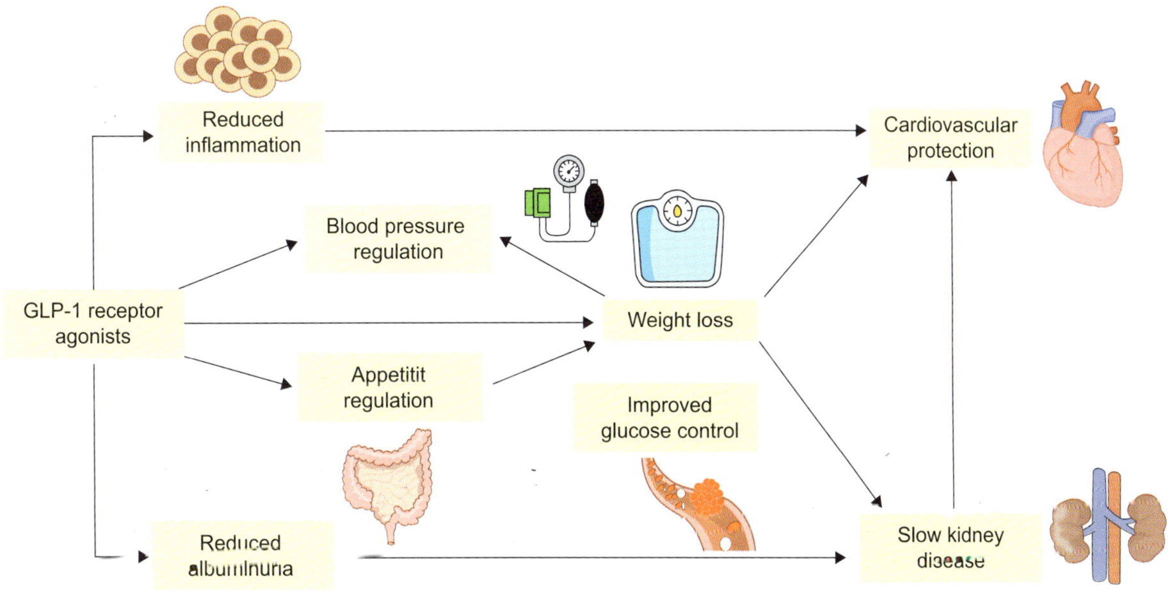

Fig. 5: Effects of GLP-1RA on important clinical outcomes in T2DM and CKD patients.[24]

Atherosclerosis and Semaglutide

Atherosclerosis is a chronic inflammatory vascular condition associated with dyslipidemia, low-grade inflammation, and macrophage accumulation in T2DM. SC semaglutide reduced carotid intima-media thickness (cIMT) by 13% over 4 months ($p < 0.001$), with consistent effects across early (<10 years), intermediate (10–15 years), and long-standing (>15 years) diabetes stages, supporting its role in attenuating subclinical atherosclerosis and providing CV protection.[22]

Heart Failure with Preserved Ejection Fraction and Semaglutide

The therapeutic benefits of semaglutide in heart failure with preserved ejection fraction (HFpEF) are attributed to both weight-dependent and weight-independent mechanisms.[26] N-terminal pro-B-type natriuretic peptide (NT-proBNP) is released from the myocardium in response to congestion-related stretch (wall stress). Patients with HF and higher NT-proBNP levels have more severe HF with greater risk of hospitalization and death. Decongestion lowers filling pressure and reduces wall stress, which lowers NT-proBNP. In phase 2 trials of HFpEF, agents that reduce NT-proBNP have been shown to reduce clinical events, consequently GLP-1RA therapies can contribute to reducing and/or preventing the incidence of CV events.[22] Semaglutide has demonstrated significant benefits in patients with obesity-HFpEF, a common heart failure phenotype.[27] The pooled STEP-HFpEF and STEP-HFpEF DM trials demonstrated that semaglutide markedly improved HF symptoms, physical limitations, and exercise capacity compared to placebo

TABLE 3: Landmark CVOTs of semaglutide.

Trial	*Population (n)*	*Semaglutide regimen*	*Primary endpoint*	*Main findings*	*Duration*
SELECT trial (2023)	*N* = 17,604 patients with overweight/ obesity, established CVD, nondiabetic	SC 2.4 mg weekly	3-point MACE	↓ MACE by 20% (HR 0.80, *p* <0.001); ↓ all-cause mortality by 19%; ↓ HF events by 18%; mean weight ↓ 9.4%	39.8 months
SUSTAIN-6 trial (2016)[25]	*N* = 3,297 patients with T2DM, 83% with CVD/renal disease	SC 0.5 or 1.0 mg weekly	3-point MACE	↓ MACE by 26% (HR 0.74); strong effect on stroke; ↓ nephropathy	25 months
PIONEER-6 trial (2019)	*N* = 3,183 patients with T2DM at high CV risk	Oral 14 mg daily	3-point MACE	Noninferior to placebo (HR 0.79); ↓ CV death (–51%); ↓ all-cause mortality (–49%) *P* < 0.001	15.9 months
SOUL trial (2024)	*N* = 9,650 patients with T2DM + either ASCVD or CKD or both	Oral 14 mg daily	3-point MACE	↓ MACE by 14% (HR 0.86); largest effect on MI; consistent benefit with/without SGLT2i, *P* = 0.006	47.5 months
FLOW trial (2024)	*N* = 3,533 patients with T2DM + CKD	SC 1.0 mg weekly	3-point MACE	↓ CV death/MI/stroke by 18% (*P* = 0.03); ↓ HF hospitalization/ CV death by 27%; ↓ all-cause mortality by 20%, *P* = 0.01	40 months (stopped early for positive efficacy)

3-Point MACE: A composite of CV death, Nonfatal myocardial infarction (MI), or Nonfatal stroke

TABLE 4: Landmark trials of semaglutide in CKD.

Trial (Year)	*Population (n)*	*Primary outcome*	*Conclusion*	*Key points*
FLOW trial (2024, NEJM)[24]	CKD (mild–moderate) + T2DM *N* = 3,534	CKD progression dialysis, transplantation, or an eGFR of <15 mL/ min/1.73 m^2 or CV death	24% ↓ risk of kidney outcomes. *P* = 0.0003	• First GLP-1RA showing kidney protection • Semaglutide reduced the risk of clinically important kidney outcomes and death from cardiovascular causes in patients with T2DM and CKD
SOUL trial[31]	ASCVD/CKD + T2DM *N* = 9650	MACE	Oral semaglutide reduced MACE, *P* = 0.66	MACE risk independent of SGLT2i use, and the combination was safe

(P = 0.0064).[28] Improvements in Kansas City Cardiomyopathy Questionnaire Clinical Summary Score (KCCQ-CSS) were 7.8 points (P < 0.001) in nondiabetic and 7.3 points (P < 0.001) in diabetes patients,[29] with greater benefit in those with higher NT-proBNP.[26] Exercise capacity improved significantly, with 6-Minute Walk Distance (MWD) gains of 20.3 m (P < 0.001) and 14.3 m (P = 0.008) in nondiabetic and diabetic cohorts, respectively.[29] Improved cardiac remodeling reductions in LA and RV volumes and better diastolic parameters were observed independent of age, gender, BMI, diabetes, or atrial fibrillation.[28]

Renal Outcomes in Patients with Chronic Kidney Disease and Semaglutide

Its renoprotective actions extend beyond glucose control, involving inhibition of oxidative stress and inflammation, induction of natriuresis, and reduction of intraglomerular pressure.[24] Semaglutide significantly delayed CKD progression in T2DM patients.[23] SUSTAIN-6 trial **Table 4** shows that the semaglutide lowered the risk of a composite kidney outcome versus placebo, while the FLOW trial showed a 24% reduction in kidney failure ≥50% eGFR decline, or kidney/CV death.[24] Semaglutide also slowed eGFR decline and limited UACR rise, with greater effects in high-risk groups.[30] Refer **Table 4** for the landmark trials evaluating semaglutide in CKD.

Natriuresis and Semaglutide

Semaglutide's renal benefits combine direct natriuretic mechanisms with indirect effects from metabolic and hemodynamic improvements.

Glucagon-like peptide-1 receptor agonists generally promote acute natriuresis via sodium-hydrogen exchanger 3 (NHE3) inhibition reducing proximal tubular sodium reabsorption, activating tubuloglomerular feedback, lowering glomerular pressure, and contributing to blood pressure reduction.[32] Long-term studies with semaglutide in T2DM showed decreased corticomedullary sodium gradient (MCR by −9%) and urine sodium/creatinine ratio (UNACR, −35%) versus placebo.[33] In semaglutide trial-specific findings, GLP-1RAs confer kidney protection through natriuresis, blood pressure lowering, weight reduction, anti-inflammatory effects, and improved endothelial function, contributing to reduced albuminuria and renal risk.[34]

Cardiovascular Kidney Metabolic Syndrome and Semaglutide

Cardiovascular kidney metabolic syndrome, defined by the AHA (2023), involves metabolic, CV, and renal risk factor interplay, leading to multiorgan dysfunction. Semaglutide provides integrated benefits across CKM stages achieving 14.9% weight loss in obesity (STEP 1 trial),[35] 31% reduction in CV death or HF, and 14% lower MACE in high-risk T2DM. In HFpEF with obesity, it reduced weight by 13.3% and improved function, while in T2DM with CKD (FLOW trial), it cut primary renal/CV events by 24% and CV mortality by 29%. Hence, agent like semaglutide are recommended for T2DM with ASCVD, CKD, or HF.[36]

SEMAGLUTIDE CLINICAL EFFECTS ON OTHER SYSTEMS

Dementia and Semaglutide

Emerging evidence indicates that semaglutide may offer neuroprotective and anti-inflammatory benefits relevant to Alzheimer's disease (AD) prevention and progression.[37] As T2DM and obesity are major adjustable risk factors for AD in a real-world study of over 1 million T2DM patients, semaglutide use was linked to a 40–70% lower risk of first-time AD diagnosis, strongest versus insulin (HR 0.33) and moderate versus other GLP-1RAs (HR 0.59), with greater benefits in women (HR 0.22) and adults ≥60 years. Semaglutide may reduce amyloid-beta(Aβ)-induced neurotoxicity, enhance autophagy, improve cerebral glucose uptake, and attenuate Aβ plaques and tau tangles via GLP-1 receptors on neurons, astrocytes, and microglia, modulating inflammatory pathways.[38] EVOKE and EVOKE+ are ongoing phase 3 trials assess oral semaglutide (14 mg daily) in amyloid-positive adults with mild cognitive impairment or early AD.[39]

Obstructive Sleep Apnea and Semaglutide

For obstructive sleep apnea (OSA), a weight reduction of ≥10–15% is recommended, as such loss is associated with substantial improvements in metabolic and CV outcomes. In clinical studies from the STEP program, semaglutide demonstrated robust efficacy about 70% of participants achieved ≥10% weight loss, and nearly 50% achieved ≥15%, highlighting its strong potential for managing obesity and related comorbidities.[18]

Osteoarthritis and Semaglutide

Osteoarthritis (OA) is a common, progressive joint disorder strongly associated with obesity, characterized by joint stress, inflammation, and cartilage damage.[40] Following semaglutide treatment, weight loss was associated with improved joint function. By lowering mechanical stress on knee joints and reducing systemic inflammation, semaglutide alleviates pain and enhances physical function, highlighting its dual benefit in managing obesity and OA.[18] A retrospective cohort study data (2020–2023) evaluated with obesity. A 10–15% weight reduction is recommended in OSA, as it significantly improves metabolic and CV parameters.[40]

Nonalcoholic Fatty Liver Disease and Semaglutide

A systematic review and meta-analysis of eight studies ($n = 2413$) found that 24 weeks of semaglutide treatment significantly reduced ALT by −14.07 U/L and AST by −6.89 U/L ($p < 0.001$), with major reductions in liver fat content (−4.97%) and liver stiffness (−0.96 kPa). In nonalcoholic fatty liver disease (NAFLD)/NASH patients, it also improves the lipid profile and HbA1c. It typically shows significant improvements in the liver and metabolism in NAFLD/NASH.[41]

ADVERSE EFFECTS

Semaglutide, administered orally or subcutaneously, is most commonly associated with gastrointestinal adverse effects, particularly nausea, diarrhea, vomiting, and constipation, which are generally mild to moderate and occur during dose escalation. Hypoglycemia may occur when combined with insulin or sulfonylureas. Key safety concerns include pancreatitis, dehydration with potential renal impairment, delayed gastric emptying, worsening diabetic retinopathy, a possible increased risk of nonarteritic anterior ischemic optic neuropathy (NAION) with semaglutide, modest heart rate increases, and an elevated fracture risk in elderly patients receiving high-dose therapy.[42] Gastrointestinal events are classified as very common (nausea and diarrhea) and common (vomiting, abdominal pain, abdominal distension, constipation, dyspepsia, belching, flatulence, GERD, and gastritis), while acute pancreatitis and delayed gastric emptying are uncommon; no rare or very rare events have been reported, and intestinal obstruction is of unknown frequency.[43] Discontinuation due to adverse events, predominantly gastrointestinal, was higher with semaglutide than placebo across major trials, including SELECT,[44] SOUL,[45] SUSTAIN-6,[46] and PIONEER,[43] whereas nongastrointestinal adverse events occurred at rates comparable to placebo.[43]

Key Safety Findings

Thyroid C-cell tumors: Semaglutide as an FDA boxed warning regarding the possible risk of thyroid C-cell tumors [including medullary thyroid carcinoma (MTC)], patients with a personal or family history of MTC or MEN2 should not take this medication.[8,10]

Tachycardia: In terms of CV safety, semaglutide is associated with a mild rise in resting heart rate (mean 1–4 beats/min vs. placebo), warranting periodic monitoring for tachycardia.[43]

Though the risk of hypoglycemia is typically minimal, but it may rise when combined with insulin or sulfonylureas.[7]

Diabetic retinopathy: Complications were slightly higher in SUSTAIN-6 trials (3.0% vs. 1.8%; HR 1.76; $P = 0.02$), possibly related to rapid HbA1c reduction, while PIONEER trials showed similar rates to placebo since patients with advanced proliferative disease were excluded.[47] Data also suggest an increased risk of NAION with long-term use.[45,48]

The incidence of acute pancreatitis was low and comparable to placebo across studies, including SOUL SELECT and SUSTAIN-6 trials.[44] Gallbladder disorders occurred slightly more often with semaglutide, e.g., 2.8% versus 2.3% in SELECT trial ($p < 0.001$).[44] In cases of mild or moderate renal or hepatic impairment, no dose adjustment is necessary; however, in cases of severe impairment, careful monitoring is recommended.[47]

Mitigating AEs: To reduce GI side effects and minimize the risk of diabetic retinopathy worsening, semaglutide treatment should follow a gradual dose-escalation regimen. For the oral formulation, this typically involves 4-week increments, e.g., 3 mg→7 mg→14 mg maximum dose).[43] When semaglutide is coadministered with insulin or sulfonylureas, adjustment of these agents may be necessary to reduce the risk of hypoglycemia. Emerging concerns include potential loss of lean muscle mass with rapid weight reduction and the risk of pulmonary aspiration during surgical procedures in patients on GLP-1RA.[49]

GUIDELINES AND RECOMMENDATIONS

According to the AACE 2023 algorithm, GLP-1RA is a first-line treatment, particularly for patients with CKD, heart failure, or ASCVD. It can be initiated at an early stage, first treatment either before metformin or become second line after metformin, and in high-risk patients. It is still the recommended supplement to metformin or in combination therapy for high A1c (>9–10%) in individuals without CKD, heart failure, or ASCVD. Semaglutide provides demonstrated CV and renal protection in addition to glucose management, which is consistent with the complications-centric treatment approach of AACE.[50]

According to the Obesity and Weight Management for the Prevention and Treatment of Diabetes: Standards of Care in Diabetes—2026 (ADA), semaglutide is recommended for long-term weight management in people with T2DM who are overweight or obese because of its effectiveness and additional health benefits.[51] Treatment should continue even after weight goals are achieved, as discontinuation often leads to weight regain. Dosing and titration should be individualized to balance efficacy and tolerability.[44]

The ADA Consensus Report indicates that semaglutide is associated with improvements in hepatic steatosis, steatohepatitis, and fibrosis regression, with a potential role in reducing fibrosis progression.[52]

ESC guidelines highlight semaglutide as a key GLP-1RA for obesity management, recommending its use in overweight patients with T2DM, and endorsing SC semaglutide in T2DM with ASCVD to reduce major CV events regardless of HbA1c. The guidelines also recommend semaglutide in overweight chronic coronary syndrome patients without diabetes to lower the risk of CV death, MI, or stroke.[53]

CONCLUSION

Semaglutide with predictable pharmacokinetic profile and including potent glycemic control, significant weight loss and robust CV, and renal protection position it as an indispensable treatment option in the current therapeutic arsenal for patients with T2DM, obesity, and associated CV diseases. Ongoing and upcoming research on semaglutide covers a broad spectrum of indications. The PIONEER PLUS trial is assessing higher oral doses (25 mg and 50 mg compared with 14 mg) in T2DM patients. The EVOKE and

EVOKE+ trials are evaluating oral semaglutide in early AD, alongside investigations into its potential benefits in OSA and PCOS for improved metabolic and hormonal outcomes. Future programs, such as the Phase 3 STEP UP trials, aim to optimize weight loss and metabolic control through combination therapies with SGLT2i and higher-dose (7.2 mg) formulations, with the STEP UP T2DM trial focusing on individuals with obesity and T2DM. Moreover, an oral formulation for chronic weight management is under regulatory review, while the Cagri Semaglutide combination (Semaglutide + Cagrilintide) a systematic review and meta-analysis has demonstrated superior efficacy in weight reduction in obese individuals.

REFERENCES

1. Mahapatra MK, Karuppasamy M, Sahoo BM. Semaglutide, a glucagon-like peptide-1 receptor agonist with cardiovascular benefits for management of type 2 diabetes. Rev Endocr Metab Disord. 2022;23(3):521-39.
2. Zhou Q, Li G, Hang K, et al. Weight loss blockbuster development: a role for unimolecular polypharmacology. Annu Rev Pharmacol Toxicol. 2025;65(1):191-213.
3. Brunton S. GLP-1 receptor agonists vs. DPP-4 inhibitors for type 2 diabetes: is one approach more successful or preferable than the other? Int J Clin Pract. 2014;68(5): 557-67.
4. Dhokte S, Czaja K. Visceral Adipose Tissue: The Hidden Culprit for Type 2 Diabetes. Nutrients. 2024;16:1015.
5. Yadav U, Kumar N. Role of obesity related inflammation in pathogenesis of peripheral artery disease in patients of type 2 diabetes mellitus. J Diabetes Metab Disord. 2023;22:175-88.
6. Pou KM, Massaro JM, Hoffmann U, et al. Visceral and subcutaneous adipose tissue volumes are cross-sectionally related to markers of inflammation and oxidative stress: The Framingham Heart Study. Circulation. 2007;116: 1234-41.
7. Holst JJ, Madsbad S. Semaglutide seems to be more effective than other GLP-1RAs. Ann Transl Med. 2017;5(24):505.
8. FDA. (2017). Highlights Of Prescribing Information of Ozempic® (Semaglutide). [online] Available from https://www.accessdata.fda.gov/drugsatfda_docs/label/2025/209637s025lbl.pdf [Last accessed January, 2026].
9. FDA. (2017). Highlights Of Prescribing Information Wegovy® (Semaglutide) [online] Available from https://www.accessdata.fda.gov/drugsatfda_docs/label/2025/215256s024lbl.pdf [Last accessed January, 2026].
10. FDA. (2017). Highlights Of Prescribing Information Rybelsus® (Semaglutide). [online] Available from https://www.accessdata.fda.gov/drugsatfda_docs/label/2025/213051Orig1s020,213051Orig1s021lbl.pdf [Last accessed January, 2026].
11. Jensen L, Helleberg H. Absorption, metabolism and excretion of the GLP-1 analogue Semaglutide in humans and nonclinical species. Eur J Pharm Sci. 2017;104:31-41.
12. Kalra S, Das S. A review of oral Semaglutide available evidence: A new era of management of diabetes with peptide in a pill form. Indian J Endocr Metab. 2022;26(2):98-105.
13. Alorfi NM, Algarni AS. Clinical impact of Semaglutide, a glucagon-like peptide-1 receptor agonist, on obesity management: a review. Clin Pharmacol. 2022;14:61-7.
14. Yang XD, Yang YY. Clinical pharmacokinetics of Semaglutide: a systematic review. Drug Des Devel Ther. 2024;18:2555-70.
15. Papakonstantinou I, Tsioufis K. Spotlight on the mechanism of action of Semaglutide. Curr Issues Mol Biol. 2024;46(12):14514-41.
16. Nauck MA, Niedereichholz U. Glucagon-like peptide-1 inhibition of gastric emptying outweighs its insulinotropic effects in healthy humans. Am J Physiol. 1997;273(5):E981-E988.
17. Ryan DH, Lingvay I. Semaglutide effects on cardiovascular outcomes in people with overweight or obesity (SELECT) rationale and design. Am Heart J. 2020;229:61-9.
18. Zhou L, He S, Li C. Two birds with one stone—Semaglutide's impacts on obesity and knee osteoarthritis: From weight loss to pain relief. Innov Med. 2025;3(1):100110.
19. Davies MJ, Aroda VR. Management of hyperglycemia in type 2 diabetes, 2022: a consensus report by the ADA and the EASD. Diabetes Care. 2022;45(11):2753-86.
20. Wadden TA, Bailey TS. Effect of subcutaneous Semaglutide vs placebo as an adjunct to intensive behavioral therapy on body weight in adults with overweight or obesity: the STEP 3 randomized clinical trial. JAMA. 2021;325(14):1403-13.
21. Rubino D, Abrahamsson N. Effect of Continued Weekly Subcutaneous Semaglutide vs Placebo on Weight Loss Maintenance in Adults With Overweight or Obesity: The STEP 4 Randomized Clinical Trial. JAMA. 2021;325(14):1414-25.
22. Patti AM, Giglio RV. Effect of Semaglutide on Subclinical Atherosclerosis and Cardiometabolic Compensation: A Real-World Study in Patients With Type 2 Diabetes. Biomedicines. 2023;11(5):1362.
23. Deanfield J, Verma S, Scirica BM, et al. Semaglutide and cardiovascular outcomes in patients with obesity and prevalent heart failure: a prespecified analysis of the SELECT trial. Lancet. 2024;404(10454):773-86.
24. Kotwal SS, Perkovic V. Effects of Semaglutide on CKD in Patients With Type 2 Diabetes. Kidney Int Rep. 2025;10(2):287-90.
25. Tuttle KR, Cherney DZ. Effects of Once-Weekly Semaglutide on Kidney Disease Outcomes by KDIGO Risk Category in the SUSTAIN 6 Trial. Kidney Int Rep. 2024;9(7):2006-15.
26. Petrie MC, Borlaug BA, Butler J, et al. Semaglutide and NT-proBNP in Obesity-Related HFpEF: Insights From the STEP-HFpEF Program. J Am Coll Cardiol. 2024;84(1): 27-40.

27. Borlaug BA, Kitzman DW, Davies MJ, et al. Semaglutide in HFpEF Across Obesity Class and by Body Weight Reduction: A Prespecified Analysis of the STEP-HFpEF Trial. Nat Med. 2023;29(9):2358-65.
28. Solomon SD, Ostrominski JW, Wang X, et al. Effect of Semaglutide on cardiac structure and function in patients with obesity-related heart failure. J Am Coll Cardiol. 2024;84(17):1587-602.
29. Kosiborod MN, Abildstrøm SZ, Borlaug BA, et al. Semaglutide in Patients with Heart Failure with Preserved Ejection Fraction and Obesity. N Engl J Med. 2023;389(12):1069-84.
30. Perkovic V, Tuttle KR. Effects of Semaglutide on Chronic Kidney Disease in Patients with Type 2 Diabetes. N Engl J Med. 2024;391:109-21.
31. Marx N, Deanfield JE. Oral Semaglutide and Cardiovascular Outcomes in People With Type 2 Diabetes, According to SGLT2i Use: Prespecified Analyses of the SOUL Randomized Trial. Circulation. 2025;151(23):1639-50.
32. Yu JH, Park SY. GLP-1 receptor agonists in diabetic kidney disease: current evidence and future directions. Kidney Res Clin Pract. 2022;41(2):136-49.
33. Gullaksen S, Vernstrøm L. The effects of Semaglutide, empagliflozin and their combination on the kidney sodium signal from magnetic resonance imaging: A prespecified, secondary analysis from a randomized, clinical trial. J Diabetes Complications. 2024;38(2):108673.
34. Heerspink HJL, Apperloo E. Effects of Semaglutide on albuminuria and kidney function in people with overweight or obesity with or without type 2 diabetes: exploratory analysis from the STEP 1, 2, and 3 trials. Diabetes Care. 2023;46(4):801-10.
35. Wilding JPH, Batterham RL. Once-Weekly Semaglutide in Adults with Overweight or Obesity. N Engl J Med. 2021;384:989-1002.
36. Mutruc V, Bologa C. Cardiovascular–Kidney–Metabolic Syndrome: A New Paradigm in Clinical Medicine or Going Back to Basics? J Clin Med. 2025;14:2833.
37. Atri A, Feldman HH. evoke and evoke+: design of two large-scale, double-blind, placebo-controlled, phase 3 studies evaluating the neuroprotective effects of Semaglutide in early Alzheimer's disease. Alzheimers Dement. 2022;18(Suppl 10):e062415.
38. Wang W, Wang QQ. Associations of Semaglutide with first-time diagnosis of Alzheimer's disease in patients with type 2 diabetes: target trial emulation using nationwide real-world data in the US. Alzheimers Dement. 2024;20:8661-72.
39. Daly T, Imbimbo BP. Targeting dementia prevention with Semaglutide: The case for APOE4 homozygotes. Alzheimers Dement. 2025;21(6):e70422.
40. Baser O, Isenman L. Impact of Semaglutide on osteoarthritis risk in patients with obesity: A retrospective cohort study. Obes Sci Pract. 2024;e762.
41. Bandyopadhyay S, Das S. Role of Semaglutide in the treatment of nonalcoholic fatty liver disease or non-alcoholic steatohepatitis: A systematic review and meta-analysis. Diabetes Metab Syndr. 2023;17(10):102849.
42. European Medicines Agency. Summary of Product Characteristics. [online] Available from https://www.ema.europa.eu/en/glossary-terms/summary-product-characteristics [Last accessed January, 2026].
43. Thethi TK, Pratley R. Efficacy, safety and cardiovascular outcomes of once-daily oral Semaglutide in patients with type 2 diabetes: The PIONEER programme. Diabetes Obes Metab. 2020;22(8):1263-77.
44. Lincoff AM, Brown-Frandsen K. Semaglutide and cardiovascular outcomes in obesity without diabetes. N Engl J Med. 2023;389:2221-32.
45. McGuire DK, Marx N. Oral Semaglutide and cardiovascular outcomes in high-risk type 2 diabetes. N Engl J Med. 2025;392:2001-12.
46. Marso SP, Bain SC. Semaglutide and cardiovascular outcomes in patients with type 2 diabetes. N Engl J Med. 2016;375:1834-44.
47. McGuire DK, Pop-Busui RP. Effects of oral Semaglutide on cardiovascular outcomes in individuals with type 2 diabetes and established atherosclerotic cardiovascular disease and/or chronic kidney disease: Design and baseline characteristics of SOUL, a randomized trial. Diabetes Obes Metab. 2023;25(7):1932-41.
48. Grauslund J, Abou Taha A. Once-weekly Semaglutide doubles the five-year risk of nonarteritic anterior ischemic optic neuropathy in a Danish cohort of 424,152 persons with type 2 diabetes. Int J Retina Vitreous. 2024;10:97.
49. MacIsaac RJ. Semaglutide: a key medication for managing cardiovascular-kidney-metabolic syndrome. Future Cardiol. 2025;21(9):663-83.
50. Samson SL, Vellanki P. American Association of Clinical Endocrinology Consensus Statement: Comprehensive Type 2 Diabetes Management Algorithm - 2023 Update. Endocr Pract. 2023;29(5):305-40.
51. American Diabetes Association Professional Practice Committee for Diabetes. Obesity and Weight Management for the Prevention and Treatment of Diabetes: Standards of Care in Diabetes—2026. Diabetes Care. 2026;49(Suppl 1):S166-S182.
52. Cusi K, Abdelmalek MF, Apovian CM, et al. Metabolic Dysfunction–Associated Steatotic Liver Disease (MASLD) in People With Diabetes: The Need for Screening and Early Intervention. A Consensus Report of the American Diabetes Association. Diabetes Care. 2025;48(7):1057-82.
53. Christodorescu R. (2024). Part II. Highlights from the clinical consensus statement by the European Society of Cardiology on obesity and cardiovascular disease: pharmacological and bariatric treatment strategies. [online] Available from https://www.escardio.org/communities/councils/cardiology-practice/education/cardiopractice/part-II-highlights-from-the-clinical-consensus-statement-by-the-european-society/ [Last accessed January, 2026].

108

CHAPTER

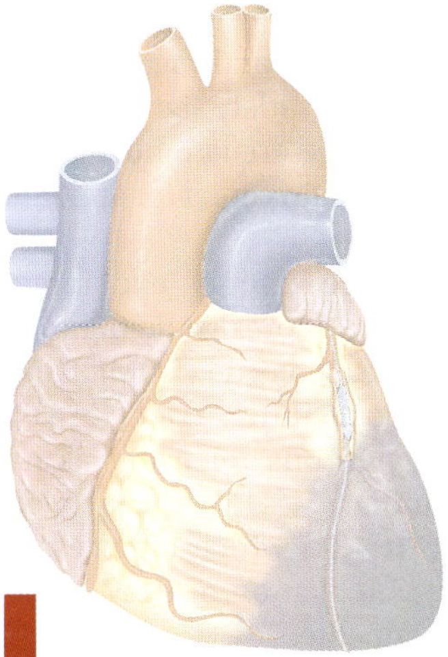

Semaglutide and Appetite Regulation: Central and Peripheral Mechanisms

Arati Dave Lalchandani, Taruni Lalchandani

INTRODUCTION

The rising incidence of obesity globally has made it an epidemic disease or a major cause of many fatal diseases, making it imperative to control it and thus prevent huge expenses on the control of many widespread metabolic noncommunicable diseases in the world.

With widespread research on obesity, it is now recognized that obesity is not just a lifestyle disease or an offshoot of mental disorders, but due to complex interplay of environmental, genetic, metabolic, neural, and endocrine factors.

Obesity is not merely an increase in body weight or imbalance of intake and output of energy but a complex biological and metabolic jumble of energy and caloric homeostasis.

In all this, the most important substance hormone called incretin, glucagon-like peptide-1 (GLP-1), secreted from L cells in the colon and distal small intestine after meal ingestion, plays the main role, and research on this and other related substances has provided the key to mechanisms causing obesity and hence its control, prevention, and maintenance.

This led to the development of GLP-1 receptor agonists (GLP-1RAs), which mimic the action of GLP-1, and the discovery of a revolutionary molecule, called semaglutide the latest generation of GLP-1 RA, long acting and with profound effects on weight reduction while influencing metabolic functions causing chronic weight gain in a positive way.[1]

Semaglutide could become the answer to combating obesity with results of large-scale clinical and field trials as well as research studies along with high-level deliberations from all over the world especially on central and peripheral mechanisms of action related to appetite regulation.

PERIPHERAL MECHANISM IN APPETITE REGULATION

Peripheral action of semaglutide is related to the gut–pancreas axis as the drug exerts powerful effects on the gastrointestinal system and pancreas even before signals activate brain receptors. The feeling of fullness and satiety after a meal to quench the appetite results from incretin effects on glucose metabolism; it is here that semaglutide acts to suppress appetite. Semaglutide's effects on pancreas are by activating GLP-1R on pancreatic islet cells which cause indirect effect on appetite. It stimulates secretion on insulin from beta cells of pancreas which is dependent on glucose levels. After a meal when glucose levels are elevated, insulin secretion peaks. When glucose level is low, then GLP-1RA stimulation is reduced thereby protecting against hypoglycemia.[2]

Semaglutide suppresses the secretion of glucagon by acting on pancreatic alpha cells. Glucagon has a counter-regulatory effect on insulin raising the glucose levels by increasing glucose production from the liver. Semaglutide's effect on glucagon suppression wanes when glucose levels fall, thus reducing chances of hypoglycemia and intermittent hunger pangs.

Effect of semaglutide on GIT: It slows gastric emptying and retains the food in the stomach longer. This causes gastric distention and hence satiety, overall resulting in lesser food consumption. These effects of semaglutide may not be observed for prolonged periods, as was seen in 20-week study, where it was observed that there was no significant difference in gastric emptying between semaglutide and placebo groups.[3]

This suggests that the peripheral mechanism causes appetite suppression and possibly side effects like nausea only during initiation of treatment but gastric motility returns to baseline by physiological adaptation over a period of time. This raises the question that this peripheral mechanism does not explain sustained weight loss over months and years of use. Therefore, it follows that semaglutide may have additional effects on brain's appetite control centers. The answer may lie with its effect on central mechanisms of appetite regulation.

Overall central and peripheral effects of semaglutide result in a significant reduction of energy intake as proven in randomized controlled trials. After treatment with semaglutide, subjects showed a decreased intake and consumption of food calories and energy, as much as 35% reduction.[3,4]

Central Mechanisms in Appetite Regulation with Semaglutide

Semaglutide acts on the central nervous system on the chief energy regulation and balance centers in the brain influencing the homeostatic settings of body weight. Semaglutide only partially accesses the blood-brain barrier. It utilizes specific anatomical gateways in the brain which are mainly two in number discovered by studies with labeled semaglutide, the first being through circumventricular organs (CVOs) which function as chemosensory areas in contact with the blood. The area postrema (AP) in the brain stem is rich in GLP-1 receptors which is a CVO with CNS neurons.[5]

The second gateway for semaglutide is via the vagus nerve which provides a link between the brain stem and the GI system. GLP-1 receptors on the lining of GI tract communicate with the afferent sensory fibers of the vagus which transmit signals of satiety to the brain stem.[5]

Signals are also received from arcuate nucleus of the hypothalamus which influences the action of semaglutide. From the CNS, it is communicated to the nuclei in hypothalamus, pons, cerebellum, and medulla oblongata.

The nucleus of the solitary tract (NST) integrates all the impulses to the brain stem from the AP and vagal afferent nerves received from the peripheral satiety signals. From the NST, signals are conveyed to the arcuate nucleus of hypothalamus (ARH) which is the main center for appetite control and energy balance.

The neurons which manage energy exchange, conservation, and expenditure are anorexigenic neurons that release peptides pro-opiomelanocortin (POMC) and cocaine- and amphetamine-regulated transcript (CART). Semaglutide activates these neurons releasing alpha melanocyte-stimulating hormone (MSH) which acts on melanocortin 4 receptors (MC4Rs) which suppresses appetite and expends energy. Activation of POMC and MC4R results in extinguished appetite.

ARH also has orexigenic (appetite stimulating) neurons that release neuropeptide Y (NPY) and agouti-related peptide (AgRP) which cause pangs of hunger and quest for food. Semaglutide inhibits NPY and AgRP neurons killing appetite.

There is also activation of satiety signals such as from lateral parabrachial nucleus (PBN) and the paraventricular nucleus (PVN) of hypothalamus. In the brain, GLP-1 producing neurons are called preproglucagon (PPG) located in NST. These neurons release GLP-1 from brain to produce satiety and stop food intake.

Semaglutide may not activate PPG NST but still causes suppressed appetite. This could mean that peripheral GLP-1 system and central GLP-1 system may have separate gut-brain circuits.[5,6]

Semaglutide may have some other powerful anorexigenic pathway which may be highly efficacious in influencing appetite and energy balance in obesity.

There may be parallel pathways which may be pharmacologically and metabolically involved in the possession of obesity.

With increasing researches on pleiotropic effects of GLP-1, the importance and application of semaglutide in appetite regulation could reveal many dimensions.[7]

LIMITATIONS

Semaglutide has been found to have a drastic influence on CNS homeostatic and hedonic pathways with a synergistic interplay with significant conversion to hidden clinical benefits. The benefits of semaglutide through its multifarious actions remain to be explored in human subjects especially with regard to adipose tissue conversions, anti-inflammatory effects, and regulation of autophagy **(Table 1)**. The central action of semaglutide on brain stem and hypothalamus through mesolimbic

TABLE 1: Brain regions, key nuclei, neuron types, and mechanisms involved in the regulation of appetite and the effects of GLP-1 receptor signaling.

Brain region	*Key nucleus/area*	*Primary neuron type(s) involved*	*Mechanism of access*	*Primary effect on appetite*
Brain stem	Area postrema (AP)	GLP-1R-expressing neurons	Direct access from circulation (CVO)	Senses circulating semaglutide; relays signal to NST; involved in nausea response
	Nucleus of the solitary tract (NST)	GLP-1R-expressing neurons (non-PPG); POMC neurons	Input from AP and vagal afferents	Integrates peripheral satiety signals; relays anorexigenic signals to hypothalamus
	Dorsal vagal complex (DVC)	ADCYAP1+ neurons	Direct access and vaginal input	Mediates semaglutide's effects on energy balance without inducing nausea
Hypothalamus	Arcuate nucleus (ARH)	POMC/CART neurons (anorexigenic); NPY/AgRP neurons (orexigenic)	Direct access at median eminence; input from NST	Activates POMC neurons (suppresses appetite); inhibits NPY/AgRP neurons (suppresses hunger)
	Paraventricular nucleus (PVN)	MC4R-expressing neurons	Input from ARH (alpha-MSH)	Major site for melanocortin-driven satiety reduces food intake
Limbic system/ reward	Ventral tegmental area (VTA)	Dopaminergic and GABAergic neurons expressing GLP-1R	Ascending projections from NST; potential direct access	Modulates dopamine signaling; reduces the motivational drive for palatable food
	Nucleus accumbens (NAc)	Dopamine–receptive neurons expressing GLP-1R	Dopaminergic input from VTA	Reduces the hedonic (pleasurable) impact of food consumption
	Amygdala	GLP-1R-expressing neurons	Input from NST and other limbic structures	Reduces brain response to food cues; modulates emotional aspects of eating

circuits could dampen the food noise, thus reducing hedonic drive for tasty foods.[8]

CONCLUSION

Semaglutide, a GLP 1 analogue, with further researches of its role involving neurometabolism, diabetology, gastrohepatic metabolism, and psychosomatic disorders, may prove to be a great innovation marking the dawn of a new era of human intervention in body modeling.

REFERENCES

1. Blundell J, Finlayson G, Axelsen M, et al. Effects of once-weekly semaglutide on appetite, energy intake, control of eating, food preference and body weight in subjects with obesity. Diabetes Obes Metab. 2017;19(9):1242-51.
2. Alorfi NM, Algarni AS. Clinical impact of semaglutide, a glucagon-like peptide-1 receptor agonist, on obesity management: a review. Clin Pharmacol. 2022;14:61-7.
3. Gibbons C, Blundell J, Hoff ST, et al. Effects of oral semaglutide on energy intake, food preference, appetite, control of eating and body weight in subjects with type 2 diabetes. Diabetes Obes Metab. 2021;23(2):581-8.
4. Friedrichsen M, Breitschaft A, Tadayon S, et al. The effect of semaglutide 2.4 mg once weekly on energy intake, appetite, control of eating, and gastric emptying in adults with obesity. Diabetes Obes Metab. 2021;23(3):754-62.
5. Gabery S, Salinas CG, Paulsen SJ, et al. Semaglutide lowers body weight in rodents via distributed neural pathways. JCI Insight. 2020;5(6):e133429.
6. Miller GD. Appetite regulation: hormones, peptides, and neurotransmitters and their role in obesity. Am J Lifestyle Med. 2017;13(6):586-601.
7. Papakonstantinou I, Tsioufis K, Katsi V. Spotlight on the mechanism of action of semaglutide. Curr Issues Mol Biol. 2024;46(12):14514-41.
8. European Association for the Study of Diabetes. (2025). Semaglutide may silence the food noise in your head. [online] Available from https://www.sciencedaily.com/releases/2025/09/250915202846.htm. [Last accessed December, 2025].

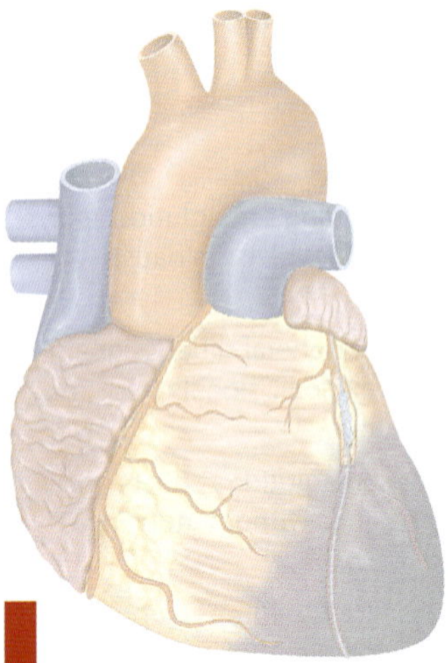

109

CHAPTER

Lifestyle Interventions Combined with Semaglutide Therapy

Dharmendra Jain, Pratap Kumar, Vikash Kumar Maurya

INTRODUCTION

Obesity is a major global public health challenge, affecting individuals across all age groups and socioeconomic strata. According to the World Health Organization (WHO), the global prevalence of obesity has nearly tripled since 1975, with over 650 million adults classified as obese in 2016, and current trends indicate a continued rise.[1] In 2022, >1 billion people worldwide were living with obesity, including 650 million adults, 340 million adolescents, and 39 million children.[2]

Obesity contributes substantially to morbidity, mortality, and health care costs. It is a leading risk factor for noncommunicable diseases (NCDs) such as type 2 diabetes mellitus, cardiovascular disease, certain cancers, and musculoskeletal disorders.[3,4] The prevalence is rising not only in high-income but also in low- and middle-income countries, driven by urbanization, sedentary lifestyles, and increased consumption of calorie-dense foods.[5]

Tackling this evergrowing problem of obesity requires health strategies focused on prevention, early intervention, and promoting a healthy environment. There have been a lot of advances in the treatment of obesity in recent years. Lifestyle interventions and GLP-1 receptor agonists form the backbone of obesity management. This chapter presents an overview of the lifestyle interventions and the glucagon-like peptide-1 receptor agonist (GLP-1 RA), semaglutide, for the management of obesity.

LIFESTYLE INTERVENTIONS IN THE MANAGEMENT OF OBESITY

Lifestyle interventions include a combination of dietary modifications, physical activity, and behavioral therapy. They are the first line of treatment for obesity and are an integral part of all other forms of therapy for obesity—medical or surgical. Once the target weight loss is achieved, they become more important in order to maintain a stable weight and retain the health benefits of treatments. **Figure 1** gives a basic summary of the lifestyle interventions in the management of obesity.[6]

Dietary Modifications

The aim of dietary modification is to maintain a calorie deficit through structured meal planning and balanced macronutrient distribution. Guidelines recommend calorie deficit plans of 500–750 kilocalories daily or estimated intakes of 1,200–1,500 kilocalories daily for women and men, respectively.[7] Calorie-restricted diets (500–750 kcal/day deficit) have been shown to achieve 5–10% weight loss within 6 months, which is associated with significant cardio-metabolic benefits, such as improved glycemic control and lipid profiles.[8,9] While maintaining the calorie deficit, an adequate supply of macronutrients also should also be taken care of.

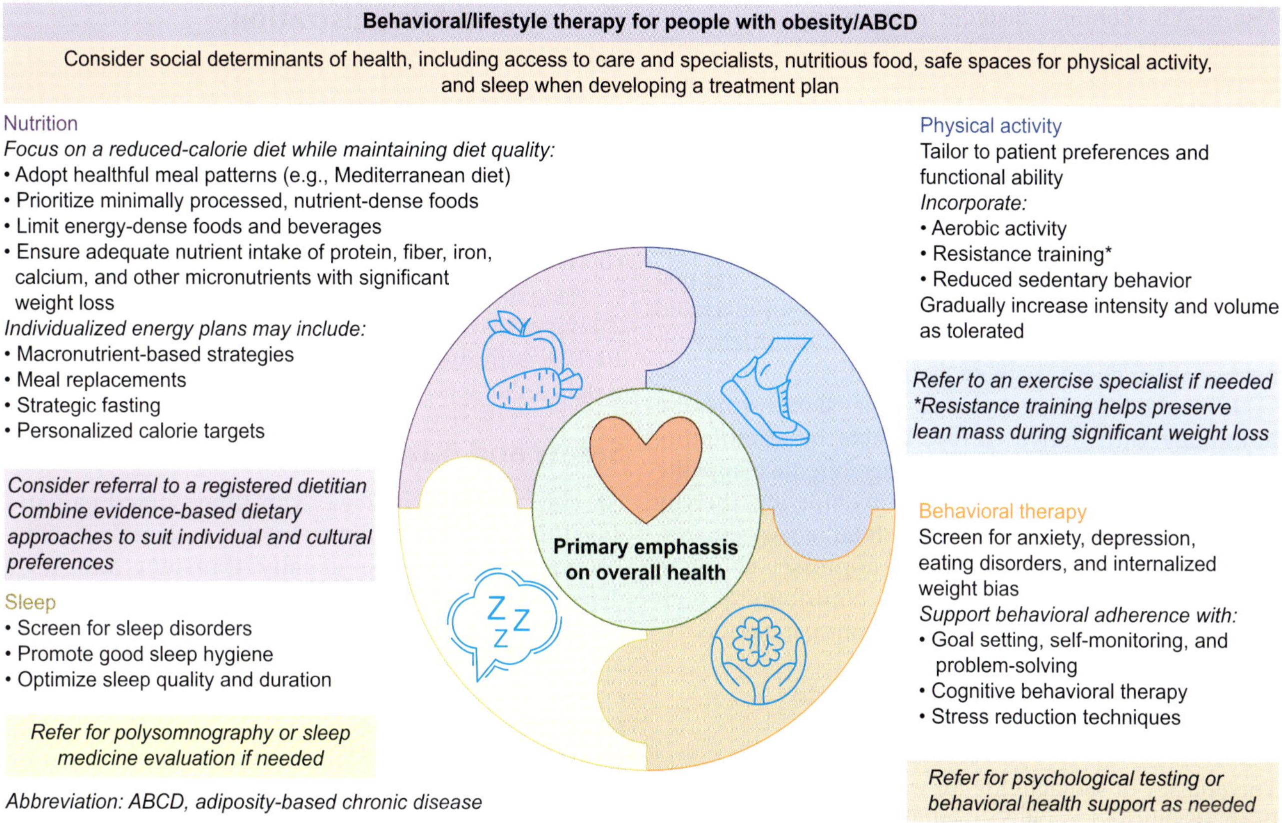

Fig. 1: AACE, 2025 algorithm for lifestyle therapy in patients with obesity.[6]

The American Association of Clinical Endocrinology (AACE)[6] suggests several key guiding points:

- Optimize and prioritize nutrient-dense carbohydrates, such as vegetables, beans/pulses, and fruits.
- Prioritize lean protein
- Consider multivitamin supplementation to include iron and calcium.
- Flexible use of meal replacements.

Physical Activity

Physical activity includes aerobic activity, resistance/strength training, reduced sedentary time, and an increase in nonexercise activity thermogenesis. Various guidelines suggest an eventual goal is ≥150 min/week of moderate-intensity physical activity, such as brisk walking, or ≥75 min/week of high-intensity physical activity, such as high-intensity interval training. Frequent and higher volumes of physical activity are required for maintenance of weight reduction. Retention of lean mass via resistance training during active weight reduction serves to preserve resting metabolic rate and overall energy expenditure.[10]

Behavioral Therapy

Depression, anxiety, and binge eating disorder are more prevalent among people with obesity compared with the general population.[11] These issues can require immediate intervention in some patients to assure that the therapeutic plan can be effective. Consultation with trained professionals for psychological screening and cognitive behavioral therapy should be considered as part of long-term follow-up for people with internal weight bias.

Sleep

Suboptimal sleep duration (<7–8 hours per night) and poor sleep quality can promote dysregulated energy intake, metabolic perturbations, and obesity.[12,13] Inadequate sleep and circadian disruption are associated with increased appetite, increased energy intake, decreased energy expenditure, and cardiometabolic disease risk.[14] For those with short sleep duration, individualized sleep hygiene counselling intended to extend sleep duration may reduce energy intake and increase weight reduction.

Also, OSA is a common disorder frequently associated with obesity and having adverse health impact. A person with obesity should be screened for this disorder and treated appropriately.

SEMAGLUTIDE IN THE MANAGEMENT OF OBESITY

Semaglutide, a once-weekly GLP-1 receptor agonist originally developed for diabetes, has demonstrated unprecedented weight loss efficacy in individuals with overweight or obesity without diabetes.[15]

It is a modified GLP-1 analogue that shares structural homology with native GLP-1. It acts by stimulating GLP-1 receptors in the hypothalamus to reduce appetite and energy intake and delays gastric emptying, thereby promoting satiety.[16,17] Peripherally, it enhances glucose-dependent insulin secretion and suppresses glucagon secretion. These effects collectively contribute to both weight reduction and improved metabolic parameters.[18]

Clinical Evidence for Semaglutide in Obesity

The efficacy of semaglutide for weight management has been established in the Semaglutide Treatment Effect in People with Obesity (STEP) trials. Some of the major trials and their inference have been listed below:

- *Step 1:* In adults with obesity without diabetes, semaglutide 2.4 mg weekly plus lifestyle modification led to a mean weight reduction of 14.9% compared to 2.4% with placebo at 68 weeks.[15]
- *Step 2:* In patients with type 2 diabetes, semaglutide 2.4 mg resulted in a mean weight loss of 9.6% versus 3.4% with placebo, along with improved glycemic control.[19]
- *Step 3:* Combining semaglutide with intensive behavioral therapy produced a mean weight reduction of 16%.[20]
- *Step 4:* Withdrawal of semaglutide after initial weight loss resulted in substantial weight regain, emphasizing the need for continued therapy to maintain benefits (21).
- *Step 5:* Long-term data (2 years follow-up) demonstrated sustained weight loss of approximately 15% at 104 weeks.[22]
- SELECT trial: Evaluated semaglutide 2.4 mg in individuals with overweight or obesity and established cardiovascular disease but without diabetes. It included over 17,000 participants, followed up for 40 months. Semaglutide reduced the risk of major adverse cardiovascular events by 20% compared to placebo.[23]

Dosing and Administration

Semaglutide is approved for obesity at a maintenance dose of 2.4 mg subcutaneously once weekly.[24] Treatment begins at 0.25 mg weekly, escalating every 4 weeks through 0.5 mg, 1.0 mg, 1.7 mg, and finally 2.4 mg, to minimize gastrointestinal side effects.[24] Weight loss is typically observed within the first few months and plateaus by 60–70 weeks.

Meta-analyses of STEP trials indicate that semaglutide 2.4 mg yields an average placebo-adjusted weight loss of 10–12%, with 70–75% of participants achieving ≥10% body weight reduction.[25]

Safety and Adverse Effects

GI side effects (nausea, vomiting, diarrhea, and constipation) predominate in the patients receiving Semaglutide and are usually transient and dose dependent.[24] Other notable safety considerations include pancreatitis, gallstone disease, thyroid C-cell tumors, and psychiatric illness. It is contraindicated in patients with a personal/family history of medullary thyroid carcinoma or multiple endocrine neoplasia type 2 (MEN-2).[24]

Clinical Use and Practical Considerations

Semaglutide is indicated for adults with body mass index (BMI) ≥30 kg/m^2 or ≥27 kg/m^2 with at least one weight-related comorbidity.[24] Ongoing lifestyle modification remains essential for optimal results. Because weight regain commonly occurs after discontinuation, long-term treatment is recommended if benefits persist and side effects are manageable.[21,22] Cost and availability remain major barriers to access in many regions.[26]

CONCLUSION

Semaglutide 2.4 mg once weekly has brought revolution in the treatment of obesity. It achieves weight loss, improves cardiometabolic health, and significantly reduces cardiovascular events in high-risk patients. Lifestyle interventions go hand in hand with the drug therapy to achieve target weight loss, prevent relapses, and maintain health benefits. Clinicians need to promote the use of Semaglutide for obesity treatment, particularly those with obesity related complications and diseases.

REFERENCES

1. World Health Organization. Obesity and overweight. [Online] Available from https://www.who.int/news-room/fact-sheets/detail/obesity-and-overweight [Last accessed January 202].

2. World Health Organization. World Obesity Day 2022: Accelerating action to stop obesity. WHO; 2022.
3. Ng M, Fleming T, Robinson M, et al. Global, regional, and national prevalence of overweight and obesity in children and adults 1980–2013: a systematic analysis. Lancet. 2014;384(9945):766-81.
4. Hruby A, Hu FB. The epidemiology of obesity: a big picture. Pharmacoeconomics. 2015;33(7):673-89.
5. Popkin BM, Adair LS, Ng SW. Global nutrition transition and the pandemic of obesity in developing countries. Nutr Rev. 2012;70(1):3-21.
6. Nadolsky K, Garvey WT, Agarwal M, et al. American Association of Clinical Endocrinology Consensus Statement: Algorithm for the Evaluation and Treatment of Adults with Obesity/Adiposity-Based Chronic Disease - 2025 Update. Endocr Pract. 2025;31(11):1351-94.
7. Garvey WT, Mechanick JI, Brett EM, et al. American Association of Clinical Endocrinologists and American College of Endocrinology Comprehensive clinical practice guidelines for medical care of patients with obesity. Endocr Pract. 2016;22(Suppl 3):1-203.
8. Jensen MD, Ryan DH, Apovian CM, et al. 2013 AHA/ACC/TOS guideline for the management of overweight and obesity in adults. J Am Coll Cardiol. 2014;63(25 Pt B): 2985-3023.
9. Hall KD, Kahan S. Maintenance of lost weight and long-term management of obesity. Med Clin North Am. 2018;102(1):183-97.
10. Oppert JM, Bellicha A, van Baak MA, et al. Exercise training in the management of overweight and obesity in adults: synthesis of the evidence and recommendations from the European Association for the Study of Obesity Physical Activity Working Group. Obes Rev. 2021;22 (Suppl 4):e13273.
11. Dawes AJ, Maggard-Gibbons M, Maher AR, et al. Mental health conditions among patients seeking and undergoing bariatric surgery: a meta-analysis. JAMA. 2016;315(2):150-63.
12. Zhu B, Shi C, Park CG, et al. Effects of sleep restriction on metabolism-related parameters in healthy adults: a comprehensive review and meta-analysis of randomized controlled trials. Sleep Med Rev. 2019;45:18-30.
13. Lin J, Jiang Y, Wang G, et al. Associations of short sleep duration with appetite-regulating hormones and adipokines: a systematic review and meta-analysis. Obes Rev. 2020;21(11):e13051.
14. Chaput J-P, McHill AW, Cox RC, et al. The role of insufficient sleep and circadian misalignment in obesity. Nat Rev Endocrinol. 2023;19(2):82-97.
15. Wilding JPH, Batterham RL, Calanna S, et al. Once-weekly semaglutide in adults with overweight or obesity. N Engl J Med. 2021;384(11):989-1002.
16. Nauck MA, Meier JJ. Incretin hormones: their role in health and disease. Diabetes Obes Metab. 2018;20(Suppl 1):5-21.
17. van Can J, Sloth B, Jensen CB, et al. Effects of the once-daily GLP-1 analogue liraglutide on gastric emptying, appetite, and energy metabolism. Int J Obes. 2014;38(6):784-93.
18. Astrup A, Carraro R, Finer N, et al. Safety, tolerability, and sustained weight loss over 2 years with liraglutide 3.0 mg. Int J Obes. 2012;36(6):843-54.
19. Davies M, Færch L, Jeppesen OK, et al. Semaglutide 2.4 mg once a week in adults with overweight or obesity and type 2 diabetes (STEP 2). Lancet. 2021;397(10278):971-84.
20. Wadden TA, Bailey TS, Billings LK, et al. Effect of subcutaneous semaglutide vs placebo as adjunct to intensive behavioural therapy on body weight. JAMA. 2021;325(14):1403-13.
21. Rubino DM, Greenway FL, Khalid U, et al. Effect of continued weekly subcutaneous semaglutide vs withdrawal on weight maintenance. JAMA. 2021;325(14):1414-25.
22. Wadden TA, Hollander P, Klein S, et al. Sustained weight loss with once-weekly semaglutide 2.4 mg over 104 weeks (STEP 5). Nat Med. 2022;28(10):2082-91.
23. Lincoff AM, Bhopalwala HM, Nicholls SJ, et al. Semaglutide and cardiovascular outcomes in obesity without diabetes (SELECT). N Engl J Med. 2023;389(21):1903-16.
24. Novo Nordisk. Wegovy (semaglutide) prescribing information. 2024.
25. Jastreboff AM, Aronne LJ, Ahmad NN, et al. Tirzepatide once weekly for the treatment of obesity. N Engl J Med. 2022;387(3):205-16.
26. Garvey WT, Mechanick JI. Obesity pharmacotherapy barriers: access, coverage, and cost. Endocr Pract. 2023;29(2):121-9.

110

CHAPTER

Obesity, Cardiovascular Disease, and Semaglutide: A Structured Review of the SELECT Trial

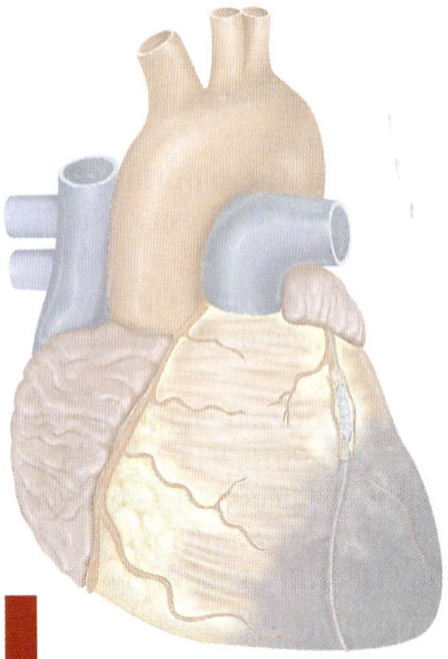

Mrinal Kanti Das

INTRODUCTION

Obesity is a global epidemic affecting over 650 million adults worldwide and a major risk factor for cardiovascular disease (CVD), the leading cause of mortality worldwide. Excess adiposity drives metabolic dysfunction, inflammation, and vascular damage, culminating in increased risk of myocardial infarction, stroke, and heart failure.[1] Traditional lifestyle interventions often fail to achieve sustained weight loss, highlighting the need for pharmacological therapies. Semaglutide offers a novel therapeutic approach, with evidence from the SELECT trial supporting its cardiovascular benefits.[2]

OBESITY–CARDIOVASCULAR DISEASE AXIS

There is a complex interplay of different mechanisms by which obesity majorly results in CVD. These are:

- *Endothelial dysfunction:* Obesity reduced nitric oxide bioavailability, increased adhesion molecules.
- *Atherosclerosis:* Obesity leads to lipid accumulation and plaque formation.
- *Hypertension:* Increased sympathetic tone and vascular stiffness caused by obesity results in hypertension.
- *Insulin resistance:* Obesity also promotes dyslipidemia and accelerates vascular damage.
- *Cardiac remodeling:* This is the fundamental step of different spectrum of heart failure. It initially causes left ventricular hypertrophy and diastolic dysfunction, which when unabated and influenced by other risk factors like inflammation may turn to systolic dysfunction.

HOW GLP-1 RECEPTOR AGONISM WORKS

This is presently a well-talked about originally an anti-diabetic genre of molecules, demonstrating significant anti-obesity activity even in absence of diabetes. The following are the mechanisms of action of GLP-1 RA:

- *GLP-1 receptor activation:* Enhances insulin secretion, suppresses glucagon, and slows gastric emptying.
- *Weight reduction:* Enhancing adipokines specially leptins via hypothalamic pathways causes appetite suppression.
- *Anti-inflammatory effects:* Reduces proinflammatory cytokines (TNF-α, IL-6).
- *Cardiovascular effects:* Improves endothelial function, lowers blood pressure, and reduces atherogenesis.

The SELECT trial, obesity, and cardiovascular outcome:[3,4]

The SELECT trial was a multicenter, randomized, double-blind, placebo-controlled study involving over 17,000 participants with obesity (BMI ≥30 kg/m^2) and established CVD but without diabetes. Participants were randomized to receive once-weekly subcutaneous semaglutide 2.4 mg or placebo. The primary endpoint was the occurrence of MACE, defined as cardiovascular death, nonfatal myocardial infarction, or nonfatal stroke. Secondary endpoints included changes in body weight, blood pressure, and hospitalization rates **(Tables 1 to 5)**.

DISCUSSION

Obesity-cardiometabolic axis is ominous. Breaking the axis was an insightful and sincere approach for long time.

TABLE 1: Participant characteristics.

Characteristic	*Semaglutide group*	*Placebo group*
Number of participants	8,500	8,500
Mean age (years)	61	61
Mean BMI (kg/m^2)	34.5	34.5
Male (%)	*72*	*72*

TABLE 2: Primary outcome.

Outcome	*Semaglutide*	*Placebo*	*Hazard ratio (95% CI)*
Major adverse cardiovascular events (MACE)	7.8%	9.7%	0.80 (0.72–0.88)

TABLE 3: Secondary outcome.

Outcome	*Semaglutide*	*Placebo*
Mean weight reduction (%)	9.4	1.3
Systolic blood pressure reduction (mmHg)	−6.2	−0.5
HbA1c reduction (%)	−0.5	−0.1
Hospitalizations for heart failure	Reduced	*Not specified*

TABLE 4: Summary of MACE reduction.

Subgroup	*Hazard ratio (95% CI)*	*Interpretation*
Age <65 years	0.78 (0.68–0.89)	Significant reduction
Age ≥65 years	0.82 (0.73–0.92)	Significant reduction
Male	0.79 (0.70–0.89)	Significant reduction
Female	0.83 (0.72–0.95)	Significant reduction

TABLE 5: Summary (MACE event-free survival).

Time (months)	*Semaglutide event-free survival (%)*	*Placebo event-free survival (%)*
0	100	100
12	95	93
24	91	87
36	88	83

But the previous molecules had significant adverse effects that resulted in their withdrawal. The SELECT trial provides compelling evidence that GLP-1 RA semaglutide significantly reduces cardiovascular risk in patients with obesity and established CVD. The mechanisms underlying these benefits include weight loss, improved glycemic control, reduced blood pressure, and anti-inflammatory effects. Importantly, these outcomes were achieved in a nondiabetic population, expanding the therapeutic scope of semaglutide. The trial underscores the importance of targeting obesity pharmacologically to mitigate cardiovascular risk. The landmark article by Gerstein HC et al. published in Lancet 2025, presents the SELECT trial, a life-changing study evaluating the cardiovascular benefits of semaglutide in patients with obesity and established cardiovascular disease but without diabetes. The trial's robust design, involving over 17,000 participants, provides strong evidence that semaglutide significantly reduces the risk of major adverse cardiovascular events by 20% relative to placebo. Secondary benefits include substantial weight loss, improved blood pressure, and better glycemic control, even in nondiabetic patients.

The study highlights the multifaceted mechanisms by which semaglutide exerts cardiovascular protection, including weight reduction, anti-inflammatory effects, and metabolic improvements. The findings are particularly important as they extend the use of GLP-1 receptor agonists beyond diabetic populations to those with obesity and cardiovascular risk alone.

Overall, the SELECT trial represents a significant advancement in obesity and cardiovascular disease management, supporting semaglutide as an effective pharmacological intervention to reduce cardiovascular morbidity and mortality in this high-risk population. The article is well-structured, comprehensive, and provides valuable insights for clinicians and researchers alike.

CONCLUSION

Semaglutide represents a promising advancement in the management of obesity and its cardiovascular complications. The SELECT trial confirms its efficacy in reducing MACE and improving cardiometabolic parameters. Future research should explore long-term outcomes and potential benefits in broader populations.

REFERENCES

1. Jastreboff AM, Aronne LJ, Ahmad NN, et al. Obesity as a disease: the obesity society position statement. Obesity (Silver Spring). 2015.
2. Buse JB, Rosenstock J, Sargent J, et al. Semaglutide in adults with overweight or obesity. N Engl J Med. 2020.
3. Gerstein HC, Colhoun HM, Dagenais GR, et al. Semaglutide and cardiovascular outcomes in patients with obesity: SELECT trial. Lancet. 2025.
4. Nicholls SJ, Ryan DH, Deanfield J, et al. Semaglutide and hospitalizations in patients with obesity and established cardiovascular disease: SELECT trial analysis. JAMA Cardiol. 2025:e254824.

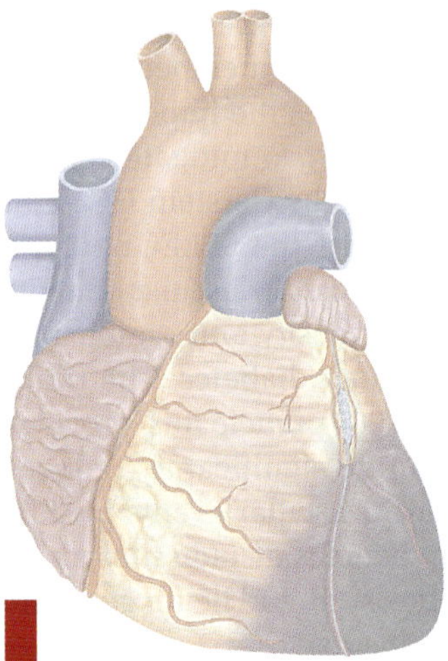

CHAPTER 111

Trials of Semaglutide in Weight Management

AK Pancholia, HK Chopra

INTRODUCTION

For individuals with overweight or obesity, lifestyle modification is the guideline-recommended foundation of treatment,[1-4] but weight loss is modest and is often regained on discontinuation.[5] Pharmacological treatments for obesity provide a valuable adjunct to lifestyle interventions, but until recently, the available agents only offered moderate weight loss over that achieved with lifestyle intervention.[6] Semaglutide is a potent long-acting glucagon-like peptide-1 (GLP-1) analog that requires once-weekly administration.[7] The Semaglutide Treatment Effect in People with Obesity (STEP) clinical trial development program is evaluating once-weekly subcutaneous semaglutide 2.4 mg in people with overweight or obesity. Based on data from the STEP trials, once-weekly subcutaneous semaglutide 2.4 mg has been approved in Canada, Europe, the UK, and the USA for chronic weight management in adults with overweight (with weight-related comorbidities) or obesity.[8-11]

TRIALS OF SEMAGLUTIDE FOR WEIGHT LOSS

STEP Program

STEP 1

STEP 1 was the largest randomized trial of semaglutide 2.4 mg weekly. In this 68-week trial, nondiabetic, obese participants were randomly assigned weekly subcutaneous semaglutide or matching placebo along with low-calorie diet.[12] At week 68, semaglutide-treated participants lost an average of 14.9% of baseline weight, compared with 2.4% for those assigned to placebo, along with improvements in several cardiometabolic risk factors, including waist circumference, systolic and diastolic blood pressure, and glycated hemoglobin A1c (HbA1c), with favorable safety and efficacy data.

STEP 2

STEP 2 was a 68-week trial of obese adults with type 2 diabetes who were assigned to once-weekly semaglutide 2.4 mg, semaglutide 1.0 mg, or matching placebo.[13] At week 68, participants treated with semaglutide 2.4 mg, semaglutide 1.0 mg, and placebo lost a mean of 9.6, 7.0, and 3.4% of baseline body weight, respectively. Thus, the 2.4 mg dose significantly increased weight loss, compared to 1.0 mg and placebo, with reduction in HbA1c, systolic and diastolic blood pressure, and other cardiometabolic risk factors.

STEP 3[14]

It was a 68-week trial that compared once-weekly subcutaneous semaglutide 2.4 mg with placebo as an adjunct to intensive behavioral therapy (IBT) and an initial low-calorie meal-replacement diet for all participants. Participants who received IBT along with semaglutide 2.4 mg lost 16.0% of body weight at week 68.

STEP 4[15]

It was a 68-week withdrawal trial, designed to assess the effect on weight change of continuing versus discontinuing once-weekly subcutaneous semaglutide

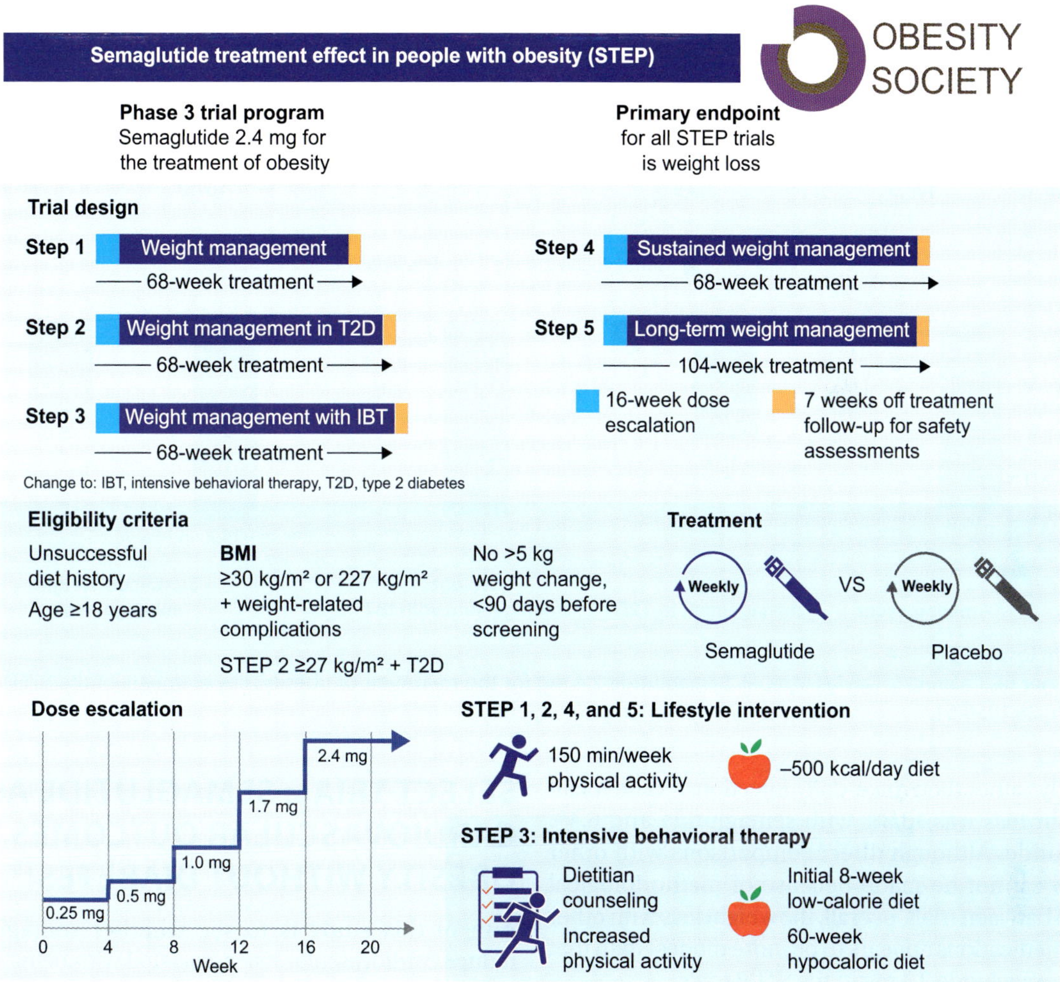

Fig. 1: Key elements of the STEP program.

Source: Kushner RF, Calanna S, Davies M, et al. Semaglutide 2.4 mg for the treatment of obesity: key elements of the STEP trials 1 to 5. Obesity. 2020;28:1050-61.

2.4 mg after an initial 20-week semaglutide run-in period. After 48 weeks of randomization, participants assigned to remain on semaglutide lost an additional 7.1 kg, resulting in a net 17.4% reduction in baseline weight. Placebo-treated participants, by contrast, gained 6.1 kg after randomization. Thus, results of STEP 4 reveal that weight regain is likely when semaglutide is terminated **(Figs. 1 and 2)**.

STEP 5[16]

This is the longest trial of the STEP program (104 weeks), where obese participants with or without diabetes were randomized to receive once-weekly subcutaneous semaglutide 2.4 mg or matching placebo.[16] Compared with 2.6% weight loss in placebo group, the semaglutide arm had 15.2% weight loss with greater improvement in cardiometabolic risk factors.

STEP 6[17]

It was a 68-week trial in adults from East Asia with a body mass index (BMI) of ≥27.0 kg/m^2 with ≥2 weight-related comorbidities or a BMI of ≥35.0 kg/m^2 with ≥1 weight-related comorbidity (one comorbidity had to be either hypertension, dyslipidemia, or, in Japan only, type 2 diabetes). Participants were randomized to semaglutide 2.4 mg, 1.7 mg, or placebo. The average decrease in body weight at week 68 was 13.2% in the semaglutide 2.4 mg group and 9.6% in the semaglutide 1.7 mg group versus 2.1% in the placebo group.

STEP 8

It is the first direct comparison of semaglutide with another weight-management medication, liraglutide, in a randomized trial. Semaglutide 2.4 mg demonstrated better efficacy than liraglutide, offering more convenient

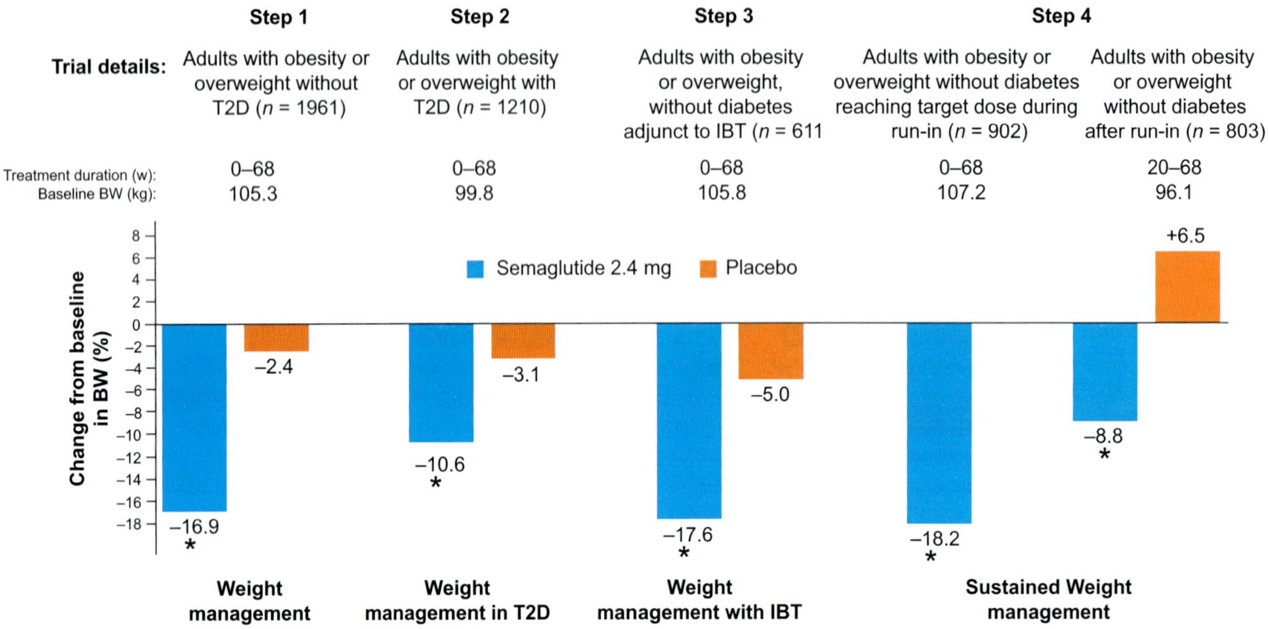

Fig. 2: Weight loss in STEP 1–4.
Source: Kushner RF, Calanna S, Davies M, et al. Semaglutide 2.4 mg for the treatment of obesity: key elements of the STEP trials 1 to 5. Obesity. 2020;28:1050-61.

once-weekly rather than once-daily injections.[18] The mean body weight loss was 15.8% with semaglutide and 6.4% with liraglutide. Although direct comparisons with other treatments cannot be made because of methodological differences between trials, overall, the weight loss with other approved medications appears to be more modest than that seen with semaglutide 2.4 mg in the STEP trials.

Efficacy Outcome

All the trials in the STEP program met the primary endpoint. Across the 68-week-long trials in individuals with overweight or obesity but without type 2 diabetes (STEP 1, 3, 4, and 8), semaglutide 2.4 mg was associated with a mean weight loss of 14.9–17.4% from baseline.[14,15,18] Furthermore, >84% participants were receiving the full dose of semaglutide at week 68.

Contraindications

- Medullary thyroid carcinoma (MTC) and multiple endocrine neoplasia syndrome type 2 (MEN 2)
- Hypersensitivity
- Pregnancy

Adverse Effects

- Acute pancreatitis, pancreatic cancer
- Gallbladder disease
- Gastrointestinal adverse reactions

SELECT TRIAL: SEMAGLUTIDE AND CARDIOVASCULAR OUTCOMES IN OBESITY WITHOUT DIABETES[19]

Aim of this study is to see whether semaglutide can reduce cardiovascular risk associated with being overweight and obesity in the absence of diabetes. It has enrolled patients 45 years of age or older who had preexisting cardiovascular disease and a BMI of 27 or greater, but no history of diabetes. A primary cardiovascular endpoint event occurred in 5% in the semaglutide group and in 8.0% in the placebo group So to conclude, in patients with preexisting cardiovascular disease and overweight or obesity but without diabetes, weekly subcutaneous semaglutide at a dose of 2.4 mg was superior to placebo in reducing the incidence of death from cardiovascular causes, nonfatal myocardial infarction, or nonfatal stroke at a mean follow-up of 39.8 months **(Fig. 3)**.

STEP TEENS TRIAL: ONCE-WEEKLY SEMAGLUTIDE IN ADOLESCENTS WITH OBESITY[20]

This study aims to see the effect of inj. semaglutide 2.4 mg once a week in adolescents (12–18 years) who are overweight or obese and have at least one weight-related coexisting condition. Substantial reduction in BMI is seen in the active arm compared to that in placebo

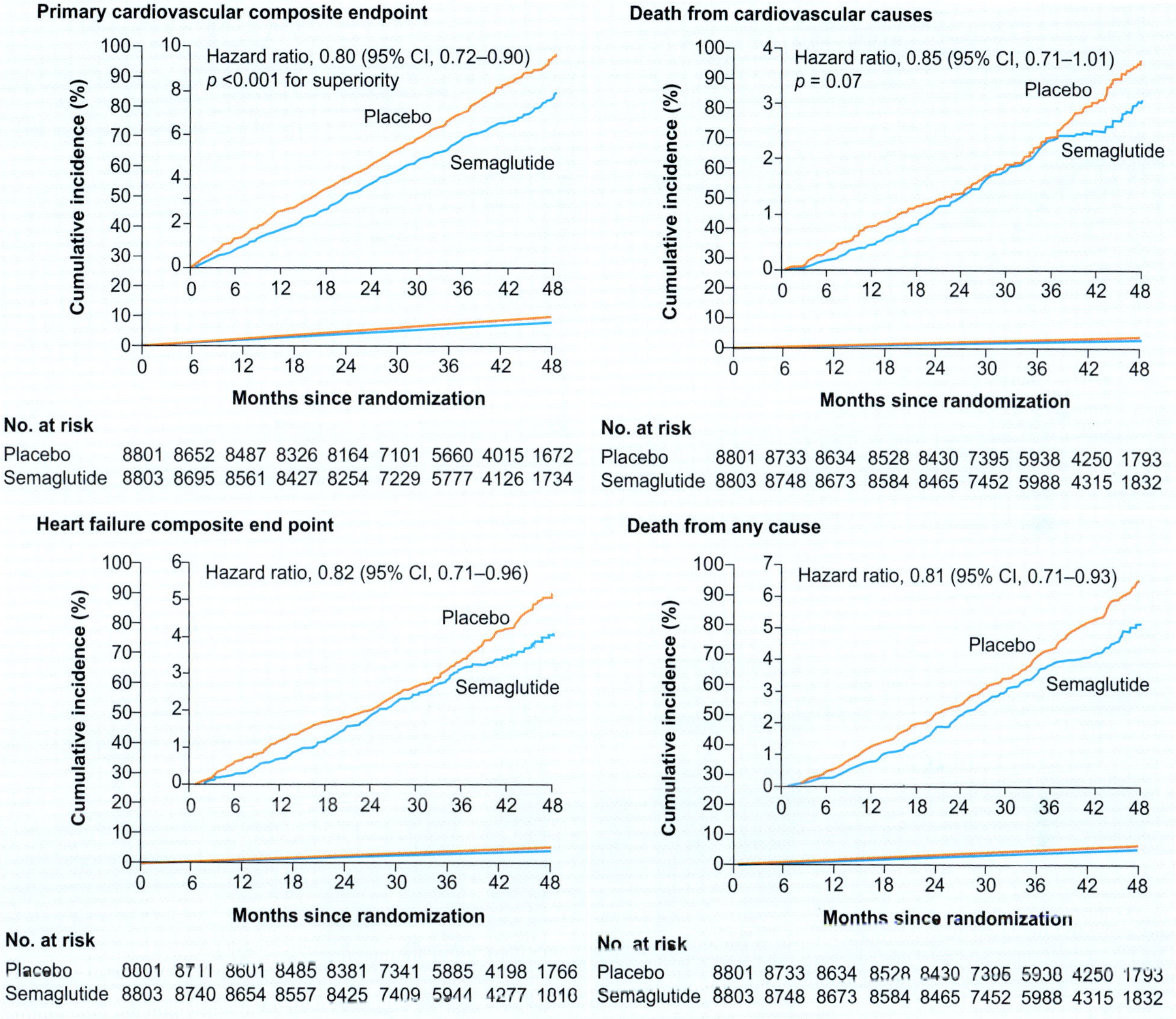

Fig. 3: Time-to-first-event analysis for primary and confirmatory secondary efficacy endpoints.
Source: Lincoff AM, Brown-Frandsen K, Colhoun HM, et al. Semaglutide and cardiovascular outcomes in obesity without diabetes. N Engl J Med. 2023;389(24):2221-32.

(–16.1 vs. 0.6%). Serious adverse events were reported in 11% of the semaglutide group and 9% of the placebo group. Thus, it is concluded that among adolescents with obesity, once-weekly treatment with a 2.4 mg dose of semaglutide plus lifestyle intervention resulted in a greater reduction in BMI than lifestyle intervention alone.

SCORE TRIAL: SEMAGLUTIDE EFFECTS ON CARDIOVASCULAR OUTCOMES IN PEOPLE WITH OVERWEIGHT OR OBESITY IN THE REAL WORLD[21]

Objective of this study was to see the effect of once-a-week inj. semaglutide 2.4 mg in individuals who are overweight or obese and have atherosclerotic cardiovascular disease (ASCVD). Over a mean follow-up of 200 days, semaglutide 2.4 mg was associated with significantly lower risks of revised MACE (myocardial infarction, stroke, and all-cause mortality). Semaglutide 2.4 mg was also associated with lower risks of all-cause mortality, cardiovascular-related mortality, and hospitalization for heart failure.

STEP UP TRIAL[22]

The objective of this study was to see the safety and efficacy of higher dose of semaglutide (7.2 mg) in people with obesity and related complications, and also to compare with 2.4 mg semaglutide once a week. After 72 weeks, the mean change in body weight was greater with

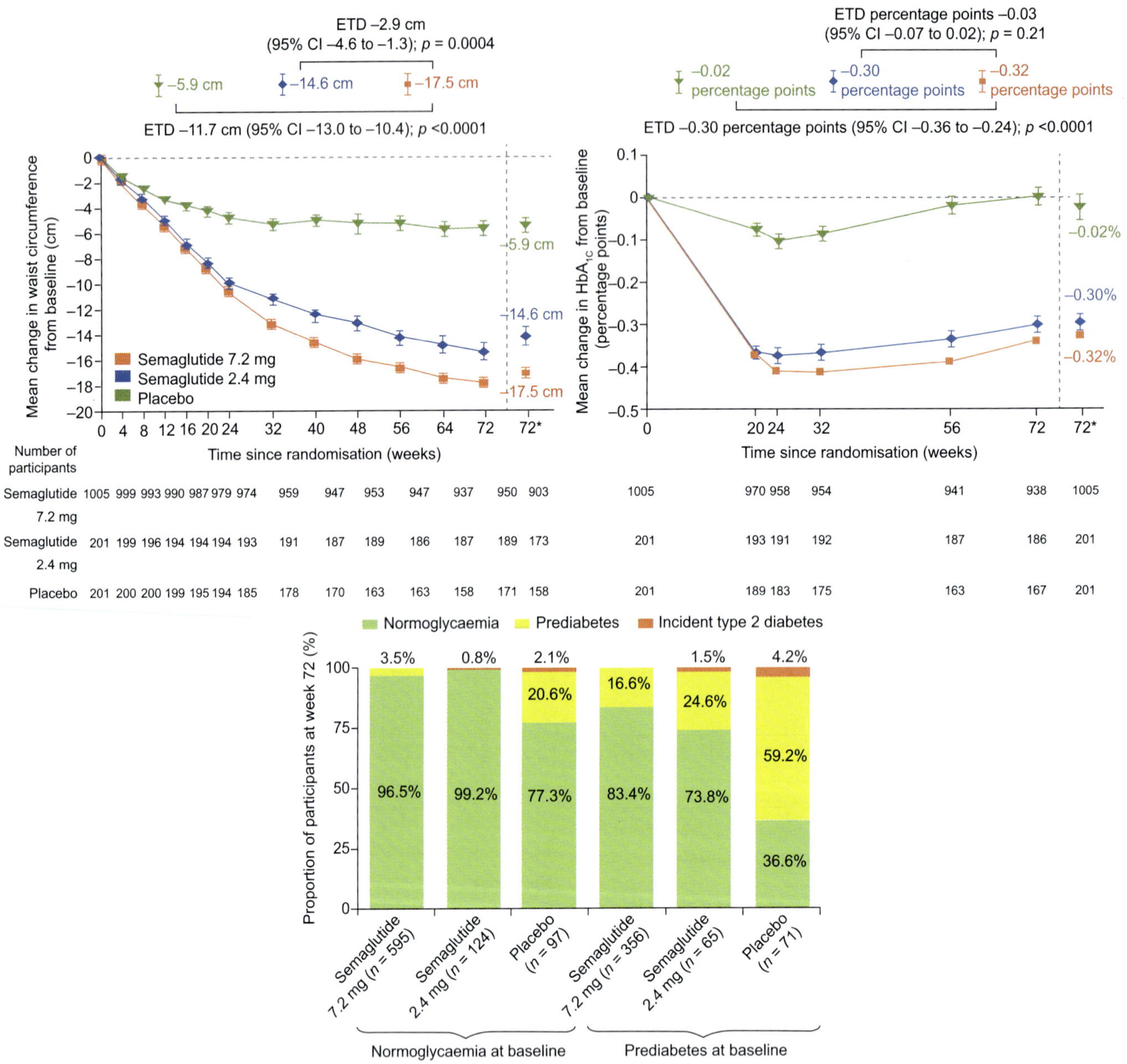

Figs. 4A to C: STEP UP trial result.

Source: Wharton S, Freitas P, Hjelmesæth J, et al. Once-weekly semaglutide 7.2 mg in adults with obesity (STEP UP): a randomised, controlled, phase 3b trial. Lancet Diabetes Endocrinol. 2025;13(11):949-63.

semaglutide 7.2 mg versus 2.4 mg (–18.7 vs. –15.6%). Gastrointestinal adverse events were more common with semaglutide 7.2 mg (70.8 vs. 61.2%) or placebo (42.8%) **(Figs. 4A to C)**.

CONCLUSION

The STEP clinical trial program has demonstrated the efficacy and tolerability of once-weekly subcutaneous semaglutide 2.4 mg in individuals with overweight or obesity with or without diabetes. Across the STEP trials, once-weekly subcutaneous semaglutide 2.4 mg was consistently associated with mean weight losses of 14.9–17.4% in participants without diabetes, and improvements in cardiometabolic risk factors, physical function, and quality of life. Furthermore, the safety profile of semaglutide 2.4 mg was comparable to that of other GLP-1RA class.

REFERENCES

1. Garvey WT, Mechanick JI, Brett EM, et al. American Association of Clinical Endocrinologists and American College of Endocrinology comprehensive clinical practice guidelines for medical care of patients with obesity. Endocr Pract. 2016;22(Suppl 3):1-203.
2. Durrer Schutz D, Busetto L, Dicker D, et al. European practical and patient-centred guidelines for adult obesity management in primary care. Obes Facts. 2019;12(1): 40-66.
3. Jensen MD, Ryan DH, Apovian CM, et al. AHA/ACC/TOS guideline for the management of overweight and obesity in adults: a report of the American College of Cardiology/ American Heart Association Task Force on Practice Guidelines and The Obesity Society. J Am Coll Cardiol. 2014;63(25 Pt B):2985-3023.
4. Yumuk V, Tsigos C, Fried M, et al. European guidelines for obesity management in adults. Obes Facts. 2015; 8(6):402-24.
5. Wadden TA, Tronieri JS, Butryn ML. Lifestyle modification approaches for the treatment of obesity in adults. Am Psychol. 2020;75(2):235-51.
6. Singh AK, Singh R. Pharmacotherapy in obesity: a systematic review and meta-analysis of randomized controlled trials of anti-obesity drugs. Expert Rev Clin Pharmacol. 2020;13(1):53-64.
7. Blundell J, Finlayson G, Axelsen M, et al. Effects of once-weekly semaglutide on appetite, energy intake, control of eating, food preference and body weight in subjects with obesity. Diabetes Obes Metab. 2017;19(9):1242-51.
8. Novo Nordisk. (2021). WEGOVY (semaglutide) highlights of prescribing information. [online] Available from https://www.novo-pi.com/wegovy.pdf [Last accessed January, 2026].
9. Medicines & Healthcare Products Regulatory Agency. (2022). Wegovy 2.4 mg, solution for injection in pre-filled pen - summary of product characteristics. [online] Available from https://mhraproducts4853.blob.core.windows.net/docs/4b161649ffc66e938bc76f4e45a4d3797af54914 [Last accessed January, 2026].
10. European Medicines Agency. (2022). Wegovy - summary of product characteristics. [online] Available from https://www.ema.europa.eu/en/medicines/human/EPAR/wegovy [Last accessed January, 2026].
11. Health Canada. (2022). Wegovy - product monograph. [online] Available from https://health-products.canada.ca/dpd-bdpp/info.do?lang=en&code=101171 [Last accessed January, 2026].
12. Wilding JPH, Batterham RL, Calanna S, et al. Once-weekly semaglutide in adults with overweight or obesity. N Engl J Med. 2021;384(11):989-1002.
13. Davies M, Færch L, Jeppesen OK, et al. Semaglutide 2.4 mg once a week in adults with overweight or obesity, and type 2 diabetes (STEP 2): a randomised, double-blind, double-dummy, placebo-controlled, phase 3 trial. Lancet. 2021;397(10278):971-84.
14. Wadden TA, Bailey TS, Billings LK, et al. Effect of subcutaneous semaglutide vs placebo as an adjunct to intensive behavioral therapy on body weight in adults with overweight or obesity: the STEP 3 randomized clinical trial. JAMA. 2021;325(14):1403-13.
15. Rubino D, Abrahamsson N, Davies M, et al. Effect of continued weekly subcutaneous semaglutide vs placebo on weight loss maintenance in adults with overweight or obesity: the STEP 4 randomized clinical trial. JAMA. 2021;325(14):1414-25.
16. Garvey WT, Batterham RL, Bhatta M, et al. Two-year effect of semaglutide 2.4 mg once-weekly in adults with overweight or obesity (STEP 5): a randomized, double-blind, placebo controlled, phase 3 trial. Nat Med. 2022;28(10):2083-91.
17. Kadowaki T, Isendahl J, Khalid U, et al. Semaglutide once a week in adults with overweight or obesity, with or without type 2 diabetes in an East Asian population (STEP 6): a randomised, double-blind, double-dummy, placebo-controlled, phase 3a trial. Lancet Diabetes Endocrinol. 2022;10(3):193-206.
18. Rubino DM, Greenway FL, Khalid U, et al. Effect of weekly subcutaneous semaglutide vs daily liraglutide on body weight in adults with overweight or obesity without diabetes: the STEP 8 randomized clinical trial. JAMA. 2022;327(2):138-50.
19. Lincoff AM, Brown-Frandsen K, Colhoun HM, et al. Semaglutide and cardiovascular outcomes in obesity without diabetes. N Engl J Med. 2023;389(24):2221-32.
20. Weghuber D, Barrett T, Barrientos-Pérez M, et al. Once-weekly semaglutide in adolescents with obesity. N Engl J Med. 2022;387(24):2245-57.
21. Smolderen KG, Mena-Hurtado C, Zhao Z, et al. Lower risk of cardiovascular events in patients initiated on semaglutide 2.4 mg in the real world: results from the SCORE study (Semaglutide Effects on Cardiovascular Outcomes in People with Overweight or Obesity in the Real World). Diabetes Obes Metab. 2025;27(11):6691-704.
22. Wharton S, Freitas P, Hjelmesæth J, et al. Once-weekly semaglutide 7.2 mg in adults with obesity (STEP UP): a randomised, controlled, phase 3b trial. Lancet Diabetes Endocrinol. 2025;13(11):949-63.

112

CHAPTER

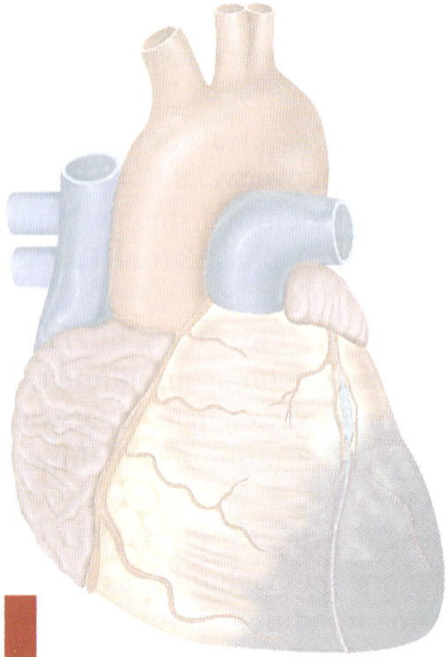

Semaglutide: A Novel Therapeutic Approach to Obesity-related HFpEF

Arjun Tandon, Aditya Kapoor

INTRODUCTION

Heart failure with preserved ejection fraction (HFpEF) has emerged as one of the most challenging syndromes in contemporary cardiology. Once considered a minority phenotype, it now accounts for nearly half of all heart failure cases worldwide, and its prevalence continues to rise in parallel with aging populations, the global obesity epidemic, and the growing burden of metabolic diseases such as type 2 diabetes mellitus (T2DM) and hypertension.[1] Unlike heart failure with reduced ejection fraction (HFrEF), where therapies such as β-blockers, ACE inhibitors, and mineralocorticoid receptor antagonists have demonstrated robust survival benefits, HFpEF has long resisted therapeutic progress. For many patients, the clinical course is characterized by persistent symptoms, impaired quality of life, frequent hospitalizations, and frustratingly limited options for disease-modifying treatment.[2]

Among the many subtypes of HFpEF, the obesity-related phenotype is particularly striking. Patients with obesity-driven HFpEF is often present at a younger age, with severe exercise intolerance, higher left atrial and ventricular filling pressures, and striking systemic congestion despite preserved systolic function. The pathophysiology is complex and multifaceted—adipose tissue promotes systemic inflammation, alters myocardial energetics, and increases epicardial fat deposition, leading to stiffness, fibrosis, and diastolic dysfunction.[3] In addition, obesity worsens associated comorbidities such as sleep apnea, hypertension, and insulin resistance, all of which amplify the hemodynamic burden on the heart. In this context, it is not surprising that conventional heart failure therapies have delivered only modest benefits in this population.[4]

This therapeutic gap has fueled interest in strategies that address the root cause—excess adiposity and its metabolic consequences. Glucagon-like peptide-1 receptor agonists (GLP-1RAs), originally developed for glucose control in T2DM, have emerged as powerful agents capable of producing double-digit weight loss, improving insulin sensitivity, and exerting favorable effects on inflammation and cardiovascular risk factors. Semaglutide, a long-acting GLP-1RA, has generated excitement due to its consistent benefits across trials of obesity and diabetes.[5]

In 2023, the STEP-HFpEF trial provided a breakthrough moment. For the first time, a pharmacological agent specifically improved symptoms, exercise capacity, and quality of life in patients with obesity-related HFpEF.[1] These findings suggest that semaglutide may represent more than a weight-loss drug—it could be the first disease-modifying therapy tailored to this challenging HFpEF phenotype. The potential to improve not just survival curves but also daily-lived experiences—breathing easier, walking further, and reclaiming quality of life—marks a new era of hope for patients long underserved by heart failure therapeutics.

PATHOPHYSIOLOGICAL LINK BETWEEN OBESITY AND HFpEF

- *Hemodynamic alterations:* In obesity, excess adiposity leads to chronic volume overload. Expanded plasma volume and higher left atrial pressures increase wall stress, while systemic hypertension amplifies afterload, straining a ventricle already vulnerable to impaired relaxation.[6]

- *Metabolic inflammation:* Adipose tissue functions as an active endocrine organ, releasing adipokines, cytokines, and free fatty acids that disrupt myocardial energetics and promote oxidative stress. Insulin resistance further compromises diastolic relaxation and enhances interstitial fibrosis.[7] These systemic changes contribute to ventricular stiffening despite preserved systolic function.
- *Epicardial adiposity and fibrosis:* Epicardial adipose tissue exerts direct paracrine effects on the myocardium, secreting proinflammatory mediators that promote myocardial steatosis and fibrosis.[8] Imaging studies demonstrate increased epicardial fat volume and adverse remodeling in obese HFpEF, correlating with worse diastolic function.
- *Impaired exercise capacity:* Patients with obesity-related HFpEF exhibit profound exercise intolerance, reflected in reduced peak VO_2 and diminished 6-minute walk distance. This limitation results from impaired diastolic filling, endothelial dysfunction, and peripheral skeletal muscle abnormalities.[9] Clinically, patients often report exertional breathlessness and fatigue during minimal activity.
- *Limited response to conventional therapy:* The obesity-HFpEF phenotype is distinct in its pathophysiology, explaining the limited efficacy of traditional heart failure therapies such as ACE inhibitors, β-blockers, and MRAs. Disease modification requires targeting adiposity and its metabolic consequences rather than neurohormonal pathways alone.[10]

SEMAGLUTIDE: MECHANISM OF ACTION RELEVANT TO HFpEF

- *Weight reduction and hemodynamic benefits:* For many patients with obesity-related HFpEF, even simple daily tasks such as climbing a flight of stairs can feel exhausting. A major driver of this limitation is the extra weight, which places constant strain on the heart. Semaglutide, a GLP-1RA, has shown an unprecedented ability to achieve sustained weight loss of 15–20% of body weight.[5] This reduction translates into less blood volume for the heart to pump, lower filling pressures, and reduced wall stress—physiological improvements that patients often experience as lighter breathing and greater stamina in daily life.
- *Improvement in metabolic homeostasis:* Obesity-related HFpEF is not only about weight; it is also about a "metabolic storm" of insulin resistance, inflammation, and abnormal lipid metabolism. Semaglutide addresses these processes at their roots. By improving insulin sensitivity and lowering blood glucose—even in patients without diabetes—it helps restore energy balance in heart muscle cells.[11] It also reduces circulating inflammatory signals from fat tissue,[12] calming the systemic inflammation that stiffens the heart. Improvements in cholesterol and triglycerides add another layer of cardiovascular protection, helping patients feel healthier beyond weight loss alone.
- *Cardiac remodeling and epicardial fat reduction:* Excess fat around the heart, called epicardial adipose tissue, is not just "silent padding"—it releases harmful signals that trigger fibrosis and stiffening of the myocardium. Semaglutide has been shown to shrink this fat depot,[13] easing both mechanical pressure and inflammatory injury to the heart. With therapy, echocardiographic and imaging data reveal healthier filling patterns and improved left atrial function, reflecting not just symptom relief but true biological reversal of disease processes.
- *Enhancement of functional capacity*: What matters most to patients is the ability to walk further, breathe easier, and live more actively. In the STEP-HFpEF trial, semaglutide improved exercise capacity—measured as higher peak VO_2 and longer 6-minute walk distances—while also boosting quality-of-life scores on the KCCQ.[1] For patients, this translates into regaining independence and confidence in daily activities.
- *Integrated mechanistic perspective*: Taken together, semaglutide targets every pillar of obesity-related HFpEF: It reduces body weight, improves metabolic balance, shrinks harmful cardiac fat, and restores physical capacity.[8] Unlike conventional therapies that only manage symptoms, semaglutide offers the first glimpse of true disease modification in this long-neglected patient group.

CLINICAL TRIALS EVIDENCE

- The GLP-1RA semaglutide has emerged as a transformative therapy for obesity, with growing evidence of benefit in HFpEF.
- *STEP Trials—proof of concept in obesity*: The STEP[14] program demonstrated that once-weekly semaglutide 2.4 mg produces sustained weight loss of 15–20% of baseline body weight in patients with or without diabetes. Beyond weight reduction, semaglutide improved blood pressure, glycemic control, and lipid profiles, thereby mitigating cardiometabolic risk factors. While not HFpEF-specific, these systemic effects suggested downstream cardiovascular benefits by reducing cardiac loading conditions, systemic inflammation, and vascular stiffness.

- *STEP-HFpEF—first disease-modifying trial in obesity-HFpEF*: Published in 2023, STEP-HFpEF[1] provided the first randomized, placebo-controlled evidence of pharmacological benefit in obese HFpEF. Over 52 weeks, semaglutide significantly improved the KCCQ-Clinical Summary Score (CSS), reflecting better symptom burden, functional status, and quality of life. Functional gains included longer 6-minute walk distances and reductions in NT-pro-BNP. Greater weight loss in the semaglutide arm reinforced the central role of adiposity reduction in mediating these improvements. Clinically, patients experienced less exertional dyspnea and greater ability to perform daily activities—clear, tangible benefits in a condition historically lacking effective medical therapies.
- *SELECT—cardiovascular outcomes in obesity with heart failure*: The SELECT trial (2024)[15] enrolled 17,604 adults with overweight/obesity and established cardiovascular disease. Semaglutide reduced major adverse cardiovascular events (MACEs), including a 28% lower risk of nonfatal myocardial infarction and a nonsignificant 15% reduction in cardiovascular death. Importantly, semaglutide decreased composite heart failure events (cardiovascular death, urgent visits, or hospitalization) by 18% and reduced all-cause mortality by 19%. These findings extend the benefit of semaglutide from weight loss and metabolic improvement to hard cardiovascular endpoints, including in patients with prevalent heart failure.
- *Future directions*: Ongoing trials are investigating semaglutide's impact on cardiac structure (e.g., left ventricular mass, diastolic filling pressures), renal outcomes, and long-term cardiovascular mortality. These studies will clarify whether the symptomatic and intermediate functional improvements observed in STEP-HFpEF translate into durable reductions in hospitalization and disease progression.

Together, the STEP and SELECT programs position semaglutide as the first therapy to target both obesity and its cardiovascular sequelae, offering a paradigm shift in the management of obesity-related HFpEF.

COMPARATIVE POSITION WITH OTHER THERAPIES

Management of HFpEF has historically been limited, with no single therapy addressing the syndrome's heterogeneous pathophysiology. Over the past few years, sodium–glucose cotransporter 2 (SGLT2) inhibitors and GLP-1RAs such as semaglutide have emerged as promising contenders, each targeting different dimensions of the disease.

Sodium–glucose Cotransporter 2 Inhibitors

Sodium-glucose cotransporter-2 inhibitors, including empagliflozin and dapagliflozin, represent the first drug class to consistently demonstrate reductions in heart failure hospitalizations and improvements in quality of life across the HFpEF spectrum, irrespective of diabetes status.[16,17] Their benefits are thought to stem from favorable effects on renal function, preload and afterload reduction, improved myocardial energetics, and reductions in systemic inflammation. Importantly, however, their weight-lowering effect is modest—typically in the range of 1–3 kg[18]—limiting their ability to directly address obesity-driven hemodynamic stress, a dominant mechanism in many HFpEF patients.

Semaglutide

In contrast, semaglutide has demonstrated unparalleled weight reduction (15–20% of baseline body weight) in obese individuals.[5] The STEP-HFpEF trial showed clinically meaningful improvements in symptoms, exercise capacity, and biomarkers of cardiac strain in patients with obesity-related HFpEF.[1] More recently, the SELECT trial extended these observations to hard outcomes, reporting reductions in MACEs and composite heart failure endpoints.[15] These effects suggest that semaglutide directly targets the obesity–HFpEF phenotype by unloading the heart through weight loss, improving metabolic profile, and reducing systemic inflammation. For many patients, this translates into tangible day-to-day improvements: Climbing stairs with less breathlessness, walking farther without fatigue, and regaining independence in daily life.

COMBINATION THERAPY: A FUTURE SYNERGY?

Given their distinct mechanisms, the combination of GLP-1RAs and SGLT2 inhibitors is an area of growing interest. Preclinical and early clinical data suggest complementary pathways: Semaglutide induces profound weight reduction and metabolic benefits, while SGLT2 inhibitors optimize hemodynamics and renal protection.[19] Together, these therapies may synergistically address both the "congestion" and the "comorbidity" dimensions of HFpEF. Trials are currently underway to assess whether such dual therapy can produce additive improvements in symptoms, functional capacity, and long-term outcomes. If proven effective, this combination could represent a paradigm shift, offering personalized therapy tailored to obesity-driven HFpEF while maintaining broad efficacy across phenotypes.

LIMITATIONS

While semaglutide represents a major advance for obesity-related HFpEF, several caveats deserve attention. First, most trial participants were obese with HFpEF, raising uncertainty about whether the benefits extend to lean HFpEF phenotypes, where mechanisms may differ. Second, the evidence base is largely medium-term. Improvements in symptoms, exercise tolerance, and biomarkers are encouraging, but whether these translate into sustained reductions in mortality or long-term morbidity remains unproven.

Practical challenges also matter. Semaglutide is costly, and its availability is uneven across regions, potentially widening gaps in care between those who can and cannot afford therapy. Adverse effects, though generally manageable, must not be overlooked: Gastrointestinal intolerance is common and rare but serious risks such as pancreatitis and gallbladder disease remain a concern.

Finally, real-world integration is still evolving. Data on how semaglutide interacts with cornerstone HF therapies—SGLT2 inhibitors, mineralocorticoid receptor antagonists, and angiotensin receptor-neprilysin inhibitors—are sparse. Patients and clinicians alike are asking whether these drugs complement one another or compete for benefit. Until head-to-head and combination trials are completed, semaglutide's precise role in the broader therapeutic armamentarium for HFpEF remains an exciting but as yet unfinished story.

LATEST GUIDELINES AND RECOMMENDATIONS

International guidance is converging on a pragmatic stance: *Use semaglutide primarily to treat obesity (and reduce CV risk) in people with HFpEF*, while formal HFpEF-specific guideline class recommendations are still evolving.

- *American College of Cardiology (ACC)*: A 2025 Expert Consensus on medical weight management for cardiovascular health recognizes *semaglutide 2.4 mg weekly* as an evidence-based option for patients with obesity and CVD, and notes *signal of benefit in obesity-related HFpEF* based on STEP-HFpEF, encouraging incorporation within multidisciplinary obesity care for HF populations. It stops short of issuing a class recommendation for HFpEF outcomes pending longer term data.[20]
- *American Diabetes Association (ADA) Standards of Care 2024/2025:* Endorse *antiobesity pharmacotherapy*—including semaglutide 2.4 mg—for adults with obesity when lifestyle therapy is insufficient, citing cardiometabolic risk reduction and recent CV-outcome data; HFpEF patients with obesity can be considered under these criteria.[21]
- *Evidence summaries for cardiology practice* (*ACC Journal* Scans) highlight that semaglutide improves *KCCQ-CSS, 6-minute walk distance, CRP, and weight* in obesity-related HFpEF, supporting clinical adoption in appropriate patients while awaiting event-driven HF endpoints.[22]
- *European Society of Cardiology (ESC):* The 2023 focused HF update predates STEP-HFpEF; ESC has *no HFpEF-specific recommendation for GLP-1 RAs yet*, but acknowledges obesity as a modifiable target in HF.[23]
- *Regulatory context:* The *FDA* added a CV-risk-reduction indication to Wegovy (semaglutide), reinforcing its role in cardiometabolic care pathways that include many HFpEF patients with obesity.[24]

CONCLUSION

- *Obesity is a key driver of HFpEF*—fueling symptoms, functional decline, and poor outcomes beyond the effects of hypertension or diabetes
- *Conventional HF therapies* (ACEi, ARNi, β-blockers, MRAs, SGLT2i) provide modest benefits but do not adequately address the obesity-HFpEF phenotype.
- *Semaglutide has changed the landscape*—inducing 15–20% weight loss, improving peak VO_2, 6-minute walk distance, NT-pro-BNP, and patient-reported quality of life.
- *STEP-HFpEF and SELECT trials* demonstrated consistent benefits across exercise capacity, symptom burden, and cardiometabolic risk, marking a paradigm shift.
- *Unanswered questions remain*—long-term mortality effects, cost, accessibility, and integration with other therapies (SGLT2i, ARNi) require further study.
- *Bottom line*: Use semaglutide to treat obesity in HFpEF, ideally alongside guideline-directed therapy; HFpEF-specific class recommendations are expected as durability and outcomes data mature.

REFERENCES

1. Kosiborod MN, Abildstrøm SZ, Borlaug BA, et al. Semaglutide in patients with heart failure with preserved ejection fraction and obesity. N Engl J Med. 2023;389(12):1069-84.
2. Borlaug BA. Evaluation and management of heart failure with preserved ejection fraction. Nat Rev Cardiol. 2020;17(9):559-73.
3. Pandey A, Golwala H, DeVore AD, et al. Trends in the use of guideline-directed therapies among dialysis patients

hospitalized with systolic heart failure: findings from the American Heart Association get with the guidelines-heart failure program. JACC Heart Fail. 2016;4(8):649-61.
4. Khayyat-Kholghi M, Oparil S, Davis BR, et al. Worsening kidney function is the major mechanism of heart failure in hypertension: the ALLHAT study. Heart Failure. 2021;9(2):100-11.
5. Wilding JP, Batterham RL, Calanna S, et al. Once-weekly semaglutide in adults with overweight or obesity. N Engl J Med. 2021;384(11):989-1002.
6. Lancellotti P, Nguyen Trung ML, Oury C, et al. Cancer and cardiovascular mortality risk: Is the die cast? Eur Heart J. 2021;42(1):110-2.
7. Paulus WJ, Tschöpe C. A novel paradigm for heart failure with preserved ejection fraction: comorbidities drive myocardial dysfunction and remodeling through coronary microvascular endothelial inflammation. J Am Coll Cardiol. 2013;62(4):263-71.
8. Packer M. Epicardial adipose tissue may mediate deleterious effects of obesity and inflammation on the myocardium. J Am Coll Cardiol. 2018;71(20):2360-72.
9. Willeit P, Kiechl S, Kronenberg F, et al. Discrimination and net reclassification of cardiovascular risk with lipoprotein (a) prospective 15-year outcomes in the Bruneck study. J Am Coll Cardiol. 2014;64(9):851-60.
10. Shah SJ, Borlaug BA, Kitzman DW, et al. Research priorities for heart failure with preserved ejection fraction: National Heart, Lung, and Blood Institute Working Group summary. Circulation. 2020;141(12):1001-26.
11. James NM, Stanford KI. Obesity and exercise: new insights and perspectives. Endocr Rev. 2025;46:763-89.
12. Kristensen SL, Rørth R, Jhund PS, et al. Cardiovascular, mortality, and kidney outcomes with GLP-1 receptor agonists in patients with type 2 diabetes: a systematic review and meta-analysis of cardiovascular outcome trials. Lancet Diabetes Endocrinol. 2019;7(10):776-85.
13. Cesaro A, De Michele G, Fimiani F, et al. Visceral adipose tissue and residual cardiovascular risk: a pathological link and new therapeutic options. Front Cardiovasc Med. 2023;10:1187735.
14. Kushner RF, Calanna S, Davies M, et al. Semaglutide 2.4 mg for the treatment of obesity: key elements of the STEP trials 1 to 5. Obesity. 2020;28(6):1050-61.
15. Lincoff AM, Brown-Frandsen K, Colhoun HM, et al. Semaglutide and cardiovascular outcomes in obesity without diabetes. N Engl J Med. 2023;389(24): 2221-32.
16. Anker SD, Butler J, Filippatos G, et al. Empagliflozin in heart failure with a preserved ejection fraction. N Engl J Med. 2021;385(16):1451-61.
17. Solomon SD, McMurray JJ, Claggett B, et al. Dapagliflozin in heart failure with mildly reduced or preserved ejection fraction. N Engl J Med. 2022;387(12):1089-98.
18. van Ruiten, Constance C. Effects of SGLT2 inhibition and GLP-1 receptor agonism on the regulation of food intake and body weight: illuminating the role of the brain; 2022.
19. DeFronzo RA. Combination therapy with GLP-1 receptor agonist and SGLT2 inhibitor. Diab Obes Metab. 2017;19(10):1353-62.
20. Heidenreich PA, Fonarow GC, Vaduganathan M, et al. 2025 ACC expert consensus decision pathway on novel therapies for cardiometabolic disease: integration of obesity, diabetes, and cardiovascular risk reduction. J Am Coll Cardiol. 2025;85(3):245-68.
21. American Diabetes Association Professional Practice Committee. 8. Obesity and weight management for the prevention and treatment of type 2 diabetes: standards of care in diabetes—2024. Diabetes Care. 2024;47(Suppl 1): S113-24.
22. Januzzi JL, Konstam MA. Semaglutide in patients with obesity-related heart failure with preserved ejection fraction. J Am Coll Cardiol. 2023;82(9):839-42.
23. McDonagh TA, Metra M, Adamo M, et al. 2023 focused update of the 2021 ESC guidelines for the diagnosis and treatment of acute and chronic heart failure. Eur Heart J. 2023;44(36):3499-599.
24. US Food and Drug Administration. FDA Approves Wegovy (semaglutide) to Reduce Risk of Cardiovascular Death, Heart Attack, and Stroke in Adults With Cardiovascular Disease and Obesity or Overweight. Silver Spring, MD: FDA; 2024. [online] Available from https://www.fda.gov/drugs/news-events-human-drugs/fda-approves-wegovy-semaglutide-reduce-risk-cardiovascular-death-heart-attack-and-stroke.

113

CHAPTER

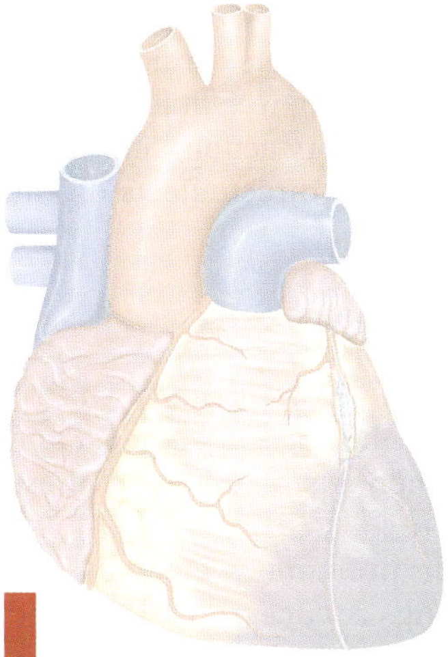

Semaglutide in Obesity with HFpEF in Women: Outcome Data

Amit Jaiswal, Roopali Khanna

INTRODUCTION

Heart failure (HF) affects approximately 64 million people worldwide, and over half of patients with HF have a preserved systolic function, which is a syndrome with substantial morbidity and mortality.[1-3] Data from epidemiological studies and RCTs in patients with heart failure with preserved ejection fraction (HFpEF) indicate that the yearly mortality rate is approximately 10–20%.[4,5] Overweight and obesity are common in the majority of patients with HFpEF (60–80%).[6,7] Obesity is a well-established risk factor for the development of HFpEF and also worsens the prognosis.[8,9] The pathophysiology of obese HFpEF comprises a combination of inflammatory, structural, hemodynamic, and metabolic mechanisms. Obese HFpEF is commonly associated with multiple comorbidities such as T2DM, hypertension, AF, renal disease, and OSA. These are the main causes of systemic inflammation leading to endothelial dysfunction, myocardial fibrosis, impaired nitric oxide pathway, increased cardiomyocyte stiffness, and diastolic dysfunction.[10,11] Epicardial adipose tissue also promotes fibrosis, impaired LV relaxation, and diastolic dysfunction.[10,11] Neurohormonal activation, such as RAAS, SNS activation, and increased production of ROS, leads to adverse cardiac remodeling and multiorgan failure in obese patients with HFpEF.[12] Whereas an increase in plasma volume expansion and cardiac output due to adipose tissue leads to elevated left ventricular diastolic filling pressures and left atrial pressure.[13] These elevated left-sided filling pressures and hypoxia from obesity associated OSA lead to pulmonary vascular remodeling and pulmonary arterial hypertension. Although the exact pathophysiology of obese HFpEF is not yet well understood, new mechanisms continue to emerge investigating the correlation between HFpEF and obesity.

OBESITY WITH HFpEF IN WOMEN

Obese HFpEF is a specific clinical phenotype, more common in younger individuals, predominantly females, and is related to worse quality of life compared to HFpEF from other causes.[14,15] Although gender differences are present in various aspects of HFpEF, including prevalence, incidence, risk factors, hemodynamics, pathophysiology, and outcomes, the scarcity of gender specific studies constrains our present understanding. However, the global prevalence of obesity is higher in females compared to males, and the severity of obesity is a strong predictor of the risk of future heart failure hospitalization.[16] Data from epidemiological studies indicate that HFpEF is more prevalent in females (67%) than in males (42%), and heart failure hospitalization also occurs more frequently in females compared to males.[17-19] However, women are more prone to develop hypertension, arterial stiffness, and concentric LVH as compared to men. PURSUIT-HFpEF study showed that female sex is independently associated with more diastolic dysfunction and worse prognosis in patients with HFpEF.[20]

MANAGEMENT OF OBESITY WITH HFpEF IN WOMEN

The management of obesity associated with HFpEF among women is still a substantial challenge due to phenotypic heterogeneity and multifaceted pathogenesis. Unlike heart failure with reduced ejection fraction (HFrEF), where traditional HF therapies, including ACEi/ARB/ARNI, beta blockers, and MRA, have proven effective, HFpEF is less responsive to these treatments. HFpEF is commonly associated with multiple comorbidities, all of which play an important role in its pathogenesis and progression. A comprehensive treatment approach should be initiated after diagnosis of HFpEF, including addressing associated comorbidities and using non-pharmacological and pharmacological therapeutic strategies. There is an insufficiency of effective therapy in the management of obesity coexisting with HFpEF in women, potentially due to the diverse clinical presentation and complex pathophysiology. SGLT2i is the only disease-modifying therapy recommended for HFpEF today. SGLT2i are recommended as a Class IIA indication in the management of HFpEF by the AHA/ACC guidelines.[21] Whereas the European Society of Cardiology (ESC) has recommended SGLT2i as a Class IA indication in the management of HFpEF.[22] Recent advances in understanding the underlying pathophysiology of HFpEF have led to the development of novel treatment approaches targeting both cardiac and systemic contributors. A GLP-1 agonist, primarily used in T2DM and obesity, is emerging as a treatment option for HFpEF.

SEMAGLUTIDE IN OBESITY WITH HFpEF IN WOMEN

FDA-approved GLP-1 RAs are broadly classified into two categories, which include the following:

- *Human GLP-1 backbone:*
  - Dulaglutide
  - Liraglutide
  - Semaglutide
- *Exendine-4 backbone:*
- Exenatide
- Tirzepatide

Semaglutide was assigned a US FDA product label in December 2017 for lowering the risk of CV death, MI, and stroke in patients with type 2 diabetes with or at high ASCVD risk based on SUSTAIN-6 and PIONEER-6 trials.[23,24] These two trials revealed a substantial 21–26% relative reduction in the risk of MACE, a composite of cardiovascular death, nonfatal MI, and stroke in patients with T2DM with or at high ASCVD risk.[23,24] However, recent studies have shown that semaglutide is associated with a larger reduction in HF-related symptoms and inflammation, greater improvements in exercise capacity, and enhanced quality of life, along with greater weight loss in patients with HFpEF, especially in obese patients with HFpEF in female patients. Semaglutide is a long-acting glucagon-like peptide-1 (GLP-1) agonist that offers cardiovascular benefits by multiple effects, including weight loss, blood pressure reduction, anti-inflammatory actions, improved endothelial function, and possible direct effects on the heart and kidneys **(Fig. 1)**.

MECHANISM OF ACTION

Semaglutide mimics the action of intrinsic GLP-1, activating GLP-1 receptors in the brain, pancreas, and gut. It offers cardiovascular benefits by following these mechanisms:

- *Weight loss:* Semaglutide promotes weight loss by delayed gastric emptying, reduces appetite, and increases satiety (by acting on the hypothalamic center), thus reducing caloric intake.[25] Weight loss leads to decreased plasma volume expansion and cardiac output due to adipose tissue, which lowers blood pressure, LA pressure, pulmonary congestion, and LV hypertrophy and stiffness.[26]
- *Improvement in diastolic dysfunction:* It reduces myocardial fat infiltration and systemic inflammation, which leads to improvement in ventricular compliance and diastolic relaxation, thus it reduces dyspnea, improves exercise tolerance, and quality of life (QoL).[26]
- *Anti-inflammatory action:* It reduces proinflammatory cytokines such as IL-6, TNF-α by GLP-1 receptor activation, which reduces cardiac fibrosis and cardiac remodeling, leading to structural and functional improvements in myocardium.[26,27]
- *Improved endothelial function:* It enhances nitric oxide availability and reduces oxidative stress, which improves endothelial function and hypertension by reducing afterload and improving myocardial perfusion.[26,28]

TRIAL EVIDENCE (TABLE 1)

SUSTAIN-6 Trial[23]

This study included 3297 patients with T2DM and high CV risk who were on standard care to assess the cardiovascular safety (noninferiority) of once-weekly semaglutide (0.5 mg or 1mg). In this study, 40.1% patients were female, the mean body weight was 92 kg, and 83.0% had confirmed CV disease, CKD, or both. The primary endpoint was a composite of the first MACE event. Over a median follow-up period of 106 weeks, semaglutide significantly reduced the risk of MACE by 26%; among components, it reduced nonfatal stroke by 39% and nonfatal MI by 26%. This study confirmed the CV safety of semaglutide.

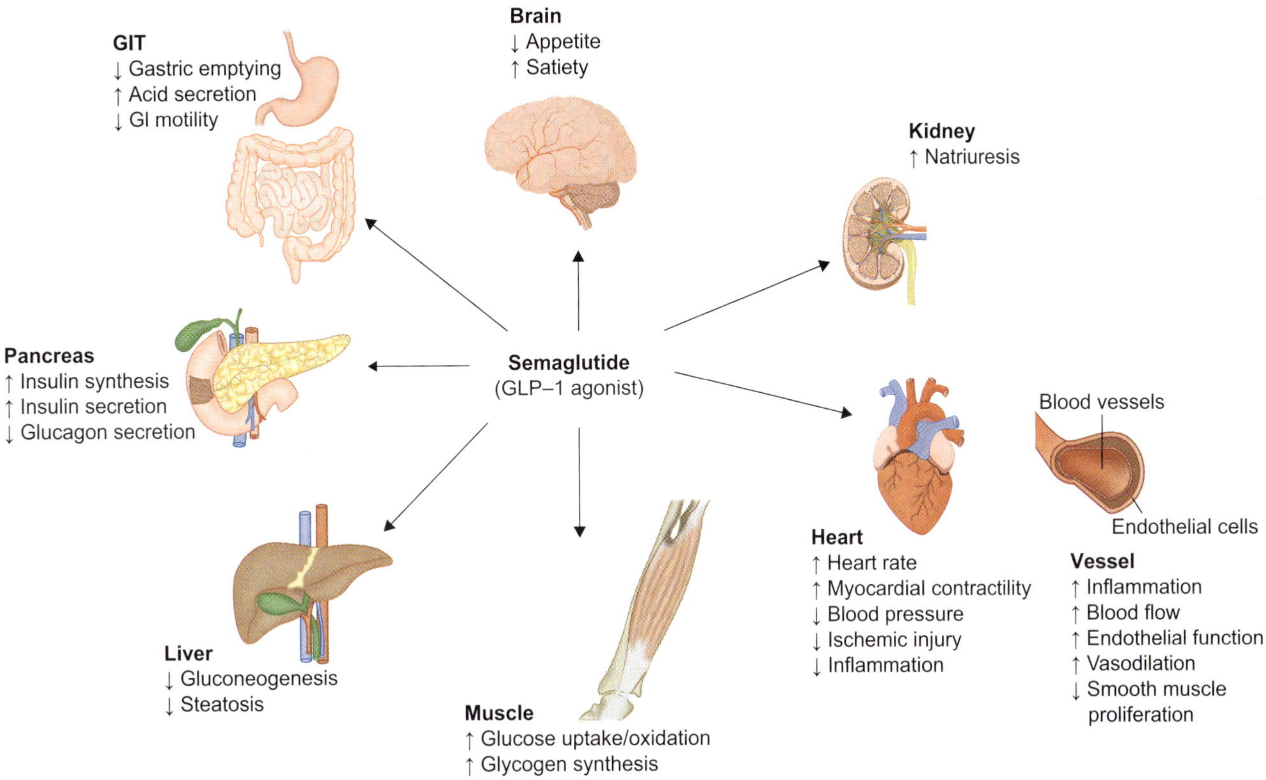

Fig. 1: Mechanism of action of semaglutide.

SELECT Trial[29]

This study aimed to assess the CV benefits of injection semaglutide (2.4 mg, s.c. once a week) in overweight and obese patients without T2DM. This RCT included 17,604 patients with established CV disease. In this study, 37.8% of patients were female, with a mean BMI of 33 kg/m^2. The primary CV endpoint was a composite of MACE. Over 39.8 months of follow-up, semaglutide reduced MACE by 20%. This study showed that semaglutide is superior to placebo in reducing the risk of a composite of death from CV causes, nonfatal MI, or stroke (MACE).

STEP-HFpEF Trial[30]

This randomized controlled trial aimed to compare the safety and efficacy of injection semaglutide (2.4 mg, s.c. once weekly) in obese or overweight patients with HFpEF without diabetes. It included 529 patients with LVEF ≥45% and BMI ≥30 kg/m^2, of whom 56.1% were women. The primary endpoints were changes in KCCQ-CSS and body weight. Whereas secondary endpoints were the change in 6MWD from baseline and the change in the CRP level. Over 52 weeks of follow-up semaglutide significantly improved KCCQ-CSS score by 16.6 points as compared to 8.7 points in placebo; weight dropped by 13.3% versus 2.6% in placebo; 6MWD increased by 21.5 m with semaglutide versus 1.2 m with placebo; CRP level decreased by 43.5% with semaglutide versus 7.3% with placebo and less serious adverse events were noted with semaglutide as compared to placebo. In this study, semaglutide led to clinically meaningful improvement in HF-related symptoms, physical function, and higher weight loss in obese patients with HFpEF without diabetes.

STEP-HFpEF DM Trial[31]

This trial aimed to compare the safety and efficacy of injection semaglutide (2.4 mg, s.c. once weekly) in obese patients with HFpEF and diabetes. It included 616 patients with LVEF of ≥45%, BMI of ≥30 kg/m^2 with type 2 diabetes mellitus, and 44.3% patients were female. Primary endpoints included changes in KCCQ-CSS and body weight. Secondary endpoints included changes in 6MWD from baseline and CRP levels. Over 52 weeks of follow-up, semaglutide significantly improved the KCCQ-CSS score by 13.7 points as compared to 6.4 points in placebo; weight dropped by 9.8% versus 3.4% in placebo; 6MWD increased by 12.7 m with semaglutide versus a small decline in placebo; CRP level decreased by 42% with

TABLE 1: Summary of randomized controlled trials on semaglutide.

Trial name	*SUSTAIN-6*[23]	*SELECT*[29]	*STEP-HFpEF*[30]	*STEP-HFpEF DM*[31]	*SOUL*[32]
Year of publication	2016	2023	2023	2024	2024
No. of patients	2,735	17,604	529	616	9,650
Female patients	40.1%	37.8%	56.1%	44.3%	33.3%
Mean weight or BMI	92 kg	33 kg/m^2	37 kg/m^2	36.9 kg/m^2	31.1 kg/m^2
Trial-population	T2DM, high CV risk	Obese or overweight with CVD, noT2DM	Obese or overweight, with HFpEF, no T2DM	Obese or overweight, with HFpEF, with T2DM	Type 2 DM, CVD or CKD
Intervention and comparator	Inj. Semaglutide (0.5 or 1 mg, s.c. once weekly) vs. placebo	Inj. Semaglutide (2.4 mg, s.c. once weekly) vs. placebo	Inj. Semaglutide (2.4 mg, s.c. once weekly) vs. placebo	Inj. Semaglutide (2.4 mg, s.c. once weekly) vs. placebo	Oral Semaglutide (14 mg once daily) vs. placebo
Mean follow-up duration	109 weeks	39.8 months	52 weeks	52 weeks	47.5 months
Primary endpoint	3-point MACE	3-point MACE	KCCQ, body weight, 6MWD	KCCQ, body weight, 6MWD	3-point MACE
Key findings	↓ MACE by 26 %, ↓ stroke, MI	↓ MACE by 20%	↑KCCQ, ↓weight, ↑6MWD, ↓ CRP	↑ QoL, ↑KCCQ, ↓weight, ↑6MWD, ↓ CRP, ↓ HbA1C	↓ MACE by 14%

semaglutide versus 12.8% with placebo. Other findings included improvements in HbA1C and a reduction in NT-proBNP levels, along with fewer HF hospitalizations, with semaglutide compared to placebo. In this study, semaglutide led to clinically meaningful improvement in HF-related symptoms, physical function, and higher weight loss in obese patients with HFpEF and diabetes.

SOUL Trial[32]

This trial was designed to assess the efficacy of oral semaglutide (14 mg once daily) in patients with type 2 diabetes and established ASCVD and/or CKD. This study included 9,650 patients aged 50 years and above with a mean BMI of 31.1 kg/m^2, and women were 33.3%. The primary endpoint was a composite of MACE, and the secondary endpoints included major kidney disease events and major adverse limb events. Over 47.5 months of follow-up, MACE was significantly decreased by 14% as compared to placebo, and secondary endpoints did not differ significantly between the two groups. This trial suggested that oral semaglutide was associated with a substantial reduction in MACE without any major adverse events.

LIMITATIONS

Studies have demonstrated that semaglutide has a good safety profile and is not associated with any serious adverse events. The most frequently reported adverse events resulting in discontinuation of semaglutide were gastrointestinal symptoms, including nausea, vomiting, decreased appetite, constipation, and diarrhea.[23,29-32] These gastrointestinal events can cause volume depletion which may lead to acute kidney injury. Regular monitoring of kidney function, electrolyte and blood glucose level are required, particularly during the early phase of gradual dose escalation, which occurs every 4 weeks. When gastrointestinal adverse effects are prominent, dose adjustment of diuretics, antihypertensive agents, and antihyperglycemic agents should be done as indicated.

RECOMMENDATION

Studies have shown that semaglutide is associated with improvements in HF symptoms and functional capacity but there are insufficient evidence to conclude that semaglutide can reduce HF events and mortality in women with HFpEF and obesity.

CONCLUSION

Semaglutide is the new emerging therapy in management of obesity-related HFpEF in women. Though data suggests that it significantly improves quality of life and functional capacity in obesity with HFpEF, further studies are warranted for long-term mortality benefit, comparative effectiveness as compared to SGLT2i and other HFpEF therapies, combination strategies (e.g., SGLT2 inhibitors and semaglutide) in high-risk phenotypes, and in lean HFpEF (HFpEF with BMI <30 but high visceral adiposity).

REFERENCES

1. GBD 2019 Diseases and Injuries Collaborators. Global burden of 369 diseases and injuries in 204 countries and territories, 1990-2019: a systematic analysis for the Global Burden of Disease Study 2019. Lancet. 2020;396(10258):1204-22.
2. Savarese G, Becher PM, Lund LH, et al. Global burden of heart failure: a comprehensive and updated review of epidemiology. Cardiovasc Res. 2023;118(17): 3272-87.
3. Dunlay SM, Roger VL, Redfield MM. Epidemiology of heart failure with preserved ejection fraction. Nat Rev Cardiol. 2017;14(10):591-602.
4. Redfield MM, Borlaug BA. Heart Failure with Preserved Ejection Fraction: A Review. 2023;329(10):827-38.
5. Dhingra A, Garg A, Kaur S, et al. Epidemiology of heart failure with preserved ejection fraction. Curr Heart Fail Rep. 2014;11(4):354-65.
6. Kitzman DW, Brubaker P, Morgan T, et al. Effect of Caloric Restriction or Aerobic Exercise Training on Peak Oxygen Consumption and Quality of Life in Obese Older Patients with Heart Failure with Preserved Ejection Fraction: A Randomized Clinical Trial. JAMA. 2016; 315(1):36-46.
7. Shah SJ, Kitzman DW, Borlaug BA, et al. Phenotype-Specific Treatment of Heart Failure with Preserved Ejection Fraction: A Multiorgan Roadmap. Circulation. 2016;134(1):73-90.
8. Kim SE, Yoo BS. Obesity and heart failure with preserved ejection fraction: focus on new drugs and future direction in medical treatment. Korean J Intern Med. 2025;40(3):357-70.
9. van Dalen BM, Chin JF, Motiram PA, et al. Challenges in the diagnosis of heart failure with preserved ejection fraction in individuals with obesity. Cardiovasc Diabetol. 2025;24(1):71.
10. Stoicescu L, Crişan D, Morgovan C, et al. Heart Failure with Preserved Ejection Fraction: The Pathophysiological Mechanisms behind the Clinical Phenotypes and the Therapeutic Approach. Int J Mol Sci. 2024;25(2): 794.
11. Kitzman DW, Lam CSP. Obese Heart Failure with Preserved Ejection Fraction Phenotype: From Pariah to Central Player. Circulation. 2017;136(1):20-23.
12. Da Young Lee. Obesity and heart failure with preserved ejection fraction: pathophysiology and clinical significance. Cardiovasc Prevent Pharmacother. 2022; 4(2):70-4.
13. Obokata M, Reddy YNV, Pislaru SV, et al. Evidence Supporting the Existence of a Distinct Obese Phenotype of Heart Failure with Preserved Ejection Fraction. Circulation. 2017;136(1):6-19.
14. Tromp J, MacDonald MR, Tay WT, et al. Heart Failure with Preserved Ejection Fraction in the Young. Circulation. 2018;138(24):2763-73.
15. Reddy YNV, Lewis GD, Shah SJ, et al. Characterization of the Obese Phenotype of Heart Failure with Preserved Ejection Fraction: A RELAX Trial Ancillary Study. Mayo Clin Proc. 2019;94(7):1199-1209.
16. Maddury J. Heart Failure in Women. Indian J Cardiovasc Dis Women. 2022;7(3):162-174.
17. Campbell P, Rutten FH, Lee MM, et al. Heart failure with preserved ejection fraction: everything the clinician needs to know. Lancet. 2024;403(10431):1083-92.
18. Savarese G, Vasko P, Jonsson Å, et al. The Swedish Heart Failure Registry: a living, ongoing quality assurance and research in heart failure. Ups J Med Sci. 2019; 124(1):65-9.
19. Pandey A, Omar W, Ayers C, et al. Sex and Race Differences in Lifetime Risk of Heart Failure with Preserved Ejection Fraction and Heart Failure with Reduced Ejection Fraction. Circulation. 2018;137(17):1814-23.
20. Sotomi Y, Hikoso S, Nakatani D, et al. PURSUIT-HFpEF Investigators. Sex Differences in Heart Failure with Preserved Ejection Fraction. J Am Heart Assoc. 2021;10(5):e018574.
21. Kittleson MM, Panjrath GS, Amancherla K, et al. 2023 ACC Expert Consensus Decision Pathway on Management of Heart Failure with Preserved Ejection Fraction: A Report of the American College of Cardiology Solution Set Oversight Committee. J Am Coll Cardiol. 2023;81(18):1835-78.
22. McDonagh TA, Metra M, Adamo M, et al. 2023 Focused Update of the 2021 ESC Guidelines for the diagnosis and treatment of acute and chronic heart failure. Eur Heart J. 2023;44(37):3627-39.
23. Marso SP, Bain SC, Consoli A, et al. Semaglutide and Cardiovascular Outcomes in Patients with Type 2 Diabetes. N Engl J Med. 2016;375(19):1834-44.
24. Husain M, Birkenfeld AL, Donsmark M, et al. PIONEER 6 Investigators. Oral Semaglutide and Cardiovascular Outcomes in Patients with Type 2 Diabetes. N Engl J Med. 2019;381(9):841-51.
25. Friedrichsen M, Breitschaft A, Tadayon S, et al. The effect of semaglutide 2.4 mg once weekly on energy intake, appetite, control of eating, and gastric emptying in adults with obesity. Diabetes Obes Metab. 2021; 23(3):754-62.
26. Withaar C, Meems LMG, Nollet EE, et al. The Cardioprotective Effects of Semaglutide Exceed Those of Dietary Weight Loss in Mice with HFpEF. JACC Basic Transl Sci. 2023;8(10):1298-314.
27. Tan SA, Tan L. liraglutide and semaglutide attenuate inflammatory cytokines interferon-gamma, tumor necrosis factor-alpha, and interleukin-6: possible mechanism of decreasing cardiovascular risk in diabetes mellitus. J Am Coll Cardiol. 2019;73(9S1):1866
28. Korakas E, Kountouri A, Pavlidis G, et al. Semaglutide Concurrently Improves Vascular and Liver Indices in Patients with Type 2 Diabetes and Fatty Liver Disease. J Endocr Soc. 2024;8(8):bvae122.

29. Lincoff AM, Brown-Frandsen K, Colhoun HM, et al. Semaglutide and Cardiovascular Outcomes in Obesity without Diabetes. N Engl J Med. 2023;389(24):2221-32.
30. Kosiborod MN, Abildstrøm SZ, Borlaug BA, et al. STEP-HFpEF Trial Committees and Investigators. Semaglutide in Patients with Heart Failure with Preserved Ejection Fraction and Obesity. N Engl J Med. 2023;389(12):1069-84.
31. Kosiborod MN, Petrie MC, Borlaug BA, et al. STEP-HFpEF DM Trial Committees and Investigators. Semaglutide in Patients with Obesity-Related Heart Failure and Type 2 Diabetes. N Engl J Med. 2024;390(15): 1394-1407.
32. McGuire DK, Busui RP, Deanfield J, et al. Effects of oral semaglutide on cardiovascular outcomes in individuals with type 2 diabetes and established atherosclerotic cardiovascular disease and/or chronic kidney disease: Design and baseline characteristics of SOUL, a randomized trial. Diabetes Obes Metab. 2023;25(7):1932-41.

114
CHAPTER

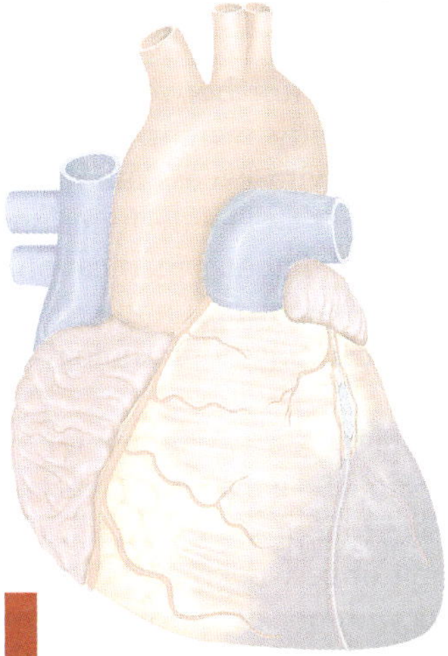

Comparison of Semaglutide versus Tirzepatide in Management of Obesity, Diabetes, and Cardiovascular Benefits: Recent Outcome Trials

Mangesh Tiwaskar, Suhas Erande

INTRODUCTION

The landscape of metabolic disease management has undergone a revolutionary transformation with the introduction of incretin-based therapies. Semaglutide, a glucagon-like peptide-1 receptor agonist (GLP-1 RA), and tirzepatide, a dual glucose-dependent insulinotropic polypeptide (GIP) and GLP-1 receptor agonist, represent the vanguard of pharmacological interventions for type 2 diabetes mellitus (T2DM) and obesity. These medications have demonstrated unprecedented efficacy in glycemic control, weight reduction, and cardiovascular risk modification, fundamentally altering treatment paradigms for millions of patients worldwide.[1,2] This chapter provides a comprehensive comparison of these two agents, examining their mechanisms of action, clinical efficacy, safety profiles, and the latest evidence from cardiovascular outcome trials conducted through 2025.

MECHANISMS OF ACTION

Semaglutide: Glucagon-like Peptide-1 Receptor Agonism

Semaglutide functions as a selective GLP-1 receptor agonist with 94% structural homology to native human GLP-1. The molecule has been engineered with specific modifications to extend its half-life to approximately 1 week, enabling once-weekly subcutaneous administration.[2] GLP-1 receptors are widely distributed throughout the body, including pancreatic beta cells, the gastrointestinal tract, cardiovascular tissues, and central nervous system regions involved in appetite regulation.

The therapeutic effects of semaglutide are mediated through multiple mechanisms. In pancreatic beta cells, GLP-1 receptor activation stimulates glucose-dependent insulin secretion, ensuring that insulin release occurs primarily in response to elevated blood glucose levels, thereby minimizing hypoglycemia risk. Concurrently, semaglutide suppresses glucagon secretion from pancreatic alpha cells in a glucose-dependent manner, reducing hepatic glucose output when it is inappropriately elevated.[3] In the gastrointestinal tract, GLP-1 receptor activation delays gastric emptying, contributing to improved postprandial glycemic control and enhanced satiety. Central nervous system effects include activation of appetite-regulating neurons in the hypothalamus and brainstem, leading to reduced food intake and sustained weight loss.[4]

Tirzepatide: Dual GIP/GLP-1 Receptor Agonism

Tirzepatide represents a novel therapeutic approach as the first dual GIP and GLP-1 receptor agonist approved for clinical use. This unimolecular agent activates both incretin receptors simultaneously, with particular affinity for the GIP receptor and additional GLP-1 receptor agonist activity.[5] The addition of GIP receptor agonism provides complementary and potentially synergistic metabolic effects beyond those achieved with GLP-1 receptor activation alone.

Glucose-dependent insulinotropic polypeptide, secreted by enteroendocrine K cells in the small intestine, plays crucial roles in glucose homeostasis, lipid metabolism, and energy balance. GIP re-enhances activation in pancreatic beta cells, enhancing glucose-dependent insulin secretion, with effects that may be additive or synergistic with GLP-1-mediated insulin release. Unlike GLP-1, GIP does not suppress glucagon secretion under hypoglycemic conditions, potentially offering a safety advantage.[6] Emerging evidence suggests that GIP receptor activation may influence adipose tissue biology, promoting nutrient storage in subcutaneous rather than visceral depots and enhancing insulin sensitivity. The combined GIP and GLP-1 receptor agonism in tirzepatide appears to produce superior weight loss compared to selective GLP-1 receptor agonists, possibly through enhanced effects on energy expenditure, adipose tissue metabolism, and central appetite regulation.[7,8]

EFFICACY IN DIABETES MANAGEMENT

Glycemic Control

Both semaglutide and tirzepatide have demonstrated remarkable efficacy in improving glycemic control in patients with T2DM. In the SUSTAIN clinical trial program, semaglutide at doses of 0.5 and 1.0 mg once-weekly consistently achieved HbA1c reductions ranging from 1.4 to 1.8% across diverse patient populations, including treatment-naive individuals and those with inadequate control on existing therapies.[2] The proportion of patients achieving HbA1c targets below 7.0% ranged from 67 to 79%, with many patients reaching even more stringent targets below 6.5%.

The SURPASS clinical trial program evaluated tirzepatide at three dose levels: 5, 10, and 15 mg once weekly. Across these trials, tirzepatide demonstrated dose-dependent HbA1c reductions ranging from 1.87 to 2.59%, representing some of the largest glycemic improvements observed with any diabetes medication to date.[6] The highest dose of tirzepatide (15 mg) consistently outperformed semaglutide 1.0 mg in head-to-head comparisons, with additional HbA1c reductions of approximately 0.4–0.5%. In the SURPASS-2 trial, which directly compared tirzepatide to semaglutide, 51% of patients receiving tirzepatide 15 mg achieved HbA1c levels below 5.7%, effectively reaching nondiabetic glycemic levels.[1]

The superior glycemic efficacy of tirzepatide likely reflects the additive effects of dual incretin receptor agonism on beta cell function, insulin sensitivity, and glucose homeostasis. Both medications achieve their glucose-lowering effects with minimal hypoglycemia risk, as their mechanisms are inherently glucose dependent.[6,9]

Weight Loss Outcomes

Perhaps the most striking distinction between these agents lies in their effects on body weight. Obesity and T2DM are intimately linked, with excess adiposity contributing to insulin resistance, beta cell dysfunction, and cardiovascular risk. Traditional diabetes medications often cause weight gain or are weight-neutral, limiting their utility in addressing the fundamental pathophysiology of T2DM in most patients.[10]

In the SUSTAIN trials, semaglutide 1.0 mg achieved mean weight reductions of 4.5 to 6.5 kg over 30–56 weeks of treatment.[2] The STEP clinical trial program specifically evaluated semaglutide 2.4 mg once weekly for chronic weight management in adults with obesity or overweight with weight-related comorbidities. In the landmark STEP 1 trial, participants without diabetes achieved a mean weight loss of 14.9% of body weight over 68 weeks, compared to 2.4% with placebo.[3] Among participants with T2DM in the STEP 2 trial, semaglutide 2.4 mg produced a mean weight loss of 9.6%, significantly exceeding the 7.0% reduction achieved with semaglutide 1.0 mg.[5]

Tirzepatide has demonstrated even more substantial weight loss across clinical trials. In the SURPASS program, weight reductions ranged from 7.6 kg with the 5 mg dose to 12.9 kg with the 15 mg dose over approximately 40 weeks in patients with T2DM.[1] The SURMOUNT clinical trial program evaluated tirzepatide specifically for chronic weight management. In SURMOUNT-1, adults with obesity or overweight without diabetes achieved mean weight reductions of 15.0, 19.5, and 20.9% with tirzepatide 5, 10, and 15 mg, respectively, compared to 3.1% with placebo over 72 weeks.[7] In SURMOUNT-2, which enrolled participants with both obesity and T2DM, tirzepatide produced weight reductions of 12.8–15.7% across the three doses, substantially exceeding placebo.[11] These results represent the most substantial weight loss achieved with any pharmacological intervention short of bariatric surgery.

The mechanisms underlying the superior weight loss with tirzepatide remain under investigation but are likely to involve enhanced effects on appetite suppression, energy expenditure, and adipose tissue metabolism conferred by the addition of GIP receptor agonism to GLP-1 receptor activation.[8]

Cardiovascular Outcomes

Cardiovascular disease represents the leading cause of morbidity and mortality in patients with T2DM and obesity. Regulatory requirements and clinical imperatives have driven extensive investigation of cardiovascular effects of diabetes medications through large-scale outcome trials. Both semaglutide and tirzepatide have been subjected to rigorous cardiovascular outcome trials that have established their roles not merely as glucose-lowering or weight loss agents, but as medications that reduce cardiovascular risk.[8,12]

Semaglutide Cardiovascular Evidence

The SUSTAIN-6 trial provided initial evidence of cardiovascular benefits with semaglutide in patients with T2DM at high cardiovascular risk. This trial demonstrated a 26% reduction in the primary composite outcome of major adverse cardiovascular events (MACE), including cardiovascular death, nonfatal myocardial infarction, and nonfatal stroke (hazard ratio 0.74; 95% CI: 0.58–0.95; $p = 0.02$).[2] This benefit was driven primarily by reductions in nonfatal stroke (39% reduction) and nonfatal myocardial infarction (26% reduction), with a numerical but nonsignificant reduction in cardiovascular death.

Building on this evidence, the SELECT trial, published in 2023, specifically evaluated semaglutide 2.4 mg in adults with established cardiovascular disease and overweight or obesity without diabetes. This landmark trial demonstrated a 20% reduction in MACE (hazard ratio 0.80; 95% CI: 0.72–0.90; $p < 0.001$) over a median follow-up of 3.4 years.[12] The cardiovascular benefits appeared to extend across diverse patient populations and were observed regardless of baseline body weight or degree of weight loss achieved, suggesting that semaglutide may confer cardioprotective effects beyond those mediated by weight reduction alone.[4,9]

RECENT 2025 CARDIOVASCULAR OUTCOME TRIALS

The year 2025 has witnessed the culmination of several landmark cardiovascular outcome trials that have substantially expanded our understanding of the cardiovascular effects of both semaglutide and tirzepatide.

SOUL Trial: Oral Semaglutide Cardiovascular Outcomes

The SOUL (Semaglutide Cardiovascular Outcomes Trial) trial, published in March 2025, evaluated oral semaglutide in 9,650 participants aged 50 years or older with type 2 diabetes, HbA1c levels between 6.5 and 10.0%, and established atherosclerotic cardiovascular disease, chronic kidney disease, or both. The trial demonstrated a 14% reduction in MACE with oral semaglutide compared to placebo, with a hazard ratio of 0.86 (95% CI: 0.77–0.96; $p = 0.006$).[13] This 14% risk reduction aligns with pooled results from eight previous trials involving injectable GLP-1 receptor agonists, establishing the oral formulation on par with injectable preparations for cardiovascular benefit.

Over a median follow-up of 49.5 months, a primary outcome event occurred in 12.0% of participants receiving oral semaglutide compared to 13.8% in the placebo group.[13] The 26% reduction in nonfatal myocardial infarction was the primary driver of the improvement in the composite primary endpoint, while nonfatal strokes were reduced by 12% and cardiovascular death by 7%. Importantly, the incidence of serious adverse events was lower in the oral semaglutide group (47.9%) compared to placebo (50.3%), with gastrointestinal disorders occurring in 5.0 and 4.4%, respectively.[13]

A prespecified analysis from the SELECT trial examining relationships between adiposity measures and cardiovascular outcomes revealed that approximately 33% of the observed MACE benefit was mediated through waist circumference reduction, suggesting that cardioprotective effects extend beyond simple weight loss and may involve more fundamental changes in body composition and metabolic health.[9,12]

SURPASS-CVOT: Tirzepatide Cardiovascular Outcomes

The SURPASS-CVOT (A Study of Tirzepatide Compared with Dulaglutide on Major Cardiovascular Events) trial, with results announced in July 2025, represents the largest and longest study of tirzepatide conducted to date. This trial enrolled 13,299 participants across 640 sites in 30 countries, randomizing them to receive either tirzepatide (maximum tolerated dose of 5, 10, or 15 mg) or dulaglutide 1.5 mg once weekly, with follow-up extending over 4.5 years.[14]

The primary analysis demonstrated that MACE was 8% less common with tirzepatide compared to dulaglutide (HR 0.92; 95% CI 0.83–1.01), meeting prespecified criteria for noninferiority. While the trial did not achieve statistical superiority for the primary MACE endpoint, tirzepatide demonstrated significantly better outcomes in several key secondary endpoints, including all-cause mortality (16% reduction), improvements in kidney function, and greater reductions in HbA1c.[14]

Treatment with tirzepatide led to greater improvements in cardiovascular biomarkers compared to dulaglutide, including lipid profiles and systolic blood pressure. The safety profiles of both medications were generally consistent with their established patterns, with gastrointestinal adverse events being the most reported for both treatments, typically mild to moderate in severity and resolving after dose escalation completion.

Discontinuation rates due to adverse events were 13.3% for tirzepatide and 10.2% for dulaglutide.[14]

Prior to the full SURPASS-CVOT results, a prespecified meta-analysis of cardiovascular events across the SURPASS program had already suggested cardiovascular benefits, with tirzepatide demonstrating a 20% reduction in cardiovascular death, nonfatal myocardial infarction, and nonfatal stroke compared to placebo and active comparators (hazard ratio 0.80; 95% CI: 0.57–1.11).[8]

Head-to-Head Comparison: Real-world Evidence

In the absence of direct randomized controlled trials comparing semaglutide and tirzepatide for cardiovascular outcomes, a major real-world trial emulation study presented at the American Heart Association Scientific Sessions 2025 assessed cardiovascular outcomes in patients with elevated cardiovascular risk, obesity, and type 2 diabetes enrolled in US insurance programs between 2018 and 2025. The study emulated both SUSTAIN-6 and SURPASS-CVOT trials to benchmark their methodology before directly comparing the two medications. The analysis demonstrated that treatment with semaglutide and tirzepatide showed similar levels of benefit on cardiovascular outcomes in individuals at elevated cardiovascular risk with obesity and diabetes.[15]

This real-world evidence is particularly valuable as it reflects clinical practice patterns and outcomes in heterogeneous patient populations outside the controlled environment of randomized trials. The finding that both medications confer similar cardiovascular benefits provides reassurance to clinicians and patients that either agent represents a viable option for cardiovascular risk reduction in appropriate populations.[15]

Safety and Tolerability

Both semaglutide and tirzepatide are generally well-tolerated, with most adverse events being mild to moderate in severity and predominantly gastrointestinal in nature. The most commonly reported side effects include nausea, vomiting, diarrhea, constipation, and abdominal discomfort. These symptoms typically occur during dose escalation and tend to diminish over time with continued treatment.[3,7]

In clinical trials, gastrointestinal adverse events led to treatment discontinuation in approximately 4–7% of patients receiving semaglutide and 5–10% of patients receiving tirzepatide, with higher rates observed at the highest doses.[5,11] The gradual dose titration strategies employed in clinical practice can help minimize these effects and improve treatment persistence.

Serious adverse events, including pancreatitis, have been reported with both medications, though the absolute incidence remains low. In the SUSTAIN-6 trial, acute pancreatitis occurred in 0.3% of semaglutide-treated patients compared to 0.2% with placebo.[2] In the SELECT trial, pancreatitis rates were similarly low at 0.4% with semaglutide 2.4 mg versus 0.3% with placebo.[12] Regulatory warnings include potential risks of thyroid C-cell tumors based on rodent studies, though no causal relationship has been established in humans. Both medications are contraindicated in patients with a personal or family history of medullary thyroid carcinoma or multiple endocrine neoplasia syndrome type 2.[2,8]

Cases of diabetic retinopathy complications have been observed in patients with preexisting retinopathy who experience rapid improvement in glycemic control. In SUSTAIN-6, diabetic retinopathy complications occurred more frequently with semaglutide (3.0%) compared to placebo (1.8%),[2] highlighting the importance of ophthalmologic monitoring in high-risk patients. Hypoglycemia risk remains minimal when these agents are used as monotherapy or in combination with medications that do not independently cause hypoglycemia, though risk increases when combined with insulin or sulfonylureas.[1,3]

In the SOUL trial, the safety profile of oral semaglutide was consistent with previous trials, with serious adverse events actually occurring less frequently in the oral semaglutide group (47.9%) compared to placebo (50.3%).[13] This finding is reassuring and suggests that the cardiovascular benefits are not offset by increased serious adverse events.

CLINICAL CONSIDERATIONS AND PATIENT SELECTION

The choice between semaglutide and tirzepatide should be individualized based on multiple factors, including treatment goals, patient preferences, comorbidities, cost considerations, and insurance coverage.[10] For patients with T2DM requiring substantial glycemic improvement, tirzepatide may offer advantages given its superior HbA1c reduction across clinical trials. The magnitude of difference, while statistically significant, translates to an additional 0.4–0.5% reduction in HbA1c with the highest tirzepatide dose compared to semaglutide 1.0 mg.[1]

For weight management, tirzepatide has demonstrated superior efficacy, with mean weight reductions exceeding those achieved with semaglutide 2.4 mg by approximately 5–6% points in head-to-head comparisons.[1,7] This distinction may be particularly relevant for patients in whom weight loss is a primary therapeutic objective or for those with obesity-related comorbidities such as obstructive sleep apnea, osteoarthritis, or nonalcoholic fatty liver disease.[11]

From a cardiovascular perspective, both medications have established benefits in reducing MACE in appropriate patient populations. The consistency of cardiovascular benefits across different formulations (subcutaneous and oral semaglutide) and different GLP-1 receptor agonists suggests a class effect,[13] with tirzepatide demonstrating noninferior cardiovascular protection to an established GLP-1 receptor agonist in SURPASS-CVOT.[14] The real-world evidence suggesting similar cardiovascular benefits between semaglutide and tirzepatide provides additional reassurance.[15]

Practical considerations include route of administration and dosing frequency. Both medications are administered once weekly via subcutaneous injection, though oral semaglutide provides an alternative for patients with needle aversion, requiring daily administration with specific timing relative to meals.[13] Cost and insurance coverage often represent significant barriers to access, with both medications carrying substantial price tags and variable coverage across different insurance plans.

FUTURE DIRECTIONS AND EMERGING RESEARCH

The therapeutic landscape for incretin-based therapies continues to evolve rapidly. Ongoing trials are evaluating these medications in expanded indications, including heart failure with preserved ejection fraction, chronic kidney disease, obstructive sleep apnea, and nonalcoholic steatohepatitis.[8] The SUMMIT trial is specifically examining tirzepatide in patients with heart failure with preserved ejection fraction and obesity, potentially expanding the cardiovascular indications for this medication.

Novel formulations and delivery systems are under development, including extended-release preparations and combination therapies. Research into the mechanisms underlying the cardiovascular benefits of these agents continues, with investigations focusing on effects beyond glycemic control and weight loss, including direct effects on vascular endothelium, inflammation, oxidative stress, and myocardial metabolism.[4,12]

The potential role of these medications in preventing progression from prediabetes to overt diabetes represents another area of active investigation. Early intervention in high-risk populations could potentially modify long-term cardiovascular trajectories and reduce the burden of metabolic disease.[9] Additionally, understanding the mechanisms by which weight loss and metabolic improvements translate to cardiovascular benefits—including the contribution of waist circumference reduction and visceral adiposity changes—will inform optimal patient selection and treatment strategies.

CONCLUSION

Semaglutide and tirzepatide represent transformative advances in the management of type 2 diabetes and obesity, offering unprecedented efficacy in glycemic control, weight reduction, and cardiovascular risk modification. While both medications share the common mechanism of GLP-1 receptor agonism, tirzepatide's additional GIP receptor agonist activity confers superior efficacy for glycemic control and weight loss, with comparable cardiovascular protection.[1,7]

The 2025 cardiovascular outcome trials, including SOUL and SURPASS-CVOT, have established robust evidence for the cardiovascular safety and efficacy of both oral and injectable formulations across diverse patient populations with varying levels of cardiovascular risk.[13,14] Real-world evidence suggests similar cardiovascular benefits between the two medications when used in clinical practice,[15] providing clinicians with confidence in either therapeutic choice.

As our understanding of these medications continues to expand, they are poised to play an increasingly significant role in comprehensive cardiometabolic disease management. The choice between semaglutide and tirzepatide should be individualized, considering patient-specific factors, treatment goals, tolerability, and practical considerations. Both medications offer powerful tools for addressing the interconnected epidemics of obesity, diabetes, and cardiovascular disease, with the potential to meaningfully improve outcomes and quality of life for millions of patients worldwide.

REFERENCES

1. Frías JP, Davies MJ, Rosenstock J, et al. Tirzepatide versus semaglutide once weekly in patients with type 2 diabetes. N Engl J Med. 2021;385(6):503-15.
2. Marso SP, Bain SC, Consoli A, et al. Semaglutide and cardiovascular outcomes in patients with type 2 diabetes. N Engl J Med. 2016;375(19):1834-44.
3. Wilding JPH, Batterham RL, Calanna S, et al. Once-weekly semaglutide in adults with overweight or obesity. N Engl J Med. 2021;384(11):989-1002.
4. Ryan DH, Lingvay I, Colhoun HM, et al. Semaglutide effects on cardiovascular outcomes in people with overweight or obesity (SELECT) rationale and design. Am Heart J. 2020;229:61-9.
5. Davies MJ, Aronne LJ, Caterson ID, et al. Liraglutide and cardiovascular outcomes in adults with overweight or obesity: a post hoc analysis from SCALE randomized controlled trials. Diabetes Obes Metab. 2018;20(3):734-9.

6. Rosenstock J, Wysham C, Frías JP, et al. Efficacy and safety of a novel dual GIP and GLP-1 receptor agonist tirzepatide in patients with type 2 diabetes (SURPASS-1): a double-blind, randomised, phase 3 trial. Lancet. 2021;398(10295):143-55.
7. Jastreboff AM, Aronne LJ, Ahmad NN, et al. Tirzepatide once weekly for the treatment of obesity. N Engl J Med. 2022;387(3):205-16.
8. Sattar N, McGuire DK, Pavo I, et al. Tirzepatide cardiovascular event risk assessment: a pre-specified meta-analysis. Nat Med. 2022;28(3):591-8.
9. Lingvay I, Brown-Frandsen K, Colhoun HM, et al. Semaglutide for cardiovascular event reduction in people with overweight or obesity: SELECT study baseline characteristics. Obesity. 2023;31(1):111-22.
10. Davies M, Færch L, Jeppesen OK, et al. Semaglutide 2.4 mg once a week in adults with overweight or obesity, and type 2 diabetes (STEP 2): a randomised, double-blind, double-dummy, placebo-controlled, phase 3 trial. Lancet. 2021;397(10278):971-84.
11. Garvey WT, Frias JP, Jastreboff AM, et al. Tirzepatide once weekly for the treatment of obesity in people with type 2 diabetes (SURMOUNT-2): a double-blind, randomised, multicentre, placebo-controlled, phase 3 trial. Lancet. 2023;402(10402):613-26.
12. Lincoff AM, Brown-Frandsen K, Colhoun HM, et al. Semaglutide and cardiovascular outcomes in obesity without diabetes. N Engl J Med. 2023;389(24):2221-32.
13. McGuire DK, David JP, Inzucchi SE, et al. Oral semaglutide and cardiovascular outcomes in high-risk type 2 diabetes. N Engl J Med. 2025;393(7):592-604.
14. Nicholls SJ, Bhatt DL, Buse JB, et al. Comparison of tirzepatide and dulaglutide on major adverse cardiovascular events in participants with type 2 diabetes and atherosclerotic cardiovascular disease: SURPASS-CVOT design and baseline characteristics. Am Heart J. 2024;268:1-11.
15. Krüger N, Schneeweiss S, Desai RJ, et al. Cardiovascular outcomes of semaglutide and tirzepatide for patients with type 2 diabetes in clinical practice. Nat Med. 2025. doi: 10.1038/s41591-025-04102-x.

115

CHAPTER

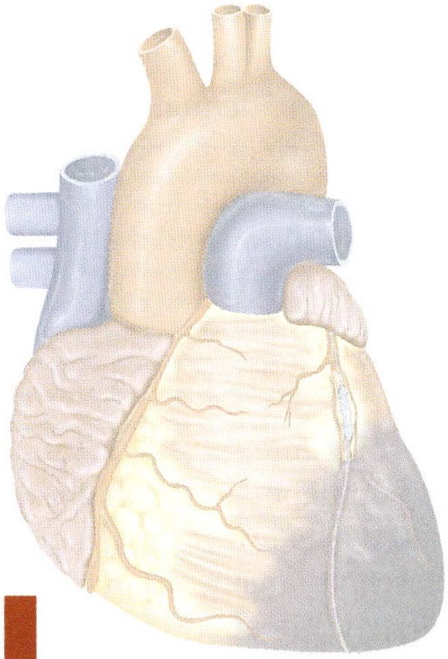

Role of Semaglutide in Pediatric and Adolescent Obesity

IB Vijayalakshmi

INTRODUCTION

The obesity in pediatric and adolescent has become a major global public health problem, with long-term complications of cardiometabolic syndrome (CMS). The CMS is well recognized as a disease entity by the World Health Organization (WHO) and the American Society of Endocrinology (ASE).[1] The CMS is also known as "insulin resistance syndrome" or "metabolic syndrome X". It was recognized as a combination of metabolic disorders or risk factors that essentially include a combination of central obesity, diabetes mellitus (DM), systemic arterial hypertension (HT), and hyperlipidemia.[2] Traditional strategies focused on lifestyle modification often produce modest or suboptimal benefits. Hence, there is a growing interest in semaglutide—a glucagon-like peptide-1 receptor agonist (GLP-1RA)—originally developed to treat type 2 diabetes in adults. Semaglutide has now emerged as the most promising and effective drug for weight management in obese adolescents. In clinical trials, it is shown to be safe and effective in reducing body mass index (BMI). It is very essential to know the pathophysiology of adolescent obesity, the pharmacology of semaglutide, and clinical evidence of its efficacy, safety, and tolerability. And also to know the current regulatory and clinical guidance, controversies, cost, challenges, and the need for future research.

BACKGROUND

Burden of Pediatric Obesity

Over the past few decades, the incidence of obesity among children and adolescents has increased tremendously all over the world. In the United States, nearly 1 in 5 adolescents aged 12–19 years is identified as obese. Childhood obesity in India is also growing rapidly,[3] leading to health crisis, particularly in urban areas, mainly due to increased consumption of junk food, sugary drinks, inactivity, and increased screen time. The present trend indicate millions are going to be affected by 2030 and thus making India a major contributor to the global burden of obesity. The present data indicate that obesity in youth is a strong predictor of an early onset of type 2 diabetes, dyslipidemia, HT, and metabolic dysfunction-associated steatotic liver disease (MASLD).[4]

Traditional obesity management emphasizes on lifestyle intervention; that includes reduction in intake of caloric diet, increase physical activities, and exercise with only modest and unsustained BMI reductions. These trends highlight the urgent need for effective and long-term strategies much beyond just lifestyle counseling. Hence, need for safe and effective pharmacological approach has increased. Now the semaglutide is at the forefront of this effort.

SEMAGLUTIDE: MECHANISM OF ACTION AND PHARMACOLOGY

Semaglutide is a synthetic analog of glucagon-like peptide-1 (GLP-1), an incretin hormone that enhances glucose-dependent insulin secretion. It suppresses glucagon release, slows gastric emptying, and also reduces appetite through central and peripheral pathways. The semaglutide's influence on appetite control involves modulation of hypothalamic circuits that control hunger and satiety center, leading to reduced caloric intake and subsequent weight loss. Originally, semaglutide was approved for type 2 diabetes in adults. But semaglutide's higher-dose (2.4 mg) once-weekly subcutaneous injection was developed for reduction of weight in adults. As it has prolonged half-life, once in a week dose is adequate, and its actions on appetite and energy intake lead to control of obesity.

But in pediatric obesity, appetite regulation and energy balance involve complex interactions between growth hormone and neurodevelopmental factors. Although the core GLP-1 mechanisms are same as in adults, pediatric patients may differ in absorption, distribution, and response, hence require dedicated clinical study rather than simple extrapolation from the data in adult.

CLINICAL EVIDENCE IN ADOLESCENTS

STEP TEENS Trial

The crucial evidence for semaglutide in adolescents with obesity came from the STEP TEENS trial,[5] a randomized double-blind, placebo-controlled study, which evaluated 2.4 mg semaglutide once-weekly plus lifestyle intervention versus placebo plus lifestyle intervention over 68 weeks. Eligible participants were obese adolescents aged 12–18 years with (BMI ≥95th percentile for age and sex). The notable findings of this study were: (1) significant 16.1% mean reduction in BMI was seen with semaglutide compared to a 0.6% increase in the placebo group, indicating a significant effect on cardiometabolic health that is the primary endpoint. (2) The weight loss was ≥5% in about 73% of treated adolescents compared to just 18% with placebo. (3) According to American College of Cardiology about 90% of participants completed the study, indicating good treatment adherence in a very challenging clinical population. (4) Cardiometabolic outcomes showed favorable reduction in waist circumference, glycemic markers, and liver enzymes. Thus, STEP TEENS trial definitely demonstrated the robust efficacy of semaglutide in reducing BMI and body weight when combined with lifestyle modifications in adolescents with obesity.

Comparative Effectiveness

Network meta-analyses comparing semaglutide with other GLP-1RAs (e.g., liraglutide, exenatide, and dulaglutide) in pediatric and adolescent populations[6] indicate that semaglutide produces the greatest reductions in BMI, weight, and BMI z-score versus placebo and other agents. These analyses also show a similar safety profile to other GLP-1RAs, with common gastrointestinal (GI) symptoms without significant increase in serious adverse effects or events.[7] A broader meta-analysis of antiobesity medications (AOMs) further demonstrate that semaglutide is better than other pharmacologic options in pediatric weight reduction, though some alternatives (e.g., phentermine-topiramate) may show similar efficacy in certain endpoints.

Safety and Tolerability in Adolescents

The safety and tolerability of semaglutide 2.4 mg, administered once a week in nondiabetic overweight or obese individuals in adults, are well known.[8] The safety profile of semaglutide in adolescents largely mirrors what has been observed in adults.[8] Hence in adolescents, also semaglutide has consistently shown reduction of weight and also mortality, as shown in meta-analyses of large randomized controlled trials (RCTs) affirming significant benefits across different groups of patients.[9] In addition, it can also improve cardiometabolic risk factors such as blood pressure, glycemia, inflammation, and lipid profiles, with a well-tolerated safety profile. Most importantly, semaglutide does not adversely affect growth or pubertal development of children and adolescents.

Adverse Events

The benefits of semaglutide are countered by adverse effects, such as pancreatitis, GI complications, gallbladder disorders, bone resorption, erectile dysfunction, visual disturbances, and thyroid and kidney dysfunction, necessitating careful monitoring. GI symptoms (nausea, vomiting, and diarrhea) are the most common adverse events (70%), typically mild to moderate, and often resolve with dose adjustment. Often thyroid dysfunction is seen in DM and obesity.

Long-term Safety Considerations

At present few trials in adolescents, including the 68-week STEP TEENS follow-up,[5] provide only limited information on long-term safety. Especially about cholelithiasis and gallbladder disease, which may be associated with rapid loss of weight. Though the risk of pancreatitis is low in trials, still it is serious enough to keep vigilance. The long-term mental health effects, including mood fluctuations or eating behaviors, which require careful monitoring, especially in adolescents. Nutritional impact, especially micronutrients, and loss of lean body mass require dietary supplements and counseling for aversion to exercise are needed. The specific safety monitoring guidelines for children and adolescents are evolving; hence, clinicians must balance between benefits of substantial BMI reduction and potential risk factors.

Regulatory and Clinical Practice Guidance

Regulatory Approvals

Semaglutide got regulatory approvals by the FDA, US for long-term weight management in pediatric patients aged above12 years with obesity, along with a low-calorie diet and high physical activity. The approval was supported by the STEP TEENS trial evidence. In global regulatory contexts, approvals differ from region to region but generally semaglutide is permitted to use in adolescents with obesity.

Clinical Recommendations

Clinical recommendations emphasize that semaglutide should be used only after complete change in lifestyle is tried and should be reserved for adolescents with BMI ≥95th percentile despite optimal nonpharmacological methods. Semaglutide is recommended as part of a multidisciplinary approach including diet regulations, increased physical activity and psychosocial counseling. Due to complexity of obesity, treatment goals include reduction in BMI, improvement in quality of life with cardiometabolic risk and long-term health.

PRACTICAL CONSIDERATIONS FOR CLINICIANS

The practical considerations for clinicians include:

- The proper selection of patients with severe obesity and related significant comorbidities despite complete lifestyle intervention program along with family support and conducive psychosocial environments. The contraindications are past history of pancreatitis, preexisting carcinoma of medullary thyroid, and any eating disorders.
- *Dosing and escalation:* Standard dose of semaglutide is to begin with a lower dose, which is titrated over weeks till 2.4 mg once weekly is tolerated. Reduced dose of 1.7 mg may be tried if patient is not tolerating high dose and persistent adverse effects occur.
- *Monitoring and follow-up:* Monitoring include growth and development parameters, BMI and body composition trends, GI symptoms, and other adverse events with cardiometabolic markers (glucose, lipids, and liver enzymes).
- *Nutritional assessments:* It is very essential to have periodic evaluation and assess nutrition of the patient frequently while increasing the dose.

CONTROVERSIES AND CHALLENGES

Long-term Efficacy and Safety

Though short-term data show impressive reductions in BMI, sustained benefits on growth, skeletal maturation; still long-term outcomes are uncertain.

Access and Equity

Despite regulatory approval, semaglutide is not uniformly available globally, insurance coverage is limited, high cost, and availability of specialists is lacking. Reports show increasing semaglutide use among US teens, yet many are denied despite meeting obesity criteria. Hence it appears that there is a gross demand to supply mismatch.

Ethical and Social Considerations

The introduction of weight reducing medicine in adolescents raises ethical debates about medicines versus holistic social, behavioral, and environmental, interventions in obesity. Critics warn against promoting medications as substitutes for lifestyle management including, increased physical activities and socioeconomic determinants of obesity in adolescents.

FUTURE DIRECTION

The new research possibilities include: (1) Long-term studies to assess safety, sustainability, and effects on health outcomes in children and adolescents. (2) The possible combination therapies, like cagrilintide plus semaglutide (CagriSema), are being evaluated in adolescents with obesity to increase efficacy. (3) The trials in younger children (<12 years). (4) The global data and registry studies to include diverse clinical settings. (5) Further investigations in biomarkers to predict response and optimize individualized treatment. (6) Future research on semaglutide to explore its use beyond diabetes and weight loss in conditions such as heart failure, nonalcoholic fatty liver disease (NAFLD/NASH), chronic kidney disease (CKD), polycystic ovary syndrome (PCOS), sleep apnea, and neurodegenerative disorders such as Alzheimer's and Parkinson's disease. (7) Evaluate the use of semaglutide in nondiabetic patients, with ongoing trials assessing cardiovascular and microvascular benefits, and exploring potential anticancer effects and strategies to prevent weight regain after stopping the treatment.[10]

CONCLUSION

The semaglutide indicates a major advancement in the medical management of obesity in children and adolescents. The clinical evidence shows remarkable reductions in BMI and weight compared to just lifestyle intervention or with placebo. Hence, it is a safe, effective, and an important way for clinicians to treat severe obesity in youth. One review demonstrated that after stopping the medicine, there was a rapid weight regain and reversal of beneficial effects on cardiometabolic markers.[10] Therefore, clinicians should and must carefully weigh the benefits against long-term safety. Hence complete care that involves alteration in lifestyle, psychosocial, and medical strategies are important. In future, continued long-term research and careful guidelines are needed for optimal results with semaglutide in treatment of obesity in children and adolescents.

REFERENCES

1. Srivastava AK. Challenges in the treatment of cardiometabolic syndrome. Indian J Pharmacol. 2012;44(2):155-6.
2. Grundy SM, Cleeman JI, Daniels SR, et al. Diagnosis and management of the metabolic syndrome: an American Heart Association/National Heart, Lung, and Blood Institute Scientific Statement. Circulation. 2005;112:2735-52.
3. Singha S, Awasthia S, Kapoor V, et al. Childhood obesity in India: A two-decade meta-analysis of prevalence and socioeconomic correlates. Clin Epidemiol Glob Health. 2023;23:101390.
4. Anton-Păduraru DT, Mindru DE, Stănescu RS, et al. Unraveling Metabolic Syndrome in Youth: The Obesity Epidemic's Hidden Complication. Children (Basel). 2025;12(4):482.
5. Weghuber D, Barrett T, Barrientos-Pérez M, et al. Once-Weekly Semaglutide in Adolescents with Obesity. N Engl J Med. 2022;387(24):2245-57.
6. Nunns M, Febrey S, Buckland J, et al. The quantity, quality and findings of network meta-analyses evaluating the effectiveness of GLP-1 RAs for weight loss: a scoping review. Southampton (UK): National Institute for Health and Care Research; 2025.
7. Nunns M, Febrey S, Buckland J, et al. The quantity, quality and findings of network meta-analyses evaluating the effectiveness of GLP-1 RAs for weight loss: a scoping review. Health Technol Assess. 2025:1-73.
8. Qin W, Yang J, Deng C, et al. Efficacy and safety of semaglutide 2.4 mg for weight loss in overweight or obese adults without diabetes: An updated systematic review and meta-analysis including the 2-year STEP 5 trial. Diabetes Obes Metab. 2024;26(3):911-23.
9. Fahim SA, Attia YM, Messiha A, et al. Comparative safety and side effects of semaglutide and tirzepatide: Implications for clinical decision-making in obesity management. Biomed Pharmacother. 2025;193: 118731.
10. West S, Scragg J, Aveyard P, et al. Weight regain after cessation of medication for weight management: systematic review and meta-analysis. BMJ. 2026;392:e085304.

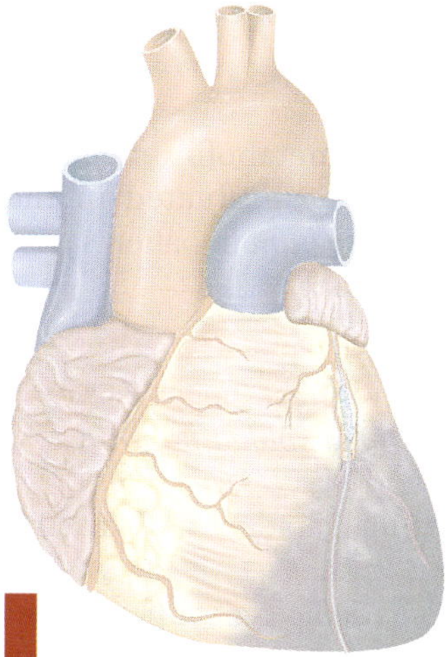

116

CHAPTER

Tirzepatide in Obesity: Indications, Contraindications, Uniqueness, CVOT, and Adverse Effects

HK Chopra, Prachi Gupta, Sunil Raheja, Rajesh Meena

INTRODUCTION

Obesity is a chronic metabolic disorder characterized by excess adiposity and is a major contributor to cardiovascular morbidity and mortality. It plays a central role in the development of atherosclerotic cardiovascular disease (ASCVD), hypertension, heart failure, and type 2 diabetes mellitus (T2DM).[1] Sustained weight reduction through lifestyle measures alone remains challenging for most individuals, leading to increased reliance on pharmacological interventions.[2] In recent years, therapies targeting incretin pathways have substantially improved obesity management. Tirzepatide, a dual agonist of glucose-dependent insulinotropic polypeptide (GIP) and glucagon-like peptide-1 (GLP-1) receptors, has emerged as a highly effective agent for weight reduction with favorable effects on cardiometabolic risk.[1]

MECHANISM OF ACTION AND THERAPEUTIC UNIQUENESS

Tirzepatide is the first therapeutic agent designed to simultaneously activate both *GIP and GLP-1 receptors*, earning the designation of a dual incretin or "twincretin."[3] It mimics the action of both endogenous incretin hormones as illustrated in **Flowchart 1**.

- *GLP-1 receptor agonism:* It enhances glucose-dependent insulin secretion, suppresses glucagon release, delays gastric emptying, and reduces appetite.[3]
- *GIP receptor agonism:* It improves insulin sensitivity, enhances adipocyte lipid handling, and may reduce nausea associated with GLP-1 therapy.[4]

The combined activation of these two incretin pathways results in superior reductions in body weight and metabolic risk markers when compared with therapies that target GLP-1 alone, establishing tirzepatide as a distinct and potent anti-obesity agent.[1]

Flowchart 1: Mechanism of action (MOA) of tirzepatide.

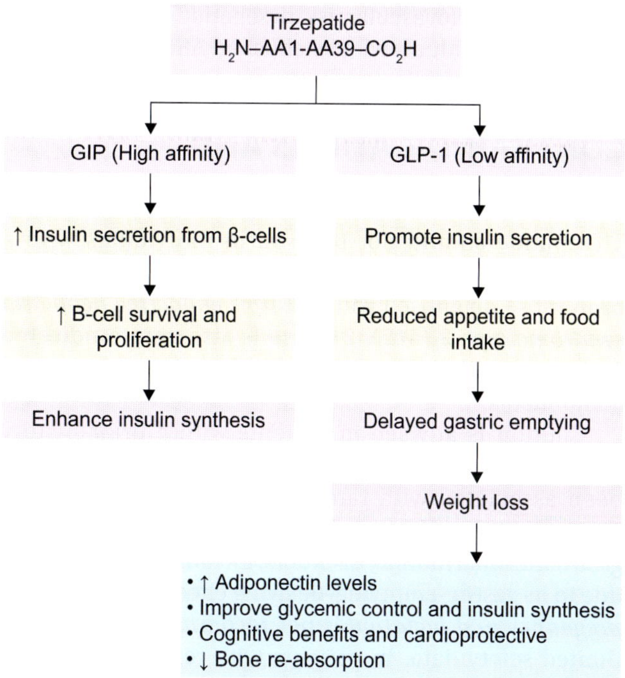

Source: Sweta, Gupta S, Bansal S, et al. Tirzepatide a novel anti diabetic molecule unfold dual action. Discov Public Health. 2024;21:75.

Unique Features

- *Dual incretin action* leading to synergistic metabolic effects
- *Greater weight reduction* compared to GLP-1 receptor agonists alone
- *Improved insulin sensitivity and lipid metabolism*
- *Once-weekly subcutaneous administration*
- Sustained reductions in body weight, HbA1c, and cardiometabolic risk markers

INDICATIONS IN OBESITY MANAGEMENT

Tirzepatide is indicated for long-term weight management in adults with:

- *Obesity*, defined as a body mass index (BMI) of ≥30 kg/m^2, or
- *Overweight* (BMI ≥27 kg/m^2) in the presence of at least one obesity-associated comorbidity such as hypertension, dyslipidemia, T2DM, or obstructive sleep apnea.[1]

Clinical studies have demonstrated consistent and substantial weight reduction, with average losses ranging from *15% to over 20% of baseline body weight*, surpassing outcomes seen with other approved pharmacotherapies for obesity.[1]

Given the strong association between excess body weight and cardiovascular risk, tirzepatide offers particular benefit in individuals with established ASCVD or those at high cardiometabolic risk.[4]

CONTRAINDICATIONS AND PRECAUTIONS

Tirzepatide should not be used in individuals with a personal or familial history of *medullary thyroid carcinoma* or in those diagnosed with *multiple endocrine neoplasia syndrome type 2 (MEN 2)*.[3] Use is also contraindicated in patients with known hypersensitivity to the drug or its components.

Caution is advised in patients with a prior history of *acute pancreatitis*, as incretin-based therapies have been associated with rare pancreatic adverse events.[4] Tirzepatide should be avoided in individuals with severe gastrointestinal motility disorders, including gastroparesis, due to its gastric-emptying–delaying effects. Its use during *pregnancy and lactation* is not recommended owing to limited safety data. In patients with renal impairment, no routine dose adjustment is required; however, careful monitoring is advised, particularly in the presence of significant gastrointestinal adverse effects that may predispose to volume depletion.[5]

CARDIOVASCULAR OUTCOME EVIDENCE

The cardiovascular safety and metabolic effects of tirzepatide have been extensively evaluated in the *SURPASS phase III clinical trial program* in patients with T2DM and high cardiovascular risk.[3,5]

Key findings include:

- Significant reductions in *body weight (up to 22.5%)*.
- Marked improvements in *HbA1c, blood pressure, and lipid parameters.*
- Reduction in inflammatory markers such as C-reactive protein.

SURPASS-CVOT is an ongoing dedicated cardiovascular outcomes trial comparing tirzepatide with dulaglutide in patients with T2DM and established CVD.

Preliminary and pooled analyses suggest:

- *Non-inferiority for major adverse cardiovascular events (MACE)*
- Trends toward reduced cardiovascular events driven by weight loss, glycemic control, and metabolic improvement.[4]

Implications for Obesity-related Cardiovascular Disease

Although a dedicated CVOT in non-diabetic obesity is awaited, the profound weight reduction and favorable cardiometabolic effects suggest potential benefits in reducing long-term cardiovascular risk.

The magnitude of weight loss and improvement in cardiometabolic parameters observed with tirzepatide suggest a potential for long-term cardiovascular risk reduction, although definitive outcome data in non-diabetic obese populations are still awaited.[2]

ADVERSE EFFECTS AND SAFETY PROFILE

The adverse effect profile of tirzepatide is largely consistent with other incretin-based therapies. *Gastrointestinal symptoms* are the most frequently reported adverse events and include nausea, vomiting, diarrhea, and constipation, particularly during treatment initiation and dose escalation.[3] These effects are generally mild to moderate in intensity and tend to diminish with continued therapy and gradual dose titration.

Less common adverse effects include injection-site reactions, dyspepsia, and fatigue.[5] Rare but clinically relevant events such as *pancreatitis* and *gallbladder disease* have been reported, with the latter likely related to rapid weight reduction rather than a direct pharmacologic effect.[4]

Importantly, current clinical data do not indicate an increased risk of heart failure exacerbation, arrhythmias, or ischemic cardiovascular events associated with tirzepatide use.[3]

LIMITATIONS

Despite its robust efficacy, several limitations warrant consideration. Long-term cardiovascular outcome data in individuals with obesity without diabetes remain limited. Additionally, the high cost of therapy and restricted availability in certain regions may limit widespread adoption. Gastrointestinal intolerance, though usually transient, may affect treatment adherence in some patients.[2]

CONCLUSION

Tirzepatide represents a significant therapeutic advance in the pharmacological management of obesity. Through dual activation of GIP and GLP-1 receptors, it achieves substantial and sustained weight loss while favorably influencing multiple cardiovascular risk factors. Although ongoing studies will further define its long-term cardiovascular benefits, current evidence supports the use of tirzepatide as an effective option for obesity management, particularly in individuals with elevated cardiometabolic risk.[1,4]

REFERENCES

1. Jastreboff AM, Aronne LJ, Ahmad NN, et al. Tirzepatide once weekly for the treatment of obesity. N Engl J Med. 2022;387:205-16.
2. Wilding JPH, Batterham RL, Calanna S, et al. Weight loss with incretin-based therapies and cardiovascular outcomes. Lancet Diabetes Endocrinol. 2023;11: 42-55.
3. Frias JP, Davies MJ, Rosenstock J, et al. Tirzepatide versus semaglutide once weekly in patients with type 2 diabetes. N Engl J Med. 2021;385:503-15.
4. Sattar N, McGuire DK. Pathways to cardiorenal protection with incretin-based therapies. Circulation. 2022;146: 1187-201.
5. Ludvik B, Giorgino F, Jodar E, et al. Once-weekly tirzepatide versus insulin glargine in type 2 diabetes. Lancet. 2021;398:583-98.

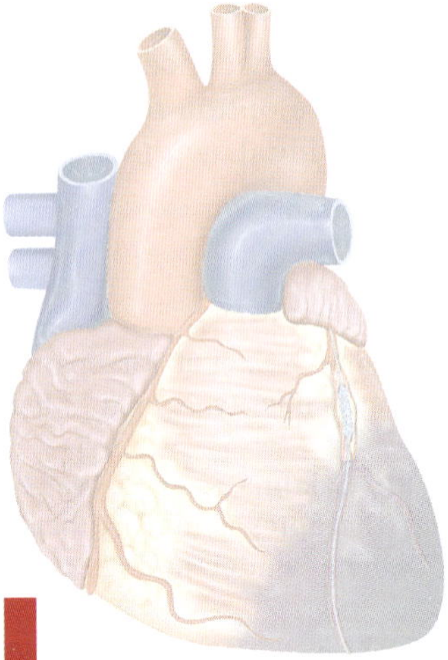

117

CHAPTER

Comparison of Tirzepatide with Semaglutide in Obesity and Diabetes with Cardiovascular Disease

Kavita Tyagi, Manikanth Vivek

INTRODUCTION

Systemic metabolic disorder (SMD) comprises a cluster of metabolic abnormalities affecting multiple organs, leading to increased morbidity and mortality from both cardiovascular and noncardiovascular causes. Atherosclerotic cardiovascular disease (ASCVD) is the leading cause of morbidity and mortality in people with diabetes.[1] Diabetes itself confers independent ASCVD risk, and among people with diabetes, all major cardiovascular risk factors, including hypertension, hyperlipidemia, and obesity, are clustered and common.[2] Diabetes is also an important risk factor for incident heart failure, which is at least twofold more prevalent in people with diabetes compared with those without diabetes and is a major cause of morbidity and mortality.[3]

Obesity is a chronic disease defined by the presence of abnormal or excessive adipose accumulation that negatively affects health outcomes, including increased risk of heart failure (HF), coronary artery disease (CAD), and stroke.[4] For individuals with HF with preserved ejection fraction (HFpEF), intentional weight loss to treat obesity is associated with improved health status and lower event rates in clinical trials. Obesity confers increased risks of HF, CAD, and stroke, and weight loss can reduce cardiovascular disease (CVD) risk.[5,6]

Epicardial adipose tissue (EAT) is a modifiable risk factor which can affect cardiac function through increased inflammation, fibrosis, and autonomic dysregulation. In addition, increased EAT volume can impair ventricular relaxation through a mechanical effect, as observed in obesity.

Therapies studied in HF include the GLP-1 receptor agonists [GLP-1 RAs (i.e., *semaglutide*)] and the GLP-1/GIP dual receptor agonist (i.e., *tirzepatide*), alternatively termed nutrient-stimulated hormone therapies (*NuSH*). Both these drugs demonstrate improved cardiovascular outcomes in individuals with type 2 diabetes mellitus (T2DM) without and with high cardiovascular risk or established disease as well as a reduction in incident HF events. Furthermore, the benefit of these therapies extends to those without T2DM but with CVD and HFpEF.

INDIVIDUAL RESULTS OF SEMAGLUTIDE AND TIRZEPATIDE

Diabetes drives interconnected risks—namely ASCVD, HF, and chronic kidney disease—all largely linked to metabolic dysfunction, often arising from obesity. As blood sugar rises (higher A1C), the likelihood of these overlapping conditions increases. This combination is known as cardiovascular-kidney-metabolic (CKM) or cardiorenal metabolic disease, reflecting their common origins and frequent coexistence.

Based on the long-term data in the randomized controlled trials (RCTs), GLP-1 RAs are approved for T2DM and obesity as they reduce HbA1c and body weight. Two major trials, *SUSTAIN-6* and *SOUL,* have established the efficacy of injectable and oral semaglutide, respectively, in terms of reduction of MACE. In patients with HFpEF and obesity, semaglutide led to greater improvement in symptoms, exercise function, and weight loss as compared to placebo (STEP-HFpEF). The same effect was seen even in patients of T2DM (STEP-HFpEF DM). In the SELECT trial comprising 17,604 individuals with CVD and BMI >27 kg/m^2, semaglutide was associated with 10.2% weight loss over 208 weeks, as well as a reduction in the primary composite end point of cardiovascular death, myocardial infarction (MI), and stroke.

In a recent meta-analysis published in *The Lancet*,[7] GLP-1 RAs resulted in a 13% reduction of MACE events, 14% reduction in cardiovascular death, 10% reduction in nonfatal MI, 10% reduction in hospitalization for HF, and 12 % reduction in the risk of death due to any cause.

Tirzepatide, a GLP-1/GIP dual receptor agonist, has better glycemic control, more weight loss, and fewer gastrointestinal (GI) adverse effects as compared to semaglutide. In patients with obesity and HFpEF (SUMMIT), tirzepatide led to lower risk of a composite of death from cardiovascular causes or worsening HF than placebo and improved health status. In the SUMMIT CMR substudy, it was seen that tirzepatide reduced LV mass and paracardiac adipose tissue and change in LV mass paralleled body weight loss.

COMPARISON BETWEEN SEMAGLUTIDE VERSUS TIRZEPATIDE

Although prospective RCTs comparing tirzepatide and semaglutide are yet to be conducted, some data are available. In a retrospective cohort analysis[8] of T2DM patients with BMI ≥25 kg/m^2, treatment with tirzepatide was associated with lower primary composite outcomes of acute MI, ischemic stroke, and all-cause mortality. The number of patients who developed new onset AF and HbA1c <7% was significantly lower in the tirzepatide group as compared to the semaglutide group.

In a phase 3b, open-label controlled trial (SURMOUNT-5), among participants with obesity but without T2DM, treatment with tirzepatide was superior to treatment with semaglutide with respect to reduction in body weight and waist circumference at week 72.[9] In a post hoc analysis of the SURMOUNT-5 trial, the average predicted 10-year CVD risk score before treatment was 9.3%. Treatment with tirzepatide was associated with significantly greater reduction in predicted 10-year CVD risk compared with semaglutide (absolute reduction from baseline of 2.4 and 1.4%, respectively; $p < 0.001$). This post hoc analysis suggests that tirzepatide treatment may provide greater benefit in primary prevention of CVD than semaglutide in people with obesity and overweight.[10]

A cohort study was conducted in T2DM patients with obesity who received tirzepatide versus semaglutide, which showed that use of tirzepatide was associated with significantly greater weight loss than semaglutide with similar rates of GI adverse effects.[11] Another retrospective cohort study was done to identify differences in cardiovascular outcomes between patients with diabetes treated with tirzepatide as compared to semaglutide. Patients were matched for age, race, gender, and ethnicity. After a 3-year follow-up, tirzepatide was associated with statistically significantly fewer MACE outcomes compared to semaglutide for each of the individual end points as well as the overall composite end point over the 3-year follow-up period, suggesting that tirzepatide offers superior cardiovascular protection for primary prevention compared to semaglutide, warranting further investigation in future studies and clinical trials.[12]

Therefore, based on many studies and meta-analyses, tirzepatide robustly improves weight, glycemic, and cardiometabolic parameters, with trends toward reduced MACE in diabetes and obesity populations. The incidence of GI side effects and discontinuation rates was less as compared to semaglutide.

LIMITATIONS

There is paucity of data available with tirzepatide regarding whether it is superior to GLP-1 RAs in terms of reduction of MACE events. Tirzepatide was compared to dulaglutide in a phase 3b randomized trial (SURPASS-CVOT), a GLP-1 RA with proven cardiovascular benefit (REWIND), in patients with T2DM and established ASCVD and were followed up for nearly ~5 years. The primary end point was reduction in MACE events—a composite of cardiovascular death, heart attack, or stroke. Tirzepatide was noninferior to dulaglutide in terms of primary endpoint but had greater improvements in A1C, weight, and cardiovascular biomarkers, including lipids and systolic blood pressure, compared to dulaglutide. In terms of safety, both had mild-to-moderate GI adverse effects with tirzepatide having slightly more discontinuation rates than dulaglutide (13.3 vs. 10.2%).

The ongoing SURMOUNT-MMO trial will investigate the effect of tirzepatide on the reduction of morbidity and mortality in adults living with obesity and provide additional evidence for the potential clinical benefits of tirzepatide in this population. Direct head-to-head

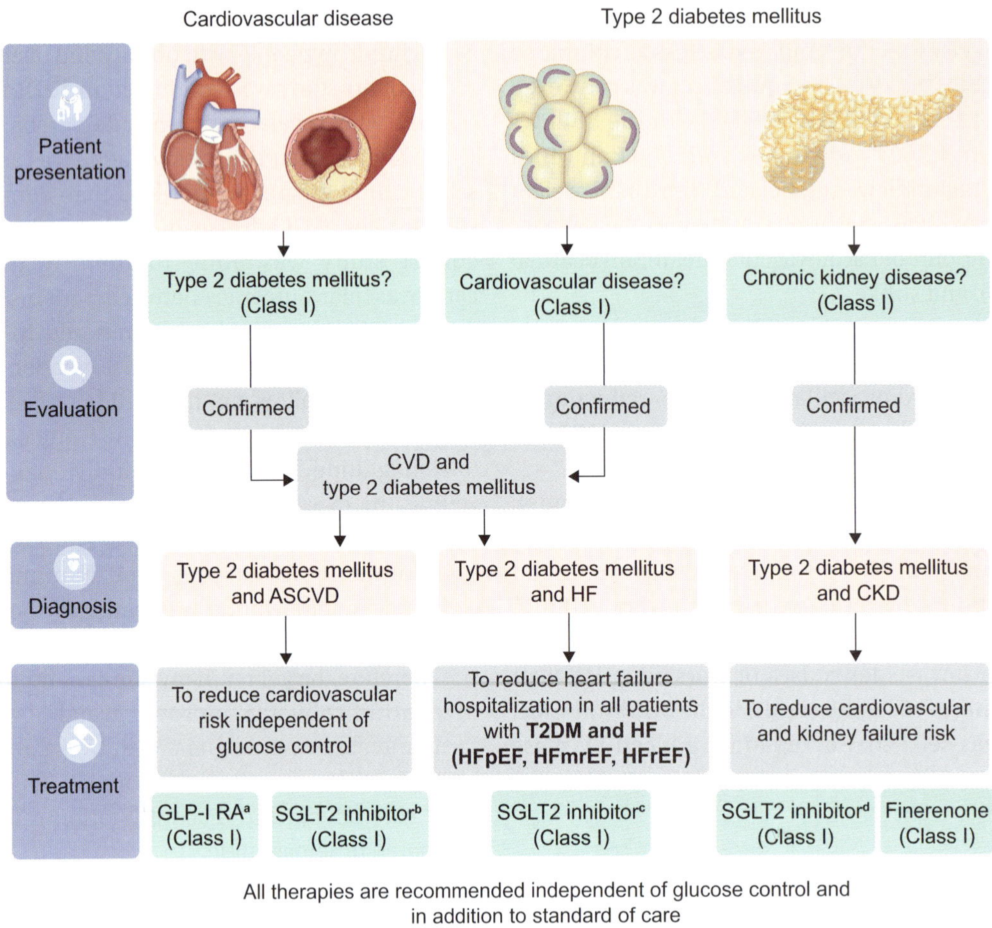

Fig. 1: 2023 ESC Guidelines for the management of cardiovascular disease in patients with diabetes.
[a]GLP-1 RAs with proven cardiovascular benefit: liraglutide, semaglutide s.c., dulaglutide, efpeglenatide.
[b]SGLT2 inhibitors with proven cardiovascular benefit: empagliflozin, canagliflozin, dapagliflozin, sotagliflozin.
[c]Empagliflozin, dapagliflozin, sotagliflozin in HFrEF; empagliflozin, dapagliflozin in HFpEF and HFmrEF.
[d]Canagliflozin, empagliflozin, dapagliflozin.

comparison trials are needed to confirm the superiority/noninferiority of tirzepatide as compared to other GLP-1 RAs in terms of CVD reduction.

GLP-1 receptor agonists, particularly semaglutide, were found to have serious ocular side effects besides GI adverse effects. In a retrospective matched observational cohort study where semaglutide versus non-GLP-1 RA were given for either T2DM or obesity, the cumulative incidence of nonarteritic anterior ischemic optic neuropathy (NAION) for the semaglutide versus non-GLP-1 RA cohorts over 36 months was 6.7 and 0.8%, respectively.[13] In another retrospective cohort study where GLP-1 RAs were given for at least 6 months or longer, the use of GLP-1 RAs among patients with diabetes was associated with a twofold higher risk of incident neovascular age-related macular degeneration (nAMD) development than among similar patients with diabetes who did not receive a GLP-1 RA **(Fig. 1)**.[14]

CONCLUSION

In people with obesity and diabetes at high cardiovascular risk, tirzepatide achieves greater reductions in body weight, glucose, and cardiometabolic risk than semaglutide. Both drugs improve cardiovascular outcomes, but semaglutide has longer follow-up supporting its established safety. GI side effects are common for both, though semaglutide leads to more GI events and discontinuations. Ultimately, treatment selection should be tailored to individual patient needs and tolerability, given the evolving evidence base.

REFERENCES

1. Rawshani A, Rawshani A, Franzén S, et al. Mortality and cardiovascular disease in type 1 and type 2 diabetes. N Engl J Med. 2017;376:1407-18.
2. Weng W, Tian Y, Kong SX, et al. The prevalence of cardiovascular disease and antidiabetes treatment characteristics among a large type 2 diabetes population in the United States. Endocrinol Diabetes Metab. 2019;2:e00076.
3. Kodama S, Fujihara K, Horikawa C, et al. Diabetes mellitus and risk of new-onset and recurrent heart failure: a systematic review and meta-analysis. ESC Heart Fail. 2020;7:2146-74.
4. Phelps NH, Singleton RK, Zhou B, et al.; NCD Risk Factor Collaboration (NCD-RisC). Worldwide trends in underweight and obesity from 1990 to 2022: a pooled analysis of 3663 population representative studies with 222 million children, adolescents, and adults. Lancet. 2024;403:1027-50.
5. Kosiborod MN, Abildstrøm SZ, Borlaug BA, et al. Semaglutide in patients with heart failure with preserved ejection fraction and obesity. N Engl J Med. 2023;389:1069-84.
6. Packer M, Zile MR, Kramer CM, et al. Tirzepatide for heart failure with preserved ejection fraction and obesity. N Engl J Med. 2024;392:427-37.
7. Badve SV, Bilal A, Lee MMY, et al. Effects of GLP-1 receptor agonists on kidney and cardiovascular disease outcomes: a meta-analysis of randomised controlled trials. Lancet Diabetes Endocrinol. 2025;13:15-28.
8. Dani SS, Makwana B, Khadke S, et al. An observational study of cardiovascular outcomes of tirzepatide vs glucagon-like peptide-1 receptor agonists. JACC Adv. 2025;4(5):101740.
9. Aronne LJ, Horn DB, le Roux CW, et al. Tirzepatide as compared with semaglutide for the treatment of obesity. N Engl J Med. 2025;393(1):26-36.
10. Mamas MA, Bays H, Li R, et al. Tirzepatide compared with semaglutide and 10-year cardiovascular disease risk reduction in obesity: post-hoc analysis of the SURMOUNT-5 trial. Eur Heart J Open. 2025;5(5):oeaf117.
11. Rodriguez PJ, Goodwin Cartwright BM, Smith SR, et al. Semaglutide with tirzepatide for weight loss in adults with overweight or obesity. JAMA Intern Med. 2024;184(9):1056-64.
12. Cervantes M, Miles B, Mehta A, et al. Comparison of cardiovascular outcomes in patients with diabetes treated with tirzepatide versus semaglutide: a multi-institutional analysis. Eur Heart J. 2024;45(Supplement_1):ehae666.
13. Hathaway JT, Shah MP, Hathaway DB, et al. Risk of nonarteritic anterior ischemic optic neuropathy in patients prescribed semaglutide. JAMA Ophthalmol. 2024;142(8):732-39.
14. Shor R, Mihalache A, Noori A, et al. Glucagon-like peptide-1 receptor agonists and risk of neovascular age-related macular degeneration. JAMA Ophthalmol. 2025;143(7):587-94.

118

CHAPTER

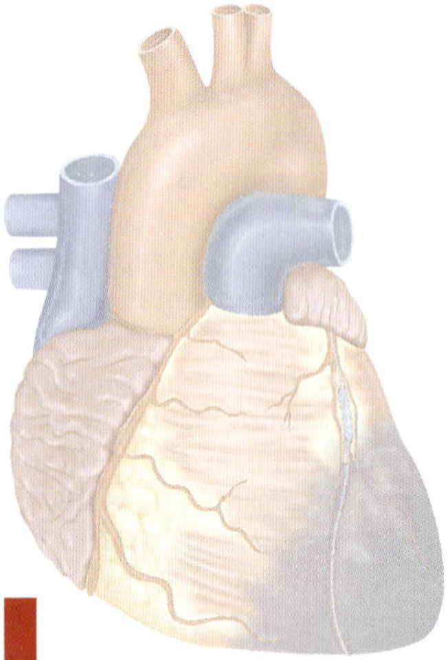

Pharmacological Profile of Tirzepatide: Dual GIP and GLP-1 Receptor Agonism and its Cardiovascular, Obesity, and Diabetes Management

Vinod Mittal, Alok Modi

INTRODUCTION

Diabetes and obesity have emerged as convergent global epidemics, together fueling cardiovascular risk through complex interactions of insulin resistance, endothelial dysfunction, and chronic inflammation.[1,2] The discovery of incretin hormones—glucagon-like peptide-1 (GLP-1) and glucose-dependent insulinotropic polypeptide (GIP)—transformed this therapeutic landscape by enabling glucose-dependent insulin release with minimal hypoglycemia.[1,3]

Tirzepatide, a first-in-class *dual GIP/GLP-1 receptor agonist*, represents a new horizon in metabolic therapy.[4-6] This 39-amino-acid acylated peptide integrates glucose lowering, weight reduction, and cardiovascular modulation—extending the concept of treatment beyond glycemia to full metabolic re-equilibration.[3,7-10] Its approval established a paradigm shift from single-pathway to dual-pathway pharmacology, achieving broader control over appetite, adiposity, and postprandial metabolism.[3,5,11-13]

MECHANISM OF ACTION

Dual Receptor Engagement and Synergistic Incretin Modulation

Tirzepatide is a unimolecular agonist with affinity for both the *glucose-dependent insulinotropic polypeptide receptor (GIPR)* and the *glucagon-like peptide-1 receptor (GLP-1R)*, producing additive and synergistic metabolic effects.[3,6] A C20 fatty-diacid side chain enables reversible albumin binding, supporting extended circulation and once-weekly administration.[3,13]

Through GIPR stimulation, tirzepatide enhances insulin sensitivity in skeletal muscle and adipose tissue, reducing ectopic fat deposition, while GLP-1R activation slows gastric emptying and promotes satiety via hypothalamic pathways.[2,3,13] Together, these actions result in pronounced reductions in HbA1c and substantial weight loss demonstrated across the SURPASS program.[4-6]

Molecular and Cellular Dynamics

Experimental data suggest GIPR signaling may potentiate GLP-1R-mediated cyclic AMP generation and sustain β-cell responsiveness.[3,14,15] This dual agonism reduces islet stress and oxidative burden, while promoting β-cell preservation and improved insulin secretory dynamics, exceeding effects achieved by GLP-1 monoagonists.[3,11]

Adiposity Modifying and Metabolic Effects

Tirzepatide significantly modulates lipid metabolism, lowering triglycerides and LDL-cholesterol (LDL-C) while modestly increasing HDL-cholesterol (HDL-C).[5,6,12] These improvements accompany double-digit kilogram weight loss, often surpassing traditional GLP-1 analogues in head-to-head comparisons.[3,7,10] Such integrated control across pancreatic, central, and hepatic pathways exemplifies the "twincretin" concept of synchronized metabolic correction **(Fig. 1)**.[3]

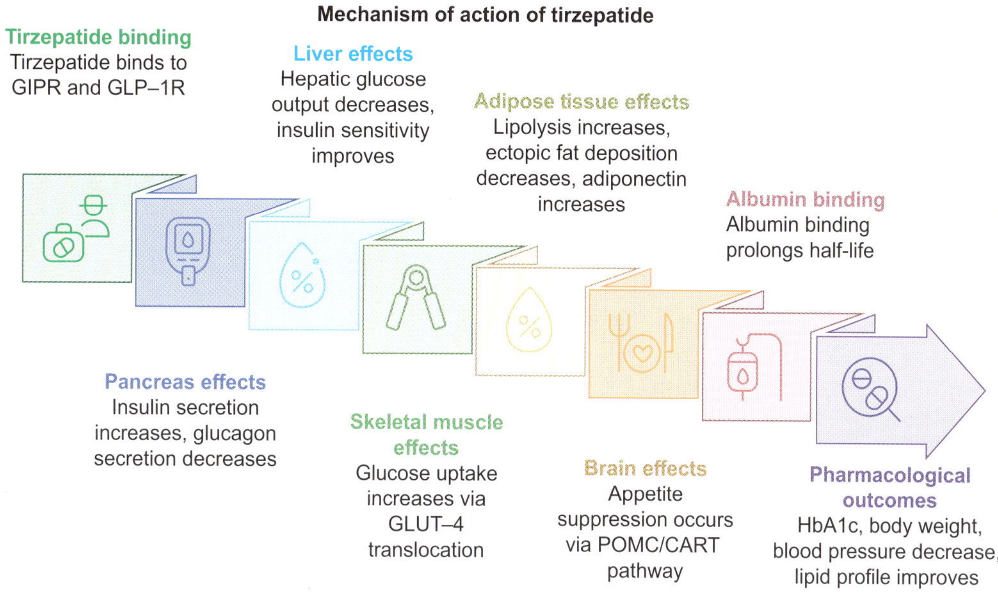

Fig. 1: Dual GIP and GLP-1 receptor engagement by tirzepatide producing integrated pancreatic, hepatic, muscular, adipose, and central metabolic effects.

PHARMACOKINETICS AND PHARMACODYNAMICS

After subcutaneous injection, tirzepatide is slowly absorbed, achieving peak plasma levels within 8–12 hours, with bioavailability around 80% and a mean half-life of approximately 116 hours.[3,13] Its albumin binding accounts for a smooth concentration profile and minimal peak-to-trough variation.[3] Metabolism proceeds through proteolytic degradation into inactive fragments, and no dosage adjustment is typically required for renal or hepatic dysfunction.[13]

Clinically, tirzepatide induces *dose-dependent reductions in fasting and postprandial glucose, HbA1c, and body weight*, consistently outperforming semaglutide 1 mg and basal insulin in SURPASS trials.[4-6] In a SURPASS-3 continuous glucose-monitoring substudy, tirzepatide increased time-in-range by >20% versus insulin degludec, reflecting its integrated modulation of insulin secretion, glucagon suppression, and gastric motility.[13]

Mechanistic modeling indicates enhanced first-phase insulin response, improved hepatic insulin sensitivity, and reduction in fasting glucagon—all partially independent of weight loss—underscoring GIPR's complementary role.[3,6] Therapeutic initiation typically begins at 2.5 mg weekly, escalating by 2.5 mg every 4 weeks to maintenance doses of 5–15 mg as tolerated, with gastrointestinal events mitigated by slow titration **(Table 1)**.[4,6,7]

CLINICAL EFFICACY

Tirzepatide's clinical performance has been validated across the *SURPASS-1-5* trials, enrolling >6,000 participants with type 2 diabetes.[4-6] In these studies, HbA1c reductions ranged from –1.9 to –2.6%, surpassing dulaglutide, semaglutide 1 mg, and basal insulin comparators.[4,5] Weight loss reached 7–12 kg, and up to –15 kg in the highest dose arms.[5,6] The proportion of patients achieving dual endpoints (HbA1c <6.5 and ≥10% weight reduction) exceeded 60%, a benchmark unmatched by any single-receptor agonist.[4,7]

In *SURPASS-2*, tirzepatide 15 mg achieved HbA1c –2.3% versus –1.9% for semaglutide 1 mg, with nearly twice the weight loss.[4,6] *SURPASS-3* demonstrated superiority over insulin degludec for both glycemic and weight endpoints, accompanied by lower incidence of hypoglycemia.[6,13] In *SURPASS-5*, combination therapy with insulin glargine yielded further HbA1c reductions (–2.4%) without excess hypoglycemia.[5,6]

Efficacy was consistent across demographic and renal subgroups, including patients ≥65 years and those with mild-to-moderate CKD.[5,13] Continuous glucose-monitoring analyses revealed enhanced time-in-range and fewer nocturnal lows.[13] Indirect comparisons suggest tirzepatide's glycemic and weight outcomes may rival surgical interventions in metabolic magnitude **(Fig. 2)**.[6,11]

TABLE 1: Comparative glycemic and weight outcomes of tirzepatide versus GLP-1 receptor agonists in major clinical trials.

Parameter	*Tirzepatide 5 mg*	*Tirzepatide 10 mg*	*Tirzepatide 15 mg*	*Semaglutide 1 mg*	*Dulaglutide 1.5 mg*	*Insulin degludec*
Mean HbA1c reduction (%)	−2.0 ± 0.3	−2.3 ± 0.4	−2.5 ± 0.5	−1.9 ± 0.4	−1.5 ± 0.3	−1.3 ± 0.4
Body-weight reduction (kg)	−7.0 ± 1.8	−9.5 ± 2.4	−11.5 ± 2.8	−5.9 ± 1.7	−3.0 ± 1.2	+1.8 ± 1.1
Percentage achieving HbA1c <7.0%	81%	86%	92%	79%	67%	62%
Percentage achieving ≥10% weight loss	36%	49%	57%	28%	14%	–
Systolic BP reduction (mm Hg)	−4.1 ± 1.2	−5.8 ± 1.3	−6.6 ± 1.4	−4.5 ± 1.1	−3.0 ± 1.0	−2.5 ± 0.9
Nausea incidence (%)	14	17	18	20	16	6
Hypoglycemia (<70 mg/dL, %)	0.8	0.9	1.0	0.7	0.6	2.4

Note: Comparative outcomes derived from *SURPASS-1–5* and head-to-head studies of tirzepatide versus GLP-1 receptor agonists and basal insulin. All values represent mean change from baseline at 40–52 weeks. Tirzepatide demonstrates *dose-dependent superiority* in both glycemic and weight endpoints, with low hypoglycemia risk.
(BP: blood pressure; HbA1c: glycated hemoglobin; SURPASS: Study of Tirzepatide versus Placebo or Active Comparator in Type 2 Diabetes)

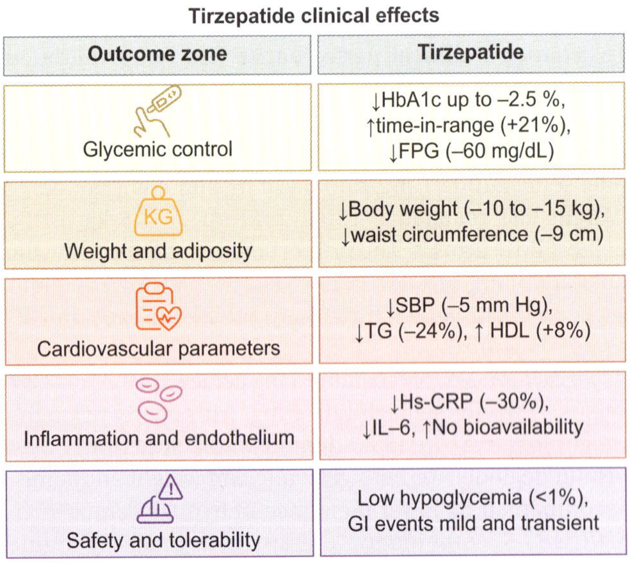

Fig. 2: Tirzepatide delivers concurrent improvements in glycemic control, weight reduction, lipid and inflammatory markers, and blood pressure—demonstrating a unified cardiometabolic benefit driven by dual GIP and GLP-1 receptor agonism.

CARDIOVASCULAR OUTCOMES

Beyond glycemic efficacy, tirzepatide confers broad cardiometabolic benefit, modulating surrogate and exploratory cardiovascular markers.[5,11,12] Across pooled analyses, systolic blood pressure decreased 4–6 mm Hg, diastolic ≈2 mm Hg, and pulse-wave velocity improved, indicating enhanced arterial compliance.[12,13]

Lipid indices demonstrate triglyceride reduction ≈ –24%, LDL-C –12%, and HDL-C +8%, complementing improvements in apoB and non-HDL-C.[2,6,12] Biomarker studies reveal decreases in hs-CRP and IL-6, implicating anti-inflammatory mechanisms beyond glucose lowering.[11,12] Echocardiographic and MRI subanalyses suggest favorable changes in left-ventricular mass index and E/E' ratio, pointing toward improved diastolic function.[6,11,12]

The ongoing *SURPASS-CVOT* trial (NCT04255433) compares tirzepatide versus dulaglutide on major adverse cardiovascular events (MACE). Preliminary reports indicate hazard ratios <1 for MACE, with full results awaited.[11,12] Early data from the *SURMOUNT* obesity trials mirror these findings, demonstrating weight-induced improvements in systolic pressure and lipid metabolism that could translate into downstream CV benefit.[2,6,10]

Mechanistically, dual GIP/GLP-1 agonism may improve myocardial energetics and endothelial nitric-oxide signaling while reducing adipose-derived inflammation.[1,3,11] The convergence of glucose, weight, and lipid modulation differentiates tirzepatide from earlier incretin analogues, situating it at the frontier of integrated cardiometabolic therapy **(Fig. 3)**.[2,6,11]

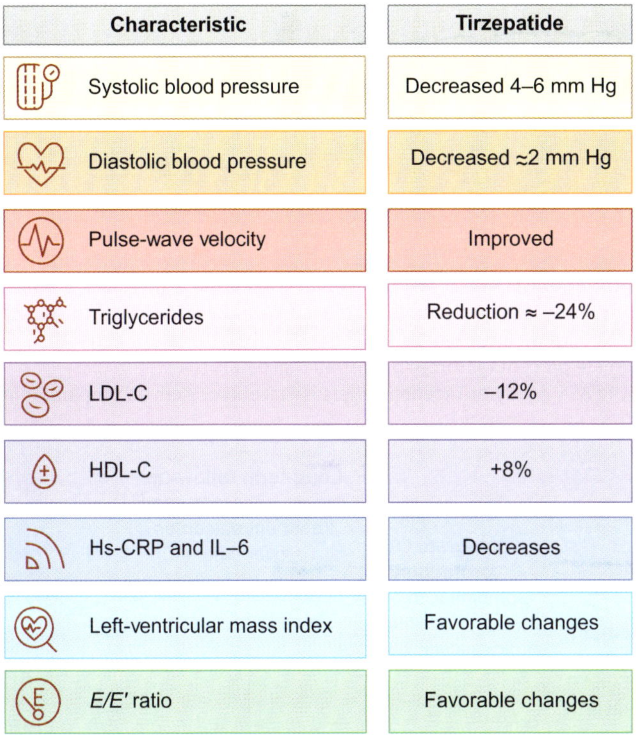

Fig. 3: Tirzepatide's cardiometabolic benefits—changes observed in key cardiovascular and metabolic parameters across pooled analyses from SURPASS and SURMOUNT trials. (DBP: diastolic blood pressure; *E*/*E*′: ratio of early diastolic transmitral flow velocity to mitral annular velocity; HDL-C: high-density lipoprotein cholesterol; hs-CRP: high-sensitivity C-reactive protein; IL-6: interleukin-6; LDL-C: low-density lipoprotein cholesterol; SBP: systolic blood pressure)

SAFETY AND ADVERSE EVENTS

Across the SURPASS and SURMOUNT programs, tirzepatide exhibited a *tolerability profile comparable to GLP-1 RAs*, with gastrointestinal symptoms as the most frequent adverse events.[4-6] Nausea, diarrhea, and transient appetite reduction typically occurred during dose escalation and subsided with continued therapy.[4,7] Discontinuation due to GI effects was ≤6%, lower than with higher dose semaglutide in several comparisons.[4-6]

Hypoglycemia incidence remained low (<1%) when tirzepatide was used without insulin or sulfonylureas, reflecting its glucose-dependent mechanism.[6,13] Modest increases in heart rate (2–4 beats per minute) were consistent with other incretin therapies.[6,13] No signal for pancreatitis, medullary thyroid carcinoma, or retinopathy progression has emerged to date, though long-term surveillance continues.[6,12,13]

Mild increases in amylase and lipase were observed but without clinical sequelae.[6,13] Injection-site reactions were infrequent and nonserious.[5,6] Adverse-event frequency was dose-dependent, underscoring the rationale for gradual titration starting at 2.5 mg.[4,6]

Safety in special populations—including the elderly and those with hepatic or renal impairment—has remained reassuring, with no excess adverse outcomes.[5,13] Overall, tirzepatide's dual-incretin mechanism provides high efficacy while maintaining safety margins comparable to established GLP-1 receptor agonists **(Table 2)**.[6,13]

TABLE 2: Summary of adverse events reported across major SURPASS trials.

Adverse event category	*Tirzepatide 5 mg*	*Tirzepatide 10 mg*	*Tirzepatide 15 mg*	*Comparator (GLP-1 RA/insulin/placebo)*
Any adverse event (%)	63	68	71	59
Serious adverse event (%)	5.0	5.4	5.7	5.2
Discontinuation due to AE (%)	4.3	5.8	6.1	4.7
Gastrointestinal disorders (%)				
• Nausea	14	17	18	20
• Diarrhea	11	13	14	10
• Vomiting	6	8	9	7
Appetite decreased (%)	8	10	11	5
Injection-site reactions (%)	3	4	4	3
Hypoglycemia (<70 mg/dL, %)	0.8	0.9	1.0	1.2
Severe hypoglycemia (events per 100 patient-years)	<0.1	<0.1	<0.1	0.3
Pancreatitis (events per 100 patient-years)	<0.1	<0.1	<0.1	<0.1

Contd...

Contd...

Adverse event category	*Tirzepatide 5 mg*	*Tirzepatide 10 mg*	*Tirzepatide 15 mg*	*Comparator (GLP-1 RA/insulin/placebo)*
Amylase/lipase elevation (%)	3	4	5	3
Heart-rate increase (beats per minute)	+2 ± 1	+3 ± 1	+4 ± 1	+2 ± 1
Gallbladder-related events (%)	0.5	0.7	0.9	0.6
Retinopathy progression (%)	0.2	0.3	0.4	0.2

Note: Adverse-event profile of tirzepatide compared with GLP-1 receptor agonists, basal insulin, or placebo across SURPASS-1–5 trials. Gastrointestinal events were the most frequent but generally mild and transient. Hypoglycemia incidence was low and similar to that of comparators, reflecting the glucose-dependent mechanism of action. No significant excess risk of pancreatitis, thyroid malignancy, or retinopathy progression was observed. Values represent pooled or approximate percentages from published trial data.

(AE: adverse event; GLP-1 RA: glucagon-like peptide-1 receptor agonist; SURPASS: Study of Tirzepatide versus Placebo or Active Comparator in Type 2 Diabetes)

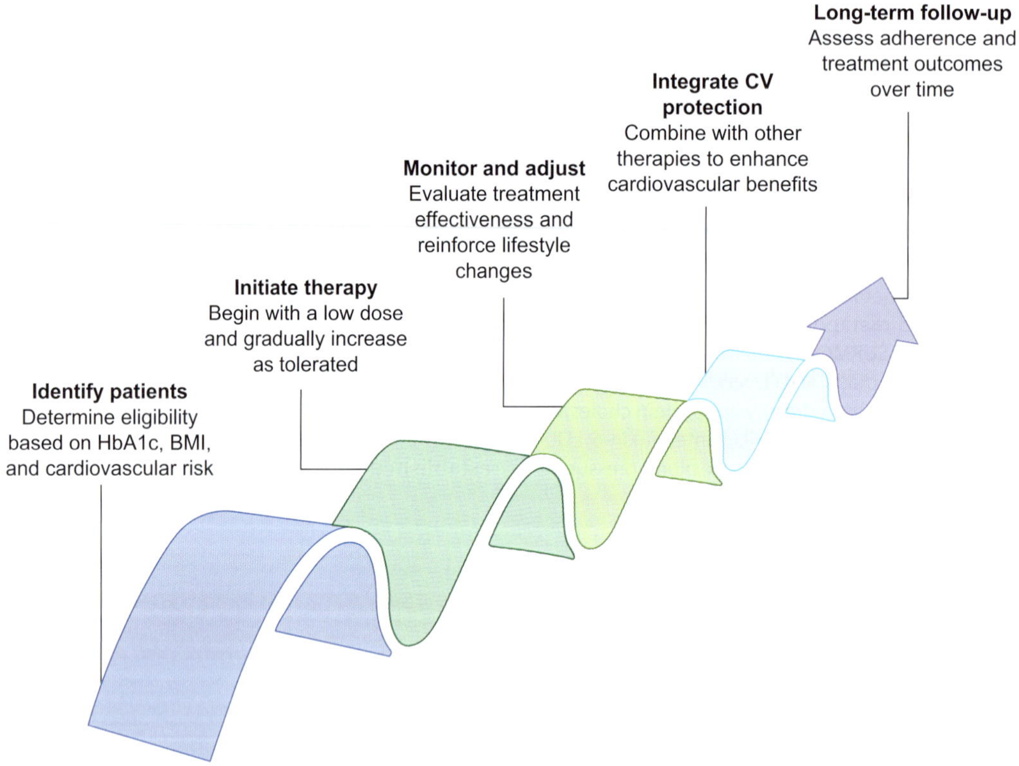

Fig. 4: Tirzepatide treatment framework—stepwise clinical algorithm illustrating practical implementation of tirzepatide therapy in type 2 diabetes and obesity management. (BMI: body mass index; CV: cardiovascular; HbA1c: glycated hemoglobin)

LIMITATIONS

Despite its robust evidence base, several limitations temper the interpretation of tirzepatide data. Most published trials were of *relatively short duration (40–104 weeks)* and lacked cardiovascular endpoint adjudication.[6,11,12] The ongoing *SURPASS-CVOT* will clarify whether the glycemic and weight benefits translate into definitive reductions in *MACE*.[11,12]

Real-world experience remains limited, particularly in *South Asian populations*, where β-cell reserve, adiposity phenotype, and socioeconomic barriers may alter response and accessibility.[5,13] Cost and cold-chain requirements pose further implementation challenges in resource-constrained settings.[5,13]

Mechanistically, unanswered questions persist regarding the *long-term interaction of GIPR and GLP-1R signaling* within adipose, hepatic, and central pathways, and whether chronic dual stimulation could induce receptor desensitization or tachyphylaxis.[3,15] Likewise, definitive data on cardiovascular and renal outcomes, bone metabolism, and combination use with SGLT2 inhibitors remain awaited.[6,11,12]

GUIDELINES/ALGORITHM/SUMMARY ILLUSTRATION

Tirzepatide is increasingly recognized within *professional consensus statements* as a preferred agent for patients with *type 2 diabetes, obesity, and high cardiovascular risk*, when not contraindicated.[4-6]

The following stepwise framework integrates evidence from SURPASS and SURMOUNT programs:

- *Step 1—identify eligible patients:* Those with HbA1c >7%, BMI ≥30 kg/m^2 (or ≥27 kg/m^2 with comorbidities), or established atherosclerotic cardiovascular disease[4,5]
- *Step 2—initiate therapy:* Start at 2.5 mg subcutaneously once weekly for 4 weeks. Escalate by 2.5 mg every 4 weeks as tolerated to 5–15 mg.[4,6,7]
- *Step 3—monitor and adjust:* Evaluate HbA1c, body weight, gastrointestinal tolerance, and blood pressure at 12–16 weeks. Reinforce diet and physical activity.[4-6]
- *Step 4—integrate cardiovascular protection:* For patients on GLP-1 RA or SGLT2i therapy, consider sequential or combinational strategies guided by CV risk profile and renal status.[11-13]
- *Step 5—long-term follow-up:* Assess adherence, adverse events, and treatment affordability every 6 months; discontinue only if persistent intolerance or lack of efficacy **(Fig. 4)**.[5,13]

Pragmatically, tirzepatide occupies the "*metabolic core*" of modern multimodal therapy—addressing glucose, weight, blood pressure, and lipids simultaneously, aligning with the current cardiometabolic care continuum.[5,6,11,12]

CONCLUSION

Tirzepatide represents a *paradigm shift in metabolic medicine*, uniting the complementary actions of GIP and GLP-1 within a single molecule.[1,3] Its capacity to deliver *unprecedented HbA1c reduction, clinically meaningful weight loss*, and promising *cardiometabolic improvements* positions it as a cornerstone for the next decade of diabetes and obesity care.[4-6]

Beyond efficacy, tirzepatide embodies a new pharmacological philosophy—*restoring metabolic harmony* rather than merely correcting hyperglycemia.[3,15] While pending long-term cardiovascular and real-world outcome data will refine its ultimate role, present evidence already affirms its transformational potential.[6,11-13]

In the evolving landscape of incretin-based therapy, tirzepatide stands not merely as another drug, but as a *blueprint for integrated cardiometabolic control*—a molecule where science, precision, and human hope intersect.[6,7,11]

REFERENCES

1. Liu QK. Mechanisms of action and therapeutic applications of GLP-1 and dual GIP/GLP-1 receptor agonists. Front Endocrinol (Lausanne). 2024;15:1431292.
2. Sztanek F, Tóth LI, Pető A, et al. New developments in pharmacological treatment of obesity and type 2 diabetes—beyond and within GLP-1 receptor agonists. Biomedicines. 2024;12(6):1320.
3. Campbell JE, Müller TD, Finan B, et al. GIPR/GLP-1R dual agonist therapies for diabetes and weight loss—chemistry, physiology, and clinical applications. Cell Metab. 2023;35(9):1519-29.
4. Min T, Bain SC. The role of tirzepatide, dual GIP and GLP-1 receptor agonist, in the management of type 2 diabetes: the SURPASS clinical trials. Diabetes Ther. 2021;12(1):143-57.
5. Karagiannis T, Avgerinos I, Liakos A, et al. Management of type 2 diabetes with the dual GIP/GLP-1 receptor agonist tirzepatide: a systematic review and meta-analysis. Diabetologia. 2022;65(7):1251-61.
6. Nauck MA, D'Alessio DA. Tirzepatide, a dual GIP/GLP-1 receptor co-agonist for the treatment of type 2 diabetes with unmatched effectiveness regarding glycaemic control and body weight reduction. Cardiovasc Diabetol. 2022;21:169.
7. Gallwitz B. Clinical perspectives on the use of the GIP/GLP-1 receptor agonist tirzepatide for the treatment of type-2 diabetes and obesity. Front Endocrinol (Lausanne). 2022;13:1004044.
8. Rizvi AA, Rizzo M. The emerging role of dual GLP-1 and GIP receptor agonists in glycemic management and cardiovascular risk reduction. Diabetes Metab Syndr Obes. 2022;15:1023-30.
9. Pelle MC, Provenzano M, Zaffina I, et al. Role of a dual glucose-dependent insulinotropic peptide (GIP)/glucagon-like peptide-1 receptor agonist (twincretin) in glycemic control: from pathophysiology to treatment. Life (Basel). 2022;12(1):29.
10. Chavda VP, Ajabiya J, Teli D, et al. Tirzepatide, a new era of dual-targeted treatment for diabetes and obesity: a mini-review. Molecules. 2022;27(13):4315.
11. Fisman EZ, Tenenbaum A. The dual glucose-dependent insulinotropic polypeptide (GIP) and glucagon-like peptide-1 (GLP-1) receptor agonist tirzepatide: a novel cardiometabolic therapeutic prospect. Cardiovasc Diabetol. 2021;20:225.

12. Taktaz F, Fontanella RA, Scisciola L, et al. Bridging the gap between GLP-1 receptor agonists and cardiovascular outcomes: evidence for the role of tirzepatide. Cardiovasc Diabetol. 2024;23:242.
13. Scheen AJ. Dual GIP/GLP-1 receptor agonists: new advances for treating type-2 diabetes. Ann Endocrinol (Paris). 2023;84(2):316-21.
14. Sweta, Gupta S, Bansal S, et al. Tirzepatide: a novel antidiabetic molecule unfolding dual action. Discover Public Health. 2024;21:75.
15. Nowak M, Nowak W, Grzeszczak W. Tirzepatide—a dual GIP/GLP-1 receptor agonist—a new antidiabetic drug with potential metabolic activity in the treatment of type 2 diabetes. Endokrynol Pol. 2022;73(4):745-55.

CHAPTER 119

Mechanisms of Cardiovascular Benefit: Emerging Insights Anti-inflammatory, Metabolic, and Vascular Effects of Tirzepatide

Parv Kamra, Rohit Tandon, Arvind Sharma

INTRODUCTION

Tirzepatide, a novel once-weekly dual glucose-dependent insulinotropic polypeptide (GIP) and glucagon-like peptide-1 (GLP-1) receptor agonist, has emerged as a transformative therapeutic agent in metabolic medicine. This unique dual mechanism enables tirzepatide to deliver significant improvements in glycemic control as well as substantial and sustainable weight loss among individuals with type 2 diabetes. Beyond these established benefits, tirzepatide is garnering increasing attention for its emerging cardiovascular advantages, reflecting its potential as a comprehensive therapy in metabolic and cardiovascular disease management.

Tirzepatide is a synthetically engineered peptide consisting of 39 amino acids, specifically designed to activate both the GIP and GLP-1 receptors. This innovative "twincretin" therapy represents a significant advancement in the incretin-based treatment landscape, offering superior efficacy compared to selective GLP-1 receptor agonists through its unique dual receptor activation mechanism.[1]

The mechanisms underlying tirzepatide's cardiovascular benefits appear to involve complex, interconnected pathways encompassing potent anti-inflammatory effects, comprehensive metabolic improvements, and direct vascular protective mechanisms. Understanding these mechanisms is crucial for optimizing therapeutic applications and identifying patient populations most likely to derive cardiovascular benefit from this transformative therapy **(Fig. 1)**.[2]

ANTI-INFLAMMATORY MECHANISMS

The anti-inflammatory actions of tirzepatide form a central pillar of its cardiovascular benefits, with growing evidence demonstrating that it reliably and substantially lowers key inflammatory biomarkers closely associated with cardiovascular risk.

Systematic Inflammatory Biomarker Reduction

A recent systematic review and meta-analysis of seven randomized clinical trials and one observational study demonstrated that tirzepatide achieves remarkable anti-inflammatory effects, with a pooled 32.9% reduction in high-sensitivity C-reactive protein (hsCRP) compared to placebo. This effect was consistently dose-dependent, with the 15 mg dose achieving the maximum 32.9% hsCRP reduction, while even the 5 mg dose produced a clinically significant 20.3% reduction.[3]

The rapid onset of anti-inflammatory effects is particularly noteworthy, with significant reductions in hsCRP, YKL-40, and intercellular adhesion molecule-1 (ICAM-1) observed within 4 weeks of treatment initiation. YKL-40, a proinflammatory cytokine associated with endothelial dysfunction and atherosclerosis, demonstrated dose-dependent reductions, with the 15 mg tirzepatide dose achieving up to 30% reductions compared to placebo. Similarly, ICAM-1, a critical marker of endothelial activation and dysfunction, showed progressive dose-dependent reductions ranging from 4.5% with the 5 mg dose to 11.2% with the 15 mg dose.[4]

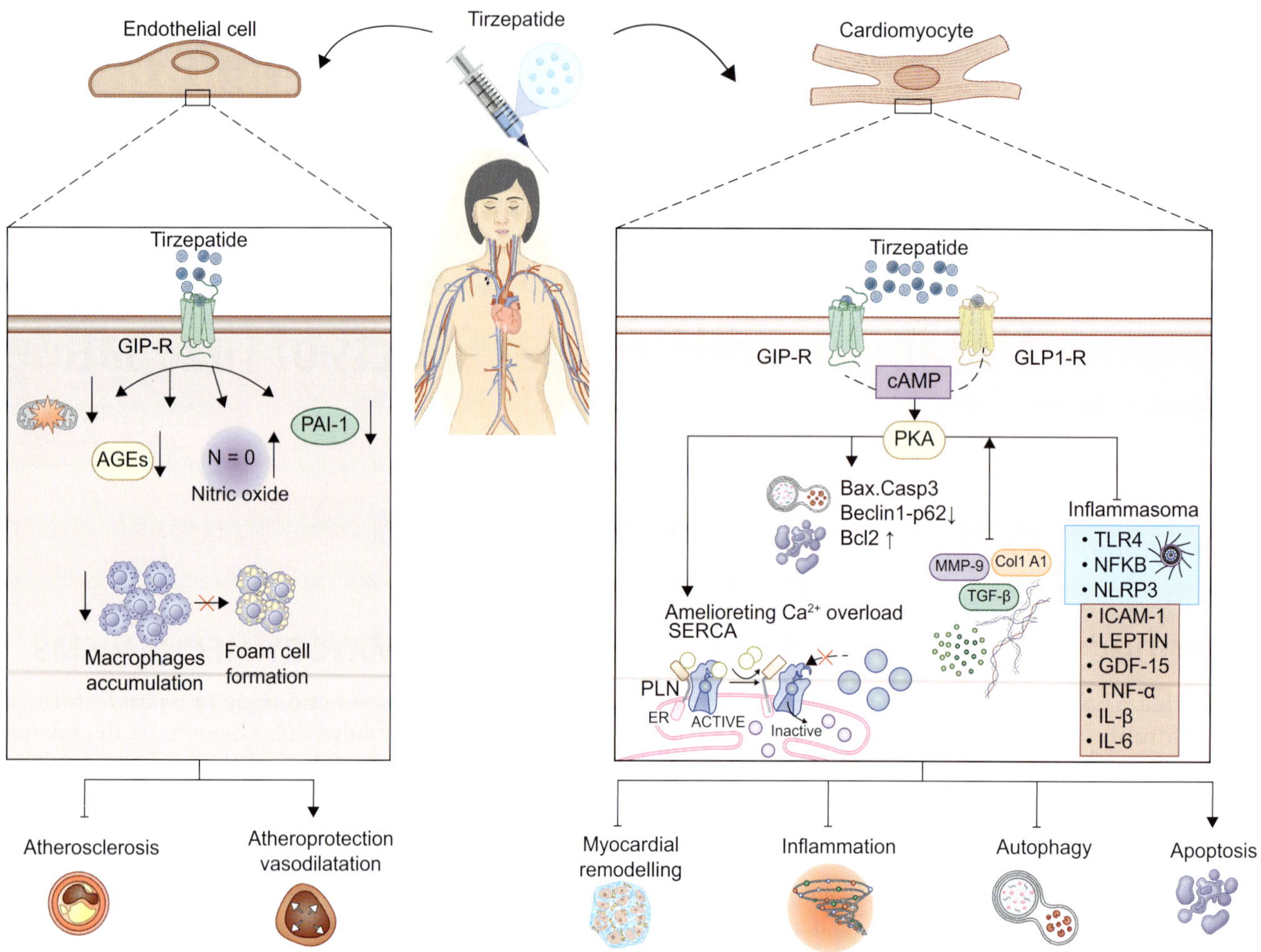

Fig. 1: Updated mechanisms of cardiovascular benefit of tirzepatide: Evidence-based anti-inflammatory, metabolic, and vascular effects.

Interleukin-6 and Cytokine Modulation

The meta-analysis also revealed significant reductions in interleukin-6 (IL-6), a key proinflammatory cytokine, with tirzepatide achieving a 17.8% reduction compared to placebo. This effect was consistent across all dose levels, with the 5, 10, and 15 mg doses producing 18.8, 17.9, and 16.8% reductions in IL-6 levels, respectively. The consistency of IL-6 reduction across different doses suggests that anti-inflammatory mechanisms may be activated at relatively low concentrations of tirzepatide.[3]

Molecular Anti-Inflammatory Pathways

The anti-inflammatory effects of tirzepatide appear to involve direct suppression of key inflammatory signaling cascades, particularly the nuclear factor-κB (NF-κB) pathway and NLRP3 inflammasome activation. Both GIP and GLP-1 receptors are expressed on various immune cells, and their activation leads to downstream suppression of proinflammatory cytokine production, including tumor necrosis factor-α (TNF-α) and interleukin-1β (IL-1β).[5]

Weight-Independent Anti-Inflammatory Effects

Importantly, mediation analyses have revealed that tirzepatide's anti-inflammatory effects are only partially explained by weight loss, suggesting substantial weight-independent mechanisms. For hsCRP, body weight change explained 0% of the variability in the pooled tirzepatide groups, compared to 13% with dulaglutide, indicating that tirzepatide's anti-inflammatory effects may be mediated through direct receptor-mediated mechanisms rather than solely through weight reduction **(Fig. 2)**.[4]

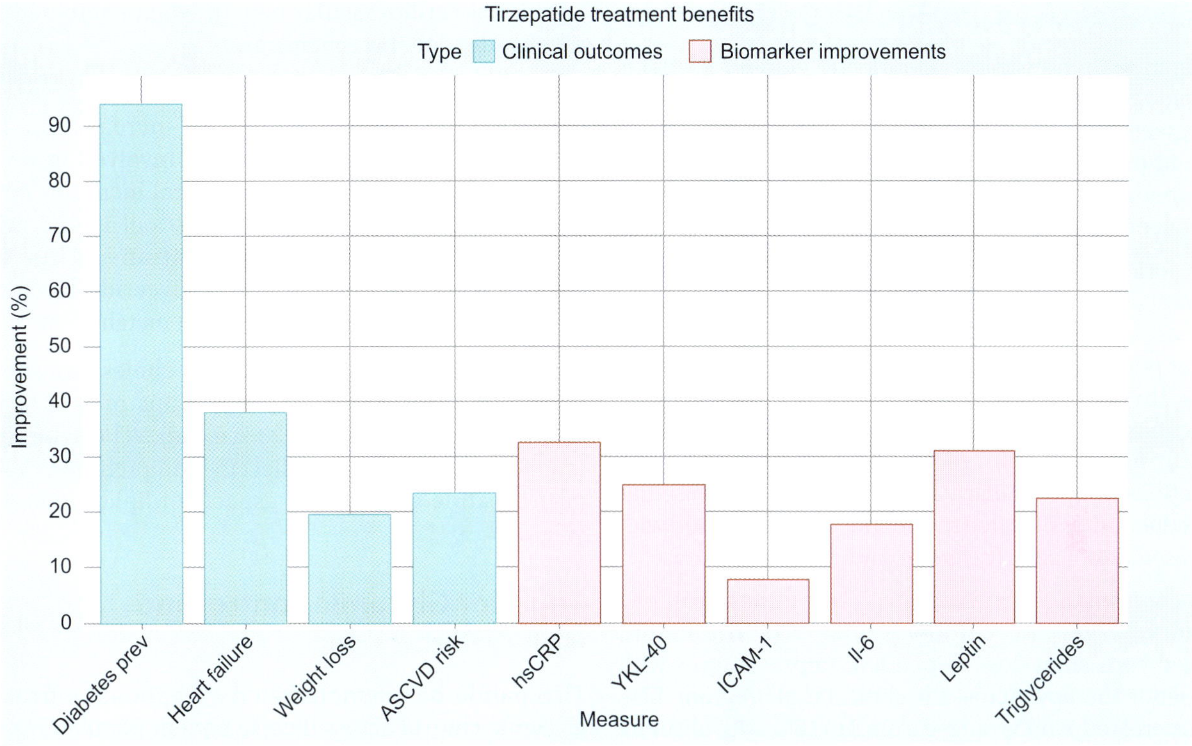

Fig. 2: Clinical outcomes and biomarker improvements with tirzepatide treatment.

METABOLIC EFFECTS

Tirzepatide's metabolic benefits represent a cornerstone of its cardiovascular protective effects, encompassing unprecedented weight loss efficacy, comprehensive improvements in body composition, and beneficial effects on hepatic and adipose tissue metabolism.

Sustained Weight Loss and Body Composition

In the SURPASS-3 trial, which included patients with type 2 diabetes receiving metformin with or without SGLT2 inhibitors, once-weekly tirzepatide resulted in notable decreases in body weight. At 52 weeks, patients randomized to the 5 mg dose lost an average of 9.8 kg, while those on the 15 mg dose achieved a mean weight loss of 15.2 kg versus insulin degludec. This demonstrates clear superiority over standard basal insulin therapy in affecting weight alongside glycemic improvement.[6]

The SURPASS-5 trial studied tirzepatide as an add-on to insulin glargine in patients with type 2 diabetes. In this 40-week study, the 5 mg weekly dose led to a mean reduction of 7.1 kg and the 15 mg dose to 10.5 kg, substantially outperforming placebo. These findings are particularly significant because insulin-based regimens are otherwise prone to cause weight gain.[7]

The quality of weight loss with tirzepatide is particularly noteworthy, with preferential reduction in adipose tissue while preserving lean muscle mass. In the SURMOUNT-1 study, tirzepatide achieved a 33.9% reduction in total body fat mass compared to only 8.2% with placebo, with improvements in the fat-to-lean mass ratio suggesting beneficial changes in body composition. The reduction in visceral adipose tissue is particularly significant from a cardiovascular perspective, as visceral fat is a potent source of inflammatory cytokines and contributes directly to insulin resistance and cardiovascular risk.[6]

Hepatic Metabolic Effects

Tirzepatide demonstrates profound beneficial effects on hepatic metabolism, with particular relevance to metabolic dysfunction-associated steatotic liver disease (MASLD). The SURPASS-3 MRI substudy demonstrated significant liver fat content (LFC) reduction with tirzepatide compared to insulin degludec treatment, with estimated treatment differences of –4.71%.[8]

Comprehensive Lipid Profile Optimization

Tirzepatide demonstrates remarkable beneficial effects on lipid metabolism that extend well beyond what would be expected from weight loss alone. The drug's effects on lipid parameters are dose-dependent and sustained, contributing significantly to cardiovascular risk reduction through multiple lipid pathways.

Triglyceride reduction: Tirzepatide achieves substantial triglyceride reductions across all clinical trials, with decreases ranging from 15 to 50% depending on dose, patient population, and baseline levels. In the SURMOUNT trials involving patients with obesity, triglyceride reductions of 27.4–66.4 mg/dL were observed, representing clinical improvements of 15–38%. These triglyceride reductions are particularly important for cardiovascular risk reduction, as elevated triglycerides are associated with increased risk of atherosclerotic cardiovascular disease.[6]

LDL cholesterol improvements: LDL cholesterol, the primary target for cardiovascular risk reduction, showed consistent dose-dependent improvements with tirzepatide therapy. Across the clinical trial program, LDL cholesterol reductions ranged from 3 to 15%, with absolute decreases of 3.9–19.3 mg/dL. While these reductions may appear modest compared to statin therapy, they represent additional cardiovascular benefit when combined with tirzepatide's other mechanisms.[6]

HDL cholesterol enhancement: Importantly, tirzepatide treatment resulted in beneficial increases in HDL cholesterol, the "good cholesterol" involved in reverse cholesterol transport. HDL cholesterol increases ranged from 4 to 15%, with absolute increases of 1.9–7.7 mg/dL across different patient populations. This HDL improvement, combined with triglyceride reduction, suggests improved overall lipoprotein metabolism.[6]

Total cholesterol optimization: Total cholesterol showed consistent dose-dependent reductions of 4–12%, with absolute decreases of 7.7–23.2 mg/dL. These improvements in total cholesterol reflect the comprehensive effects of tirzepatide on multiple aspects of lipid metabolism **(Fig. 3)**.[6]

Superior Glycemic Control and HbA1c Reduction

Tirzepatide has demonstrated exceptional efficacy in glycemic control across diverse patient populations with type 2 diabetes mellitus (T2DM), consistently achieving superior HbA1c reductions compared to existing therapies.

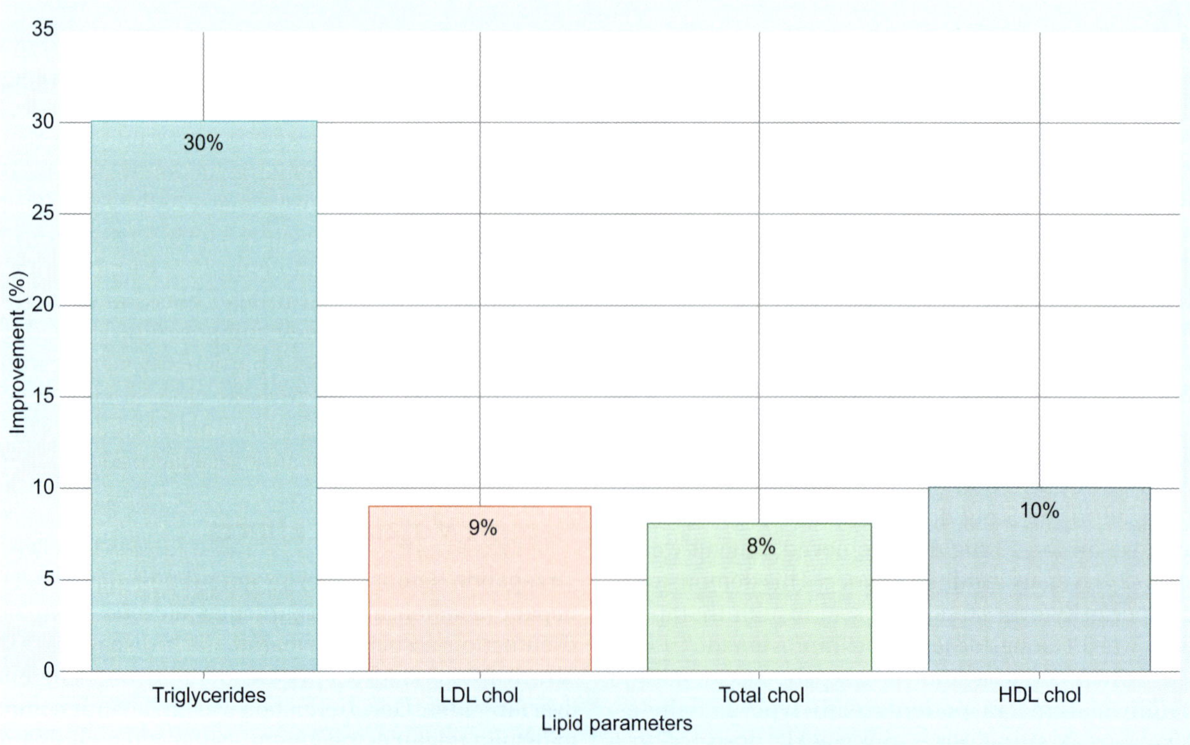

Fig. 3: Lipid profile improvements with tirzepatide treatment (dose-dependent effects).

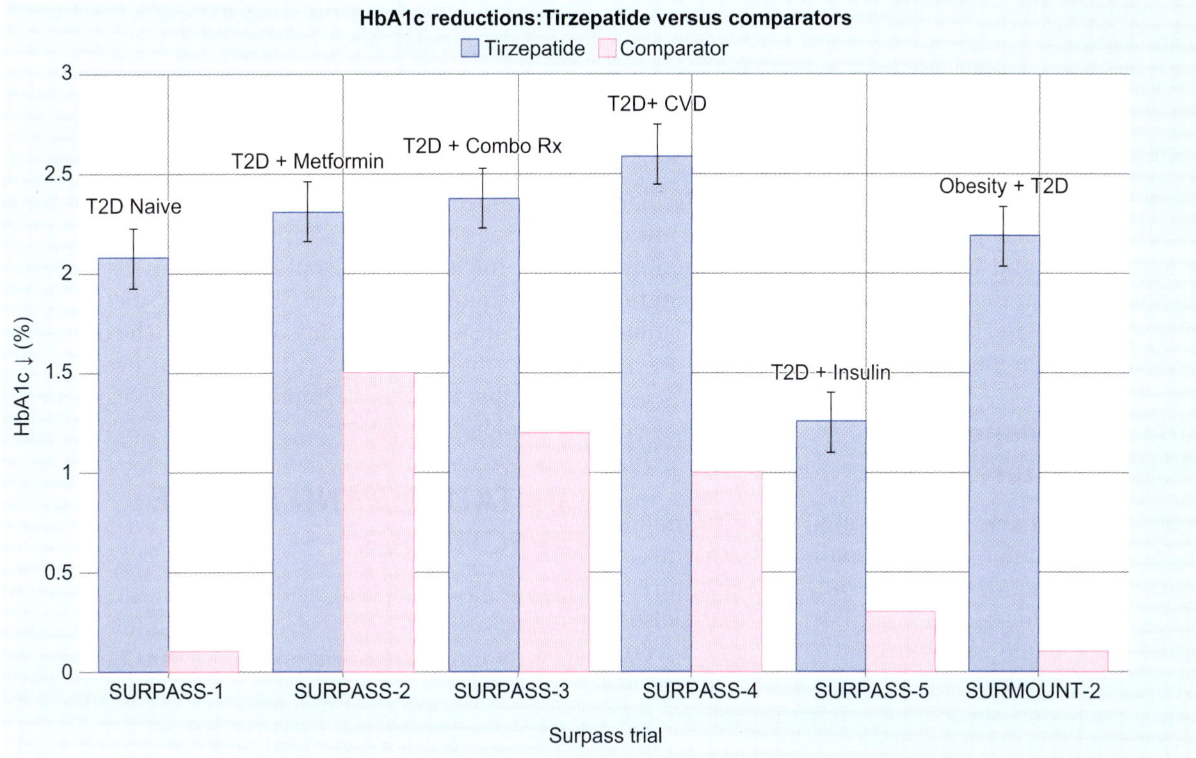

Fig. 4: HbA1c reduction with tirzepatide across major clinical trials.

The SURPASS-1 trial in treatment-naive patients with T2DM showed HbA1c reductions of 1.87% to 2.07% with tirzepatide compared to placebo. More impressively, in SURPASS 2, tirzepatide demonstrated superiority over semaglutide 1 mg, achieving HbA1c reductions of 2.01–2.30% compared to 1.86% with semaglutide. The SURPASS-3 trial, comparing tirzepatide to insulin degludec, showed remarkable HbA1c reductions of 1.93–2.37%, significantly superior to insulin therapy.[6]

Most notably, in SURPASS-4, which enrolled patients with established cardiovascular disease, tirzepatide achieved the highest HbA1c reductions observed in the program, ranging from 2.04 to 2.58% compared to insulin glargine. This superior glycemic control in high-risk cardiovascular patients has direct implications for cardiovascular risk reduction, as intensive glycemic control has been associated with reduced microvascular complications and potential macrovascular benefits **(Fig. 4)**.[6]

VASCULAR EFFECTS

Tirzepatide's direct vascular effects contribute significantly to its cardiovascular benefits through improvements in endothelial function, blood pressure regulation, and microvascular perfusion.

Blood Pressure Effects and Hemodynamic Benefits

Clinical trials consistently demonstrate significant blood pressure reductions with tirzepatide treatment, with dose-dependent effects on both systolic and diastolic blood pressure. Pooled estimates show average reductions of approximately 4.8 mm Hg in systolic and 1.7 mm Hg in diastolic readings, whether used alone or added to background treatment.

Greater effects have been reported in Japanese cohorts with type 2 diabetes; at 15 mg weekly, mean declines reached approximately 11.0 mm Hg systolic and 5.6 mm Hg diastolic from baseline. The basis for this amplified response in Asian populations remains under investigation. In adults with obesity without diabetes, the SURMOUNT-1 ambulatory blood pressure monitoring substudy documented significant 24-hour systolic blood pressure reductions at all tested doses by week 36, with diastolic lowering evident at the lower doses. A dose-related rise in 24-hour heart rate was observed; however, current evidence does not indicate an increased risk of atrial fibrillation.[6]

Endothelial Function and Microvascular Benefits

Both GIP and GLP-1 receptors are expressed in vascular endothelium, and their activation leads to enhanced nitric oxide production and improved endothelial function. Tirzepatide has been shown to enhance endothelial nitric oxide synthase activity, leading to improved vasodilation and reduced vascular inflammation.[5]

Arterial Compliance and Vascular Structure

Clinical studies have demonstrated improvements in arterial compliance with tirzepatide treatment, as evidenced by reductions in pulse pressure, an indirect marker of arterial stiffness. In the SUMMIT trial mechanistic analysis, improvements in arterial compliance were associated with reduced cardiac afterload and enhanced coronary perfusion, potentially contributing to the observed cardiovascular benefits.[9]

CLINICAL OUTCOMES EVIDENCE

SUMMIT Trial: Heart Failure Breakthrough

The SUMMIT trial represents a watershed moment in cardiovascular medicine, providing the first definitive evidence that a pharmacological intervention can reduce heart failure outcomes in patients with heart failure with preserved ejection fraction (HFpEF) and obesity. Tirzepatide achieved a 38% reduction in the composite endpoint of cardiovascular death or worsening heart failure events (9.9 vs. 15.3% with placebo), with the benefit driven primarily by a significant reduction in worsening heart failure events.[10]

SURMOUNT Program: Comprehensive Cardiometabolic Benefits

The SURMOUNT program has provided robust evidence of tirzepatide's comprehensive cardiometabolic benefits across diverse patient populations. Post hoc analyses using validated risk prediction models demonstrated significant reductions in predicted 10-year atherosclerotic cardiovascular disease (ASCVD) risk, with relative risk reductions ranging from 16.4 to 23.5% compared to a 12.7% risk increase with placebo.[7]

SURPASS Program: Cardiovascular Safety and Efficacy

The prespecified meta-analysis of the SURPASS program, encompassing seven randomized controlled trials with robust cardiovascular endpoint ascertainment, demonstrated excellent cardiovascular safety with hazard ratios consistently favoring tirzepatide. The overall hazard ratio for major adverse cardiovascular events was 0.80, with upper confidence limits well below regulatory safety thresholds.[11]

LIMITATIONS AND FUTURE DIRECTIONS

Despite the compelling evidence supporting tirzepatide's cardiovascular benefits, several important limitations and areas for future investigation require consideration.

Current Evidence Limitations

While the evidence base is substantial and growing, most cardiovascular outcome data comes from post hoc analyses and meta-analyses of trials primarily designed for metabolic endpoints rather than dedicated cardiovascular outcomes. The SUMMIT trial, while providing definitive evidence in HFpEF patients with obesity, represents a specific patient population, and broader generalizability requires confirmation in diverse cardiovascular disease phenotypes.[6]

The duration of follow-up, while substantial for drug development standards, may be insufficient to capture the full magnitude of long-term cardiovascular benefits. Cardiovascular benefits of metabolic therapies often continue to accrue over extended periods, and longer term follow-up studies will be essential to understand tirzepatide's full therapeutic potential.[7]

Mechanistic Knowledge Gaps

Despite significant advances in understanding tirzepatide's mechanisms, important questions remain regarding the precise molecular pathways underlying its cardiovascular benefits. The relative contributions of weight-dependent versus weight-independent effects require further clarification, particularly in populations where weight loss may be limited or contraindicated.[3]

The optimal dosing strategies for cardiovascular benefit specifically, as opposed to metabolic outcomes, remain to be fully established. While higher doses generally provide greater metabolic benefits, the dose-response relationships for specific cardiovascular endpoints require more detailed characterization across diverse patient populations.[6]

Future Research Priorities

The ongoing SURPASS-CVOT and SURMOUNT-MMO trials will provide crucial dedicated cardiovascular outcomes data in patients with established T2DM and obesity, respectively. These trials will help establish the magnitude of cardiovascular benefit and identify optimal patient populations for cardiovascular risk reduction.[6]

Investigation of combination therapies represents an important frontier, as tirzepatide's mechanisms suggest potential synergistic effects with established cardiovascular protective agents, including SGLT2 inhibitors, ACE inhibitors, and statins. Understanding these interactions will be crucial for optimizing comprehensive cardiovascular risk reduction strategies.[2]

The development of predictive biomarkers to identify patients most likely to derive cardiovascular benefit from tirzepatide represents a critical area for future research. Such biomarkers could help optimize treatment selection and improve clinical outcomes while minimizing unnecessary exposure and healthcare costs.[4]

CONCLUSION

Tirzepatide represents a transformative advancement in cardiovascular medicine, offering unprecedented benefits through the integration of potent anti-inflammatory effects, comprehensive metabolic improvements, and direct vascular protective mechanisms. The dual GIP/GLP-1 receptor agonism provides synergistic effects that address fundamental pathophysiological processes underlying cardiovascular disease, extending far beyond traditional glucose control paradigms. The evidence base supporting tirzepatide's cardiovascular benefits continues to expand rapidly, with landmark achievements including the first proven pharmacological therapy for HFpEF with obesity and unprecedented diabetes prevention efficacy. The consistent improvements in inflammatory biomarkers, cardiovascular risk factors, and clinical outcomes across diverse patient populations suggest broad therapeutic potential with implications for cardiovascular disease prevention and management. The remarkable 94% reduction in diabetes progression risk and 38% reduction in heart failure events represent paradigm-shifting achievements that will likely influence cardiovascular medicine practice for years to come. As our understanding of tirzepatide's complex mechanisms continues to evolve through ongoing research, the drug is positioned to play an increasingly central role in comprehensive cardiovascular risk management.

REFERENCES

1. Sardar MB, Nadeem ZA, Babar M. Tirzepatide: a novel cardiovascular protective agent in type 2 diabetes mellitus. Curr Probl Cardiol. 2024;49(5):102489.
2. Taktaz F, Fontanella RA, Scisciola L, et al. Bridging the gap between GLP1-receptor agonists and cardiovascular outcomes: evidence for the role of tirzepatide. Cardiovasc Diabetol. 2024;23(1):242.
3. Anti-inflammatory effects of tirzepatide: a systematic review and meta-analysis of randomized controlled trials and observational studies. Diabetes Res Clin Pract. 2024;216:111845.
4. Wilson JM, Lin Y, Luo MJ, et al. The dual glucose-dependent insulinotropic polypeptide and glucagon-like peptide-1 receptor agonist tirzepatide improves cardiovascular risk biomarkers in patients with type 2 diabetes: a post hoc analysis. Diabetes Obes Metab. 2022;24(1):148-53.
5. Alharbi SH. Anti-inflammatory role of glucagon-like peptide 1 receptor agonists and its clinical implications in the treatment of diabetes. Biomed Pharmacother. 2024;171:116091.
6. Sattar N, García-Pérez LE, Rodríguez A, et al. Tirzepatide and cardiometabolic parameters in obesity: summary of current evidence. Diabetes Obes Metab. 2025;27(10):5386-92.
7. Jastreboff AM, le Roux CW, Stefanski A, et al. Tirzepatide for obesity treatment and diabetes prevention. N Engl J Med. 2025;392(10):958-71.
8. Tirzepatide in metabolic dysfunction-associated steatotic liver disease and type 2 diabetes mellitus. Explor Dig Dis. 2024;3(5):289-307.
9. Packer M, Zile MR, Kramer CM, et al. Effects of tirzepatide on circulatory overload and end-organ congestion in heart failure with preserved ejection fraction and obesity. Nat Med. 2024;30(11):3291-9.
10. Packer M, Zile MR, Kramer CM, et al. Tirzepatide for heart failure with preserved ejection fraction and obesity. N Engl J Med. 2025;392:427-37.
11. Sattar N, McGuire DK, Pavo I, et al. Tirzepatide cardiovascular event risk assessment: a pre-specified meta-analysis. Nat Med. 2022;28(3):591-8.

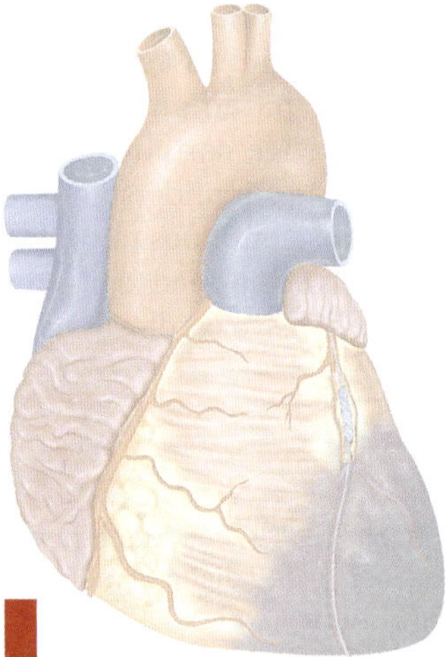

120

CHAPTER

Effects of Tirzepatide on Endothelial Function, Arterial Stiffness, and Vascular Health

Shishu Shankar Mishra, Asharam Panda, Biswaranjan Mishra

INTRODUCTION

Cardiovascular disease (CVD) remains the leading cause of morbidity and mortality globally, with endothelial dysfunction and arterial stiffness serving as central pathophysiological drivers of atherosclerosis, heart failure, and hypertension. The endothelium regulates vascular tone, thrombosis, inflammation, and permeability. Early impairment, often termed "endothelial dysfunction", predicts adverse outcomes across multiple cardiovascular conditions. Similarly, increased arterial stiffness, typically assessed via carotid-femoral pulse-wave velocity, is an independent predictor of cardiovascular mortality.[1]

Glucagon-like peptide-1 receptor agonists (GLP-1RAs) have demonstrated cardiovascular benefit in outcome trials, partly attributed to improved vascular function. Tirzepatide, the first-in-class dual GIP/GLP-1 receptor agonist, provides superior glycemic control and weight loss compared to GLP-1RAs alone.[2] Whether these effects translate into superior endothelial and vascular outcomes remains an area of active investigation.

This review examines tirzepatide's potential vascular effects, integrating mechanistic, biomarker, and clinical evidence, while highlighting existing knowledge gaps.

MECHANISTIC BASIS FOR VASCULAR BENEFITS

Glucagon-like Peptide-1 Receptor-mediated Endothelial Effects and Receptor Modulation

Glucagon-like peptide-1 receptor activation promotes endothelial nitric oxide synthase (eNOS) phosphorylation, enhancing nitric oxide (NO) bioavailability and vasodilation.[3] Preclinical studies demonstrate reductions in oxidative stress, vascular inflammation, and endothelial apoptosis with GLP-1R agonists.[4] These mechanisms provide a biologically plausible rationale for tirzepatide's vascular benefits. While less well understood, GIP receptor stimulation may augment adipose tissue metabolism and exert anti-inflammatory effects **(Fig. 1)**. Experimental data suggest that GIP activation modulates lipid handling and macrophage polarization, potentially complementing GLP-1R-driven endothelial benefits.[5]

Anti-inflammatory and Oxidative Stress Pathways

Tirzepatide reduces circulating inflammatory cytokines (e.g., IL-6, CRP) and oxidative stress markers, mechanisms known to impair vascular function.[6,7] Proteomic analyses further indicate reductions in atherogenic proteins linked to endothelial dysfunction.[8]

INDIRECT EFFECTS: WEIGHT LOSS, GLYCEMIA, AND LIPIDS

Perhaps the strongest determinant of vascular improvement is tirzepatide's unparalleled effect on weight loss (10–20% body weight reduction in SURMOUNT trials).[9] Weight loss improves insulin sensitivity, lowers systemic inflammation, and reduces blood pressure. These indirect benefits substantially relieve vascular burden.

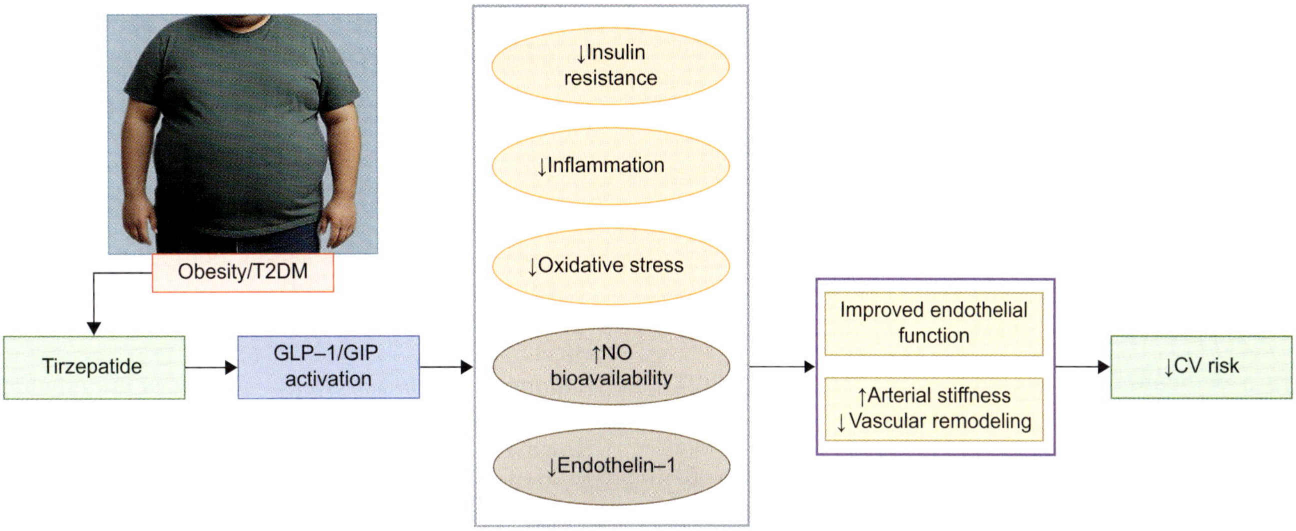

Fig. 1: Schematic presentation of mechanisms of action of tirzepaptide in patients with obesity/diabetes in different molecular pathways leading to improved vascular health that is reflected in decreases cardiovascular (CV) risk.

VASCULAR ENDOTHELIAL–GLYCEMIC INTERFACE

Hyperglycemia impairs endothelial function by generating advanced glycation end products (AGEs), increasing reactive oxygen species, and blunting NO signaling. Tirzepatide improves glycemic control to a greater extent than selective GLP-1RAs, often achieving HbA1c reductions >2% in T2DM.[10] Improved glycemic control itself is strongly linked to better endothelial-dependent vasodilation, as demonstrated in intensive glycemic control studies in diabetes.[11] Thus, tirzepatide's superior glucose-lowering effect likely contributes to endothelial recovery.

LIPID METABOLISM AND VASCULAR BIOLOGY

Atherogenic dyslipidemia—characterized by elevated triglycerides, low HDL, and small dense LDL particles—impairs vascular homeostasis. Tirzepatide significantly reduces triglycerides (up to 20–24%) and improves ApoB/A1 ratios.[12] Lipid improvement directly reduces endothelial activation and smooth muscle proliferation. By comparison, GLP-1RAs produce modest lipid benefits, suggesting tirzepatide may confer incremental vascular advantage.

EFFECTS ON ADIPOSE TISSUE AND INFLAMMATION

Adipose tissue dysfunction drives vascular injury through adipokine secretion (TNF-α, IL-6) and systemic inflammation. Tirzepatide enhances adipose insulin sensitivity and reduces ectopic fat deposition, including hepatic steatosis.[13] Decreased visceral adiposity alleviates vascular oxidative stress and stiffness. Emerging data suggest reductions in epicardial adipose tissue volume, a known mediator of coronary endothelial dysfunction.[14]

CLINICAL TRIAL EVIDENCE

SURMOUNT Trial (Obesity)

The SURMOUNT-1 and -2 trials showed that tirzepatide achieved weight loss of 15–21% over 72 weeks.[9] Post-hoc analyses revealed parallel improvements in systolic BP, triglycerides, hs-CRP, and waist circumference—all correlates of endothelial health.[15] Importantly, reductions in CRP were dose-dependent, consistent with anti-inflammatory vascular benefit.

SURPASS Trial (Diabetes)

In head-to-head trials against insulin degludec and semaglutide, tirzepatide produced superior HbA1c reductions, weight loss, and favorable lipid effects.[10] Exploratory endpoints showed improvements in biomarkers of vascular injury such as plasminogen activator inhibitor-1 (PAI-1) and leptin/adiponectin ratios.[12] These findings suggest tirzepatide may shift the vascular milieu beyond glycemia.[16]

SUMMIT Trial (HFpEF)

The SUMMIT trial is particularly informative for vascular outcomes. Obese HFpEF is characterized by systemic endothelial dysfunction, increased vascular stiffness, and impaired arterial-ventricular coupling. Tirzepatide improved 6-minute walk distance, KCCQ scores, and NT-proBNP.[9,17] While vascular stiffness was not directly measured, improvements in exercise capacity and congestion suggest enhanced vascular compliance and endothelial-cardiac interaction.

AMBULATORY BLOOD PRESSURE SUBSTUDY

In a dedicated analysis, tirzepatide reduced 24-hour systolic BP by ~7 mm Hg and diastolic BP by ~4 mm Hg over 40 weeks.[18] Ambulatory measures are stronger predictors of vascular outcomes than office BP, reinforcing the likelihood of downstream stiffness reduction. No adverse increase in heart rate was observed, in contrast to some GLP-1RAs.

EVIDENCE FROM BIOMARKERS AND OMICS

Proteomic profiling in tirzepatide-treated patients demonstrated reductions in proteins linked to vascular remodeling, including matrix metalloproteinases, angiopoietin-like proteins, and inflammatory chemokines.[8] Such changes are biologically consistent with improved endothelial barrier integrity and reduced arterial stiffness.Metabolomic studies further suggest tirzepatide enhances ketone body utilization and fatty acid oxidation, which may reduce endothelial oxidative stress.[13]

PREDICTED ASCVD RISK

Modeling studies show tirzepatide lowers predicted 10-year ASCVD risk by simultaneously improving glycemia, weight, blood pressure, and lipid parameters.[7] This underscores its potential as a vascular protective agent.

EVIDENCE ON ENDOTHELIAL FUNCTION AND ARTERIAL STIFFNESS

Despite encouraging surrogate and indirect outcomes, direct studies evaluating FMD, cfPWV, or central aortic pressures with tirzepatide are scarce.[19,20] By contrast, GLP-1RAs have more robust evidence demonstrating improved endothelial responsiveness and reduced arterial stiffness. Whether tirzepatide surpasses GLP-1RAs in vascular effects due to dual agonism remains unproven.

COMPARATIVE EFFECTIVENESS: TIRZEPATIDE VERSUS GLUCAGON-LIKE PEPTIDE-1 RECEPTOR AGONISTS

While both GLP-1RAs and tirzepatide improve endothelial function, tirzepatide's dual receptor agonism offers additional pathways:

- *Greater weight loss* → larger hemodynamic and inflammatory improvements
- *Stronger lipid modulation* → greater anti-atherogenic effect
- *Enhanced insulin sensitivity* → reduced endothelial glucotoxicity

However, tirzepatide lacks the robust FMD and cfPWV trial evidence that GLP-1RAs have accumulated.[21] Until such data are available, superiority claims remain inferential.

GUIDELINE AND CLINICAL PRACTICE IMPLICATIONS

Recent ADA/EASD consensus (2023) and ESC cardiovascular prevention guidelines (2024) emphasize GLP-1RAs and tirzepatide as preferred therapies in patients with T2DM and obesity at high cardiovascular risk.[22,23] While endothelial outcomes are not specifically listed, guideline authors highlight vascular biomarkers (BP, CRP, and lipids) as surrogate evidence of benefit. For clinical practice:

- Tirzepatide may be prioritized in patients with *obesity, hypertension, and metabolic syndrome,* where vascular dysfunction is prominent.
- Careful titration is needed in those with low baseline BP or on multiple antihypertensives to avoid hypotension.
- Monitoring CRP, lipid panels, and ambulatory BP may help assess vascular response.

LIMITATIONS OF CURRENT EVIDENCE

- *Lack of direct mechanistic RCTs:* Few trials have measured endothelial function or arterial stiffness endpoints with tirzepatide.
- *Attribution challenge:* It remains unclear whether vascular improvements are direct drug effects or secondary to weight loss.
- *Short trial duration:* Many available studies assess biomarkers or hemodynamics over short follow-up, limiting insights into long-term vascular remodeling.
- *Population heterogeneity:* Studies span diabetes, obesity, and HFpEF cohorts, complicating generalizability.

CLINICAL IMPLICATIONS

- Tirzepatide should be expected to improve vascular risk profiles in clinical practice via indirect mechanisms (weight, BP, glycemia, and lipids).
- Clinicians should monitor blood pressure and volume status, as substantial improvements may necessitate antihypertensive adjustments.
- While direct endothelial benefits are biologically plausible, they remain unconfirmed by gold-standard physiologic measures.

FUTURE DIRECTIONS

- Randomized mechanistic trials assessing FMD, cfPWV, and arterial compliance are needed.
- Comparative trials with GLP-1RAs at equivalent weight loss will help determine whether dual GIP/GLP-1 agonism provides unique vascular benefits.
- Advanced imaging (PET and MRI) and proteomic profiling may clarify how tirzepatide alters vascular biology.

CONCLUSION

Tirzepatide represents a paradigm shift in cardiometabolic therapy. By targeting dual incretin pathways, it delivers unmatched improvements in weight, glycaemia, and cardiometabolic biomarkers. Collectively, these changes are expected to enhance endothelial function and reduce arterial stiffness, thereby lowering vascular risk. However, direct mechanistic evidence remains sparse and claims of endothelial protection should be considered plausible but unproven. Dedicated vascular outcome studies will determine whether tirzepatide confers a direct endothelium-specific benefit beyond its metabolic effects. Its role in contemporary CVD prevention appears promising, especially for obese and high-risk diabetic patients.

REFERENCES

1. Prabhakaran D, Jeemon P, Roy A. Cardiovascular diseases in India: Current epidemiology and future directions. Circulation. 2016;133:1605-20.
2. Bin Abdul Malik MH, Khan NN, Chowdhari MJ, et al. Evaluating the Impact of Tirzepatide on Clinical Outcomes. Cureus. 2025 Apr 11;17(4):e82118.
3. Nature Communications Review. Mechanisms of GLP-1R signalling in vascular biology. Nat Commun. 2024.
4. GLP-1 receptor cardiovascular protection mechanisms. Nat Rev Endocrinol. 2024.
5. Taktaz F, Fontanella RA, Scisciola L, et al. Bridging the gap between GLP-1 RAs and dual agonists. Cardiovasc Diabetol. 2024;23(1):242.
6. Sardar MB, Nadeem ZA, Babar M. Tirzepatide: A novel cardiovascular protective agent. Cardiovasc Diabetol. 2024;49(5):102489.
7. Hankosky ER, Wang H, Neff LM, et al. Tirzepatide reduces predicted 10-year ASCVD risk. Diabetes Obes Metab. 2024;26(1):319-28.
8. Wilson J, et al. Tirzepatide improves cardiovascular risk biomarkers. Lancet Diabetes Endocrinol. 2021.
9. Borlaug BA, et al. SUMMIT: Tirzepatide in HFpEF with obesity. Nat Med. 2024.
10. Frías JP, Davies MJ, Rosenstock J, et al. Tirzepatide versus semaglutide once weekly in patients with type 2 diabetes. N Engl J Med. 2021;385:503-15.
11. Ceriello A, Esposito K, Piconi L et al. Oscillating glucose is more deleterious to endothelial function than sustained hyperglycemia in type 2 diabetes. Diabetes. 2008;57:1349-54.
12. Hartman ML, Sanyal AJ, Loomba R, et al. Effects of tirzepatide on lipid parameters and adipokines in patients with obesity and T2DM. Diabetes Obes Metab. 2023;25:1024-33.
13. Gastaldelli A, Cusi K, Pettiti M, et al. Mechanisms of action of tirzepatide on insulin sensitivity and lipid metabolism. J Clin Endocrinol Metab. 2023;108:e143-55.
14. Iacobellis G, Mohseni M, Bianco SD, et al. Epicardial fat and coronary artery disease: Role of adipokines in vascular inflammation. Curr Atheroscler Rep. 2021;23:50.
15. Krumholz HM, et al. Tirzepatide and ambulatory blood pressure. Hypertension. 2024.
16. Observational CV outcome analysis of tirzepatide. JACC. 2024.
17. SUMMIT extension findings: HF outcomes. Nat Med. 2025.
18. Ambulatory BP substudy: SURMOUNT. Hypertension. 2024.
19. Ahn Y. Methods for measuring endothelial function. Vasc Med. 2024.
20. Systematic review of vascular measures with GLP-1RA/tirzepatide. J Diabetes Res. 2024.
21. Frontiers Mini-review. GLP-1 receptor agonists and endothelial function. Front Cardiovasc Med. 2025.
22. Davies MJ, Aroda VR, Collins BS, et al. Management of hyperglycemia in type 2 diabetes, 2023. ADA–EASD consensus report. Diabetes Care. 2023;46:2753-86.
23. Visseren FL, Mach F, Smulders YM, et al. 2024 ESC Guidelines on cardiovascular disease prevention in clinical practice. Eur Heart J. 2024;45:210-83.

121

CHAPTER

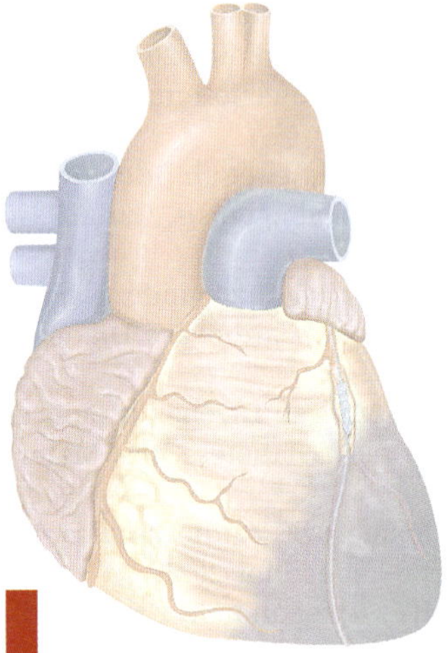

Cardiovascular Safety Profile and Adverse Event Monitoring with Tirzepatide

VK Katyal, Deepinder Singh, Bijender Singh

INTRODUCTION

Obesity has acquired epidemic proportions worldwide and is associated with serious health issues in individuals affected by it. It is a major risk factor for metabolic disorders including diabetes mellitus (DM), hyperlipidemia, metabolic liver disease, cardiovascular disorders, viz., coronary heart disease, heart failure, atrial fibrillation, sudden cardiac arrest, stroke, and several cancers. Higher BMI is associated with higher all-cause mortalities and accounts for 4 million deaths worldwide, of which cardiovascular disease (CVD) accounts for two thirds of cases. While overweight is defined as BMI 25–30, obesity is labeled if BMI is >30; however, in Asians, lower levels are said to define overweight and obesity: 23–27.5 and >27.5, respectively. Higher waist circumference is said to be a marker of abdominal obesity which carries higher cardiometabolic risk. Sustained weight loss of >10% is associated with improvement in obesity-related diseases including DM, fatty liver disease, obstructive sleep apnea, hypertension, and reduction in risk from CVDs.[1] Management of obesity includes diet control, physical exercise, anti-obesity medications, bariatric surgery, and behavioral interventions. If lifestyle modifications fail to achieve results in weight loss, anti-obesity medications are indicated. However, effective and safe drugs are necessary to achieve weight loss goals to reduce cardiovascular morbidity and mortality. Several novel anti-obesity drugs demonstrate improved cardiovascular outcomes in individuals with type 2 diabetes mellitus (T2DM), both without and with high cardiovascular risk or established CV disease.[2] FDA has approved five categories of weight-loss medications, viz., tirzepatide (a dual glucose-dependent insulinotropic polypeptide (GIP)/glucagon-like peptide-1 (GLP-1) receptor coagonist, semaglutide and liraglutide [GLP-1 receptor agonists (RAs)], orlistat, and two combination therapies (naltrexone/bupropion and phentermine/topiramate).[3] Cardiovascular safety of weight loss drugs is essential before these are approved for use, as laid down by the FDA and the European Medicines Agency.

TIRZEPATIDE

This anti-obesity drug, approved in 2022 for weight loss, is a "twincretin" due to its dual action on the GIP and GLP-1 receptors. It constitutes 39 amino acids to which native GIP is added with a 20-carbon fatty diacid component, which prolongs its half-life to 5 days, thereby allowing once-weekly administration. Both GIP and GLP-1 RAs act synergistically. GIP inhibits gastric secretion activity, stimulates insulin secretion, and has insulin-like action on adipose tissue inhibiting lipolysis and promoting lipogenesis.[3,4] GLP-1 augments insulin secretion and suppresses glucagon release; it slows gastric emptying and induces a sense of early satiety resulting in better control of blood glucose levels, weight loss by decreasing food consumption due to delayed gastric emptying, and fat loss percentage. This benefits T2DM patients as observed in phase III trials, viz., SURPASS and SURMOUNT. Tirzepatide has also been shown to improve blood pressure (BP) and to reduce low-density lipoprotein (LDL) cholesterol and triglycerides. Tirzepatide efficacy and safety were assessed in a phase III SURPASS 1–5 clinical trial program.[5]

Glucagon-like Peptide-1 and Glucose-dependent Insulinotropic Polypeptide Receptor Agonists

Long-acting GLP-1 RAs such as liraglutide and semaglutide have been extensively used in clinical practice and provide cardiovascular benefits in diabetes patients. It is a preproglucagon generated by L cells in the small intestine and functions to increase postprandial insulin production and lower blood glucose. On the other hand, GIP isolated from intestinal extract has a potent insulinotropic effect. However, these effects are inhibited in hyperglycemic states. It is largely responsible for control of postprandial hyperglycemic state in T2DM. GLP-1 and GIP work in tandem with GLP-1 inhibiting glucagon expression when blood glucose levels are high, and GIP acts to lower blood glucose concentrations. Dual GLP-1/GIP RAs were introduced in 2013 because of antihyperglycemic, insulinotropic efficacy, and weight loss effect. Based on these findings, a coagonist molecule, tirzepatide, having glucose-lowering potential along with weight loss capabilities, was approved for T2DM in 2022.[5]

CARDIOMETABOLIC AND SAFETY PROFILE OF TIRZEPATIDE (FIG. 1)

Hb1AC

Tirzepatide produced strong Hb1Ac-decreasing effect as depicted in the SURPASS-2[5] study, in which patients received 5–15 mg of tirzepatide for 40 weeks. It reduced Hb1Ac by 2.09–2.46% (vs. semaglutide—1.86%) and similarly over 52 weeks in the SURPASS-3[6] trial, Hb1Ac reduction was from 1.93 to 2.37% vis-à-vis dulaglutide which resulted in 1.34% reduction.

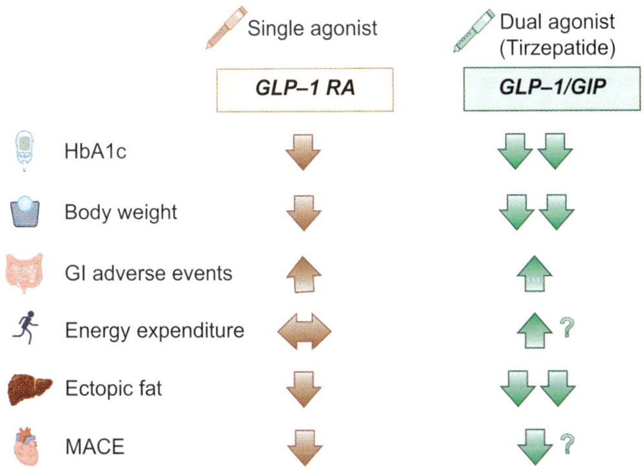

Fig. 1: Comparison between GLP-1 RA and GLP-1/GIP dual agonists (tirzepatide).

Body Weight

Obesity is a major risk factor for the development of CVDs and DM. Tirzepatide reduces weight up to 20% as shown in various trials, viz., SURPASS-3 and SURPASS-5. Body weight was reduced by 9.8 kg with 5 mg weekly dose, and 15.2 kg with 15 mg dose in SURPASS-3 and 7.1 to 10.5 kg by 5 and 15 mg doses in SURPASS-5 trials. In the SURMOUNT-1 trial, where one comorbidity was associated with DM, tirzepatide in weekly SC doses of 5, 10, and 15 mg reduced weight by 15, 19.5, and 20.9%, respectively, over 72 weeks. The percentage of patients who lost >20% of their body weight was over 50% in the tirzepatide 10- and 15-mg groups. Tirzepatide caused mild GIT side effects and 2.6% withdrew the drug. It also reduced liver fat content as measured by MRI–proton fat density fraction, as seen in the SURPASS-3 study.[7] Apart from decreasing food intake, tirzepatide also increased energy expenditure. The reduction in body weight achieved with tirzepatide may also improve cardiovascular risk factors, as observed in clinical trials.

Lipid Profile

Tirzepatide has been shown to affect lipids favorably in various studies. In the SURPASS-4 trial versus insulin glargine, tirzepatide reduced TC, LDL, and TG by 5.6, 7.9, and 22.5% in T2DM patients and also increased HDL by 10.5%, respectively. Similar results were observed in the SURPASS-5 trial, thereby improving atherogenic dyslipidemia in T2DM. Activation of the GIP receptor increases adipose tissue blood flow and promotes adipose tissue lipid uptake. GIP receptor agonism in adipocytes may be a key regulator of postprandial lipid clearance and overall lipid homeostasis.[8] Further studies on how GLP-1/GIP dual agonism improves atherogenic dyslipidemia are needed.

Blood Pressure

Tirzepatide has also been observed to reduce BP in clinical trials. There were significantly lower systolic and diastolic BP measurements compared with patients in the control group, regardless of whether tirzepatide was used as a monotherapy or add-on therapy. Tirzepatide treatment reduced systolic and diastolic BP by 4.8 and 1.7 mm Hg, respectively. Tirzepatide appears to have a more significant impact on BP in Japanese individuals with T2DM. At a dose of 15 mg, tirzepatide reduced systolic BP by 11.0 mm Hg and diastolic BP by 5.6 mm Hg from baseline.

The effect of tirzepatide on 24-hour ambulatory blood pressure monitoring (ABPM) parameters in patients with obesity without T2DM has been evaluated

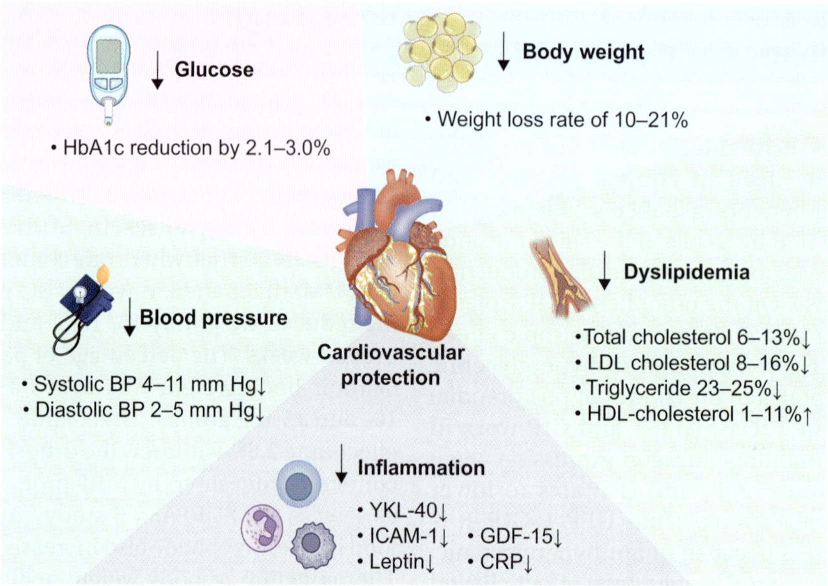

Fig. 2: Potential mechanisms by which tirzepatide effects cardiovascular benefits.

in the SURMOUNT-1 ABPM substudy.[9] After 36 weeks of treatment, tirzepatide was associated with statistically significant reductions in the mean 24-hour systolic BP at all doses and reduced diastolic BP at the two lower doses. Simultaneously, tirzepatide treatment was associated with a dose-dependent increase in the mean 24-hour HR.

Inflammatory Markers

Glucose-dependent insulinotropic polypeptide and GLP-1 have anti-inflammatory properties resulting in decreased inflammation—a marker of increased CV risk.[10] In post hoc analysis, inflammation, endothelial dysfunction, and cellular stress biomarkers were measured before and after 26 weeks of tirzepatide treatment at doses of 10 and 15 mg, resulting in decreasing the levels of YKL-40 (also known as chitinase-3-like protein-1), intercellular adhesion molecule-1 (ICAM-1), leptin, and growth differentiation factor 15 compared with baseline **(Fig. 2)**.[11]

Major Adverse Cardiovascular Events

Over the past two decades, high exposure to CV risks and outcomes has led to postapproval withdrawals of AOMs (fenfluramine, sibutramine, and more recently, lorcaserin) and diabetes medications (rosiglitazone and muraglitazar). Therefore, the preapproval evaluation of these drugs and their effects on major adverse cardiovascular events (MACE) and, in some cases, postapproval surveillance procedures are recommended by the FDA.[12]

In patients with DM with atherosclerotic cardiovascular diseases (ASCVD), several GLP-1 RAs have been observed to provide macrovascular protection by decreasing the major adverse CV events (MACE-CV death, myocardial infarction, or stroke). Therefore, GLP-1 RAs are now approved and recommended for the treatment of T2DM with ASCVD.[13] It has been recently observed that the metabolic effects of GLP-1 RA can be enhanced by combining these with GIP and/or glucagon. Apart from beneficial effects on glucose and lipid metabolism, this combination provides beneficial effects on body weight, BP, and inflammatory markers. Tirzepatide, one of such combinations, has been tried in SURPASS trials.

In the SURPASS-CVOT trial, tirzepatide was demonstrated to be noninferior to dulaglutide for MACE in DM patients with established ASCVD.[14] The SURPASS-CVOT results show that tirzepatide preserved the cardioprotective benefit of a GLP-1 RA while providing additional benefits, including greater kidney protection, reduced overall risk of death apart, and additional benefits of improvements in Hb1AC and body weight. A prespecified meta-analysis of MACE (*MACE-4*) (*i.e., cardiovascular death, myocardial infarction, stroke, and hospitalization for unstable angina)* in patients with DM in seven SURPASS trials[15,16] to evaluate potential benefits of "twincretins," i.e., tirzepatide and control groups over 26 weeks, the hazard ratios were 0.80 [95% confidence interval (CI), 0.57–1.11] for MACE-4, 0.90 (95% CI, 0.50–1.61) for cardiovascular death, and 0.80 (95% CI, 0.51–1.25) for all-cause death.[17]

Side-effects Profile of Tirzepatide

- >10%—blood glucose <54 mg/dL (added to basal insulin) (14–19%), nausea (12–18%), diarrhea (12–17%), decreased appetite (5–11%), serum lipase/amylase increased, and injection site reactions (3.2%)
- 1–10%—vomiting (5–9%), dyspepsia (5–8%), constipation (5–7%), abdominal pain (5–6%), injection site reactions (3.2%), hypersensitivity reactions (3.2%), severe hypoglycemia (add-on to basal insulin) (1–2%)
- <1%—acute gallbladder disease (0.6%), visual problems

Black Box Warnings

Risk of thyroid C-cell tumors:

- Contraindicated in patients with a personal or family history of MTC or in patients with multiple endocrine neoplasia syndrome type 2
- Advise patients of potential risk for MTC and possible symptoms of thyroid tumors (e.g., a mass in the neck, dysphagia, dyspnea, and persistent hoarseness)

Drug Interactions—Monitor Closely

Cyclosporine, dienogest/estradiol valerate, digoxin, divalproex sodium, glimepiride, glipizide, glyburide, insulin aspart, insulin degludec, insulin degludec/insulin aspart, insulin detemir, insulin glargine, insulin glulisine, insulin lispro, insulin regular human, levothyroxine, lithium, phenytoin, tacrolimus, theophylline, valproic acid, and warfarin.

CONCLUSION

Glucagon-like peptide-1 receptor agonists are now approved for prevention and treatment of atherovascular disease in patients having T2DM. However, it has been observed in SURPASS trials that additional cardiovascular and metabolic effects can be obtained in these patients if GLP-1 and GIP RAs are combined. One such drug, tirzepatide, tested in diverse situations in SURPASS, is now recommended primarily for weight reduction, glycemic control, and several markers associated with CV involvement in T2DM.

Tirzepatide is the best among various anti-obesity drugs approved. Tirzepatide has the greatest weight reduction effect, strong antihypertensive impact, moderate reduction in triglycerides, best fasting glucose, and glycosylated Hb reduction. Its CV outcomes are noninferior to once-weekly GLP-1 RA dulaglutide. Side-effect profile is nearly identical to other GLP-1 RAs. Therefore, tirzepatide appears to be the way forward for cardiovascular complications, namely, HFpEF, reduction in macrovascular MACE, viz., heart failure, hospitalization for coronary events, atrial fibrillation, sudden death, and stroke after first CV episode, and tirzepatide should be prioritized, particularly in individuals with weight-related complications and comorbidities.

REFERENCES

1. Liu L, Li Z, Ye W, et al. Safety and effects of anti-obesity medications on weight loss, cardiometabolic, and psychological outcomes in people living with overweight or obesity: a systematic review and meta-analysis. EClinicalMedicine. 2024;79:103020.
2. Kittleson MM, Benjamin EJ, Blumer V, et al. 2025 ACC scientific statement on the management of obesity in adults with heart failure: a report of the American College of Cardiology. J Am Coll Cardiol. 2025;86:1953-75.
3. Dahl D, Onishi Y, Norwood P, et al. Effect of subcutaneous tirzepatide vs placebo added to titrated insulin glargine on glycemic control in patients with type 2 diabetes: the SURPASS-5 randomized clinical trial. JAMA. 2022;327:534-45.
4. Jastreboff AM, Aronne LJ, Ahmad NN, et al. Tirzepatide once weekly for the treatment of obesity. N Engl J Med. 2022;387:205-16.
5. Cho YK, Lee YL, Jung CH, et al. The cardiovascular effect of tirzepatide: a glucagon-like peptide-1 and glucose-dependent insulinotropic polypeptide dual agonist. J Lipid Atheroscler. 2023;12(3):213-22.
6. Frías JP, Davies MJ, Rosenstock J, et al. Tirzepatide versus semaglutide once weekly in patients with type 2 diabetes. N Engl J Med. 2021;385:503-15.
7. Ludvik B, Giorgino F, Jódar E, et al. Once-weekly tirzepatide versus once-daily insulin degludec as add-on to metformin with or without SGLT2 inhibitors in patients with type 2 diabetes (SURPASS-3): a randomised, open-label, parallel-group, phase 3 trial. Lancet. 2021;398:583-98.
8. Nauck MA, Quast DR, Wefers J, et al. The evolving story of incretins (GIP and GLP-1) in metabolic and cardiovascular disease: a pathophysiological update. Diabetes Obes Metab. 2021;23(Suppl 3):5-29.
9. Lemos JA. Abstract 10370: effects of tirzepatide on 24-hour ambulatory blood pressure and heart rate in adults with obesity—results from the SURMOUNT-1 ambulatory blood pressure monitoring sub-study. Circulation. 2022;146(Suppl_1):A10370.
10. Sharif S, Van der Graaf Y, Cramer MJ, et al. Low-grade inflammation as a risk factor for cardiovascular events and all-cause mortality in patients with type 2 diabetes. Cardiovasc Diabetol. 2021;20:220.
11. Wilson JM, Lin Y, Luo MJ, et al. The dual glucose-dependent insulinotropic polypeptide and glucagon-like peptide-1 receptor agonist tirzepatide improves cardiovascular risk biomarkers in patients with type 2 diabetes: a post hoc analysis. Diabetes Obes Metab. 2022;24:148-53.
12. Alobaida M, Alrumayh A, Oguntade AS, et al. Cardiovascular safety and superiority of anti-obesity

medications. Diabetes Metab Syndr Obes Targets Ther. 2021;14:3199-208.

13. Davies MJ, Aroda VR, Collins BS, et al. Management of hyperglycemia in type 2 diabetes, 2022. A consensus report by the American Diabetes Association (ADA) and the European Association for the Study of Diabetes (EASD). Diabetes Care. 2022;45:2753-86.
14. ElSayed NA, Aleppo G, Aroda VR, et al. Pharmacologic approaches to glycemic treatment: standards of care in diabetes-2023. Diabetes Care. 2023;46(Suppl 1):S140-57.
15. Cosentino F, Grant PJ, Aboyans V, et al. 2019 ESC guidelines on diabetes, pre-diabetes, and cardiovascular diseases developed in collaboration with the EASD. Eur Heart J. 2020;41:255-323.
16. Das SR, Everett BM, Birtcher KK, et al. 2018 ACC expert consensus decision pathway on novel therapies for cardiovascular risk reduction in patients with type 2 diabetes and atherosclerotic cardiovascular disease: a report of the American College of Cardiology Task Force on expert consensus decision pathways. J Am Coll Cardiol. 2018;72:3200-23.
17. Sattar N, McGuire DK, Pavo I, et al. Tirzepatide cardiovascular event risk assessment: a pre-specified meta-analysis. Nat Med. 2022;28:591-8.

122

CHAPTER

Potential Role of Tirzepatide in Atherosclerosis Regression and Plaque Stabilization

Shraddha Ranjan, Manish Bansal, Ravi R Kasliwal, HK Chopra

INTRODUCTION

Traditional isolated glucagon-like peptide-1 (GLP-1) receptor agonists (GLP-1 RAs) such as semaglutide and liraglutide have demonstrated robust efficacy in reducing glycosylated hemoglobin (HbA1c), promoting weight loss, and improving cardiovascular outcomes in patients with type 2 diabetes mellitus (T2DM). Tirzepatide is a new dual incretin receptor agonist, also referred to as "twincretin," which refers to its complementary metabolic actions on these two endogenous incretin hormones that play key roles in glucose homeostasis, insulin secretion, and energy balance. It is administered subcutaneously once a week due to its prolonged half-life (~5 days). Clinical trials have shown that tirzepatide produces significant reductions in HbA1c (up to 2.4–2.6%) and body weight loss up to 15–20% in diabetics and obese patients. This effect was superior to most existing GLP-1 RAs. Tirzepatide has strong indirect and mechanistic plausibility to slow atherosclerosis progression and to favor more stable plaque biology (through weight loss, better glycemia, lipid and blood-pressure effects, and anti-inflammatory/endothelial benefits). The favorable effects on lipid profile, blood pressure, and inflammatory biomarkers predict its role as an atherosclerosis-reversing and cardiovascular protective drug.

Direct evidence for plaque regression or stabilization in humans is still limited as it will require histopathology, which is not a feasible option. Advanced imaging is the next best method to assess atherosclerosis, and several imaging trials (CCTA/IVUS/NIRS) are underway or planned (e.g., T-PLAQUE). Large hard-outcome (MACE/atherosclerotic events) randomized trials specifically powered to show a reduction in atherosclerotic events versus standard care are not yet available.

PHARMACOLOGY OF TIRZEPATIDE

Glucagon-like peptide-1 and GIP are gut-derived peptides secreted by enteroendocrine cells of intestinal mucosa in response to nutrient intake, which augments insulin secretion from pancreatic beta cells ultimately. This results in the "incretin effect," whereby oral ingestion of glucose stimulates insulin secretion more potently than a matched increase in plasma glucose achieved by intravenous glucose administration.[1] GLP-1 is produced by L-cells, which are particularly abundant in the ileum and colon, and GIP is produced by K-cells, mainly in the duodenum and upper jejunum. It functions as a dual agonist of the GIP receptor (GIPR) and the GLP-1 receptor (GLP-1R). The GLP-1 component leads to enhanced glucose-dependent insulin secretion, glucagon suppression, delayed gastric emptying, appetite reduction, and weight loss (a mechanism shared with GLP-1R agonists). The GIPR activity appears to add further benefits in weight loss, fat-mass reduction, and possibly direct metabolic effects beyond those of GLP-1R alone **(Fig. 1)**.[1,2]

Although the reduced food intake stimulated by tirzepatide is considered to be the main contributor to the reduced body weight, many other mechanisms are still not fully understood. One theory is that increased energy expenditure induced by tirzepatide may contribute to the reduced body weight and liver fat content.

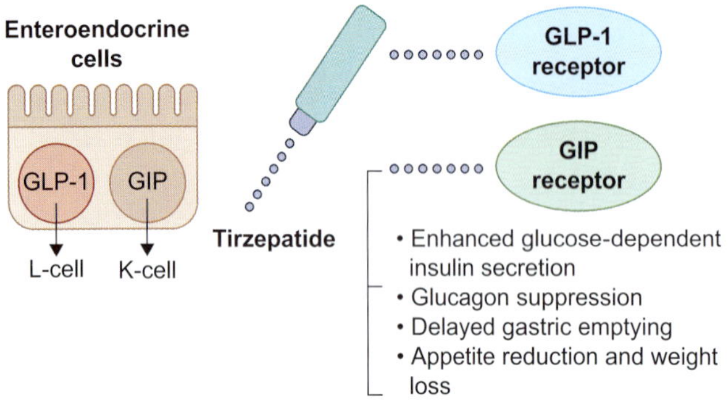

Fig. 1: Pharmacology of tirzepatide.

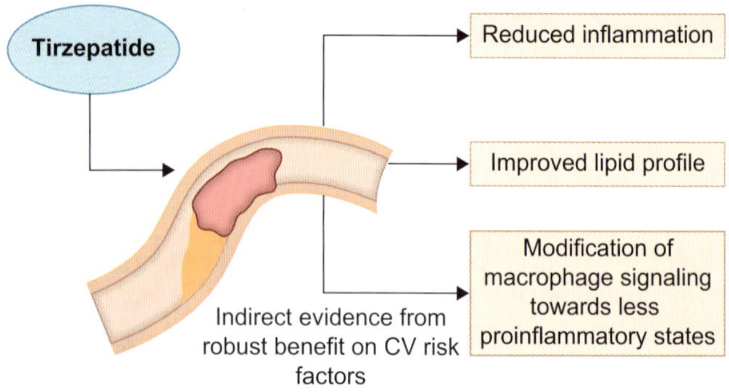

Fig. 2: Proposed pathways for plaque stabilization by tirzepatide.

CARDIOVASCULAR EFFECTS OF TIRZEPATIDE[3-8]

- Once-weekly subcutaneous administration of a tirzepatide dose-dependently reduced HbA1c levels across all studies. The results of the SURPASS trials (phase 3) showed that individuals who had established T2DM and were treated with tirzepatide experienced a reduction in HbA1c levels ranging from 2.0 to 3.0%. This proved to be a much stronger HbA1c-lowering effect when compared with placebo or drugs including GLP-1 RA and basal insulin.
- Tirzepatide has also been shown to significantly reduce body weight in clinical trials. In the SURPASS-3 and SURPASS-5 trials, once-weekly subcutaneous tirzepatide administration significantly reduced body weight compared to insulin in patients with T2DM. In the SURMOUNT-1 trial, a phase 3 trial including only obese patients, the weight loss rates in patients who received tirzepatide at doses of 5, 10, and 15 mg were 15, 19.5, and 20.9%, respectively. This was significantly higher than the 3.1% weight loss rate observed in patients who received placebo.
- Besides its profound body weight-reducing effect, tirzepatide also showed a significant ability to reduce liver fat content. These data provide additional evidence on the metabolic effects of this novel GLP-1/GIP dual RA.
- Tirzepatide has also been shown to reduce BP in clinical studies. The patients treated with tirzepatide showed significantly lowered systolic and diastolic BP compared with patients in the control group, regardless of whether tirzepatide was used as a monotherapy or add-on therapy. The effect of tirzepatide was measured during 24-hour ambulatory BP monitoring (ABPM) in individuals living with obesity without T2DM in the SURMOUNT-1 ABPM substudy, which showed statistically significant and clinically meaningful reductions after 36 weeks of treatment.
- Tirzepatide has been shown to improve lipid profiles in clinical studies. In SURPASS-4 and 5, tirzepatide, whether used as monotherapy or add-on therapy, lowered the percentage change of total cholesterol (TC), low-density lipoprotein cholesterol (LDL-C), and triglycerides (TGs) and significantly increased high-density lipoprotein cholesterol (HDL-C). Although GLP-1 RAs have been shown to reduce the production of lipoproteins, chylomicrons, and postprandial TGs, the effect of chronic treatment with GIP RAs on plasma lipids is not completely understood.
- Low-grade inflammation has been identified as a significant risk factor for cardiovascular diseases. Tirzepatide treatment has been shown to have favorable effects on inflammatory markers in clinical trials. In a 26-week phase 2 study involving patients with obesity and T2DM, treatment with tirzepatide dose-dependently decreased the circulating levels of specific biomarkers of inflammation and endothelial dysfunction previously associated with cardiovascular events, suggesting a net improvement in the cardiovascular risk profile of these patients.
- Tirzepatide action on a few of the above mechanisms promises to have a favorable effect on plaque stabilization **(Fig. 2)**.

LOCAL VASCULAR EFFECT OF TIRZEPATIDE PROMOTING PLAQUE STABILIZATION

As discussed above, tirzepatide significantly improves metabolic milieu and cardiovascular risk-factor modulation. This is the indirect way this drug causes plaque stabilization. Beyond systemic effects, tirzepatide may exert more direct vascular wall benefits that support plaque stabilization.

Glucagon-like peptide-1 receptor agonists have been shown to improve endothelial function (e.g., increased

TABLE 1: Stabilizing the unstable atherosclerotic plaque—role of tirzepatide.

Pathophysiological feature	*Effect on unstable plaque*	*Potential stabilizing role of tirzepatide*
Large lipid/necrotic core	Expanded atherogenic lipid and necrotic core volume	Improves insulin resistance, reduces triglycerides/VLDL, increases HDL, and limits lipid deposition
Thin fibrous cap	Cap thinning and ECM degradation	Reduces MMP activity and inflammation, promotes collagen synthesis and cap thickening
Macrophage/foam-cell infiltration	Proinflammatory cytokine release	Shifts macrophages from M1 to M2 phenotype, enhances efferocytosis, and decreases inflammation
Endothelial dysfunction	Leukocyte adhesion and prothrombotic state	Enhances NO bioavailability, reduces oxidative stress and vascular inflammation
Plaque neovascularization	Fragile microvessels and intraplaque hemorrhage	Reduces oxidative stress, stabilizes microvessels
Prothrombotic surface	Tissue factor exposure and platelet activation	Improves endothelial integrity, decreases thrombogenicity

nitric oxide (NO) production, reduced adhesion-molecule expression). Improved endothelial NO release reduces leukocyte adhesion, platelet activation, and promotes vasodilatation—all of which contribute to a less thrombogenic plaque surface and slower lesion progression.[9]

In unstable plaques, macrophages are predominantly of the M1 (proinflammatory) phenotype, secreting MMPs, TNF-α, IL-1β, IL-6, and promoting ECM degradation and necrotic core formation. On the other hand, M2 macrophages promote resolution of inflammation, efferocytosis (clearance of dead cells), and tissue repair. Tirzepatide can shift macrophage populations toward less proinflammatory states (M2) or reduce macrophage activation, making the plaque less vulnerable.

Uptake of oxidized LDL (via lower circulating LDL/VLDL and perhaps reduced macrophage activation) is reduced, and efferocytosis is enhanced, causing the necrotic core to be stabilized or shrunk. Additionally, reduced adipose tissue-derived inflammation and improved insulin sensitivity reduce advanced glycation endproducts and oxidative stress, thereby reducing foam-cell formation.

A key hallmark of stabilized plaque is a thick fibrous cap rich in collagen, produced by smooth-muscle cells (SMCs), and low MMP activity. Improved metabolic control leads to reduced SMC apoptosis, reduction in neovascularization, intraplaque hemorrhage, and thrombogenic surface.[10,11]

Unstable or vulnerable plaques have been a region of interest, and the understanding of their pathophysiology has led to targeting the pathways by newer drugs such as tirzepatide. **Table 1** summarizes the effect of this drug on unstable plaque.

CURRENT DATA

No definitive randomized trial has yet shown that tirzepatide causes atherosclerotic plaque regression or reduces hard ischemic events specifically via plaque modification. Mechanistic human tissue data are sparse. Most direct evidence about plaque cell biology comes from animal/preclinical or surrogate human biomarker studies. Translating that to clinically meaningful plaque stabilization in humans needs advanced imaging and histology data. Several randomized imaging studies are active or planned to measure direct plaque effects by imaging, such as coronary CT angiography, IVUS, and NIRS.

A notable example is the T-PLAQUE design, a randomized trial assessing changes in coronary atheroma volume by MDCTA/CTCA in people with T2D and atherosclerosis. It is a multicenter, randomized, double-blind, placebo-controlled, parallel-group phase 4 study evaluating the effects of tirzepatide on atherosclerotic plaque progression assessed by coronary computed tomography angiography (CCTA) in participants with a diagnosis of T2DM and atherosclerosis. Study will assess changes in coronary atheroma volume comparing tirzepatide 15 mg/week plus standard of care (SOC), as compared to placebo plus SOC.[12]

Another proof-of-principle trial is assessing coronary plaque composition by NIRS/IVUS and microvascular function in obese people with CAD over 52 weeks. These trials will provide direct evidence on plaque burden and composition.[13]

This research methodology has its limitations because of heterogeneity of effects. The magnitude of effect on plaque may vary by baseline disease (e.g., diabetes vs. obesity vs. established CAD), concomitant statin/PCSK9 use, and duration of treatment.

Studies using vascular biopsy or advanced PET/targeted imaging for inflammation (e.g., 18F-FDG PET) before/after therapy are planned to get better insight.

DISCUSSION

In the evolving landscape of cardiometabolic therapeutics, tirzepatide stands out as a promising agent that bridges the metabolic-vascular interface. If future research confirms its role in plaque stabilization, it may represent a paradigm shift in how we treat atherosclerosis—not only by slowing its progression but by actively converting the plaque to a safer, more stable state. For clinicians, the implication is that tirzepatide offers more than glucose/weight control—it may serve as a vascular-protective agent, especially in patients with established atherosclerosis and high risk.

The SURPASS and SURMOUNT phase 3 clinical development programs were designed to demonstrate the efficacy and safety of tirzepatide to enable regulatory approval for T2D and obesity, respectively. The results showed that the risk was not increased with tirzepatide, and thus proved its safety. A cardiovascular meta-analysis of all studies from the SURPASS program indicated that tirzepatide did not increase the risk of MACEs in participants with T2DM compared with controls.[14]

Careful patient selection, monitoring, early initiation, and integration with standard cardiovascular therapies will maximize benefit. At present, the high cost of tirzepatide is a major barrier to its uptake. Like other new, effective agents for T2D and obesity, the availability of tirzepatide is limited to high-income countries, with its use largely based on financial means rather than clinical needs.

CONCLUSION

Tirzepatide is the first dual GIP/GLP-1 receptor coagonist approved for T2DM and obesity. It has profound effects on glycemic control, body weight reduction, and improvements in cardiovascular risk factors with safety and tolerability comparable to selective GLP-1RAs. The concept of plaque stabilization by tirzepatide is scientifically plausible and supported by compelling indirect clinical evidence. Nevertheless, the evidence base is not yet definitive: human imaging/histology data are lacking, causality remains unproven, and the exact contribution of plaque stabilization versus systemic risk-factor reduction is unresolved. Going forward, dedicated imaging/biomarker studies, mechanistic research, and long-term outcome trials are key to validating the concept and guiding clinical application.

REFERENCES

1. Elrick H, Stimmler L, Hlad CJ Jr, et al. Plasma insulin response to oral and intravenous glucose administration. J Clin Endocrinol Metab. 1964;24:1076-82.
2. Campbell JE, Drucker DJ. Pharmacology, physiology, and mechanisms of incretin hormone action. Cell Metab. 2013;17(6):819-37.
3. Rosenstock J, Wysham C, Frías JP, et al. Efficacy and safety of a novel dual GIP and GLP-1 receptor agonist tirzepatide in patients with type 2 diabetes (SURPASS-1): a double-blind, randomized, phase 3 trial. Lancet. 2021;398(10300):143-55.
4. Frías JP, Davies MJ, Rosenstock J, et al. Tirzepatide versus semaglutide once weekly in patients with type 2 diabetes (SURPASS-2). N Engl J Med. 2021;385(6):503-15.
5. Ludvik B, Škrha J, Cariou B, et al. Once-weekly tirzepatide versus titrated insulin degludec in participants with type 2 diabetes (SURPASS-3): a randomised, open-label, parallel-group, phase 3 trial. Lancet. 2021;398(10300):117-29.
6. Del Prato S, Pratley R, Almeida J, et al. Once-weekly tirzepatide versus titrated insulin glargine in people with type 2 diabetes (SURPASS-4): a randomized, open-label, phase 3 trial. Lancet. 2021;398(10300):547-58.
7. Dahl D, Onishi Y, Norwood P, et al. Effect of subcutaneous tirzepatide vs placebo added to titrated insulin glargine on glycaemic control in patients with type 2 diabetes: the SURPASS-5 randomised clinical trial. JAMA. 2022;327(6):534-45.
8. Jastreboff AM, Aronne LJ, Ahmad NN, et al. Tirzepatide once weekly for the treatment of obesity. N Engl J Med. 2022;387:205-16.
9. Drucker DJ. The cardiovascular biology of glucagon-like peptide-1. Cell Metab. 2016;24(1):15-30.
10. Sharif S, Van der Graaf Y, Cramer MJ, et al. Low-grade inflammation as a risk factor for cardiovascular events and all-cause mortality in patients with type 2 diabetes. Cardiovasc Diabetol. 2021;20:220.
11. Wilson JM, Lin Y, Luo MJ, et al. The dual glucose-dependent insulinotropic polypeptide and glucagon-like peptide-1 receptor agonist tirzepatide improves cardiovascular risk biomarkers in patients with type 2 diabetes: a post hoc analysis. Diabetes Obes Metab. 2022;24:148-53.
12. Hamidi H, Bagheri M, Benzing T, et al. Rationale and design of the trial: effect of tirzepatide on progression of coronary atherosclerosis using MDCT—the T-PLAQUE randomized-controlled trial. Am Heart J. 2024;278:24-32.
13. Eli Lilly and Company. (2025). Effect of tirzepatide on coronary atheroma volume comparing tirzepatide 15 mg/week plus standard of care versus placebo plus standard of care. [online] Available from https://clinicaltrials.gov/study/NCT05708859 [Last accessed January, 2026].
14. Sattar N, McGuire DK, Pavo I, et al. Tirzepatide cardiovascular event risk analysis. Diabetes Care. 2022;45(5):1222-30.

CHAPTER 123

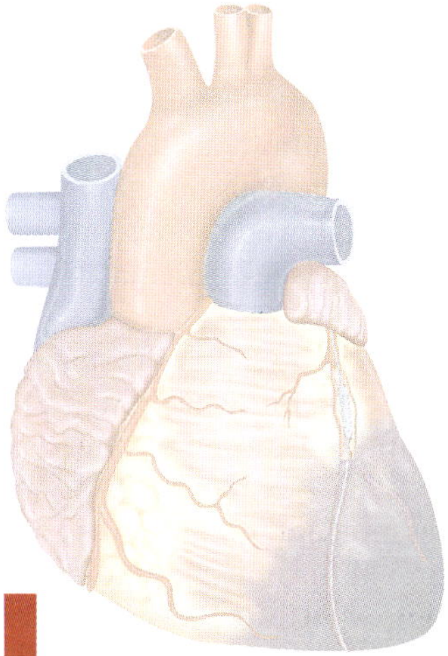

Comparison of Tirzepatide versus Semaglutide in Obesity with Heart Failure

Vivek Tandon, Milan Bhardwaj

INTRODUCTION

Obesity is both a risk factor and a disease modifier in heart failure (HF). Obesity causes increased cardiac workload, which over time can lead to left ventricular hypertrophy and diastolic dysfunction. Obesity causes low-grade inflammation, insulin resistance, renin–angiotensin–aldosterone system (RAAS), and sympathetic activation, which then contribute to HF progression. Obstructive sleep apnea is also more common with obesity, worsening pulmonary hypertension, and right ventricular (RV) strain. Heart failure with preserved ejection fraction (HFpEF) is the phenotype most strongly linked to obesity, and weight loss therapies show the clearest benefit. Heart failure with reduced ejection fraction (HFrEF) is not directly caused by obesity, but obesity can worsen outcomes in HFrEF. Sustained intentional weight loss (through fat loss, not cachexia) improves symptoms, exercise capacity, and quality of life in HFpEF. In HFrEF, weight management is still recommended (especially for comorbid diabetes, obstructive sleep apnea, and hypertension), but robust randomized controlled trial (RCT) evidence for weight loss therapies is awaited.

Semaglutide, a glucagon-like peptide-1 receptor agonist (GLP-1 RA), improves glucose-dependent insulin secretion, decreases glucagon secretion, delays gastric emptying, and increases pancreatic β-cell proliferation. Its interaction with GLP-1 receptors in the hypothalamus may mitigate hunger sensation, decrease food cravings, and enhance feelings of satiety.[1] Semaglutide was approved by the US FDA for obesity in June 2021. The recommended dosage for weight loss is 0.25 mg injected subcutaneously once weekly, initially for the first 4 weeks, which is then increased to 0.5 mg for the next 4 weeks. This is followed by 1 mg for the next 4 weeks and then increased to maintenance dose of either 1.7 or 2.4 mg (after 4 weeks of 1.7 mg dose).

Based on the favorable results observed in the SUSTAIN and PIONEER trials, the US FDA has approved injectable and oral semaglutide for enhancing glycemic control in adults with T2DM. Following the positive outcomes observed in the Semaglutide Treatment Effect in People with Obesity (STEP) trials, the US FDA has approved the use of subcutaneous semaglutide at 2.4 mg weekly for chronic weight management in adult patients who are obese (BMI >30 kg/m^2) or overweight (BMI >27 kg/m^2) with at least one weight-related condition such as hypertension, T2DM, dyslipidemia, or obstructive sleep apnea. The mean weight loss in these patients with 2.4 mg dose was around 15% and this was sustained with continued treatment. The STEP TEENS trial demonstrated the safety and efficacy of semaglutide in adolescents aged 12–17 years.[2-9]

In the STEP-HFpEF trial, obese patients with HFpEF (LVEF >45%) without diabetes received weekly semaglutide 2.4 mg for 52 weeks. Significant improvements were observed in symptoms, physical function, and exercise capacity, alongside substantial weight loss, and reductions in CRP and NT-proBNP levels. The mean change in the Kansas City Cardiomyopathy Questionnaire Clinical Summary Score (KCCQ CSS) was 16.6 points with semaglutide versus 8.7 points with placebo, and mean body weight reduction was 13.3% versus 2.6%. The 6-minute walk distance improved by 21.5 m versus 1.2 m.

However, the trial was limited to 1 year and was not powered for hard outcomes such as mortality or major HF hospitalization.[10] Similarly, the STEP-HFpEF DM trial evaluated 616 adults with HFpEF, obesity, and T2DM over 52 weeks. Semaglutide led to greater reductions in HF-related symptoms and improved physical limitations alongside weight loss compared to placebo.[11] The FLOW study demonstrated that a lower dose of semaglutide (1 mg weekly) reduced the risk of clinically significant kidney outcomes and first HF events in patients with T2DM and chronic kidney disease (CKD).[12]

The SELECT trial evaluated semaglutide in 17,604 overweight or obese adults with preexisting cardiovascular disease (CVD) (prior MI, stroke, or peripheral artery disease) but without diabetes. Weekly subcutaneous semaglutide (up to 2.4 mg) resulted in a 20% reduction in cardiovascular death, nonfatal myocardial infarction, and nonfatal stroke compared to placebo over a median follow-up of 40 months, and benefits appeared early in the study period.[13] The SELECT trial demonstrates that semaglutide can significantly reduce the risk of major cardiovascular events even in people without diabetes, if they have obesity with preexisting CVD. These trials highlighted that treating obesity itself provides meaningful cardiovascular benefits, and obesity in HFpEF is not merely a comorbidity but a modifiable driver of disease pathology.

The SUSTAIN-6 trial demonstrated the safety of injectable semaglutide in adults with T2DM and high cardiovascular risk. Nonfatal stroke risk was significantly lower, while rates of nonfatal myocardial infarction were reduced but not statistically significant.[14] The SOUL trial assessed oral semaglutide in high-risk T2DM patients with a history of atherosclerotic cardiovascular disease (ASCVD), CKD, or both and found a 14% reduction in major adverse cardiovascular events (MACE) over an average 4-year follow-up.[15] The OASIS trials showed that oral semaglutide 25–50 mg was effective for weight loss and comparable to injectable doses. It may provide an alternative treatment option to injectable semaglutide in patients who prefer oral administration.[16,17]

Pooled analyses of SELECT, FLOW, STEP-HFpEF, and STEP-HFpEF DM trials indicated that semaglutide reduces the risk of combined cardiovascular death or worsening HF events in HFpEF, though its effect on cardiovascular death alone was not significant.[18] Semaglutide has strong evidence for significant and sustained (>10%) weight loss in patients with and without diabetes. It also has strong evidence for cardiovascular benefit in people with obesity and established ASCVD (SELECT trial) and also improved symptoms/functional outcomes in HFpEF trials—but hard mortality outcome benefits are less consistent across.

Tirzepatide, approved by the FDA for T2DM in May 2022 and for obesity in November 2023, is a dual agonist for glucose-dependent insulinotropic polypeptide (GIP) and GLP-1 receptors, with greater affinity for GIP.[19] It is administered once weekly via subcutaneous injection with initial dose of 2.5 mg for 4 weeks, followed by incremental dosage adjustments of 2.5 mg every 4 weeks to a maximum dose of 15 mg weekly.

The SURPASS program demonstrated that tirzepatide reduces HbA1c (1.87–3.02%) and body weight (5.4–12.9 kg) and improves multiple cardiometabolic risk factors (including reduction in liver fat, new-onset macroalbuminuria, blood pressure, and lipids) across the T2DM spectrum.[20] FDA approval for obesity was based on the SURMOUNT-1 and SURMOUNT-2 trials, which reported weight reductions up to 20.9% after 72 weeks.[21,22] In the recently published SURMOUNT-5 trial among participants with obesity but without diabetes, treatment with maximum tolerated doses of tirzepatide was superior to treatment with maximum tolerated doses of injectable semaglutide with respect to reduction in body weight and waist circumference at week 72. The mean percent change in weight at week 72 was −20.2% with tirzepatide and −13.7% with semaglutide. Hence, at maximum tolerated doses, tirzepatide seems to be more efficacious than semaglutide for weight loss.[23] A post hoc analysis by Mamas et al. estimated a greater reduction in predicted 10-year CVD risk with tirzepatide, suggesting superiority in primary prevention of CVD in adults with obesity but without diabetes.[24]

In the SUMMIT trial, 731 patients with HFpEF and obesity received tirzepatide (up to 15 mg weekly) or placebo for 52 weeks. Death from cardiovascular causes or a worsening heart-failure event occurred in 9.9% patients in the tirzepatide group versus 15.3% in the placebo group. Worsening heart-failure events occurred in 8.0% in the tirzepatide group compared to 14.2% in the placebo arm. At 52 weeks, the mean change in the KCCQ CSS was 19.5 in the tirzepatide group as compared with 12.7 in the placebo group. Tirzepatide significantly reduced HF-related events and improved quality of life, exercise tolerance, and weight loss in obese patients with HFpEF. Benefit was primarily driven by reduction in HF events, not CV death.[25] The SURPASS-CVOT (Cardiovascular Outcomes Trial) evaluated the cardiovascular safety and efficacy of tirzepatide compared to dulaglutide in patients with T2DM and ASCVD. This trial directly compares two incretin-based therapies—tirzepatide, a dual GIP/GLP-1 RA, and dulaglutide, a GLP-1 RA—with established cardiovascular benefits. MACE were 8% less common with tirzepatide, and the rates of all-cause mortality, improvements in kidney function, and reductions in HbA1c were significantly better with tirzepatide.[26]

Some observational/real-world datasets, such as the STEER study, suggest semaglutide may show stronger short-term reductions in major adverse CV events versus tirzepatide in nonrandomized comparisons.[27] The STEER study was a retrospective observational study using the Komodo Research Database comparing the cardiovascular outcomes of patients >45 years with established ASCVD, with overweight or obesity, and without diabetes who were treated with tirzepatide or semaglutide. The results showed that semaglutide was associated with a 57% greater reduction in the risk of MACE, such as heart attack, stroke, or death, compared to tirzepatide in patients without diabetes who had no treatment gaps longer than 30 days. The study, sponsored by Novo Nordisk, was presented at the European Society of Cardiology Congress in August 2025. This was a nonrandomized observational study with limitations of short follow-up, low event counts, adherence sensitivity, and residual confounding. Another real-world study published in JAMA included data from US Healthcare claims from 2018 to 2024 and included patients with cardiometabolic HFpEF, and follow-up was up to 52 weeks.[28] They compared new users of semaglutide, tirzepatide, and sitagliptin (sitagliptin being used as a "placebo-proxy" since it has little known effect on HF outcomes) in three cohorts. These findings were benchmarked against results from the STEP-HFpEF DM and SUMMIT trials. In patients with cardiometabolic HFpEF, semaglutide and tirzepatide showed >40% risk reduction for the composite of hospitalization for HF or all-cause mortality compared with a placebo proxy. Tirzepatide showed no meaningful benefit over semaglutide.

LIMITATIONS

Head-to-head randomized trials comparing tirzepatide versus semaglutide for HF hard outcomes are absent, and indirect comparisons drive much inference. Follow-up duration in many studies is ~1–2 years, and long-term efficacy and mortality benefits need confirmation. Real-world studies are helpful but subject to bias, and they should not replace randomized evidence. Most RCTs are in patients with HFpEF with obesity, and generalizability to HFrEF or nonobese HF should not be presumed. Although weight loss and metabolic improvements may help HFrEF patients with obesity, caution should be maintained for GI side effects and early symptomatic volume/orthostatic changes, which can complicate therapy. Also, potential concerns such as a modest increase in resting heart rate with GLP-1 RAs could be undesirable in some HFrEF patients. Both semaglutide and tirzepatide show robust benefits in HFpEF but cannot currently be recommended for HFrEF due to lack of supportive evidence, especially in advanced disease. There are gaps in evidence on how much incremental benefit they provide on top of SGLT2 inhibitors and which effects are weight-independent versus weight-mediated.

CONCLUSION

Magnitude of weight loss is larger with maximal tolerated dose of tirzepatide versus semaglutide in head-to-head trial comparison (SURMOUNT-5). Weight loss likely mediates part of the HF symptom improvements, and a post hoc analysis predicted a greater long-term reduction in cardiovascular risk with tirzepatide. Tirzepatide (SUMMIT) reduced the risk of a composite of CV death or worsening heart-failure events versus placebo (≈38% relative risk reduction) in adults with HFpEF and obesity and also improved symptoms and quality of life. The risk of CV death alone, however, was not reduced. Semaglutide (STEP trials) improved symptoms, physical function (6-minute walk), and quality of life and produced substantial weight loss (~9–11%), but its trials were underpowered for hard CV endpoints (no consistent large signal for CV death reduction). However, in obese and overweight patients without diabetes and with preexisting CVD, including HF, the SELECT trial demonstrated that semaglutide can significantly reduce the risk of major cardiovascular events. Hence, the choice of therapy should consider weight loss magnitude, side-effect profile, patient preference, administration route, cost, and comorbidities, as no statistically significant superiority for primary HF outcomes has been demonstrated conclusively between tirzepatide and semaglutide. Gastrointestinal (GI) side effects are common for both and contribute to significant discontinuation rates.

REFERENCES

1. Drucker DJ. Mechanisms of action and therapeutic application of glucagon-like peptide-1. Cell Metab. 2018;27:740-56.
2. Wilding JPH, Batterham RL, Calanna S, et al. Once-weekly semaglutide in adults with overweight or obesity. N Engl J Med. 2021;384:989-1002.
3. Davies M, Færch L, Jeppesen OK, et al. Semaglutide 2.4 mg once a week in adults with overweight or obesity, and type 2 diabetes (STEP 2): a randomised, double-blind, double-dummy, placebo-controlled, phase 3 trial. Lancet. 2021;397:971-84.
4. Wadden TA, Bailey TS, Billings LK, et al. Effect of subcutaneous semaglutide vs placebo as an adjunct to intensive behavioral therapy on body weight in adults with overweight or obesity: the STEP 3 randomized clinical trial. JAMA. 2021;325:1403-13.

5. Rubino D, Abrahamsson N, Davies M, et al. Effect of continued weekly subcutaneous semaglutide vs placebo on weight loss maintenance in adults with overweight or obesity: the STEP 4 randomized clinical trial. JAMA. 2021;325:1414-25.
6. Garvey WT, Batterham RL, Bhatta M, et al. Two-year effects of semaglutide in adults with overweight or obesity: the STEP 5 trial. Nat Med. 2022;28:2083-91.
7. Rubino DM, Greenway FL, Khalid U, et al. Effect of weekly subcutaneous semaglutide vs daily liraglutide on body weight in adults with overweight or obesity without diabetes: the STEP 8 randomized clinical trial. JAMA. 2022;327:138-50.
8. Kadowaki T, Isendahl J, Khalid U, et al. Semaglutide once a week in adults with overweight or obesity, with or without type 2 diabetes in an East Asian population (STEP 6): a randomised, double-blind, double-dummy, placebo-controlled, phase 3a trial. Lancet Diabetes Endocrinol. 2022;10:193-206.
9. Weghuber D, Barrett T, Barrientos-Pérez M, et al. Once-weekly semaglutide in adolescents with obesity. N Engl J Med. 2022;387:2245-57.
10. Kosiborod MN, Abildstrøm SZ, Borlaug BA, et al. Semaglutide in patients with heart failure with preserved ejection fraction and obesity. N Engl J Med. 2023;389:1069-84.
11. Kosiborod MN, Petrie MC, Borlaug BA, et al. Semaglutide in patients with obesity-related heart failure and type 2 diabetes. N Engl J Med. 2024;390:1394-407.
12. Perkovic V, Tuttle KR, Rossing P, et al. Effects of semaglutide on chronic kidney disease in patients with type 2 diabetes. N Engl J Med. 2024;391:109-21.
13. Lincoff AM, Brown-Frandsen K, Colhoun HM, et al. Semaglutide and cardiovascular outcomes in obesity without diabetes. N Engl J Med. 2023;389:2221-32.
14. Marso SP, Bain SC, Consoli A, et al. Semaglutide and cardiovascular outcomes in patients with type 2 diabetes. N Engl J Med. 2016;375:1834-44.
15. McGuire DK, Marx N, Mulvagh SL, et al. Oral semaglutide and cardiovascular outcomes in high-risk type 2 diabetes. N Engl J Med. 2025;392:2001-12.
16. Knop FK, Aroda VR, do Vale RD, et al. Oral semaglutide 50 mg taken once per day in adults with overweight or obesity (OASIS 1): a randomised, double-blind, placebo-controlled, phase 3 trial. Lancet. 2023;402:705-19.
17. Wharton S, Lingvay I, Bogdanski P, et al. Oral semaglutide at a dose of 25 mg in adults with overweight or obesity. N Engl J Med. 2025;393:1077-87.
18. Kosiborod MN, Deanfield J, Pratley R, et al. Semaglutide versus placebo in patients with heart failure and mildly reduced or preserved ejection fraction: a pooled analysis of the SELECT, FLOW, STEP-HFpEF, and STEP-HFpEF DM randomised trials. Lancet. 2024;404:949-61.
19. Willard FS, Douros JD, Bn Gabe M, et al. Tirzepatide is an imbalanced and biased dual GIP and GLP-1 receptor agonist. JCI Insight 2020;5:e140532.
20. Sinha R, Papamargaritis D, Sargeant JA, et al. Efficacy and safety of tirzepatide in type 2 diabetes and obesity management. J Obes Metab Syndr. 2023;32:25-45.
21. Jastreboff AM, Aronne LJ, Ahmad NN, et al. Tirzepatide once weekly for the treatment of obesity. N Engl J Med. 2022;387:205-16.
22. Garvey WT, Frias JP, Jastreboff AM, et al. Tirzepatide once weekly for the treatment of obesity in people with type 2 diabetes (SURMOUNT-2): a double-blind, randomised, multicentre, placebo-controlled, phase 3 trial. Lancet. 2023;402:613-26.
23. Aronne LJ, Horn DB, le Roux CW, et al.; SURMOUNT-5 Trial Investigators. Tirzepatide as compared with semaglutide for the treatment of obesity. N Engl J Med. 2025; 393:26-36.
24. Mamas MA, Bays H, Li R, et al. Tirzepatide compared with semaglutide and 10-year cardiovascular disease risk reduction in obesity: post-hoc analysis of the SURMOUNT-5 trial. Eur Heart J Open. 2025;5(5): oeaf117.
25. Packer M, Zile MR, Kramer CM, et al. Tirzepatide for heart failure with preserved ejection fraction and obesity. N Engl J Med. 2025;392:427-37.
26. Nicholls SJ, Bhatt DL, Buse JB, et al. Comparison of tirzepatide and dulaglutide on major adverse cardiovascular events in participants with type 2 diabetes and atherosclerotic cardiovascular disease: SURPASS-CVOT design and baseline characteristics. Am Heart J. 2024;267:1-11.
27. Wilson L, Zhao Z, Divino V, et al. Semaglutide is associated with a lower risk of cardiovascular events compared with tirzepatide in patients with overweight or obesity and ASCVD and without diabetes in routine clinical practice (results from the STEER study). Presented at: the European Society of Cardiology (ESC) Congress together with World Congress of Cardiology; 2025 Aug 29–Sep 1; Madrid.
28. Krüger N, Schneeweiss S, Fuse K, et al. Semaglutide and tirzepatide in patients with heart failure with preserved ejection fraction. JAMA. 2025;334(14):1255-66.

124

CHAPTER

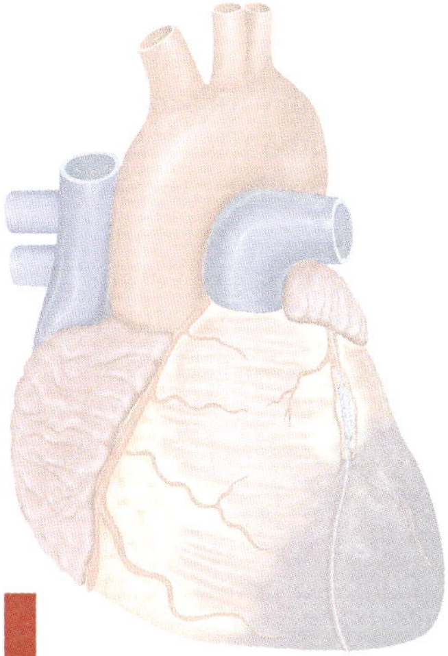

Efficacy, Safety, and Tolerability of Tirzepatide in Obese Patients without Diabetes: Current Status

Sudhir Kumar Mathi, Andru Krishna Vamsi, Rohit Walia

INTRODUCTION

Obesity is a massive global health problem with profound implications for cardiovascular and metabolic dysfunction. Tirzepatide can achieve weight loss outcomes comparable to bariatric surgery and was approved by FDA for chronic weight management.[1] This chapter provides a comprehensive review of tirzepatide in nondiabetic patients.

OBESITY AND THE RISK: PATHOPHYSIOLOGY

Abdominal obesity is crucial factor for cardiovascular disease and metabolic syndrome. There is complex interaction between adipose tissue dysfunction, chronic low-grade inflammation, insulin resistance, and metabolic dysfunction contributing to cardiovascular risk. Visceral adiposity leads to adipokine dysregulation, increased inflammatory mediators, and altered lipid metabolism, which promote endothelial dysfunction and atherosclerosis.[2-4]

CLINICAL INDICATIONS

Body mass index (BMI) ≥30 kg/m^2 or 27 kg/m^2 with comorbidities such as hypertension, dyslipidemia, atherosclerotic cardiovascular disease, prediabetes, insulin resistance, and obstructive sleep apnea not improving on lifestyle measures can benefit from tirzepatide.[2-8] Though it is also used in diabetes mellitus (DM) and effective reducing the progression of prediabetes to overt diabetes in this chapter we focus on nondiabetic patients.

TIRZEPATIDE: MECHANISM OF ACTION, PHARMACOKINETICS, AND PHARMACODYNAMICS

Tirzepatide is a 39 amino acid peptide functioning as a twincretin by acting dual agonist for glucagon-like peptide-1 (GLP-1) and glucose-dependent insulinotropic polypeptide (GIP) receptors. GLP-1 receptor activation stimulates glucose-dependent insulin secretion, suppresses glucagon release when glucose levels are elevated, delays gastric emptying, reduces appetite, and promotes satiety. GIP receptor activation enhances postprandial insulin secretion, improves beta cell function, modulates adipose metabolism, and synergistically enhances weight loss with GLP-1 effects. It has 80% bioavailability, a 5 day half-life for weekly dosing, and a primary elimination via proteolytic cleavage, amide hydrolysis and beta oxidation, while the cytochrome P450 enzymes are not involved in elimination so neither hepatic nor renal impairment affects tirzepatide pharmacokinetics.[2]

CLINICAL EVIDENCE: TRIALS

The SURMOUNT-1 trial investigated doses of 5 mg, 10 mg, and 15 mg s.c. once weekly in nondiabetic individuals with obesity (BMI >30 or BMI >27 and weight-related complication) and showed dose-dependent weight loss up to 20.9% at 72 weeks. There were significant BMI, fat mass, HbA1c, cardiovascular risk factor, and quality of life improvements.[3] The SURMOUNT-2 trial investigated doses of 10 mg and 15 mg s.c. once weekly in patients with overweight (BMI >27) and diabetes (DM) and reported a weight loss of 14.7% for the high dose treatment arm after 72 weeks compared to a weight loss of 3.2% following placebo treatment.[4]

The SURPASS-1 trial reported a reduction in total body fat mass of 26% for all tirzepatide doses pooled (5 mg, 10 mg, and 15 mg tirzepatide s.c. once weekly groups) compared to placebo.[5] The SURPASS-2 trial compared all doses of tirzepatide to 1 mg s.c once weekly of semaglutide and reported that 15 mg dose tirzepatide on average resulted in absolute reduction in body weight of 6.6% more than semaglutide.[5] Tirzepatide also has favorable effects on total cholesterol and triglycerides, decreased LDL increase in HDL, decrease in systolic, and diastolic blood pressure. It also has cardioprotective effect postmyocardial infarction.[6]

Tirzepatide has shown reductions in both body fat mass and lean body mass.

MRI analysis of body composition in a subset of participants from the SURPASS-3 study revealed a larger decrease in muscle fat infiltration than anticipated. However, it also indicated an overall reduction in fat-free muscle mass.[7,9] In clinical trials, tirzepatide has been demonstrated to elicit substantial weight reduction, with less weight loss in trial participants with diabetes (T2D) compared to participants without T2D. In the SURMOUNT-2 trial, participants with T2D achieved a mean weight loss of up to 14.7% from baseline after 72 weeks as compared to the SURMOUNT-1 trial with a similar dose-escalation and involving slightly younger and more overweight participants without T2D, a mean weight loss of up to 20.9% from baseline was reported after 72 weeks.[3,4,6] A mean weight reduction of 24.5% after 72 weeks of treatment with tirzepatide in nondiabetic obese adults with weight-related comorbidities was reported for the SURMOUNT-3 trial.[3] The SURMOUNT-4 trial reported 26% weight reduction in overweight or obese participants without T2D over 88 weeks of treatment. There seems to be reduced glucoregulatory effects of both GLP-1 and GIP observed in patients with T2D compared to age- and BMI-matched controls without T2D.[8] Weight loss plateaus typically within 24–36 weeks depending on dose and patient factors.

SAFETY AND TOLERABILITY

Most adverse events (AE) are gastrointestinal in nature and most pronounced during the dose-escalation phase and are transient lasting for 2–4 days. Gradual dose escalation improves tolerability. Frequency of AE was 77–82% in the SURMOUNT trials, and up to 95% was reported in an Asian-Pacific population with a lower mean body weight in the SURPASS-AP-combo trial. Comparing the SURMOUNT-1 and -2 trials (similar duration and demographics but participants with and without T2D), nausea was reported by 31% (non-T2D) versus 23% (T2D) of participants during treatment with the highest tirzepatide dose (15 mg). Diarrhea was reported by 23% (non-T2D) versus 19% (T2D) of participants treated with tirzepatide 15 mg. Collectively, AEs in participants without T2D were reported in up to 82% of participants with 4–7% of participants discontinuing due to AEs. Serious AEs consisting of acute cholecystitis and acute pancreatitis were rare.[8,10-12]

OTHER USEFUL EFFECTS

Tirzepatide improves both markers of beta cell function and insulin sensitivity, alcohol dependence, has been proven beneficial in heart failure with preserved ejection fraction (HFpEF), Alzheimer, obstructive sleep apnea (OSA), doxorubicin-induced cardiomyopathy, diabetic kidney disease, steatohepatitis, and congenital generalized lipodystrophy. Tirzepatide also has neuroprotective and cerebrovascular benefits in obese patients and decreases incidence of dementia and stroke. The CMR substudy of the SUMMIT trial demonstrated that tirzepatide therapy in obesity-related HFpEF led to reduced LV mass and pericardiac adipose tissue compared to placebo and LV mass change with patient's weight loss. These physiological changes may contribute to reduction in heart failure events. GLP1 and GIP receptors are widely expressed in the central nervous system and insulin significantly regulates synaptic and cognitive functions. It has been shown that dysregulation of the expression of the GLP1 and GIP receptors and impairment of insulin receptor substrate 1 (IRS1) are implicated in the development and progression of neurodegenerative diseases such as Alzheimer's disease. Long-term tirzepatide improves renal function in patients with obesity, chronic renal disease, and HFpEF.[9,11-16]

CONCLUSION

Tirzepatide has revolutionized the obesity pharmacotherapy. Studies with combination with other drugs acting on multiple receptors may come out in future. It also has potential to benefit diseases other than obesity and future trials are needed to explore these effects. Awaited SURMOUNT CVOT and SURMOUNT-MMO results will shed further light in this regard.

REFERENCES

1. Jastreboff AM, Aronne LJ, Ahmad NN, et al. Tirzepatide once weekly for the treatment of obesity. N Engl J Med. 2022;387(3), 205-16.
2. Rosenstock J, Wysham C, Frías JP, et al. Efficacy and safety of a novel dual GIP and GLP-1 receptor agonist tirzepatide in patients with type 2 diabetes (SURPASS-1): a double-blind, randomised, phase 3 trial. Lancet. 2021;398(10295):143-55.
3. Hankosky ER, Wang H, Neff LM, et al. Tirzepatide reduces the predicted risk of atherosclerotic cardiovascular disease and improves cardiometabolic risk factors in adults with obesity or overweight: SURMOUNT-1 post hoc analysis. Diabetes Obes Metab. 2024;26(1):319-28.
4. Garvey WT, Frias JP, Jastreboff AM, et al. Tirzepatide once weekly for the treatment of obesity in people with type 2 diabetes (SURMOUNT-2): a double-blind, randomised, multicentre, placebo-controlled, phase 3 trial. Lancet. 2023;402(10402):613-26.
5. Frías JP, Davies MJ, Rosenstock J, et al; SURPASS-2 Investigators. Tirzepatide versus Semaglutide Once Weekly in Patients with Type 2 Diabetes. N Engl J Med. 2021;385(6):503-15.
6. Wadden TA, Chao AM, Machineni S, et al. Tirzepatide after intensive lifestyle intervention in adults with overweight or obesity: the SURMOUNT-3 phase 3 trial. Nat Med. 2023;29(11):2909-18.
7. Aronne LJ, Sattar N, Horn DB, et al. Continued Treatment with Tirzepatide for Maintenance of Weight Reduction in Adults with Obesity: The SURMOUNT-4 Randomized Clinical Trial. JAMA. 2024;331(1):38-48.
8. Safwan M, Bourgleh MS, Alotaibi SA, et al. Gastrointestinal safety of semaglutide and tirzepatide vs. placebo in obese individuals without diabetes: a systematic review and meta analysis. Ann Saudi Med. 2025;45(2):129-43.
9. Alshehri GH, Al-Kuraishy HM, Waheed HJ, et al. Tirzepatide: a novel therapeutic approach for Alzheimer's disease. Metab Brain Dis. 2025;40(5):221.
10. Packer M, Zile MR, Kramer CM, et al; SUMMIT Trial Study Group. Tirzepatide for Heart Failure with Preserved Ejection Fraction and Obesity. N Engl J Med. 2025;392(5): 427-37.
11. Loomba R, Hartman ML, Lawitz EJ, et al; SYNERGY-NASH Investigators. Tirzepatide for Metabolic Dysfunction-Associated Steatohepatitis with Liver Fibrosis. N Engl J Med. 2024;391(4):299-310.
12. Gastaldelli A, Cusi K, Fernández Landó L, et al. Effect of tirzepatide versus insulin degludec on liver fat content and abdominal adipose tissue in people with type 2 diabetes (SURPASS-3 MRI): a substudy of the randomised, open-label, parallel-group, phase 3 SURPASS-3 trial. Lancet Diabetes Endocrinol. 2022;10(6):393-406.
13. Kramer CM, Borlaug BA, Zile MR, et al; SUMMIT Trial Study Group. Tirzepatide Reduces LV Mass and Paracardiac Adipose Tissue in Obesity-Related Heart Failure: SUMMIT CMR Substudy. J Am Coll Cardiol. 2025;85(7): 699-706.
14. Beccuti G, Bioletto F, Parasiliti-Caprino M, et al. Estimating Cardiovascular Benefits of Tirzepatide in Sleep Apnea and Obesity: Insight from the SURMOUNT-OSA Trials. Curr Obes Rep. 2024;13(4):739-42.
15. Kanbay M, Copur S, Siriopol D, et al. Effect of tirzepatide on blood pressure and lipids: A meta-analysis of randomized controlled trials. Diabetes Obes Metab. 2023;25(12):3766-78.
16. Packer M, Zile MR, Kramer CM, et al; SUMMIT Trial Study Group. Interplay of Chronic Kidney Disease and the Effects of Tirzepatide in Patients with Heart Failure, Preserved Ejection Fraction, and Obesity. The SUMMIT Trial. J Am Coll Cardiol. 2025;85(18):1721-35.

125

CHAPTER

Combination of Tirzepatide with Lifestyle Interventions: Diet and Exercise Synergies

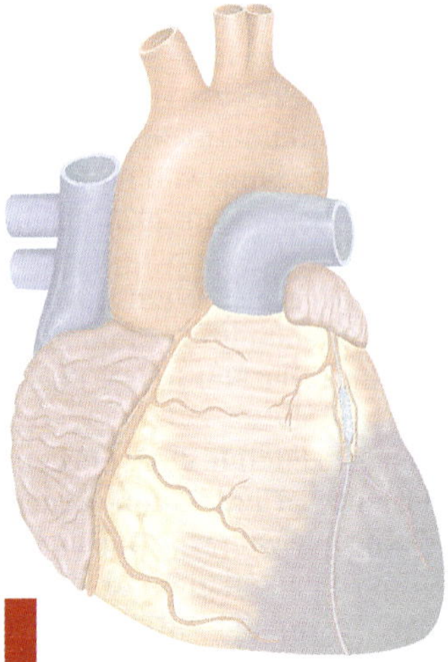

SB Gupta

INTRODUCTION

Approximately 1 out of 10 Americans has diabetes, and among these, 90–95% have type 2 diabetes mellitus (T2DM).[1] Uncontrolled diabetes is known for leading to serious complications such as ischemic heart disease, kidney damage, and vision impairment.

Other highly prevalent conditions worldwide are overweight and obesity, both of which are chronic diseases and precursors for several complications, including diabetes mellitus.

Lifestyle interventions such as caloric restrictions in diet and exercising regularly are the cornerstone of the management of overweight and obesity. It is always challenging to sustain weight loss by lifestyle interventions alone.

Anti-obesity drugs have been used for a number of years; however, earlier generations of such drugs were not well tolerated because of their side effects and had only modest weight loss.

Tirzepatide, a synthetic polypeptide, is a dual agonist for the glucose-dependent insulinotropic polypeptide (GIP) and glucagon-like peptide-1 (GLP-1) receptors. Tirzepatide leads to significant improved glycemic control, having similar benefits like GLP-1 receptor agonist, semaglutide. The US Food and Drug Administration (FDA) approved tirzepatide, a novel medication for treating T2DM, in May 2022. Tirzepatide is administered once weekly subcutaneously with incremental dosage adjustments.

The SURPASS-1 trial,[2] a double-blind, placebo-controlled phase 3, 40-week study, showed that in patients with HbA1c ≥7.5% and ≤9.5% received tirzepatide subcutaneously once weekly at doses of 5 mg (n = 121), 10 mg (n = 121), or 15 mg (n = 121), or placebo (n = 115), had significant reduction in HbA1c, fasting glucose and body weight compared to placebo. Nearly 90% of patients reached an HbA1c goal of <7% and approximately 50% reached an HbA1c <5.7%. Patients lost –7.0, –7.8, and –9.5 kg of weight in the 5, 10, and 15 mg tirzepatide groups, respectively, compared to –0.7 kg with placebo.

The SURPASS-4 trial,[3] an open-label, randomized, parallel-group phase 3 study, compared tirzepatide subcutaneously 5, 10, or 15 mg weekly versus insulin glargine in 1,878 adults with HbA1c ≥7.5% and ≤10.5% with 1:1:1:3 randomization. Patients receiving tirzepatide 10 mg showed –2.34% HbA1c reduction, –2.58% reduction with 15 mg, and –1.44% reduction with insulin glargine at 52 weeks. Body weight reduction of ≥10% was achieved in 36% of the individuals in the 5 mg tirzepatide group, 53% with 10 mg tirzepatide, and 66% with 15 mg tirzepatide compared to 2% in the insulin glargine group. Reduction in the weight was sustained over 104 weeks. Hypoglycemia was noted more frequently with insulin glargine (19%) versus tirzepatide (6–9%). However, gastrointestinal (GI) side effects were more frequently reported in the tirzepatide group in comparison to insulin glargine.

The SURPASS-5 clinical trial[4] enrolled 475 adults, randomized in a 1:1:1:1 ratio, on tirzepatide 5 mg (n = 116), 10 mg (n = 119), or 15 mg (n = 120) subcutaneously weekly or insulin glargine (n = 120), 44% women with a mean age of 60.6 years and mean HbA1c 8.31% over 40 weeks. A total of 451 patients completing the trial reported a –2.11% reduction in HbA1c levels at 5 mg, –2.40% with 10 mg, and –2.34% with 15 mg weekly dosing as compared to –0.86% with insulin glargine. Mean weight reduction of –5.4 kg

Similar to VAT, ectopic cardiac adipose tissue accumulation was found to be associated with the development of metabolic and cardiac complications, including coronary artery disease. Although the long-term relationship between ectopic cardiac adipose tissue accumulation (in any depot) and coronary artery disease is largely unknown, a few cross-sectional studies have reported a potential association between excess ectopic cardiac adipose tissue and coronary artery disease. Cardiac fat depots, including pericardial and epicardial fat, have been associated with coronary events in the general population independent of traditional cardiovascular risk factors.[1]

Pericardial adipose tissue was associated with an increased risk of all-cause CVD and atherosclerosis burden. Excess epicardial adipose tissue deposition measured by ultrasound, CT, and MRI has been related to abnormal myocardial flow reserve, coronary plaque vulnerability, coronary artery calcification, and coronary artery disease severity. Epicardial adipose tissue-derived adipocytokines, inflammation, and systemic mediators such as reactive oxygen species may favor the development of a local proatherogenic environment by paracrine and vasocrine mechanisms, thus promoting the pathogenesis of coronary artery disease.

Besides effects on atherosclerosis in larger arteries, excess adiposity is linked to abnormalities in the coronary microvasculature—a key regulator of coronary flow reserve. Coronary microvascular disease is related to endothelial dysfunction and small-vessel remodeling in responses to neural, mechanical, and metabolic factors. Microvascular disease is independently associated with BMI and provides prognostic information regarding cardiovascular risk among individuals with obesity.

Visceral Adiposity, Ectopic Fat, and Heart Failure

Obesity is a major risk factor for heart failure—an association not fully explained by obesity-related cardiovascular risk factors. Individuals with obesity are 2× more at risk of developing heart failure than those who have normal body weight. According to the Framingham Heart Study, each BMI increment by 1 unit is associated with a 5% increased heart failure risk in men and 7% in women after adjusting for other cardiovascular risk factors, and the risk of heart failure was found to be increased across the entire spectrum of BMI. In a meta-analysis looking at the association between obesity and heart failure incidence, each 10-cm increase in waist circumference was associated with an increased incidence of heart failure, with higher incidence for heart failure starting in the overweight BMI range.

Approximately 50% of individuals with obesity have heart failure with preserved ejection fraction (HFpEF), which means that the usual clinical parameter (left ventricular ejection fraction) is normal, posing a substantial challenge in clinical practice. Although left ventricular ejection fraction has generally been found to be preserved in patients with obesity, many investigators have found evidence of subclinical myocardial dysfunction when sensitive cardiac imaging measurements such as myocardial strain are used. The prevalence of abnormal subclinical myocardial function (i.e., abnormal myocardial strain) in obesity has been reported to range from 37% to 54%. Abnormal subclinical myocardial function in asymptomatic obese patients with diabetes mellitus has been associated with the progression of adverse CVD. Longer duration of obesity and its severity (BMI ≥40 kg/m^2) have been identified as major factors predisposing to cardiac dysfunction and heart failure. Surgical treatment of obesity prevents development of heart failure and improves established heart failure, including HFpEF. Although the relationship between obesity and incident heart failure may involve hemodynamic and anatomic cardiac changes related to excess adiposity, evidence suggests that the relationship is also mediated by obesity-related metabolic, inflammatory, and hormonal changes.

Incretin-based Therapies

Incretins are hormones that are secreted from enteroendocrine cells in the gut mucosa after a meal. They are potent stimulators of postprandial insulin secretion under hyperglycemic conditions and contribute to approximately 70% of the physiological postprandial insulin secretion. The so-called incretin effect describes this phenomenon and also explains that orally ingested glucose leads to a higher insulin response than intravenously administered glucose leading to isoglycemic glucose excursions compared to oral glucose. In man, the peptides glucagon-like peptide-1 (GLP-1) and glucose-dependent insulinotropic polypeptide (GIP) are the major incretin hormones. While GIP loses its insulinotropic effect in T2DM with chronic hyperglycemia, GLP-1 is still able to stimulate insulin secretion. Parenteral administration of pharmacological doses of GLP-1 is able to normalize plasma glucose by stimulating insulin secretion and simultaneously inhibiting glucagon secretion in subjects with T2DM and hyperglycemia. Native GLP-1 is not suitable for treatment, since the peptide is degraded rapidly within minutes by the enzyme dipeptidyl-peptidase-IV (DPP-4). Utilizing

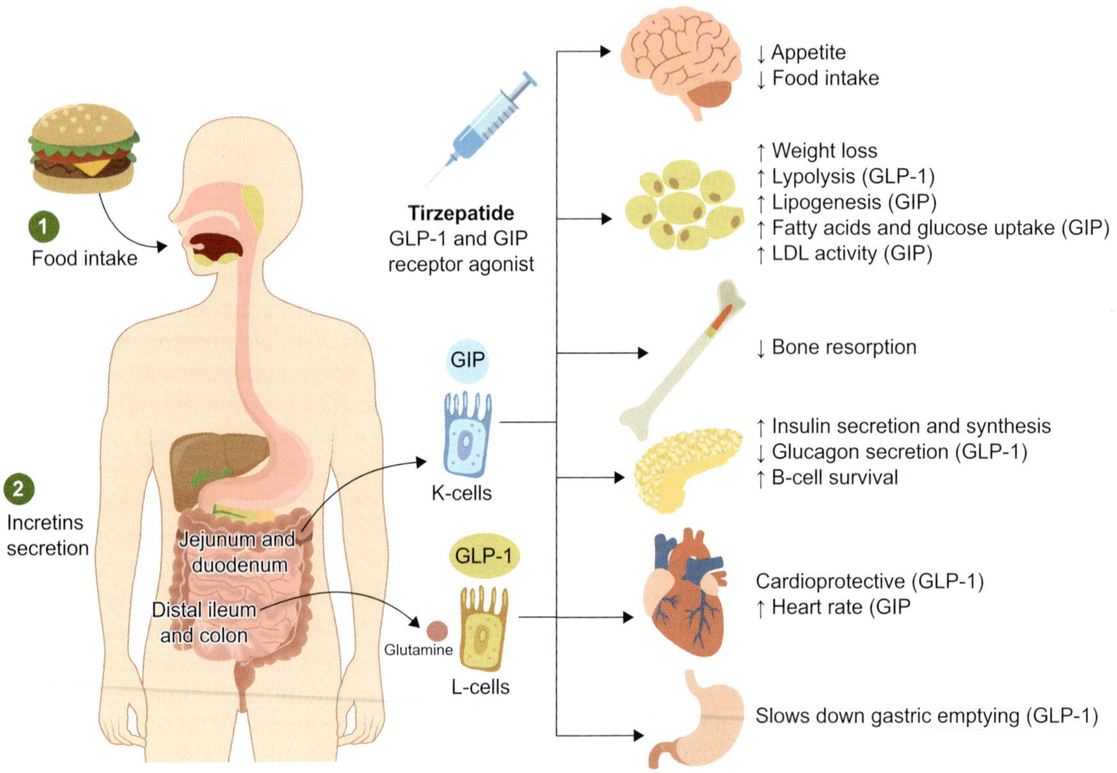

Fig. 3: Mechanism of action and systemic effects of tirzepatide.

the concept of elevating GLP-1 concentrations, DPP-4 inhibitors as oral agents and synthetic injectable, DPP-4-resistant GLP-1 receptor agonists (GLP-1RA) were introduced as treatment options for T2DM therapy. GLP-1RA provides strong and effective glycemic control and also lower body weight and systolic blood pressure. They have a low risk of causing hypoglycemia and also promote satiety by central nervous system effects and by slowing gastric emptying.

GLP-1 RA has been placed prominently in the international recommendations for the treatment of T2DM as the first injectable agent before insulin due to the advantageous outcomes in cardiovascular safety studies that demonstrated a reduction of the combined cardiovascular endpoint three-component major adverse cardiovascular event (MACE-3; cardiovascular death, nonfatal myocardial infarct, nonfatal stroke) for the GLP-1 RA albiglutide, efpeglenatide, dulaglutide, liraglutide, and semaglutide **(Fig. 3)**.[2,3]

TIRZEPATIDE

Tirzepatide, also referred to as a "twincretin", is a novel dual GLP-1/GIP receptor agonist and the first medication designed as a single molecule to bind to both GIP and GLP-1 receptors. Once-weekly tirzepatide offers dosing flexibility ranging from 2.5 to 15 mg per 0.5 mL injection. Its unique molecular structure contributes to its favorable pharmacokinetic profile, with a linear peptide backbone consisting of 39 amino acids with an acyl fat-chain conjugation designed to enhance albumin binding and extend its half-life. Tirzepatide shows a high bioavailability of 81%, with peak plasma concentrations attained at 48 hours post administration. Notably, its half-life of 117 hours, approximately 5 days, supports its once-weekly dosing regimen. While the approved indication for tirzepatide is only as an adjunct treatment to improve glycemic control in adults with T2DM, clinical trials have demonstrated significant reductions in body weight across all dosage groups, among other interesting metabolic improvements along with cardiovascular benefits, especially among patients with HFpEF.[4,5]

Metabolic Effects of Tirzepatide

Multiple studies have investigated the effect of tirzepatide on various metabolic outcomes. Two clinical trial programs have investigated the efficacy and safety of tirzepatide, with SURMOUNT trials focusing mainly on its effects on body weight. The SURMOUNT-1 trial assessed

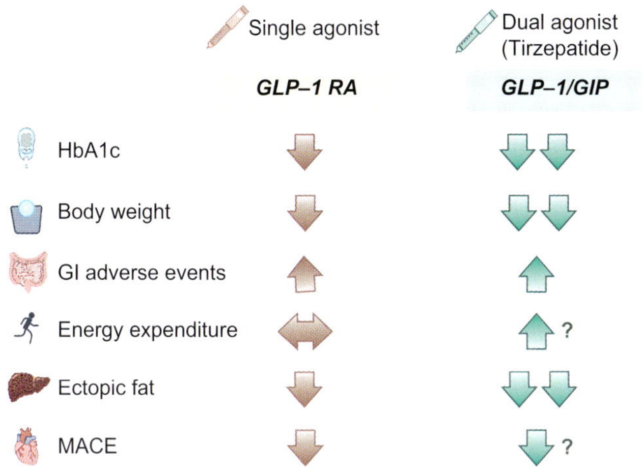

Fig. 4: Comparative metabolic and cardiovascular effects of GLP-1 receptor agonists and dual GLP-1/GIP receptor agonism.

the weight-reducing potential of tirzepatide in obese participants (BMI > 30 or >27 kg/m^2 with weight-related complications) not having T2DM. Notably, a subgroup of 1,032 participants (40.6%) had prediabetes, defined as having an HbA1c level of 5.7–6.4% (39–47 mmol/mol). Meanwhile, the SURMOUNT-2 trial targeted weight loss in participants with T2DM and overweight status (BMI >27 kg/m^2). The effects of tirzepatide were examined across doses of 5, 10, and 15 mg subcutaneously once weekly in SURMOUNT-1, while SURMOUNT-2 only examined the 10 and 15 mg doses **(Fig. 4)**.

In the SURMOUNT-1 trial, a reduction in body weight of up to 20.9% after 72 weeks of treatment with the 15 mg dose of tirzepatide was reported, while placebo exhibited a 3.1% weight loss. Similarly, in the SURMOUNT-2 trial, placebo treatment experienced a weight loss of 3.2%, whereas participants in the 15 mg treatment dose experienced a weight reduction of 14.7% after 72 weeks. The SURMOUNT-3 clinical trial tested the effect of using tirzepatide after a successful intensive lifestyle intervention in adults with overweight or obesity and at least one weight-related complication. The participants experienced an 18.5% weight loss after 72 weeks of tirzepatide injections, while placebo had a 2.5% weight loss [treatment difference of 20.8%; 95% confidence interval (CI), –23.2%, –18.5%; $p < 0.001$]. The trial also found that 87.5% of participants lost more than 5% additional weight loss with tirzepatide, while 16.5% of the participants receiving placebo met that threshold.

Additionally, findings from the SURPASS trials which investigated the effect of tirzepatide in participants with T2DM revealed weight reductions ranging from 5% to 14% across doses of tirzepatide. Additionally, in the SURPASS-2 trial, all doses of tirzepatide were compared to a once-weekly subcutaneous injection of 1 mg semaglutide. The trial findings indicated that, on average, the 15 mg tirzepatide dose resulted in a 6.6% greater absolute reduction in body weight compared to semaglutide. The SURPASS-3 trial revealed that tirzepatide doses decreased body weight by 7.5 to 12.9 kg from baseline, while insulin degludec increased body weight by 2.3 kg. SURPASS-5 and SURPASS-6 also showed that the addition of tirzepatide to insulin glargine resulted in a significant weight loss ranging from –7.1 to –10.5 kg compared to placebo and –12.2 kg compared to addition of insulin lispro.

A recent network meta-analysis including 47 randomized controlled trials with 17,163 subjects showed tirzepatide to be the most effective FDA-approved GLP-1 RA in weight reduction, resulting in a mean weight loss of 8.47 kg (95% CI –9.68 to –7.26), with high confidence in presented evidence. Tirzepatide also resulted in the most significant reduction in BMI by –2.85 kg/m^2 (95% CI, –3.70 to –2.01) and waist circumference by –6.77 cm (95%, CI –8.97 to –4.57). Additionally, an interesting subgroup analysis by Ma et al.[8] included 235 T2DM patients with normal body weight by BMI indicator (<25 kg/m^2) at baseline and showed that tirzepatide doses 5, 10, and 15 mg resulted in significant reductions in body weight by –3.5 kg (5.5%), –6.8 kg (10.8%), and –6.1 kg (9.8%), respectively.[6]

Weight-loss Maintenance/Weight Regain

The SURMOUNT-4 phase 3 randomized withdrawal clinical trial investigated the effect of tirzepatide, with diet and physical activity, on the maintenance of weight reduction. The trial included adults with a BMI ≥ 30 or ≥ 27 kg/m^2 with weight-related complications, excluding T2DM. Participants received once-weekly subcutaneous tirzepatide at the maximum tolerated dose (10 or 15 mg) for 36 weeks open-label, followed by a 52-week double-blind, placebo-controlled period. Afterward, 670 out of 783 participants were randomized (1:1) to either continue receiving tirzepatide ($n = 335$) or switch to placebo ($n = 335$) for the subsequent 52 weeks.

The primary endpoint was the mean percent change in weight from week 36 to week 88. Another secondary endpoint was the proportion of participants at week 88 maintaining at least 80% of weight lost during the lead-in period. Results showed that participants completing the lead-in period experienced a mean weight reduction of 20.9%. From week 36 to week 88, continuing tirzepatide resulted in a mean percent weight change of –5.5%, which is significantly lower than the 14.0% increase observed with placebo. Additionally, 89.5% of participants on tirzepatide maintained at least 80% of the weight loss, compared to only 16.6% on placebo. This indicates that continued treatment of tirzepatide maintains and augments weight reduction, whereas discontinuation results in significant regain of weight lost. This raises the question about the termination point of tirzepatide, with the potential of being a lifelong treatment instead of a temporary therapy for weight loss. Following lifestyle interventions, a substantial portion ranging from 30% to 50% of lost body weight is typically regained within a year, while over half of patients revert to their initial body weight within 5 years post-treatment initiation. Altogether, the prevention of weight regain subsequent to weight loss stands out as a big challenge in obesity management.

Appetite regulation plays a crucial role in weight loss maintenance due to its impact on controlling food intake and energy balance. Tirzepatide exerts a multifaceted influence on appetite regulation and food intake through its activation of GIP and GLP-1 receptors energy intake during a buffet lunch significantly decreased from baseline, in contrast to the placebo group. This calorie intake was significantly lower with tirzepatide compared to placebo (–309.8 kcal; 95% CI, –423.0, –196.6; $p<0.001$). Moreover, the reduction in energy intake with tirzepatide was numerically higher compared to a 1 mg semaglutide dose, although not statistically significant.

The study also found that by week 28, both tirzepatide and semaglutide elicited a reduction in appetite compared to baseline, as evidenced by higher overall appetite scores that did not show a significant change. This effect on appetite was again comparable between tirzepatide and semaglutide.

Glycemic Control

The completed clinical trial program, known as SURPASS, was primarily designed to assess the glucose-lowering efficacy of tirzepatide in participants with T2DM. These trials utilized mean change in HbA1c as the primary endpoint, with weight loss outcomes evaluated as secondary measures. Tirzepatide was investigated both as monotherapy in the SURPASS-1 trial and as an add-on to various glucose-lowering therapies, including metformin, insulin, SGLT2 inhibitors, sulfonylurea, or combinations thereof. Notably, the SURPASS-2 trial compared tirzepatide to semaglutide 1 mg subcutaneously once weekly, while in the "SURPASS J-Mono" trial it was compared against dulaglutide 0.75 mg subcutaneously once weekly. The SURPASS trials showed significant reductions in HbA1c levels, ranging from 20.4 mmol/mol with the 5 mg dose to 28.2 mmol/mol with the 15 mg dose, after treatments lasting between 40 and 52 weeks.

A recent network meta-analysis showed that tirzepatide significantly reduced HbA1c, with a mean difference of –2.10% (95%) pooled from all studies involving tirzepatide. This reduction marked the most significant compared to all other GLP-1 RA. Tirzepatide was also the most effective in reducing fasting blood glucose [mean difference –3.12 mmol/L (95% CI –3.59 to –2.66)], proving to be the most effective GLP-1 RA drug for glycemic control.

Inflammation

Chronic inflammation is a common underlying factor in various metabolic disorders, including obesity, T2DM, and non-alcoholic fatty liver disease (NAFLD). These conditions are characterized by persistent low-grade inflammation, which contributes to their pathogenesis and progression. Certain blood parameters such as mean platelet volume (MPV), prognostic nutritional index (PNI), and uric acid-to-HDL cholesterol ratio (UHR) can serve as potential indicators of inflammation, metabolic syndrome, and disease progression in patients with T2DM, obesity, prediabetes, NAFLD, and diabetic kidney disease.

Recent studies have demonstrated that tirzepatide possesses anti-inflammatory properties that may beneficially impact these metabolic disorders. Tirzepatide can reduce inflammation in cardiac tissues, suggesting potential protective effects against diabetes-related cardiac dysfunction. Additionally, tirzepatide has been shown to alleviate oxidative stress and inflammation by modulating lipid metabolism pathways, which could be advantageous in managing NAFLD and related conditions. Moreover, tirzepatide has been associated with reductions in key inflammatory markers. A post hoc analysis of a phase 2 trial found that treatment with tirzepatide led to significant decreases in biomarkers such as YKL-40, intercellular adhesion molecule 1 (ICAM-1), C-reactive protein (CRP), leptin, and growth differentiation factor 15 over 26 weeks. These findings underscore the potential anti-inflammatory effects of tirzepatide **(Fig. 5)**.

Lipid Profile

Tirzepatide demonstrates significant effects on lipid profile parameters, as evidenced by data from various clinical trials. Across different trials, total cholesterol exhibited reductions ranging from 2.2% to 15.4%, while low-density lipoprotein cholesterol levels decreased by 5.3–19.3%, with the exception of findings from the SURMOUNT-2 trial, which reported a modest increase of 2.3–3.2% in LDL-C. Notably, high-density lipoprotein cholesterol levels showed improvements, with increases ranging from 0.9% to 10.8%.

Magnetic resonance imaging investigations conducted as part of the SURPASS-3 trial elucidated the impact of tirzepatide on liver fat content. Participants with a fatty liver index ≥60 demonstrated a substantial absolute reduction

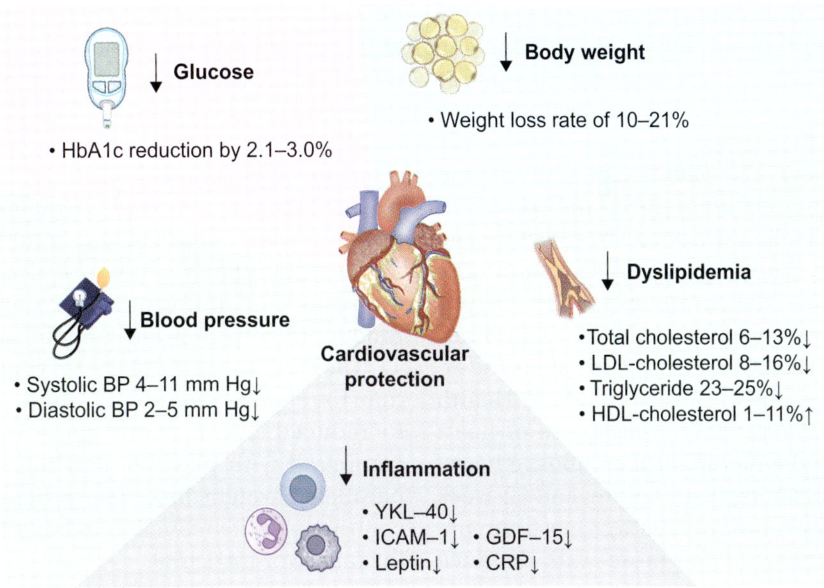

Fig. 5: Multisystem cardiometabolic benefits contributing to cardiovascular protection.

of 8.1% in liver fat content from baseline following treatment with pooled 10 and 15 mg doses of tirzepatide, compared to a 3.4% reduction observed in participants treated with insulin degludec. Additionally, a network meta-analysis revealed that tirzepatide significantly lowered triglyceride levels by an average of –0.89 mmol/L (95% CI, –1.64 to –0.13) compared to placebo. These findings, although may be primary driven from the weight loss seen in these trials, underscore the favorable impact of tirzepatide on lipid parameters and thereafter its impact on cardiovascular health.

Blood Pressure

Tirzepatide has also been shown to reduce BP in clinical studies. The patients treated with tirzepatide showed significantly lowered systolic and diastolic BP compared with patients in the control group, regardless of whether tirzepatide was used as a monotherapy or add-on therapy. Overall, tirzepatide treatment reduced systolic and diastolic BP by 4.8 and 1.7 mm Hg, respectively.

Tirzepatide appears to have a more significant impact on BP in Japanese individuals with T2DM. At a dose of 15 mg, tirzepatide reduced systolic BP by 11.0 mm Hg and diastolic BP by 5.6 mm Hg from baseline.

The effect of tirzepatide on 24-hour mean systolic BP, diastolic BP, and heart rate (HR) measured during 24-hour ambulatory BP monitoring (ABPM) in individuals living with obesity without T2DM has been evaluated in the SURMOUNT-1 ABPM substudy. After 36 weeks of treatment, tirzepatide was associated with statistically significant and clinically meaningful reductions in the mean 24-hour systolic BP at all doses and reduced diastolic BP at the two lower doses. Simultaneously, tirzepatide treatment was associated with a dose-dependent increase in the mean 24-hour HR. Fortunately, there is no clear evidence that tirzepatide increases the risk of AF.

The effect of tirzepatide treatment on cardiovascular events has been studied in SURPASS-4, a trial involving patients with known coronary, peripheral arterial, or cerebrovascular diseases or those who were at a high risk of these diseases. In this study, no tirzepatide dose numerically increased the risk of cardiovascular events. Instead, for patients treated with the highest dose of tirzepatide (15 mg/wk), the risk of developing any MACE (e.g., MI, stroke, hospitalization for angina, or all-cause death) was estimated to be 0.50 (95% CI, 0.26–0.95). Collectively, tirzepatide did not increase the risk of MACEs in participants with T2DM compared with controls.[7-10]

Although most patients with heart failure have preserved ejection fraction (HFpEF) rather than reduced ejection fraction (HFrEF), treatment options for HFpEF remain limited. Previous trials using the GLP-1 agonist semaglutide—STEP HFpEF and STEP HFpEF Diabetes, which enrolled patients with HFpEF and obesity, showed improvements in quality of life, physical limitations, and weight loss. These studies were not powered for a reduction in major clinical outcomes.

The SUMMIT trial is the first trial to investigate the efficacy of tirzepatide, a long-acting dual agonist of GLP-1 and GIP receptors on a composite outcome of death from cardiovascular causes or a worsening heart failure event.

It randomized (double-blind) trial, a total of 731 patients with class II to IV heart failure, ejection fraction ≥50%, and BMI ≥ 30 kg/m^2 were assigned to tirzepatide (titrated up to 15 mg SC weekly; $n = 364$) or placebo ($n = 367$) added to background therapy for a median of 104 weeks (quartile 1, 66; quartile 3, 126 weeks). The primary end points were whether tirzepatide reduced the combined risk of cardiovascular death or worsening heart failure and improved Kansas City Cardiomyopathy Questionnaire Clinical Summary Score. The current expanded analysis included sensitivity analyses of the primary end points, 6-minute walk distance, EQ-5D-5L health state index, Patient Global Impression of Severity Overall Health score, New York Heart Association class, use of heart failure medications, and a hierarchical composite based on all-cause death, worsening heart failure, and 52-week changes in Kansas City Cardiomyopathy Questionnaire Clinical Summary Score and 6-minute walk distance **(Figs. 6A and B)**.[7,8,11]

Compared with placebo, tirzepatide produced a consistent beneficial effect across all composites of death and worsening heart failure events, analyzed as time to first event (hazard ratios, 0.41–0.67). At 52 weeks, tirzepatide increased the Kansas City Cardiomyopathy Questionnaire Clinical Summary Score by 6.9 points (95% CI, 3.3–10.6; $p < 0.001$) **(Figs. 7A and B)**, 6-minute walk distance 18.3 m (95% CI, 9.9–26.7; $p < 0.001$) **(Figs. 8A and B)**, and EQ-5D-5L 0.06 (95% CI, 0.03–0.09; $p < 0.001$). The tirzepatide group shifted to a more favorable Patient Global Impression of Severity Overall Health score [proportional odds ratio, 1.99 (95% CI, 1.44–2.76)] **(Figs. 9A and B)** and New York Heart Association class [proportional odds ratio, 2.26 (95% CI, 1.54–3.31); both $p < 0.001$] and required fewer heart failure medications ($p = 0.015$) **(Figs. 10A and B)**. The broad spectrum of effects was reflected in benefits on the hierarchical composite [win ratio, 1.63 (95% CI, 1.17–2.28); $p = 0.004$].

Tirzepatide produced a comprehensive, meaningful improvement in heart failure across multiple complementary domains; enhanced health status, quality of life, functional capacity, exercise tolerance, and well-being; and reduced symptoms and medication burden in patients with HFpEF and obesity **(Fig. 11)**.

The favorable effects of tirzepatide on HF may be related to an amelioration of the blood volume expansion that characterizes obesity-related HF, and the decrease in adipocyte mass would be expected to minimize the antinatriuretic effects of secreted adipocytokines (particularly leptin and aldosterone). In addition, shrinkage of fat depots would diminish the proinflammatory phenotype of hypertrophied fat cells; this inflammatory response is manifest both systemically and locally by virtue of deleterious paracrine influence of epicardial adipose tissue. The lessened secretion of inflammatory adipocytokines might act to alleviate coronary endothelial inflammation with secondary beneficial effects on microvascular rarefaction and myocardial fibrosis, two important mechanisms in the pathogenesis of HFpEF. It is noteworthy that glucose-dependent insulinotropic polypeptide receptors are abundant in epicardial adipocytes, and the action of tirzepatide on glucose-dependent insulinotropic polypeptide receptors may produce incremental anti-inflammatory effects.

The CMR substudy of the SUMMIT trial demonstrated that tirzepatide therapy in obesity-related HFpEF led to reduced LV mass and paracardiac adipose tissue compared with placebo, and the changes in LV mass paralleled weight loss. These beneficial changes may contribute to the reduction in heart failure events seen in the main SUMMIT trial.

Tirzepatide in Heart Failure with Reduced Ejection Fraction

All-Cause Mortality and Cardiovascular Outcomes with Tirzepatide in Patients with Type 2 Diabetes and Heart Failure with Reduced Ejection Fraction. Aravinthan Vignarajah, et.al. studies **(Fig. 12)**.

In this retrospect analysis, primary and secondary outcomes were composite and individual for heart failure exacerbation, all-cause mortality, and hospitalization. Secondary outcomes also included MI, AF/atrial flutter, and ventricular tachycardia/fibrillation (VT/VF) assessed over 1 year.

They identified 1,298 patients after propensity score matching. Tirzepatide user group was linked to lower odds compared with the control group for the composite outcome (0.38, 032–0.46; $p < 0.001$), all-cause mortality (0.11, 0.07–0.18, $p < 0.001$), hospitalization (0.43, 0.37–0.51; $p < 0.001$), heart failure exacerbation (0.24, 0.19–0.31; $p < 0.001$), MI (027, 0.22–0.34, $p < 0.001$), AF (0.66, 0.55–0.78; $p < 0.001$), and VT/VF (0.56, 0.19–0.31; 0.001).

Tirzepatide significantly improves CV outcomes in diabetic HFrEF patients, strongly supporting its use as an alternative to GLP1 RA.

In a study, "Cardiovascular Outcomes with Tirzepatide versus Dulaglutide in Type 2 Diabetes (SURPASS-CVOT 2025)," Nicholls et al.[7] conducted an active-comparator-controlled, double-blind, noninferiority trial in which patients with T2DM and atherosclerotic cardiovascular disease were randomly assigned in a 1:1 ratio to receive a weekly subcutaneous injection of tirzepatide (up to 15 mg) or dulaglutide (1.5 mg), an agent that has been shown to reduce the incidence of cardiovascular events. The primary

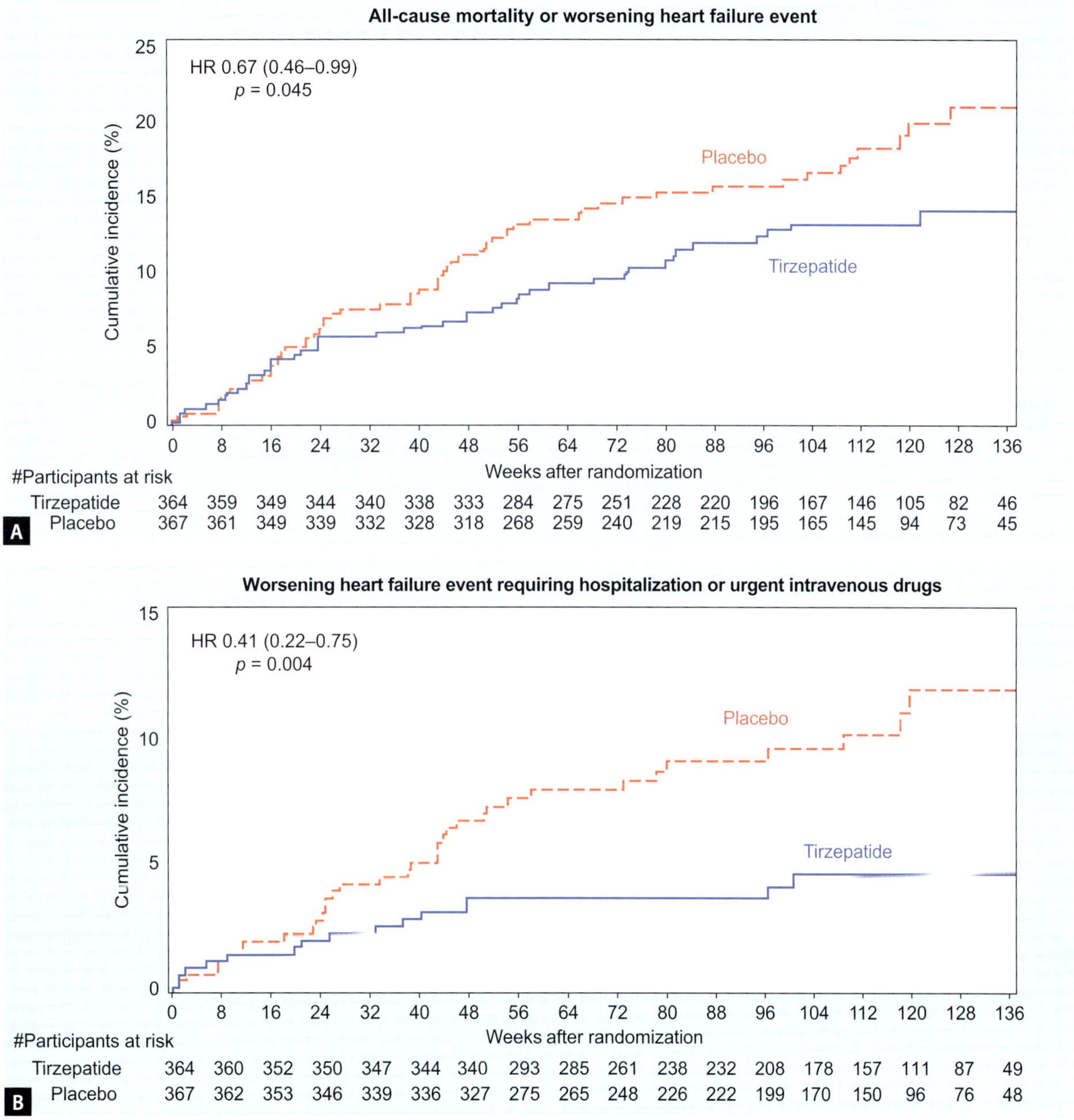

Figs. 6A and B: Effects of tirzepatide on fatal and heart failure (HF) events. (A) Effect of tirzepatide on time to first all-cause death or worsening HF event. In an intention-to-treat analysis, tirzepatide significantly reduced this end point by 33% compared with placebo [hazard ratio (HR), 0.67 (95% CI, 0.45–0.99); $p = 0.045$]. Worsening HF event was defined as worsening symptoms of HF requiring hospitalization, intravenous therapy in an urgent care setting, or oral diuretic intensification; (B) Effect of tirzepatide on time to first HF event (excluding oral diuretic intensification). In an intention-to-treat analysis, tirzepatide significantly reduced this end point by 59% compared with placebo [HR, 0.41 (95% CI, 0.22–0.75); $p = 0.004$].

end point was a composite of death from cardiovascular causes, MI, or stroke and was tested for noninferiority of tirzepatide to dulaglutide.

A total of 13,299 patients underwent randomization; 134 were subsequently excluded because they did not meet inclusion criteria. The modified intention-to-treat population thus included 6,586 patients in the tirzepatide group and 6,579 in the dulaglutide group. The mean (±SD) age of the patients was 64.1 ± 8.8 years. 29.0% were women. The mean BMI (the weight in kilograms divided

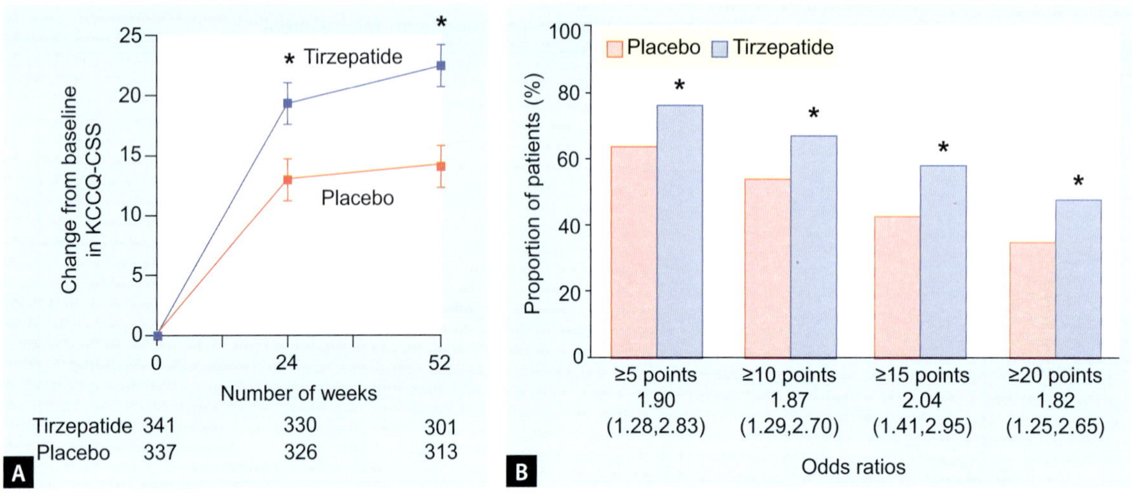

Figs. 7A and B: (A) KCCQ-CSS at 24 and 52 weeks; (B) Proportion of patients achieving KCCQ-CSS threshold change at 52 weeks.

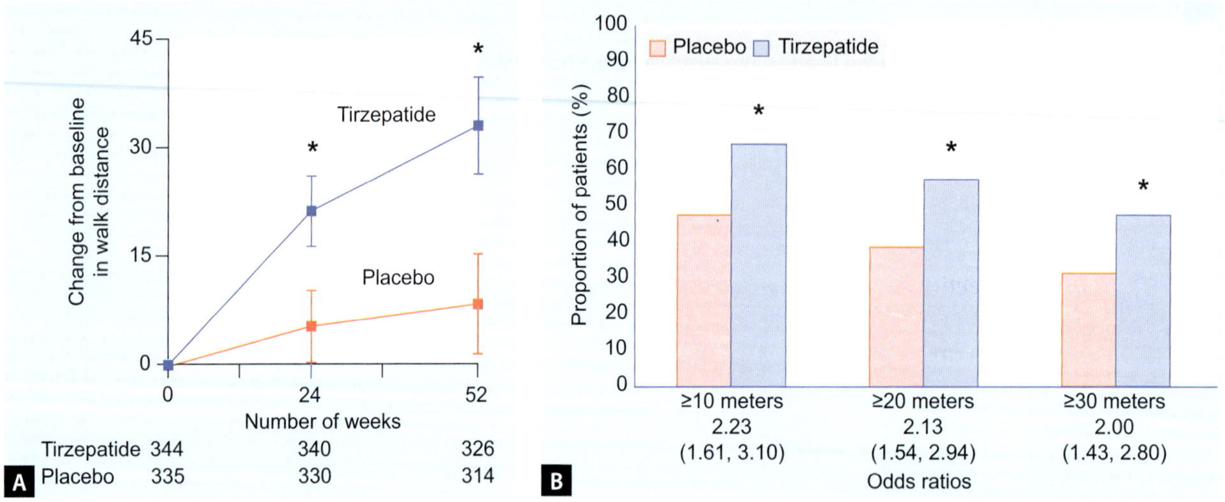

Figs. 8A and B: (A) 6-Minute walk distance at 24 and 52 weeks; (B) Proportion of patients achieving walk distance threshold change at 52 weeks.

by the square of the height in meters) was 32.6 ± 5.5, the mean glycated hemoglobin level was 8.4 ± 0.9%, and the mean duration of diabetes was 14.7 ± 8.8 years. A primary end-point event occurred in 801 patients (12.2%) in the tirzepatide group and 862 (13.1%) in the dulaglutide group (hazard ratio, 0.92; 95.3% CI, 0.83–1.01; $p = 0.003$ for noninferiority; $p = 0.09$ for superiority). The incidence of adverse events appeared to be similar in the two groups, although more gastrointestinal adverse events were observed in the tirzepatide group.

Among patients with T2DM and atherosclerotic cardiovascular disease, tirzepatide was noninferior to dulaglutide with respect to a composite of death from cardiovascular causes, MI, or stroke.

In a study Semaglutide and Tirzepatide in Patients with Heart Failure with Preserved Ejection Fraction, Krugar et al.[11] concluded that patients initiating semaglutide or tirzepatide had a more than 40% lower risk of hospitalization for heart failure or all-cause mortality compared with sitagliptin (a glucose-lowering drug with no effect on heart failure end points). In a head-to-head comparison, tirzepatide showed no meaningful benefit over semaglutide.

These findings complement early results from small clinical trials and support the use of semaglutide and tirzepatide in patients with cardiometabolic heart failure with preserved ejection fraction.

In a study titled "Outcomes of Tirzepatide vs Semaglutide in Patients with Type 2 Diabetes and Heart

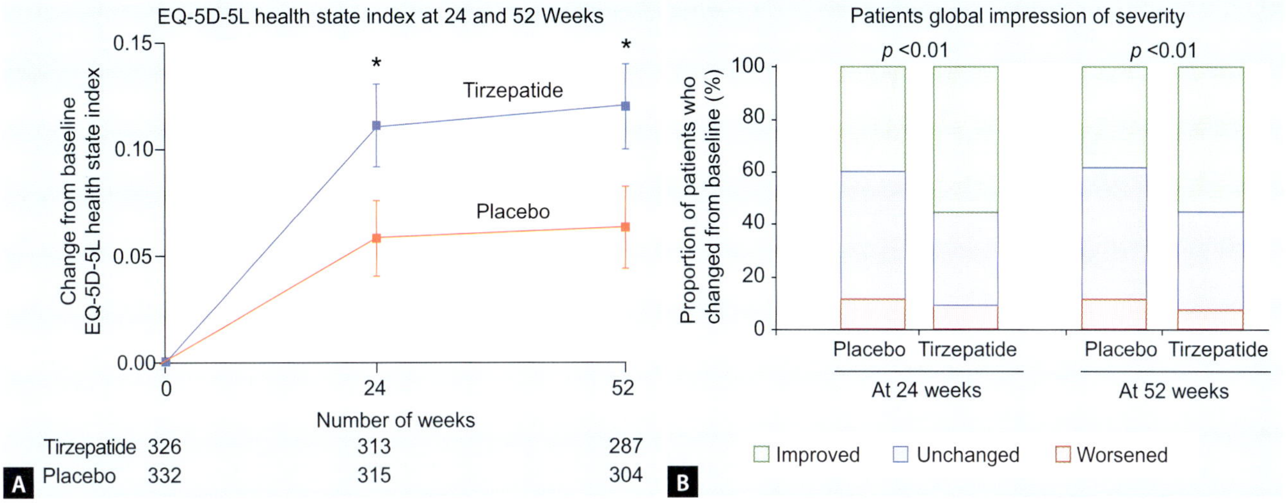

Figs. 9A and B: Effect of tirzepatide on change from baseline in EQ-5D-5L health state index and Patient Global Impression of Severity (PGIS) overall health. (A) Effect of tirzepatide on change from baseline in EQ-5D-5L health state index. At 52 weeks, in an intention-to-treat analysis, tirzepatide increased EQ-5D-5L health state index with a between-group difference of 0.06 (95% CI, 0.033–0.087; $p < 0.001$); (B) Effect of tirzepatide on change in PGIS overall health. At 24 weeks, the tirzepatide group by intention to treat was more likely to show improvement in PGIS overall health (55.2% vs. 40.4%) and less likely to report worsening in PGIS overall health (9.1% vs. 11.5%). Proportional odds ratio (OR) for improvement in PGIS overall health with tirzepatide versus placebo was 1.68 (95% CI, 1.22–2.29; $p = 0.001$). At 52 weeks, tirzepatide group by intention to treat was more likely to show improvement in PGIS overall health (55.2% vs. 38.5%) and less likely to report worsening in PGIS overall health (7.4% vs. 11.3%). Proportional OR for improvement in PGIS overall health with tirzepatide versus placebo was 1.99 (95% CI, 1.44–2.76; $p < 0.001$). $^*p < 0.001$, tirzepatide versus placebo.

Failure with Preserved Ejection Fraction: A Retrospective Cohort Analysis", Murshid et al.[12] studied 14,157 patients on semaglutide and 2,222 on tirzepatide. 2,222 matched pairs were analyzed. All-cause mortality occurred in 81 patients treated with tirzepatide versus 108 in the semaglutide group (3.7% vs. 4.9%; risk difference –1.2%; 95% CI, –2.4 to –0.0; $p = 0.046$). There were no significant differences in new-onset AF/atrial flutter (3.3% vs. 3.4%; $p = 0.908$), hospitalizations (3.1% vs. 3.0%; $p = 0.574$), acute-on-chronic diastolic HF episodes (3.3% vs. 3.3%; $p = 0.944$), and intravenous diuretic use (4.4% vs. 5.4%; $p = 0.116$) It was concluded that tirzepatide was associated with a statistically significant reduction in all-cause mortality compared to semaglutide, without significant differences in other clinical outcomes. These findings support the potential cardiovascular benefit of tirzepatide in this population and highlight the need for prospective studies to validate its long-term effects.

In the study "Tirzepatide compared with semaglutide and 10-year cardiovascular disease risk reduction in obesity: *post-hoc* analysis of the SURMOUNT-5 trial," Mamas et al.[8] found that "treatment with tirzepatide was associated with greater predicted 10-year CVD risk reduction compared with semaglutide." This post hoc analysis suggests that tirzepatide treatment may provide greater benefit in primary prevention of CVD than semaglutide in people with obesity and overweight.

Adherence and Adverse Effects of Tirzepatide

The use of tirzepatide has been linked with gastrointestinal adverse effects, occasionally presenting with severity. A network meta-analysis showed a significantly higher odds ratio of discontinuation due to adverse events compared with placebo (2.30), which reflects the adherence level to medication. The analysis also found a positive association with diarrhea, a significantly elevated odds ratio of nausea, and a higher risk of vomiting than placebo. However, to increase patient adherence to medication, findings from a 12-week phase 2 clinical trial using moderate dose-escalation protocols have demonstrated promising insights into enhancing gastrointestinal tolerability. Thus, within the trial programs, tirzepatide administration was initiated at a dosage of 2.5 mg once weekly, with subsequent incremental increases of 2.5 mg every 4 weeks. This approach to dose escalation suggests a potential for mitigating adverse reactions associated with tirzepatide therapy, thereby enhancing patient adherence. Individuals

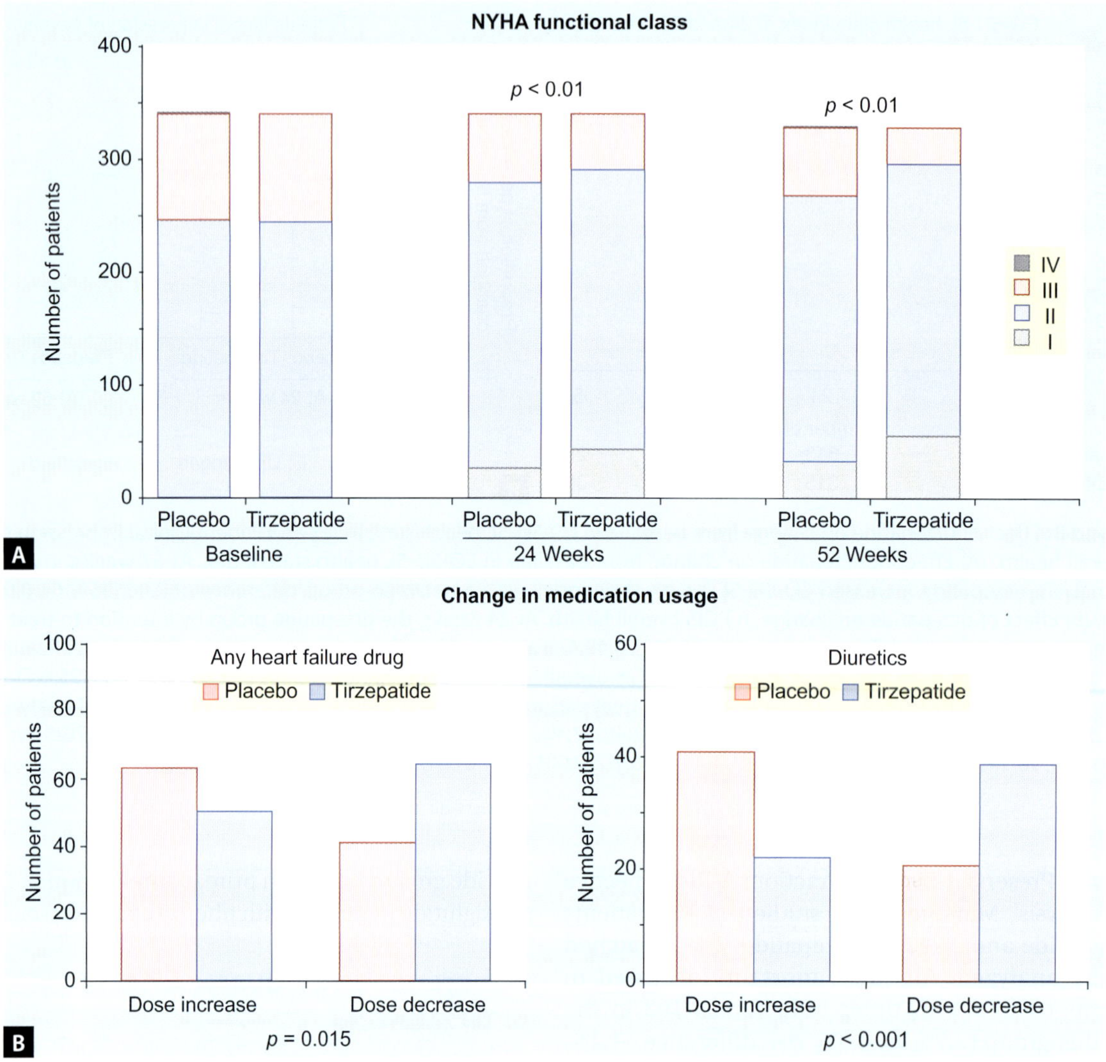

Figs. 10A and B: (A) NYHA functional class; (B) Change in medication usage.

with severe gastrointestinal disorders, encompassing conditions such as severe gastroparesis, are advised against the use of tirzepatide due to potential exacerbation of symptoms as per the. Multiple comorbid populations are advised to be cautious when using tirzepatide. Patients with renal impairment are at risk of acute kidney injury, particularly as gastrointestinal side effects like nausea and diarrhea can lead to dehydration. Pregnant women should only be prescribed tirzepatide when the benefits outweigh potential risks, given animal studies showing malformations and the lack of human data on its teratogenicity. Additionally, patients on insulin or sulfonylureas may experience a dose-dependent risk of hypoglycemia, especially at higher doses. Therefore, careful dosing adjustments and monitoring for adverse events are essential when using tirzepatide in these populations. Finally, patients with hepatic impairment should practice caution with tirzepatide treatment, as cases of cholelithiasis and cholecystitis have been reported, likely due to the rapid weight loss induced by tirzepatide.

CONCLUSION

Tirzepatide has been found to be a powerful drug in HF management with multiple favorable features:

- *Reduced clinical events:* Tirzepatide, as shown in the SUMMIT trial, is associated with lower all-cause mortality and reduced heart-failure–related hospitalization compared with placebo.
- *Improved quality of life:* Tirzepatide is found to be associated with enhanced physical tolerance and reduced

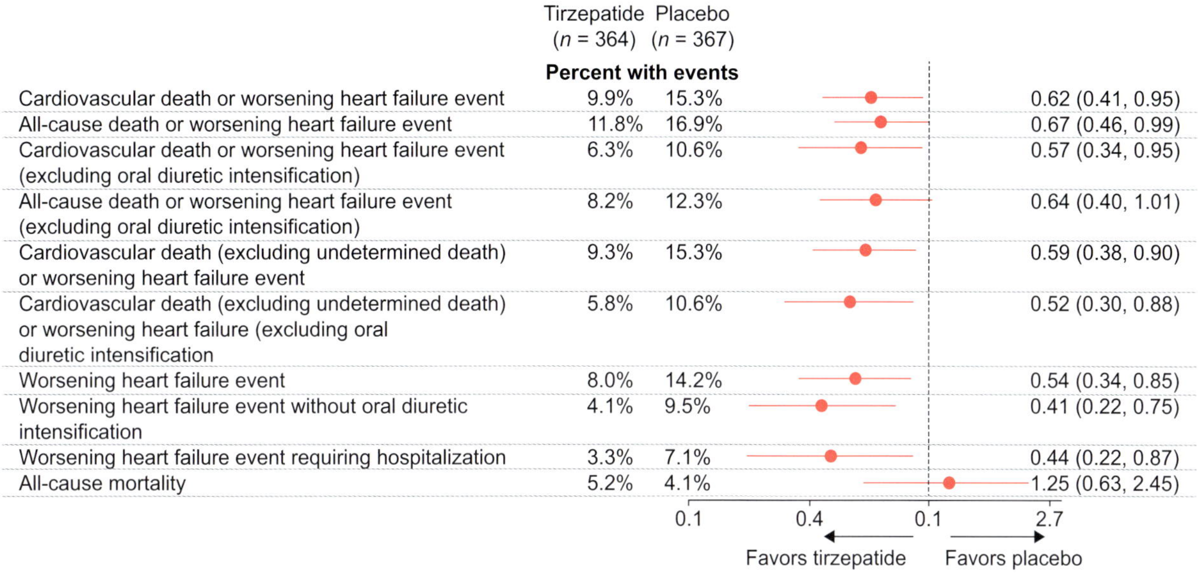

Fig. 11: Sensitivity analyses of the primary composite endpoint in patients with HFpEF.

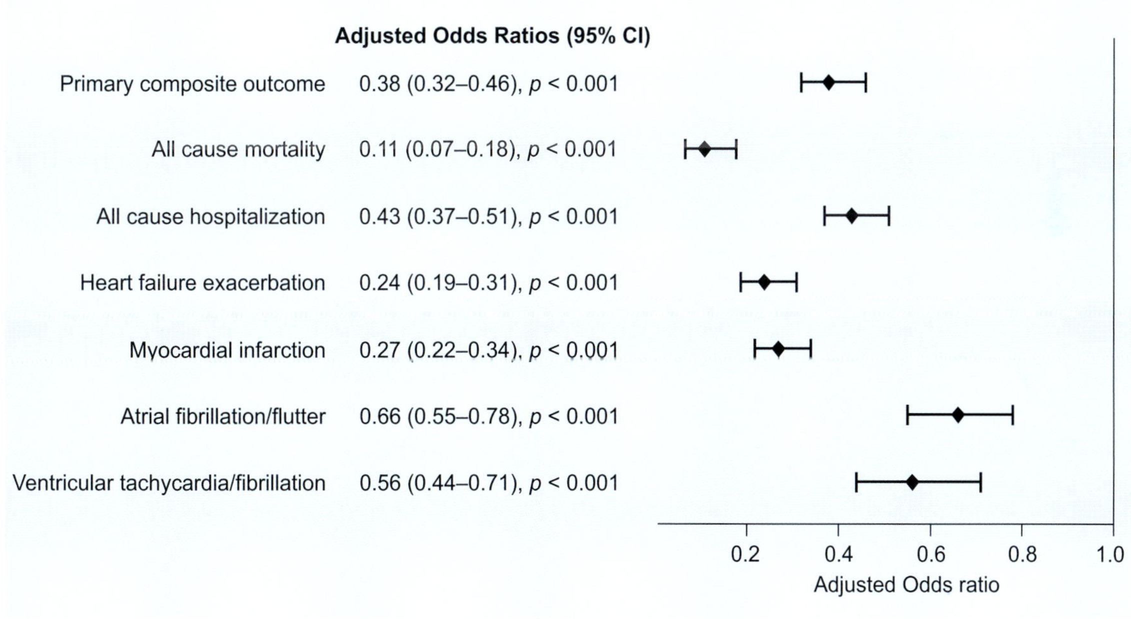

Fig. 12: Association of tirzepatide therapy with major clinical outcomes in HFpEF.

symptoms, such as improvement in the Kansas City Cardiomyopathy Questionnaire (KCCQ) score.

- *Weight loss*: Use of tirzepatide is associated with significant (average ~11–03%) weight loss and reduced inflammation. The reductions in LV mass and pericardiac adipose tissue parallel weight loss, levering of blood pressure and reduction in inflammation (evidenced by reduced hs-CRP) are the major underlying mechanisms.
- *Safety profile:* Tirzepatide is a reasonably well tolerated drug. Major side effects related to the gastrointestinal system can be mitigated by gradual dose escalation.
- The role of tirzepatide in heart failure and cardiovascular disease needs to be further defined in large cohorts of population so as to make it one of the essential therapies in patients with obesity and heart failure, with or without diabetes mellitus.

REFERENCES

1. Piche ME, Tchernof A, Despres JP. Obesity phenotypes, diabetes and cardiovascular disease. Circ Res. 2020; 126:1477-500.
2. Cho YK, Lee YL, Jung CH. The Cardiovascular effect of tirzepatide: A Glucagon-like peptide-1 and glucose-dependent insulinotropic polypeptide dual agonist. J Lipid Atheroscler. 2023;12(3):213-22.
3. Sokary S, Bawadi H. The promise of tirzepatide: A narrative review of metabolic benefits. Primary Care Diabetes. 2025;19:229-37.
4. Galindo RJ, Cheng AYY, Longuet C, et al. Insights into the Mechanism of Action of Tirzepatide: A Narrative Review. Diabetes Ther. 2025;17(1):19-40..
5. Gallwitz B. Clinical perspectives on the use of the GIP/GLP-1 receptor agonist tirzepatide for the treatment of type-2 diabetes and obesity. Front Endocrinol. 2022;13:1004044.
6. Aronne LJ, Horn DB, le Roux CW, et al. Tirzepatide as compared with semaglutide for the treatment of obesity. N Engl J Med. 2025;393:26-36.
7. Nicholls SJ, Pavo I, Bhatt DL, et al. Cardiovascular Outcomes with Tirzepatide versus Dulaglutide in Type 2 Diabetes. N Engl J Med. 2025;393:2409-20.
8. Mamas MA, Bays H, Li R, et al. Tirzepatide compared with semaglutide and 10-year cardiovascular disease risk reduction in obesity: post-hoc analysis of the SURMOUNT-5 trial. Eur Heart J Open. 2025;5(5):oeaf117.
9. Zile MR, Borlaug BA, Kramer CM, et al. Effects of tirzepatide on the clinical trajectory of patients with heart failure, preserved ejection fraction, and obesity. Circulation. 2025;151:656-68.
10. Idris I. Tirzepatide shown to improve clinical outcomes for patients with heart failure with preserved ejection fraction (HFpEF) and obesity. Diabetes Obes Metab. 2024;2:e70008.
11. Krüger N, Schneeweiss S, Fuse K, et al. Semaglutide and tirzepatide in patients with heart failure with preserved ejection fraction. JAMA. 2025;334;(14):1255-66.
12. Murshid A, Awad M, Ahmad S, et al. Outcomes of Tirzepatide vs Semaglutide in Patients with Type 2 Diabetes and Heart Failure with Preserved Ejection Fraction: A Retrospective Cohort Analysis. Circulation. 2025;152 (Suppl_3). https://doi.org/10.1161/circ.152.suppl_3.437088.

127

CHAPTER

Future Directions: Biomarkers and Personalized Therapy in Heart Failure Patients Treated with Tirzepatide

Vineet Bhatia, Vidit Bhatia, Parneesh Arora

INTRODUCTION

Enhanced longevity has led to the accumulation of risk factors for heart failure (HF) in the general population. Heart failure with preserved ejection fraction (HFpEF) accounts for 50% of all patients of HF. Obesity is highly prevalent in this subset of HF (two thirds of HFpEF patients are obese).[1] The American Heart Association regards obesity-related HFpEF as an advanced form of cardiovascular-kidney-metabolic disease characterized by expansion of circulatory volume, pressure overload, and chronic inflammation.[2] These eventually lead to hypertension, chronic kidney disease (CKD), and blood volume expansion—the three hallmarks that best differentiate obesity-related HFpEF from asymptomatic individuals with obesity but no HF.[3]

Obese HFpEF patients exhibit enhanced expression of the several biomarkers of endothelial injury and chronic inflammation. Albuminuria, elevated levels of troponin, and N-terminal proBNP (NT-proBNP) levels are common in such patients. These biomarkers are positively correlated with the degree of cardiac dysfunction, systemic congestion, poor functional capacity, and enhanced risk of hospitalization for HF.[4]

The LIFE-Heart study looked at certain novel biomarkers in HFpEF patients.[5] Those studied included adrenomedullin, a biomarker of volume expansion; thrombospondin-2 (THBS2), a marker of fibrosis; and Galectin-9, TRAIL-R2, and CD4, markers of inflammation. These biomarkers are elevated in the obesity HFpEF group and found to be lower in the frail HFpEF, obese non-HF groups.

As the quest for precision medicine expands, newer molecules which deliver targeted therapy are seeing the light of the day. One such drug is tirzepatide, a long-acting glucose-dependent insulinotropic polypeptide receptor and glucagon-like peptide-1 receptor agonist. The drug has shown promising results in the landmark SUMMIT trial in reducing the risk of worsening HF as compared to placebo in patients with obesity and HFpEF.[6] It is postulated that the drug targets the cardiovascular-kidney-metabolic disease axis and dampens the effects of circulatory volume-pressure overload and systemic inflammation.

A WORD ABOUT THE SUMMIT TRIAL: TRIAL DESIGN AND KEY FINDINGS

In total, 129 centers spread across 9 nations enrolled 731 patients with obesity HFpEF in the trial over a period of 2 years. 364 patients were assigned to the tirzepatide arm and 367 to the placebo arm. The patients had high body mass index (>38 kg/m^2), increased waist circumference, and a higher prevalence of coronary artery disease and atrial fibrillation. The mean Kansas City Cardiomyopathy Questionnaire Clinical Summary Score (KCCQ-CSS) was high at 54 and the mean 6-minute walk distance (6MWD) was a dismal 303 m. Nearly 50% of the participants had evidence of worsening HF in the preceding year which prompted either hospitalization or emergency room visits. Biomarkers evaluated included high-sensitivity troponin I, C-reactive protein (CRP), and microalbuminuria. A little above 40% had elevated troponin I levels, 66% had elevated CRP, while 26.5% had microalbuminuria. Hypertension was common and so was renal dysfunction (50% had CKD stage 3, 26.5% had microalbuminuria, and 6.1% had macroalbuminuria).

When the drug effect on blood pressure was evaluated, the curves were found to diverge as early as 4 weeks as compared to placebo and this continued until 24 weeks and was maintained at 52 weeks. This was primarily due to the effect of the drug on systolic blood pressure as the effect on diastolic blood pressure was negligible. The pulse pressure which is a marker of aortic stiffness showed a progressive decline [estimated treatment difference (ETD) –3.9 mm Hg, CI –5.6 to –2.2; $p < 0.001$].

The drug also had a significant positive impact on the blood volume and plasma volume with an ETD of -0.58 and -0.32 L, respectively, at the end of 52 weeks. Similar trends were noted in the CRP levels with a significant -37.2% decline from baseline values at the end of 52 weeks. Thus, effects on blood volume, plasma volume, and CRP were highly favorable.

Tirzepatide also had a promising positive influence on the biomarkers of cardiac and kidney injury. The ETD in troponin I levels was -9.8 and -10.4% at 24 and 52 weeks, respectively, while the NT-proBNP levels showed an ETD of -9.7 and -10.5% in a similar time frame, respectively.

Although a reduction of eGFR was noted at 12 weeks (–1.1 mL/min/m^2), it did not reach statistical significance. However, after 52 weeks of therapy, the eGFR in fact improved (ETD 2.9 mL/min/m^2). As compared with placebo, tirzepatide decreased the urine albumin-creatinine ratio (UACR) at 24 weeks (ETD –25%, 95% CI –35.5 to –12.7; $p = 0.051$).

Another group of parameters which showed improvement were the KCCQ-CSS score, reduction in body weight, and 6MWD. The ETDs were 6.9 points, 11.6%, and 18.3 m, respectively. All were statistically significant.

The SUMMIT trial showed a 38% reduction in death from cardiovascular causes or a worsening HF and a 46% reduction in worsening HF.

DISCUSSION OF THE FINDINGS OF THE TRIAL AND HOW TO VIEW THE BIOMARKER CHANGES

The SUMMIT trial has positioned tirzepatide as a vital drug in the armamentarium of physicians in the management of obesity associated HFpEF. As we enter an era of evidence-based medicine, this drug provides us very satisfying proof about the mechanisms by which it offers relief in this group of patients. Several parameters point to HFpEF as a cardiovascular-kidney-metabolic disease. The drug effectively and positively impacts several biomarkers (circulatory volume, pressure overload, renal dysfunction, and cardiac injury) concerned with which reflect the disease process.

Tirzepatide reduces the blood and plasma volume early in the course of treatment. This helps reduce the diastolic filling pressures and eventually leads to improvements in exercise capacity and KCCQ-CSS scores. Also, volume expansion may occur secondary to elevated levels of substances like leptin and aldosterone released by the adipocytes. These promote sodium and water retention and expansion of circulatory volume.[7] The drug by negating these effects may bring about marked clinical improvement.

Positive impact is noted on systolic blood pressure while the diastolic blood pressures are largely unaffected. This may indicate reduced circulatory volume. Also, pulse pressure which reflects arterial stiffness is positively impacted. The aortic stiffness which is an indicator of elevated filling pressures is also reduced.

Chronic kidney disease is common in HFpEF patients and may be due to volume expansion (leading to hyperfiltration by the glomeruli) or renal injury and fibrosis secondary to the release of leptin and aldosterone by the adipocytes.[7] Tirzepatide by suppressing these adipocytokines and reducing the blood volume may lead to decline in the progression curve of renal dysfunction and reduce albuminuria. This is a welcome feature and may be related to a decline in interglomerular hypertension. The initial decline in eGFR (at 12 weeks) may be secondary to the initial fall in systolic blood pressure and blood volume while the subsequent improvement (at 24 and 52 weeks) may be due to the favorable effect of tirzepatide on eGFR and UACR. The subsequent beneficial effect may be potentially mediated by long-term decrease in fat mass and the suppression of adipocytokines, improvements in blood pressure, and reduced inflammation.

Troponin I elevations in HFpEF are believed to be indicators of myocardial injury and higher levels are associated with a higher risk of hospitalization for worsening HF.[8] Such patients also have higher filling pressures, ventricular vascular stiffness, lower myocardial stress reserve, and poor exercise capacity. Tirzepatide is known to lower troponin levels and this mirrors the fall in CRP levels. This may be due to anti-inflammatory effects of the drug. Lowered CRP levels also correlate well with an improvement in the 6-minute walk test capability.[9] These improvements may be due to previously mentioned mechanisms or improvement in skeletal muscle functioning or oxygen uptake which are more than often an issue in HFpEF patients.

A biomarker which deserves special mention is NT-proBNP. The levels of this marker in HFpEF–obesity group are usually normal or lower[10,11] than what levels are used to qualify patients to enroll in large-scale HFpEF trials. The median NT-proBNP levels in SUMMIT trial were <200 pg/mL as compared to the trials like STEP-HFpEF (Research Study to Investigate How Well Semaglutide Works in People Living with Heart Failure and Obesity) (median 470 pg/mL) and other large outcome trials (median levels 900–1,400 pg/mL). Obese patients who undergo bariatric surgery or intense anti-obesity dietary caloric restriction with subsequent weight loss often exhibit a two- to fivefold rise in their NT-proBNP levels.[12,13] This is possibly related to relief of adiposity-related cardiac chamber constraints which in turn leads to greater ventricular distensibility.[14] The rise in the NT-proBNP levels may explain the natriuresis noted after weight loss.[15] On the contrary, this rise is not seen in HFpEF if treatment produces a notable improvement in HF. The tirzepatide-treated arm despite a weight loss of 11.6% and a reduced diuretic use showed only a 10% reduction in the NT-proBNP levels.

SUMMIT CMR SUBSTUDY: TIRZEPATIDE REDUCES LV MASS AND PARACARDIAC ADIPOSE TISSUE IN OBESITY-RELATED HEART FAILURE[16]

Patients with obesity-related HFpEF exhibit an increased total heart volume and epicardial adipose tissue (EAT). The pericardial adipose tissue along with the EAT is often referred to as paracardiac adipose tissue. The EAT may play a role in pathogenesis of HF by secreting proinflammatory adipocytokines locally. Also, the epicardial and pericardial fat may lead to impaired filling of the heart due to external compression and the consequent reduced cardiac chamber distention. The latter causes reduced release of natriuretic peptides which promotes HF. While semaglutide has not shown promising data when it comes to reduction of LV mass or EAT, it does cause desirable reductions in left atrial dimensions. Tirzepatide in the SUMMIT trial CMR arm showed favorable outcomes when it comes to LV mass and EAT. A total of 175 patients had a baseline cardiac MR at the start of the study while 106 had a follow-up CMR at 52 weeks. There was a decrease in LV mass of 11 g while the paracardiac mass was reduced by 45 g. The decrease in LV mass correlated with changes in body weight, blood pressure, waist circumference, left ventricular and left atrial end diastolic and end systolic volume. These may translate into the final clinical benefits seen at the end of the trial.

PERSONALIZED MANAGEMENT FOR OBESITY—HEART FAILURE WITH PRESERVED EJECTION FRACTION

Heart failure with preserved ejection fraction is a heterogeneous disorder with several phenotypes. Unbiased clustering methods (based on machine learning and latent class analysis) help to classify patients on the basis of clinical characteristics, echocardiographic observations, and biomarker concentrations into several phenotypes. One such distinct phenotype is the obesity HFpEF group. In this subgroup, the leptin–aldosterone–neprilysin axis activation is postulated to play an important role in the pathogenesis leading to sodium retention, plasma volume expansion, and regional (such as myocardial) and systemic inflammation and fibrosis.[17] There is also an acceleration in the accumulation and inflammation of epicardial fat.[18] The mineralocorticoid antagonist eplerenone is found to be beneficial in HFpEF patients with central obesity. With tirzepatide found to act on similar target pathways, it may have a vital role in such phenotypes of HFpEF. The SUMMIT CMR substudy has already shown beneficial effect of tirzepatide on EAT, as discussed above. Proteomics—the large-scale study of proteins—in the LIFE-Heart study targeting biomarkers has shown improvement in the obesity HFpEF phenotypes. So there seems to be a role of personalized therapy based on phenotyping of HFpEF patients.

CONCLUSION

At the present time, tirzepatide has been shown to positively affect several biomarkers. These include biomarkers of cardiac stress and injury (troponin I, NT-proBNP), systemic inflammation (hsCRP), and cardiac remodeling (LV mass and paracardiac adipose tissue). These biomarkers may help us guide therapy and identify a subset of patients who are likely to benefit from tirzepatide. AI-based techniques may help classify HFpEF phenotypes likely to benefit from targeted therapy.

REFERENCES

1. Borlaug B, Zile MR, Kramer CM, et al. Effects of tirzepatide on circulatory overload and end-organ damage in heart failure with preserved ejection fraction and obesity: a secondary analysis of the SUMMIT trial. Nat Med. 2025;31:544-51.
2. Ndumele CE, Rangaswami J, Chow SL, et al. Cardiovascular-kidney-metabolic health: a presidential advisory from the American Heart Association. Circulation. 2023;148:1606-35.

3. Katz DH, Burns JA, Aguilar FG, et al. Albuminuria is independently associated with cardiac remodelling, abnormal right and left ventricular function, and worse outcomes in heart failure with preserved ejection fraction. JACC Heart Fail. 2014;2:586-96.
4. Obokata M, Reddy YNV, Melenovsky V, et al. Myocardial injury and cardiac reserve in patients with heart failure and preserved ejection fraction. J Am Coll Cardiol. 2018;72:29-40.
5. Kresoja KP, Rommel KP, Wachter R, et al. Proteomics to improve phenotyping in obese patients with heart failure with preserved ejection fraction. Eur J Heart Fail. 2021;23:1633-44.
6. Packer M, Zile MR, Kramer CM, et al. Tirzepatide for heart failure with preserved ejection fraction and obesity. N Engl J Med. 2025;392:427-37.
7. Packer M. Leptin–aldosterone–neprilysin axis: identification of its distinctive role in the pathogenesis of the three phenotypes of heart failure in people with obesity. Circulation. 2018;137:1614-31.
8. Fudim M, Ambrosy AP, Sun JL, et al. High-sensitivity troponin I in hospitalized and ambulatory patients with heart failure with preserved ejection fraction: insights from the Heart Failure Clinical Research Network. J Am Heart Assoc. 2018;7:e010364.
9. Tada A, Doi S, Harada T, et al. Autoimmune disorders in heart failure with preserved ejection fraction. JACC Heart Fail. 2024;12:1257-69.
10. Kosyakovsky LB, Liu EE, Wang JK, et al. Uncovering unrecognized heart failure with preserved ejection fraction among individuals with obesity and dyspnea. Circ Heart Fail. 2024;17:e011366.
11. Reddy YNV, Rikhi A, Obokata M, et al. Quality of life in heart failure with preserved ejection fraction: importance of obesity, functional capacity, and physical inactivity. Eur J Heart Fail. 2020;22:1009-18.
12. Abrahamsson N, Engström BE, Sundbom M, et al. Gastric bypass surgery elevates NT-Pro BNP levels. Obes Surg. 2013;23:1421-6.
13. Kistorp C, Bliddal H, Goetze JP, et al. Cardiac natriuretic peptides in plasma increase after dietary induced weight loss in obesity. BMC Obes. 2014;1:24.
14. Obokata M, Reddy YNV, Melenovsky V, et al. Uncoupling between intravascular and distending pressures leads to underestimation of circulatory congestion in obesity. Eur J Heart Fail. 2022;24:353-61.
15. Docherty NG, Fändriks L, le Roux CW, et al. Urinary sodium excretion after gastric bypass surgery. Surg Obes Relat Dis. 2017;13:1506-14.
16. Kramer CM, Borlaug BA, Zile MR, et al. Tirzepatide reduces LV mass and paracardiac adipose tissue in obesity-related heart failure: SUMMIT CMR substudy. J Am Coll Cardiol. 2025;85:699-706.
17. Uijl A, Savarese G, Vaartjes I, et al. Identification of distinct phenotypic clusters in heart failure with preserved ejection fraction. Eur J Heart Fail. 2021;23:973-82.
18. Lacobellis G, Petramala L, Marinelli C, et al. Epicardial fat thickness and primary aldosteronism. Horm Metab Res. 2016;48:238-41.

128

CHAPTER

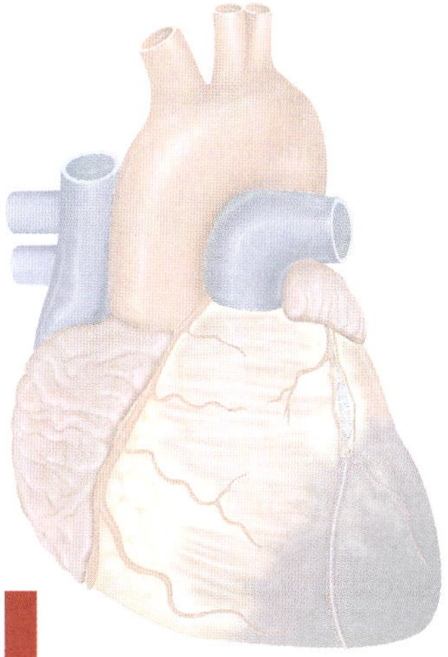

Effects of Tirzepatide on Blood Pressure and Arterial Stiffness

Mansi Kaushik, Manish Bansal, Ravi R Kasliwal

INTRODUCTION

Tirzepatide, a novel dual glucose-dependent insulinotropic polypeptide (GIP) and glucagon-like peptide-1 (GLP-1) receptor agonist, has emerged as a groundbreaking therapeutic agent for type 2 diabetes mellitus and obesity management. Beyond its primary metabolic effects, mounting evidence suggests that tirzepatide exerts significant cardiovascular benefits, particularly in the regulation of blood pressure and improvement of arterial stiffness. This chapter explores the mechanisms and clinical evidence surrounding tirzepatide's cardiovascular effects, with specific focus on its impact on blood pressure control and arterial compliance.

VASCULAR AGING, ARTERIAL STIFFNESS, AND HYPERTENSION

Globally, cardiovascular illnesses are the primary cause of morbidity and mortality. Vascular aging and related increase in arterial stiffness are the main underlying causes of cardiovascular disorders. Both structural and functional artery wall alterations brought on by endothelial dysfunction and tunica media remodeling are characteristics of arterial stiffness.[1-4] It is one of the first indicators of vascular aging, and is followed by a loss of elasticity of big cushioning arteries, particularly the aorta, with resultant loss of Windkessel effect **(Fig. 1)**.[5] Numerous processes, such as inflammation, calcification, elastin crosslinking, and the buildup of collagens, in addition to the production of reactive oxygen species (ROS), result in an overall increase in arterial stiffness.[1] Another important factor is endothelial dysfunction, which is a proinflammatory state with decreased vasodilatory capacity and prothrombotic characteristics. This is primarily brought on by the lack of nitric oxide (NO) and the increased production of chemokines.[6]

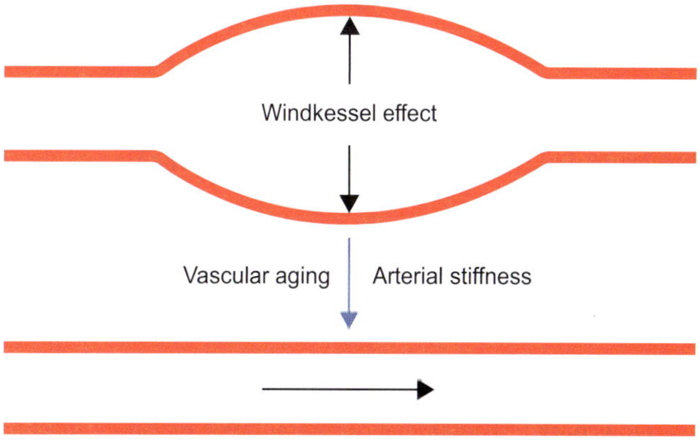

Fig. 1: The effects of vascular stiffness on hemodynamics: Large artery stiffening and vascular ageing are linked to a number of detrimental hemodynamic effects, such as loss of Windkessel function.

Long-standing hypertension has long been thought to be the cause of arterial stiffness. However, recent investigations have suggested that arterial stiffness may contribute to the pathogenesis of hypertension. Mice given a diet high in fat and sugar (HFHS) developed microalbuminuria, oxidative stress, insulin resistance (IR), and chronic inflammation, changes that are seen in obese people.[7] On the HFHS diet, aortic pulse wave velocity (PWV) rose in 1–2 months while blood pressure remained stable. This was followed by an increase in blood pressure at 6 months, suggesting that aortic wall stiffening preceded the rise in mean arterial pressure (MAP) and pulse pressure (PP). Within 2 months, tissue transglutaminase-2 activity—a NO-sensitive enzyme that aids in matrix protein crosslinking increased while aortic NO availability decreased. Aortic stiffness may be modulated by increased crosslinking by tissue transglutaminase-2 due to decreased NO bioavailability. An increase in aortic inflammation was demonstrated by elevated TNF-α, MCP-1, and macrophage inflammatory protein-1α expression. Weight, PWV, and blood pressure all returned to normal in 2 months when HFHS mice were fed a regular diet, suggesting that the mechanisms causing aortic stiffness and high blood pressure were reversible in this paradigm.[8]

DIABETES, ARTERIAL STIFFNESS, AND HYPERTENSION

Insulin resistance, the hallmark of type 2 diabetes is an established cause of hypertension in adults. Various mechanisms are involved in the development of hypertension in patients with IR **(Flowchart 1)**.

Advanced Glycation End Products

The process of adding carbohydrates to a protein, lipid, or DNA is known as glycation. Glycation is often used to describe enzymatic glycation, such as forming a glycosidic bond while employing a sugar donor during glycoprotein synthesis.[9] As a result of glycation, protein function in tissues, such as blood vessels, skin, and tendons, are lost with resultant loss of elasticity. The glycation process is significantly enhanced in presence of IR.[10] Oxidative stress that results from a biological system's inability to detoxify ROS after an imbalance in their synthesis and accumulation in cells and tissues, is increased leading to hypertension. AGEs also cause endothelial dysfunction and decrease endothelial cells' production of NO, which results in vasoconstriction and an increase in total peripheral resistance.[11] Additionally, the AGEs increase the activity of the renin-angiotensin-aldosterone system (RAAS).[12]

Systemic Inflammation

Important aspects of hypertension that are critical to vascular aging and contribute to vascular stiffness include fibrosis, perivascular inflammation, and vascular calcification.[13]Adipocytokines such TNF-α, IL-6, and hs-CRP are known to be produced by visceral adipocytes. IR and Met S have been linked to chronic inflammatory processes, according to several studies.[14] The complex process of inflammation, which has frequently been connected to high blood pressure, involves a variety of cell types and released molecules. ROS production is elevated in dendritic cells from hypertensive patients, which results in T-lymphocyte activation.[15] T-cells directly contribute to endothelial cell dysfunction and renal injury.

Flowchart 1: Diagrammatic representation of various mechanisms that lead to hypertension in patients with insulin resistance.

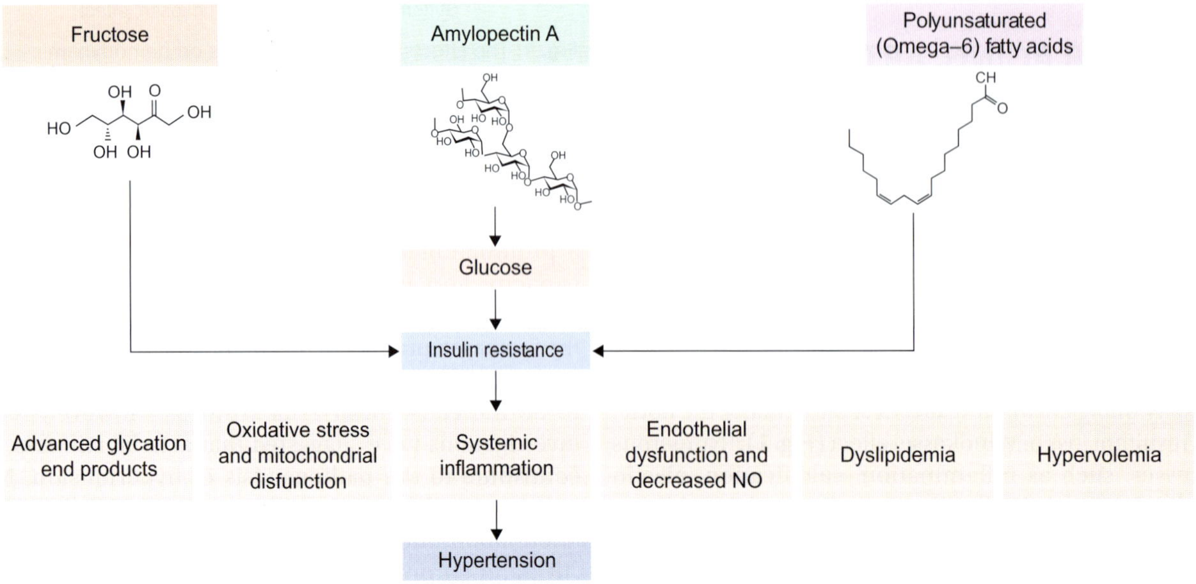

Hypervolemia

Insulin increases Na reabsorption as angiotensin II (AII) through certain receptors on the renal tubules. Angiotensinogen, which can be transformed into AI, is also secreted by adipocytes. ACEs convert AI to AII, which in turn causes the zona glomerulosa of the adrenal cortex to produce more aldosterone. Through increased blood volume and total peripheral resistance, RAAS activation raises arterial blood pressure. It has long been known that insulin affects the entire nephron. Bourdeau et al. showed that insulin is deposited in the proximal tubule using the radioisotope technique.[16]

Research on the signal transduction mechanism of insulin led to the discovery of insulin receptor substrate (IRS) 1.[17] Significantly, IRS1-specific signaling anomalies have often been associated with IR.[18] Thus, by promoting salt retention in an IRS1-independent way, hyperinsulinemia may be a major factor in the pathogenesis of IR-associated hypertension.

Therefore, a pharmaceutical intervention that tackles diabetes, obesity, and its subsequent effects on blood pressure, low-grade systemic inflammation and vascular stiffness may provide a comprehensive approach to the management.

Tirzepatide treatment has been shown to significantly lower excess body weight, improve blood pressure, and lower inflammatory and vascular endothelial dysfunction markers.

TIRZEPATIDE

Tirzepatide is a dual agonist used to treat obesity and type II diabetes mellitus. It operates on both GLP-1 and GIP receptors. The GIP and GLP-1 receptors, which are the targets of native GIP and GLP-1, are both specifically bound to and activated by tirzepatide. It is a modified peptide consisting of 39 amino acids with a C20 fatty diacid moiety that increases the half-life and allows albumin binding. Tirzepatide decreases glucagon levels and increases insulin secretion in both the first and second phases in a glucose-dependent way.[19]

Apart from reducing fasting and postprandial glucose concentrations in type 2 diabetes patients, tirzepatide also reduces body weight, food consumption, and delays gastric emptying. The first dose causes the maximum delay, which eventually declines. Tirzepatide lowers postprandial hyperglycemia by slowing the absorption of post meal glucose.

Mechanisms of Action on Cardiovascular Parameters

According to studies, tirzepatide may lower the risk of atherosclerotic cardiovascular disease (CVD) and improve cardiometabolic risk factors. Blood pressure, cholesterol, and persistent inflammation are some of these risk factors.[20]

Preclinical and clinical studies have demonstrated that GLP1 receptor agonists (GLP1RA) can slow the onset and progression of atherosclerosis.[21,22] Tirzepatide reduced the 10-year estimated risk of ASCVD in obese patients according to SURMOUNT-1 data analysis. It has been demonstrated to reduce the risk of ASCVD by lowering blood pressure, waist circumference, lipid, glucose, and HbA1c levels. It is interesting to note that tirzepatide medication dramatically reduced risk in patients with higher baseline ASCVD risk.[20]

Tirzepatide appears to improve arterial compliance through several mechanisms. The medication's anti-inflammatory properties help reduce vascular inflammation, a key contributor to arterial stiffening. Chronic low-grade inflammation promotes collagen deposition and elastin degradation in arterial walls, processes that tirzepatide may help reverse.

Glucose-dependent insulinotropic polypeptide demonstrates protective vascular and anti-inflammatory effects via following mechanisms.

Endothelial Protection

At physiological concentrations (50 pM), GIP protects blood vessel cells (endothelial cells) from oxidative damage caused by advanced glycation end-products (AGEs), which are harmful compounds elevated in diabetes. It reduces expression of AGE receptors (preventing cellular damage signals) decreases ROS production and lowers proatherogenic factors like PAI-1 (which promotes blood clots and atherosclerosis).[23]

Broader Anti-inflammatory Effects

GIP reduces inflammatory cytokines and oxidative stress in both visceral fat tissue and endothelial cells.[24]

According to preclinical research, GLP1RAs, like tirzepatide, may have a direct effect on the vasculature by improving endothelial function and reducing inflammation, both of which are critical for preventing atherosclerosis.[25] Clinical trials have demonstrated that tirzepatide lowers the risk of cardiovascular events at different doses, indicating a possible therapy option for patients who are overweight or obese.[26]

Endothelial function improvement represents another pathway through which tirzepatide enhances arterial compliance. The drug promotes NO bioavailability and reduces oxidative stress, leading to improved endothelium-dependent vasodilation and reduced arterial stiffness. Weight loss associated with tirzepatide therapy also contributes to improved arterial elasticity, as obesity is closely linked to increased arterial stiffness.

Mechanisms of Blood Pressure Reduction

The blood pressure-lowering effects of tirzepatide appear to be multifactorial, involving both direct and indirect mechanisms. The compound's dual agonist activity at GIP and GLP-1 receptors triggers a cascade of physiological responses that collectively contribute to improved hemodynamic parameters.

Antiobesity treatments like tirzepatide may have cardioprotective effects because obesity is known to raise the risk of cardiovascular illness, including heart failure.[27] According to the SURPASS-2 trial, semaglutide, a GLP-1 R agonist, which is taken once a week at a dose of 1 mg, is less effective at lowering blood pressure than tirzepatide, which is taken once a week at doses of 10 or 15 mg.[28] Tirzepatide's GIP agonism and stronger capacity for stimulating weight loss may be the cause of the variation in efficacy. For semaglutide, tirzepatide 15 mg, and tirzepatide 10 mg, the mean systolic blood pressure drop was 5.3 mm Hg, 6.5 mm Hg, and 3.6 mm Hg, respectively. Tirzepatide is thought to lower blood pressure due to a number of variables, including weight loss, natriuresis, vasodilation, concomitant medication, and extracellular volume decrease.[29] It has been demonstrated that tirzepatide lowers blood pressure, either as a result of enhanced endothelial function or reduced inflammation.

In *SURPASS-4*, tirzepatide demonstrated dose-dependent reductions in systolic blood pressure compared to insulin glargine. The reductions ranged from approximately -3 to -5 mm Hg depending on the dose, with weight-loss independent effects explaining 33–57% of the difference between tirzepatide and insulin glargine groups.[30]

This trial enrolled participant with established CVD, 94% were already receiving antihypertensive medications at baseline.

The blood pressure reduction with tirzepatide was mediated through both weight-loss dependent and weight-loss independent pathways. Approximately 43–67% of the blood pressure lowering effect appeared to be weight-loss independent, suggesting direct vascular or other mechanisms beyond weight reduction alone.

Consistency Across Studies

Blood pressure reductions with tirzepatide were not dependent on concomitant antihypertensive medications, as similar reductions were observed whether participants were receiving them or not.[31]

Overall Cardiometabolic Benefits

Favorable changes were seen in blood pressure, heart rate, and lipid concentrations with tirzepatide compared to glargine, as part of an overall improvement in cardiovascular risk factors.

The blood pressure-lowering effect of tirzepatide represents an important secondary benefit beyond its primary effects on glycemic control and weight reduction in this high-risk population.[30]

A weekly dose of tirzepatide at 15 mg effectively lowered systolic blood pressure by up to 12.6 mm Hg, according to the SURPASS program, which comprised five investigational studies.[31] In comparison, long-term GLP-1RA dosage may only marginally raise systolic blood pressure by 2 mm Hg.[32] According to vasodilatory effect studies, smooth muscle cells and endothelial arterioles contain GIPR and GLP1R, which may have a cardioprotective impact through endothelium-dependent vasodilation.[33] In a trial with 16 T2DM patients and 12 nondiabetic controls, GLP1 infusion of 0.4 pmoL/kg/min during a 2-hour hyperglycemic clamp improved flow-mediated vasodilation in both groups.[34] It has been suggested that GIP promotes vasodilation through NO secretion and controls inflammation and leukocyte adhesion through endothelin 1.[35]

Researchers have found that GIP plays a critical role in controlling lipid metabolism and cardiac and vascular function. GIP may have a major effect on the cardiovascular system because it affects not only endothelial cells but also adipose tissue and circulating lipids. This theory is supported by research that links polymorphisms in the GIPR gene to features of the metabolic syndrome and CVD.[36] Tirzepatide's combined action on GIP and GLP-1 receptors may help improve cardiovascular and metabolic regulation **(Fig. 2)**.

To fully comprehend tirzepatides' impact on vasodilation and its specific effects on cardiovascular function, more research is needed.

Safety Considerations

The cardiovascular benefits of tirzepatide occur within an acceptable safety profile. With the highest dose of tirzepatide (15 mg per week), the risk of experiencing any major adverse cardiovascular event MACE-4 and MACE-3 (including myocardial infarction, stroke, hospitalization for angina, and all-cause death) has been estimated at 0.50 (0.26–0.95) in SURPASS 4, which was designed to provide preliminary evidence of tirzepatide's cardiovascular safety.[37]

CLINICAL IMPLICATIONS AND FUTURE DIRECTIONS

Tirzepatide's cardiovascular advantages go beyond managing diabetes and obesity, which is its main indication. The drug's ability to simultaneously address

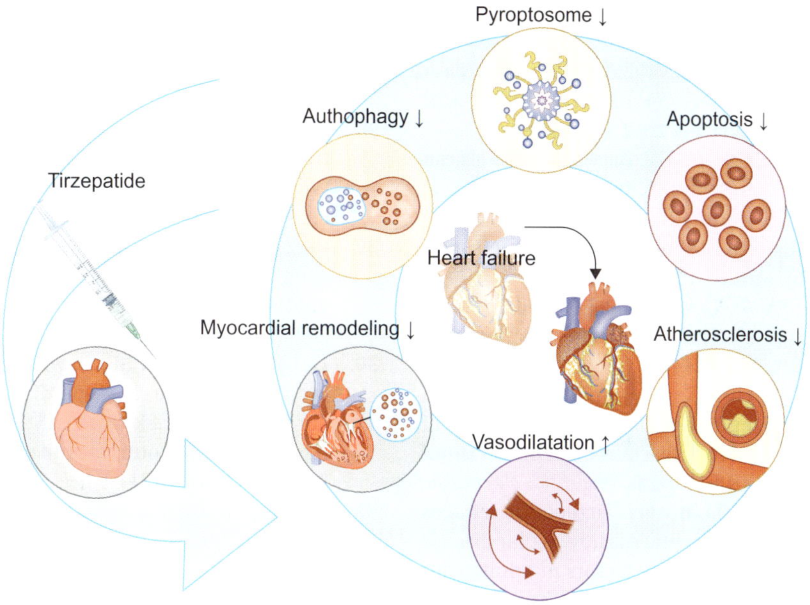

Fig. 2: Cardiovascular effects of tirzepatide.

multiple cardiovascular risk factors including blood pressure, arterial stiffness, weight, and glycemic control, makes it a promising option for holistic patient management. For patients with metabolic syndrome who need to reduce their cardiovascular risk, tirzepatide is a valuable therapeutic option because of these effects.

To determine tirzepatide's role in primary and secondary cardiovascular prevention, future research should focus on specific cardiovascular outcome trials. Long-term studies concentrating on arterial stiffness parameters and their correlation with hard cardiovascular endpoints will provide valuable insights into the drug's cardioprotective mechanisms.

CONCLUSION

Tirzepatide's positive effects on blood pressure and arterial stiffness constitute a major breakthrough in the management of cardiovascular risk. The medication's dual receptor action offers distinct cardiovascular protection routes, leading to improvements in vascular health indicators that are clinically significant. As our understanding of tirzepatide's cardiovascular effects continue to evolve, it may emerge as a key treatment for patients requiring comprehensive metabolic and cardiovascular risk reduction.

REFERENCES

1. Zieman SJ, Melenovsky V, Kass DA. Mechanisms, pathophysiology, and therapy of arterial stiffness. Arterioscler Thromb Vasc. Biol. 2005;25:932-43.
2. Peng X, Haldar S, Deshpande S. Wall stiffness suppresses Akt/eNOS and cytoprotection in pulse-perfused endothelium. Hypertension. 2003;41:378-81.
3. Duprez DA. Arterial stiffness and endothelial function. Hypertension. 2010;55:612-3.
4. Wang M, Monticone RE, McGraw KR. Proinflammatory arterial stiffness syndrome: a signature of large arterial aging. J Vasc Res. 2018;55:210-23.
5. Cavalcante JL, Lima JAC, Redheuil A, et al. Aortic stiffness. J Am Coll Cardiol. 2011;57:1511-22.
6. Endemann DH, Schiffrin EL. Endothelial dysfunction. J Am Soc Nephrol. 2004;15:1983.
7. Weisbrod RM, Shiang T, Al Sayah L, et al. Arterial stiffening precedes systolic hypertension in diet-induced obesity. Hypertension. 2013;62:1105-10.
8. Kaess BM, Rong J, Larson MG, et al. Aortic stiffness, blood pressure progression, and incident hypertension. JAMA. 2012;308:875-81.
9. Reily C, Stewart TJ, Renfrow MB, et al. Glycosylation in health and disease. Nat Rev Nephrol. 2019;15:346-66.
10. Thornalley PJ. Dicarbonyl intermediates in the maillard reaction. Ann NY Acad Sci. 2005;1043:111-7.
11. Alp NJ, Channon KM. Regulation of endothelial nitric oxide synthase by tetrahydrobiopterin in vascular disease. Arter Thromb Vasc Biol. 2004;24:413-20.
12. Cheng CL, Tang Y, Zheng Z, et al. Advanced glycation end-products activate the renin angiotensin system through the rage/pi3-k signaling pathway in podocytes. Clin Investig Med. 2012;35:18701.
13. Guzik TJ, Skiba DS, Touyz RM, et al. The role of infiltrating immune cells in dysfunctional adipose tissue. Cardiovasc Res. 2017;113:1009-23.
14. Bersch-Ferreira ÂC, Sampaio GR, Gehringer MO, et al. Association between plasma fatty acids and inflammatory

markers in patients with and without insulin resistance and in secondary prevention of cardiovascular disease, a cross-sectional study. Nutr J. 2018;17:26.
15. Loperena R, Harrison DG. Oxidative stress and hypertensive diseases. Med Clin. 2017;101:169-93.
16. Bourdeau JE, Chen ER, Carone FA. Insulin uptake in the renal proximal tubule. Am J Physiol. 1973;225:1399-404.
17. Sun XJ, Rothenberg P, Kahn CR, et al. Structure of the insulin receptor substrate IRS-1 defines a unique signal transduction protein. Nature. 1991;352:73-7.
18. Carvalho E, Jansson PA, Axelsen M, et al. Low cellular IRS 1 gene and protein expression predict insulin resistance and NIDDM. FASEB J. 1999;13:2173-8.
19. Cosku T, Sloop KW, Loghin C, et al. LY3298176, a novel dual GIP and GLP-1 receptor agonist for the treatment of type 2 diabetes mellitus: From discovery to clinical proof of concept. Mol Metab. 2018;18:3-14.
20. Hankosky ER, Wang H, Neff LM, et al. Tirzepatide reduces the predicted risk of atherosclerotic cardiovascular disease and improves cardiometabolic risk factors in adults with obesity or overweight: SURMOUNT-1 post hoc analysis. Diabetes Obes Metab. 2024;26(1):319-28.
21. Marso SP, Daniels GH, Brown-Frandsen K, et al. Liraglutide and cardiovascular outcomes in type 2 diabetes. N Engl J Med. 2016;375(4):311-22.
22. Rizzo M, Nikolic D, Patti AM, et al. GLP-1 receptor agonists and reduction of cardiometabolic risk: potential underlying mechanisms. Biochim Biophys Acta Mol Basis Dis. 2018;1864(9 Pt B):2814-21.
23. Ojima A, Matsui T, Maeda S, et al. Glucose-dependent insulinotropic polypeptide (GIP) inhibits signaling pathways of advanced glycation end products (AGEs) in endothelial cells via its antioxidative proper ties. Horm Metab Res. 2012;44(7):501-5.
24. Nauck MA, Quast DR, Wefers J, et al. The evolving story of incretins (GIP and GLP-1) in metabolic and cardiovascular disease: a pathophysiological update. Diabetes Obes Metab. 2021;23(Suppl 3):5-29.
25. Kaneko S. Tirzepatide: a Novel, once-weekly dual GIP and GLP-1 receptor agonist for the treatment of type 2 diabetes. touchrev Endocrinol. 2022;18(1):10-9.
26. Sattar N, McGuire DK, Pavo I, et al. Tirzepatide cardiovascular event risk assessment: a pre-specified meta analysis. Nat Med. 2022;28(3):591-8.
27. Berglund LM, Lyssenko V, Ladenvall C, et al. Glucose-dependent Insulinotropic Polypeptide stimulates Osteopontin expression in the vasculature via Endothelin-1 and CREB. Diabetes. 2016;65(1):239-54.
28. Frías JP, Davies MJ, Rosenstock J, et al.; SURPASS-2 Investigators. Tirzepatide versus Semaglutide Once Weekly in Patients with Type 2 Diabetes. N Engl J Med. 2021;385(6):503-15.
29. Kido K, Carey B, Caccamo M, et al. Call to action for drug interactions between tirzepatide and heart failure guideline-directed medical therapy. J Am Pharm Assoc. 2024;64(1):169-73.
30. Del Prato S, Kahn SE, Pavo I, et al. Tirzepatide versus insulin glargine in type 2 diabetes and increased cardiovascular risk (SURPASS-4): a randomised, open-label, parallel-group, multicentre, phase 3 trial. Lancet. 2021;398(10313):1811-24.
31. Lingvay I, Brown-Frandsen K, Colhoun HM, et al. Semaglutide for cardiovascular event reduction in people with overweight or obesity: SELECT study baseline characteristics. Obes (Silver Spring). 2023;31(1): 111-22.
32. Goud A, Zhong J, Peters M, et al. GLP-1 agonists and blood pressure: a review of the evidence. Curr Hypertens Rep. 2016;18(2):16.
33. Koffert J, Honka H, Teuho J, et al. Effects of meal and incretins in the regulation of splanchnic blood flow. Endocr Connect. 2017;6(3):179-87.
34. Ceriello A, Esposito K, Testa R, et al. The possible protective role of glucagon-like peptide 1 on endothelium during the meal and evidence for an endothelial resistance to glucagon-like peptide 1 in diabetes. Diabetes Care. 2011;34(3):697-702.
35. Bowker N, Hansford R, Burgess S, et al. Genetically predicted glucose-dependent Insulinotropic polypeptide (GIP) levels and Cardiovascular Disease Risk are driven by distinct causal variants in the GIPR Region. Diabetes. 2021;70(11):2706-19.
36. Saxena R, Hivert MF, Langenberg C, et al. Genetic variation in GIPR influences the glucose and insulin responses to an oral glucose challenge. Nat Genet. 2010;42(2):142-8.
37. Min T, Bain SC. The role of Tirzepatide, dual GIP and GLP-1 receptor agonist, in the management of type 2 diabetes: the SURPASS clinical trials. Diabetes Ther. 2021;12(1):143-57.

CHAPTER 129

Safety and Cardiovascular Adverse Events Associated with Tirzepatide

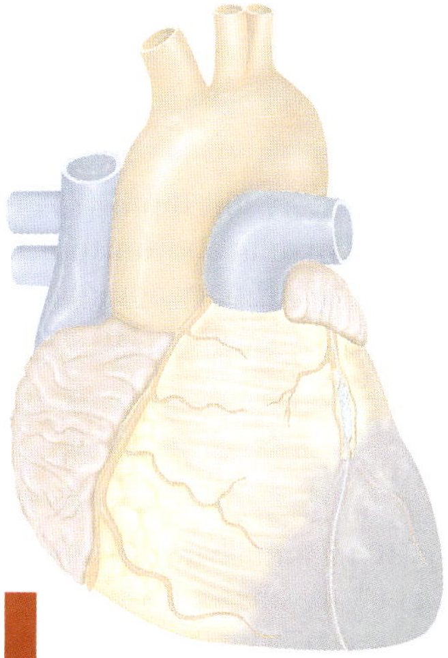

Kiron Varghese

INTRODUCTION

Cardiovascular (CV) disease is a leading cause of death in people with type 2 diabetes (T2D). Similarly, individuals with obesity without diabetes are at higher risk for a variety of illnesses. In particular, obesity is increasingly being recognized as a major risk factor for heart failure with preserved ejection fraction (HFpEF) and about two-thirds of patients with HFpEF have obesity.[1]

Tirzepatide is a once-weekly dual agonist of glucose-dependent insulinotropic polypeptide (GIP) and glucagon-like peptide-1 (GLP-1) receptors, now widely used for T2D and obesity.

Since the 2008 US Food and Drug Administration (FDA) guidance, new glucose-lowering therapies have been required to demonstrate that they do not unacceptably increase major adverse CV events.

This article focuses specifically on CV safety and adverse events associated with tirzepatide.

META-ANALYSES AND SYSTEMATIC REVIEWS OF CARDIOVASCULAR EVENTS

Multiple meta-analyses have assessed CV outcomes and arrhythmias with tirzepatide:

All seven randomized controlled trials with a duration of at least 26 weeks from the tirzepatide T2D clinical development program, SURPASS were included in a prespecified CV meta-analysis. The analysis showed that tirzepatide treatment was not associated with increased risk of the MACE-4 outcome [hazard ratio (HR) of 0.80 (95% CI: 0.57–1.11)], CV death [HR = 0.90 (95% CI: 0.50–1.61)], myocardial infarction (MI) [HR = 0.76 (95% CI: 0.45–1.28)], stroke [HR = 0.81 (95% CI: 0.39–1.68)] and hospitalized unstable angina [HR = 0.46 (95% CI: 0.15–1.41)] compared to the pooled comparator group, indicating no increase in CV risk and a point estimate compatible with potential benefit.[2]

The meta-analysis explored outcomes by tirzepatide dose (5, 10, and 15 mg) and found no signal of excess MACE at higher doses; HR estimates were numerically below 1.0 across various doses, but event numbers were modest and CIs were wide. Overall, these findings satisfied regulatory expectations that tirzepatide does not increase MACE risk compared with active or placebo controls in T2D.[2]

Despite favorable effects of tirzepatide on a range of CV risk factors, to date its CV safety has been reported from results of only a single trial, SURPASS-4.

SURPASS-4: High CV-Risk T2D versus Insulin Glargine

SURPASS-4 enrolled adults with T2D and high CV risk—established CVD, chronic kidney disease, or multiple risk factors—and randomized them to once-weekly tirzepatide (5/10/15 mg) or titrated basal insulin glargine for a median of 85–104 weeks.[3]

This trial, which compared tirzepatide treatment to insulin glargine treatment in people with T2D at increased CV risk, suggested no significant difference in the incidence of major CV events.

In SURPASS-4, the notable side effects were nausea (12–23%), diarrhea (13–22%), reduced appetite (9–11%), and vomiting (5–9%) which were more common with tirzepatide than glargine (nausea 2%, diarrhea 4%, decreased appetite <1%, and vomiting 2%, respectively). However, in most cases, these side effects were mild-to-moderate in severity and occurred during the dose-escalation phase. The number of subjects with hypoglycemia (glucose <54 mg/dL) was lower with tirzepatide (6–9%) compared to glargine (19%), especially in those not on sulfonylureas (tirzepatide 1–3% vs. glargine 16%). MACE-4 events (CV death, MI, stroke, and hospitalization for unstable angina) occurred in 109 participants and were not higher with tirzepatide compared with glargine (HR: 0.74, 95% CI: 0.51–1.08). 60 deaths [n = 25 (3%) tirzepatide; n = 35 (4%) glargine], thus excluding a major harm signal and suggesting a nonsignificant trend to fewer events. The point estimates for individual components (CV death, MI, and stroke) were all in favor of tirzepatide or were neutral, although numbers were small and CIs crossed 1.0. Similarly, hospitalization for heart failure (HHF) and other serious CV adverse events were similar or numerically lower with tirzepatide than with insulin glargine.[3]

Other SURPASS Phase 3 Trials

In the broader SURPASS-1, -2, -3 and -5 population (generally lower baseline CV risk), CV events were infrequent, and none of the individual trials was powered for MACE.

Across these studies, serious CV adverse events and MACE occurred in *low single-digit percentages*, with similar or numerically fewer events in tirzepatide versus placebo, insulin, or glucagon-like peptide-1 receptor agonist (GLP-1RA) comparator. No trial individually showed a clear numerical excess of MI, stroke, or HF with tirzepatide.[4]

Non-MACE Cardiovascular Safety Findings within RCTs

Beyond MACE, several other CV-relevant parameters were studied, and favorable effects have been noted on blood pressure, heart rate, and lipids with no signal of harm.[5]

Arrhythmias were uncommon and generally balanced between arms in SURPASS trials. In a meta-analysis studying the effect of tirzepatide on the risk of atrial fibrillation (AF) in patients with T2D, pooled data from SURPASS-2 to -5 showed that tirzepatide compared with placebo or an active comparator did not significantly increase the risk of AF (risk ratio = 1.59; 95% CI: 0.46–5.47). The authors concluded that tirzepatide "does not increase the risk for AF in patients with T2D."[4]

Cardiovascular Adverse Events in Obesity and Heart Failure Trials

SUMMIT Trial: HFpEF and Obesity

The SUMMIT trial randomized patients with HFpEF (LVEF ≥50%) and obesity to tirzepatide or placebo on top of guideline-directed HF therapy.[6] The primary composite endpoint was time to first CV death or worsening HF event (HF hospitalization or urgent HF visit).

Over a median follow-up of ~2 years, tirzepatide significantly reduced the primary endpoint: HR approximately 0.62 versus placebo (95% CI around 0.41–0.95), driven mainly by fewer HF hospitalizations/urgent visits, with a trend toward fewer CV deaths.

From a safety standpoint, SUMMIT showed no excess of arrhythmias or ischemic events with tirzepatide versus placebo and instead suggests a favorable HF event profile. Adverse events (mainly gastrointestinal) leading to discontinuation of the trial drug occurred in 23 patients (6.3%) in the tirzepatide group and in five patients (1.4%) in the placebo group.[6]

SURMOUNT Obesity Trials

In SURMOUNT-1 and related obesity trials (participants with obesity, with and without diabetes), serious CV adverse events and MACE were systematically collected but were infrequent. Serious CV events occurred in a low proportion of participants and were similar or numerically lower with tirzepatide compared to placebo, with no consistent signal for excess MI, stroke, HF, or arrhythmias.

A majority of participants in both tirzepatide and placebo groups reported at least one adverse event during the treatment period (78.9–81.8% with tirzepatide vs. 72.0% with placebo). Serious adverse events were reported by 6.3% participants with similar percentages in the tirzepatide and placebo groups. The most common adverse events with tirzepatide were gastrointestinal, including nausea, vomiting, diarrhea, and constipation, were mild-to-moderate in severity and noted mainly during dose escalation. Treatment discontinuation due to adverse events occurred in 4.3%, 7.1%, 6.2%, and 2.6% of participants receiving 5-mg, 10-mg, and 15-mg tirzepatide doses and placebo, respectively.[7]

REAL-WORLD CARDIOVASCULAR OUTCOMES AND ADVERSE EVENTS

T2D Cohorts: Tirzepatide versus GLP-1RAs

The largest real-world study to date, a TriNetX-based cohort analysis of 140,308 adults with T2D, compared tirzepatide with GLP-1RAs over a median follow-up of

~10.5 months. After propensity matching, tirzepatide use was associated with lower all-cause mortality: adjusted HR of 0.58 (95% CI: 0.45–0.75), lower MACE: HR of 0.80 (95% CI: 0.71–0.91), and lower composite of MACE + all-cause mortality and fewer kidney events, including acute kidney injury.[8]

Subgroup analyses showed consistent benefit across strata of baseline CVD, kidney function, BMI, and other comorbidities. While residual confounding is inevitable, these findings are reassuring and suggest at least comparable, and possibly superior, CV outcomes versus GLP-1RAs in routine practice.

JACC Advances 2025 Observational Study

Dani et al. conducted a retrospective cohort analysis of adults ≥40 years with T2D, BMI ≥25 kg/m^2, and preexisting ischemic heart disease treated with tirzepatide or GLP-1RAs using real-world claims/registry data and propensity score matching.[9] Tirzepatide was associated with better composite CV outcomes, with lower adjusted hazards for MACE and HF hospitalization, broadly concordant with the RCT meta-analysis and the Chuang cohort.[8,9]

Gastrointestinal symptoms were significantly less common with tirzepatide compared to GLP-1RA: HR of 0.687 (95% CI: 0.564–0.837) p value <0.001.

Pancreatitis and Gallbladder or Biliary Disease

Zeng et al. conducted a systematic review and meta-analysis to analyze the available data from clinical trials and assess the safety issues of tirzepatide (pancreatitis and gallbladder or biliary disease) in T2D and obesity.[10]

When compared to all control groups consisting of basal insulin (glargine or degludec), selective GLP-1RA (dulaglutide or semaglutide once weekly), and placebo, there was no significantly increased risk of pancreatitis associated with tirzepatide (RR: 1.46, 95% CI: 0.59–3.61; $I^2 = 0.0\%$, $p = 0.436$). However, for gallbladder or biliary disease, the composite of gallbladder or biliary disease was significantly associated with tirzepatide compared with placebo or basal insulin (RR: 1.97, 95% CI: 1.14–3.42; $I^2 = 0.0\%$, $p = 0.558$), but not with the risk of cholelithiasis, cholecystitis, or biliary diseases.

Nassar et al. assessed the recurrence of acute pancreatitis over a 5-year period in a retrospective cohort study using the TriNetX platform, encompassing 258,238 individuals with T2D or obesity who had a history of acute pancreatitis. GLP-1RA users had significantly lower recurrence rates of acute pancreatitis, with a recurrence rate of 13.8% in GLP-1RA users without risk factors compared to 40.9% for nonusers. Semaglutide and tirzepatide showed the most favorable outcomes; semaglutide users had lower recurrence rates than exenatide (10.1% vs. 27%) and slightly lower than dulaglutide (13.6% vs. 15.4%), though not statistically significant with dulaglutide. Tirzepatide users displayed the lowest recurrence risk (6.2% vs. 11.7%) compared to semaglutide.[11]

Heart Failure and Atrial Fibrillation Real-World Data

In AF populations, a 2025 observational study (Wu et al.) reported that tirzepatide may be associated with *reduced AF burden* and fewer AF-related interventions compared with other therapies in patients with T2D, though this is hypothesis-generating and vulnerable to confounding by indication and channeling bias.[12]

Overall, real-world data so far *align with RCT evidence*, suggesting no emergent CV harm signal and potential benefit for MACE and HF outcomes; however, observational designs cannot prove causality, and duration of follow-up remains modest.

PHARMACOVIGILANCE DATA AND CASE REPORTS

Food and Drug Administration Adverse Event Reporting System and Other Spontaneous-reporting Analyses

A real-world data analysis of tirzepatide in the FDA adverse event reporting system (FAERS) database attempted to evaluate the potential association between tirzepatide and adverse drug reactions (ADRs).[13] The study identified several previously unrecognized ADRs that may manifest in patients using tirzepatide, including elevated thyroid hormones, abdominal rigidity, and feeding disorders. However, controlling for confounding variables poses a significant challenge. Moreover, the true incidence rates of each adverse event could not be assessed due to the absence of comprehensive data on the total number of patients using tirzepatide in real-world settings. It is worth noting that spontaneous reporting is limited by under-reporting, stimulated reporting, lack of denominators, and confounding, and hence, it may not be possible to establish a causal relationship between tirzepatide and ADRs using such studies.

Case Reports of Cardiovascular Adverse Events

A small but important body of case reports has described severe CV events temporally linked to tirzepatide.

The best-documented example is a life-threatening ventricular fibrillation episode reported by Kammaripalle et al. in 2025: a middle-aged man developed severe vomiting and diarrhea after high-dose tirzepatide, leading to profound electrolyte disturbances and subsequent ventricular fibrillation requiring resuscitation. The authors concluded that electrolyte derangements secondary to gastrointestinal toxicity were the likely precipitating factor, rather than a direct proarrhythmic effect of tirzepatide, but emphasized the need for careful electrolyte monitoring in high-risk patients.[14]

Other case series and reports have mentioned palpitations, tachycardia, or nonspecific CV symptoms in tirzepatide-treated patients, but causality is difficult to establish, and many involve concomitant factors such as dehydration, preexisting heart disease, or interacting medications.

Overall, case reports highlight *rare but serious potential CV complications*, often secondary to non-CV adverse events (e.g., severe GI loss), and support a cautious monitoring approach in susceptible individuals.

Integration with Overall Safety Profile: Non-CV Adverse Events and Cardiovascular Risk

Tirzepatide's adverse-event profile is dominated by gastrointestinal symptoms—nausea, vomiting, diarrhea, and reduced appetite—especially during dose escalation.[3] In most patients, these events are mild-to-moderate and transient, but in some, they can lead to dehydration, orthostatic hypotension, and electrolyte imbalances. These, in turn, can indirectly increase CV risk, as illustrated by the ventricular fibrillation case where severe GI losses led to marked electrolyte abnormalities and malignant arrhythmia.[14]

At the same time, tirzepatide produces *favorable changes* in multiple CV risk modifiers: Large, sustained reductions in body weight (often >15% in obesity trials), clinically meaningful reductions in blood pressure and improvements in lipids and improved glycemic control and, in some settings, reduced albuminuria and slower eGFR decline, which have downstream CV implications.[4]

Hypoglycemia is uncommon with tirzepatide monotherapy but can occur when combined with insulin or sulfonylureas. In SURPASS-4, hypoglycemia was significantly less frequent with tirzepatide than with insulin glargine, but episodes still occurred and, in vulnerable patients, hypoglycemia is a known trigger for arrhythmias and ischemic events.[3]

Thus, the overall CV safety profile reflects a *balance* between indirect risks from severe GI toxicity or hypoglycemia and substantial improvements in CV risk factors, with current evidence suggesting the latter predominates in most patients.

CLINICAL INTERPRETATION: MANAGING CARDIOVASCULAR RISK WITH TIRZEPATIDE

Data from RCTs, meta-analyses, and real-world studies collectively indicate that tirzepatide is *CV-safe*, with no increase in MACE and emerging evidence of benefit in selected populations (e.g., HFpEF with obesity and high-risk T2D).

When initiating tirzepatide, clinicians should pay particular attention to:

- *Higher-risk patients:* Those with established HF (especially HFpEF with congestion), prior ventricular arrhythmias, significant coronary artery disease, advanced age, CKD, or concomitant diuretic/RAAS-blocker therapy.[6]
- *Monitoring needs:* Baseline and periodic measurement of blood pressure, heart rate, renal function, and electrolytes, particularly if GI adverse events are prominent or if the patient is on diuretics or has marginal volume status (Barry Borlaug).
- *Concomitant therapies:* Adjustment of insulin or sulfonylurea doses to minimize hypoglycemia risk, and careful titration of antihypertensives when large BP reductions occur.[2]

In patients where CV risk is the primary therapeutic concern, tirzepatide should be considered alongside established cardioprotective agents:

- For *atherosclerotic CVD (ASCVD)*, GLP-1RAs with proven CV benefit and SGLT2 inhibitors remain first-line; existing data suggest that tirzepatide is at least noninferior and possibly favorable in this context, but dedicated CV outcomes trials (e.g., SURPASS-CVOT) are awaited.[15]
- For *HFpEF with obesity*, SUMMIT provides strong evidence that tirzepatide reduces HF events and improves quality of life, making it as a promising therapeutic option in such patients.[6]

Pragmatically, tirzepatide can be integrated into cardiometabolic care as a potent weight-loss and glucose-lowering agent with a reassuring safety profile, provided that volume status, GI tolerance, and comorbid heart disease are actively monitored.

KNOWLEDGE GAPS AND FUTURE DIRECTIONS

Despite rapidly expanding evidence, several important questions remain:

- *Long-term CV safety and benefit:* Existing RCT and observational follow-up is mostly ≤2–3 years. Longer-term data are needed to determine whether MACE reduction emerges overtime and to confirm durability of HF benefits.
- *Dedicated CV outcome trials:* Full peer-reviewed results from large CVOTs such as *SURPASS-CVOT* will be critical to define tirzepatide's place relative to established GLP-1RAs and SGLT2 inhibitors for secondary CV prevention.
- *Arrhythmia risk:* Although AF meta-analysis and early observational data are reassuring, more granular data on AF burden, ventricular arrhythmias, and sudden death are needed, particularly in older and structurally abnormal hearts.
- *Mechanistic insights:* Further work is required to unravel how rapid weight loss, autonomic changes, and structural cardiac remodeling interact with CV events in tirzepatide-treated patients.
- *Targeted pharmacovigilance* focusing specifically on CV adverse events, using active surveillance and linkage with outcome registries, will be essential as global use expands.[1]

CONCLUSION

Current evidence from randomized trials, meta-analyses, real-world cohorts, and pharmacovigilance indicates that *tirzepatide does not increase MACE* and may reduce HF events in patients with HFpEF and obesity, while improving multiple cardiometabolic risk factors.

The most common side effects of tirzepatide are gastrointestinal issues such as nausea, diarrhea, and decreased appetite, which usually lessen over time

Post-marketing data and case reports reveal rare but potentially serious CV events, typically secondary to severe non-CV adverse events such as GI-induced electrolyte disturbances, underscoring the need for careful monitoring in high-risk individuals. As use of tirzepatide increases, vigilant patient selection, active surveillance, and integration with proven cardioprotective therapies will be key to maximizing benefit while minimizing adverse effects.

REFERENCES

1. Borlaug BA, Zile MR, Kramer CM, et al. Effects of tirzepatide on circulatory overload and end-organ damage in heart failure with preserved ejection fraction and obesity: a secondary analysis of the SUMMIT trial. Nat Med. 2025;31:544-51.
2. Sattar N, McGuire DK, Pavo I, et al. Tirzepatide cardiovascular event risk assessment: a pre-specified meta-analysis. Nat Med. 2022;28(3):591-8.
3. Del Prato S, Kahn SE, Pavo I, et al. Tirzepatide versus insulin glargine in type 2 diabetes and increased cardiovascular risk (SURPASS-4). Lancet. 2021;398(10313):1811-24.
4. Forzano I, Varzideh F, Avvisato R, et al. Tirzepatide: a systematic update. Int J Mol Sci. 2022;23(23):14631.
5. Taktaz F, Fontanella RA, Scisciola L, et al. Bridging the gap between GLP1-receptor agonists and cardiovascular outcomes: evidence for the role of tirzepatide. Cardiovasc Diabetol. 2024;23:242.
6. Packer M, Zile MR, Kramer CM, et al. Tirzepatide for heart failure with preserved ejection fraction and obesity. N Engl J Med. 2025;392(5):427-37.
7. Jastreboff AM, Aronne LJ, Ahmad NN, et al. Tirzepatide once weekly for the treatment of obesity. N Engl J Med. 2022;387:205-16.
8. Chuang MH, Chen JY, Wang HY, et al. Clinical outcomes of tirzepatide or GLP-1 receptor agonists in individuals with type 2 diabetes. JAMA Netw Open. 2024;7(8):e2427258.
9. Dani SS, Makwana B, Khadke S, et al. An observational study of cardiovascular outcomes of tirzepatide vs glucagon-like peptide-1 receptor agonists. JACC Adv. 2025;4(5):101740.
10. Zeng Q, Xu J, Mu X, et al. Safety issues of tirzepatide (pancreatitis and gallbladder or biliary disease) in type 2 diabetes and obesity: a systematic review and meta-analysis. Front Endocrinol. 2023;14:1214334.
11. Nassar M, Nassar O, Abosheaishaa H, et al. Decreased risk of recurrent acute pancreatitis with semaglutide and tirzepatide in people with type 2 diabetes or obesity with a history of acute pancreatitis: A propensity matched global federated TriNetX database-based retrospective cohort study. Diabetes Metab Syndr. 2024;18(9):103116.
12. Wu JY, Tseng KJ, Kao CL, et al. Clinical effectiveness of tirzepatide for patients with atrial fibrillation and type 2 diabetes. Diabetes Res Clin Pract. 2025;225:112279.
13. Liu L. A real-world data analysis of tirzepatide in the FDA adverse event reporting system (FAERS) database. Front Pharmacol. 2024;15:1397029.
14. Kammaripalle TKC, Giordano JR, Rana H, et al. Life-threatening ventricular fibrillation linked to high-dose tirzepatide-induced gastrointestinal side effects. Cureus. 2025;17(6):e85366.
15. Sumithran P, Russell AW, Zoungas S. Cardiovascular effects of tirzepatide. J Endocrinol. 2025;264(2):e240259.

130 CHAPTER

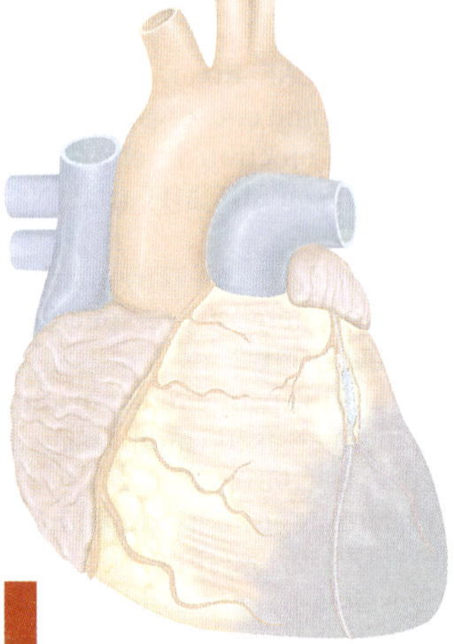

Future Perspectives: Tirzepatide in Cardioprotection and Heart Disease Prevention

Ranjan Modi, Sunil Modi

INTRODUCTION

Cardiovascular disease (CVD) remains the leading cause of mortality worldwide, often driven by modifiable cardiometabolic risk factors including type 2 diabetes mellitus (T2DM), obesity, dyslipidemia, and hypertension. With the global rise in obesity and insulin resistance, there is an urgent need for therapeutic agents that target these interrelated conditions while simultaneously offering cardiovascular protection.

Tirzepatide, a first-in-class dual glucose-dependent insulinotropic polypeptide (GIP) and glucagon-like peptide-1 (GLP-1) receptor agonist, has emerged as a groundbreaking agent initially developed for T2DM and obesity. However, its profound effects on metabolic, inflammatory, and hemodynamic pathways make it a compelling candidate for CVD prevention and treatment. The ongoing evolution of tirzepatide from a metabolic drug to a cardiometabolic therapeutic marks a significant paradigm shift in modern medicine.

MECHANISM OF ACTION AND PLEIOTROPIC EFFECTS

Tirzepatide simultaneously activates GIP and GLP-1 receptors, enhancing insulin secretion, suppressing glucagon release, and slowing gastric emptying. This dual-incretin approach produces superior glycemic control compared to GLP-1 receptor agonists alone, while also yielding substantial weight loss and improvements in lipid profiles and inflammatory markers.[1]

Glucose-dependent insulinotropic polypeptide receptors are expressed in various tissues including adipose, heart, and vasculature, where they may exert additional benefits such as anti-inflammatory, lipolytic, and vasodilatory effects.[2] Meanwhile, GLP-1 receptor agonism has already been associated with reduced cardiovascular events in large randomized controlled trials (RCTs) like LEADER and SUSTAIN-6.[3,4] The combination may offer additive or synergistic effects, translating into robust cardioprotective properties.

METABOLIC RISK FACTOR REDUCTION: THE FOUNDATION FOR CARDIOPROTECTION

Tirzepatide's impact on modifiable cardiovascular risk factors is striking:

- *Weight loss:* In the SURMOUNT-1 trial, patients with obesity but without diabetes experienced up to 22.5% weight reduction with tirzepatide, surpassing results seen with GLP-1 RAs.[5] Weight loss itself leads to reduced blood pressure, improved lipid profiles, and lower left ventricular (LV) wall stress.
- *Blood pressure reduction:* Tirzepatide has been shown to reduce systolic blood pressure by 5–10 mm Hg in multiple studies, a clinically meaningful change associated with lower cardiovascular risk.[6]
- *Lipid modulation:* Reductions in triglycerides, LDL-C, and increases in HDL-C have been observed, improving the atherogenic lipid profile.[7]
- *Inflammatory markers:* Decreases in C-reactive protein (CRP) and interleukin-6 levels suggest that tirzepatide exerts systemic anti-inflammatory effects, relevant in atherosclerosis and vascular remodeling.[8]

These risk factor improvements provide a strong mechanistic basis for cardiovascular event reduction, even before definitive outcomes data are published.

CARDIOVASCULAR OUTCOME TRIALS: PRESENT EVIDENCE AND WHAT IS AHEAD

While GLP-1 receptor agonists like liraglutide and semaglutide have proven cardiovascular benefit, tirzepatide's data are currently preliminary but promising.

SURPASS-4 Trial

The SURPASS-4 trial enrolled patients with T2DM and high cardiovascular risk and compared tirzepatide to insulin glargine. While not powered to assess MACE, tirzepatide showed a neutral to favorable cardiovascular safety profile and superior improvements in glycemic control and weight.[9] The study demonstrated no increase in MACE and fewer adverse cardiovascular outcomes in the tirzepatide group, although formal conclusions await larger trials.

SURPASS-CVOT

The SURPASS-CVOT (NCT04255433) is a pivotal cardiovascular outcomes trial comparing tirzepatide with dulaglutide in patients with established CVD. With over 13,000 participants enrolled, this large RCT will provide conclusive evidence regarding MACE reduction and is expected to report results in 2026. Given dulaglutide's already proven cardiovascular benefit, tirzepatide must demonstrate noninferiority or superiority to establish its role in cardiovascular prevention.

TIRZEPATIDE BEYOND DIABETES: A PRIMARY PREVENTION TOOL?

A particularly exciting prospect is the use of tirzepatide in people without diabetes, particularly those with obesity or metabolic syndrome. The SURMOUNT trials have already demonstrated that tirzepatide leads to massive reductions in weight and cardiometabolic parameters in nondiabetic individuals.[5] This opens the door for its potential primary prevention use—similar to how statins are employed in individuals with elevated LDL but without existing heart disease.

A large portion of cardiovascular events occurs in patients without diagnosed diabetes but with insulin resistance, visceral adiposity, and subclinical inflammation. Tirzepatide could serve as a disease-modifying agent in this high-risk, underserved population.

EMERGING ROLE IN HEART FAILURE: ESPECIALLY HEART FAILURE WITH PRESERVED EJECTION FRACTION

Heart failure with preserved ejection fraction (HFpEF) is a growing epidemic closely linked with obesity, T2DM, and metabolic syndrome. Traditional heart failure therapies have limited efficacy in this subgroup. GLP-1 RAs have shown mixed results in heart failure, but tirzepatide—with its dual action and significant weight loss—may hold unique promise.

Preclinical studies suggest both GIP and GLP-1 agonism improve myocardial glucose utilization, reduce fibrosis, and enhance diastolic function.[10] Additionally, tirzepatide-induced reductions in LV mass, epicardial fat, and systemic inflammation could positively impact HFpEF pathophysiology.

Ongoing trials are evaluating tirzepatide's role in HFpEF specifically, and early imaging studies already suggest beneficial structural remodeling.

SYNERGISTIC POTENTIAL WITH OTHER CARDIOPROTECTIVE AGENTS

Another future direction is combination therapy. Tirzepatide could be paired with:

- *SGLT2 inhibitors:* Known for their heart failure and kidney protection, SGLT2i may complement tirzepatide's metabolic and anti-inflammatory effects.
- *Statins:* Dual therapy could aggressively address both dyslipidemia and insulin resistance.
- *Antihypertensives:* Tirzepatide's BP-lowering effects could reduce the need for multiple agents.

Such combinations may define the future of comprehensive cardiometabolic care, especially in patients with multiple overlapping risk factors.

LIMITATIONS AND FUTURE CONSIDERATIONS

Despite its promise, several barriers must be addressed before tirzepatide becomes a routine cardiovascular prevention agent:

- *Long-term safety:* Though well-tolerated in trials, longer term surveillance is needed to rule out pancreatic, thyroid, or gallbladder complications.
- *Cost and access:* As a biologic, tirzepatide may be expensive and not easily accessible in low-resource

settings. Health systems must evaluate their cost-effectiveness in preventing costly cardiovascular events.

- *Patient adherence:* Injectable therapies may face resistance among patients. Oral formulations or longer acting injectables could help improve adherence.
- *Regulatory approval:* At present, tirzepatide is approved for T2DM and obesity. Its expansion into cardiovascular indications will depend on the results of ongoing outcome trials.

CONCLUSION

Tirzepatide represents one of the most exciting developments in cardiometabolic therapeutics. With its ability to significantly improve glycemic control, promote weight loss, and favorably modulate multiple cardiovascular risk factors, it is uniquely positioned to play a transformative role in heart disease prevention.

Ongoing cardiovascular outcomes trials like SURPASS-CVOT will be critical in defining tirzepatide's place in future guidelines. If proven effective in reducing MACE, tirzepatide could shift from a metabolic agent to a cornerstone therapy for both primary and secondary cardiovascular prevention, especially in populations with obesity, insulin resistance, and HFpEF.

In the coming years, tirzepatide may not only change how we treat diabetes and obesity—it could reshape the prevention and management of heart disease as we know it.

REFERENCES

1. Frias JP, Davies MJ, Rosenstock J, et al. Tirzepatide versus semaglutide once weekly in patients with type 2 diabetes. N Engl J Med. 2021;385(6):503-15.
2. Finan B, Ma T, Ottaway N, et al. Unimolecular dual incretins maximize metabolic benefits in rodents, monkeys, and humans. Sci Transl Med. 2013;5(209):209ra151.
3. Marso SP, Daniels GH, Brown-Frandsen K, et al. Liraglutide and cardiovascular outcomes in type 2 diabetes. N Engl J Med. 2016;375(4):311-22.
4. Marso SP, Bain SC, Consoli A, et al. Semaglutide and cardiovascular outcomes in patients with type 2 diabetes. N Engl J Med. 2016;375(19):1834-44.
5. Jastreboff AM, Aronne LJ, Ahmad NN, et al. Tirzepatide once weekly for the treatment of obesity. N Engl J Med. 2022;387(3):205-16.
6. Gastaldelli A, Cusi K, Fernandez L, et al. Effects of tirzepatide versus insulin glargine on blood pressure and lipid profiles in type 2 diabetes: SURPASS-4. Lancet Diabetes Endocrinol. 2021;9(12):878-90.
7. Sattar N, McGuire DK, Pavo I, et al. Tirzepatide's cardiometabolic potential: a review of mechanisms and clinical data. Cardiovasc Diabetol. 2022;21(1):1-12.
8. Nauck MA, Quast DR, Wefers J, et al. GLP-1 receptor agonists in the treatment of type 2 diabetes—state-of-the-art. Mol Metab. 2021;46:101102.
9. Del Prato S, Kahn SE, Pavo I, et al. Tirzepatide versus insulin glargine in type 2 diabetes and increased cardiovascular risk (SURPASS-4). Lancet. 2021;398(10313):1811-24.
10. Lee DS, Park J, Kwon JE, et al. GIP and GLP-1 receptor dual agonist ameliorates cardiac function and remodeling in obese mice. J Endocrinol Invest. 2023;46(5):1117-27.

131

CHAPTER

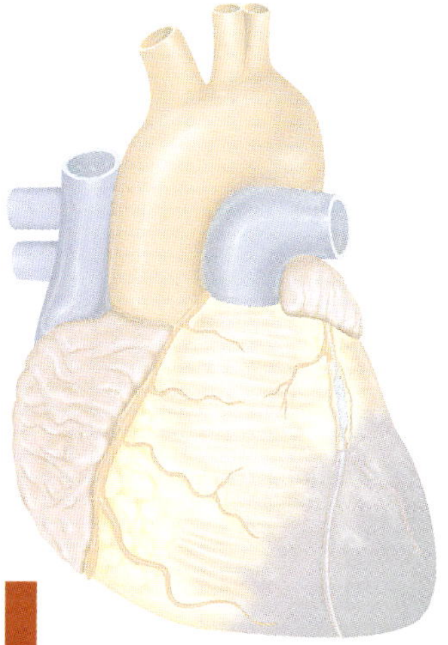

Morbidity and Mortality Benefits of Tirzepatide in Patients with HFpEF

Preeti Gupta, Dikshant Jain

INTRODUCTION

Heart failure with preserved ejection fraction (HFpEF) represents approximately 50% of all heart failure cases globally, with obesity emerging as a critical phenotype-defining comorbidity.[1,2] The obesity-related HFpEF phenotype is characterized by younger age at presentation, female predominance, metabolic dysregulation, and disproportionate symptoms relative to hemodynamic derangement.[3] Despite significant advances in heart failure therapeutics, treatment options for HFpEF have historically been limited, with sodium-glucose cotransporter-2 (SGLT2) inhibitors being the primary disease-modifying therapy until recently.[4]

Tirzepatide, a novel dual glucose-dependent insulinotropic polypeptide (GIP) and glucagon-like peptide-1 (GLP-1) receptor agonist, has demonstrated unprecedented weight loss efficacy in obesity trials (10–15% body weight reduction). Given the intersection between obesity, metabolic syndrome, and HFpEF pathophysiology—encompassing systemic inflammation, epicardial adiposity, circulatory congestion, and left ventricular remodeling—tirzepatide emerged as a promising therapeutic candidate.[5] The SUMMIT trial (semaglutide and tirzepatide in HFpEF with morbid obesity), presented at the American Heart Association Scientific Sessions 2024 and published in the New England Journal of Medicine, provided definitive evidence for tirzepatide role in this population.[1]

This chapter collates the current evidence on morbidity and mortality benefits of tirzepatide in obesity-related HFpEF, provides mechanistic insights, addresses implementation challenges, and offers practical guidance for healthcare individuals managing this complex patient population.

THE DRUG

The SUMMIT Trial: Landmark Evidence

The SUMMIT trial was a multicenter, randomized, double-blind, placebo-controlled phase III study enrolling 731 patients with obesity-related HFpEF **(Flowchart 1)**.[6] Patients had body mass index (BMI) ≥30 kg/m^2, left ventricular ejection fraction (LVEF) ≥50%, New York Heart Association (NYHA) class II-IV symptoms, and elevated natriuretic peptides. Participants received once-weekly subcutaneous tirzepatide (titrated to maximum tolerated dose of 5, 10, or 15 mg) or placebo for a median follow-up of 104 weeks.[6] Baseline demographic and clinical characteristics of the study population, as well as key efficacy and safety outcomes, are summarized in **Table 1**.

Primary composite endpoint: The trial demonstrated a 38% relative risk reduction in the primary composite outcome of cardiovascular death or worsening heart failure events (hazard ratio [HR] 0.62; 95% confidence interval [CI], 0.41-0.95; P = 0.026).[1] This composite included heart failure hospitalizations, urgent heart failure visits requiring intravenous therapy, and oral diuretic intensification.

Individual components:

- *Worsening heart failure events* occurred in 36 patients (9.9%) in the tirzepatide group versus 56 patients (15.3%) in the placebo group (HR: 0.62; 95% CI: 0.41–0.95).[1]
- *Cardiovascular deaths* occurred in 8 patients (2.2%) in the tirzepatide group versus 5 patients (1.4%) in the

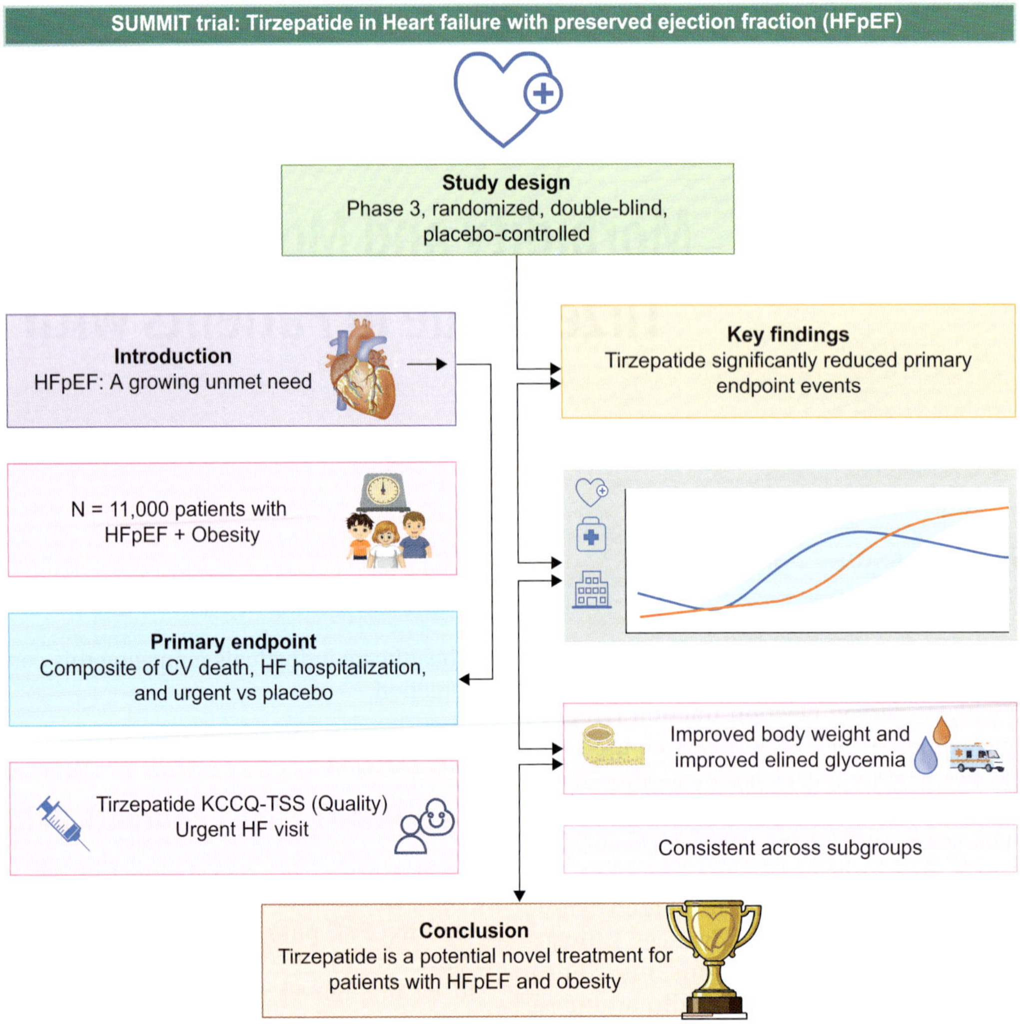

Flowchart 1: SUMMIT trial design and key results. Flowchart depicting study design (randomization schema, inclusion criteria BMI ≥30, LVEF ≥50%, NYHA II-IV) with forest plot showing primary composite endpoint (HR: 0.62; 95% CI: 0.41–0.95; *P* = 0.026) and individual components. Include key secondary endpoints: KCCQ-CSS improvement (+6.9 points), 6MWD increase (+30.5 meters), and weight reduction (–11.6% vs. –3.2%).

placebo group (HR: 1.58; 95% CI: 0.52–4.83), though this component was not statistically powered.[1]

- *All-cause mortality* showed no significant difference, with events occurring in 17 tirzepatide-treated patients versus 10 placebo patients.[1]

Functional Capacity and Quality of Life Improvements

Beyond hard cardiovascular outcomes, tirzepatide demonstrated clinically meaningful improvements in patient-centered outcomes:[1,3]

Kansas City Cardiomyopathy Questionnaire (KCCQ-CSS): At 52 weeks, tirzepatide improved KCCQ clinical summary score by a mean of 19.5 points compared to 12.7 points with placebo [estimated treatment difference (ETD) 6.9 points; 95% CI: 3.3–10.6; *P* <0.001). This exceeded the 5-point threshold for clinical significance.[1]

Six-minute walk distance (6MWD): Tirzepatide increased 6MWD by a mean of 31.6 meters compared to 1.2 meters with placebo (ETD 30.5 meters; 95% CI: 21.9–39.1; *P* <0.001), representing substantial functional improvement.[1]

EuroQol-5D-5L (EQ-5D-5L): Health-related quality of life improved significantly across all five domains (mobility, self-care, usual activities, pain/discomfort, and anxiety/depression).[1]

Weight reduction: Mean body weight decreased by 11.6% with tirzepatide versus 3.2% with placebo at 52 weeks, with greater weight loss correlating with larger improvements in functional and quality-of-life measures.[1,5]

Mechanistic Insights: Reverse Cardiac Remodeling

Secondary analyses from SUMMIT provide mechanistic understanding of tirzepatide cardiovascular benefits:[2,4]

Cardiac magnetic resonance (CMR) substudy: Among 256 patients undergoing serial CMR imaging, tirzepatide reduced:

- Left ventricular mass by 11 g ($P < 0.001$), suggesting favorable reverse remodeling[4]
- Paracardiac adipose tissue volume by 45 mL ($P < 0.001$)[4]
- The magnitude of LV mass reduction paralleled the degree of weight loss, indicating a dose-response relationship[4,5]

Hemodynamic and volumetric effects: At 52 weeks, tirzepatide reduced:

- Systolic blood pressure (ETD—5.8 mm Hg; $P < 0.001$)[2]
- Estimated plasma volume (ETD—3.8%; P<0.001)[2]
- High-sensitivity C-reactive protein (CRP) (ETD—35.2%; $P < 0.001$), reflecting reduced systemic inflammation[2]
- N-terminal pro-B-type natriuretic peptide (NT-proBNP) levels, indicating reduced cardiac wall stress[2]

Adiposity-mediated pathways: Greater reductions in waist circumference and waist-to-hip ratio correlated with larger improvements in exercise capacity and symptoms, supporting the central role of visceral adiposity in HFpEF pathophysiology.[5] Patients with higher baseline BMI and central adiposity demonstrated more severe HF phenotypes but achieved consistent benefits from tirzepatide across the adiposity spectrum.[5]

Safety Profile and Adverse Events

Tirzepatide's safety profile in HFpEF mirrored that observed in obesity and diabetes trials:[1,6]

- *Gastrointestinal effects:* The most common adverse events were nausea (17% vs. 7% placebo), diarrhea (15% vs. 9%), and vomiting (10% vs. 4%).[1] These were predominantly mild-to-moderate, occurring during dose titration, and rarely led to discontinuation.
- *Hypoglycemia:* Rates were low and similar between groups in patients without diabetes. In diabetic patients receiving concurrent glucose-lowering therapy, vigilant monitoring and medication adjustment were required.[1]
- *Serious adverse events:* Overall serious adverse event rates were comparable between tirzepatide (32%) and placebo (36%).[1] Notably, hospitalizations for worsening heart failure—the most clinically relevant serious adverse event—were reduced in the tirzepatide group.[3]
- *Discontinuations:* Treatment discontinuation rates were 13% for tirzepatide versus 9% for placebo, with gastrointestinal intolerance being the primary driver.[1]

Subgroup Analyses and Phenotype-specific Considerations

Post-hoc analyses revealed important phenotypic considerations:[3,5]

- *BMI and central adiposity:* Benefits were consistent across BMI categories (30–34.9, 35–39.9, ≥40 kg/m^2), though patients with higher BMI at baseline experienced greater absolute improvements in functional parameters.[5] Waist-to-hip ratio (WHR) emerged as an important modifier; patients with elevated WHR but lower BMI exhibited greater baseline kidney dysfunction and exercise impairment, yet still benefited from therapy.[5]
- *Diabetes status:* Approximately 50% of SUMMIT participants had type 2 diabetes.[6] Benefits on the primary endpoint and quality-of-life measures were consistent regardless of diabetes status, suggesting mechanisms beyond glycemic control contribute to therapeutic efficacy.[1,5]
- *NYHA class:* Most patients (>80%) were NYHA class II at enrollment.[6] While class III patients were underrepresented, available data suggest proportional benefit across symptom severity.[3]

Comparison with Other GLP-1 Receptor Agonists

Prior to SUMMIT, the STEP-HFpEF and STEP-HFpEF-DM trials established proof-of-concept for GLP-1 receptor agonist therapy in HFpEF using semaglutide.[7] SUMMIT extends these findings with several notable distinctions:

- *Dual agonism:* Tirzepatide's GIP receptor activity may provide additional metabolic benefits, insulin sensitivity, and potentially enhanced weight loss compared to selective GLP-1 agonists.
- *Hard cardiovascular outcomes:* SUMMIT uniquely demonstrated reduction in worsening heart failure events, whereas STEP trials focused on symptom/functional endpoints.[1,7]
- *Magnitude of effect:* Weight loss and functional improvements with tirzepatide numerically exceeded those with semaglutide, though direct comparative trials are lacking.[1,7,8]

LIMITATIONS

Trial-specific Limitations

Mortality statistical power: SUMMIT was powered for the composite endpoint, not individual mortality.[6] The numerical imbalance in cardiovascular deaths (8 vs. 5) and all-cause mortality (17 vs. 10), though not statistically significant, warrants longer-term surveillance in postmarketing studies and real-world registries.[1]

Follow-up duration: Median 104-week follow-up may be insufficient to capture long-term cardiovascular remodeling effects and mortality differences.[1] HFpEF is a chronic progressive disease; multi-year data are needed.[9]

Generalizability: SUMMIT enrolled a highly selected population (BMI ≥30, median 38 kg/m^2) with predominantly NYHA class II symptoms and stringent exclusion criteria.[6] Applicability to:

- Leaner HFpEF phenotypes (BMI <30)
- Advanced HF (NYHA IV, recent decompensation)
- Older adults (mean age 65; limited representation of ≥80 years)
- Nonobese HFpEF phenotypes (atrial fibrillation-dominant, ischemic, etc.) remain uncertain[9,10]

Racial and geographic diversity: While multinational, enrollment predominantly consisted of white participants from North America and Europe; data in Asian, Black, and Hispanic populations are limited.[6]

Clinical Implementation Challenges

Cost and access: Tirzepatide's high acquisition cost (approximately $1,000–1,500 per month) and variable insurance coverage create significant access barriers, particularly in resource-limited settings and for uninsured/underinsured patients.

Gastrointestinal tolerability: Up to 17% experience nausea, requiring careful patient selection, dose titration, and potentially excluding patients with severe gastroparesis, inflammatory bowel disease, or prior bariatric surgery.[1]

Frailty and sarcopenia: Concerns exist regarding accelerated muscle loss in elderly or frail HFpEF patients.[11] The trial excluded severely malnourished patients; clinical vigilance for sarcopenia with nutritional counseling and resistance exercise is essential.[11]

Drug-drug interactions: Delayed gastric emptying may affect absorption of oral medications. Critical medications (levothyroxine, anticoagulants, and antiseizure drugs) may require monitoring and dose adjustment.

Knowledge Gaps

- *Combination therapy:* Optimal sequencing and combination with SGLT2 inhibitors (standard of care in HFpEF) requires study; observational data suggest additive benefits, but prospective trials are lacking.[8]
- *Duration of therapy:* Appropriate treatment duration and consequences of discontinuation (weight regain, symptom recurrence) are unknown.
- *Phenotype-specific response:* Predictors of response beyond BMI (e.g., inflammatory biomarkers, adipokine profiles, and genetic markers) need identification to personalize therapy.[5]
- *Reduced EF transition:* Whether Tirzepatide prevents progression from HFpEF to HFrEF is speculative.[12]

GUIDELINES/ALGORITHM/SUMMARY ILLUSTRATION

Current Guideline Context (2024-2025)

ACC Expert Consensus on HFpEF Management (2023): Emphasizes comorbidity-directed therapy as cornerstone. It recommends:

- SGLT2 inhibitors for all HFpEF patients (class 1, level A)
- Weight loss for obese patients (class 1, level B)
- Optimal BP control, diabetes management, and treatment of atrial fibrillation

ESC Position on Obesity in CVD (2024): Acknowledges GLP-1 receptor agonists promote weight loss and cardiovascular benefits in obesity. Recommends their use in overweight/obese patients with T2DM to promote weight reduction (class IIa, level B). Post-SUMMIT, tirzepatide specifically for HFpEF is anticipated to receive stronger recommendations.

AHA/ACC/HFSA HF Guidelines (2022): Predate SUMMIT and STEP trials; recommend weight management but do not specify pharmacotherapy.[4] Updates expected in 2025-2026 guideline revisions.

Proposed Clinical Algorithm for Tirzepatide in HFpEF (Fig. 1)

STEP 1: Identify eligible patients

- Confirmed HFpEF (LVEF ≥50%, symptoms, and elevated natriuretic peptides)[4]
- BMI ≥30 kg/m^2 (or ≥27 kg/m^2 with high waist circumference/metabolic syndrome)[5,6]
- NYHA class II-III symptoms despite guideline-directed medical therapy[4]

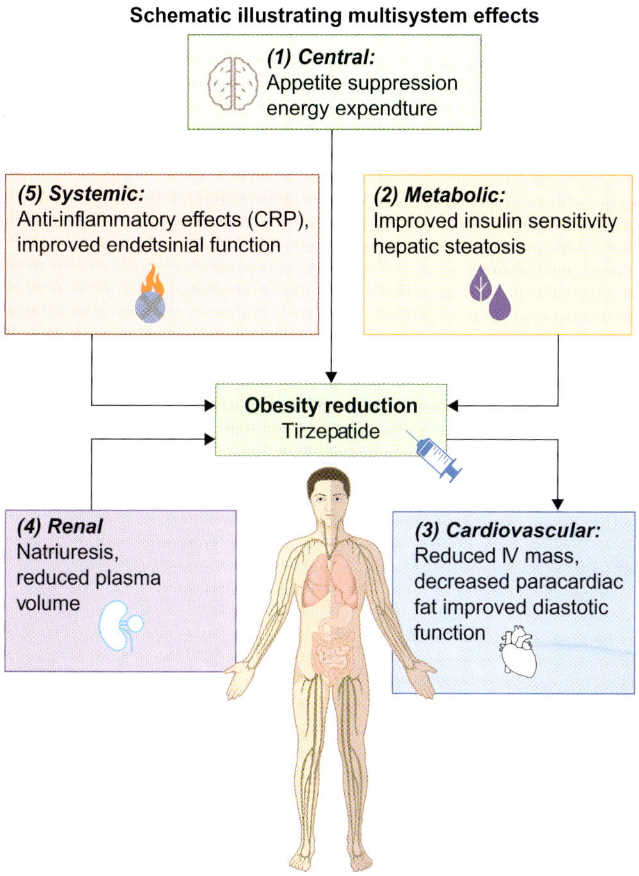

Fig. 1: Mechanistic pathways of tirzepatide in HFpEF. Schematic illustrating multisystem effects: (1) Central—appetite suppression and energy expenditure; (2) Metabolic—improved insulin sensitivity and reduced hepatic steatosis; (3) cardiovascular—reduced LV mass, decreased paracardiac fat, and improved diastolic function;[4,13] (4) Renal—natriuresis and reduced plasma volume;[2] (5) systemic—anti-inflammatory effects (↓CRP) and improved endothelial function.[2] Arrows connecting obesity reduction to each pathway.

- Absence of contraindications: Medullary thyroid cancer, MEN-2 syndrome, severe gastroparesis, active pancreatitis, and severe kidney disease (eGFR <30)

STEP 2: Optimize foundational HFpEF therapy

- Initiate/maximize SGLT2 inhibitor (dapagliflozin 10 mg or empagliflozin 10 mg daily).[4]
- Control hypertension (target SBP <130 mm Hg): Diuretics, ARNi/ARB, and MRA.[4]
- Manage diabetes (target HbA1c <7–8%).
- Treat atrial fibrillation (rate/rhythm control and anticoagulation).[4]
- Address OSA (CPAP if indicated).

STEP 3: Initiate tirzepatide

- Start 2.5 mg subcutaneously once weekly.[6]
- Titrate every 4 weeks: 2.5 → 5 → 7.5 → 10 → 15 mg based on tolerability.[6]
- Counsel on GI side effects, dietary modifications (small frequent meals, avoid high-fat foods).[1]
- Adjust concurrent diabetes medications to prevent hypoglycemia.[1]

STEP 4: Monitor response and safety

- Assess at 1, 3, 6, 12 months, then every 6 months:
  - Weight, vital signs, and symptoms (NYHA class, KCCQ)[1]
  - Functional capacity (6MWT if available)[1]
  - Natriuretic peptides, renal function, and HbA1c[2]
  - Adverse effects (GI symptoms, hypoglycemia, and pancreatitis symptoms)[1]
- Nutritional assessment (screen for sarcopenia and protein intake)[11]
- Resistance exercise prescription to preserve lean mass[11]

STEP 5: Long-term management

- Continue therapy if clinical benefit (symptom improvement, weight loss ≥5%, and reduced HF events)[3]
- Reassess if plateau or intolerance; consider dose reduction before discontinuation.
- Monitor for weight regain and symptom recurrence if therapy stopped.

CONCLUSION

The SUMMIT trial marks a paradigm shift in obesity-related HFpEF management, establishing tirzepatide as the first pharmacotherapy to demonstrate morbidity reduction in this difficult-to-treat phenotype.[1] The 38% relative risk reduction in the composite of cardiovascular death or worsening heart failure events, coupled with unprecedented improvements in functional capacity, quality of life, and cardiac reverse remodeling, positions tirzepatide as a foundational therapy alongside SGLT2 inhibitors.[1,3,4]

Mechanistic insights reveal multifaceted benefits extending beyond weight loss alone, encompassing reduced systemic inflammation, decreased adiposity-related cardiac stress, favorable hemodynamic remodeling, and improved metabolic health.[2,4,5,13] The consistency of benefit across diabetes status, BMI categories, and baseline functional capacity strengthens the generalizability of findings within the obesity-HFpEF phenotype.[5]

However, important caveats temper enthusiasm. The numerical imbalance in mortality events, though statistically nonsignificant, necessitates cautious interpretation and extended surveillance.[1] Cost, access

TABLE 1: Baseline characteristics and outcomes in SUMMIT.

Characteritic		*Tirzepatide (n = 364)*	*Placebo (n = 367)*
Demographics and comorbidities			
Age (years)		65 ± 11	65 ± 11
Female (%)	58%	38 ± 5	60 ± 11
BMI (kg/m^2)	58%	38 ± 6	38 ± 10
Hypertension (%)	90%	30 ± 6	320 ± 50
T2DM (%)	90%	320 ± 50	320 ± 50
Hypertertion (%)	30%	55 ± 5	55 ± 5
Atrial fibrillation (%)			

Baseline measurements		*Outcomes*	
KCCQ-CSS	45 ± 10	12%	18%
KCCQ-CSS	45 ± 10	12%	↓
Primary endpoint events			
Hospitalizations	+10	+1%	32
KCQQ change (points)	+2	↑	↑
6MWD change (meters)	+5	↑	
Adverse events (%)	70%	60	⚠

Note: Two-column table comparing tirzepatide (n = 364) versus placebo (n = 367): Demographics (age 65 ± 11 years, 58% female, BMI 38 ± 6 kg/m^2),[6] comorbidities (T2DM 50%, HTN 90%, atrial fibrillation 30%),[6] baseline KCCQ-CSS, 6MWD, LVEF. Outcomes: primary endpoint events, hospitalizations, KCCQ/6MWD changes, and adverse events.[1]

barriers, gastrointestinal tolerability, and potential sarcopenia risk require individualized assessment.[11] Optimal integration with SGLT2 inhibitors, appropriate patient selection beyond BMI cut-offs, and long-term durability of benefit remain active research questions.[8]

Looking forward, tirzepatide exemplifies the promise of phenotype-specific HFpEF therapeutics.[10,12] As obesity prevalence escalates globally, and HFpEF incidence rises in parallel, tirzepatide addresses a critical unmet need.[9,14] Forthcoming guideline updates will likely incorporate tirzepatide as a class IIa or I recommendation for obesity-related HFpEF, fundamentally reshaping clinical practice. Clinicians should familiarize themselves with appropriate patient selection, dosing protocols, and monitoring strategies to optimize outcomes while minimizing risks.

In the evolving landscape of HFpEF management—moving from "one-size-fits-all" approaches toward precision, phenotype-guided therapy—tirzepatide stands as a testament to translating mechanistic understanding into tangible clinical benefit.[12,15] For the obese patient with HFpEF, struggling with dyspnea, exercise intolerance, and impaired quality of life despite conventional therapy, tirzepatide offers genuine hope for improved morbidity and restored functional capacity.[1,3]

REFERENCES

1. Kosiborod MN, Abildstrøm SZ, Borlaug BA, et al. Tirzepatide for Heart Failure with Preserved Ejection Fraction and Obesity. N Engl J Med. 2024;391(23):2203-12.
2. Borlaug BA, Zile MR, Kramer CM, et al. Effects of Tirzepatide on circulatory overload and end-organ damage in heart failure with preserved ejection fraction and obesity: a secondary analysis of the SUMMIT trial. Nat Med. 2024;30(12):3649-56.
3. Neuen BL, Cherney DZI, Kosiborod MN, et al. Effects of Tirzepatide on the Clinical Trajectory of Patients With Heart Failure, Preserved Ejection Fraction, and Obesity. Circulation. 2025;151(2):112-22.
4. Abbasi J, Lundberg GP, Ferdinand KC. Tirzepatide Reduces LV Mass and Paracardiac Adipose Tissue in

Obesity-Related Heart Failure: SUMMIT CMR Substudy. J Am Coll Cardiol. 2024;84(25):2503-17.
5. Kosiborod MN, Petrie MC, Borlaug BA, et al. Impact of Body Mass Index, Central Adiposity, and Weight Loss on the Benefits of Tirzepatide in HFpEF: The SUMMIT Trial. J Am Coll Cardiol. 2025;86(4):242-55.
6. Kosiborod MN, Abildstrøm SZ, Borlaug BA, et al. Design and Baseline Characteristics of SUMMIT: Semaglutide and Tirzepatide in HFpEF with Morbid Obesity. JACC Heart Fail. 2023;11(8 Pt 2):1024-38.
7. Kosiborod MN, Petrie MC, Borlaug BA, et al. Semaglutide in Patients with Obesity-Related Heart Failure and Type 2 Diabetes. N Engl J Med. 2024;390(15):1394-407.
8. Sharma A, Vaishnav AS, Ezekowitz JA, et al. GLP-1 Receptor Agonists Along With SGLT2 Inhibitors in Heart Failure With Preserved Ejection Fraction. JACC Heart Fail. 2024;12(11):1814-26.
9. Dunlay SM, Roger VL, Redfield MM. Epidemiology of heart failure with preserved ejection fraction. Nat Rev Cardiol. 2017;14(10):591-602.
10. Heidenreich PA, Bozkurt B, Aguilar D, et al. 2022 AHA/ACC/HFSA Guideline for the Management of Heart Failure. Circulation. 2022;145(18):e895-1032.
11. Kitzman DW, Brubaker P, Morgan T, et al. Effect of Caloric Restriction or Aerobic Exercise Training on Peak Oxygen Consumption and Quality of Life in Obese Older Patients With Heart Failure With Preserved Ejection Fraction. JAMA. 2016;315(1):36-46.
12. Borlaug BA, Redfield MM. Diastolic and systolic heart failure are distinct phenotypes within the heart failure spectrum. Circulation. 2011;123(18):2006-13.
13. Borlaug BA, Kass DA. Ventricular-vascular interaction in heart failure. Cardiol Clin. 2011;29(3):447-59.
14. Vaduganathan M, Claggett BL, Jhund PS, et al. Projected Burden of Heart Failure with Preserved Ejection Fraction. JACC Heart Fail. 2022;10(10):715-25.
15. Virani SS, Newby LK, Arnold SV, et al. 2023 AHA/ACC/ACCP/ASPC/NLA/PCNA Guideline for the Management of Patients with Chronic Coronary Disease. Circulation. 2023;148(9):e9-119.

132

CHAPTER

Metabolic Benefits, Weight Loss, and Safety Data of Tirzepatide in SURMOUNT Trials 1–5

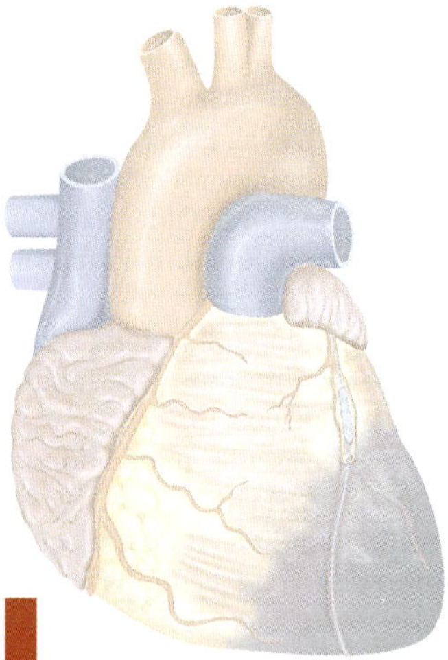

Jugal Kishor Sharma, Pooja Khosla, Vinus Taneja

INTRODUCTION

A significant development in the pharmacologic treatment of metabolic disorders is tirzepatide, a novel dual agonist of the glucose-dependent insulinotropic polypeptide (GIP) and glucagon-like peptide-1 (GLP-1) receptors. When compared to conventional single-pathway therapies, its special "twincretin" mechanism allows for the synergistic activation of both incretin pathways, producing better improvements in glycemic control, weight loss, and cardiovascular health. Tirzepatide is a synthetic 39-amino acid peptide that is structurally derived from the native GIP backbone. Its pharmacokinetic stability and duration of action are improved by lipidation, terminal amidation, and selective amino acid substitutions.

Clinically significant decreases in body weight, blood pressure, and cardiometabolic risk are achieved by tirzepatide's potent effects on glucose regulation, appetite suppression, and energy metabolism through its dual-receptor activity. Tirzepatide is positioned as a transformative therapy in the continuum of managing cardiovascular and metabolic diseases due to its effectiveness in a variety of clinical populations, including those with type 2 diabetes, obesity, metabolic syndrome, and heart failure.

STRUCTURE

Overview

Tirzepatide is a synthetic 39-amino-acid peptide engineered to activate both GIP and GLP-1 receptors. This dual action improves glycemic control and induces profound weight loss in type 2 diabetes and obesity.[1]

Peptide Backbone

Modeled after native human GIP, tirzepatide incorporates strategic modifications from semaglutide and GLP-1 to enhance metabolic activity. Two α-aminoisobutyric acid (Aib) residues at positions 2 and 13 confer resistance to dipeptidyl peptidase-4 (DPP-4) degradation, improving stability and pharmacokinetics.[2]

Lipidation

A γ-glutamate and bis-aminodiethoxyacetyl spacer links a C20 fatty diacid chain (eicosanedioic acid) to lysine-20, enabling albumin binding and extending the elimination half-life to permit once-weekly dosing.[1]

Terminal Modification

C-terminal amidation enhances molecular stability and minimizes enzymatic degradation.[1]

MECHANISM OF ACTION

Glucose-dependent Insulinotropic Polypeptide Receptor Agonism

Tirzepatide binds to GIPR with high affinity (Kd ≈ 0.135 nM). It enhances glucose-stimulated insulin secretion and improves adipose tissue insulin sensitivity. Blockade studies confirm that GIPR signaling is central to tirzepatide's insulinotropic and glucose-lowering effects.[3]

Glucagon-like Peptide-1 Receptor Agonism

Tirzepatide is a *biased agonist* at GLP-1R (Ki ≈4.2 nM), favoring cAMP signaling while limiting β-arrestin recruitment, thereby reducing receptor desensitization. This leads to sustained insulin release, reduced glucagon secretion, slowed gastric emptying, and appetite suppression.[3,4]

Synergistic Dual-receptor Activation

Simultaneous GIPR and GLP-1R stimulation yields additive benefits in glycemic control and body-weight reduction beyond those achieved with selective GLP-1 agonists. Dual activation increases adiponectin (~26%), improving lipid handling and insulin sensitivity.[1,4]

Pharmacokinetics:[3,4]

- *Bioavailability*: ~80% (SC)
- *Albumin binding*: ~99%
- *Volume of distribution*: ~10 L
- T_{max}: 8–72 hours
- $t_{½}$: ~5 days (supports weekly dosing)

Metabolism occurs via proteolytic cleavage and β-oxidation; tirzepatide bypasses CYP450 pathways, with metabolites excreted in urine and feces.

Structural insight: Cryo-EM imaging reveals dual-site receptor binding that promotes Gs-protein activation. The lipidated Lys20 enhances reversible albumin binding, while Aib residues slow enzymatic degradation, prolonging action.[1,2]

ROLE IN HYPERTENSION

Clinical Evidence

In the *SURMOUNT-1 trial*, tirzepatide lowered systolic BP by ~6.8 mm Hg and diastolic BP by ~4.2 mm Hg versus placebo over 72 weeks.[5]

Mechanistic Basis

Weight loss is the main mediator, explaining ~70% of BP reduction (r = 0.31; p < 0.0001). Decreases in circulating volume and improved vascular compliance also contribute. Data from *SUMMIT* showed sustained reductions in systolic BP (–5 mm Hg) and blood volume (–0.6 L) with parallel improvements in exercise capacity, reflecting better hemodynamics and cardiac efficiency.[5]

Clinical and Regulatory Status

Although not yet approved as an antihypertensive, tirzepatide (FDA-approved for *type 2 diabetes* and *chronic weight management*) consistently lowers BP in diverse populations, supporting its role as a cardiometabolic therapy.

Major Trials

- *SURMOUNT-1*: Reduced prevalence of stage 2 hypertension from 16% → 7% among obese, nondiabetic adults.[5]
- *SUMMIT*: In HFpEF with obesity, tirzepatide cut cardiovascular death or worsening HF by 38%, with consistent benefits across CKD subgroups.[6]
- *Real-world studies*: Among >140,000 patients, tirzepatide reduced major adverse cardiovascular events (MACE) by 20% (HR 0.80 vs. GLP-1 monotherapy).[7]

Safety and Implications

Mild dizziness (4–5%) was the most frequent BP-related adverse event; severe hypotension was rare (0.2%). Tirzepatide's ability to lower BP, body weight, and insulin resistance simultaneously suggests it may evolve into a frontline therapy for obesity-associated hypertension pending outcome-trial validation.[5]

ROLE IN CARDIOMETABOLIC HEALTH

Comprehensive Effects

Through dual GIP–GLP-1 activation, tirzepatide improves multiple cardiometabolic domains: Glycemia, lipid profile, inflammation, liver health, and adiposity distribution. It acts beyond glucose lowering to modify cardiovascular and renal risk physiology.[8]

Lipid Profile Modulation

Meta-analyses of randomized trials demonstrate dose-dependent improvements in all lipid parameters: Triglyceride reductions up to 22%, LDL decrease, total-cholesterol decline, and HDL increase. Tirzepatide also reduces atherogenic lipoproteins (ApoB, ApoC-III) while elevating protective adiponectin levels, reflecting improved lipid handling and endothelial function.[9]

Insulin Sensitivity and Pancreatic Function

Tirzepatide substantially lowers fasting insulin and HOMA2-IR indices, with only 20–40% of its effect attributable to weight loss alone. Beta-cell recovery is evident from HOMA2-B increases (~100%) and large decreases in proinsulin levels (–50%) and proinsulin/C-peptide ratios, indicating restored insulin synthesis and improved secretory efficiency.[10]

Body Composition and Visceral Fat

Dual-energy X-ray studies (SURMOUNT-1 DXA) revealed selective fat reduction: ~75% of weight loss from fat mass with preservation of lean tissue. Visceral and hepatic fat declined significantly, accompanied by improved muscle composition and reduced intramuscular lipid infiltration.[11]

Metabolic Syndrome Reduction

In pooled analyses ($n \approx 7{,}800$), the prevalence of metabolic syndrome declined from 82 to 51%, corresponding to a 72% reduction in risk. Individual parameters improved across BP, triglycerides, HDL-C, and waist circumference, emphasizing its holistic metabolic correction.[8]

Hepatic and Anti-inflammatory Benefits

Tirzepatide demonstrated substantial efficacy in metabolic-associated steatotic liver disease (MASLD). The SYNERGY-NASH trial showed steatohepatitis resolution in >70% of patients at high doses, reducing liver fat by >50% and improving fibrosis markers. Anti-inflammatory effects include reductions in hs-CRP, YKL-40, ICAM-1, and leptin levels within weeks, paralleling improvements in adipokine balance and endothelial function **(Fig. 1)**.[12]

TIRZEPATIDE AND WEIGHT MANAGEMENT

In Obesity without Diabetes

In SURMOUNT-1 (72 weeks), tirzepatide achieved unprecedented pharmacologic weight loss: Mean 16, 21, and 22.5% reductions with 5, 10, and 15 mg doses, compared with 2.4% for placebo. Up to 57% of participants lost ≥20% of body weight. SURMOUNT-5 confirmed superiority over semaglutide (20.2 vs. 13.7% weight loss at 72 weeks). These represent the largest recorded effects from any medication-based obesity therapy.[13]

In Obesity with Type 2 Diabetes

Across the SURPASS program, tirzepatide produced dose-dependent reductions in both weight and HbA1c. In SURPASS-1, mean losses were 7.0 kg (5 mg), 7.8 kg (10 mg), and 9.5 kg (15 mg), versus 0.7 kg with placebo. SURPASS-2 showed superiority to semaglutide 1 mg.[14]

Real-world Effectiveness

In a 1,896-patient analysis, tirzepatide induced 7.3 kg mean weight loss over ~10 months. Compared with semaglutide, tirzepatide produced superior outcomes (>5% loss: 49 vs. 26%; >15% loss: 10 vs. 3%). Efficacy was greater in nondiabetic individuals, confirming the strength of its appetite-regulating and metabolic effects.[15]

Long-term Maintenance and Discontinuation

The SURMOUNT-4 trial demonstrated ongoing therapy necessity for sustained results: Only 5% of those switched

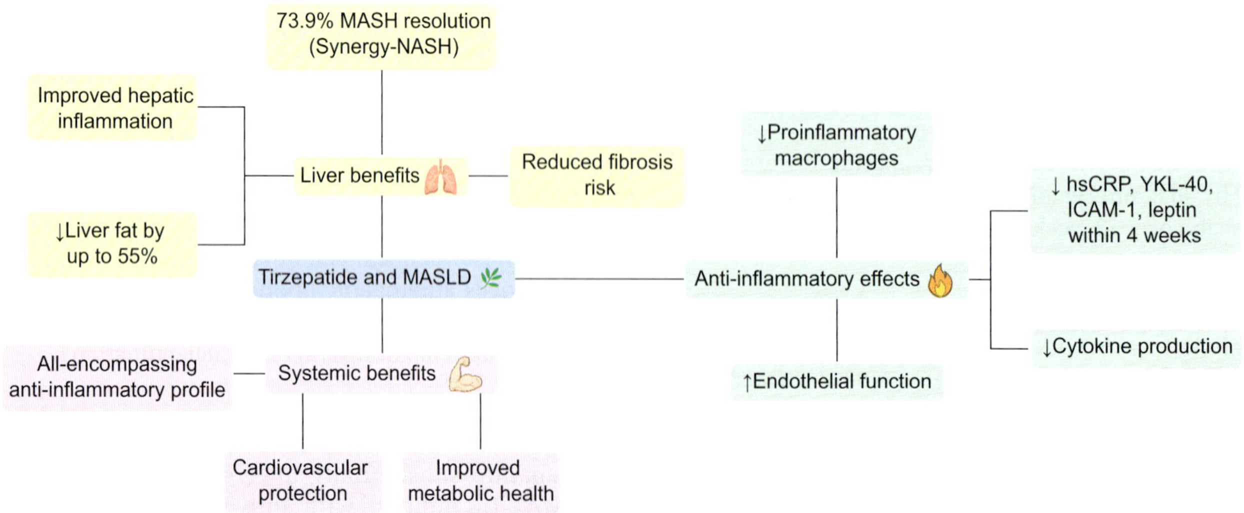

Fig. 1: Comprehensive effects of tirzepatide on liver and systemic inflammation.

to placebo maintained ≥25% weight loss at 88 weeks versus 55% of continuous-dose recipients. Discontinuation led to partial regain and reduced quality of life **(Fig. 2)**.[16,17]

TIRZEPATIDE'S ROLE IN HYPOGONADISM

Tirzepatide demonstrates potential as a nonhormonal therapy for obesity-related hypogonadism. In a pilot trial involving men with functional hypogonadism, 2 months of treatment yielded greater improvements in body weight, endogenous testosterone, and erectile function compared with testosterone replacement or lifestyle modification. The drug enhanced LH, FSH, and SHBG levels, leading to sustained recovery of the hypothalamic–pituitary–gonadal axis and normalization of testosterone in most subjects after prolonged therapy. Improvements in erectile function correlated with vascular and metabolic restoration, underscoring tirzepatide's capacity to reverse the underlying pathophysiology rather than provide exogenous hormonal substitution.[18,19]

SAFETY DATA OF TIRZEPATIDE IN SURMOUNT AND SURPASS TRIALS

Tirzepatide showed a good and well-tolerated safety profile that was on par with other GLP-1 receptor agonists in the SURPASS (type 2 diabetes) and SURMOUNT (obesity/overweight without diabetes) trials. The majority of side effects were mild to moderate in intensity, dose-dependent, and mostly gastrointestinal in nature, including constipation, diarrhea, and nausea. The low frequency of serious adverse events (SAEs) and their rates of occurrence compared to placebo or active comparators support tirzepatide's excellent general safety and tolerability in a range of patient populations.

Safety Data Comparison Across SURMOUNT Trials 1–4

Study Population Overview

The SURMOUNT trials evaluated tirzepatide in different populations:

- *SURMOUNT-1*: Obesity/overweight without diabetes
- *SURMOUNT-2*: Obesity with type 2 diabetes
- *SURMOUNT-3*: Obesity/overweight after intensive lifestyle intervention
- *SURMOUNT-4*: Weight maintenance after initial tirzepatide treatment

Any Adverse Events

Adverse event rates were consistently higher with tirzepatide across all trials, ranging from 77 to 87% versus 71 to 77% with placebo **(Table 1)**.[16,20-22]

Gastrointestinal Side Effects

SURMOUNT-4 (maintenance phase) showed the lowest GI adverse event rates, likely due to patients being already established on treatment **(Table 2)**.[16]

Treatment Discontinuation due to Adverse Events

Discontinuation rates were highest in SURMOUNT-1 and SURMOUNT-2, with the 10 mg dose showing consistently higher discontinuation rates across trials **(Table 3)**.[16,20]

Serious Adverse Events

Serious adverse event rates were generally similar between tirzepatide and placebo across all trials, indicating no increased risk of serious complications **(Table 4)**.[16,20,21]

Mortality by Trial

No deaths were attributed to tirzepatide by investigators across all trials **(Table 5)**.[16,20]

Special Safety Concerns

- *Pancreatitis*: The incidence was <0.5% in SURMOUNT-1, 0% in SURMOUNT-2, 0.3% in both tirzepatide and placebo groups in SURMOUNT-3, and 0% in adjudicated cases in SURMOUNT-4.[16,20,21]
- *Cholelithiasis/cholecystitis*: Tirzepatide was associated with slightly higher rates (1–2% in SURMOUNT-1, 1.4 vs. 1.0% in SURMOUNT-3), whereas SURMOUNT-4 reported 0.3% in both groups, suggesting a mild but discernible class effect.[16,20,21]

Key Safety Patterns Across Trials

Throughout trials, tirzepatide has demonstrated a reliable and positive safety profile. The risk of hypoglycemia was low in participants without diabetes, whereas the rates of serious events were comparable in diabetic cohorts but slightly higher overall. As tolerability improved over time, adverse events were lowest during maintenance phases. The 10 mg dose had the highest discontinuation rates and gastrointestinal side effects, which were most prevalent during dose escalation but lessened with continued use. Safety results were dose-dependent. Tirzepatide's long-term tolerability and clinical safety were supported by its overall stable safety across populations, which showed no new safety signals or elevated cardiovascular risk.[16,20,21]

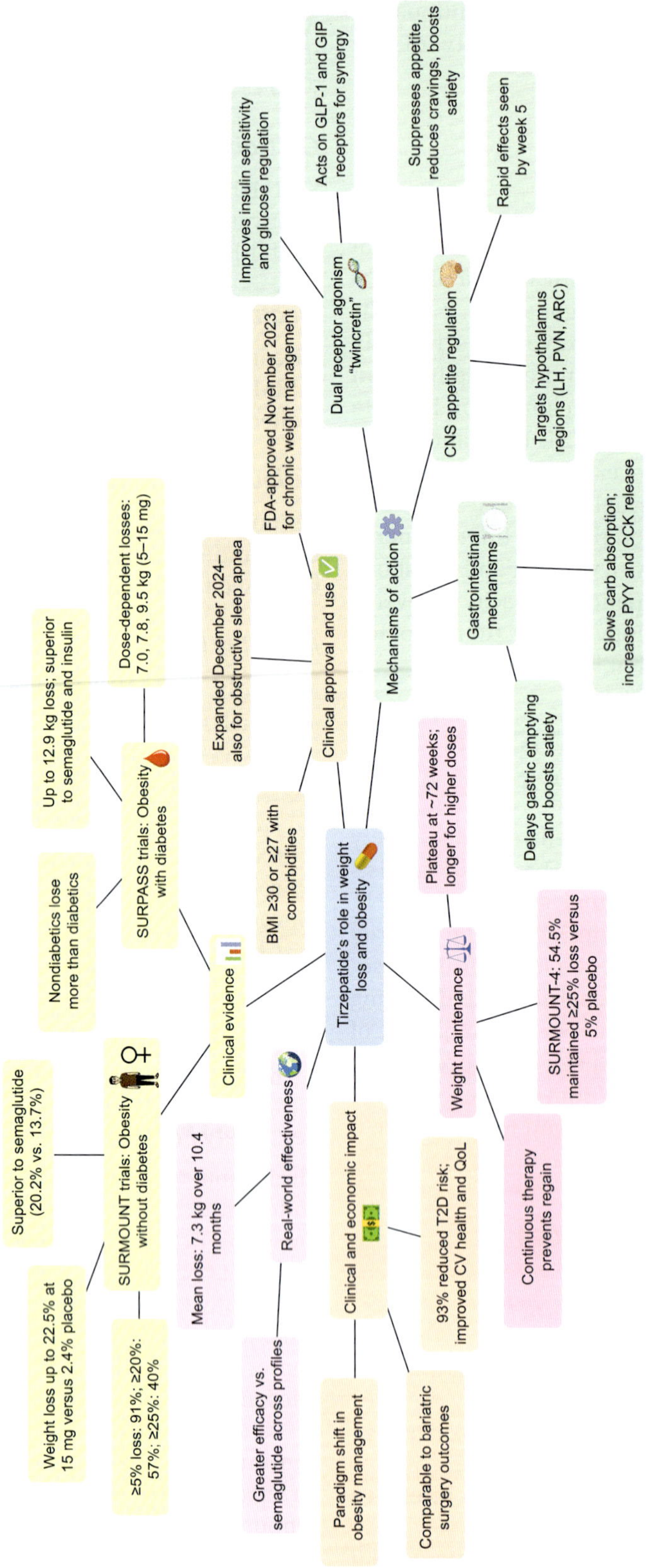

Fig. 2: Tirzepatide's role in weight loss and obesity management.

TABLE 1: SURMOUNT trials any adverse event summary.

Trial	*Population*	*Tirzepatide 5 mg*	*Tirzepatide 10 mg*	*Tirzepatide 15 mg*	*Placebo/control*
SURMOUNT-1	Obesity without DM	81%	82%	79%	72%
SURMOUNT-2	Obesity with T2DM	Not specified	77.8%	80.5%	71.2%/71.0%
SURMOUNT-3	Postlifestyle intervention	87.1%	–	–	76.7%
SURMOUNT-4	Maintenance phase	–	26.3%	–	10.4%

TABLE 2: SURMOUNT trial gastrointestinal adverse event summary.

Trial	*Event*	*Tirzepatide 5 mg*	*Tirzepatide 10 mg*	*Tirzepatide 15 mg*	*Placebo*
SURMOUNT-1	Nausea	25%	33%	31%	10%
	Diarrhea	19%	21%	23%	7%
	Vomiting	8%	11%	12%	2%
SURMOUNT-2	Nausea	–	31%	36%	9%/6%
	Diarrhea	–	23%	24%	9%/8%
	Vomiting	–	13%	16%	2%/1%
SURMOUNT-3	Nausea	27.2%	–	–	6.8%
	Diarrhea	Not specified	–	–	Not specified
	Vomiting	Not specified	–	–	Not specified
SURMOUNT-4	Nausea	–	8.1%	–	2.7%
	Diarrhea	–	10.7%	–	4.8%
	Vomiting	–	5.7%	–	1.2%

TABLE 3: Discontinuation rate by trials.

Trial	*Population*	*Tirzepatide 5 mg*	*Tirzepatide 10 mg*	*Tirzepatide 15 mg*	*Placebo*
SURMOUNT-1	Obesity without DM	4.3%	7.1%	6.2%	2.6%
SURMOUNT-2	Obesity with T2DM		6.1%	7.3%	3.0%/3.2%
SURMOUNT-3	Postlifestyle	Not specified	–	–	Not specified
SURMOUNT-4	Maintenance	–	1.8%	–	0.9%

TABLE 4: Serious adverse events rate by trials.

Trial	*Tirzepatide 5 mg*	*Tirzepatide 10 mg*	*Tirzepatide 15 mg*	*Placebo*
SURMOUNT-1	6%	7%	5%	7%
SURMOUNT-2	–	6.5%	5.4%	6.6%/6.5%
SURMOUNT-3	5.9%	–	–	4.8%
SURMOUNT-4	–	3.0%	–	3.0%

TABLE 5: Death reported in SURMOUNT trials.

Trial	*Tirzepatide deaths*	*Placebo deaths*	*Causes*
SURMOUNT-1	7 total (4 in 5 mg, 2 in 10 mg, 1 in 15 mg)	0	COVID-19, trauma, hepatic failure, homicide, stroke
SURMOUNT-2	2 (both in 10 mg)	0	Smoke inhalation, cardiorespiratory arrest
SURMOUNT-3	1 (myocardial infarction)	1 (myocardial infarction)	Neither considered drug-related
SURMOUNT-4	1 (congestive heart failure)	1 (colon adenocarcinoma)	Neither considered drug-related

TABLE 6: SURPASS trial safety summary.

Parameter	SURPASS-1 (monotherapy)	SURPASS-2 (vs. semaglutide)	SURPASS-3 (vs. insulin degludec)	SURPASS-4 (CVOT background)	SURPASS-5 (add-on to insulin glargine)
Population	T2DM, drug-naïve	T2DM on metformin	T2DM on metformin	T2DM with CVD risk factors	T2DM on insulin glargine
Common GI AEs (nausea/diarrhea/vomiting)	27/21/10%	31/23/13%	35/25/15%	29/22/12%	33/24/16%
Discontinuation due to AEs	5.2%	6.8%	7.5%	6.3%	8.1%
Serious AEs	3.5%	4.1%	5.0%	4.6%	5.8%
Hypoglycemia (severe/overall)	Rare (<1%/ <5%)	Rare (<1%/<4%)	Rare (<1%/<4%)	Rare (<1%/<3%)	2%/12% (with insulin background)
Pancreatitis	<0.5%	<0.5%	<0.5%	<0.5%	<0.5%
Gallbladder disease	1.2%	1.4%	1.5%	1.3%	1.6%
Injection site reactions	2.8%	3.1%	3.4%	3.0%	3.5%
Deaths	None drug-related	None drug-related	None drug-related	None drug-related	None drug-related

Comparative Safety Profile of Tirzepatide in SURPASS-1 to SURPASS-5 Trials

Tirzepatide continuously showed a good safety profile in the five pivotal SURPASS trials for type 2 diabetes. The majority of adverse effects were mild and temporary gastrointestinal symptoms that were dose-dependent, like nausea or diarrhea. Serious side effects were rare and happened at rates comparable to those of other diabetes treatments. Severe hypoglycemia was rare and mostly happened when tirzepatide was taken with sulfonylureas or high-dose insulin.[16,20,21]

Important findings from the SURPASS trials demonstrate tirzepatide's excellent general safety and tolerability. The most frequent gastrointestinal side effects, which were primarily nausea, vomiting, and diarrhea, occurred during dose escalation, particularly at the 15 mg dose, and usually went away with time. From 5.2% in SURPASS-1 to 8.1% in SURPASS-5—the latter because it was used with insulin—treatment discontinuations were rare.[16,20]

Except in cases where tirzepatide was used in conjunction with sulfonylureas or high-dose insulin, where rates reached roughly 12% in SURPASS-5, severe hypoglycemia was extremely uncommon (<1%). There were no new safety concerns found, and SAEs, such as pancreatitis, happened in <0.5–5% of cases, which is comparable to other treatments. Crucially, even in patients with high cardiovascular risk, tirzepatide was not linked to any deaths, confirming its good safety record in a variety of clinical contexts **(Tables 6 and 7)**.[16,20,21]

TABLE 7: Current limitations and missing data for tirzepatide.

Aspect	Key limitations/missing data
Long-term safety and tolerability	Safety data limited beyond 2 years; long-term risks (pancreatitis, medullary thyroid carcinoma, cancer, CV outcomes) not fully established
Real-world effectiveness and adherence	Trial outcomes may not reflect real-world settings; discontinuation and AE rates may differ
Comparative efficacy and positioning	No definitive evidence for MACE reduction; ongoing CVOTs versus semaglutide/SGLT2i; uncertain benefit of combination therapy
Special populations	Insufficient data in renal/hepatic impairment, pregnancy, pediatrics, elderly ≥75 years, transplant recipients, prior pancreatitis
Durability of weight loss and benefits	Weight regain after discontinuation (SURMOUNT-4); unclear long-term maintenance strategy
Affordability, access, and health system integration	High cost; limited insurance coverage; unclear cost-effectiveness for long-term obesity care

CONCLUSION

In the treatment of metabolic and cardiometabolic disorders, tirzepatide represents a paradigm shift. It tackles the multifactorial nature of type 2 diabetes and obesity by combining strong glycemic control, significant weight loss, and all-encompassing cardiovascular benefits into a single agent. Its superior efficacy, favorable safety profile, and potential to improve long-term cardiovascular outcomes are consistently demonstrated by clinical evidence from the SURPASS and SURMOUNT programs.

Current data support tirzepatide's role as a cornerstone therapy for patients with metabolic and obesity-related diseases, even though ongoing trials like SURPASS-CVOT will further clarify its impact on morbidity and mortality. By bridging the gap between glucose control, weight management, and cardiovascular protection, tirzepatide may redefine the standards of cardiometabolic care with further research, optimization of dosing strategies, and long-term surveillance.

REFERENCES

1. Chavda VP, Ajabiya J, Teli D, et al. Tirzepatide, a new era of dual-targeted treatment for diabetes and obesity: a mini-review. Molecules. 2022;27(13):4315.
2. Zhao F, Zhou Q, Cong Z, et al. Structural insights into multiplexed pharmacological actions of tirzepatide and peptide 20 at the GIP, GLP-1 or glucagon receptors. Nature Commun. 2022;13(1):1057.
3. PDB101. Diabetes Mellitus: Tirzepatide. [online] Available from https://pdb101.rcsb.org/global-health/diabetes-mellitus/drugs/incretins/drug/tirzepatide/tirzepatide. [Last accessed January, 2026].
4. Farzam K, Patel P. Tirzepatide. Treasure Island: StatPearls; 2024.
5. Krumholz HM, de Lemos JA, Sattar N, et al. Tirzepatide and blood pressure reduction: stratified analyses of the SURMOUNT-1 randomised controlled trial. Heart. 2024;110:heartjnl-324170.
6. Packer M, Zile MR, Kramer CM, et al. Tirzepatide for heart failure with preserved ejection fraction and obesity. N Engl J Med. 2025;392(5):427-37.
7. Chuang MH, Chen JY, Wang HY, et al. Clinical outcomes of tirzepatide or GLP-1 receptor agonists in individuals with type 2 diabetes. JAMA Network Open. 2024;7(8): e2427258.
8. Sattar N, García-Pérez L-E, Rodríguez A, et al. Tirzepatide and cardiometabolic parameters in obesity: summary of current evidence. Diabetes Obes Metabo. 2025;27(10):5386-92.
9. Corrao S, Pollicino C, Maggio D, et al. Tirzepatide against obesity and insulin-resistance: pathophysiological aspects and clinical evidence. Front Endocrinol (Lausanne). 2024;15:1402583.
10. Thomas MK, Nikooienejad A, Bray R, et al. Dual GIP and GLP-1 receptor agonist tirzepatide improves beta-cell function and insulin sensitivity in type 2 diabetes. J Clin Endocrinol Metab. 2020;106(2):388-96.
11. Lee CJ, Mao H, Thieu VT, et al. Tirzepatide as monotherapy improved markers of beta-cell function and insulin sensitivity in type 2 diabetes (SURPASS-1). J Endocr Soc. 2023;7(5):bvad056.
12. American College of Gastroenterology. (2024). Tirzepatide Produces NASH Resolution and Decreases Fibrosis: Results from the SYNERGY-NASH Trial. [online] Available from https://gi.org/journals-publications/ebgi/rich_jul2024/. [Last accessed January, 2026].
13. Ard J, Lee CJ, Gudzune K, et al. Weight reduction over time in tirzepatide-treated participants by early weight loss response: post hoc analysis in SURMOUNT-1. Diabetes Obes Metab. 2025;27(9):5064-71.
14. American Diabetes Association. (2021). Latest Data From SURPASS Trials Demonstrate Tirzepatide Provided Meaningful Blood Sugar Reductions. [online] Available from https://diabetes.org/newsroom/latest-data-from-SURPASS-trials-demonstrate-tirzepatide-provided-blood-sugar-reductions-weight-loss. [Last accessed January, 2026].
15. Kelly MS, Scopelliti EM, Goodson KE, et al. Real-world evaluation of the effects of tirzepatide in patients with type 2 diabetes mellitus. Diabetes Obes Metabo. 2024;26(12):5661-8.
16. Aronne LJ, Sattar N, Horn DB, et al. Continued treatment with tirzepatide for maintenance of weight reduction in adults with obesity: the SURMOUNT-4 Randomized Clinical Trial. JAMA. 2024;331(1):38-48.
17. Gibble TH, Cao D, Murphy M, et al. Tirzepatide associated with improved health-related quality of life in adults with obesity or overweight in SURMOUNT-4. Obesity (Silver Spring). 2025;33(11):2076-92.
18. Tucker ME. (2025). Tirzepatide Tops TRT for Men With Hypogonadism and Obesity. [online] Available from https://www.medscape.com/viewarticle/tirzepatide-tops-trt-men-hypogonadism-and-obesity-2025a1000jga. [Last accessed January, 2026].
19. Cowart K, Murphy C, Carris N. Association of tirzepatide with erectile dysfunction in people with type 2 diabetes. J Diabetes Complicat. 2025;39(10):109116.
20. Wadden TA, Chao AM, Machineni S, et al. Tirzepatide after intensive lifestyle intervention in adults with overweight or obesity: the SURMOUNT-3 phase 3 trial. Nat Med. 2023;29(29):1-10.
21. Sinha R, Papamargaritis D, Sargeant JA, et al. Efficacy and safety of tirzepatide in type 2 diabetes and obesity management. J Obes Metab Syndr. 2023;32(1):25-45.
22. Hunter Gibble T, Cao D, Zhang XM, et al. Tirzepatide was associated with improved health-related quality of life in adults with obesity or overweight and type 2 diabetes: results from the phase 3 SURMOUNT-2 trial. Diabetes Ther. 2025;16(5):977-91.

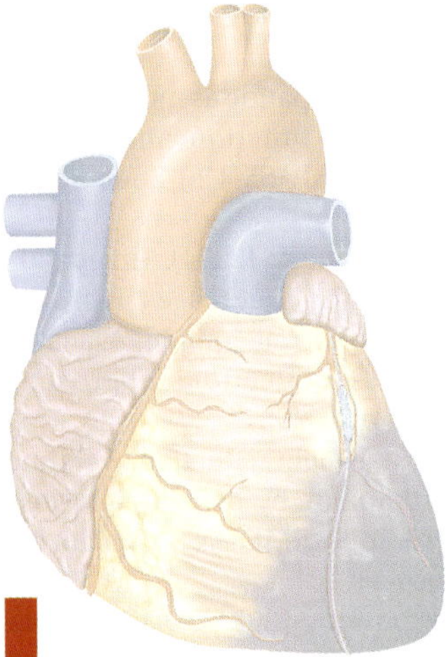

133
CHAPTER

Head-to-Head Comparison of Tirzepatide (10 mg and 15 mg) versus Semaglutide (1.7 mg and 2.4 mg) in Obesity with or without Diabetes

Sanjay Mittal, Aparajita Kumar, Abhishek Kumar Tiwari

INTRODUCTION

Obesity is a complex, progressive, and relapsing adiposity-related disease, which has emerged as a global health crisis affecting over 650 million adults. Although it is debatable on whether to classify obesity as a disease or a mere lifestyle choice, the incidence is rapidly increasing causing adverse impact on metabolic health, cardiovascular disease (CVD) incidence, and mortality globally. The advent of glucagon-like peptide-1 receptor agonists (GLP-1RAs) has revolutionized the pharmacological management of obesity, of which semaglutide and tirzepatide represent the most potent options currently available. These agents have demonstrated clinical benefit in specific high-risk patient groups such as atherosclerotic cardiovascular disease (ASCVD), heart failure with preserved ejection fraction (HFpEF), metabolic dysfunction-associated steatohepatitis, obstructive sleep apnea, osteoarthritis, and diabetes mellitus.

Tirzepatide 10–15 mg and semaglutide 1.7–2.4 mg are both highly effective incretin-based therapies for obesity, with or without type 2 diabetes (T2D). Tirzepatide provides greater weight loss and broader metabolic effects, with emerging evidence for favorable cardiac remodeling, whereas semaglutide has the most cardiovascular outcomes data to date. This comprehensive review examines the comparative efficacy, safety, and clinical applications of these agents in obesity management, both with and without concomitant diabetes.

DIFFERENCES IN MECHANISM OF ACTION

Semaglutide is a selective long-acting GLP-1RA having 94% structural homology with human GLP-1 and has demonstrated substantial efficacy in weight management through enhanced glucose-dependent insulin secretion, delayed gastric emptying, and reduced appetite. It has structural modifications that enhance albumin binding and provide resistance to dipeptidyl peptidase-4 (DPP-4) degradation, resulting in an extended half-life of approximately 7 days. Upon GLP-1 receptor activation, semaglutide initiates a signaling cascade involving adenylyl cyclase activation and increased intracellular cyclic AMP levels. The therapeutic effects include glucose-dependent insulin secretion from pancreatic β cells, suppression of glucagon release, delayed gastric emptying, and direct central nervous system effects that reduce appetite and food intake.

On the other hand, tirzepatide has a novel "twincretin mechanism", being the first dual glucose-dependent insulinotropic peptide (GIP)/GLP-1RA. Dual agonism enhances anorectic, insulinotropic and adipocytic signaling, translating into larger reductions in body weight, glycemia, and ectopic adiposity at comparable gastrointestinal tolerability compared to semaglutide in head-to-head clinical trials, offering potentially superior metabolic benefits in obesity management **(Table 1)**.

Semaglutide 2.4 mg has been evaluated extensively in the STEP and SELECT programs, demonstrating robust GLP-1-mediated effects on appetite, caloric intake, weight loss, blood pressure, and atherogenic lipoproteins, as well as a 20% relative risk reduction in major adverse cardiovascular events (MACEs) in patients with established ASCVD and obesity without diabetes. Semaglutide 1.0 mg has previously demonstrated a 26% relative risk reduction in MACE versus placebo in high-risk T2D in SUSTAIN6, with neutral effects on heart

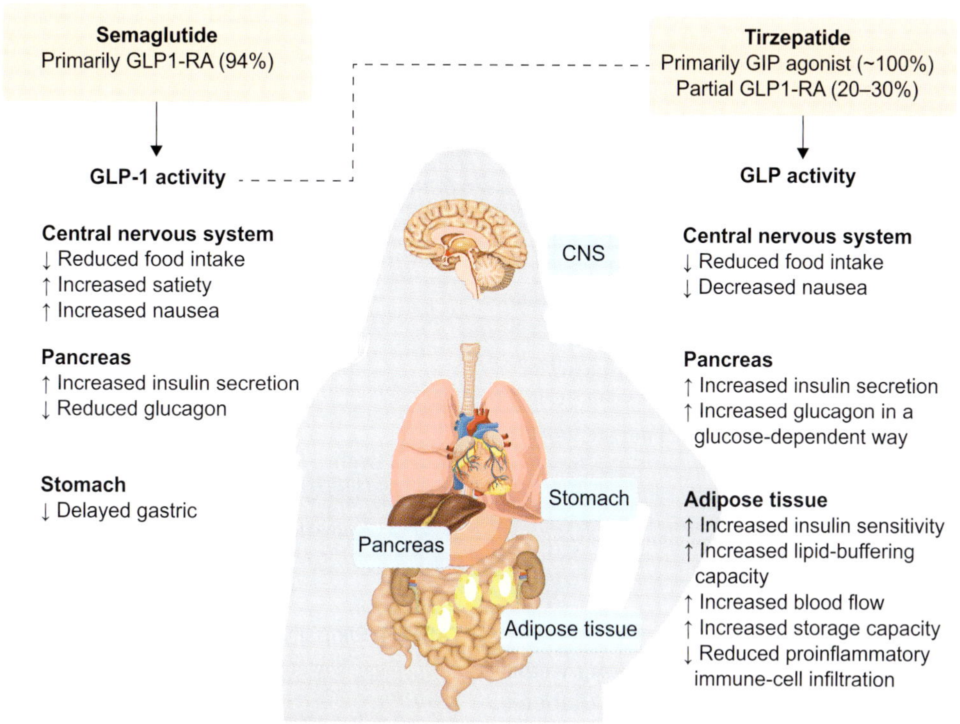

Fig. 1: Comparative mechanisms of action of semaglutide and tirzepatide across organ systems.

TABLE 1: Mechanistic differences.

Feature	*Tirzepatide*	*Semaglutide*
Receptor activity	Dual GIP + GLP-1 agonist	GLP-1 agonist only
Appetite and satiety	Strong	Strong
Energy expenditure and adipose effects	GIP-mediated effects contribute to greater fat loss	Limited to GLP 1 pathways

failure hospitalization but has noted improvements in nephropathy **(Fig. 1)**.

DOSE AND ADMINISTRATION

Both semaglutide and tirzepatide have a half-life of nearly 1 week, hence administered as once weekly subcutaneous injection. For treatment of obesity, semaglutide is indicated in the dose of 1.7–2.4 mg subcutaneous injection every week; whereas tirzepatide is prescribed in once weekly doses of 10–15 mg subcutaneously. Semaglutide is also available as oral formulation initiated at 3 mg dose once daily, with dose uptitrated to 14 mg daily, though weight loss was lesser than the injectable form.

Both therapeutic agents are initiated at small doses, and recommended to be gradually escalated every 4 weeks to achieve the target dose. The entire process of dose uptitration should usually take 16–20 weeks. The adoption of slow dose escalation helps to minimize gastrointestinal side effects and improved tolerability. The following chart describes the differential dosing of both agents **(Table 2)**.

TIRZEPATIDE VERSUS SEMAGLUTIDE IN ADULTS WITH OBESITY WITHOUT DIABETES: THE EVIDENCE

Evidence for Tirzepatide: The SURMOUNT Program

The SURMOUNT trials evaluated tirzepatide in nondiabetic obese individuals. SURMOUNT-1 demonstrated dose-dependent mean weight loss of approximately 15%, 19.5%, and 20.9% with 5 mg, 10 mg, and 15 mg doses, respectively over 72 weeks, representing the largest weight reductions reported in obesity pharmacotherapy to date.

SURMOUNT-3 demonstrated that tirzepatide produced substantial additional weight loss coupled with intensive lifestyle intervention, while SURMOUNT-4 confirmed that treatment discontinuation led to significant regain, but continuation-maintained weight loss exceeding 25% from baseline.

Notably, 30–36% of participants receiving higher dose tirzepatide achieved ≥20% weight loss—approximately double the proportion seen with semaglutide 2.4 mg administered subcutaneously.

TABLE 2: Dose schedule of tirzepatide versus semaglutide.

Time period	*Tirzepatide*	*Semaglutide*
Starting dose	2.5 mg S/C weekly for 4 weeks	0.25 mg S/C weekly for 4 weeks
First dose escalation	5 mg S/C weekly for 4 weeks	0.5 mg S/C weekly for 4 weeks
Second dose escalation	7.5 mg S/C weekly for 4 weeks	1 mg S/C weekly for 4 weeks
Third dose escalation	10 mg S/C weekly for 4 weeks	1.7 mg S/C weekly for 4 weeks
Final dose escalation	15 mg S/C weekly for 4 weeks	2.4 mg S/C weekly for 4 weeks
Maintenance dose	10–15 mg S/C weekly	1.7–2.4 mg S/C Weekly

Evidence for Semaglutide: The STEP Program

The STEP program evaluated semaglutide 2.4 mg weekly in adults with obesity or overweight without diabetes. In STEP-1, mean body weight reduction at 68 weeks was approximately 15%, compared with 2–3% with placebo. Subsequent trials confirmed robustness across different settings:

- STEP-3 showed additive benefit when combined with intensive behavioral therapy
- STEP-4 demonstrated substantial weight regain following drug withdrawal, reinforcing obesity as a chronic disease
- STEP-5 provided 2-year data, confirming durability of ~15% weight loss with continued therapy.

Across STEP trials, roughly half of participants achieved ≥15% weight loss, and 15–20% achieved ≥20% loss.

The comparison of STEP and SURMOUNT trials in nondiabetic population shows that across comparable durations, tirzepatide produces ~5–7 percentage points greater mean weight loss than semaglutide 2.4 mg **(Table 3)**. Moreover, tirzepatide *doubles the likelihood of ≥20% weight loss*, a threshold associated with major cardiometabolic and functional benefits **(Table 4)**.

Duration of Treatment

Based on evidence from clinical trials evaluating the effects of withdrawal of both drugs after attaining initial weight loss; namely STEP-4 for semaglutide and SURMOUNT-4 for tirzepatide, both drugs require *long-term continuation.* Tirzepatide leads to *greater absolute regain* if stopped as compared to semaglutide—probably owing to greater initial weight loss. This signals that obesity is a chronic disease likely to relapse once the therapy is withdrawn **(Table 5)**.

TABLE 3: Evidence-based comparison between tirzepatide and semaglutide for weight loss in nondiabetics (mean percentage weight loss).

Trial (population: obesity, no diabetes)	*Drug and dose*	*Duration*	*Mean weight loss*
SURMOUNT-1	Tirzepatide 5 mg	72 weeks	~15%
	Tirzepatide 10 mg	72 weeks	~19.5%
	Tirzepatide 15 mg	72 weeks	~20.9%
STEP-1	Semaglutide 2.4 mg	68 weeks	~14.9%
STEP-3 (with intensive lifestyle)	Semaglutide 2.4 mg	68 weeks	~16.0%
STEP-5 (2-year data)	Semaglutide 2.4 mg	104 weeks	~15.2%

TABLE 4: Clinically meaningful thresholds.

Outcome	*Tirzepatide (SURMOUNT-1) dose 10–15 mg/week*	*Semaglutide (STEP-1/3/5) dose 2.4 mg/week*
≥10% weight loss	~75–85%	~65–70%
≥15% weight loss	~50–57%	~45–55%
≥20% weight loss	~30–36%	~15–20%

TABLE 5: Durability and withdrawal.

Trial	*Design*	*Key finding*
SURMOUNT-4	Tirzepatide run-in → withdrawal	Continued therapy maintained ~25% loss; *withdrawal led to ~14% regain* in 1 year
STEP-4	Semaglutide run-in → withdrawal	Continued therapy maintained loss; *withdrawal led to ~6–7% regain*

TIRZEPATIDE VERSUS SEMAGLUTIDE IN ADULTS WITH DIABETIC OBESITY (DIABESITY): THE EVIDENCE

Tirzepatide has been extensively tested in people with T2D and obesity. The program was group of five SURPASS trials, testing various aspects in diabetic obese individuals. Semaglutide on the other hand has also been tested extensively in diabetic population in a host of trials under STEP program. STEP 1, STEP 6, STEP 11, STEP HFpEF DM, and STEP UP trials. Tirzepatide (SURPASS 1–5) achieved greater HbA1c reduction and generally greater weight loss than standard dose semaglutide (STEP-2/6/11). High-dose semaglutide (STEP-UP T2D, 7.2 mg) substantially improves weight loss and narrows the gap. The comparative summary of the trials has been given in **Table 6**.

The head-to-head clinical outcomes signals in people with diabetic obesity are given below in **Table 7**.

Thus, people with diabesity show better glycemic control with tirzepatide, almost akin to insulin, with greater weight loss as compared to semaglutide 2.4 mg. Weight loss in T2D is attenuated versus nondiabetics for both drugs, but tirzepatide consistently yields larger weight loss at approved doses. High-dose semaglutide (7.2 mg) meaningfully improves weight outcomes and approaches dual-agonist magnitude. Tirzepatide also works well with basal insulin and in high cardiovascular risk cohorts. Semaglutide shows added value in HFpEF with diabetes with regards to symptomatology and improved quality of life.

HEAD-TO-HEAD OBESITY DATA: SURMOUNT-5

SURMOUNT-5 is a pivotal phase IIIb head-to-head trial enrolling adults with obesity or overweight plus at least one weight-related comorbidity (without diabetes), randomized to maximum tolerated tirzepatide 10 or 15 mg versus semaglutide 1.7 or 2.4 mg for 72 weeks. Tirzepatide achieved mean weight reduction of 20.2% versus 13.7% with semaglutide, corresponding to approximately 47% greater relative weight loss and a statistically significant advantage in all prespecified categorical weight-loss thresholds. Beyond weight loss, tirzepatide

TABLE 6: Trials comparing outcomes with use of tirzepatide versus semaglutide in diabetic obese population.

Program	*Trial*	*Population (T2DM and obesity)*	*Drug (weekly dose)*	*Comparator*	*Duration*	*HbA1c change*	*Weight change*	*≥10% weight loss*
SURPASS	*1*	Early T2D, drug-naïve (many overweight/obese)	Tirzepatide 5–15 mg	Placebo	40 weeks	–1.9 to –2.1%	–7 to –9.5 kg	~35–45%
	2	T2DM on metformin	Tirzepatide 5 mg	*Semaglutide 1.0 mg*	40 weeks	–2.0%	–7.6 kg	~40%
			Tirzepatide 10 mg			–2.2%	–9.3 kg	~50%
			Tirzepatide 15 mg			–2.3%	–11.2 kg	~60%
	3	T2D on metformin	Tirzepatide 10–15 mg	Insulin degludec	52 weeks	–2.4 to –2.6%	–10 to –12.9 kg	~55–65%
	4	T2D, high CV risk	Tirzepatide 10–15 mg	Insulin glargine	52 weeks	–2.3 to –2.6%	–8 to –11.7 kg	~50–60%
	5	T2D on basal insulin	Tirzepatide 10–15 mg (on insulin)	Placebo	40 weeks	–2.1 to –2.4%	–7 to –8.8 kg	~45–55%
STEP	*2*	Obesity and T2DM	Semaglutide 2.4 mg	Placebo (±1.0 mg arm)	68 weeks	–1.6%	–9.6% (~–9–10 kg)	~25–30%
	6	East Asian obesity and T2DM	Semaglutide 2.4 mg	Placebo	68 weeks	–1.4%	–13.2%	~35–40%
	11	Obesity with early dysglycemia/T2DM	Semaglutide 2.4 mg	Placebo	68 weeks	–1.3%	–14–15%	~40–45%
	HFpEF DM	Obesity, HFpEF, and T2DM	Semaglutide 2.4 mg	Placebo	52 weeks	–1.2%	–9.8%	~30%
	UP T2D	Obesity and T2DM	Semaglutide 7.2 mg	Placebo	72 weeks	–1.8%	~17%	~55–60%

TABLE 7: Head-to-head trials and patterns.

Aspect	Tirzepatide (SURPASS)	Semaglutide (STEP)
HbA1c lowering	Greater (≈ −2.2 to −2.6%)	Moderate (≈ −1.3 to −1.8%)
Weight loss (standard dose)	Greater absolute kg loss	Less than tirzepatide at standard dose
Weight loss (high dose)	10–15 mg already high	7.2 mg (STEP-UP) narrows gap
On insulin	Effective without weight gain	Data limited
CV-risk populations	Strong efficacy in high-risk T2D	Symptom/QoL benefit in HFpEF DM
Hypoglycemia	Low (↑ only with insulin)	Low

in SURMOUNT-5 produced larger improvements in secondary cardiometabolic endpoints, including waist circumference, systolic blood pressure, and glycemic markers, although detailed subgroup analyses by baseline CVD, heart failure, or chronic kidney disease have not yet been fully reported. Gastrointestinal adverse events (nausea, vomiting, and diarrhea) occurred in both groups with similar qualitative profiles, but emerging comparative meta-analytic data suggest numerically fewer treatment discontinuations with tirzepatide 10–15 mg than with semaglutide 2.4 mg. The results are summarized in **Table 8**.

TABLE 8: Surmount 5 trial results: tirzepatide versus semaglutide—head-to-head comparison for weight loss at 72 weeks.

Parameter	Tirzepatide 15 mg/week	Semaglutide 2.4 mg/week
Mean % weight loss	~20.2%	~13.7%
≥10% weight loss	~80%	~60%
≥15% weight loss	~65%	~40%
≥20% weight loss	~45%	~20%
≥25% weight loss	~30%	~12%

Absolute difference: ~6.5 percentage points in favor of tirzepatide, relative advantage ~47% greater weight loss.

CARDIOVASCULAR OUTCOMES AND HARD ENDPOINTS: THE EVIDENCE

Semaglutide was tested in nondiabetic people with obesity and CVD in SELECT trial. The SELECT trial evaluated once-weekly semaglutide 2.4 mg versus placebo in 17,604 adults with established CVD, body mass index (BMI) ≥27 kg/m^2, and no diabetes, demonstrating a 20% relative risk reduction in three-point MACE (cardiovascular death, nonfatal myocardial infarction, and nonfatal stroke). Secondary endpoints included favorable trends in cardiovascular and all-cause mortality, with significant reductions in nonfatal myocardial infarction and a composite of cardiovascular death or heart failure hospitalization (HR: 0.82; 95% CI: 0.71–0.96). Crucially, SELECT decoupled cardiovascular benefit from glycemic control. Unlike earlier GLP-1RA cardiovascular outcomes trials, where glucose lowering was a potential mediator, SELECT demonstrates event reduction in a nondiabetic population. This finding underscores obesity itself—through inflammation, hemodynamic stress, dyslipidemia, and ectopic fat deposition—as a modifiable driver of CVD.

The degree of weight loss observed in SELECT (~9–10% on average) was more modest than in earlier obesity-focused trials such as STEP-1. This likely reflects the older age, higher comorbidity burden, and longer follow-up of the SELECT population. Yet cardiovascular benefit emerged early and was sustained over time, suggesting that mechanisms beyond absolute weight reduction are operative. Improvements in inflammatory markers, blood pressure, lipoprotein profiles, and possibly vascular function may contribute meaningfully to risk reduction.

As far as the data on CV outcomes regarding tirzepatide is concerned, SURPASS-CVOT trial proves it at best noninferior to dulaglutide (another GLP1-RA) in diabetic population. SURPASS-CVOT was a large cardiovascular outcomes trial designed to evaluate the cardiovascular safety of tirzepatide compared with an established GLP-1RA (dulaglutide) in patients with T2D at high cardiovascular risk.

The available evidence of CV safety and efficacy is compared in **Table 9**.

The Implication of the contrast:

Question	Answered by SELECT?	Answered by SURPASS-CVOT?
Does treating obesity reduce CV events?	*Yes*	No
Can CV benefit occur without diabetes?	*Yes*	No
Is dual incretin therapy CV-safe?	Not tested	*Yes*
Does more weight loss mean more CV benefit?	Suggested	Not addressed

TABLE 9: CV efficacy of semaglutide versus tirzepatide.

Feature	*SELECT*	*SURPASS-CVOT*
Population	Obesity, *no T2DM*, established ASCVD	T2DM with established/ high CV risk
Intervention	Semaglutide 2.4 mg	Tirzepatide 5–15 mg
Comparator	Placebo	Dulaglutide (active GLP-1 RA)
Primary aim	*Superiority* for CV event reduction	*Noninferiority* for CV safety
Primary result	*~20% MACE reduction*	*Noninferior* to dulaglutide
Key implication	Obesity Rx = CV risk modification	Dual incretin therapy is CV-safe

STRUCTURAL AND CARDIOMETABOLIC EFFECTS

In obesity without diabetes, tirzepatide 10–15 mg drives larger improvements in blood pressure, glycemic indices, and atherogenic lipids than semaglutide 2.4 mg in indirect comparisons of SURMOUNT-1 and STEP-1 and in the direct SURMOUNT-5 head-to-head trial. Given the log-linear relationship between blood pressure, glycemia, and atherosclerotic risk, these differences may translate into incremental long-term cardiovascular benefit, although this has not yet been definitively tested in a dedicated cardiovascular outcome trial.

The SUMMIT imaging substudy demonstrates that tirzepatide favorably remodels the heart and pericardial adipose depots in obesity-related HFpEF, reducing left ventricular mass and paracardiac adipose volume, and mitigating markers of circulatory volume overload and systemic inflammation. In contrast, semaglutide's most compelling cardiovascular data is derived from macrovascular MACE reductions in SUSTAIN-6 and SELECT, with less direct evidence for reverse remodeling but robust demonstration of risk reduction in established coronary, cerebrovascular, and peripheral arterial disease.

Semaglutide in Heart Failure with Preserved Ejection Fraction (STEP-HF Trial)

The STEP-HF trial evaluated whether semaglutide 2.4 mg once weekly improves symptoms, function, and weight in patients with HFpEF and obesity, with and without diabetes.

In STEP-HFpEF (without diabetes), 530 nondiabetic patients with HFpEF (EF >45%) and obesity were randomized to receive 2.4 mg S/C of semaglutide weekly versus placebo. Over a period of 52 weeks semaglutide showed 13.3% weight loss, 16 points improvement in KCC-CSS, 25 meters increase in 6-minute-walk distance and marked reduction in the inflammatory marker—CRP.

In STEP-HFpEF DM (with diabetes), nearly 600 diabetic patients with HFpEF and obesity were randomized to receive 2.4 mg S/C of semaglutide weekly or placebo. Over a period of 52 weeks semaglutide showed 9.8% weight loss, 13 points improvement in KCC-CSS, significant improvement in effort tolerance, and HbA1c reduction 1–1.2%.

STEP-HFpEF trials show that semaglutide 2.4 mg produces meaningful weight loss and large improvements in symptoms, quality of life, and functional capacity in obese HFpEF patients—with or without diabetes—without compromising heart failure safety.

Based on data for cardiovascular safety and efficacy, semaglutide stands above tirzepatide as of now. Nevertheless, tirzepatide has ample data with regards to cardiovascular safety and concomitant cardiovascular risk factor modification.

SAFETY, TOLERABILITY, AND PRACTICAL CONSIDERATIONS

Both agents share a predominantly gastrointestinal side effect profile, including nausea, vomiting, and diarrhea, which are dose-dependent and mitigated by gradual uptitration. Serious adverse events related to gastrointestinal complications and gallbladder disease are infrequent but clinically relevant; semaglutide has been associated with increased retinopathy complications in rapid glycemic improvement settings in SUSTAIN-6, while tirzepatide has not shown a disproportionate signal to date, though comparative data are limited.

Both semaglutide and tirzepatide carry boxed warnings regarding the potential risk of thyroid C-cell tumors, based on rodent studies showing dose-dependent thyroid C-cell tumors at clinically relevant exposures. Both medications are contraindicated in patients with a personal or family history of medullary thyroid carcinoma (MTC) or Multiple Endocrine Neoplasia Syndrome type 2 (MEN 2). Patients should be counseled about symptoms of thyroid tumors, including neck mass, dysphagia, or persistent hoarseness.

Both agents carry risks of hypoglycemia when combined with insulin or sulfonylureas, necessitating dose adjustments of concomitant glucose-lowering medications. Rare but serious adverse events include acute pancreatitis, acute kidney injury (particularly with volume depletion from gastrointestinal effects), and severe allergic reactions.

Dose-escalation strategies in SURMOUNT and STEP mirror clinical practice and are essential to maintain tolerability at maintenance doses of tirzepatide 10–15 mg and semaglutide 2.4 mg, with high overall treatment adherence and low rates of permanent discontinuation in both programs. Current comparative evidence suggests that, despite more potent weight loss, tirzepatide does not incur a materially higher burden of severe gastrointestinal adverse events than semaglutide 2.4 mg and may be associated with slightly fewer discontinuations in network meta-analyses.

CONCLUSION

Obesity guidelines emphasize a personalized comprehensive approach, with a focus on risk reduction over mere weight loss, incorporating social and family support systems, along with behavioral, dietary, and pharmacological interventions for sustained results. Incorporating ethnicity-specific BMI, along with measures of central adiposity and adiposity-related complications should be assessed to guide the need for pharmacotherapy.

For patients with obesity (with or without T2D) in whom maximal weight loss and regression of ectopic adiposity are central goals—such as in HFpEF, severe left ventricular hypertrophy, or high cardiometabolic burden—tirzepatide 10–15 mg currently offers superior weight reduction and more pronounced improvements in multiple risk factors than semaglutide 1.7–2.4 mg, supported by SUMMIT data for structural and symptomatic benefit in HFpEF. In contrast, for patients with established ASCVD and obesity without diabetes, semaglutide 2.4 mg is the only dose with proven MACE reduction in a large outcomes trial (SELECT), complementing prior SUSTAIN-6 data at 1 mg in high-risk T2D.

Data from dedicated cardiovascular outcome trials directly comparing tirzepatide and semaglutide agent will be instrumental in obesity pharmacotherapy selection, balancing the more mature atherosclerotic event-reduction evidence for semaglutide against the superior weight loss and HFpEF-related structural benefits of tirzepatide, individualized by predominant phenotype (ASCVD versus obesityHFpEF), glycemic status, tolerability, access, and therapeutic goals.

BIBLIOGRAPHY

1. Ahmad O, Ibrahim R, Pham HN, et al. Early glucagon-like peptide-1 receptor agonist use after myocardial infarction in patients with type 2 diabetes. Int J Cardiol. 2026;445:134042.
2. Aronne LJ, Horn DB, le Roux CW, et al. Tirzepatide as Compared with Semaglutide for the Treatment of Obesity. N Engl J Med. 2025;393(1):26-36.
3. Aronne LJ, Sattar N, Horn DB, et al. Continued Treatment With Tirzepatide for Maintenance of Weight Reduction in Adults With Obesity: The SURMOUNT-4 Randomized Clinical Trial. JAMA. 2024;331(1):38-48.
4. Bray GA, Kim KK, Wilding JPH, et al. Obesity: a chronic relapsing progressive disease process. A position statement of the World Obesity Federation. Obes Rev. 2017;18(7):715-23.
5. Davies M, Færch L, Jeppesen OK, et al. Semaglutide 2·4 mg once a week in adults with overweight or obesity, and type 2 diabetes (STEP 2): a randomised, double-blind, double-dummy, placebo-controlled, phase 3 trial. Lancet. 2021;397(10278):971-84.
6. Hamza M, Papamargaritis D, Davies MJ. Tirzepatide for overweight and obesity management. Expert Opin Pharmacother. 2025;26(1):31-49.
7. Holst JJ. The physiology of glucagon-like peptide 1. Physiol Rev. 2007;87(4):1409-39.
8. Horn DB, Kahan S, Batterham RL, et al. Time to weight plateau with tirzepatide treatment in the SURMOUNT-1 and SURMOUNT-4 clinical trials. Clin Obes. 2025;15(3):e12734.
9. Jastreboff AM, Aronne LJ, Ahmad NN, et al. Tirzepatide Once Weekly for the Treatment of Obesity. N Engl J Med. 2022;387(3):205-16.
10. Madsbad S, Holst JJ. The promise of glucagon-like peptide 1 receptor agonists (GLP-1RA) for the treatment of obesity: a look at phase 2 and 3 pipelines. Expert Opin Investig Drugs. 2025;34(3):197-215.
11. Marso SP, Bain SC, Consoli A, et al. Semaglutide and Cardiovascular Outcomes in Patients with Type 2 Diabetes. N Engl J Med. 2016;375(19):1834-44.
12. NCD Risk Factor Collaboration (NCD-RisC). Trends in adult body-mass index in 200 countries from 1975 to 2014: a pooled analysis of 1698 population-based measurement studies with 19·2 million participants. Lancet. 2016;387(10026):1377-96. Erratum in: Lancet. 2016;387(10032):1998.
13. Pedersen SD, Manjoo P, Dash S, et al. Pharmacotherapy for obesity management in adults: 2025 clinical practice guideline update. CMAJ. 2025;197(27):E797-E809.
14. Rubino D, Abrahamsson N, Davies M, et al. Effect of Continued Weekly Subcutaneous Semaglutide vs Placebo on Weight Loss Maintenance in Adults With Overweight or Obesity: The STEP 4 Randomized Clinical Trial. JAMA. 2021;325(14):1414-25.

15. Sinha R, Papamargaritis D, Sargeant JA, et al. Efficacy and Safety of Tirzepatide in Type 2 Diabetes and Obesity Management. J Obes Metab Syndr. 2023;32(1):25-45.
16. Trocchio LL, Peters F. Taking back control: The experience of adults using semaglutide and tirzepatide for obesity treatment - A qualitative study. Obes Pillars. 2025;17:100237.
17. Wadden TA, Chao AM, Machineni S, et al. Author Correction: Tirzepatide after intensive lifestyle intervention in adults with overweight or obesity: the SURMOUNT-3 phase 3 trial. Nat Med. 2024;30(6):1784. Erratum for: Nat Med. 2023;29(11):2909-18.
18. Wharton S, Lau DCW, Vallis M, et al. Obesity in adults: a clinical practice guideline. CMAJ. 2020;192(31):E875-E891.

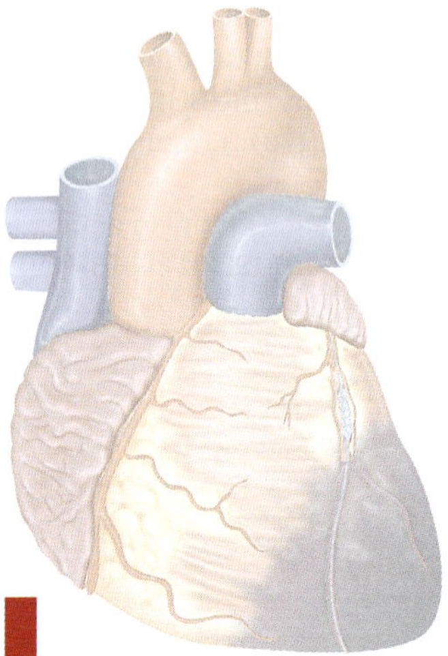

134

CHAPTER

GLP-1 Agonists and Dual Incretin Agonists (GIP/GLP-1) in Obesity and Cardiovascular Disease

Krishna Rao, Nikhila Sri Rao, Nilesh Sai Rao

INTRODUCTION

Obesity has emerged as one of the most important drivers of rising global cardiovascular disease (CVD) burden. According to the Global Burden of Disease (GBD) 2023 analysis, metabolic risk factors such as high body mass index account for a substantial and growing proportion of disability-adjusted life years (DALYs) attributable to CVD worldwide.[1] Specifically, high body mass index and high fasting plasma glucose have shown the greatest proportional increase in DALYs attributable to CVD in comparison to all risk factors.[1] With rising obesity prevalence, cardiovascular morbidity and mortality remain increased despite advances in cardiovascular management and therapies, thus underscoring the evident need for addressing metabolic risks in a multifactorial fashion.

EPIDEMIOLOGY OF OBESITY AND CARDIOVASCULAR RISK

The GBD 2023 analysis highlights high BMI as a leading metabolic risk factor contributing to CVD burden globally, with rising attributable DALYs over the past three decades.[1] This burden spans atherosclerotic cardiovascular disease (ASCVD), heart failure (HF), and cardiometabolic conditions that amplify cardiovascular risk. Significantly, the impact of obesity is not confined to high-income countries; obesity prevalence and associated cardiovascular burden are accelerating across low- and middle-income regions, reflecting shifts in dietary patterns, urbanization, and physical activity levels.[1,2] It is projected that nearly one in two adults in the United States will have obesity by 2030.[3] Globally, there are >1 billion people living with obesity, with prevalence rising in most countries.[2] NCD-risk analyses demonstrate that obesity has replaced undernutrition as the dominant nutritional challenge in many regions, which pose implications for future cardiovascular morbidity and mortality.[2]

PATHOPHYSIOLOGIC LINKS BETWEEN OBESITY AND CARDIOVASCULAR DISEASE

Obesity contributes to cardiovascular morbidity and mortality through both direct and indirect mechanisms. Ectopic fat and adipose tissue deposition in visceral regions augment inflammation, oxidative stress, and endothelial dysfunction, which are fundamental processes in atherosclerotic progression.[4] Obesity also contributes directly to cardiovascular pathology through adverse effects on myocardial structure, vascular biology, and hemodynamic changes that result in renin-angiotensin-aldosterone activation.[4] Indirectly, obesity predisposes patients to type 2 diabetes mellitus, insulin resistance, hypertension, kidney disease, and dyslipidemia, all of which are recognized risk factors of CVD.

Lifestyle-based weight reduction has long been accepted as the cornerstone of obesity management. While effective for modest weight loss and improvements in cardiometabolic risk factors, large, and randomized trials have shown that even intensive lifestyle interventions have failed to produce significant reductions in major adverse cardiovascular events (MACEs) in high-risk populations, as observed from the Look AHEAD multicenter, randomized clinical trial.[5] Post-hoc secondary analyses demonstrated that greater magnitude of weight loss was associated with lower CVD incidence; however, the benefits were not uniformly achieved across the population.[6] Lifestyle interventions certainly remain an imperative component of obesity management in mitigating cardiovascular risk and strengthening cardiometabolic fitness. At the same time, these findings reinforce the biological complexity of obesity as a chronic, relapsing disease that goes beyond a condition of simple caloric excess. Optimal obesity management and associated cardiovascular benefit require robust adjunctive approaches, particularly in the pharmacologic realm.

OBESITY WONDER DRUGS—GLP-1 RECEPTOR AGONISTS AND DUAL INCRETIN AGONISTS (GLP-1/GIP)

Glucagon-like peptide-1 (GLP-1) and glucose-dependent insulinotropic peptide (GIP) are naturally occurring metabolic hormones known as incretins. Incretins are produced in the gastrointestinal (GI) tract and bind to their respective receptors to promote a variety of effects on insulin secretion, glucose regulation, and more metabolic processes.

Glucagon-like peptide-1 agonists are "incretin mimetics", a class of medications that bind GLP-1 receptors to lower blood sugar, promote weight loss, and boost glucose-dependent insulin release from pancreatic beta cells.[7] Dual incretin agonists have complementary action, activating both GIP and GLP-1 receptors to further enhance glycemic control. These wonder drugs, developed as therapeutic agents for type 2 diabetes, are simultaneously heralding a new era in the management of obesity with great potential to change the natural history of this otherwise recalcitrant metabolic disease.

The three FDA approved agents for obesity from the class of GLP-1/dual incretin agonists are semaglutide and liraglutide (GLP-1 receptor agonist), and tirzepatide (dual GLP-1/GIP receptor agonist). They exert their effects through multiple complementary pathways. Effects of GLP-1/dual incretin agents include resetting the brain's center for satiety and appetite regulation, improving insulin sensitivity, delaying gastric emptying, and promoting sustained weight loss preferentially in visceral regions **(Fig. 1)**.

INCRETIN-BASED THERAPIES AND CARDIOVASCULAR BENEFIT (TABLE 1)

The *SELECT* trial demonstrated that in patients with overweight or obesity and established CVD (prior MI 76%, prior CVA 23%, and PAD) without diabetes, once weekly semaglutide was associated with a decreased risk of MACE (CV death, nonfatal MI, and stroke) compared with placebo (6.5% vs. 8.0% HR 0.8 CI 0.7–0.9, <0.001) at a mean follow-up of 39.8 months.[8] The *STEP-HFpEF* showed that in patients with HFpEF and obesity, treatment with semaglutide (2.4 mg) led to larger reductions in symptoms (mean point change of 7.8) and physical limitations, and greater weight loss (–10.7% points) than placebo over 52 weeks.[9]

The *SUMMIT* trial treatment of patients with HFpEF and obesity with tirzepatide led to a lower risk of composite of death from CV causes or worsening HF and improved health status compared with placebo.[10] A systematic review and meta-analysis (*PROSPERO* study) of 99,599 patients treated with several GLP-1R agonists demonstrated reduced mortality and MACE in high-risk populations, demonstrating benefits beyond glycemic control, although at the expense of increased GI side effects.[11]

The *SURPASS-CVOT* trial confirmed the noninferiority of tirzepatide compared with semaglutide with respect to a composite of death from CV causes, myocardial infarction, or stroke.[12] The *SURMOUNT-5* trial compared tirzepatide (Zepbound) and semaglutide (Wegovy) head-to-head phase and showed that tirzepatide outperformed semaglutide in sustained weight reduction over 72 weeks in adults with obesity or overweight with comorbidities.[13]

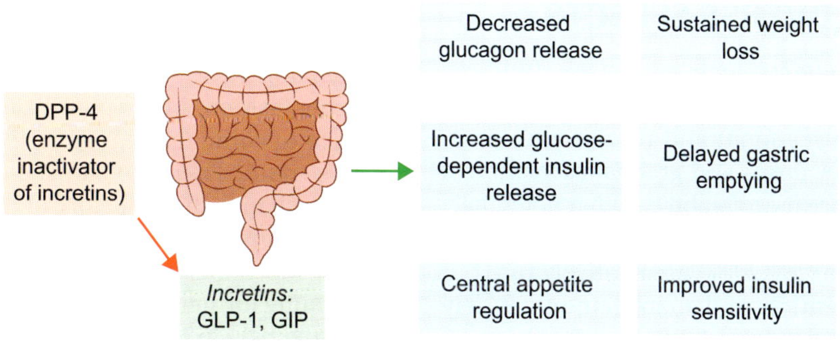

Fig. 1: Effects of GLP-1 agonists and dual incretin agents (GIP/GLP-1).

TABLE 1: Key randomized trials of incretin-based therapies in obesity and CVD.[8-11,14]

Clinical trial	Population studied	Agent	Key outcomes
SELECT[8]	• Preexisting CVD and obesity (BMI ≥27 kg/m^2) • No history of diabetes • Prediabetes 66 (9)%	Semaglutide • 1 × weekly semaglutide injection (0.24–2.4 mg)	• Semaglutide superior to placebo • Reduced incidence of (MACE) death from CV causes, nonfatal MI, and nonfatal stroke
STEP-HFpEF[9]	• HFpEF • Obesity	Semaglutide • Once weekly injections 52 weeks follow-up	• Greater reduction in HF symptoms • Greater weight loss than placebo
SUMMIT trial[10]	• HFpEF • Obesity (BMI at least 30 kg/m^2) • Follow-up 2 years	Tirzepatide • Maximum dose 15 mg per week or placebo	• Improved CV outcomes and survival • Improved health status (KCCQ-CSS) compared with placebo
FLOW study[14]	Type 2 diabetes and CKD	Semaglutide • 1 mg weekly injections	Reduced risk of kidney outcomes and CV mortality
PROSPERO systematic review and meta-analysis[11]	99,599 high-risk patients treated	GLP-1R agonists	Reduced mortality and MACE

COMPARING CLINICAL EFFICACY (WEIGHT LOSS AND GLYCEMIC CONTROL)

Semaglutide (Ozempic, Wegovy, and Rybelsus)

Based on STEP trials, ~15% sustained weight loss at 2 years with strong evidence for durable glycemic control and CV benefit in diabetes populations led to new approval for CV and CKD benefit in January 2025.

Tirzepatide (Zepbound and Mounjaro)

Based on SURMOUNT/SURPASS, peak weight loss is expected at 72–88 weeks, greater than semaglutide across most dose comparisons, followed by plateau. The dual GLP-1 and GIP mechanism likely yields superior HgA1c reduction and weight loss in head-to-head comparative analysis from RCTs.

GLP-1 AND DUAL GIP/GLP-1 SAFETY PROFILE AND ADVERSE EFFECTS

Gastrointestinal side effects such as nausea, fullness, and early satiety are the most common, but they occur in the initial stages of treatment and resolve with time. Initiating therapy in low doses and gradual escalation is recommended to enhance the tolerability. Other potentially serious adverse effects such as pancreatitis (0.3%) and gallbladder disease (1.5–2.5%) are relatively rare but require prompt recognition and management. Rarely reported, thyroid C-cell tumor risk is primarily observed in rodents and not in human subjects as demonstrated in millions of patientyears follow-up; however, this would require close surveillance and long-term follow-up.

LIMITATIONS AND UNANSWERED QUESTIONS

Majority of the studies did not include patient populations from different demographics; therefore, results could be biased. Low- and middle-income countries are sharing most of the burden of obesity and CV diseases and this population was not adequately represented in the studies. In addition, studies have included different BMI criteria and failed to use waist to hip ratio, which could be a more reliable metric, as it represents visceral adiposity. Affordability and side effects could be the limiting factors for widespread use of antiobesity agents. There is considerable variation and tolerability of these medications by patients and therefore individualization of treatment is necessary. The prohibitive cost of these medications is a limiting factor even in high income countries and this will have to be addressed at multiple levels. Medical community, pharmaceutical industry, healthcare policy makers, and governing bodies will have to collaborate and come up with solutions to lower costs and enhance accessibility to patients to use them in an equitable fashion. Many pharmaceutical companies are in a race to come up with generic versions and this is a positive trend. Then, we can see a real impact of these agents to change the trajectory of obesity and CV burden. Secondary analyses suggest reductions in plasma volume as a key mechanism, though effects on skeletal muscle mass require further research; particularly due to potential sarcopenia risks in HFpEF populations.

CONCLUSION

The therapeutic armamentarium for HFpEF has expanded considerably. Mineralocorticoid receptor antagonists including finerenone (nonsteroidal MRA) accorded class 2b indication while SGLT2 inhibitors received class 2a indication. The GLP1 receptor agonists (semaglutide) and GLP1/GIP dual agonists (tirzepatide) have now shown promising results in HFpEF and obesity. Metabolic factors including obesity are the prime driving forces for the global CV burden and rising incidence of HFpEF. Mitigating the threat of obesity is of paramount importance to reduce CV morbidity and mortality. Behavioral modification including lifestyle interventions in conjunction with pharmacologic therapies involving "incretin mimetics" could change the trajectory of obesity associated CV diseases. Evidence from STEPHFpEF and SUMMIT trials demonstrated substantial weight loss, improved quality of life, reduced cardiovascular events, and decreased mortality in patients with HFpEF and obesity. Future HF guidelines are expected to formally incorporate these antiobesity pharmacotherapies as recommended treatments for obesity-related HFpEF.

REFERENCES

1. Global Burden of Cardiovascular Diseases and Risks 2023 Collaborators. Global, Regional, and National Burden of Cardiovascular Diseases and Risk Factors in 204 Countries and Territories, 1990-2023. J Am Coll Cardiol. 2025;86(22):2167-243.
2. NCD Risk Factor Collaboration (NCD-RisC). Worldwide trends in underweight and obesity from 1990 to 2022: a pooled analysis of 3663 population representative studies with 222 million children, adolescents, and adults. Lancet 2024;403(10431):1027-50.
3. Ward ZJ, Bleich SN, Cradock AL, et al. Projected U.S. State-Level Prevalence of Adult Obesity and Severe Obesity. N Engl J Med. 2019;381(25):2440-2450.
4. Powell-Wiley TM, Poirier P, Burke LE, et al. Obesity and Cardiovascular Disease: A Scientific Statement From the American Heart Association. Circulation. 2021;143(21):e984-1010.
5. Look AHEAD Research Group; Wing RR, Bolin P, Brancati FL, et al. Cardiovascular effects of intensive lifestyle intervention in type 2 diabetes. N Engl J Med. 2013;369(2):145-54.
6. Look AHEAD Research Group; Gregg EW, Jakicic JM, Blackburn G, et al. Association of the magnitude of weight loss and changes in physical fitness with long-term cardiovascular disease outcomes in overweight or obese people with type 2 diabetes: a post-hoc analysis of the Look AHEAD randomised clinical trial. Lancet Diabetes Endocrinol. 2016;4(11):913-21.
7. Liu QK. Mechanisms of action and therapeutic applications of GLP-1 and dual GIP/GLP-1 receptor agonists. Front Endocrinol (Lausanne). 2024;15:1431292.
8. Lincoff AM, Brown-Frandsen K, Colhoun HM, et al. Semaglutide and Cardiovascular Outcomes in Obesity without Diabetes. N Engl J Med. 2023;389(24):2221-32.
9. Kosiborod MN, Abildstrøm SZ, Borlaug BA, et al. Semaglutide in Patients with Heart Failure with Preserved Ejection Fraction and Obesity. N Engl J Med. 2023;389(12):1069-84.
10. Packer M, Zile MR, Kramer CM, et al. Tirzepatide for Heart Failure with Preserved Ejection Fraction and Obesity. N Engl J Med. 2025;392(5):427-37.
11. Galli M, Benenati S, Laudani C, et al. Cardiovascular Effects and Tolerability of GLP-1 Receptor Agonists: A Systematic Review and Meta-Analysis of 99,599 Patients. J Am Coll Cardiol. 2025;86(20):1805-19.
12. Nicholls SJ, Pavo I, Bhatt DL, et al. Cardiovascular outcomes with tirzepatide versus dulaglutide in type 2 diabetes. N Engl J Med. 2025;393:2409 20.
13. Aronne LJ, Horn DB, le Roux CW, et al. Tirzepatide as compared with semaglutide for the treatment of obesity. N Engl J Med. 2025;393(1):26-36.
14. Perkovic V, Tuttle KR, Rossing P, et al. Effects of Semaglutide on Chronic Kidney Disease in Patients with Type 2 Diabetes. N Engl J Med. 2024;391(2):109-21.

135

CHAPTER

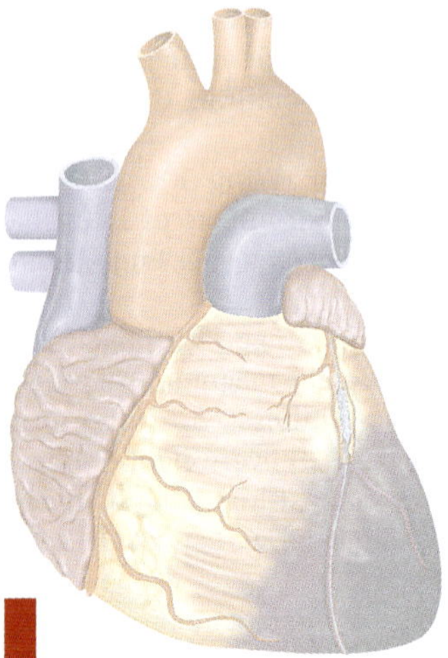

Comparison of Tirzepatide versus Semaglutide in Obesity with Cardiovascular Disease

Tripti Deb, Ramya Pechetty

INTRODUCTION

Obesity and cardiovascular disease (CVD) pose significant global health challenges. With obesity rates projected to affect half of US adults by the end of this decade, the need for effective treatments has never been more urgent.[1] According to the National Family Health Survey (NFHS-5, 2019–2021), around 24% of women and 23% of men in India are overweight or obese. A more recent nationwide study by the Indian Council of Medical Research (ICMR) found that among adults over 20 years, one in every four people has generalized obesity.[2] Incretin-based therapies, specifically *semaglutide* (a GLP-1 receptor agonist) and *tirzepatide* (a dual GIP/GLP-1 receptor agonist), have revolutionized this field. These medications not only promote substantial weight loss but also show promise in reducing major adverse cardiovascular events (MACE).[3,4] This analysis provides a concise comparison of their mechanisms, efficacy, safety, and clinical roles in patients with obesity and established CVD.

MECHANISMS OF ACTION

Semaglutide: GLP-1 Receptor Agonist

Semaglutide mimics the GLP-1 hormone and acts on multiple pathways: It reduces appetite in the brain, delays gastric emptying to promote fullness, and enhances glucose-dependent insulin secretion.[3,4] This multifaceted action leads to weight loss and improved metabolic parameters.

Tirzepatide: Dual-agonist Advantage

Tirzepatide is a novel "twin-cretin" that activates both GIP and GLP-1 receptors. The *GLP-1* component provides benefits similar to semaglutide, while the *GIP* component offers unique advantages. GIP receptors on fat cells (adipocytes) are involved in fat metabolism, and their nonoverlapping effects on the central nervous system contribute to tirzepatide's superior weight loss efficacy.[3,5] This dual action on both appetite and metabolism is key to its potent effects.

EFFICACY IN WEIGHT LOSS

Head-to-head trials consistently show *tirzepatide is more effective for weight loss* than semaglutide.[5-7]

- *Semaglutide's performance:* In the *STEP 1* trial, semaglutide 2.4 mg resulted in an average weight reduction of approximately *15%* over 68 weeks.
- *Tirzepatide's unprecedented results*: The *SURMOUNT-1* trial showed that tirzepatide's 15 mg dose leads to a remarkable *20.9%* weight reduction. A direct comparison in the *SURMOUNT-5* trial found that the tirzepatide patients lost an average of *20.2%* of their body weight versus *13.7%* for those on semaglutide.[5,7] This 47% greater relative weight loss with tirzepatide is significant, as greater weight loss is linked to more pronounced improvements in cardiovascular risk factors.

CARDIOVASCULAR OUTCOME DATA

The evidence for cardiovascular benefits differs in maturity between the two drugs, but both are highly promising.

Semaglutide: Established by *SELECT* Trial

Semaglutide's cardioprotective role is definitively established by the *SELECT* trial.[8,9] This landmark study on over 17,600 nondiabetic patients with obesity and established CVD demonstrated that semaglutide reduced the risk of MACE (cardiovascular death, nonfatal MI, or nonfatal stroke) by a significant *20%*.[8] This evidence has led to a cardiovascular indication for semaglutide, making it a cornerstone for secondary prevention in this population. Semaglutide also shows promise in improving the outcomes for patients with *obesity-related heart failure with preserved ejection fraction (HFpEF)*.[10]

Tirzepatide: Emerging Evidence

While the definitive CV outcomes trial for tirzepatide in nondiabetic obese patients (*SURMOUNT-MMO*) is ongoing, other trials and real-world data are very encouraging.[11]

- *SURPASS-CVOT:* In this trial, done in patients with *type 2 diabetes* confirmed tirzepatide's cardioprotective effect, by showing a significant *8% lower risk of MACE* compared with dulaglutide.[8]
- *Real-world data:* Recent observational studies suggest that tirzepatide may be associated with favorable cardiovascular outcomes, including lower rates of heart failure exacerbations and acute kidney injury.[11] A real-world cohort study showed that tirzepatide users had a lower hazard of CVD events than semaglutide users.[9]
- *SUMMIT trial:* This study demonstrated a significant reduction in the risk of death from cardiovascular causes or worsening heart failure in obese patients with HFpEF.[10]

SAFETY PROFILE AND TOLERABILITY

Both medications share a similar safety profile, with *gastrointestinal side effects* (nausea, vomiting, diarrhea) being the most common, especially during dose escalation.[8] Head-to-head data from the *SURMOUNT-5* trial showed that semaglutide was associated with a higher discontinuation rate due to GI issues compared to tirzepatide, although tirzepatide had more injection-site reactions.[5] Both drugs carry a boxed warning about the risk of thyroid C-cell tumors based on animal studies.

PATIENT AND ECONOMIC CONSIDERATIONS

Both semaglutide and tirzepatide are *once-weekly subcutaneous injections* with gradual dose escalation. The choice between them should be a shared decision.

Tirzepatide may be preferred for patients prioritizing maximum weight loss due to its superior efficacy.

Semaglutide offers the advantage of established, long-term cardiovascular outcomes data from the SELECT trial, making it a robust choice for patients with a history of CVD.

The *high cost* of both drugs remains a significant barrier to access.[8] Insurance coverage varies, though the SELECT trial results have expanded coverage for semaglutide in some cases.[9] The high cost has also led to the availability of unapproved compounded versions, which carry safety risks.

LIMITATIONS

The primary limitations in comparing these drugs include the *lack of a direct head-to-head randomized controlled trial (RCT)* comparing their cardiovascular outcomes in a nondiabetic population. Much of the evidence for tirzepatide in this group is from ongoing studies (like SURMOUNT-MMO) or observational data, which are susceptible to various biases.

CONCLUSION

The comparative analysis of tirzepatide and semaglutide reveals significant advancements in the management of obesity, particularly in the context of CVD. Tirzepatide is consistently associated with greater weight loss compared to semaglutide. This superiority is observed across different doses and durations of treatment, with higher doses and longer durations yielding more pronounced weight reduction. This enhanced weight loss has significant implications for improving cardiometabolic risk factors.

Semaglutide has a well-established role in cardiovascular risk reduction, especially for patients with established CVD. The SELECT trial definitively demonstrated a 20% reduction in MACE in overweight or obese patients with established CVD without diabetes, securing semaglutide's approval for a cardiovascular indication. Furthermore, both semaglutide and tirzepatide show promise in patients with obesity-related HFpEF, improving symptoms, functional capacity, and reducing the risk of worsening heart failure events, as evidenced by studies such as STEP-HFpEF and SUMMIT.

For tirzepatide, while *positive cardiovascular outcomes* in patients with type 2 diabetes and preexisting CVD have been confirmed by the *SURPASS-CVOT trial* (demonstrating noninferiority to dulaglutide and significant reductions in MACE and all-cause mortality), the definitive head-to-head cardiovascular outcomes data in nondiabetic obese populations (from the SURMOUNT-MMO trial) are still awaited. However, promising real-world data and the SUMMIT trial results for HFpEF patients suggest strong potential.

Overall, these therapies represent a *paradigm shift* in cardiometabolic medicine, offering potent tools to combat the intertwined epidemics of obesity and CVD. The choice between tirzepatide and semaglutide should be personalized, considering the patient's specific weight loss goals, cardiovascular history, and tolerability to side effects. Continued research, particularly long-term head-to-head randomized clinical trials, is crucial to further refine our understanding of their sustained benefits, safety profiles, and optimal integration into clinical practice.

REFERENCES

1. Wong ND, Karthikeyan H, Fan W. US population eligibility and estimated impact of tirzepatide treatment on obesity prevalence and cardiovascular disease events. Cardiovasc Drugs Ther. 2025;39(4):837-47.
2. Ahirwar R, Mondal PR. Prevalence of obesity in India: a systematic review. Diabetes Metab Syndr. 2019;13(1): 318-21.
3. Di Odoardo LAF, Zucchetti O, Sciatti E, et al. Obesity update: cardiovascular risk and therapeutic innovations (focus on semaglutide and tirzepatide). Eur Heart J Suppl. 2025;27(Suppl 3):iii137-42.
4. Sawami K, Tanaka A, Node K, et al. Updated evidence on cardiovascular and renal effects of GLP-1 receptor agonists and combination therapy with SGLT2 inhibitors and finerenone: a narrative review and perspectives. Cardiovasc Diabetol. 2024;23:410.
5. Rodriguez P, Goodwin Cartwright B, Gratzl S, et al. Semaglutide vs tirzepatide for weight loss in adults with overweight or obesity. JAMA Intern Med. 2024;184: 1056-64.
6. Aamir A, Latif R, Alqoofi J, et al. Comparative efficacy of tirzepatide vs. semaglutide in reducing body weight in humans: a systematic review and meta-analysis of clinical trials and real-world data. J Clin Med Res. 2025;17:285-96.
7. Munawar M, Ali N, Nazeer H, et al. Tirzepatide versus semaglutide for weight loss in overweight and obese adults: a systematic review and meta-analysis of direct comparative studies. Cureus. 2025;17:e86080.
8. Chaphalkar S, Cheriyedath S. (2024). Tirzepatide beats semaglutide in lowering diabetes risk and cardiovascular events in obesity patients. [online] Available from https://www.news-medical.net/news/20240828/Tirzepatide-beats-semaglutide-in-lowering-diabetes-risk-and-cardiovascular-events-in-obesity-patients.aspx#. [Last accessed January, 2026].
9. Baser O, Samayoa G, Yapar N, et al. Semaglutide and tirzepatide use and reduction of cardiovascular risks in adults with overweight and obesity. Med Res Arch. 2024;12:1-12.
10. Kittleson M, Benjamin E, Blumer V, et al. 2025 ACC scientific statement on the management of obesity in adults with heart failure: a report of the American College of Cardiology. J Am Coll Cardiol. 2025;86(20):1953-75.
11. Dani S, Makwana B. An observational study of cardiovascular outcomes of tirzepatide vs glucagon-like peptide-1 receptor agonists. JACC Adv. 2025;4:101740.

136

CHAPTER

Angiotensin Receptor–Neprilysin Inhibitor in the Management of Obesity-associated Heart Failure

Atul Kaushik, Vivudh Pratap Singh

INTRODUCTION

Obesity-associated heart failure (HF) is a growing public health concern due to rising prevalence of obesity globally. Obesity is a well-known risk factor for HF and it has a bidirectional impact. It not only increases the incidence of HF but also worsens prognosis once HF develops. It usually manifests as heart failure with preserved ejection fraction (HFpEF), but heart failure with reduced ejection fraction (HFrEF) is also seen.[1,2]

Angiotensin receptor-neprilysin inhibitors (ARNIs), particularly sacubitril/valsartan, have emerged as a significant advancement in HF therapy, especially for HFrEFs.[3]

PATHOPHYSIOLOGY OF OBESITY-ASSOCIATED HEART FAILURE

There are several mechanisms proposed that link obesity with HF:

- *Increased blood volume and cardiac output*, causing left ventricular (LV) hypertrophy[4]
- *Insulin resistance and metabolic syndrome*, which contribute to myocardial fibrosis and diastolic dysfunction[5]
- *Neurohormonal activation*, including the renin-angiotensin-aldosterone system (RAAS) and sympathetic nervous system[6]
- *Adipokines and inflammation*, with cytokines such as leptin, resistin, and TNF-α contributing to myocardial remodeling.[7]

All these mechanisms make obesity-associated HF a challenge to tackle. But ARNI contains two classes of drugs such as sacubitril/valsartan. *Sacubitril*, a neprilysin inhibitor, which increases levels of natriuretic peptides, bradykinin, and adrenomedullin, leading to vasodilation, natriuresis, and inhibition of fibrosis.[3] *Valsartan*, an angiotensin II receptor blocker (ARB), inhibits the deleterious effects of RAAS activation. Together, they offer a dual mechanism, reducing adverse neurohormonal effects while enhancing beneficial natriuretic peptide pathways.

EVIDENCE SUPPORTING ANGIOTENSIN RECEPTOR–NEPRILYSIN INHIBITOR USE IN OBESITY-ASSOCIATED HEART FAILURE

The PARADIGM-HF trial demonstrated that sacubitril/valsartan significantly reduced cardiovascular death and HF hospitalization compared to enalapril in HFrEF patients. In patients across various BMI categories, including obese individuals (BMI ≥30 kg/m^2), the relative risk reduction for the primary outcome was consistent. The hazard ratio for the composite endpoint (cardiovascular death or HF hospitalization) was 0.80 (95% CI: 0.73–0.87; p <0.001).[8]

Post-hoc analyses and registry data suggest obese patients may derive similar or greater benefits from ARNI therapy in terms of symptom improvement, reverse remodeling, and biomarker reduction.[9,10] In the

REAL.IT study, nearly 40% of patients showed ≥30% NT-proBNP reduction, and more than half improved LVEF by ≥5% after 1 year of ARNI therapy.[11]

In the PARAGON-HF trial, sacubitril/valsartan did not significantly reduce the primary endpoint in the overall population. However, subgroup analysis showed possible benefit in those with EF at the lower end of the HFpEF spectrum (45–57%), many of whom were obese. In patients with higher adiposity (as measured by waist-to-height ratio), the benefits were more pronounced, with a relative risk reduction of 22% in centrally obese patients.[12,13]

So, ARNI offers some advantages in obese HF patients by:

- *Enhanced natriuresis* to counteract fluid retention common in obesity[3]
- *Antifibrotic and anti-inflammatory effects* are beneficial in obesity-induced myocardial remodeling.[14]
- *Blood pressure reduction* without excessive hypotension is often well-tolerated in obese patients with higher baseline pressures.[8]
- *Weight-neutral profile*, unlike some other HF medications.[15]

But there are some challenges to the use of ARNI in obese patients like obese individuals may require individualized dosing due to altered pharmacokinetics.[16] Though generally well-tolerated, hypotension and renal function must be monitored, especially in patients with comorbid hypertension or CKD.[8] Though promising, evidence in HFpEF remains less conclusive than in HFrEF.[12] Obesity often coexists with diabetes, sleep apnea, and hypertension, requiring comprehensive management beyond ARNI therapy.[2,5]

Ongoing studies such as PARAGLIDE-HF and further analyses from PARAGON-HF may clarify ARNI's role in obesity-associated HFpEF. Moreover, combining ARNI therapy with metabolic interventions (e.g., GLP-1 receptor agonists or bariatric surgery) may improve overall outcomes in obese HF patients.[17]

CONCLUSION

Angiotensin receptor–neprilysin inhibitors, particularly sacubitril/valsartan, represent a potent therapeutic option in the management of HF in obese individuals. While robust evidence supports their use in HFrEF regardless of BMI, their role in obesity-associated HFpEF is promising but requires further validation. Considering the unique pathophysiological features of obesity-associated HF, ARNI therapy may offer dual benefits by targeting both hemodynamic and metabolic pathways.

REFERENCES

1. Kenchaiah S, Evans JC, Levy D, et al. Obesity and the risk of heart failure. N Engl J Med. 2002;347(5):305-13.
2. Pandey A, Patel KV, Vaduganathan M, et al. Physical activity, fitness, and obesity in heart failure with preserved ejection fraction. JACC Heart Fail. 2018;6(12):975-82.
3. McMurray JJ, Packer M, Desai AS, et al. Angiotensin–neprilysin inhibition versus enalapril in heart failure. N Engl J Med. 2014;371(11):993-1004.
4. Abel ED, Litwin SE, Sweeney G. Cardiac remodeling in obesity. Physiol Rev. 2008;88(2):389-419.
5. Paulus WJ, Tschöpe C. A novel paradigm for heart failure with preserved ejection fraction. J Am Coll Cardiol. 2013; 62(4):263-71.
6. Doehner W, Frenneaux M, Anker SD. Metabolic impairment in heart failure: the myocardial and systemic perspective. J Am Coll Cardiol. 2014;64(13):1388-400.
7. Van Linthout S, Tschope C. Inflammation—cause or consequence of heart failure or both? Curr Heart Fail Rep. 2017;14(4):251-65.
8. McMurray JJ, Solomon SD, Inzucchi SE, et al. PARADIGM-HF: a randomized trial of LCZ696 vs enalapril. N Engl J Med. 2014;371(11):993-1004.
9. Dewan P, Docherty KF, McMurray JJ. Sacubitril/valsartan in Asian patients with heart failure with reduced ejection fraction. Eur J Heart Fail. 2020;22(5):779-83.
10. Januzzi JL, Prescott MF, Butler J, et al. Association of change in N-terminal pro–B-type natriuretic peptide following initiation of sacubitril–valsartan treatment with cardiac structure and function in patients with HFrEF. JAMA. 2019;322(11):1085-95.
11. Rosano GM, Seferovic P, Savarese G, et al. Real-world use of sacubitril/valsartan in the management of HFrEF: results from the REAL.IT study. ESC Heart Fail. 2023;10(1):147-56.
12. Solomon SD, McMurray JJ, Anand IS, et al. PARAGON-HF trial: sacubitril/valsartan in patients with HFpEF. N Engl J Med. 2019;381(17):1609-20.
13. Packer M, Lam CSP, Lund LH, et al. Impact of obesity on the response to sacubitril/valsartan in HFpEF: a subgroup analysis of PARAGON-HF. Circulation. 2021;143(9):877-88.
14. Von Lueder TG, Sangaralingham SJ, Wang BH, et al. Renin-angiotensin blockade combined with natriuretic peptide system augmentation: novel approach to heart failure therapy. Hypertension. 2013;61(2):290-8.
15. Seferovic PM, Petrie MC, Filippatos GS, et al. Type 2 diabetes mellitus and heart failure: a position statement from the Heart Failure Association of the European Society of Cardiology. Eur J Heart Fail. 2018;20(5):853-72.
16. Sharma A, Zhao D, Hammill BG, et al. Trends in nonadherence to evidence-based heart failure therapies in Medicare beneficiaries. JACC Heart Fail. 2018;6(7):561-9.
17. Vaduganathan M, Januzzi JL, Pitt B, et al. Initiation, titration, and sequencing of foundational drugs for heart failure with reduced ejection fraction. Lancet. 2020;396(10255):489-502.

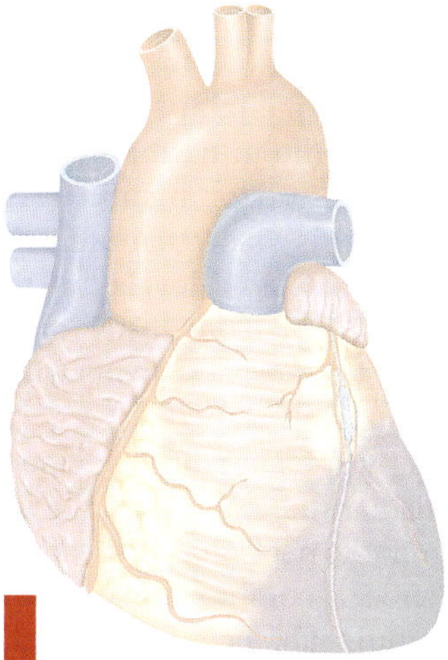

137

CHAPTER

Angiotensin Receptor Blockers and Neprilysin Inhibitors and Blood Pressure Control in Obese Patients

Shitij Chaudhary, Neha Chopra, Nirmal Ghati

INTRODUCTION

Obesity and systemic hypertension are worldwide problems and have continued to grow over the last decade. Mechanistically, both are intertwined, and when associated with type 2 diabetes mellitus, they constitute the metabolic syndrome. Obesity predisposes to systemic hypertension by various mechanisms that include sympathetic overactivity, plasma volume expansion, activation of the renin–angiotensinogen–aldosterone system (RAAS), and increased risk of obstructive sleep apnea.[1] While obese patients are more likely to develop systemic hypertension, they are also more likely to have treatment-resistant hypertension. They may require more antihypertensive medications for blood pressure (BP) control.[2-5] While there is a paucity of data specifically about BP control in obese patients, the metabolic side effects of antihypertensive drugs, viz., weight gain and worsening insulin sensitivity, are particularly relevant in this population. Similarly, antihypertensive drugs like angiotensin receptor blockers and neprilysin inhibitors (ARNi), which have been shown to improve insulin sensitivity in individuals with obesity and hypertension, may be promising in this population.[6]

MECHANISM OF ACTION OF ARNi

Sacubitril–valsartan, the first-in-class angiotensin receptor–neprilysin inhibitor (ARNi), is one of the four pillars of therapy for the management of heart failure with reduced ejection fraction (HFrEF), following the overwhelming benefits in the form of decreased mortality and heart failure hospitalizations observed in the PARADIGM-HF trial.[7] It combines angiotensin receptor blockade by valsartan along with neprilysin inhibition by sacubitril. Neprilysin is a metallopeptidase that hydrolyzes natriuretic peptides, namely atrial natriuretic peptide (ANP), B-type natriuretic peptide (BNP), and C-type natriuretic peptide (CNP). Natriuretic peptides lead to diuresis, natriuresis, peripheral vasodilation, and sympatholytic effects, which translate into the BP-lowering and reverse cardiac remodeling effects seen with ARNi **(Flowchart 1)**.[8] Thus, while ARNi has been utilized as a breakthrough treatment in HFrEF, its use as an antihypertensive has not been extensively studied and

Flowchart 1: Mechanism of action of ARNi.

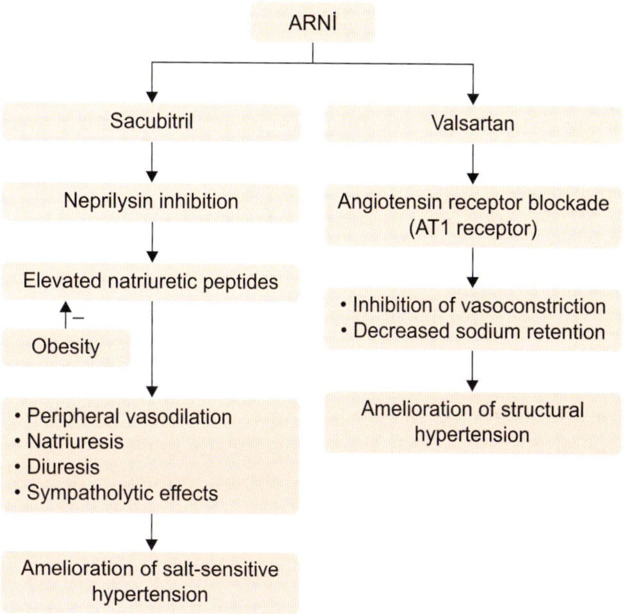

remains underutilized. The following section reviews the available data on ARNi as an antihypertensive agent with a special focus on obese patients.

EFFICACY OF ARNi IN TREATMENT-NAÏVE HYPERTENSION

Various studies have looked at the BP-lowering effects of ARNi in treatment-naïve hypertensive patients. Ruilope et al. studied 1,328 patients with mild-to-moderate hypertension and showed a mean reduction in sitting diastolic BP of −2.17 mm Hg (95% CI: −3.28 to −1.06; p <0.0001) versus the appropriate comparator dose of valsartan.[9] A meta-analysis of randomized controlled trials of sacubitril–valsartan versus angiotensin receptor blockers (ARBs) alone (olmesartan or valsartan) by Zhao et al.,[10] showed sacubitril–valsartan lowered mean systolic BPs by −5.43 mm Hg [95% confidence interval (CI): −6.36 to −4.49 mm Hg; $p < 0.001$], and mean diastolic BP by −2.34 mm Hg (95% CI: −2.67 to −2.01 mm Hg; $p < 0.001$), over and above ARBs. The average reductions in systolic BP achieved by sacubitril–valsartan in dosages of 100, 200, and 400 mg daily translate to around 14, 18, and 20 mm Hg, respectively, reflecting the dose-dependent reductions in systolic BP with ARNi. The average reduction in diastolic BP achieved by sacubitril–valsartan translates to around 9–10 mm Hg.[10] These reductions are equal to or even greater than what is achieved by a combination of two antihypertensive drug classes at standard doses.[11] Sacubitril–valsartan was also shown to reduce the need for additional antihypertensive agents for adequate BP control compared to ARBs at 52 weeks.[12] In total, 32% patients in the ARNi arm and 47% patients in the ARB arm required additional antihypertensive agents (calcium channel blocker/thiazide diuretic) ($p < 0.002$) for adequate BP control at 52 weeks.[12]

In all these studies, sacubitril–valsartan was well-tolerated, with no major adverse side effects. Nasopharyngitis, upper respiratory tract infections, and dizziness are the most commonly reported side effects in some of the studies.[13,14] While head-to-head trials with other antihypertensives other than ARBs are lacking, sacubitril–valsartan is a promising option as an antihypertensive in treatment-naïve patients. The long-term efficacy and outcome data are also lacking, with the longest follow-up of 52 weeks in two studies.[12,14] None of the studies discussed above specifically dealt with obese hypertensive patients. Some of the inferences from these studies might favor the use of ARNi as an antihypertensive agent, specifically in this population:

- Sacubitril–valsartan has been shown to enhance insulin sensitivity in obese hypertensive patients compared to amlodipine.[6] In the post hoc analysis of the PARADIGM-HF trial, ARNi led to a greater HbA1c reduction compared to enalapril after 1 and 3 years of follow-up. Also, the initiation of new oral antihyperglycemic drugs and/or insulin was lower in the ARNi group.[15] This was attributed to higher glucagon-like peptide 1 (GLP-1) levels due to decreased degradation with ARNi. Thus, ARNi may offer additional benefits in hypertensive patients with metabolic syndrome and insulin resistance.
- Thiazide diuretics, particularly at higher doses, worsen lipid and glucose metabolism, resulting in hyperglycemia and dyslipidemia. Similarly, beta-blockers lead to weight gain and dyslipidemia. A combination of both these drugs has the maximum diabetogenic potential. Thus, ARNi may be an alternative to these drug classes by virtue of its insulin-sensitizing effects.
- Obese hypertensives may have associated left ventricular systolic dysfunction with or without coronary artery disease. ARNi has already been shown to reduce mortality and heart failure hospitalizations in the HFrEF population and, therefore, should be the first-line antihypertensive agent in patients with associated left ventricular systolic dysfunction. In patients with HFrEF not tolerating ARNi due to hypotension, drugs such as calcium channel blockers and nitrates, which do not have any mortality benefit in this population, must be discontinued, and ARNi must be uptitrated to maximally tolerated doses.
- Obesity is a state of "natriuretic peptide deficiency," attributed to both decreased production of natriuretic peptides and increased clearance, through an adiposity-associated clearance receptor, NPR3.[16] Natriuretic peptide deficiency in obesity is hypothesized to increase the susceptibility to cardiometabolic diseases.[17] ARNi increases natriuretic peptide levels and thus may target this basic pathophysiology in obese hypertensive patients.
- Obese and overweight hypertensive patients have been shown to require a greater number of antihypertensive agents for BP control compared to those with normal weight (mean number of antihypertensive agents 1.73, 1.88, and 1.96 in the normal weight, overweight, and obese categories, respectively).[3] ARNi, by virtue of its greater BP-lowering effects, may decrease the need for additional antihypertensive agents and their subsequent side effects.

EFFICACY OF ARNi IN RESISTANT HYPERTENSION

Resistant hypertension is defined as BP above goal despite treatment with three antihypertensives with complementary mechanisms of action, including a diuretic at maximally tolerated doses or BP at goal requiring at least four antihypertensives.[18] Data on how to specifically manage obese patients with resistant hypertension are lacking, and recommendations are largely derived from hypertension trials with a significant proportion of obese patients. A few inferences from these studies suggest a possible role of ARNi in this population:

- The efficacy of spironolactone in patients with true resistant hypertension points to a possible role of aldosterone in the pathophysiology of resistant hypertension.[19] In the same study, patients with a higher waist circumference had a better response to spironolactone. ARNi inhibits RAAS by virtue of angiotensin receptor blockade along with neprilysin inhibition. This dual mechanism of action might prove beneficial in patients with resistant hypertension.
- ARNi has been shown to significantly lower BP in patients with heart failure with preserved ejection fraction (HFpEF) and apparent resistant and apparent mineralocorticosteroid antagonist (MRA) resistant hypertension.[20] Thus, ARNi may be a useful antihypertensive agent in patients who have elevated BP despite treatment with four antihypertensive agents, including an MRA.

Antihypertensive Pharmacotherapy in Obesity

The goal of antihypertensive therapy in obesity is to effectively lower BP without increasing the metabolic risks associated with obesity. As discussed above, beta-blockers and thiazide diuretics may worsen glucose and lipid metabolism; therefore, their BP-lowering efficacy has to be balanced against the metabolic side effects in obese patients. Additionally, obese patients require a greater number of antihypertensive agents for adequate BP control. Thus, the current hypertension guidelines do not recommend any antihypertensive agent over the other, nor do they discourage the use of beta-blockers and thiazide diuretics due to metabolic side-effects, since a combination of drugs is often required for BP control in this population. This is also supported by the subanalysis of the ACCOMPLISH trial, in which the cardiovascular outcomes did not differ between the obese patients treated with an ACEi, either combined with a CCB or a diuretic.[21]

Therefore, ARNi may prove to be a superior agent for BP control, especially in obese patients with HFrEF and apparent MRA-resistant hypertension. It may also be an alternative to thiazide diuretics and beta-blockers in obese patients with dyslipidemia and/or diabetes (**Flowchart 2**). The only drawback of this drug class in today's world

Flowchart 2: Suggested algorithm for the use of ARNi as an antihypertensive in obese patients.

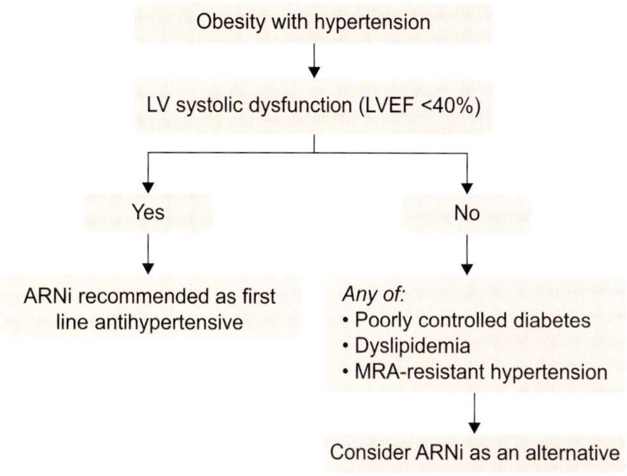

would be cost-effectiveness compared to other cheaper alternative drugs that are readily available.

While we suggest ARNi as a viable option for BP control in these subgroups of patients, head-to-head trials and long-term outcome data with ARNi in hypertension are required.

CONCLUSION

ARNi has shown promise as an antihypertensive in both treatment-naïve and resistant hypertension. Its effects might be more relevant in the obese population due to its beneficial metabolic effects, besides the superior BP-lowering effects. Head-to head comparisons with other antihypertensive agents and long-term outcome data in hypertension are the need of the hour to establish this promising yet underutilized drug for hypertension.

REFERENCES

1. Jordan J, Toplak H, Grassi G, et al. Joint statement of the European Association for the Study of Obesity and the European Society of Hypertension: obesity and difficult to treat arterial hypertension. J Hypertens. 2016;34(9):1678-88.
2. Bramlage P, Pittrow D, Wittchen H-U, et al. Hypertension in overweight and obese primary care patients is highly prevalent and poorly controlled. Am J Hypertens. 2004;17(10):904-10.
3. Reisin E, Graves JW, Yamal J-M, et al. Blood pressure control and cardiovascular outcomes in normal-weight, overweight, and obese hypertensive patients treated with three different antihypertensives in ALLHAT. J Hypertens. 2014;32(7):1503.
4. Bhan V, Yan RT, Leiter LA, et al. Relation between obesity and the attainment of optimal blood pressure and lipid

targets in high vascular risk outpatients. Am J Cardiol. 2010;106(9):1270-6.
5. Lloyd-Jones DM, Evans JC, Larson MG, et al. Differential control of systolic and diastolic blood pressure: factors associated with lack of blood pressure control in the community. Hypertension. 2000;36(4):594-9.
6. Jordan J, Stinkens R, Jax T, et al. Improved insulin sensitivity with angiotensin receptor neprilysin inhibition in individuals with obesity and hypertension. Clin Pharmacol Ther. 2017;101(2):254-63.
7. McMurray JJV, Packer M, Desai AS, et al. Angiotensin-neprilysin inhibition versus enalapril in heart failure. N Engl J Med. 2014;371(11):993-1004.
8. Azizi M, Rossignol P, Hulot JS. Emerging drug classes and their potential use in hypertension. Hypertension. 2019;74(5):1075-83.
9. Ruilope LM, Dukat A, Böhm M, et al. Blood-pressure reduction with LCZ696, a novel dual-acting inhibitor of the angiotensin II receptor and neprilysin: a randomised, double-blind, placebo-controlled, active comparator study. Lancet. 2010;375:1255-66.
10. Zhao Y, Yu H, Zhao X, et al. The effects of LCZ696 in patients with hypertension compared with angiotensin receptor blockers: a meta-analysis of randomized controlled trials. J Cardiovasc Pharmacol Ther. 2017;22(5):447-57.
11. Wang B, Mo X, Wu Z, et al. Systematic review and meta-analysis of the correlation between plasma homocysteine levels and coronary heart disease. J Thorac Dis. 2022;14(3):646-53.
12. Williams B, Cockcroft JR, Kario K, et al. Effects of sacubitril/valsartan versus olmesartan on central hemodynamics in the elderly with systolic hypertension: the PARAMETER study. Hypertension. 2017;69(3):411-20.
13. Kario K, Sun N, Chiang FT, et al. Efficacy and safety of LCZ696, a first-in-class angiotensin receptor neprilysin inhibitor, in Asian patients with hypertension. Hypertension. 2014;63(4):698-705.
14. Supasyndh O, Sun N, Kario K, et al. Long-term (52-week) safety and efficacy of sacubitril/valsartan in Asian patients with hypertension. Hypertens Res. 2017;40(5):472-6.
15. Seferovic JP, Claggett B, Seidelmann SB, et al. Effect of sacubitril/valsartan versus enalapril on glycaemic control in patients with heart failure and diabetes: a post-hoc analysis from the PARADIGM-HF trial. Lancet Diabetes Endocrinol. 2017;5(5):333-40.
16. Parcha V, Patel N, Musunuru K, et al. Natriuretic peptide deficiency in obese individuals. JACC. 2021;77(24):3138-40.
17. Wang TJ, Larson MG, Levy D, et al. Impact of obesity on plasma natriuretic peptide levels. Circulation. 2004;109(5):594-600.
18. Writing Committee Members; Jones DW, Ferdinand KC, et al. 2025 AHA/ACC/AANP/AAPA/ABC/ACCP/ACPM/AGS/AMA/ASPC/NMA/PCNA/ SGIM guideline for the prevention, detection, evaluation and management of high blood pressure in adults: a report of the American College of Cardiology/American Heart Association Joint Committee on Clinical Practice Guidelines. Circulation. 2025;152(11):e114-218.
19. de Souza F, Muxfeldt E, Fiszman R, et al. Efficacy of spironolactone therapy in patients with true resistant hypertension. Hypertension. 2010;55(1):147-52.
20. Jackson AM, Jhund PS, Anand IS, et al. Sacubitril-valsartan as a treatment for apparent resistant hypertension in patients with heart failure and preserved ejection fraction. Eur Heart J. 2021;42(36):3741-52.
21. Weber MA, Jamerson K, Bakris GL, et al. Effects of body size and hypertension treatments on cardiovascular event rates: subanalysis of the ACCOMPLISH randomised controlled trial. Lancet. 2013;381(9866):537-45.

CHAPTER 138

Angiotensin Receptor–Neprilysin Inhibitor and the Gut Microbiome in Obesity and Cardiovascular Disease

Preeti Gupta, Dikshant Jain

INTRODUCTION

In daily practice, we confront a recurring triad: obesity, cardiometabolic dysfunction, and heart failure (HF). Angiotensin receptor-neprilysin inhibition (ARNI; sacubitril/valsartan) transformed HF management by combining renin-angiotensin-aldosterone system (RAAS) blockade with neprilysin (NEP) inhibition, augmenting natriuretic peptides and other vasoactive hormones. Beyond the usual hemodynamic improvement, ARNI also touches pathways central to obesity biology—adipose lipolysis, browning, insulin signaling—and, intriguingly, enteroendocrine peptides that are degraded by NEP (e.g., GLP-1). In parallel, the gut microbiome has emerged as a mechanistic nexus connecting diet, adiposity, inflammation, and atherosclerosis via metabolites (e.g., TMAO), endotoxemia (LPS), and bile-acid/short chain fatty acids (SCFA) signaling. Recent preclinical data and post-hoc clinical analyses invite a question we often ponder at the bedside: Can ARNI favorably intersect with gut-metabolic axes that drive obesity and cardiovascular disease (CVD)? **Figure 1** provides an overview of these integrated gut-adipose-heart interactions, while **Figure 2** details the key molecular and microbial pathways involved. In this chapter, we collect and understand the mechanistic and clinical evidence, highlighting the translational implications, and propose practical, testable algorithms for integrating ARNI into cardiometabolic care while awaiting definitive human microbiome data.

ANGIOTENSIN RECEPTOR–NEPRILYSIN INHIBITION

Neprilysin Biology at the Cardiometabolic Interface

Neprilysin (membrane zinc metalloprotease) degrades natriuretic peptides (ANP/BNP), bradykinin, substance P, GLP-1, glucagon, and others. NEP inhibition amplifies NP-cGMP signaling, which in adipose tissue promotes lipolysis, mitochondrial biogenesis, and "beige"/brown fat programming via NPR-A and PKG pathways, improving substrate handling and energy expenditure.[1-3] The NP–NPR-A–cGMP–PKG adipocyte pathway is shown in **Figure 2A**. Obesity features a "natriuretic handicap", with lower NP bioactivity and higher clearance through NPR-C in adipose tissue; restoring NP signaling is metabolically salutary.[2,4] Experimental work also shows NEP inhibition can augment GLP-1-dependent insulin secretion in β-cell dysfunction and modulate glucagon dynamics, underscoring complex glycemic effects that may depend on route of stimulus and metabolic state.[5-7] This endocrine crosstalk is depicted in **Figure 2B**.

Key mechanistic takeaways:

1. Neprilysin inhibition ↑NP signaling → lipolysis, browning, and improved oxidative capacity.[1-3]
2. NEP inhibition interacts with incretin biology (GLP-1), potentially improving β-cell responsiveness but with context-dependent effects on glucose and glucagon.[5-7]
3. In obesity, altered NP receptor expression (↑NPR-C) blunts NP actions; ARNI may partially overcome this.[4]

Gut Microbiome in Obesity and Cardiovascular Disease

Obesity and HF associate with dysbiosis—reduced diversity, altered firmicutes/bacteroidetes balance, and expansion of pathobionts—leading to metabolic endotoxemia (circulating LPS), impaired barrier function, and systemic inflammation.[8-12] Microbial metabolites shape cardiovascular risk: *TMAO* (produced from dietary choline/carnitine) correlates with incident coronary events, stroke, HF risk, and mortality in many cohorts (though not all), while SCFAs (acetate, propionate, and butyrate) generally support barrier integrity, GLP-1 secretion, and blood-pressure regulation.[13-18] These contrasting microbial pathways are summarized in **Figure 2C**. In HF, the "gut–heart axis" encompasses congestion-induced barrier injury, uremic milieu, bile-acid shifts, and drug–microbe interactions that can alter efficacy and toxicity.[9,10,19] Key microbiome-derived biomarkers relevant to cardiometabolic care, including TMAO, SCFAs, LPS, and bile acids, along with their clinical interpretation and assay methods, are summarized in **Figure 3**.

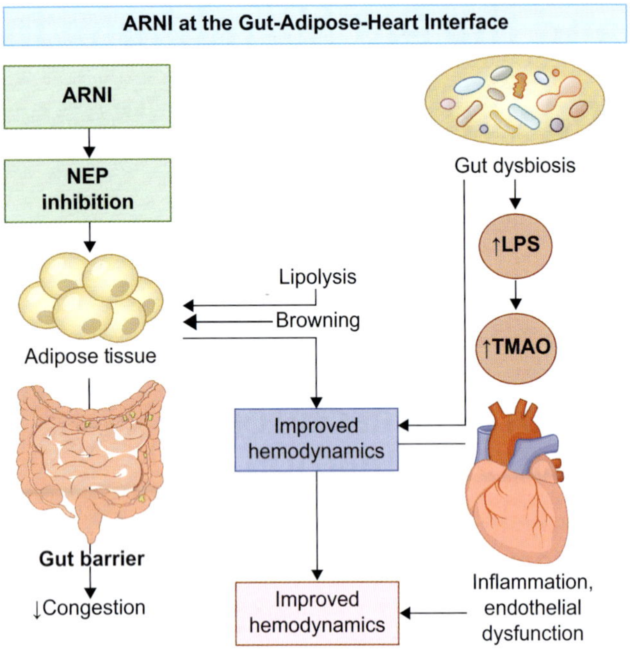

Fig. 1: Mechanistic schematic—ARNI at the gut–adipose–heart axis showing NEP inhibition → ↑NP–cGMP signaling (adipose lipolysis/browning), potential ↑GLP-1 bioactivity, improved hemodynamics; overlay with gut dysbiosis → ↑LPS/TMAO → inflammation/endothelial dysfunction; hypothesized ARNI-mediated attenuation.

Clinical relevance: Elevated TMAO and biomarkers of intestinal permeability predict adverse outcomes in CAD/HF; attenuating endotoxemia and restoring eubiosis may improve cardiometabolic profiles.[13-16,18,20]

Evidence that ARNI Touches Gut–metabolic Pathways

Glycemic control: In PARADIGM-HF post-hoc analyses, sacubitril/valsartan reduced HbA1c modestly versus enalapril and delayed insulin initiation among HFrEF patients with diabetes; pooled HF analyses suggest a small but consistent HbA1c reduction not clearly modified by LVEF.[21,22] These clinical effects and their effect sizes relative to comparators are summarized in **Figure 4**. These clinical signals align with NEP–incretin interactions observed in experimental models.[5-7]

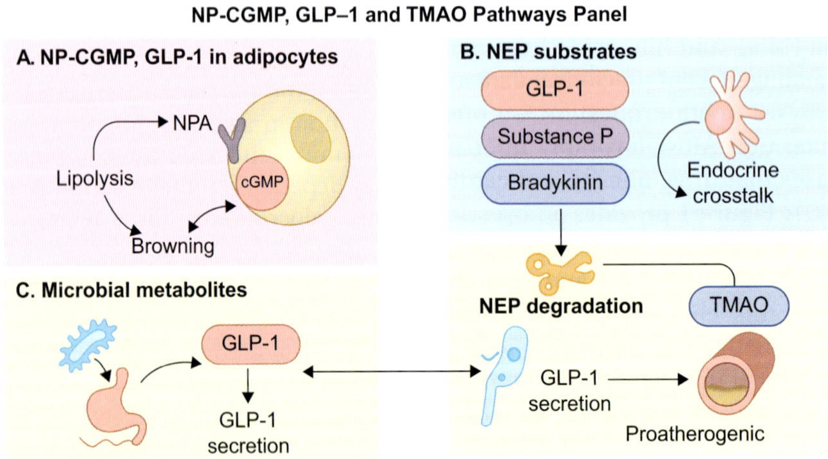

Figs. 2A to C: Pathways panel—(A) NP–NPR-A–cGMP–PKG in adipocytes; (B) NEP substrates (GLP-1, substance P, and bradykinin) and endocrine crosstalk; (C) Microbial metabolites (SCFAs ↑GLP-1; TMAO proatherogenic).

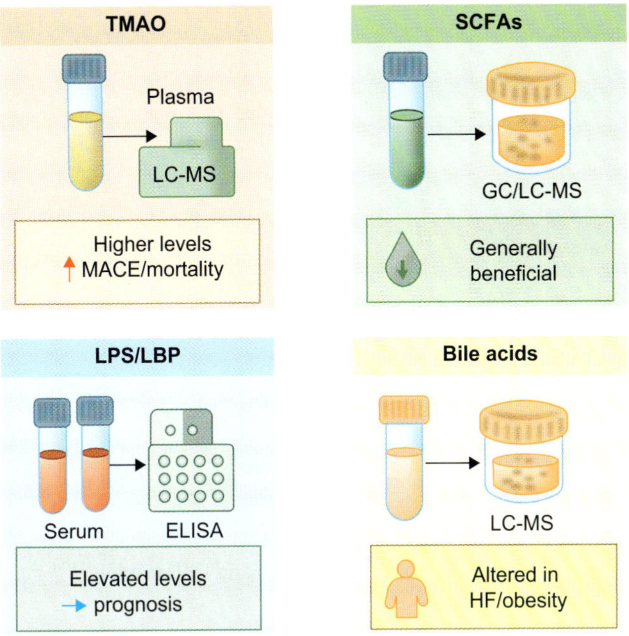

Fig. 3: Summary of microbiome endpoints relevant to cardiometabolic care (TMAO, SCFAs, LPS, and bile acids) with assay methods and clinical interpretation. (GC-MS: gas chromatography-mass spectrometry; HF: heart failure; LBP: LP-5-binding protein; LC-MS: liquid chromatography-mass spectrometry; LPS: lipopolysaccharide; SCFAs: short-chain fatty acids; TMAO: trimethylamine N-oxide)

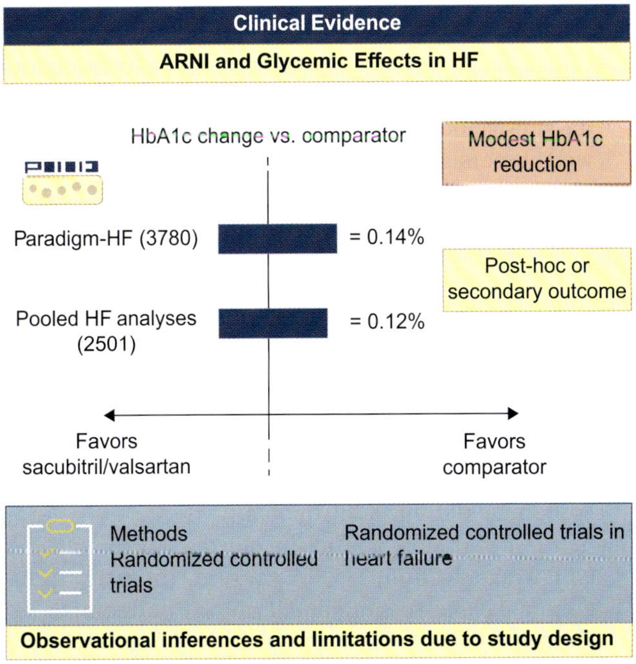

Fig. 4: Clinical evidence forest—bar/forest plot of HbA1c changes versus comparators from PARADIGM-HF and pooled HF analyses;[21,22] annotate effect sizes.

Microbiome modulation (preclinical): In a murine model of chronic intermittent hypoxia (a sleep-apnea proxy linked to obesity), sacubitril/valsartan mitigated dysbiosis and vascular injury, suggesting ARNI can indirectly normalize gut microbial composition under cardiometabolic stress.[23] In diabetic kidney disease mice, sac/val improved renal fibrosis *and* shifted gut microbiota composition, hinting at systemic benefits through gut pathways.[24] Genus-level microbial shifts observed in these models are visualized as heatmaps in **Figure 5**.

Adipose and energy balance biology: Translational work shows enhancing NP signaling increases lipolysis and browning, with favorable effects on whole-body glucose homeostasis.[1-3,24] Given ARNI increases NP bioactivity, this pathway plausibly contributes to weight-neutral or weight-beneficial effects in HF populations with fluid-weight confounding; robust dedicated weight endpoints remain limited.

Integration with endotoxemia: While no human trial shows ARNI lowers TMAO or LPS directly, by improving HF hemodynamics (congestion and perfusion) and possibly enhancing GLP-1/SCFA axes, ARNI could indirectly decrease barrier injury and systemic inflammation. This remains a hypothesis requiring targeted human studies anchored in microbiome endpoints.[9,10,13,19]

FROM MECHANISMS TO CLINIC: WHERE MIGHT ARNI FIT?

In patients with obesity, diabetes, and HF (HFrEF or some HFpEF phenotypes), ARNI is already guideline-concordant for HF outcomes; its *added metabolic advantages*—modest HbA1c lowering, improved insulin dynamics in experimental models, and NP-mediated adipose effects—are clinically welcome.[21,22] For cardiometabolic patients without guideline indications for ARNI, data are insufficient to justify off-label use solely for obesity or dysbiosis. Instead, ARNI should be embedded in a *bundle*: sodium restriction, high-fiber Mediterranean-style diet, structured exercise, sleep-apnea management, and (in select cases) GLP-1RA/SGLT2i, all of which synergize with ARNI's hemodynamic and metabolic footprint and may rebalance the gut ecosystem.[9,13-16,19]

RESEARCH LANDSCAPE AND GAPS

- *Direct human microbiome endpoints:* Few trials assess ARNI's impact on α/β-diversity, SCFAs, bile acids, TMAO, LPS, and barrier markers.
- *Phenotype-specific effects:* Obese HFpEF versus HFrEF, OSA-predominant patients, and NAFLD/CAD overlap

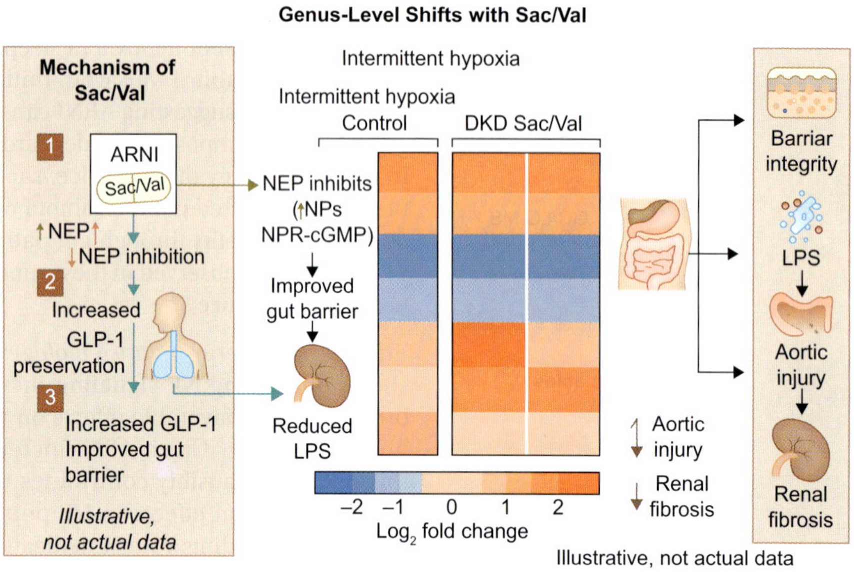

Fig. 5: Preclinical microbiome data—heatmap of genus-level shifts with Sac/Val in intermittent hypoxia and DKD models.[23,24]

- *Combination strategies:* ARNI + GLP-1RA or SGLT2i may converge on gut-metabolic benefits; head-to-head microbiome readouts are lacking.
- *Causality:* Distinguishing hemodynamic improvement effects from true microbiome modulation is essential.

LIMITATION

There are several constraints when translating these insights to the ward:

- *Sparse human microbiome data with ARNI:* Evidence of direct microbiome modulation is largely preclinical.[23,24]
- *Context-dependent glycemic effects:* NEP inhibition interacts with GLP-1 and glucagon; human studies show small HbA1c benefits but mixed signals on incretin dynamics and occasional hypoglycemia reports, particularly in diabetes cohorts with intensive background therapy.[6,7,21-23]
- *Confounding by HF improvement:* Better perfusion/decongestion itself can normalize gut barrier function, complicating attribution to NEP-specific mechanisms.[9,10]
- *Heterogeneity in microbiome literature:* TMAO associations vary across populations; causality is stronger in experimental than in primary-prevention human cohorts.[13-18]
- *Generalizability beyond HF:* Using ARNI primarily for obesity or NAFLD without HF evidence is not yet supported by randomized data.

GUIDELINES/ALGORITHM/SUMMARY ILLUSTRATION

Algorithm: "Cardio-Metabolic-Microbiome ARNI Pathway"

1. *Identify phenotype:* HF (HFrEF; HFpEF with obesity/OSA), obesity (BMI ≥30), T2D, NAFLD, CAD with metabolic endotoxemia markers (TMAO/LPS if available).
2. *Establish foundation:* Mediterranean-style high-fiber diet (↑prebiotics), 150–300 min/week aerobic + 2 days resistance, OSA screening and CPAP if indicated, weight management, SGLT2i ± GLP-1RA per diabetes/obesity guidelines.
3. *HF optimization:* If ARNI-eligible, initiate sacubitril/valsartan (after ACEi washout if needed), uptitrate.
4. *Targeted labs (optional, research-oriented):* Baseline and 3–6-month TMAO, fasting LPS/LBP, fecal SCFAs, stool 16S (where available) to phenotype endotoxemia and response.
5. *Safety and interactions:* Monitor BP, renal function, potassium; watch for hypoglycemia with insulin/secretagogues after ARNI uptitration in T2D; coordinate diuretic adjustments.
6. *Iterate:* If persistent obesity/insulin resistance, consider GLP-1RA addition; if OSA present, intensify CPAP adherence; reassess metabolic and HF endpoints.
7. *Outcome focus:* Symptoms (KCCQ), NT-proBNP, HF hospitalizations; secondarily HbA1c, weight, waist circumference, and—if available—gut markers.

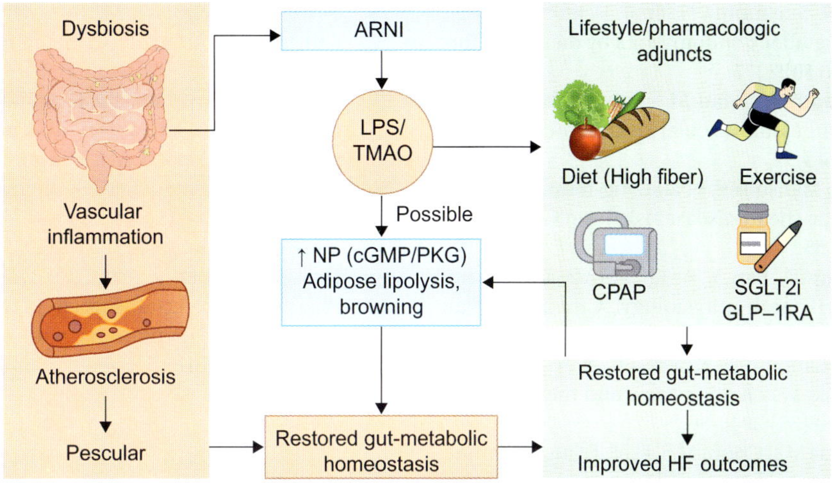

(ARNI: angiotensin receptor–neprilysin inhibition; CPAP: continuous positive airway pressure; GLP-1RA: glucagon-like peptide-1 receptor agonist; LPS: lipopolysaccharide; NEP: neprilysin; NF: heart failure; NP: natriuretic peptide; TMAO: trimethylamine N-oxide)

Summary illustration: A one-page infographic linking (A) dysbiosis → LPS/TMAO → vascular inflammation; (B) ARNI →↑NP signaling and possible ↑GLP-1 tone; (C) lifestyle/pharmacologic adjuncts that synergize to restore gut–metabolic homeostasis.

CONCLUSION

From my vantage point as a cardiologist managing obese, dysmetabolic patients with HF, ARNI delivers proven HF outcome benefits while offering plausible, modest metabolic advantages. Mechanistically, NEP inhibition enhances NP signaling in adipose tissue (lipolysis/browning) and intersects incretin biology; clinically, ARNI modestly lowers HbA1c and delays insulin initiation in HFrEF with diabetes. Preclinical studies suggest ARNI may ameliorate dysbiosis under cardiometabolic stress, but we lack definitive human data connecting ARNI to improvements in TMAO, LPS, or SCFAs. The practical path today is *integration*: deploy ARNI where indicated, layer lifestyle and microbiome-sensitive therapies (dietary fiber, weight loss, OSA treatment, and SGLT2i/GLP-1RA), and prioritize trials that embed microbiome endpoints. As our field pivots toward cardiometabolic phenotyping, I anticipate that clarifying ARNI's role in the gut–heart axis will refine therapy selection for the obese HF patient and possibly illuminate new endpoints that matter to both heart and host.

REFERENCES

1. Wu W, Tsuchida H, Kato T, et al. Enhancing natriuretic peptide signalling in adipose tissue, but not in muscle, protects against diet-induced obesity and insulin resistance. JCI Insight. 2017;2(21):e94054.
2. Madamanchi C, Alhosaini H, Sumida A, et al. Obesity and natriuretic peptides. J Am Coll Cardiol. 2014;63(17):1700-10.
3. Kimura H, Nagoshi T, Oi Y, et al. Treatment with atrial natriuretic peptide induces adipose and skeletal muscle thermogenic programming. Sci Rep. 2021;11: 17479.
4. Gentili A, Frangogiannis NG. Modulation of natriuretic peptide receptors in human adipose tissue: impact of obesity. Adipocyte. 2017;6(4):325-31.
5. Esser N, Paquot N, Scheen AJ, et al. Neprilysin inhibition improves IV but not oral glucose-mediated insulin secretion via GLP-1R signalling in β-cell dysfunction. Am J Physiol Endocrinol Metab. 2022;322(3):E307-18.
6. Esser N, Paquot N, Scheen AJ, et al. Neprilysin inhibition in mouse islets enhances insulin secretion akin to DPP-4 inhibition. Islets. 2018;10(4):e1502521.
7. Kjeldsen SAS, Gabriel-Cornu V, Hedrington MS, et al. Neprilysin inhibition increases glucagon levels in humans and mice. J Endocr Soc. 2021;5(9):bvab084.
8. Violi F, Carnevale R, Loffredo L, et al. Gut barrier dysfunction and endotoxemia in heart failure. Biochem Biophys Res Commun. 2023;640:33-43.
9. Snelson M, R Muralitharan R, Liu CF, et al. The role of gut microbiota and metabolites in heart failure. Circ Res. 2025;136(11):1382-406.
10. Zhao S, Sun Y, Zhang T, et al. Decoding the impact of gut microbiota on heart failure. Front Cardiovasc Med. 2025;12.
11. García-Jiménez C, Gutiérrez-Salmerón M, Chocarro-Calvo A, et al. Metabolic endotoxemia: a link between obesity and cardiovascular disease. J Mol Endocrinol. 2014;51(2):R51-64.

12. Fuke N, Nagata N, Suganuma H, et al. Regulation of gut microbiota and metabolic endotoxemia by dietary factors. Nutrients. 2019;11(10):2277.
13. Canyelles M, Tondo M, Cofan M, et al. Gut microbiota-derived TMAO and cardiovascular risk: narrative review. Nutrients. 2023;15(3).
14. Heianza Y, Ma W, Manson JE, et al. Long-term changes in TMAO and coronary heart disease risk. J Am Coll Cardiol. 2020;75(20):2152-65.
15. Tang WHW, Wang Z, Fan Y, et al. TMAO and related metabolites in HF pathophysiology. Circ Heart Fail. 2024;17:e011569.
16. Schiattarella GG, Sannino A, Toscano E, et al. TMAO and cardiovascular risk: systematic review and meta-analysis. Eur Heart J. 2017;38(39):2948-56.
17. Budoff MJ, Daviglus ML, Criqui MH, et al. Trimethylamine-N-oxide and risk of incident ASCVD: multi-ethnic cohort. Sci Rep. 2025;15:
18. Wang M, Wu C, Tang WHW, et al. TMAO and long-term mortality in a multi-ethnic US cohort. Front Cardiovasc Med. 2023;10:1195801.
19. Florek K, Michalska M, Boratynska-Kominek M, et al. Gut microbiota's role in heart failure. Heart Fail Rev; 2025.
20. Parantainen J, Salomaa V, Havulinna AS, et al. Biomarkers of intestinal permeability and metabolic endotoxemia predict mortality in CAD. J Nutr Biochem; 2025.
21. Seferovic JP, Claggett B, Seidelmann SB, et al. Effect of sacubitril/valsartan vs enalapril on glycemic control in HFrEF with diabetes: PARADIGM-HF post-hoc. Lancet Diabetes Endocrinol. 2017;5(5):333-40.
22. Wijkman MO, et al. Effects of sacubitril/valsartan on glycemia in HF patients with and without diabetes: pooled PARAGON-HF and PARADIGM-HF. Card Fail Rev; 2022.
23. Wang J, Xu J, Deng X, et al. Sacubitril/valsartan mitigates intermittent hypoxia-related gut microbiome alteration and aortic injury (preclinical). Sleep Breath. 2023;27.
24. Wang P, Yang Y, Li G, et al. Sacubitril/valsartan improves DKD in mice and regulates gut microbiota. Front Pharmacol. 2022;13:1025449.

139

CHAPTER

Angiotensin Receptor–Neprilysin Inhibitor and Renal Protection in Obese Patients with Cardiovascular Disease

Jayagopal PB

INTRODUCTION

Cardiovascular disease (CVD) is the leading cause of morbidity and mortality worldwide. As per the recent WHO report, CVD accounts for approximately 32% of global mortality. Among this, one fifth of the deaths are from the Indian population.[1,2] However, the presence of multimorbidity such as chronic kidney disease (CKD), diabetes mellitus (DM), and obesity in CVD will significantly increase the risk of all-cause mortality and cardiovascular mortality. The American Heart Association (AHA) termed these overlapping conditions as cardiovascular–kidney–metabolic (CKM) syndrome. CKM syndrome is highly prevalent in the UK population. Approximately one third of participants are at advanced CKM stages (stage 3 or higher).[3] About 90% of the US population has CKM syndrome, and approximately 15% of them have an advanced CKM stage. Higher CKM stage was significantly associated with an increased risk of mortality.[4] A recent study conducted among the Asian population indicates that about 71.5% have CKM syndrome.[5]

OBESITY, CHRONIC KIDNEY DISEASE, AND CARDIOVASCULAR DISEASE

Obesity is increasing worldwide, and nearly 50% of the worldwide population is overweight or obese. This is often associated with arrhythmias, diabetes, and other metabolic abnormalities. Likewise, CKD is on the rise and affects one in 10 adults. This leads to a decline in renal function, eventually leading to ESRD. However, the CVS events are the common cause of mortality. This is a combination of CKD and obesity that leads to the CKM syndrome.

Cardiovascular–kidney–metabolic syndrome conceptualizes the interconnection between metabolic risk factors (obesity and diabetes), renal disease, and cardiovascular disorders **(Fig. 1)**. The AHA's advisory classified CKM syndrome into five stages, based on their risk spectrum and pathophysiology **(Table 1)**.[6] Currently, there is no universally accepted clinical guideline or single diagnostic test for CKM syndrome.

PATHOPHYSIOLOGY

In obesity, adipokines are released, leading to activation of the inflammatory pathways. Often, there is insulin resistance and neurohormonal activation, including sympathetic and renin–angiotensin activation. This leads to an increasing cardiovascular event, especially in HFpEF **(Flowchart 1)**.

Obesity is a low-grade proinflammatory state that leads to the deposition of cytokine-laden macrophages in renal and adipose tissues. Adipokines such as leptin and TNF-α induce a proinflammatory state. The metabolic dysfunction associated with obesity leads to renal damage by RAASi activation. This leads to a relative deficiency of atrial and brain natriuretic peptides. This leads to Na^+ reabsorption, increased extracellular volume expansion, and hypertension (HTN). In addition, the obesity-related glomerulopathy increases the progression of disease in established CKD patients.

Management of CKM syndrome includes both lifestyle intervention and pharmacological treatment. SGLT-2 inhibitors, GLP-1 RAs, and nonsteroidal MRAs are currently accepted treatment options for CKM syndrome.

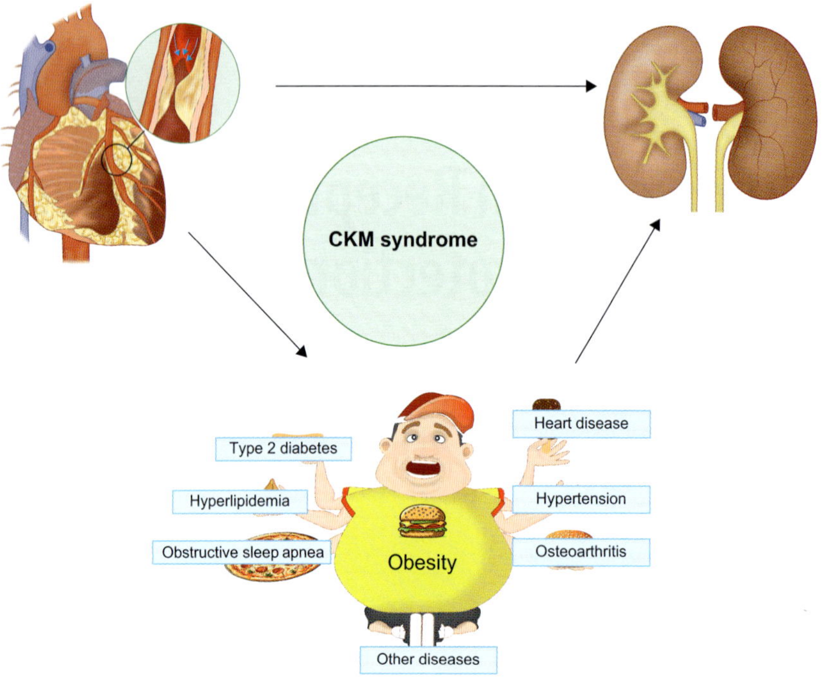

Fig. 1: Triad of CKM syndrome.

TABLE 1: Stages of CKM syndrome.

Stage	*CKM syndrome*
Stage 0	No CKM risk factors
Stage 1	Excess or dysfunctional adiposity
Stage 2	Metabolic risk factors (hypertriglyceridemia, hypertension, diabetes, metabolic syndrome) or moderate- to high-risk chronic kidney disease
Stage 3	Subclinical CVD in CKM syndrome or risk equivalents (high predicted CVD risk or very high-risk CKD)
Stage 4	Clinical CVD in CKM syndrome

Flowchart 1: Correlation between obesity, CKD, and CVD.

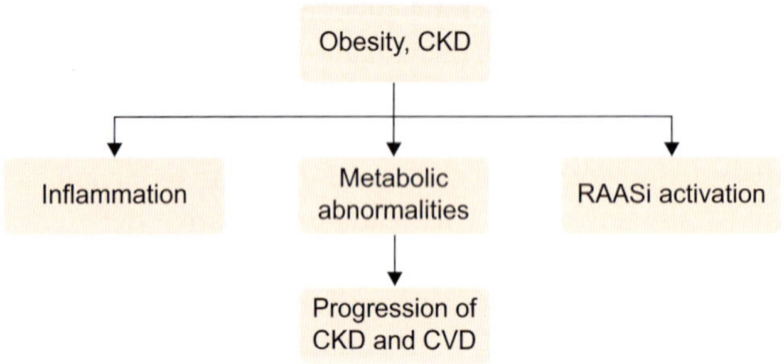

However, angiotensin receptor–neprilysin inhibitor (ARNI) has been developed as an effective therapeutic option for the management of CKM syndrome. ARNI is the cornerstone treatment for the management of heart failure, LV dysfunction, etc. The beneficial effects of ARNI in managing various comorbidities, including CKD, DM, HTN, and obesity, have also been proven.[7]

Angiotensin receptor–neprilysin inhibitor is the cornerstone treatment for heart failure, which has been proven to have a cardioprotective effect as evidenced by the PARADIGM-HF trial. The insights from the PARAGLIDE-HF trial suggest that obese patients with HFmEF and HFpEF experience a more beneficial impact from ARNI compared to patients with normal/overweight BMI.[8] Additionally, ARNI is shown to have a positive effect in Asian HFrEF patients with obesity, comparable to that in the Western population. Also, obese HFrEF patients can have better tolerability of ARNI than the general population. Overall, ARNI has shown beneficial effects on patients who have obesity, renal disease, and CVD.[9]

Angiotensin receptor–neprilysin inhibitor has both renoprotective and cardioprotective effects.[10] The results from a real-world study conducted among HFrEF patients with advanced kidney disease (stage 4/5) indicate that HF rehospitalization and mortality were comparatively lower in patients who were receiving ARNI and also showed a better eGFR and LVEF than those who were not treated with ARNI. Overall, ARNI is well tolerated by the majority of patients with HFrEF and CKD.[11] Treatment with ARNI is beneficial in heart failure patients with cardiorenal syndrome.[12]

The efficacy of ARNI has been well established in the PARADIGM trial, which compared ARNI with enalapril in HFrEF. The available BMI for the patient with KDIGO categories was only 1,910 out of 8,399 patients.[13]

The renal risk categorization has been based on eGFR rates till recently. However, the new KDIGO map also uses the urine–albumin–creatinine ratio to stratify risk into low, intermediate, and high risk for future renal events, as defined by a 40% decline in renal function or end-stage renal disease. An analysis of 1,910 participants in the PARADIGM-HF trial showed 42, 32, and 26% in the low-, medium-, and high-risk groups, respectively. The risks were highest in the highest risk categories (7.6, 9.4, and 14.9 per 100 person-years). The 25% high-risk group of patients had the maximum cardiac events. ARNI was beneficial in all heart failure patients across the entire spectrum.[13,14] When this study cohort was analyzed, the mean BMI was 29.6 ± 5.5, 29.5 ± 5.4, and 29.9 ± 5.6 in the three groups, respectively. This again proves the efficacy of ARNI in obese CKD patients.[14]

The efficacy of ARNI in HF, stratified by BMI, was analyzed in another small study. This did not provide a substantial benefit. However, in the larger SWEDISH HF registry, obese patients often received guideline-directed medical therapy (GDMT) well and in target doses. Five-year mortality and heart failure hospitalization were analyzed. All-cause mortality was 47%, and in obese individuals, mortality was 62%. Use of ARNI was associated with a lower risk for all-cause mortality.[15]

However, the CVS events and mortality in obesity are of particular interest. Obesity may have an advantage in advanced CKD patients. A study by Ladhani et al. showed that a 1 kg/m^2 increase in BMI had no impact on CVS mortality. With increasing BMI, there was a reduction in CVS mortality. The obesity paradox is quite interesting in patients with CKD. This has been seen in HF patients as well.[16]

The two drugs which have been proven to reduce mortality in HFpEF are SGLT-2 inhibitors and semaglutide. The role of RAASi is quite controversial. Obesity is well-known to produce HFpEF and diastolic dysfunction. ARNI in experimental male Zucker rats has shown improvement in diastolic function and blunted disease progression.[17]

Similarly, the analysis of the PARAGLIDE HF study in HFpEF showed that ARNI reduced NT-proBNP levels. Thus, they showed a significant clinical benefit with ARNI. This benefit has also been observed in Indian patients.[9]

CONCLUSION

Obesity is a complex disease process leading to significant cardiovascular morbidity and mortality. At present, in an elderly population, the coexistence of CKD makes it even more challenging a scenario. Use of ARNI, which has proven therapy for heart failure, has again shown benefit in this disease spectrum. Hopefully, with the newer obesity therapy, this entity can be addressed further.

REFERENCES

1. World Health Organization. (2025). Cardiovascular diseases (CVDs). [online] Available from https://www.who.int/news-room/fact-sheets/detail/cardiovascular-diseases-(cvds). [Last accessed January, 2026].
2. Shannawaz M, Rathi I, Shah N, et al. (2025). Prevalence of CVD among Indian adult population: systematic review and meta-analysis. Int J Environ Res Public Health. 2025;22(4):539.
3. Chen Y, Wu X, Long T, et al. Prevalence and mortality association of different stages of cardiovascular-kidney-metabolic syndrome. JACC Adv. 2025;4(6 Pt 2):101843.
4. Aggarwal R, Ostrominski JW, Vaduganathan M. Prevalence of cardiovascular-kidney-metabolic syndrome stages in US adults, 2011-2020. JAMA. 2024;331(21):1858-60.
5. Tsai MK, Kao JT, Wong CS, et al. Cardiovascular-kidney-metabolic syndrome and all-cause and cardiovascular mortality: a retrospective cohort study. PLoS Med. 2025;22(6):e1004629.
6. Ndumele CE, Rangaswami J, Chow SL, et al. Cardiovascular-kidney-metabolic health: a presidential advisory from the American Heart Association. Circulation. 2023; 148(20):1606-35.
7. Mittal S, Harikrishnan S, Gupta A, et al. Angiotensin receptor neprilysin inhibitor in chronic heart failure and comorbidity management: Indian consensus statement. Ther Adv Cardiovasc Dis. 2024;18:17539447241301959.
8. Grant CH, Bell S. Obesity and chronic kidney disease: the dual epidemic in cardiovascular health. Eur Cardiol. 2025;20:e28.
9. Harrington J, Mentz R, Adams K, et al. Abstract 4140480: the relationship between obesity status and change in NT-proBNP with angiotensin-neprilysin inhibition in patients with mildly reduced or preserved ejection fraction and recent worsening heart failure event: results from the PARAGLIDE-HF trial. Circulation. 2024;150(Suppl_1):A4140480.
10. Tsukamoto S, Uehara T, Azushima K, et al. Updates for cardio-kidney protective effects by angiotensin receptor-neprilysin inhibitor: requirement for additional evidence of kidney protection. J Am Heart Assoc. 2023;12(8):e029565.
11. Chang H-Y, Lin C-C, Chao C-J, et al. Real-world experience of angiotensin receptor–neprilysin inhibition in reduced ejection fraction heart failure patients with advanced kidney disease. Mayo Clin Proc. 2023;98(1):88-99.
12. Molla MA, Kumar A, Goru B, et al. Effect of angiotensin receptor neprilysin inhibitor in patients of heart failure

with reduced ejection fraction with reduced ejection fraction with cardiorenal syndrome type-1. Int J Basic Clin Pharmacol. 2022;11(6):592-6.

13. Chatur S, Neuen B, Claggett B, et al. Effects of sacubitril/valsartan across the spectrum of renal impairment in patients with heart failure. JACC. 2024;83(22):2148-59.
14. Chertow GM. Revisiting a "Paradigm" in cardiovascular and kidney disease*. JACC. 2024;83(22):2160-2.
15. Cappelletto C, Stolfo D, Orsini N, et al. Use of and association between heart failure pharmacological treatments and outcomes in obese versus non-obese patients with heart failure with reduced ejection fraction: data from the Swedish Heart Failure Registry. Eur J Heart Fail. 2023;25(5):698-710.
16. Ladhani M, Craig JC, Irving M, et al. Obesity and the risk of cardiovascular and all-cause mortality in chronic kidney disease: a systematic review and meta-analysis. Nephrol Dial Transplant. 2017;32(3):439-49.
17. Aroor AR, Mummidi S, Lopez-Alvarenga JC, et al. Sacubitril/valsartan inhibits obesity-associated diastolic dysfunction through suppression of ventricular-vascular stiffness. Cardiovasc Diabetol. 2021;20(1):80.

140

CHAPTER

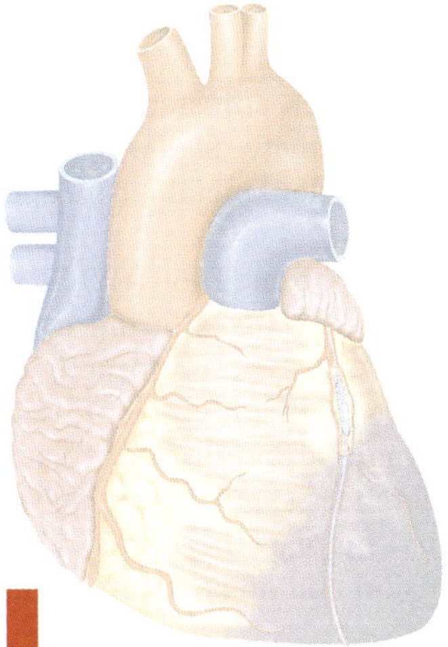

Gender Differences in Angiotensin Receptor–Neprilysin Inhibitor Response Among Obese Patients

Sanjay C Porwal, Shaik Nafeez Javed, Aditya Porwal

INTRODUCTION

Cardiovascular disease (CVD) remains the leading global cause of mortality, with obesity recognized as a significant modifiable risk factor contributing to its development and progression.[1] In recent years, angiotensin receptor-neprilysin inhibitors (ARNIs), particularly sacubitril/valsartan, have emerged as a breakthrough therapy in managing heart failure with reduced ejection fraction (HFrEF), offering superior outcomes compared to traditional renin-angiotensin-aldosterone system (RAAS) inhibitors.[2] Despite this advancement, there remains limited understanding of how gender and obesity together influence ARNI efficacy and safety.

Gender differences in cardiovascular pathophysiology are well-documented, encompassing disparities in cardiac structure, hormonal profiles, endothelial function, and neurohormonal activation.[3] Women are more likely to exhibit heart failure with preserved ejection fraction (HFpEF) and show unique responses to pharmacologic therapy, potentially due to sex-based variations in pharmacokinetics and pharmacodynamics.[4] Concurrently, obesity alters hemodynamic load and myocardial metabolism in a gender-specific manner, contributing further to heterogeneity in drug response and remodeling patterns.

Given the rising prevalence of obesity and the expanding use of ARNI therapy in heart failure management, it is critical to explore how gender modulates ARNI efficacy in obese patients.[5] A meta-analysis involving over 10 million participants demonstrated a consistent, log-linear rise in all-cause mortality with increasing body mass index (BMI) beyond 25 kg/m^2.[6] While obesity negatively impacts multiple organ systems and contributes to chronic illnesses such as cancer and kidney disease, approximately 67.5% of deaths linked to elevated BMI are due to CVD.[7] This chapter aims to examine current evidence, hypothesize potential mechanisms, and highlight gaps that warrant further clinical investigation.

OVERVIEW OF ANGIOTENSIN RECEPTOR-NEPRILYSIN INHIBITOR MECHANISM IN CARDIOVASCULAR DISEASE

Angiotensin receptor-neprilysin inhibitors represent a novel class of heart failure therapies that combine neprilysin inhibition with angiotensin II receptor blockade. Neprilysin is a neutral endopeptidase responsible for degrading natriuretic peptides, bradykinin, and other vasoactive substances. Its inhibition results in enhanced levels of these peptides, leading to vasodilation, natriuresis, diuresis, and attenuation of maladaptive cardiac remodeling. Meanwhile, angiotensin receptor blockade mitigates the detrimental effects of the RAAS, including vasoconstriction, sodium retention, and hypertrophy.[8]

The first-in-class ARNI, sacubitril/valsartan, demonstrated significant clinical benefits in the PARADIGM-HF trial, showing superiority over enalapril in reducing cardiovascular death and hospitalization in patients with HFrEF. Since then, its role has expanded across various cardiovascular conditions including hypertension and HFpEF, albeit with variable outcomes.[5]

GENDER DIFFERENCES IN CARDIOVASCULAR PHYSIOLOGY

Biological sex exerts a profound influence on cardiovascular physiology. Women tend to have smaller ventricular chamber sizes, higher left ventricular ejection fraction, and greater arterial compliance compared to men. These structural and functional distinctions contribute to gender-based variability in disease presentation and therapeutic response.[9]

Hormonal differences, particularly estrogen's cardioprotective effects, modulate vascular tone, inflammation, and lipid metabolism, which may delay the onset of CVD in premenopausal women. Postmenopause, however, this protective advantage diminishes, leading to increased cardiovascular risk. Additionally, differences in autonomic regulation and endothelial function contribute to the sex-specific pathophysiology of heart failure and hypertension.[10]

Despite these disparities, women remain underrepresented in most cardiovascular clinical trials, including those involving ARNIs, limiting the ability to draw definitive conclusions on gender-based efficacy.[11]

OBESITY-RELATED CARDIAC REMODELING AND METABOLISM

Obesity is not only a risk factor for heart failure but also a modifier of cardiac structure and function. Excess adiposity leads to hemodynamic overload, increased blood volume, and elevated cardiac output, resulting in left ventricular hypertrophy and eventual dilation. These alterations can differ by sex.

Women with obesity demonstrate increased myocardial oxygen consumption and reduced cardiac efficiency compared to men. This sex-specific metabolic response may stem from differences in substrate utilization, mitochondrial function, and hormonal influences.[12] Obesity also affects left ventricular remodeling differently: Women are more prone to concentric hypertrophy and HFpEF, whereas men more frequently develop eccentric hypertrophy and HFrEF.[13]

These divergent patterns of obesity-induced cardiac remodeling suggest that the efficacy and safety profile of ARNI therapy may not be uniform across genders in obese populations.

PHARMACOKINETIC AND PHARMACODYNAMIC GENDER VARIABILITY

Gender differences in pharmacokinetics (PK) and pharmacodynamics (PD) are well established and may significantly impact ARNI efficacy and tolerability. Women typically have a higher percentage of body fat, lower glomerular filtration rate (even when adjusted for body size), and altered hepatic enzyme activity, all of which can influence drug absorption, distribution, metabolism, and elimination.[14]

Notably, enzymes such as cytochrome P450 (CYP3A4) are more active in women, potentially altering drug metabolism. Additionally, the expression and activity of drug transporters and receptors, including neprilysin and angiotensin receptors, may be modulated by sex hormones. These PK/PD differences can result in higher plasma drug concentrations, increased sensitivity to adverse effects (e.g., hypotension and angioedema), and variations in clinical outcomes.

This variability underscores the need for sex-specific dosing strategies or monitoring protocols, particularly in obese patients where altered volume of distribution and renal clearance may further complicate pharmacological response.[11]

EVIDENCE OF GENDER-SPECIFIC ANGIOTENSIN RECEPTOR-NEPRILYSIN INHIBITOR RESPONSE

While robust clinical trial data on gender-specific ARNI responses in obese populations are currently lacking, indirect evidence points toward meaningful sex-based differences. Retrospective analyses of the PARADIGM-HF and other trials have indicated that women may experience greater quality-of-life improvement and reductions in NT-proBNP levels compared to men. However, these findings have not always reached statistical significance due to underpowered female subgroups.

Broadly, women appear more susceptible to ARNI-induced hypotension and drug intolerance, potentially due to their smaller body size and different hemodynamic responses. Yet, they may derive similar or greater therapeutic benefit when appropriately managed.

Sex hormones, particularly estrogen and testosterone, modulate neurohormonal activity, vascular reactivity, and natriuretic peptide pathways all of which are central to ARNI mechanisms. For instance, testosterone has been implicated in promoting myocardial hypertrophy and RAAS activation, while estrogen exerts antihypertrophic and anti-inflammatory effects. This hormonal influence may contribute to differing clinical phenotypes of heart failure and variable ARNI responses between men and women.[10]

In the context of obesity, which independently alters cardiac signaling and drug metabolism, these gender-specific effects may be amplified. Thus, individualized treatment strategies considering both sex and body composition are essential for optimizing ARNI therapy in heart failure patients.

Gender differences significantly impact the pharmacokinetics and clinical outcomes of ARNI therapy **(Fig. 1)**. Women typically have higher body fat, lower renal clearance, and more active hepatic enzymes (e.g., CYP3A4), leading to higher plasma drug levels and slower elimination. These factors contribute to greater sensitivity to ARNIs, with increased risks of hypotension and adverse effects such as dizziness. Hormonal influences, especially estrogen, may enhance ARNI efficacy by modulating RAAS and neprilysin pathways, while testosterone in men may promote opposing effects. Despite higher adverse event rates, some evidence suggests women may experience greater improvements in quality of life and biomarker responses. These differences underscore the need for sex-specific considerations in ARNI dosing and monitoring, particularly in obese patients **(Table 1)**.

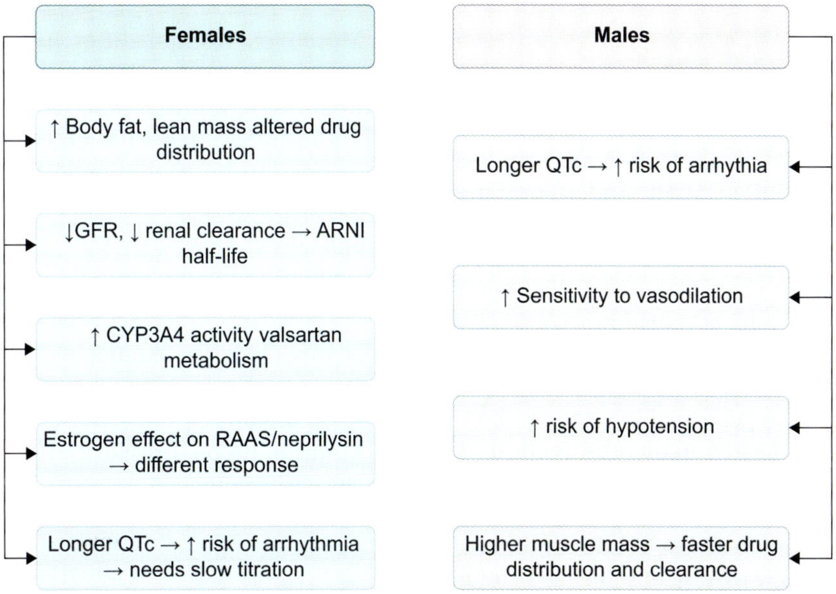

Fig. 1: Gender differences in ARNI pharmacokinetics and clinical outcomes.
(↑/↓: increased/decreased; AE: adverse effects; CYP3A4: cytochrome P450 3A4 enzyme; GFR: glomerular filtration rate; NT-proBNP: N-terminal pro b-type Natriuretic Peptide; RAAS: renin-angiotensin-aldosterone system)

TABLE 1: Summary of known gender differences in ARNI pharmacokinetics and outcomes.

Parameter	*Female*	*Male*	*Clinical implication*
Body composition	Higher body fat percentage; lower lean mass	Lower body fat percentage	Alters drug distribution; may lead to higher plasma drug levels in women
Renal clearance	Lower glomerular filtration rate (adjusted for body size)	Higher GFR	May increase ARNI half-life and risk of hypotension in women
Hepatic metabolism (CYP3A4 activity)	Generally higher activity	Lower activity	Faster metabolism of valsartan in women may affect drug exposure
Volume of distribution	Smaller volume	Larger volume	Higher peak concentrations of sacubitril/valsartan in women
Hormonal influence	Estrogen modulates RAAS and neprilysin pathways	Testosterone linked to myocardial hypertrophy and RAAS activation	Differential responses in neurohormonal blockade effectiveness
QT interval prolongation	Longer baseline QTc interval	Shorter QTc interval	Higher risk of drug induced arrhythmias in women

Contd...

Contd...

Parameter	Female	Male	Clinical implication
Blood pressure response	Greater sensitivity to vasodilation	Less sensitive	Increased incidence of ARNI-induced hypotension in women
Reported tolerability	Higher rates of adverse effects (e.g., dizziness and hypotension)	Generally, better tolerated	May require slower titration and closer monitoring in women
Clinical outcome (quality of life, NT-proBNP reduction)	Some studies suggest greater benefit	Consistent benefit	Possible enhanced therapeutic effect in women, though understudied

LIMITATIONS

Despite growing interest in personalized cardiovascular therapies, current evidence on gender-specific ARNI responses in obese patients remains limited. Most landmark ARNI trials, including PARADIGM-HF, underrepresented women and lacked stratified analysis based on sex and obesity status. Additionally, obesity is a heterogeneous condition—differences in visceral versus subcutaneous fat, metabolic profiles, and comorbidities are rarely accounted for in subgroup analyses. Pharmacokinetic and pharmacodynamic variability by sex and adiposity further complicates interpretation yet remains understudied in real-world populations. Lastly, many observations are drawn from post hoc or observational studies, limiting causal inference. Rigorous, adequately powered clinical trials specifically designed to assess gender and obesity interactions in ARNI therapy are urgently needed to inform clinical guidelines and optimize outcomes.

SUMMARY

The management of heart failure, particularly in obese patients, has been significantly advanced with the advent of ARNIs, notably sacubitril/valsartan. While their benefits in reducing morbidity and mortality in HFrEF are well established, gender-specific responses—especially in the context of obesity—remain underexplored. This chapter highlights key biological, metabolic, and pharmacological factors that may contribute to differential ARNI outcomes between obese men and women.

Women generally have preserved ejection fraction, greater arterial compliance, and distinct hormonal influences such as cardioprotective effects of estrogen. Obesity introduces additional complexity through its sex-specific impact on cardiac remodeling and myocardial metabolism. For instance, obese women exhibit higher myocardial oxygen consumption and reduced efficiency, which may influence ARNI responsiveness.

Moreover, women differ in pharmacokinetic and pharmacodynamic handling of cardiovascular drugs due to variations in body fat percentage, glomerular filtration rate, and hepatic enzyme activity. These factors may predispose to both enhanced therapeutic effects and increased sensitivity to adverse events such as hypotension. Despite these known differences, current trial designs often fail to stratify by sex and obesity, resulting in a one-size-fits-all approach to therapy.

Given this, clinicians should:

- Consider body composition and sex when initiating ARNI therapy.
- Monitor blood pressure and renal function more closely in women.
- Tailor follow-up and dose titration with attention to metabolic phenotype and tolerance.

CONCLUSION

Gender and obesity are critical, yet often overlooked, modifiers of cardiovascular drug response, including ARNI therapy. While ARNIs offer substantial benefits in heart failure management, their efficacy and safety may vary between obese men and women due to differences in cardiac remodeling, metabolism, hormonal influences, and pharmacokinetics. Current evidence remains limited, largely due to underrepresentation of women and lack of obesity-stratified analyses in clinical trials. Recognizing these gaps is essential to move toward more personalized, equitable treatment strategies. Clinicians should incorporate sex-specific and obesity-related factors when prescribing ARNIs, with careful monitoring and individualized adjustments. Future research must prioritize gender-inclusive, obesity-focused trials to optimize ARNI therapy across diverse patient populations and improve cardiovascular outcomes.

REFERENCES

1. Yusuf S, Joseph P, Rangarajan S, et al. Modifiable risk factors, cardiovascular disease, and mortality in 155 722 individuals from 21 high-income, middle-income, and low-income countries (PURE): a prospective cohort study. Lancet. 2020;395(10226):795-808.
2. Greenberg B. Angiotensin receptor-neprilysin inhibition (ARNI) in heart failure. Int J Heart Fail. 2020;2(2):73.
3. Martinez C, Rikhi R, Haque T, et al. Gender identity, hormone therapy, and cardiovascular disease risk. Current problems in cardiology. 2020;45(5):100396.
4. Beale AL, Meyer P, Marwick TH, et al. Sex differences in cardiovascular pathophysiology: why women are overrepresented in heart failure with preserved ejection fraction. Circulation. 2018;138(2):198-205.
5. Kuchulakanti PK. ARNI in cardiovascular disease: current evidence and future perspectives. Future Cardiology. 2020;16(5):505-15.
6. Global BMI Mortality Collaboration; Di Angelantonio E, Bhupathiraju ShN, Wormser D, et al. Body-mass index and all-cause mortality: individual-participant-data meta-analysis of 239 prospective studies in four continents. Lancet. 2016;388(10046):776-86.
7. GBD 2015 Obesity Collaborators. Health effects of overweight and obesity in 195 countries over 25 years. New England journal of medicine. 2017;377(1):13-27.
8. Volpe M, Tocci G, Battistoni A, et al. Angiotensin II receptor blocker neprilysin inhibitor (ARNI): new avenues in cardiovascular therapy. High Blood Press Cardiovasc Prev. 2015;22(3):241-6.
9. Zhou Q, Bei Y. Gender differences in cardiovascular diseases. J Cardiovasc Transl Res. 2020;13(1):1-2.
10. Huang CK, Lee SO, Chang EB, et al. Androgen receptor (AR) in cardiovascular diseases. J Endocrinol. 2016;229(1):R1-16.
11. Stramba-Badiale M, Priori SG. Gender-specific prescription for cardiovascular diseases? Eur Heart J. 2005;26(16):1571-2.
12. Peterson LR, Soto PF, Herrero P, et al. Impact of gender on the myocardial metabolic response to obesity. JACC Cardiovasc Imaging. 2008;1(4):424-33.
13. Coromilas E, Bello NA. Gender differences in obesity-associated cardiac remodeling. Gender Genome. 2017;1(2):76-9.
14. Stolarz AJ, Rusch NJ. Gender differences in cardiovascular drugs. Cardiovasc Drugs Ther. 2015;29(4):403-10.

141

CHAPTER

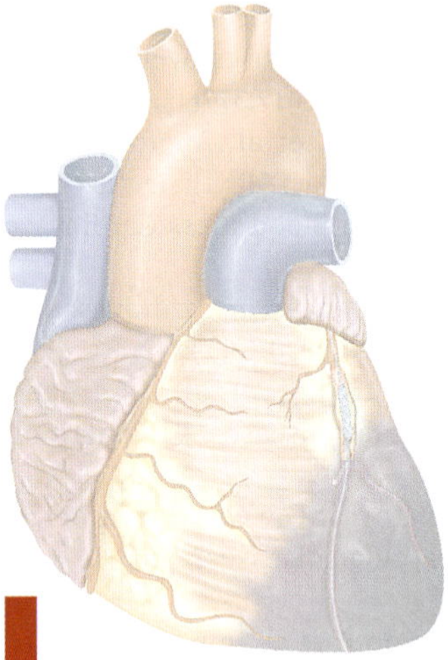

ARNI in Obesity-associated Heart Failure: Mechanistic Rationale and Evidence from Major Outcome Trials

Tapan Ghose, Pushpit Singh

INTRODUCTION

Obesity has become a key factor in the current epidemic of heart failure (HF) and is closely linked to negative effects on cardiovascular structure, function, and outcomes. Obesity-related HF patients demonstrate a distinct clinical and biological phenotype marked by plasma volume expansion, increased neurohormonal activation, low-grade systemic inflammation, insulin resistance, and a relative lack of circulating natriuretic peptides (NPs). These irregularities are especially noticeable in heart failure with preserved ejection fraction (HFpEF), but they also pertain to heart failure with reduced ejection fraction (HFrEF). By tackling both impaired NP signaling and maladaptive renin–angiotensin–aldosterone system (RAAS) activation, angiotensin receptor–neprilysin inhibitors (ARNIs), which combine neprilysin inhibition with RAAS blockade, provide a mechanism-based therapeutic strategy for this population.

OBESITY, NATRIURETIC PEPTIDE DEFICIENCY, AND HEART FAILURE PATHOPHYSIOLOGY

Obesity is consistently associated with inappropriately low circulating concentrations of B-type natriuretic peptide (BNP) and *N*-terminal pro-BNP relative to the degree of intracardiac filling pressure, a phenomenon commonly described as the "natriuretic handicap of obesity."[1,2] This state arises from multiple interrelated mechanisms, including increased expression of NP clearance receptors within adipose tissue, alterations in peptide synthesis and posttranslational processing, and enhanced neprilysin-mediated degradation.[1-3] Consequently, obese patients with HF exhibit attenuated natriuresis, impaired vasodilatory responses, and reduced antifibrotic and antihypertrophic signaling, promoting persistent volume overload and adverse myocardial remodeling.[1,4] Simultaneous activation of the RAAS and sympathetic nervous system further intensifies sodium retention, vascular dysfunction, and ventricular stiffness.[3,5]

Angiotensin receptor–neprilysin inhibitor therapy directly targets these interlinked abnormalities by restoring endogenous NP activity through neprilysin inhibition while concurrently mitigating angiotensin II–mediated effects via angiotensin receptor blockade. This dual neurohormonal modulation provides a compelling mechanistic advantage in obesity-associated HF, where suppression of NP signaling and excessive RAAS activation are central to disease progression.[1,3,6]

EVIDENCE FROM PARADIGM-HF: IMPLICATIONS FOR OBESE PATIENTS WITH HFrEF

The PARADIGM-HF trial definitively established sacubitril/valsartan as superior to enalapril in reducing both cardiovascular mortality and HF-related hospitalizations in patients with chronic HFrEF.[5] Prespecified subgroup analyses demonstrated that the relative treatment benefit of ARNI therapy was preserved across body mass index (BMI) categories, including individuals with overweight and obesity.[5] Notably, obese patients experienced a higher baseline risk of

HF events, resulting in greater absolute risk reductions despite having lower circulating concentrations of NPs at baseline.[1,2,5] These observations suggest that obesity-related impairment in NP signaling does not diminish responsiveness to ARNI therapy and may, in fact, enhance its clinical relevance by targeting a key pathophysiological deficit.[3,5]

Taken together, findings from PARADIGM-HF provide robust evidence supporting sacubitril/valsartan as a cornerstone component of guideline-directed medical therapy in obese patients with HFrEF.[5]

EVIDENCE FROM PARAGON-HF: OBESITY-DOMINANT HFpEF PHENOTYPE

The PARAGON-HF trial compared sacubitril/valsartan with valsartan in patients with HFpEF and narrowly missed its primary composite endpoint of total heart failure hospitalizations and cardiovascular death.[6] However, prespecified and post hoc analyses demonstrated clinically meaningful heterogeneity in treatment response **(Table 1)**. Patients with higher BMI, particularly those meeting criteria for obesity, experienced greater reductions in total HF hospitalizations.[4,6] Enhanced therapeutic benefit was also observed in women and in patients with left ventricular ejection fraction at the lower end of the preserved spectrum—subgroups that substantially overlap with obesity-associated HFpEF phenotypes.[4,6]

These findings suggest that neprilysin inhibition may preferentially benefit HFpEF patients in whom obesity-related NP deficiency and volume overload are dominant pathophysiological drivers, conditions characterized by heightened neprilysin activity and maladaptive neurohormonal activation.[1,3,6]

PARADISE-MI TRIAL: ROLE OF ARNI IN POSTMYOCARDIAL INFARCTION PATIENTS AND IMPLICATIONS FOR OBESITY

The PARADISE-MI trial was a large, randomized, and double-blind study designed to evaluate the efficacy of sacubitril/valsartan compared with ramipril in patients following acute myocardial infarction complicated by pulmonary congestion and/or left ventricular systolic

TABLE 1: Role of ARNI in obesity-associated heart failure—mechanisms and trial evidence.

Domain	*Obesity-associated HF abnormality*	*Effect of ARNI (sacubitril/valsartan)*	*Supporting evidence*
Natriuretic peptide signaling	Relative BNP/NT-proBNP deficiency due to increased clearance receptor expression and enhanced neprilysin activity	Neprilysin inhibition increases bioavailability and activity of endogenous natriuretic peptides	Mechanistic studies;[1-3] PARADIGM-HF;[5] PARAGON-HF[6]
Neurohormonal activation	Enhanced RAAS and sympathetic nervous system activation	Angiotensin receptor blockade suppresses maladaptive RAAS signaling	PARADIGM-HF;[5] mechanistic framework[3]
Volume overload	Plasma volume expansion and sodium retention	Improved natriuresis, reduced preload, and congestion relief	PARADIGM-HF;[5] biomarker and NP analyses[1,3]
Cardiac remodeling	Increased left ventricular hypertrophy and myocardial fibrosis	Antifibrotic effects and promotion of reverse remodeling	PARADIGM-HF echocardiographic analyses[5]
Heart failure hospitalizations	Higher baseline HF hospitalization risk in obese patients	Reduction in first and recurrent HF hospitalizations	PARADIGM-HF;[5] PARAGON-HF BMI subgroup analyses[6]
HFpEF phenotype	Obesity-driven HFpEF with congestion, inflammation, and lower preserved EF	Greater reduction in HF events in obese HFpEF subsets	PARAGON-HF subgroup analyses;[6] EF-spectrum analyses[4]
Functional status	Reduced exercise tolerance and higher NYHA functional class	Improvement in symptoms, NYHA class, and quality of life	PARADIGM-HF;[5] QoL analyses[4]
Metabolic profile	Insulin resistance and chronic low-grade inflammation	Improvement in insulin sensitivity and glycemic control	Mechanistic studies;[1-3] PARADIGM-HF post hoc analysis[7]
Blood pressure	Obesity-associated hypertension	Effective blood pressure reduction with good tolerability	PARADIGM-HF[5]
Safety and tolerability	Concerns regarding hypotension or renal dysfunction	Comparable renal safety; manageable hypotension risk	PARADIGM-HF;[5] PARAGON-HF[6]

dysfunction (left ventricular ejection fraction ≤40%).[8] The trial enrolled more than 5,600 patients and assessed a composite primary endpoint comprising cardiovascular death, hospitalization for HF, or outpatient development of symptomatic HF.

Sacubitril/valsartan did not achieve a statistically significant reduction in the primary composite endpoint compared with ramipril (hazard ratio approximately 0.90; $p = 0.06$), narrowly missing conventional thresholds for significance.[8] Nevertheless, several secondary and exploratory analyses demonstrated favorable effects of ARNI therapy on cardiac remodeling parameters, including reductions in left ventricular mass index and improvements in indices of diastolic function assessed by tissue Doppler imaging.[8] These findings suggest that neprilysin inhibition may exert beneficial effects on myocardial structure and function in the early postmyocardial infarction period, even in the absence of a clear reduction in short-term clinical events.

BODY MASS INDEX-BASED SUBGROUP ANALYSES

Given the established role of obesity as a modifier of cardiovascular risk and HF progression, prespecified and post hoc analyses of PARADISE-MI explored treatment effects across BMI categories. Patients were stratified into normal weight, overweight, obese, and severely obese groups. Event rates for the composite endpoint were lowest among patients with overweight BMI (25–29.9 kg/m^2), consistent with the widely described "obesity paradox" in cardiovascular disease.[9]

Importantly, no significant interaction was observed between BMI category and treatment assignment, indicating that the relative efficacy and safety of sacubitril/valsartan were consistent across the spectrum of adiposity.[8,9] Obese and severely obese patients derived comparable clinical benefit without an excess of adverse events, including hypotension or renal dysfunction. These findings reinforce the concept that elevated BMI does not attenuate responsiveness to ARNI therapy in postmyocardial infarction patients with left ventricular dysfunction.

Clinical Implications

Collectively, data from PARADISE-MI support the use of sacubitril/valsartan as a safe and mechanistically favorable therapeutic option following myocardial infarction in patients at high risk for HF, irrespective of BMI status. When interpreted alongside evidence from PARADIGM-HF and PARAGON-HF, these results further strengthen the rationale for ARNI therapy across a broad continuum of cardiovascular disease, including obesity-associated phenotypes characterized by heightened neurohormonal activation and adverse ventricular remodeling.

Body Mass Index-dependent Gradient of Therapeutic Benefit

Pooled analyses across the left ventricular ejection fraction spectrum indicate that the therapeutic benefit of sacubitril/valsartan progressively increases as ejection fraction declines and as neurohormonal activation becomes more pronounced.[4,6] Given that increasing adiposity is consistently associated with greater suppression of endogenous NP activity,[1,2] a biological gradient can be postulated whereby higher BMI confers enhanced responsiveness to neprilysin inhibition.[3,4] Although this interaction has not yet been conclusively demonstrated in prospective, BMI-stratified randomized trials, available subgroup and pooled analyses support the hypothesis that obesity may act as a modifier of treatment response to ARNI therapy across the HF spectrum.[4,6,10]

METABOLIC AND INFLAMMATORY EFFECTS OF ARNI IN OBESITY

Beyond hemodynamic unloading and neurohormonal modulation, ARNI therapy has demonstrated potentially favorable effects on metabolic and inflammatory pathways in both mechanistic and clinical studies. Improvements in insulin sensitivity, glycemic control, and surrogate markers of systemic inflammation have been reported following initiation of sacubitril/valsartan, effects that are biologically consistent with enhanced NP signaling and attenuation of maladaptive RAAS activity.[1-3,7] Given the close pathophysiological interplay between obesity, insulin resistance, chronic low-grade inflammation, and HF progression, these pleiotropic actions may contribute meaningfully to improved clinical outcomes in obese patients with HF.[3,4,7] However, variability in study design, patient phenotype, and assessed endpoints highlights substantial heterogeneity across existing data, underscoring the need for dedicated prospective trials specifically powered to evaluate metabolic and inflammatory outcomes in obesity-associated HF.[7]

CLINICAL IMPLICATIONS AND FUTURE DIRECTIONS

For obese patients with HFrEF, ARNI therapy should be prioritized as first-line treatment in accordance with contemporary international HF guidelines, given its well-established benefits in reducing mortality and HF-related hospitalizations.[5,11] In obesity-associated HFpEF, ARNI therapy represents a rational, phenotype-guided therapeutic strategy, particularly among patients with recurrent congestion, left ventricular ejection fraction at the lower end of the preserved spectrum, and heightened cardiometabolic risk—features commonly enriched in obese HFpEF phenotypes.[4,6,10]

Future investigations should focus on obesity-stratified randomized controlled trials, mechanistic studies examining NP kinetics, neprilysin activity, and intracardiac filling pressures, as well as large-scale real-world registries to define effectiveness across diverse populations. Such efforts are especially critical in regions experiencing a rapidly rising burden of obesity and cardiometabolic disease, where tailored HF management strategies are urgently needed.[1-3,10,12]

CONCLUSION

Heart failure associated with obesity constitutes a syndrome that is biologically distinct, characterized by impaired signaling of NPs and excessive activation of neurohormones. Research from PARADIGM-HF and PARAGON-HF, along with mechanistic and metabolic investigations, indicates that ARNI therapy successfully addresses these abnormalities and provides clinically significant advantages throughout the HF spectrum. By including obesity as a factor influencing therapeutic response, it may be possible to improve precision-based management and outcomes in this growing patient population.

REFERENCES

1. Madamanchi C, Alhosaini H, Sumida A, et al. Obesity and natriuretic peptides, BNP and NT-proBNP. Heart Fail Rev; 2014.
2. Khan AM, Cheng S, Magnusson M, et al. Cardiac natriuretic peptides, obesity, and insulin resistance: evidence from two community-based studies. J Clin Endocrinol Metab. 2011;96(10):3242-9.
3. Packer M. Leptin–aldosterone–neprilysin axis in obesity and heart failure. JACC Heart Fail; 2018.
4. Solomon SD, Vaduganathan M, Claggett BL, et al. Sacubitril/valsartan across the spectrum of ejection fraction in heart failure. Circulation. 2020;141(5):352-61.
5. McMurray JJV, Packer M, Desai AS, et al. Angiotensin-neprilysin inhibition versus enalapril in heart failure. N Engl J Med. 2014;371(11):993-1004.
6. Solomon SD, McMurray JJV, Anand IS, et al. Angiotensin-neprilysin inhibition in heart failure with preserved ejection fraction. N Engl J Med. 2019;381(17):1609-20.
7. Seferovic JP, Claggett B, Seidelmann SB, et al. Effect of sacubitril/valsartan versus enalapril on glycaemic control in patients with heart failure and diabetes: a post-hoc analysis of PARADIGM-HF trial. Lancet Diabetes Endocrinol. 2017;5(5):333-40.
8. Pfeffer MA, Claggett B, Lewis EF, et al. Angiotensin receptor–neprilysin inhibition in acute myocardial infarction. N Engl J Med. 2021;385:1845-55.
9. Lavie CJ, De Schutter A, Patel DA, et al. Body composition and survival in stable coronary heart disease: impact of lean mass index and body fat in the "obesity paradox." J Am Coll Cardiol. 2012;60:1374-80.
10. Vaduganathan M, Claggett BL, Jhund PS, et al. Estimating lifetime benefits of sacubitril/valsartan across the spectrum of ejection fraction. JAMA Cardiol; 2020.
11. McDonagh TA, Metra M, Adamo M, et al. 2021 ESC Guidelines for the diagnosis and treatment of acute and chronic heart failure. Eur Heart J. 2021;42(36):3599-726.
12. Pandey A, Patel KV, Vaduganathan M, et al. Physical activity, fitness, and obesity in heart failure with preserved ejection fraction. JACC Heart Fail. 2018;6(12):975-82.

142

CHAPTER

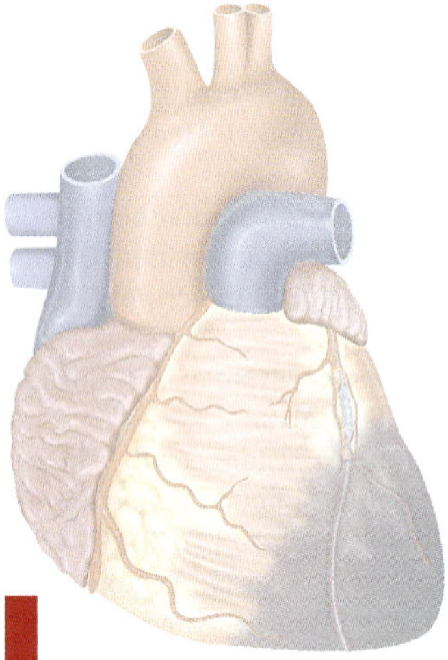

Digital Technologies to Enhance ARNI Management in Obese Patients

Bhavik S Shah, Sharvari Mahajan, Ajaykumar U Mahajan

INTRODUCTION

Obesity is a complex, multifactorial, chronic condition that increases the risk of a wide range of diseases, including heart failure. Its prevalence has almost tripled globally since 1976, with 13% of the world's population now living with obesity.[1] Obesity has been a recognized risk factor for heart failure across its spectrum, frequently complicating its treatment because of altered pharmacodynamics and increased comorbidity burden. It has been proven to worsen the prognosis in both heart failure with preserved ejection fraction (HFpEF) as well as heart failure with reduced ejection fraction (HFrEF). Today, in the era of guideline-directed medical treatment (GDMT), angiotensin receptor neprilysin inhibitors (ARNI) have become cornerstone therapy in HFrEF. However, management of ARNI in obese patients demands careful dose titration, regular monitoring, and adherence support due to complexities related to altered hemodynamics and metabolic changes.

In recent times, "telehealth" or remote healthcare delivery using digital communication tools such as mobile devices has emerged as a powerful adjunct to traditional care, offering solutions for more frequent patient engagement, better monitoring, and tailored management in chronic diseases, including heart failure. This chapter focuses specifically on the recent advances, evidence, and practical aspects of digital health interventions to enhance ARNI management in obese patients with heart failure, highlighting modalities, effectiveness, limitations, and clinical implementation.

EVOLUTION OF DIGITAL TECHNOLOGIES

- *Remote patient monitoring (RPM) for clinical parameters:* Telemonitoring with home-based devices such as Bluetooth-enabled blood pressure cuffs, weight scales, and heart rate monitors allows continuous collection of vital parameters essential for patients who have been prescribed ARNI. These tools are specifically helpful for obese patients, enabling frequent assessment of hemodynamics without repeated hospital or clinic visits, thereby facilitating early detection of fluid overload or hypotension.

  A cohort study by Nguyen et al. has demonstrated that telemonitoring interventions improved ARNI dose optimization compared to standard of care by enabling timely notifications to the clinician and interventions based on real-time data trends such as sudden weight gain or a drop in blood pressure.[2] Integration of data streams into electronic health records (EHR) supports clinical decision-making, enhancing safety and efficacy.
- *Video consultations and virtual clinics:* The recent pandemic led to the evolution of video consultation in a way that nobody had imagined in the past. Video visits allow cardiologists and multidisciplinary heart failure teams to remotely evaluate the patients' clinical status, review symptoms, and adjust medications, including ARNI. This approach overcomes barriers posed by obesity-related mobility challenges, increasing access to specialist care.[3] Virtual heart

failure clinics incorporating nurse-led or pharmacist-led telephonic or video follow-ups have demonstrated improved GDMT adherence, including ARNI initiation and dose titration with greater patient satisfaction and fewer hospitalizations.[4]

- *Mobile health (mHealth) applications:* Smartphone applications designed for heart failure and obesity management provide personalized and tailored support for medication reminders, symptom tracking, dietary guidance, and physical activity encouragement. Such applications can prompt patients to record their weight, blood pressure, and recent blood investigations and transmit these data to clinicians, facilitating proactive ARNI dose adjustments. Behavioral change techniques embedded within these applications improve lifestyle adherence relevant to weight management and heart failure outcomes.[5]
- *Artificial intelligence (AI) and algorithm-driven dose titration:* Emerging AI-enabled digital health platforms apply machine learning algorithms to integrated patient data for the target population. These data generally include clinical reports and information gathered from wearable devices, and this leads to the generation of personalized ARNI titration recommendations in obese individuals. These data can also be used to flag adverse events and notify clinicians before the decompensation of heart failure starts. Such systems reduce the workload of the clinician and enable standardized, evidence-based dose adjustments remotely. Pilot studies applying algorithm-guided dose titration have shown promise in other chronic diseases such as diabetes.[6] Similar approaches are under evaluation in heart failure and obesity cohorts to improve safety and adherence.

EFFECTIVENESS OF DIGITAL HEALTH

Various clinical studies, though limited specifically to ARNI in obesity, support broader efficacy of digital health in chronic disease management, including heart failure and obesity separately.

- Colaone et al. showed that nurse-led digital health interventions in obese or overweight individuals have demonstrated successful short-term weight loss and lifestyle changes, important contributors to improving ARNI efficacy and heart failure prognosis.[7]
- Nutritional therapy through digital health, focusing on carbohydrate restriction and personalized counseling, has resulted in sustained weight loss and potential improvement in symptoms of heart failure.[8]
- Ard et al. led real-world analysis that concluded that a digital health-delivered obesity-management program that includes pharmacotherapy, such as anti-obesity medications, shows weight loss outcomes comparable to clinical trials, supporting digital health in managing obese heart failure patients on ARNI.[9]
- Zheng et al. concluded that video-based telemedicine interventions have been associated with improved medication adherence in heart failure patients, a critical factor for optimal ARNI outcomes in obese patients.[10]

CLINICAL IMPLICATIONS

A structured clinical pathway is advisable for incorporating digital health in ARNI management in obesity **(Flowchart 1)**.

- Baseline assessment
  - Comprehensive evaluation of cardiac function, renal status, and obesity-related comorbidities
  - Digital literacy and telehealth readiness assessments
  - Initiation of wearable devices and apps for remote monitoring
- ARNI initiation and telehealth onboarding
  - Start ARNI with baseline laboratory reports and standardized education via video consultation.
  - Set up daily monitoring of weight, blood pressure, and heart rate using remote monitoring devices or wearables.
  - Provide mHealth application for symptom reporting and medication compliance.
- Remote monitoring and dose titration
  - Frequent data review by multidisciplinary team via integrated dashboard
  - AI-based alerts for abnormal parameters indicating intolerance or congestion
  - Weekly or biweekly teleconsultations for dose titration based on clinical and remote data

Flowchart 1: A streamlined algorithm for using digital technologies to enhance ARNI management in obese patients.

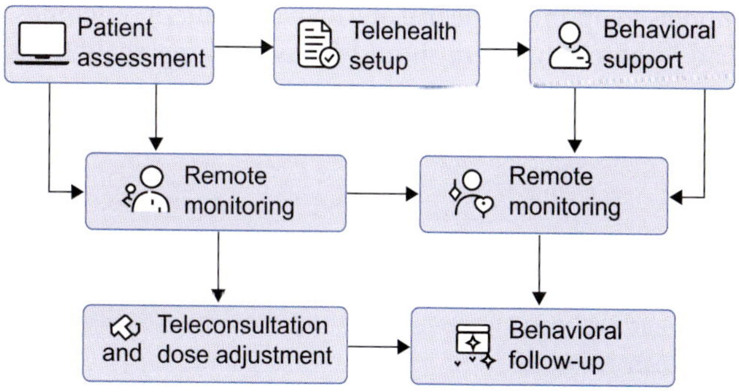

- Behavioral support and lifestyle coaching
    - Telenutrition counseling and exercise programs tailored for obese patients with heart failure
    - Motivational messaging and educational content through mobile applications
    - Psychological support via digital health for adherence barriers
- Escalation and in-person review
    - Identify patients with inadequate response, inertia, or complications.
    - Arrange hybrid care model combining telehealth and traditional visits in complex cases.

LIMITATIONS

- *Digital divide:* Limited access to technology or low digital literacy among elderly or socioeconomically disadvantaged patients impairs effectiveness.
- *Engagement fatigue:* Sustaining long-term patient engagement with telehealth platforms and self-monitoring remains challenging.
- *Lack of large-scale ARNI-specific data:* More randomized controlled studies focused on telehealth interventions in obese heart failure patients, specifically on ARNI, are needed to define best practices.
- *Privacy concerns:* Data security and confidentiality require robust safeguards and patient trust.
- *Integration challenges:* Seamless integration of wearables, applications, and electronic medical records into clinical workflows remains technical hurdle.

CONCLUSION

Digital health interventions offer a transformative opportunity to enhance ARNI management in obese heart failure patients by enabling patient-centered remote monitoring, improving medication adherence and dose titration, and addressing obesity-related lifestyle factors simultaneously. Despite challenges in access, engagement, and evidence gaps, current data support integrating digital health into comprehensive heart failure models to optimize the use of ARNI and patient outcomes. The research in future should focus on large-scale trials to refine digital health strategies tailored specifically for obesity and investigate cost-effectiveness and long-term benefits.

REFERENCES

1. Hinchliffe N, Capehorn MS, Bewick M, et al. The potential role of digital health in obesity care. Adv Ther. 2022;39(10):4397-412.
2. Nguyen HTT, Tran HB, Tran PM, et al. Effect of a telemedicine model on patients with heart failure with reduced ejection fraction in a resource-limited setting in Vietnam: cohort study. J Med Internet Res. 2025;27:e67228.
3. Yu X, Cao J, Xu J, et al. Efficacy of telemedical interventional management in patients with coronary heart disease undergoing percutaneous coronary intervention: randomized controlled trial. J Med Internet Res. 2025;27:e63350.
4. Fox DS, Zawadski N, Buss K, et al. Impact of pharmacist telehealth comanagement for heart failure. JACC Adv. 2025;4(7):101906.
5. Chiavarini M, Giacchetta I, Rosignoli P, et al. E-health and m-health in obesity management: a systematic review and meta-analysis of RCTs. Nutrients. 2025;17(13):2200.
6. Thiagarajan N, Tan HC, Rama Chandran S, et al. Web-based, algorithm-guided insulin titration in insulin-treated type 2 diabetes: pre-post intervention study. JMIR Form Res. 2025;9:e68914.
7. Colaone E, Belluzzi E, Pozzuoli A, et al. Effectiveness of telemedicine nursing interventions in the management of overweight and obesity in adults: a systematic review and meta-analysis. Curr Obes Rep. 2025;14(1):63.
8. Athinarayanan S, Bjornstad P, Shanmugam PV, et al. (2025). Effectiveness of telehealth nutritional therapy in preventing chronic kidney disease among adults with type 2 diabetes and obesity: a real-world, retrospective, propensity score–matched cohort study. [online] Available from https://www.ssrn.com/abstract=5734945 [Last accessed January, 2026].
9. Ard JD, Hong YR, Foster GD, et al. Twelve-month analysis of real-world evidence from a telehealth obesity-treatment provider using antiobesity medications. Obesity (Silver Spring). 2024;32(12):2246-54.
10. Zheng Y, Adhikari S, Li X, et al. Association between video-based telemedicine visits and medication adherence among patients with heart failure: retrospective cross-sectional study. JMIR Cardio. 2024;8:e56763.

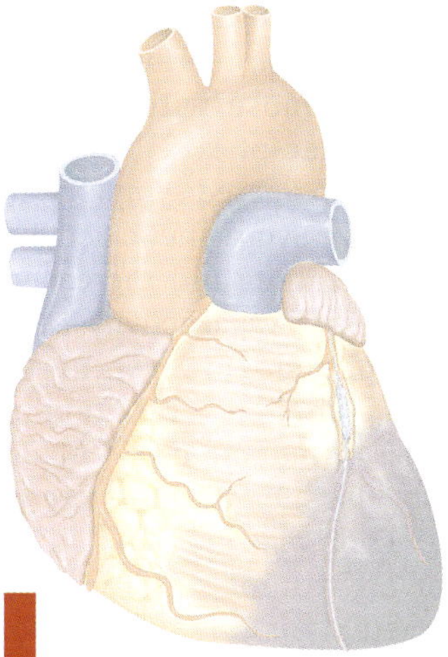

143

CHAPTER

Effects of Bisoprolol in Tachyarrhythmia with Cardiovascular Disease: Lifelong Benefits

Supratip Kundu, Srina Ray, Saumitra Ray

INTRODUCTION

Cardiac arrhythmia is a commonly encountered problem in our clinical practice; unlike myocardial infarction and ischemic stroke, incidence is higher in elderly, chronic kidney disease, and those with heart failure.[1] Sympathetic nervous system (SNS) has an important role to play in cardiovascular diseases. SNS secretes catecholamines which act on adrenoreceptors in heart and kidney, thereby promoting various physical and metabolic processes. Adrenoreceptors are of two types—alpha and beta receptors. As heart has predominance of beta receptors; hence, beta-blocker has an important role to play in cardiovascular diseases. It acts as antiarrhythmic, antianginal, and antihypertensive drugs and an important component of remodeling prevention drugs for heart failure. Effect on heart rate reduction and antianginal properties are similar for all beta-blockers whereas remodeling prevention effects are different among different beta-blockers. As antiarrhythmic drugs, beta-blockers are classified as class II antiarrhythmic according to Vaughan Williams' classification.[2] Beta-blockers can grossly be divided into selective and nonselective beta-blockers. Metoprolol, bisoprolol, and nebivolol are selective beta-blockers and rest are nonselective beta-blockers. Selective beta-blocker scores over nonselective beta-blockers due to their selective affinity toward beta-1 receptors and are safe in COPD patients. Among these selective beta-blockers, bisoprolol has more affinity toward beta-1 receptors than other selective beta-blocker.[3] In this chapter, we shall discuss the role of bisoprolol in tachyarrhythmia and cardiovascular diseases.

PROPERTY

Bisoprolol has 10,000 times more affinity to beta-1 receptor than beta-2 receptors. Bisoprolol has high oral bioavailability, with almost 80% absorbed, and first-pass metabolism is low, mainly by CYP3A4 and CYP2D6. It has low lipophilicity and very less amount crosses blood–brain barrier. So it causes less fatigue. Half-life is about 3–4 hours and it is completely eliminated in 5 days. Bisoprolol is excreted 50% through liver and 50% through kidney. Tubular secretion is the main mechanism of elimination. Bisoprolol fumarate has a long half-life of 9–12 hours and is suitable for once daily dosing.[4-9]

BETA-BLOCKERS FOR ISCHEMIC HEART DISEASE

Selective beta-blockers act specifically on beta-1 receptor and they decrease contractility. At the same time, it decreases conduction through the conducting fibers of heart. Hence, it decreases heart rate. By decreasing contractility and heart rate, it decreases myocardial oxygen demand. Hence, it decreases angina. It also reduces ischemia/reperfusion injury in myocardial infarction patients. When it starts within the first 24 hours, it reduces mortality.[10,11]

SYMPATHETIC NERVOUS SYSTEM FOR GENESIS OF ARRHYTHMIA

Sympathetic nervous system is responsible for fight or flight response when faced with some emotional or physical threat. Catecholamines secreted from SNS act on adrenoreceptors.[12,13] Normal heart function depends on smooth and coherent working of two types of cells: One is conduction system cells and the other is cardiomyocytes. The heart contains pacemaker cells throughout conduction systems. Normally, pacemaker cells in SA node act as primary pacemaker and any dysfunction of these pacemaker cells leads to activation of subsidiary pacemaker. Current propagates to cardiomyocytes which causes rhythmic contraction. Action of catecholamines stimulates a series of physical and biochemical response which leads to increased contractility, increased heart rate, increased relaxation, and arrhythmogenicity.

Adrenoreceptors are of five types: Alpha 1, alpha 2, beta 1, beta 2, and beta 3. Among these alpha-1 receptors are present in peripheral vasculature and alpha-2 receptors are present in peripheral presynaptic nerve endings. Beta-1 receptors are mainly concentrated on heart. Beta-1 receptors bind with nor epinephrine which is a G protein-coupled receptor and it stimulates protein kinase A. Activation of protein kinase A converts ATP to CAMP which in turn activates various proteins like L-type calcium channel, phospholamban resulting in cytosolic Ca influx which in turn leads to activation of excitation contraction coupling. Activation of beta-1 receptors also leads to increased calcium influx in the conducting cells of heart leading to increased speed of conduction and increased automaticity. SA node acts as pacemaker of the heart. So activation of beta-1 receptors leads to increased heart rate, increased force of contraction, increased conduction, and increased lusitropy.[14] Apart from beta-1, beta-2 receptors are for 20% of beta-receptors. Beta-2 receptors are mainly present on peripheral vasculature, bronchioles. Beta-2 receptor binds with epinephrine and it is same GPCR which activates protein kinase A and subsequently adenylyl cyclase which converts ATP to CAMP. But unlike beta-1, beta-2 activation leads to inhibition of release of stored calcium and hence peripheral vasodilation.[15] Beta-3 unlike beta-1 and beta-2 is not G protein-coupled receptor but it releases endothelium-derived relaxing factor, nitric oxide. Beta-1 and beta-2 receptors are desensitized due to overexposure and this effect is mediated by G protein-coupled kinases. But beta-3 receptors do not possess GRK site, hence their levels remain unchanged. This relative overactivation of beta-3 receptors leads to decreased contractility of ventricular myocardium. Beta-3 receptors also cause glycogenolysis leading to increased sugar level.[16,17]

The autonomic nervous system consists of both sympathetic and parasympathetic nervous system (PNS). Both SNS and PNS are responsible for arrhythmogenicity. Sympathetic efferent fibers reach the heart through paravertebral stellate ganglion. Vagal preganglionic fibers reach the heart through superior cervical, inferior cervical, and thoracic rami which anastomose with cardiac sympathetic nerves to form cardiac plexus.[18-20] Atrial fibrillation (AF) is caused by both increased sympathetic and parasympathetic overactivity.[21] Sympathetic activity increased spontaneous depolarization and increased delayed afterdepolarization. Increased vagal activity leads to shortened atrial refractory period. However, nerve fibers are not uniformly distributed, hence variation of ERP in different parts of atria sets up micro-reentry circuit. Increased sympathetic activity also increases the rate of AVNRT by increasing AV conduction velocity.

However, for ventricular arrhythmia, SNS activity is proarrhythmic and PNS activity is antiarrhythmic. SNS activity leads to increased rate of spontaneous depolarization and it also shortens ERP of ventricular musculature. However, SNS is not uniformly distributed throughout the ventricle. Hence, this difference sets up micro-reentry circuit. Moreover, ischemia and electrolyte imbalance enhance these conditions. For patient of hereditary familial arrhythmia, SNS stimulation leads to increased cytosolic calcium and hence initiation of VT.[22,23] Whereas for Brugada syndrome, parasympathetic activity is proarrhythmic because a decrease in rate leads to prolonged inactivation of sodium channels and it leads to arrhythmogenesis.[24]

ROLE OF BETA-BLOCKER IN TACHYARRHYTHMIA

Beta-blockers are useful for preventing the development of AF in surgical setting, including both CABG and non-CABG. All these studies address low rates of adverse effects with bisoprolol. However, one of these studies found bisoprolol more effective than carvedilol, and another study found it as comparable efficacy to amiodarone. Bisoprolol also reduces the rate of AF. A recent Cochrane review confirms that beta-blockers substantially reduce burden of supraventricular and ventricular arrhythmia after cardiac surgery and particularly burden of supraventricular arrhythmia after noncardiac surgery. Regarding the choice of beta-blockers, it states that bisoprolol should be the first choice if it is used before surgery.[25-30]

In a nonsurgical setting, there is a weak evidence that bisoprolol prevents recurrence postelectrical cardioversion of AF with bisoprolol being as efficient as sotalol. However, as compared to carvedilol, evidence for its efficacy is mixed. Bisoprolol when combined with propafenone has shown to more rapid in conversion of AF to sinus rhythm as compared to propafenone alone; however, percentage of patients converted to sinus rhythm remains the same in both groups. Bisoprolol is also effective in lowering heart rate in AF. Bisoprolol also improves the quality of life in paroxysmal AF. The author also concludes regarding the elimination of AF episodes in 84 patients. However, due to lack of control group, we cannot draw any conclusions.[31,32]

A meta-analysis by Nasr et al.[33] showed that taken together carvedilol, bucindolol, metoprolol, nevibolol, and bisoprolol prevent the onset of AF in heart failure. Evidence of bisoprolol mainly comes from CIBIS I and CIBIS II. Taken together, bisoprolol and metoprolol reduce the rate of new onset AF by 41%.[33]

For rhythm control strategy of AF, initially, catheter ablation was tried when antiarrhythmic drugs including one beta-blocker were ineffective. However, later, based on the results of these trials, it was concluded that catheter ablation was far more effective in rhythm control as compared to antiarrhythmic drugs (beta-blocker + one antiarrhythmic either from class I or class III). Till now, there is no specific trial which focuses on the role of bisoprolol in AF.[34,35]

In case of paroxysmal SVT, there is little but solid evidence that bisoprolol or diltiazem are less effective than catheter ablation for preventing recurrences in AVNRT. However, evidence base for AVRT and atrial tachycardia is not present.[6]

So to conclude, bisoprolol is efficient as a part of rate and rhythm control strategy in surgical patients, both cardiac as well as noncardiac patients. However, for nonsurgical patients, bisoprolol is mainly effective for rate control strategy. In the case of AVNRT, it is clearly less effective than catheter ablation.

BISOPROLOL FOR TREATMENT OF VENTRICULAR ARRHYTHMIA

Bisoprolol has been shown to be effective in reducing ventricular arrhythmia burden in both structurally normal hearts as well as structural heart diseases.

A positive impact of bisoprolol on ventricular arrhythmia reduction comes from CIBIS trial. In CIBIS I, bisoprolol reduces mortality in heart failure patients but not sudden cardiac death or death related to ventricular arrhythmia. It may be due to small sample size; however, following CIBIS II, performed on a large population of patients, there are significantly fewer sudden deaths among patients on bisoprolol.[36,37]

In patients with acute myocardial ischemia, in NSTEMI patients, early bisoprolol admission was protective for ventricular arrhythmia and MACE with few adverse effects of bisoprolol.[38]

Bisoprolol reduces PVC burden as well as significantly inhibits PVC generation. Results came from three small studies. The effect is more pronounced when heart rate is above 80 per minute.[39,40]

In patient with LQTs, there is a weak evidence that bisoprolol is both safe and effective. Fazio et al.[41] found no major adverse cardiac event in patients treated with bisoprolol. Of the 12 minor CV events, 3 occurred in the absence of treatment with nadolol and propranolol and 2 during treatment with bisoprolol. Steinberg et al.[42] in their study show that bisoprolol shortens QTc, it was well tolerated but equivalence of bisoprolol as compared to other established beta-blockers is less conclusive. Due to small sample size, these studies are less conclusive and large clinical trials are needed.[41,42]

So overall, in patients with ventricular arrhythmia, bisoprolol reduces mortality and number of hospitalizations due to severe arrhythmia in stable heart failure patients. It lowers mortality and reduces ventricular arrhythmia burden and MACE in patients with NSTEMI, and it reduces PVC burden. Its role in treating long QTs is less well established.

Limitations of these analyses are heterogeneity of evidences, which ranges from low quality to a few high-quality studies. Very few randomized clinical trial was found in this topic.

BETA-BLOCKERS IN POST-MI PATIENTS

ESC 2025 published a few trials on beta-blockers in post-MI patients with mildly reduced EF (40–49%) and without clinical features of heart failure. These trials are REBOOT-CNIC, BETAMI, DANBLOCK, and CAPITAL-RCT. Meta-analysis of these trials recruited 1,885 patients (979 patients from REBOOT, 422 patients from BETAMI, 430 patients from DANBLOCK, and 54 patients from CAPITAL RCT trial). Primary end-points consist of composite of all cause death, new onset MI, or heart failure hospitalization. Primary end-point occurs in 10.7% in beta-blocker group and 14.4% in no beta-blocker group which equals to 25% relative risk reduction. There is no heterogeneity of effect between different trials or population of different countries. Three individual components of primary end-points follow the same path as composite end-points and these components are numerically lower in beta-blocker group. Cardiac deaths, among these, are probably most significantly associated with beta-blocker treatment.

CONCLUSION

Current evidence supports the role of bisoprolol for the treatment of supraventricular arrhythmia especially for rate control during AF. It is also useful for both primary and secondary prevention of ventricular arrhythmia.

Head-to-head clinical trials comparing safety and efficacy of bisoprolol and other beta-blockers are needed in this respect.

REFERENCES

1. Khurshid S, Choi SH, Weng LC, et al. Frequency of cardiac rhythm abnormalities in a half million adults. Circ Arrhythm Electrophysiol. 2018;11:e006273.
2. Lei M, Wu L, Terrar DA, et al. Modernized classification of cardiac antiarrhythmic drugs. Circulation. 2018; 138:1879-96
3. Wiysonge CS, Bradley HA, Volmink J, et al. Beta-blockers for hypertension. Cochrane Database Syst Rev. 2012;11:Cd002003.22.
4. Lopez-Sendon J, Swedberg K, McMurray J, et al. Expert consensus document on beta-adrenergic receptor blockers. Eur Heart J. 2004;25(15):1341-62.
5. Dorow P, Bethge H, Tonnesmann U. Effects of single oral doses of bisoprolol and atenolol on airway function in nonasthmatic chronic obstructive lung disease and angina pectoris. Eur J Clin Pharmacol. 1986;31(2):143-7.
6. Neuss H, Conrad A, Mitrovic V, et al. Electrophysiologic effects of an acute beta-blockade induced by bisoprolol in patients with supraventricular tachycardia as assessed by His-bundle electrograms. J Cardiovasc Pharmacol. 1986;8 (Suppl 11):S167-70.
7. Sugimoto T, Hayakawa H, Osada H, et al. Clinical evaluation of bisoprolol in the treatment of extrasystoles and sinus tachycardia: an interim report. J Cardiovasc Pharmacol. 1986;8 (Suppl 11):S171-4.
8. Kramer B, Balser J, Stubbig K, et al. Comparison of bisoprolol with other beta adrenoceptor blocking drugs. J Cardiovasc Pharmacol. 1986;8 (Suppl 11):S46-57.
9. Leopold G. Balanced pharmacokinetics and metabolism of bisoprolol. J Cardiovasc Pharmacol. 1986;8 (Suppl 11): S16-20.
10. Pepine CJ. Effects of treatment on outcome in mildly symptomatic patients with ischemia during daily life. The Atenolol Silent Ischemia Study (ASIST). Circulation. 1994;90(2):762-8.
11. Task Force Members; Montalescot G, Sechtem U, et al. 2013 ESC Guidelines on the Management of Stable Coronary Artery Disease: the Task Force on the management of stable coronary artery disease of the European Society of Cardiology. Eur Heart J. 2013;34(38):2949-3003.
12. Brodde OE. Beta-adrenoceptors in cardiac disease. Pharmacol Ther. 1993;60:405-30.
13. Brodde OE, Michel MC. Adrenergic and muscarinic receptors in the human heart. Pharmacol Rev. 1999;51:651-90.
14. Lefkowitz RJ, Rockman HA, Koch WJ. Catecholamines, cardiac beta-adrenergic receptors, and heart failure. Circulation. 2000;101:1634-7.
15. Barki-Harrington L, Perrino C, Rockman HA. Network integration of the adrenergic system in cardiac hypertrophy. Cardiovasc Res. 2004;63:391-402.
16. Moens AL, Yang R, Watts VL, et al. Beta 3-adrenoreceptor regulation of nitric oxide in the cardiovascular system. J Mol Cell Cardiol. 2010;48:1088-95.
17. Cannavo A, Koch WJ. Targeting β3-adrenergic receptors in the heart: selective agonism and β-blockade. J Cardiovasc Pharmacol. 2017;69:71-8.
18. Hasan W. Autonomic cardiac innervation: development and adult plasticity. Organogenesis. 2013;9:176-93.
19. Benarroch EE. Parasympathetic system; overview. In: Aminoff MJ, Daroff RB (Eds). Encyclopedia of the Neurological Sciences, 2nd edition. Oxford: Academic Press; 2014. pp. 805-8.
20. Shen MJ, Zipes DP. Role of the autonomic nervous system in modulating cardiac arrhythmias. Circ Res. 2014;114:1004-21.
21. Sharifov OF, Fedorov VV, Beloshapko GG, et al. Roles of adrenergic and cholinergic stimulation in spontaneous atrial fibrillation in dogs. J Am Coll Cardiol. 2004;43:483-90.
22. Manolis AA, Manolis TA, Apostolopoulos EJ, et al. The role of the autonomic nervous system in cardiac arrhythmias: the neuro-cardiac axis, more foe than friend? Trends Cardiovasc Med. 2021;31:290-302.
23. Zhu C, Hanna P, Rajendran PS, et al. Neuromodulation for ventricular tachycardia and atrial fibrillation: a clinical scenario-based review. JACC Clin Electrophysiol. 2019;5:881-96.
24. Popa IP, Şerban DN, Mărănducă MA, et al. Brugada syndrome: from molecular mechanisms and genetics to risk stratification. Int J Mol Sci. 2023;24:3328.
25. Marazzi G, Iellamo F, Volterrani M, et al. Comparison of effectiveness of carvedilol versus bisoprolol for prevention of postdischarge atrial fibrillation after coronary artery bypass grafting in patients with heart failure. Am J Cardiol. 2011;107(2):215-9.
26. Sleilaty G, Madi-Jebara S, Yazigi A, et al. Postoperative oral amiodarone versus oral bisoprolol as prophylaxis against atrial fibrillation after coronary artery bypass graft surgery: a prospective randomized trial. Int J Cardiol. 2009;137(2):116-22.
27. Behmanesh S, Tossios P, Homedan H, et al. Effect of prophylactic bisoprolol plus magnesium on the incidence of atrial fibrillation after coronary bypass surgery: results of a randomized controlled trial. Curr Med Res Opin. 2006;22(8):1443-50.
28. Sezai A, Nakai T, Hata M, et al. Feasibility of landiolol and bisoprolol for prevention of atrial fibrillation after coronary artery bypass grafting: a pilot study. J Thorac Cardiovasc Surg. 2012;144(5):1241-8.
29. Okamura H, Arakawa M, Miyagawa A, et al. Incidence of postoperative atrial fibrillation in transdermal beta-blocker patch users is lower than that in oral beta-blocker users after cardiac and/or thoracic aortic surgery. Gen Thorac Cardiovasc Surg. 2019;67(12):1007-13.
30. Yasui T, Oka T, Shioyama W, et al. Bisoprolol transdermal patch treatment for patients with atrial fibrillation after noncardiac surgery: a single-center retrospective study of 61 patients. SAGE Open Med. 2020;8:2050312120907817.

31. Blessberger H, Kammler J, Domanovits H, et al. Perioperative beta-blockers for preventing surgery-related mortality and morbidity. Cochrane Database Syst Rev. 2018;3:CD004476.
32. Plewan A, Lehmann G, Ndrepepa G, et al. Maintenance of sinus rhythm after electrical cardioversion of persistent atrial fibrillation; sotalol vs bisoprolol. Eur Heart J. 2001;22(16):1504-10.
33. Nasr IA, Bouzamondo A, Hulot JS, et al. Prevention of atrial fibrillation onset by beta-blocker treatment in heart failure: a meta-analysis. Eur Heart J. 2007;28(4):457-62.
34. Andrade JG, Wazni OM, Kuniss M, et al. Cryoballoon ablation as initial treatment for atrial fibrillation: JACC state-of-the-art review. J Am Coll Cardiol. 2021;78(9):914-30.
35. Wazni OM, Dandamudi G, Sood N, et al. Cryoballoon ablation as initial therapy for atrial fibrillation. N Engl J Med. 2021;384(4):316-24.
36. A randomized trial of beta-blockade in heart failure. The Cardiac Insufficiency Bisoprolol Study (CIBIS). CIBIS Investigators and Committees. Circulation. 1994;90(4):1765-73.
37. The Cardiac Insufficiency Bisoprolol Study II (CIBIS-II): a randomised trial. Lancet. 1999;353(9146):9-13.
38. Maclean E, Zheng S, Nabeebaccus A, et al. Effect of early bisoprolol administration on ventricular arrhythmia and cardiac death in patients with non-ST elevation myocardial infarction. Heart Asia. 2015;7(2):46-51.
39. Kobayashi Y, Miyata A, Chiyoda K, et al. Dipyridamole suppresses catecholamine- and Ca^{++} influx-sensitive ventricular arrhythmias. Jpn Circ J. 1996;60(9):629-40.
40. Shinohara M, Fujino T, Koike H, et al. Assessment of a novel transdermal selective β1-blocker, the bisoprolol patch, for treating frequent premature ventricular contractions in patients without structural heart disease. J Cardiol. 2017;70(3):212-9.
41. Fazio G, Vernuccio F, Lo Re G, et al. Role of bisoprolol in patients with long QT syndrome. Ann Noninvasive Electrocardiol. 2013;18(5):467-70.
42. Steinberg C, Padfield GJ, Al-Sabeq B, et al. Experience with bisoprolol in long-QT1 and long-QT2 syndrome. J Interv Card Electrophysiol. 2016;47(2):163-70.

144

CHAPTER

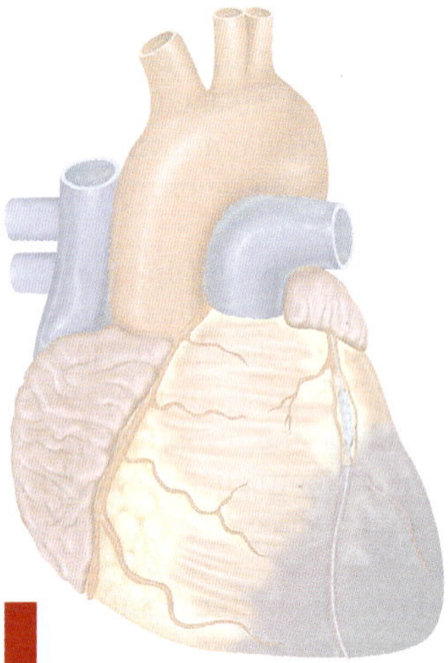

Bisoprolol in CAD (CCS, ACS, Syndrome X) with Obesity: What is New?

Sarita Rao, K Roshan Rao, Abhishek Rathore, Abhishek Nagar, Achukatla Kumar

INTRODUCTION

Cardiovascular disease (CVD) remains the foremost global health challenge, accounting for nearly 17.9 million deaths annually and driving substantial morbidity across both developed and developing nations.[1] In India, the burden of CVD has increased steeply over the past two decades, affecting increasingly younger populations. This surge is closely linked to the escalating prevalence of obesity, diabetes, smoking, poor dietary habits, and sedentary lifestyles.[2]

Coronary artery disease (CAD) is a heterogeneous and evolving disorder that is driven by multiple pathogenic mechanisms.[3] It manifests clinically across a spectrum ranging from acute coronary syndromes (ACS), including unstable angina, NSTEMI, and STEMI, to chronic coronary syndromes (CCS).[4] ACS is characterized by acute myocardial ischemia and is distinguished by clinical symptoms, ECG changes, and biomarker elevation.[5] In contrast, CCS (formerly termed stable CAD) reflects a persistent or recurrent imbalance between myocardial oxygen supply and demand, producing stable ischemic symptoms.[4]

Despite major advancements in diagnostics and therapeutics, CAD remains the leading cause of mortality worldwide.[27] A significant subset of patients, particularly women, experience classic angina symptoms and demonstrate objective ischemia despite having non-obstructive or normal epicardial coronaries on angiography.[28] This condition, historically called cardiac syndrome X, is now more precisely classified as microvascular angina (MVA) or a key component of Ischemia with No Obstructive Coronary Arteries (INOCA).[29]

Syndrome X is typically defined by exertional or atypical chest pain with normal coronary angiography findings and is especially prevalent in peri- and post-menopausal women.[30]

Previously believed to carry a benign course, contemporary research demonstrates that Syndrome X/MVA is associated with persistent angina, impaired quality of life, recurrent hospital admissions, and an elevated long-term risk of adverse outcomes such as HFpEF, myocardial infarction, and arrhythmias.[31] Hormonal dysregulation, endothelial dysfunction, chronic inflammation, and altered nociception play important roles in its pathophysiology.[29]

Obesity has emerged as a major global health threat and is a key contributor to both obstructive and non-obstructive forms of myocardial ischemia.[32] Beyond promoting traditional atherosclerosis, obesity induces coronary microvascular dysfunction, thereby mimicking or overlapping with Syndrome X and INOCA presentations.[31] Individuals with obesity often demonstrate preserved or minimally obstructed epicardial coronaries but develop ischemia due to reduced coronary flow reserve, increased microvascular resistance, endothelial dysfunction, and adverse metabolic milieu.[33] Additionally, epicardial adipose tissue (EAT) promotes local inflammation, oxidative stress, and paracrine-mediated plaque vulnerability.[34]

PATHOPHYSIOLOGY OF OBESITY IN CORONARY ARTERY DISEASE

Obesity promotes coronary artery disease through a complex interplay of metabolic, endocrine, inflammatory, and hemodynamic mechanisms.[35] Atherogenic dyslipidemia remains a central driver of obesity-related CAD, contributing to accelerated plaque formation and vascular injury.[35] Beyond lipid abnormalities, adipose tissue acts as a highly active endocrine organ, secreting a wide range of bioactive molecules, collectively known as adipocytokines, that exert potent cardiometabolic effects.[36]

Adipocytes release multiple adipokines, including adiponectin, leptin, resistin, VEGF, and several pro-inflammatory cytokines such as TNF-α, IL-1, IL-6, and monocyte chemoattractant protein-1 (MCP-1). In obesity, the endocrine profile is significantly altered.[37]

Adiponectin levels decrease, reducing its anti-inflammatory and anti-atherogenic actions. The levels of leptin, resistin, TNF-α, IL-6, and other inflammatory mediators increase, promoting endothelial dysfunction, oxidative stress, monocyte recruitment, and vascular inflammation.[38] These changes create a pro-atherogenic environment that accelerates the development and progression of CAD. Clinical studies have shown that individuals who are obese during early adulthood tend to remain obese over long-term follow-up, and successful transition to normal weight is uncommon, reinforcing the chronic nature of obesity as a cardiovascular risk factor.[39] Circulating adipokine levels have been associated with the presence and severity of CAD, making them potential biomarkers for risk stratification, early detection, and prognostication of obesity-related atherosclerosis.[40] Additionally, increased body mass elevates metabolic demand, leading to higher blood volume and cardiac output. In the early stages of "uncomplicated" obesity, this hemodynamic load often results in left ventricular hypertrophy, which represents a compensatory response to maintain cardiac efficiency.[40,41] Obesity-induced inflammation affects vascular and non-vascular tissues alike. Adipocyte-derived factors such as resistin and leptin stimulate endothelial activation, impair nitric oxide bioavailability, and promote vasoconstriction, thereby contributing to microvascular dysfunction and progression of macrovascular atherosclerosis.[41] **(Flowchart 1)**.

Clinically, obese patients frequently present with exertional chest pain, dyspnea, diminished exercise capacity, and atypical symptoms that may delay diagnosis.[42] Obesity also limits the accuracy of noninvasive stress testing; hence, modalities such as stress CMR, coronary CT angiography, PET-based flow assessment, and invasive coronary physiology may be particularly helpful in these patients.[43]

Optimal management requires a multi-dimensional approach focused on intensive lifestyle intervention, weight

Flowchart 1: Pathophysiologic mechanisms linking obesity to coronary artery disease and ischemic syndromes.

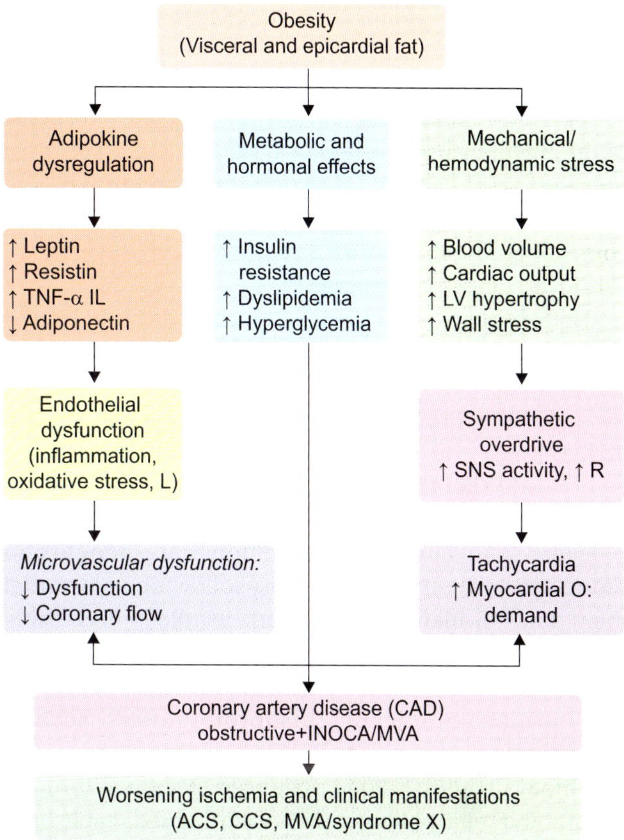

reduction, cardiometabolic risk control, lipid management, glycemic optimization, and targeted pharmacotherapies. Within this therapeutic landscape, beta-blockers such as bisoprolol, with their high β_1-selectivity, favorable metabolic profile, and hemodynamic benefits, offer important emerging advantages, especially in patients with CAD and obesity.[44]

BISOPROLOL

Bisoprolol is a highly selective β_1-adrenergic receptor blocker that is widely used in the management of hypertension, chronic stable angina, and congestive heart failure. As a cardioselective agent, it predominantly targets β_1-receptors in cardiac tissue, producing negative chronotropic and inotropic effects that lower heart rate, reduce myocardial contractility, and subsequently decrease myocardial oxygen consumption, thereby easing cardiac workload.[45] Unlike non-selective beta-blockers, bisoprolol has minimal action on β_2-receptors, avoiding unwanted bronchoconstriction or metabolic disturbances and improving overall tolerability, especially in patients with comorbid respiratory or metabolic diseases.[46]

Beyond its cardiac effects, bisoprolol also inhibits β_1-receptors in the juxtaglomerular apparatus, suppressing renin release and attenuating activation of the renin-angiotensin-aldosterone system (RAAS). This dual mechanism of cardiac rate/contractility reduction and RAAS inhibition makes bisoprolol particularly effective in controlling blood pressure and preventing downstream cardiovascular complications.[45]

Beta-blockers occupy a central position in the cardiovascular continuum, modulating excessive sympathetic nervous system (SNS) activity implicated in hypertension, CAD, acute coronary syndromes, arrhythmias, and heart failure. Bisoprolol is endorsed as first-line therapy for chronic stable angina, both as monotherapy or in combination with calcium channel blockers, and continues to demonstrate benefits in reducing morbidity and mortality following myocardial infarction.[47] Evidence also supports its role in decreasing the long-term risk of stroke and recurrent coronary events in high-risk cardiovascular populations.[45,47]

Pharmacokinetically, bisoprolol offers several advantages that support long-term use—it has high oral bioavailability (~90%), balanced clearance through hepatic and renal pathways (50% each), a predictable half-life of 10–12 hours, and low first-pass metabolism. Its low lipophilicity limits central nervous system penetration and reduces fatigue, sleep disturbances, and other CNS-related adverse effects, enabling reliable once-daily dosing.[7-18,48]

Recent guidelines have reinforced its relevance. The 2024 Indian consensus identifies beta-blockers, particularly bisoprolol, as key therapeutic agents in CAD owing to their effects on heart rate, blood pressure, ischemic burden, arrhythmia prevention, and post-MI survival, emphasizing individualized selection based on comorbidities such as hypertension and heart failure. International hypertension bodies—including the European Society of Hypertension and joint recommendations from obesity and hypertension societies—continue to support beta-blocker use in patients with both obesity and hypertension, as these individuals often exhibit heightened sympathetic drive and demonstrate a stronger blood pressure-lowering response than their leaner counterparts.[49]

In CCS, contemporary guidelines align—the 2024 ESC CCS and the 2023 AHA/ACC CCD guidelines maintain bisoprolol as a first-line anti-anginal therapy, while clarifying that long-term beta-blocker therapy is not recommended solely for event prevention in stable CAD without recent MI or left ventricular dysfunction. Importantly, in INOCA and microvascular angina (Syndrome X), beta-blockers, including bisoprolol, are now recognized as appropriate first-line agents, helping improve symptoms by lowering heart rate, enhancing diastolic perfusion time, and restoring microvascular oxygen delivery, with calcium channel blockers, nitrates, or ranolazine added based on specific endotypes.[48,50]

OBESITY–CORONARY ARTERY DISEASE–SYMPATHETIC AXIS: WHY BISOPROLOL?

Obesity promotes coronary artery disease through an integrated pathway involving metabolic dysfunction, endothelial injury, microvascular impairment, and heightened SNS activation.[51] This "Obesity–CAD–Sympathetic Axis" creates a distinctive ischemic phenotype characterized by elevated resting heart rate, increased myocardial oxygen demand, impaired coronary flow reserve, and autonomic imbalance, all of which contribute to both obstructive CAD and INOCA or microvascular angina.[52] Persistent sympathetic overactivity in obesity, driven by insulin resistance, hyperinsulinemia, leptin excess, chronic inflammation, and conditions such as sleep apnea, produces tachycardia and exaggerated myocardial workload, making heart rate control a central therapeutic goal. Bisoprolol, with its high β_1-selectivity and clean hemodynamic profile, fits precisely into this pathophysiological framework by effectively reducing heart rate, blunting sympathetic drive, lowering myocardial oxygen consumption, and prolonging diastolic perfusion time, thereby improving both epicardial and microvascular coronary flow.[53] In addition, bisoprolol mitigates the hemodynamic burden associated with obesity, such as increased blood volume, cardiac output, and left ventricular hypertrophy, while offering advantages in patients with HFpEF-like physiology, exertional dyspnea, and microvascular angina. Importantly, unlike older non-selective beta-blockers, bisoprolol is metabolically neutral and does not worsen insulin resistance, lipid profiles, or body weight, making it particularly suitable for obese patients with diabetes, metabolic syndrome, or prediabetes.[53] By targeting the sympathetic overdrive and microvascular dysfunction central to obesity-related CAD, bisoprolol provides a mechanistically aligned therapeutic option across the spectrum of ACS, CCS, and INOCA/MVA, offering improved symptom control, better ischemic protection, and enhanced quality-of-life in this increasingly prevalent patient population[53,54] **(Table 1)**.

TABLE 1: Key clinical studies.

Study/year	*Population (CAD/obesity context)*	*Design and size*	*Intervention/ comparator (bisoprolol focus where applicable)*	*Key CAD/HR outcomes*	*Obesity/metabolic notes*
BISO-CAD sub-analysis (Chen et al., 2020)[6]	Asian patients with angiographically documented CAD and comorbid hypertension; obesity not a predefined subgroup	Prospective study; subgroup analysis from BISO-CAD; several hundred CAD patients on bisoprolol	Bisoprolol titrated to resting heart-rate (RHR) target; no active non-BB comparator within this sub-analysis	Lower RHR with bisoprolol was associated with improvement in composite cardiac clinical outcomes (cardiac death, non-fatal MI, unstable angina hospitalization, HF hospitalization), independent of blood pressure change	BMI/obesity not a stratification variable; no dedicated weight or obesity-specific outcome reported
Differential β-blocker effect in CAD (Cordero et al., 2011)[19]	Stable CAD patients receiving β-blockers; mixed risk profile including patients with obesity but not analyzed separately	Observational analysis; CAD cohort treated with different β-blockers	Compared atenolol, bisoprolol, metoprolol for RHR control in CAD	β-blocker therapy significantly reduced RHR; atenolol, bisoprolol and metoprolol were more effective than other β-blockers in RHR reduction	Obesity present in real-world cohort but not reported as a modifier of bisoprolol effect
Stable angina trials—bisoprolol vs. atenolol (early RCTs)[20-22]	Patients with chronic stable, exercise-induced angina pectoris (a clinical manifestation of CAD); obesity generally not specified	Placebo-controlled or active-controlled, double-blind randomized crossover or parallel trials; sample sizes ~20–several hundred	Bisoprolol 10 mg once daily vs. atenolol 100 mg or placebo	Bisoprolol provided 24 hours anti-anginal efficacy, improved exercise capacity, and reduced frequency of ischemic episodes, with similar or better efficacy than atenolol	Trials did not report obesity-specific analyses or weight-related outcomes
TIBBS (Total Ischemic Burden Bisoprolol Study)—stable angina[23]	631 patients with stable angina and positive exercise-induced ischemia; obesity prevalence not detailed	Randomized trial: bisoprolol vs. nifedipine for 8 weeks	Bisoprolol vs. nifedipine (CCB), doses titrated; both on background anti-anginal therapy as per standard practice	Bisoprolol reduced total ischemic burden (ST-segment depression and duration) by 73% vs. 46% with nifedipine and reduced number and duration of transient ischemic episodes and morning ischemia	No dedicated obesity or weight outcomes; obesity not used for stratification
Large β-blocker effectiveness study including metabolic endpoints[24]	Patients receiving bisoprolol vs. other β-blockers, ACEi/ARB, or diuretics across cardiovascular indications (including CAD); many overweight/obese but not CAD-specific	Observational comparative effectiveness analysis with propensity-score matching	Bisoprolol cohort vs. other β-blockers and non-BB comparators; followed for incident metabolic adverse events	No major difference in dyslipidemia risk vs. ACEi/ARB; dyslipidemia risk slightly higher vs. some other β-blockers	No significant difference in risk of obesity vs. diuretics by conventional HR; subdistribution hazard suggested a trend but confidence intervals crossed null, so no clear obesity signal
CAD with obesity—non-bisoprolol focused trials[25,26]	Overweight/obese patients with stable CAD or post-ACS enrolled in contemporary secondary-prevention trials and guideline datasets	Large RCTs or observational cohorts evaluating multifactorial secondary prevention	Usually intensive lifestyle, statins, ACEi/ARB, β-blockers as a class; individual β-blockers (including bisoprolol) not always specified	Show benefits of comprehensive risk-factor control on major adverse cardiovascular events (MACE) in obese CAD populations	Obesity frequently a baseline risk factor and predictor of recurrent events, but specific signal for bisoprolol vs. other β-blockers is not isolated

CONCLUSION

Bisoprolol occupies a clinically relevant position at the intersection of obesity, CAD, and microvascular ischemia. Various studies demonstrate that bisoprolol effectively lowers heart rate, reduces myocardial oxygen demand, and mitigates the sympathetic overactivity characteristic of obesity-related CAD. Its β-selectivity, pharmacokinetic predictability, and metabolic neutrality make it suitable for patients with obesity, diabetes, or INOCA/MVA phenotypes. While existing studies have shown favorable hemodynamic and symptomatic outcomes, the evidence base is limited by the predominance of short-term observational data and reliance on surrogate markers. Larger randomized trials with long-term follow-up are needed to determine the impact of bisoprolol on major cardiovascular events and its comparative role within contemporary multimodal management of obesity-associated coronary disease.

REFERENCES

1. Roth GA, Mensah GA, Johnson CO, et al. GBD-NHLBI-JACC Global Burden of Cardiovascular Diseases Writing Group. Global burden of cardiovascular diseases and risk factors, 1990–2019: update from the GBD 2019 study. J Am Coll Cardiol. 2021;77(15):1958-9.
2. Prabhakaran D, Jeemon P, Sharma M, et al. The changing patterns of cardiovascular diseases and their risk factors in the states of India: the Global Burden of Disease Study 1990–2016. The Lancet Global Health. 2018;6(12):e1339-51.
3. Libby P. Inflammation in atherosclerosis. Arterioscler Thromb Vasc Biol. 2012;32(9):2045-51.
4. Collet JP, Thiele H, Barbato E, et al. 2020 ESC Guidelines for the management of acute coronary syndromes in patients presenting without persistent ST-segment elevation: The Task Force for the management of acute coronary syndromes in patients presenting without persistent ST-segment elevation. Eur Heart J. 2021;42(14):1289-367.
5. Thygesen K, Alpert JS, Jaffe AS, et al. Fourth Universal Definition of Myocardial Infarction (2018). Circulation. 2018;138(20):e618-51. Erratum in: Circulation. 2018;138(20):e652.
6. Chen YD, Yang XC, Pham VN, et al. Resting heart rate control and prognosis in coronary artery disease patients with hypertension previously treated with bisoprolol: a sub-group analysis of the BISO-CAD study. Chin Med J. 2020;133(10):1155-65.
7. Kobalava Z, Kvasnikov B, Burtsev Y, et al. Effectiveness and Tolerability of Bisoprolol/Perindopril Single-Pill Combination in Patients with Arterial Hypertension and a History of Myocardial Infarction: The PRIDE Observational Study. Adv Ther. 2023;40(6):2725-40.
8. Boytsov SA, Burtsev YP, Khomitskaya YV, et al. Effectiveness and Tolerability of the Single-Pill Combination of Bisoprolol and Perindopril in Patients with Arterial Hypertension and Stable Coronary Artery Disease in Daily Clinical Practice: The STYLE Study. Adv Ther. 2021;38(6):3299-313.
9. Chaturvedi S, Lipszyc DH, Licht C, et al. Cochrane in context: pharmacological interventions for hypertension in children. Evid Based Child Health. 2014;9(3):581-3.
10. Nikolic VN, Jankovic SM, Deljanin-Ilic M, et al. Population pharmacokinetic analysis of bisoprolol in patients with stable coronary artery disease. Eur J Drug Metab Pharmacokinet. 2018;43(1):35-44.
11. Tagliamonte E, Cirillo T, Rigo F, et al. Ivabradine and bisoprolol on doppler-derived coronary flow velocity reserve in patients with stable coronary artery disease: beyond the heart rate. Adv Ther. 2015;32(8):757-67.
12. Chen Y, Yang X, Nguyen Pham V, et al. Heart rate control is associated with reduced cardiovascular events in Asian patients with coronary artery disease treated with bisoprolol (BISO-CAD): results from a multi-national, real-world experience. Curr Med Res Opin. 2018;34(2):217-25.
13. Chen Y, Yang X, Huang S, et al. Occurrence of composite cardiac endpoints with change in resting heart rate among Chinese patients with coronary artery disease: Chinese cohort from the real-world BISO-CAD study. Curr Med Res Opin. 2018;34(11):1921-6.
14. Skoczylas A, Adamczak M, Chudek J, et al. Cilazapril increases plasma ghrelin concentration in obese patients with arterial hypertension. Endokrynol Pol. 2010;61(1):21-7.
15. Cheymol G, Poirier JM, Carrupt PA, et al. Pharmacokinetics of beta-adrenoceptor blockers in obese and normal volunteers. Br J Clin Pharmacol. 1997;43(6):563-70.
16. Erne P, Schoenenberger AW, Zuber M, et al. Effects of anti-ischaemic drug therapy in silent myocardial ischaemia type I: the Swiss Interventional Study on Silent Ischaemia type I (SWISSI I): a randomized, controlled pilot study. Eur Heart J. 2007;28(17):2110-7.
17. Eichwede F, Komar K, Müller R, et al. Preoperative treatment with beta-receptor blockers and isoflurane anesthesia. Hemodynamic interactions in patients with coronary disease. Anaesthesist. 1990;39(7):361-6.
18. Vinnik NI, Kaĭdashev IP. Clinical description of effectiveness of pioglitazone in a complex therapy of patients with ischemic heart disease on background of metabolic syndrome. Lik Sprava. 2011;(1-2):82-9.
19. Cordero A, Bertomeu-González V, Mazón P, et al. Differential effect of β-blockers for heart rate control in coronary artery disease. Clin Cardiol. 2011;34(12):748-54.
20. Terol I, Plaza L, Rodrigo F. Bisoprolol in the treatment of chronic stable angina pectoris. J Cardiovasc Pharmacol. 1990;16 (Suppl 5):S208-212.
21. Kohli RS, Khurmi NS, Kardash MM, et al. Efficacy of once daily bisoprolol in stable angina pectoris: an objective comparison with atenolol and long term follow-up. Eur Heart J. 1985;6(10):845-50.
22. de Muinck ED, Lie KI. Safety and efficacy of beta-blockers in the treatment of stable angina pectoris. J Cardiovasc Pharmacol. 1990;16 (Suppl 5):S123-8.
23. Von Arnim T. Medical treatment to reduce total ischemic burden: Total ischemic burden bisoprolol study (TIBBS),

a multicenter trial comparing bisoprolol and nifedipine. J Am Coll Cardiol. 1995;25(1):231-8.
24. Foch C, Allignol A, Hohenberger T, et al. Effectiveness of bisoprolol versus other β-blockers and other antihypertensive classes: a cohort study in the Clinical Practice Research Datalink. Journal of Comparative Effectiveness Research. 2022;11(6):423-36.
25. Joseph P, Swedberg K, Leong DP, et al. The evolution of β-blockers in coronary artery disease and heart failure (Part 1/5). Journal of the American College of Cardiology. 2019;74(5):672-82.
26. Virani SS, Newby LK, Arnold SV, et al. 2023 AHA/ACC/ACCP/ASPC/NLA/PCNA Guideline for the Management of Patients With Chronic Coronary Disease: A Report of the American Heart Association/American College of Cardiology Joint Committee on Clinical Practice Guidelines. Circulation. 2023;148(9):e9-119.
27. Abbafati C, Abbas KM, Abbasi M, et al. Global burden of 369 diseases and injuries in 204 countries and territories, 1990–2019: a systematic analysis for the Global Burden of Disease Study 2019. Lancet. 2020;396(10258):1204-22.
28. Sharaf BL, Pepine CJ, Kerensky RA, et al. Detailed angiographic analysis of women with suspected ischemic chest pain (pilot phase data from the NHLBI-sponsored Women's Ischemia Syndrome Evaluation [WISE] study angiographic core laboratory). American Journal of Cardiology. 2001;87(8):937-41; A3.
29. Taqueti VR, Carli MFD. Coronary Microvascular Disease Pathogenic Mechanisms and Therapeutic Options: JACC State-of-the-Art Review. J Am Coll Cardiol. 2018;72(21):2625-41.
30. Kunadian V, Chieffo A, Camici PG, et al. An EAPCI Expert Consensus Document on Ischaemia with Non-obstructive Coronary Arteries in Collaboration with European Society of Cardiology Working Group on Coronary Pathophysiology & Microcirculation Endorsed by Coronary Vasomotor Disorders International Study Group. EuroIntervention. 2021;16(13):1049-69.
31. Murthy VL, Naya M, Taqueti VR, et al. Effects of sex on coronary microvascular dysfunction and cardiac outcomes. Circulation. 2014;129(24):2518-27.
32. Li C, Liu X, Adhikari BK, et al. The role of epicardial adipose tissue dysfunction in cardiovascular diseases: an overview of pathophysiology, evaluation, and management. Front Endocrinol (Lausanne). 2023;14:1167952.
33. Moreno-Viedma V, Amor M, Sarabi A, et al. Common dysregulated pathways in obese adipose tissue and atherosclerosis. Cardiovasc Diabetol. 2016;15(1):120.
34. Lavie CJ, Arena R, Alpert MA, et al. Management of cardiovascular diseases in patients with obesity. Nat Rev Cardiol. 2018;15(1):45-56.
35. Lavie CJ, McAuley PA, Church TS, et al. Obesity and cardiovascular diseases: Implications regarding fitness, fatness, and severity in the obesity paradox. J Am Coll Cardiol. 2014;63(14):1345-54.
36. Jouy SH, Mohan S, Scichilone G, et al. Adipokines in the Crosstalk between Adipose Tissues and Other Organs: Implications in Cardiometabolic Diseases. Biomedicines. 2024;12(9):2129.
37. Lehr S, Hartwig S, Sell H. Adipokines: A treasure trove for the discovery of biomarkers for metabolic disorders. Proteomics Clin Appl. 2012;6(1-2):91-101.
38. Jayaraj RL, Aburawi EH. Mechanistic relationship between obesity-induced inflammation triggering endothelial dysfunction and the initiation of atherosclerosis development. Heart Vessels Transplant. 2025;9(Issue 1).
39. Calling S, Johansson SE, Nymberg VM, et al. Trajectories of body mass index and risk for coronary heart disease: a 38-year follow-up study. PLoS ONE. 2021;16.
40. Puchałowicz K, Kłoda K, Dziedziejko V, et al. Association of adiponectin, leptin and resistin plasma concentrations with echocardiographic parameters in patients with coronary artery disease. Diagnostics. 2021;11(10):1774.
41. Poirier P, Lavie CJ, Connelly K. Practical implications of obesity for cardiovascular diagnostics. Canadian J Cardiol. 2025;41(9):1679-98.
42. Para I, Albu A, Porojan MD. Adipokines and arterial stiffness in obesity. Medicina. 2021;57(7):653.
43. Ge Y, Steel K, Antiochos P, et al. Stress CMR in patients with obesity: insights from the Stress CMR Perfusion Imaging in the United States (SPINS) registry. Eur Heart J Cardiovasc Imaging. 2020;22(5):518.
44. Marti HP, López AAP, Schwartzmann P. Safety and tolerability of β-blockers: importance of cardioselectivity. Current Medical Research and Opinion. 2024;40(sup1):55-62.
45. Wagner L, Kenreigh C. Bisoprolol. xPharm: The Comprehensive Pharmacology Reference. 2023;1-5.
46. Godoy LC, Farkouh ME, Austin PC, et al. Association of beta-blocker therapy with cardiovascular outcomes in patients with stable ischemic heart disease. J Am Coll Cardiol. 2023;81(24):2299-2311.
47. Sharma K, Sathe S, Desai B, et al. Optimizing cardiovascular outcomes with bisoprolol: an evidence-based perspective. Cureus. 2025;17(8):e89579.
48. Leopold G. Balanced pharmacokinetics and metabolism of bisoprolol. J Cardiovasc Pharmacol. 1986:8 (Suppl 11):S16-20.
49. Chopra HK, Sethi KK, Nair T. National Consensus Statement on Role of Bisoprolol across Cardiovascular Continuum: Special Focus on Women. JAPI. 2025;74(1).
50. Vrints C, Andreotti F, Koskinas KC, et al. 2024 ESC Guidelines for the management of chronic coronary syndromes. Eur Heart J. 2024;45(36):3415-537.
51. Sorop O, Olver TD, DeWouw JV, et al. The microcirculation: a key player in obesity-associated cardiovascular disease. Cardiovascular Research. 2017;113(9):1035-45.
52. Młynarska E, Bojdo K, Frankenstein H, et al. Endothelial dysfunction as the common pathway linking obesity, hypertension and atherosclerosis. Int J Molecul Sci. 2025;26(20):10096.
53. Canale MP, Villahermosa SMD, Martino G, et al. Obesity-related metabolic syndrome: mechanisms of sympathetic overactivity. Int J Endocrinol. 2013;2013:865965.
54. Kalil GZ, Haynes WG. Sympathetic nervous system in obesity-related hypertension: mechanisms and clinical implications. Hypertens Res. 2012;35(1):4-16.

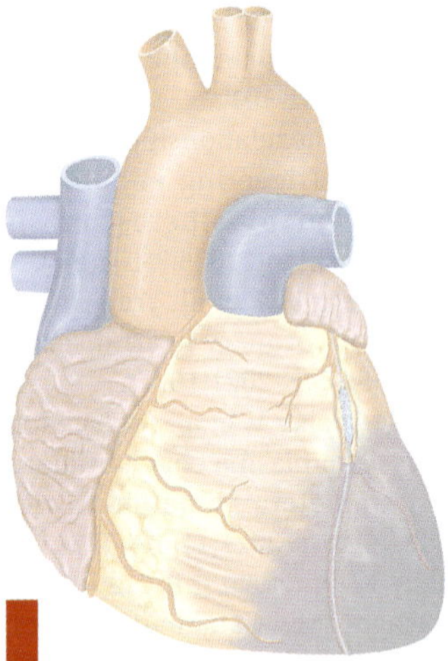

145

CHAPTER

Bisoprolol in Diabetes with Obesity: Sustained Benefits from an Endocrine Perspective

Sahana Shetty, Pankti Parikh, Kanhai Lalani

INTRODUCTION

The coexistence of type 2 diabetes mellitus (T2DM) and obesity, termed "diabesity," has become a worldwide health crisis. In India, the ICMR-INDIAB study shows diabetes (11.4%) and prediabetes (15.3%) are widespread, alongside high rates of generalized obesity (28.6%) and abdominal obesity (39.5%). Projected to 2021, this translates to ~101 million people with diabetes, 136 million with prediabetes, ~315 million with generalized obesity, and ~351 million with abdominal obesity.[1] Obesity is a major driver of type 2 diabetes, contributing to the majority of cases.[2,3]

The interrelationship between the two conditions is driven by common pathophysiological mechanisms, including insulin resistance, chronic low-grade inflammation, adipose tissue dysfunction, and neuroendocrine dysregulation. Obesity accelerates β-cell failure and glucose intolerance, while diabetes worsens lipid metabolism and promotes fat deposition, creating a vicious cycle of metabolic deterioration. This bidirectional interplay amplifies cardiovascular and renal risk, making diabesity a major contributor to global cardiovascular mortality.[2-4]

Diabesity is also associated with chronic hyperactivity of the sympathetic nervous system (SNS). The resulting persistent adrenergic drive in patients with diabesity contributes significantly to myocardial and vascular damage.[3,4]

Beta-blockers (BBs) have long been cornerstone therapy for cardiovascular conditions, particularly in postmyocardial infarction patients and those with heart failure. However, traditional BBs have historically been viewed with caution in diabetic populations due to concerns about metabolic adverse effects, including impaired insulin sensitivity, weight gain, and masking of hypoglycemic symptoms. These concerns have led to the underutilization of these life-saving medications in diabetic patients, despite robust evidence for cardiovascular benefits.[4,5]

Bisoprolol is a highly selective β_1-adrenergic receptor antagonist (β_1:β_2 ratio of 13.5) that demonstrates unique endocrine-metabolic properties that distinguish it from traditional BBs, offering sustained cardiovascular benefits while preserving crucial metabolic pathways essential for glucose homeostasis and energy balance.[6,7] Bisoprolol also exhibits low lipophilicity, which restricts its penetration across the blood–brain barrier.[8]

PATHOPHYSIOLOGICAL MECHANISMS

Beta-1 adrenergic receptors are predominantly located in cardiac tissue, where they regulate heart rate, contractility, and atrioventricular conduction. In contrast, β_2-receptors are widely distributed in metabolic tissues, including skeletal muscle, liver, and adipose tissue, where they facilitate glucose uptake, glycogenolysis, and lipolysis.

Traditional nonselective BBs antagonize both β_1 and β_2 receptors, leading to reduced skeletal muscle glucose uptake, impaired hepatic glycogenolysis, suppressed lipolysis, and consequent risks of dysglycemia and weight gain. In contrast, bisoprolol's high β_1-selectivity minimizes these metabolic disruptions while preserving cardiovascular efficacy. It maintains insulin-mediated glucose disposal, normal counter-regulatory responses, and is associated with a ~17% reduction in HOMA-IR, indicating improved insulin sensitivity.[4,6,7,9,10]

BISOPROLOL'S FAVORABLE EFFECT ON PANCREATIC B-CELL FUNCTION AND INSULIN SECRETION

Recent studies have demonstrated that bisoprolol may exert unexpectedly favorable effects on pancreatic β-cell function. At clinically relevant concentrations, bisoprolol enhanced glucose-stimulated insulin secretion in MIN6-K8 β-cells and isolated mouse islets through increased intracellular cAMP production, adenylyl cyclase activation, and subsequent PKA-mediated phosphorylation of ryanodine receptor 2 (RYR2). This facilitated calcium-induced calcium release, augmenting insulin secretory capacity. Notably, these effects were more pronounced in diabetic islets from NSY.B6-Ay/a mice, indicating potential to restore compromised β-cell function in established diabetes. The mechanism further involves TRPM5 activation, promoting sustained calcium channel activity and insulin release. Collectively, these findings challenge traditional concerns about BB therapy in diabetes and suggest that bisoprolol may support rather than impair pancreatic endocrine function.[11]

Bisoprolol enhances insulin receptor signaling without altering insulin binding, indicating a postreceptor mechanism through improved intracellular signal transduction by preserving insulin-mediated glucose uptake in skeletal muscle—the major site of insulin-dependent glucose disposal—it avoids the metabolic limitations of nonselective BBs, which impair peripheral glucose utilization via β2-receptor antagonism and reduced muscle perfusion. In the TENACITY trial, 400 postacute coronary syndrome patients treated with bisoprolol maintained stable HbA1c over 1 year (6.2 ± 0.6% vs. 6.1 ± 0.7%; $p = 0.64$) while achieving significant cardiovascular protection.[12] This evidence highlights bisoprolol's ability to preserve insulin sensitivity and glucose homeostasis in diabetic populations **(Table 1)**.

TABLE 1: Metabolic profile: Bisoprolol versus nonselective beta-blockers.

Nonselective beta-blockers	*Bisoprolol (β_1-selective)*
• $\beta_1 + \beta_2$ blockade • ↓Skeletal muscle glucose uptake • Impaired hepatic glycogenolysis • Suppressed adipose lipolysis • Weight gain, dyslipidemia • Insulin resistance risk ↑	• High β_1-selectivity • Preserves skeletal muscle glucose uptake • Maintains hepatic glucose regulation • Supports adipose lipolysis • Weight and lipid neutrality • Improved insulin sensitivity (↓ HOMA-IR) • Stable HbA1c (TENACITY study)

Adipose Tissue Metabolism and Energy Balance

Pharmacokinetic studies in obese patients reveal that bisoprolol demonstrates limited tissue distribution into adipose tissue despite its lipophilicity. This distribution pattern may contribute to its metabolic neutrality by minimizing interference with adipose tissue β_3-adrenergic receptor-mediated lipolysis and thermogenesis.[13]

Brown adipose tissue (BAT) function is critical to energy expenditure and metabolic homeostasis. Selective β_1-antagonism preserves important β_2- and β_3-mediated thermogenic pathways.[6,14] A longitudinal analysis of hypertensive patients demonstrated that while BBs as a class were associated with BMI increases, patients receiving bisoprolol and carvedilol showed significantly lower BMI values compared to those on conventional agents.[15]

Sympathetic-Metabolic Axis and Neuroendocrine Regulation

The high β_1-selectivity preserves crucial β_2-adrenergic pathways involved in metabolic regulation. These include β_2-mediated insulin-stimulated glucose uptake in skeletal muscle, β_2-dependent vasodilation that facilitates nutrient delivery to metabolically active tissues, and β_2-mediated glycogenolysis during hypoglycemic episodes.[5,6,15]

Studies contrasting bisoprolol with less selective agents demonstrate superior metabolic profiles, including preserved insulin sensitivity and reduced incidence of new-onset diabetes.[4,5,15] A comprehensive analysis of diabetic patients with systolic heart failure showed that bisoprolol therapy resulted in stable HbA1c levels (7.0 ± 0.20% to 6.9 ± 0.23%, $p = 0.92$) compared to carvedilol, which showed improvement in glycemic control but from a higher baseline.[15]

Hormonal Regulation and Metabolic Syndrome Management

Bisoprolol's impact on the renin-angiotensin-aldosterone system (RAAS) provides additional endocrine benefits relevant to metabolic syndrome management. The drug reduces renin secretion by approximately 65%, leading to decreased angiotensin II formation and aldosterone production. This RAAS modulation contributes to improved insulin sensitivity, as angiotensin II is known to impair insulin signaling and promote insulin resistance through multiple molecular mechanisms. The reduction in aldosterone also supports improved endothelial function and reduced oxidative stress, factors that contribute to insulin resistance in diabetic patients.[16,17]

Long-term Metabolic–Cardiovascular Protection

The significance of sustained therapy becomes apparent when considering the natural progression of diabetic complications. Diabetic patients face progressive β-cell dysfunction, worsening insulin resistance, and increasing cardiovascular risk over time. Bisoprolol's ability to provide cardiovascular protection while preserving or potentially enhancing insulin receptor function and pancreatic β-cell capacity positions it as an ideal long-term therapeutic choice for this population. The drug's mortality benefits, demonstrated in landmark trials like CIBIS-II (34% reduction in all-cause mortality, HR 0.66; 95% CI 0.54–0.81), occur without metabolic compromise, representing optimal integration of cardiovascular and endocrine therapeutic goals.[18,19]

LIMITATIONS

A limitation inherent to the BB drug class is that, in the absence of compelling CVD comorbidities (HF, post-MI, or angina), bisoprolol and other BBs are not typically recommended as first-line monotherapy for hypertension in T2DM/obesity patients. Guidelines generally advocate for initial therapy involving RAAS blockers, often combined with CCBs or diuretics. Therefore, bisoprolol's clinical significance is realized when a BB is medically indicated by established CVD, ensuring that its superior metabolic management can proceed concurrently with critical cardioprotective therapy.

Most mechanistic studies examining bisoprolol's effects on insulin receptor function and pancreatic β-cell secretion have been conducted in controlled laboratory settings using cell culture models or small animal studies. While these findings provide crucial mechanistic insights, translation to complex human metabolic physiology requires validation through larger clinical trials designed explicitly with endocrine endpoints.

While bisoprolol with high β_1-selectivity confers metabolic benefits, it necessitates clinical caution regarding the potential masking of hypoglycemia symptoms. BBs can attenuate the β_1-mediated tachycardia response to low blood sugar. Even though other adrenergic warning signs (like sweating and tremors) are usually preserved.

SUMMARY

The T2DM/obesity patient must possess a compelling GDMT indication for a BB, such as HFrEF, post-MI, or angina. Agents such as metoprolol (outside of specific succinate use for HF, approached cautiously) and atenolol must be avoided due to their association with worsening insulin resistance, increased risk of incident T2DM, and unfavorable lipid effects.[15,20]

If such an indication is absent, first-line therapy should prioritize RAAS blockers in combination with other classes.

Bisoprolol Initiation Strategy

- Start with a low dose (1.25 mg daily) to assess metabolic tolerance
- Target dose 5–10 mg daily
- Monitor glucose patterns during the titration period
- Assess hypoglycemia awareness and symptom recognition
- Regular evaluation of metabolic syndrome components
- Coordination with the multidisciplinary diabetes care team

CONCLUSION

Bisoprolol represents a transformative approach to cardiovascular risk management in diabetic patients with obesity. The convergence of molecular, cellular, and clinical evidence demonstrates that this highly selective β_1-adrenergic receptor antagonist provides sustained cardiovascular benefits while actively supporting rather than compromising metabolic homeostasis. The drug's unique endocrine profile—characterized by enhanced insulin receptor tyrosine kinase activity, preserved pancreatic β-cell secretory capacity, and metabolic neutrality—addresses the fundamental concerns that have historically limited BB use in diabetic populations.

The endocrine significance of bisoprolol extends beyond simple metabolic neutrality to encompass potential beneficial effects on insulin signaling pathways and glucose homeostasis. Demonstrating enhanced insulin receptor function and augmented insulin secretion in compromised pancreatic islets suggests that bisoprolol may actively contribute to metabolic improvement rather than merely avoiding metabolic harm. This represents a paradigm shift from defensive prescribing practices to therapeutic optimization that integrates cardiovascular and endocrine benefits.

For practicing endocrinologists managing diabetic patients with obesity, bisoprolol offers an evidence-based solution to the complex challenge of cardiovascular risk reduction without metabolic compromise. The drug's demonstrated mortality benefits (34% reduction in all-cause mortality from CIBIS-II) occur within a framework of preserved glucose homeostasis and insulin sensitivity, representing optimal therapeutic integration.

Future endocrinological research should focus on detailed mechanistic studies of bisoprolol's interactions with incretin-based therapies, systematically evaluating its effects on adipokine regulation and BAT function, and developing personalized dosing strategies based on individual metabolic phenotypes.

REFERENCES

1. Anjana RM, Unnikrishnan R, Deepa M, et al. Metabolic non-communicable disease health report of India: the ICMR-INDIAB national cross-sectional study (ICMR-INDIAB-17). Lancet Diabetes Endocrinol. 2023; 11(7):474-89.
2. Chandrasekaran P, Weiskirchen R. The role of obesity in type 2 diabetes mellitus—an overview. Int J Mol Sci. 2024;25:1882.
3. Zatterale F, Longo M, Naderi J, et al. Chronic adipose tissue inflammation linking obesity to insulin resistance and type 2 diabetes. Front Physiol. 2020;10:1607.
4. Drygała S, Radzikowski M, Maciejczyk M. β-blockers and metabolic modulation: unraveling the complex interplay with glucose metabolism, inflammation and oxidative stress. Front Pharmacol. 2024;15:1489657.
5. Sarafidis PA, Bakris GL. Do the metabolic effects of β-blockers make them leading or supporting antihypertensive agents in the treatment of hypertension? J Clin Hypertens. 2006;8(5):351-6.
6. Smith C, Teitler M. Beta-blocker selectivity at cloned human beta1- and beta2-adrenergic receptors. Cardiovasc Drugs Ther. 1999;13(2):123-6.
7. Owada A, Suda S, Hata T, et al. The effects of bisoprolol, a selective beta1-blocker, on glucose metabolism by long-term administration in essential hypertension. Clin Exp Hypertens. 2001;23(4):305-16.
8. Sigaroudi A, Kinzig M, Wahl O, et al. Quantification of bisoprolol and metoprolol in simultaneous human serum and cerebrospinal fluid samples. Pharmacology. 2017;101(1-2):29-34.
9. Janka HU, Ziegler AG, Disselhoff G, et al. Influence of bisoprolol on blood glucose, glucosuria, and haemoglobin A1 in noninsulin-dependent diabetics. J Cardiovasc Pharmacol. 1986;8 (Suppl 11):S96-9.
10. Lauridsen UB, Christensen NJ, Lyngsøe J. Effects of nonselective and β-1-selective blockade on glucose metabolism and hormone responses during insulin-induced hypoglycemia in normal man. J Clin Endocrinol Metab. 1983;56(5):876-82.
11. Murao N, Morikawa R, Seino Y, et al. β-adrenergic blockers increase cAMP and stimulate insulin secretion through a PKA/RYR2/TRPM5 pathway in pancreatic β-cells in vitro. Pharmacol Res Perspect. 2025;13(2):e70092.
12. Sharma K, Desai H, Sharma N, et al. To evaluate the "Real World" clinical performance of bisoprolol in post-myocardial infarction with left ventricular dysfunction: TENACITY study. J Assoc Physicians India. 2022;70(4):11-2.
13. Cheymol G, Poirier J, Carrupt P, et al. Pharmacokinetics of beta-adrenoceptor blockers in obese and normal volunteers. Br J Clin Pharmacol. 1997;43:563-70.
14. Dumont L, Caron A, Richard G, et al. The effects of the β1-adrenergic receptor antagonist bisoprolol administration on mirabegron-stimulated human brown adipose tissue thermogenesis. Acta Physiologica. 2024;240(5):e14127.
15. Poljaković HM, Tabaković M, Halilović E, et al. Beta-blockers and their impact on metabolic processes. World J Adv Res Rev. 2024;23(2):1938-47.
16. Favre GA, Esnault VLM, Van Obberghen E. Modulation of glucose metabolism by the renin-angiotensin-aldosterone system. Am J Physiol Endocrinol Metab. 2015;308(6):435-49.
17. Lastra-Lastra G, Sowers JR, Restrepo-Erazo K, et al. Role of aldosterone and angiotensin II in insulin resistance: an update. Clin Endocrinol (Oxf). 2009;71(1):1-6.
18. Stather R. CIBIS II. Inpharma Wkly. 1998;1154:13-4.
19. Erland E, Philippe L, Patricia V, et al. Results from post-hoc analyses of the CIBIS II trial: effect of bisoprolol in high-risk patient groups with chronic heart failure. Eur J Heart Fail. 2001;3(4):469-79.
20. Bakris GL, Fonseca V, Katholi RE, et al. Metabolic effects of carvedilol vs metoprolol in patients with type 2 diabetes mellitus and hypertension: a randomized controlled trial. JAMA. 2004;292(18):2227-36.

146

CHAPTER

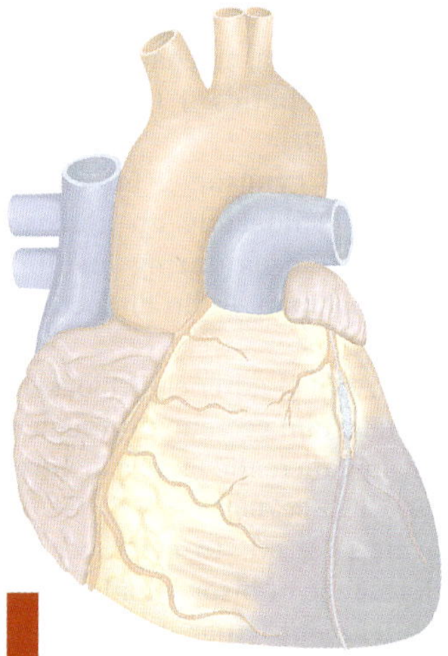

Bisoprolol in High-risk Coronary Artery Disease with Obesity in Women

Abhishek Garg, Shibba Takkar Chhabra

INTRODUCTION

Cardiovascular disease (CVD) remains the leading cause of morbidity and mortality in women worldwide, accounting for more deaths than all forms of cancer combined. Among the spectrum of CVD, coronary artery disease (CAD) contributes significantly to adverse outcomes, especially in women with high-risk features such as diabetes mellitus, hypertension, metabolic syndrome, and obesity.

Obesity, particularly central obesity, has emerged as a critical driver of cardiovascular risk. The rising prevalence of obesity in women across both developed and developing nations, including India, parallels the increasing burden of CAD. Women with obesity often exhibit a constellation of metabolic disturbances—insulin resistance, dyslipidemia, and systemic inflammation—that accelerate atherosclerosis and worsen prognosis following myocardial infarction (MI) or revascularization. Importantly, obesity modifies the clinical presentation of CAD in women, often leading to atypical symptoms, delayed diagnosis, and undertreatment.

Obese women with high-risk CAD face complex challenges due to heightened sympathetic drive, increased oxygen demand, and endothelial dysfunction, predisposing them to recurrent ischemia and heart failure (HF). Beta-blockers (BBs) are central to therapy, as they lower myocardial workload, improve angina, reduce the risk of reinfarction and enhance survival. Bisoprolol, a highly selective β_1-blocker with long action and minimal metabolic effects, is particularly useful in this group, where preserving insulin sensitivity and avoiding weight gain are vital.

This chapter will review the epidemiology, pathophysiology, and clinical implications of high-risk CAD in obese women, with a special focus on the role of bisoprolol as a therapeutic option.

EPIDEMIOLOGY AND RISK PROFILE

Obesity has become a critical public health concern worldwide. According to the World Health Organization (WHO), more than 650 million adults are obese, and the prevalence continues to rise in both developed and developing nations.[1] Among women, obesity rates have shown a consistent upward trajectory, especially in middle-aged and postmenopausal groups, where hormonal changes, sedentary lifestyle, and altered fat distribution predispose to central adiposity.[2]

In South Asia, and particularly in India, the burden is even more alarming due to the unique "Asian Indian phenotype," characterized by greater abdominal adiposity and metabolic disturbances at lower body mass index (BMI) levels compared to Caucasians.[3] Data from the ICMR–INDIAB study demonstrated high prevalence of generalized obesity and central obesity in women, with significant urban–rural differences, underlining the urgent need for targeted strategies.[4]

Obesity is closely associated with multiple cardiovascular risk factors, including hypertension, insulin resistance, dyslipidemia, and systemic inflammation, which together accelerate the development of CAD.[5] Women with obesity tend to accumulate visceral fat, which is metabolically active and promotes endothelial dysfunction, prothrombotic tendency, and adverse vascular remodeling.[6] The interplay of these mechanisms makes obese women particularly vulnerable to high-risk CAD, defined by recurrent ischemic events, extensive atherosclerosis, and progression to HF.

Importantly, women often present with CAD differently compared to men. They are more likely to have atypical or nonclassical anginal symptoms, such as dyspnea, fatigue, or epigastric discomfort, which can lead to delays in diagnosis and underutilization of evidence-based therapies.[7] Obesity further complicates this picture, as excess body weight may mask ischemic symptoms or lead to misattribution of chest pain to musculoskeletal or gastrointestinal causes. As a result, obese women with CAD are frequently diagnosed at later stages, when disease burden is already extensive.[7]

In India, women with acute MI experience nearly twice the mortality risk compared to men, despite representing a smaller fraction of acute coronary syndrome (ACS) cases. Studies have shown that women account for approximately 25–32% of ACS presentations in the country.[8,9] Postmenopausal women are particularly at risk, with some reports indicating CAD prevalence as high as 91%, largely due to the clustering of risk factors such as hypertension, obesity, dyslipidemia, and diabetes.[8,9] Beyond traditional determinants, female-specific conditions—such as menopause, pregnancy-associated complications, anemia, migraine, and depression—further heighten cardiovascular vulnerability. Women with ACS, especially those presenting with ST-elevation myocardial infarction (STEMI), more frequently demonstrate single-vessel disease, typically involving the left anterior descending artery.[10] Hence, Indian women tend to have poorer prognoses than men, with significantly elevated 1-year mortality rates after MI.

Clinical outcomes in this population are also less favorable. Procedural risks during percutaneous coronary intervention or coronary artery bypass grafting are heightened in obese women, owing to factors such as smaller vessel caliber, higher bleeding risk, and impaired wound healing.[10]

Thus, the epidemiological data clearly highlight that women with obesity constitute a high-risk subset within the CAD population. Their increased susceptibility arises not only from a higher burden of traditional risk factors but also from gender-specific pathophysiological differences and clinical challenges in diagnosis and treatment (as shown in **Table 1**).[11] Addressing this group requires both aggressive preventive measures and tailored

TABLE 1: Gender-based differences in cardiovascular disease.

Aspect	*Women*	*Men*
Anatomical differences	Smaller hearts (~25% smaller), narrower vessels, and relatively stronger contraction	Larger hearts, broader vessels
Functional characteristics	Higher heart rate, elevated peripheral resistance during stress	Greater rise in BP and peripheral resistance during stress
Aging response	Postmenopausal women show a sharper rise in BP and a greater risk of hypertension	BP rises more gradually with age
Coronary artery disease	Lower overall plaque burden, more nonobstructive CAD, and better myocardial salvage before menopause	Higher incidence of plaque rupture, more complex lesions, particularly in younger men
Heart failure	More prone to HFpEF (smaller LV chambers, stiffer arteries, diastolic dysfunction)	Higher risk of HFrEF and pathological remodeling
Hormonal impact	Estrogen improves lipid profile (↑HDL, ↓LDL), supports endothelial function, and promotes clot breakdown	Testosterone/DHEA improves lipid profile, but benefits decline with age
Postmenopause and andropause	Loss of estrogen → higher CVD risk (endothelial dysfunction, inflammation, stiff arteries)	Decline in testosterone/DHEA reduces cardiovascular protection
Mental health and CVD	Anxiety and depression are strongly linked to higher CVD risk	Mental health is less strongly associated with CVD
Risk factor patterns	Menopause, autoimmune disorders, and stress-related CVD are more frequent	Atherosclerosis, HFrEF, and adverse remodeling are more dominant
Protective influences	Premenopausal hormonal shield, favorable remodeling, and lower CVD rates before 75 years	Better established therapies for CAD and HF
Challenges in management	Less studied disease mechanisms, limited tailored therapies, and stress-related CVD are more prevalent	Clearer pathophysiology, but higher burden of severe CAD in younger males

therapeutic strategies, where agents such as bisoprolol may play a pivotal role due to their efficacy and metabolic safety.

BETA-BLOCKERS IN CORONARY ARTERY DISEASE: AN OVERVIEW

Beta-blockers are a cornerstone of cardiovascular therapeutics, with established benefits across CVD. Their primary mechanism—antagonism of adrenergic receptors—reduces the adverse effects of excessive sympathetic nervous system (SNS) activation, a pathophysiological driver of hypertension, CAD, ACS, and HF.[12] By lowering heart rate, myocardial contractility, and blood pressure, BBs effectively reduce myocardial oxygen demand, alleviate ischemia, and improve survival in high-risk populations.[10] The clinical utility of BBs extends from early intervention in hypertension to long-term secondary prevention after MI and chronic angina management.

The BB class is heterogeneous, comprising agents with distinct receptor selectivity and additional pharmacological properties. Early agents, including propranolol, timolol, and nadolol, were nonselective, blocking both β_1- and β_2-adrenoceptors. While effective, these drugs carried risks of bronchospasm and peripheral vasoconstriction due to β_2 blockade.[13] Later generations introduced cardioselective agents such as atenolol, metoprolol, bisoprolol, and nebivolol, which preferentially inhibit β_1-receptors in the myocardium, thereby reducing cardiac workload while limiting respiratory and vascular adverse effects.[13] Furthermore, certain third-generation BB, such as carvedilol and labetalol, exhibit additional vasodilatory properties through α_1-adrenergic antagonism, while nebivolol enhances nitric oxide bioavailability, offering favorable vascular effects.[13] This pharmacological diversity underpins the classification of BBs into three generations, as shown in **Table 2**.

Bisoprolol

Among the above, bisoprolol is of particular interest in high-risk CAD with obesity, due to its high β_1-selectivity, long half-life, and neutral metabolic profile, which make it especially suitable for women with comorbidities such as diabetes and obesity.[13] Distinctive pharmacological features of bisoprolol are summarized in **Table 3**.

TABLE 2: Generations of beta-blockers.

Generation	Key features	Drugs
First generation	Nonselective; act on both β_1 and β_2 receptors	Propranolol, sotalol
Second generation	Cardioselective; stronger affinity for β_1 receptors	Bisoprolol, metoprolol
Third generation	Highly β_1-selective with added vasodilatory benefits	Nebivolol, carvedilol

TABLE 3: Distinctive characteristics of bisoprolol.

Category	Key features
Cardioselectivity	Marked β_1 receptor preference (about 20 times higher than β_2). Around four to five times more β_1-selective than nebivolol
Mechanism of action	Lowers heart rate, oxygen requirement, and contractility; suppresses renin release and downregulates the renin-angiotensin system
Pharmacokinetics	• Balanced metabolism via the kidney (50%) and liver (50%). High oral bioavailability (>90%) • Predictable pharmacokinetics with low variability. Half-life of 10–12 hours enables once-daily dosing • Minimal first-pass metabolism (~10%). Food does not interfere with absorption
Pharmacodynamics	Sustained 24-hour effect. No intrinsic sympathomimetic action. Negligible membrane-stabilizing effects at therapeutic levels
Metabolic neutrality	Little to no impact on lipid or glucose metabolism
Lung and circulation	Negligible effects on respiratory function and peripheral blood flow, making it suitable for patients with COPD or peripheral vascular disease
Other benefits	No significant impact on sexual performance. Moderate protein binding (~30%) lowers drug–drug interaction risk
Clinical applications	Useful in hypertension, ischemic heart disease, chronic heart failure, and secondary prevention after myocardial infarction

Pharmacokinetics

Bisoprolol demonstrates a balanced elimination through both the liver and kidneys, with roughly equal contributions from each pathway. It has a prolonged elimination half-life of about 10–12 hours and a high oral bioavailability approaching 90%, which supports convenient once-daily administration and stable systemic concentrations. Because of its limited first-pass metabolism and relatively low lipophilicity, the drug produces fewer central nervous system-related adverse effects, contributing to better tolerance and suitability for long-term therapy.[14]

Clinical Application in Coronary Artery Disease

Bisoprolol is a highly selective β_1-adrenergic receptor antagonist that has become an integral therapy across the cardiovascular spectrum.[11] Its ability to lower morbidity and mortality, coupled with reductions in the risk of stroke and adverse cardiovascular events, reinforces its relevance in contemporary practice, particularly in women with obesity and high-risk CAD, where safety, tolerability, and metabolic neutrality are critical considerations.[11]

Blockade of β_1-adrenoreceptors is a cornerstone in the management of CAD, offering multiple therapeutic benefits. By attenuating sympathetic drive, bisoprolol and other BBs help in slowing atheromatous progression, lowering reinfarction risk, reducing infarct size, and minimizing the chance of myocardial rupture. Their effects include raising the threshold for ventricular fibrillation, reducing platelet aggregation, and lowering myocardial oxygen demand through reductions in heart rate, systolic blood pressure, and contractility. Furthermore, bisoprolol prolongs diastolic filling time, decreases circulating free fatty acids with arrhythmogenic potential, and promotes redistribution of coronary blood flow. Collectively, these actions lead to symptom relief, fewer cardiovascular events, and lower mortality in patients with CAD.[15]

The evolution of BBs evidence in CAD is well illustrated by three pivotal trials. The Beta-Blocker Heart Attack Trial (BHAT)[15] established β-blockade as a cornerstone of post-MI therapy, demonstrating significant reductions in all-cause mortality and reinfarction, thereby setting the foundation for secondary prevention. A decade later, the TIBBS trial[16] provided bisoprolol-specific data in chronic stable angina, showing superior efficacy over nifedipine in reducing ischemic burden and improving circadian ischemia control, underscoring the advantages of cardioselectivity and once-daily dosing. More recently, the TENACITY trial[17] confirmed the relevance of bisoprolol in the modern era, demonstrating improvements in left ventricular ejection fraction (LVEF), arrhythmic burden, and metabolic parameters in post-ACS patients with LV systolic dysfunction, as part of guideline-directed therapy. Collectively, these trials trace the trajectory from class-wide mortality benefit (BHAT) to bisoprolol's anti-ischemic superiority (TIBBS) and its role in contemporary multidimensional management (TENACITY), reinforcing its utility in high-risk populations such as obese women with CAD. Various studies addressing sex-specific outcomes were performed, and the consolidated findings are presented in **Table 4**.

Recently, the ABYSS trial[26] (3,698 patients; 18% women; LVEF ≥40%) examined the impact of discontinuing long-term BBs after MI. Over 3 years, stopping therapy increased the risk of a composite outcome (death, MI, stroke, or cardiovascular hospitalization) by 16% compared to continuation (23.8 vs. 21.1%). Withdrawal was also associated with rises in SBP (+3.7 mm Hg), DBP (+3.9 mm Hg), and HR (+9.8 bpm), all highly significant.

The recently published BETAMI-DANBLOCK trial[27] has renewed interest in the role of BBs in the modern post-MI era. Involving >5,500 patients with preserved LVEF (≥40%) and no clinical HF, the study demonstrated that long-term BBs were associated with a modest but significant reduction in the composite of death or major adverse cardiovascular events (MACE), primarily driven by fewer recurrent infarctions. While overall mortality did not differ significantly, the reduction in nonfatal ischemic outcomes underscores the continued protective effect of BBs, even in an era of aggressive reperfusion, dual antiplatelet therapy, and statins.

These findings reinforce the class benefit of BBs and provide contemporary support for the use of cardioselective agents such as bisoprolol, particularly in high-risk subgroups including women and obese patients, where sympathetic overactivity and recurrent ischemia remain critical therapeutic targets.

GUIDELINES REGARDING THE BISOPROLOL IN CORONARY ARTERY DISEASE

Bisoprolol has been incorporated into the 2020 International Society of Hypertension (ISH) guidelines for patients with CAD, underscoring its value in comprehensive cardiovascular risk management.[28]

The 2020 NICE review confirms that bisoprolol is widely prescribed in routine clinical practice following ACS, underscoring its continued role in secondary prevention.[29]

TABLE 4: Clinical evidence of bisoprolol in coronary artery disease.

Study	*Findings*	*Conclusion*
Kato et al.[18]	Stable angina patients showed better exercise tolerance, reduced ST-segment depression, and fewer angina episodes. Benefits noted with 5–10 mg dosing	Effective for stable angina, with added benefit when titrated from 5 to 10 mg
Wagner[19]	Exercise capacity improved, ST-segment depression reduced, sustained efficacy with 5–10 mg dosing, and minimal side effects	Provides reliable long-term management of stable angina within 5–20 mg range
Terol et al.[20]	Chronic stable angina patients had reduced angina frequency (89%), with over half becoming angina-free, low side effect rate	Once-daily bisoprolol is effective and well-tolerated for long-term angina control
von Arnim[16]	Bisoprolol reduced transient ischemic episodes and ischemia duration more effectively than nifedipine, showing circadian benefits	Superior to nifedipine in reducing ischemia burden with once-daily use
Maclean et al.[21]	Early bisoprolol in NSTEMI patients lowered ischemic burden and adverse events, protective against VA and MACE	Early therapy reduces adverse outcomes in NSTEMI
Sabiò et al.[22]	A large cohort showed reduced angina recurrence, MI, arrhythmias, and mortality with bisoprolol over 14 years; lower discontinuation rates than other β-blockers	Supports use as first-line long-term therapy in primary care for CHD
Chen et al.[23]	Bisoprolol improved outcomes in hypertensive CAD patients, with consistent HR reduction and improved composite endpoints	Effective in CAD patients with hypertension for better outcomes
Sharma et al.[17]	In post-ACS LVSD patients, bisoprolol improved LVEF, reduced HR and ST depression, stabilized HbA1c, and improved lipid profile	Useful in GDMT with benefits on LV function, arrhythmias, and lipid profile
Godoy et al.[24]	A large CAD cohort showed lower primary events and fewer HF hospitalizations with the use of bisoprolol	Associated with reduced risk of recurrent events and HF hospitalization
Maheshwari et al.[25]	Bisoprolol and metoprolol equally reduced BP and HR in stable CAD, with bisoprolol preferred for tolerance	Both are effective, but bisoprolol is favored for better tolerability

The 2023 American Heart Association (AHA) guidelines recommend BBs for patients with chronic coronary disease who have a LVEF ≤40% or a history of MI, as they significantly reduce MACE.[30]

The 2024 Indian consensus statement recognizes BBs as first-line agents for CAD, highlighting their efficacy in reducing heart rate, blood pressure, and myocardial oxygen consumption, while preventing arrhythmias and improving survival after MI. It emphasizes individualized therapy, especially in those with comorbid hypertension or HF.[10]

Uses of Bisoprolol in Females in Specific Conditions

Higher Comorbidities

Women with CVDs frequently present with multiple coexisting conditions. Owing to its β_1-selectivity and favorable tolerability, bisoprolol is a suitable therapeutic option in patients with comorbidities such as diabetes, renal or hepatic dysfunction, asthma, and COPD. Compared with less selective BBs, it has a lower risk of altering glucose metabolism or provoking respiratory complications, making it a safer agent in complex clinical scenarios.[31]

Use during Pregnancy

Bisoprolol, an FDA category C agent, may be used for blood pressure control in pregnancy from the second trimester onward with appropriate fetal monitoring. Current evidence suggests no significant increase in congenital anomalies; however, prolonged therapy has been associated with a modest rise in preterm delivery and reduced birth weight. According to the UK Teratology Information Service, potential effects on fetal growth are more likely due to maternal hypertension rather than BB therapy itself. Importantly, bisoprolol exposure is not an indication for pregnancy termination but warrants close monitoring in women with hypertensive or cardiac complications.[32]

Use in Breastfeeding

Available evidence suggests that bisoprolol can be used safely during breastfeeding, with no significant impact on infant growth or neurodevelopmental outcomes. While generally well tolerated, occasional minor effects such as drowsiness or suboptimal weight gain have been reported, highlighting the need for careful monitoring of breastfed infants.[33]

Benefits during Menopause

After menopause, women often experience a pronounced rise in systolic blood pressure and heightened sympathetic activity, both of which contribute to increased cardiovascular risk. Bisoprolol has demonstrated benefits in alleviating menopausal symptoms, particularly among women with coronary heart disease. Moreover, its use has been associated with improved bone mineral density and a reduced risk of fractures, likely through favorable effects on trabecular bone microarchitecture.[34]

CONCLUSION

Cardiovascular disease in women is shaped by unique risk factors such as hormonal influences, pregnancy complications, and menopause, contributing to delayed diagnoses, higher morbidity, and increased mortality. Despite lower early incidence compared with men, women often encounter worse long-term outcomes. Bisoprolol, a cardioselective β1-blocker, offers consistent blood pressure control and protection across the cardiovascular continuum. Its favorable safety profile makes it suitable in complex scenarios such as pregnancy (with close monitoring), breastfeeding, and menopause. Beyond cardiovascular benefits, evidence also suggests a positive role in postmenopausal women by improving bone health and reducing fracture risk.

Given the dual challenges of obesity and sex-specific risk factors, bisoprolol's cardioselectivity, metabolic neutrality, and proven efficacy across landmark and contemporary trials position it as a vital therapy for improving outcomes in obese women with CAD.

REFERENCES

1. World Health Organization. Obesity and overweight. Fact sheet. Geneva: WHO; 2021.
2. Poirier P, Giles TD, Bray GA, et al. Obesity and cardiovascular disease: pathophysiology, evaluation, and effect of weight loss. Circulation. 2006;113(6):898-918.
3. Misra A, Khurana L. The metabolic syndrome in South Asians: epidemiology, determinants, and prevention. Metab Syndr Relat Disord. 2009;7(6):497-514.
4. Anjana RM, Deepa M, Pradeepa R, et al. Prevalence of diabetes and prediabetes in 15 states of India: results from the ICMR–INDIAB study. Diabetologia. 2017;60(2):295-308.
5. Yusuf S, Hawken S, Ounpuu S, et al. Obesity and the risk of myocardial infarction in 27,000 participants from 52 countries: INTERHEART study. Lancet. 2005;366(9497):1640-9.
6. Després JP. Body fat distribution and risk of cardiovascular disease: an update. Circulation. 2012;126(10):1301-13.
7. Shaw LJ, Shaw RE, Merz CN, et al. Impact of ethnicity and gender differences on angiographic coronary artery disease prevalence and in-hospital mortality in the ACC–NCDR. Circulation. 2008;117(14):1787-801.
8. Sharma YP, Vemuri KS, Bootla D, et al. Epidemiological profile, management and outcomes of patients with acute coronary syndrome: single centre experience from North India. Indian Heart J. 2021;73(2):174-9.
9. Khan MY, Pandit S, Guha S, et al. Demographic profile, clinical characteristics and medical management patterns of Indian coronary artery disease patients: a nationwide EMR study. Expert Rev Cardiovasc Ther. 2021;19(8):769-75.
10. Vijayalakshmi IB, Nemani L, Kher M, et al. The gamut of coronary artery disease in Indian women. Indian J Cardiovasc Dis Women. 2023;8:43.
11. Chopra HK, Sethi KK, Nair T, et al. National Consensus Statement on role of bisoprolol across cardiovascular continuum: special focus on women. J Assoc Physicians India. 2025;73(5):e16-33.
12. Sipahi I, Tuzcu EM, Wolski KE, et al. β-blockers and progression of coronary atherosclerosis: pooled analysis of 4 IVUS trials. Ann Intern Med. 2007;147(1):10-8.
13. Frishman WH. Beta-adrenergic blockers: a 50-year historical perspective. Am J Ther. 2008;15(6):565-76.
14. Singh R, Prakash A, Ahmad MB, et al. Is bisoprolol underutilized in US heart failure patients? JACC Adv. 2024;3(11):101290.
15. A randomized trial of propranolol in patients with acute myocardial infarction. I. Mortality results. JAMA. 1982;247(12):1707-14.
16. von Arnim T. Medical treatment to reduce total ischemic burden: TIBBS trial comparing bisoprolol and nifedipine. J Am Coll Cardiol. 1995;25(1):231-8.
17. Sharma K, Desai H, Sharma N, et al. To evaluate the 'real world' clinical performance of bisoprolol in post-MI with LV dysfunction: TENACITY study. J Assoc Physicians India. 2022;70(4):11-2.
18. Kato K, Niitani H, Kanazawa T, et al. Clinical evaluation of bisoprolol in patients with stable angina pectoris. J Cardiovasc Pharmacol. 1986;8(Suppl 11):S154-9.
19. Wagner G. Summary of short- and long-term studies with bisoprolol in coronary heart disease. J Cardiovasc Pharmacol. 1986;8(Suppl 11):S160-6.
20. Terol I, Plaza L, Rodrigo F. Bisoprolol in the treatment of chronic stable angina pectoris. J Cardiovasc Pharmacol. 1990;16(Suppl 5):S208-12.
21. Maclean E, Zheng S, Nabeebaccus A, et al. Effect of early bisoprolol administration on ventricular arrhythmia and cardiac death in NSTEMI. Heart Asia. 2015;7(2):46-51.
22. Sabidó M, Thilo H, Guido G. Long-term effectiveness of bisoprolol in patients with angina: a real-world study. Pharmacol Res. 2019;139:106-12.

23. Chen YD, Yang XC, Pham VN, et al. Resting heart rate control and prognosis in CAD patients with hypertension on bisoprolol: BISO-CAD subgroup analysis. Chin Med J (Engl). 2020;133(10):1155-65.
24. Godoy LC, Farkouh ME, Austin PC, et al. Association of beta-blocker therapy with outcomes in stable ischemic heart disease. J Am Coll Cardiol. 2023;81(24):2299-311.
25. Maheshwari RA, Rathi P, Shah J, et al. Metoprolol and bisoprolol in coronary artery disease: an observational study. J Young Pharm. 2024;16(1):42-9.
26. Silvain J, Cayla G, Ferrari E, et al. β-blocker interruption after uncomplicated myocardial infarction: rationale and design of the ABYSS trial. Am Heart J. 2023;258:168-76.
27. Munkhaugen J, Kristensen AM, Halvorsen S, et al. Beta-blockers after myocardial infarction in patients without heart failure. N Engl J Med. 2025;393:1901-11.
28. Unger T, Borghi C, Charchar F, et al. Clinical practice guidelines. Hypertension. 2020;75:1334-57.
29. National Guideline Centre (UK). Evidence Review for Beta-blockers: Acute Coronary Syndromes. London: NICE; 2020.
30. Virani SS, Newby LK, Arnold SV, et al. 2023 AHA/ACC/ACCP/ASPC/NLA/PCNA guideline for chronic coronary disease. J Am Coll Cardiol. 2023;82(9):833-955.
31. Liu G, Xue Y, Liu Y, et al. Multimorbidity in cardiovascular disease and association with life satisfaction: a Chinese national cross-sectional study. BMJ Open. 2020;10(12):e042950.
32. Stryuk RI. Bisoprolol in treatment of arterial hypertension in pregnant women. Med Alphabet. 2019;2(27):32-4.
33. De-Haan T, Hazan A, Kaduri NB, et al. Bisoprolol during breastfeeding: a prospective case series. Neurotoxicol Teratol. 2023;98:107232.
34. Lima R, Wofford M, Reckelhoff JF. Hypertension in postmenopausal women. Curr Hypertens Rep. 2012;14(3):254-60.

PART II

Advances in Lipid Management in CVD

SECTION 22

Nonstatin Therapy and Dyslipidemia

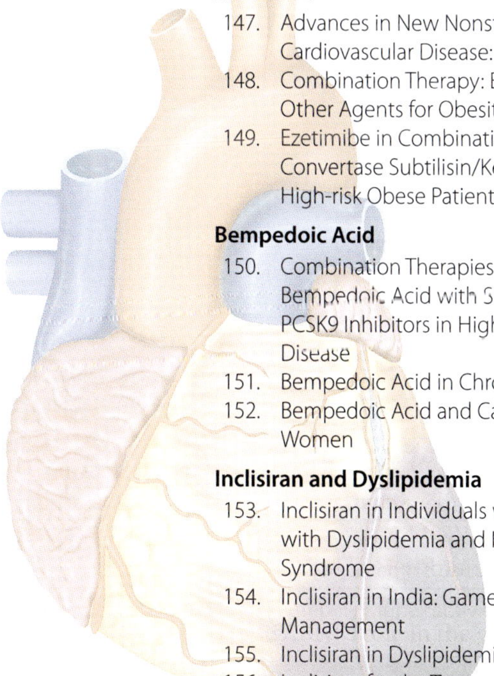

147

CHAPTER

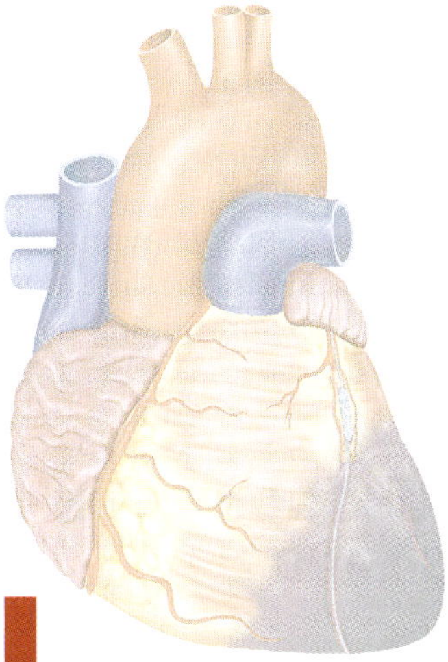

Advances in New Nonstatin Therapies in Cardiovascular Disease: Outcome Data

R Manivasagam, M Bharathkumaran

INTRODUCTION

Cardiovascular disease is one of the leading causes of death in the world. Atherosclerotic cardiovascular disease (ASCVD) is one among the important components of cardiovascular disease. ASCVD includes coronary artery disease (myocardial infarction or obstructive coronary artery disease), cerebrovascular disease (stroke, transient ischemic attack, or significant carotid artery stenosis), peripheral arterial disease (claudication or limb ischemia), aortic atherosclerotic disease, and prior coronary or arterial revascularization due to atherosclerosis. It is now undeniable that low-density lipoprotein cholesterol (LDL-C) has a causal relationship with atherosclerosis, the process that promotes the development of clinical ASCVD. A meta-analysis of 26 randomized trials found that each 1.0 mmol/L (18 mg/dl) decrease in LDL-C resulted in a 22% relative risk reduction in major vascular events (p <0.0001), further supporting the concept that lower is better when it comes to LDL-C. Statins are the cornerstone of both prevention and management of ASCVD. In 1994, the Scandinavian Simvastatin Survival Study was the first to demonstrate that statins improve outcomes in patients with coronary artery disease and hyperlipidemia **(Fig. 1)**.

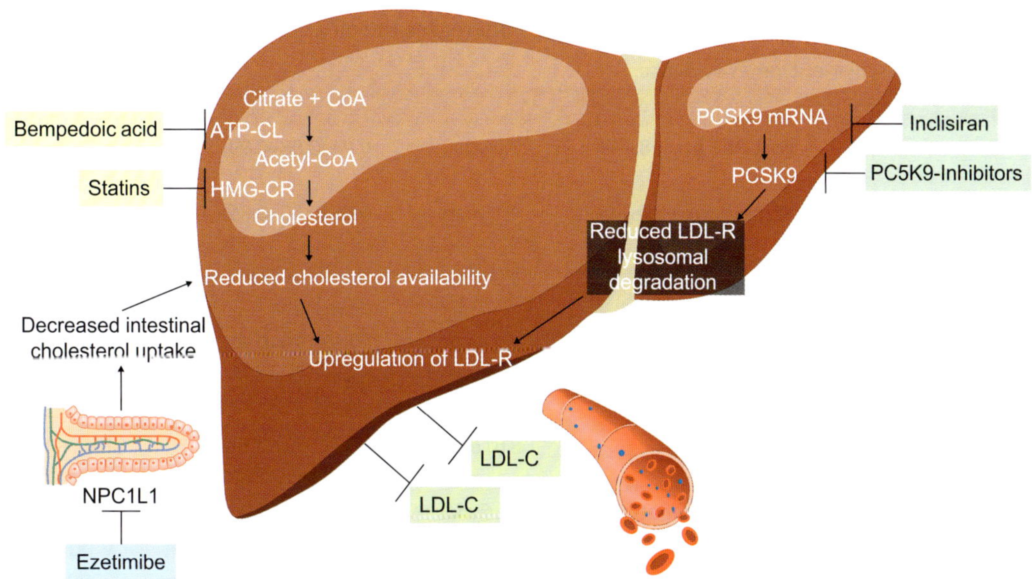

Fig. 1: Mechanisms of action of various nonstatin therapies targeting lipid metabolism in the liver and intestine.

NEED FOR NONSTATIN THERAPY DRUGS

- Despite their proven efficiency, lipid-lowering statins fail to help many patients achieve the recommended LDL-C goals and ASCVD prevention in many patients.
- Many patients still experience ASCVD events despite achieving LDL-C levels, a phenomenon referred to as "residual risk".[1]
- Many patients are often not adherent to therapy and may discontinue these drugs due to statin-associated muscle symptoms (SAMS) or fear of adverse drug effects (ADEs).[2] Nearly 55% of former statin users discontinued statins, most commonly due to muscle-related symptoms. Data recently suggests a 10–45% increased in risk of new-onset diabetes mellitus in statin users versus nonstatin users.[3] Neurocognitive effects are also one of the drivers for the development of newer nonstatin cholesterol-lowering medications.

WHEN YOU NEED NONSTATIN THERAPIES?

Indications

- Patients with statin intolerance
- High cardiovascular risk
- ASCVD events were recorded
- Genetic conditions requiring additional modification of lipid levels

Past Nonstatin Lipid-lowering Drugs

- Fibric acid derivatives (e.g., clofibrate, fenofibrate, and gemfibrozil) bind to PPAR-alpha receptors, resulting in a decrease in triglycerides, an increase in high-density lipoprotein cholesterol (HDL-C), and only a modest decrease in LDL-C.
- Niacin modulates lipolysis in adipose tissues but exhibits poor tolerability and side effects.
- Bile acid sequestrants/resins (cholestyramine and colesevelam) bind bile acids in the intestine and excrete the complex in feces, preventing their reabsorption. Tolerability and dosage formulations are limiting factors.

RECENT DRUGS AMONG NONSTATIN THERAPIES (TABLES 1 AND 2)

- Ezetimibe
- Proprotein convertase subtilisin/kexin type 9 (PCSK9 inhibitors)
- Bempedoic acid (BDA)
- Inclisiran, a small interfering RNA (siRNA) therapy

Ezetimibe

It is a drug within the class of selective cholesterol absorption inhibitors. It is now the second line of treatment of choice for the management of hypercholesterolemia in patients at high risk of ASCVD events.

Mode of Action

Ezetimibe inhibits the absorption of cholesterol by targeting a sterol transporter called Niemann-Pick C1-Like 1 (NPC1L1; SLC65A2), which is localized in the brush border cells of the small intestine and is involved in the uptake of cholesterol. This action decreases the delivery of cholesterol to the mesenteric veins and liver, and finally increases the clearance of cholesterol from the blood.

TABLE 1: Landmark cardiovascular-outcomes evidence.

Agent (trial)	*Population*	*Follow-up*	*MACE HR (95% CI)*	*Notes/Subgroups*
Ezetimibe + simvastatin (IMPROVE-IT)	Post-ACS (*n* = 18,144)	7 years	0.94 (0.88–0.99)	LDL-C 16 mg/dL lower vs. control
Ezetimibe mono ≥75 years (EWTOPIA-75)	Statin-naïve elderly	4.1 years	0.66 (0.50–0.86)	Supports primary-prevention use
Rosuvastatin + ezetimibe (RACING)	ASCVD	3 years	Noninferior to high-dose statin	Lowers discontinuations
Evolocumab (FOURIER)	ASCVD on statin	2.2 years	0.85 (0.79–0.92)	LDL-C median 30 mg/dL
Alirocumab (ODYSSEY OUTCOMES)	Recent ACS	2.8 years	0.85	Greater benefit if LDL-C ≥100 mg/dL
Inclisiran (ORION-9/10/11 pooled)	HeFH/ASCVD	510 days	LDL-C surrogate only; outcomes ongoing	ORION-4, VICTORION pending
Bempedoic acid (CLEAR Outcomes)	Statin-intolerant high-risk	40.6 months	0.87 (0.79–0.96)	MI ↓23%, Revasc ↓19%
Evinacumab (ELIPSE-HoFH)	HoFH	24 weeks	Outcome data not yet powered; LDL-C ↓50%	CV-outcome trials needed

TABLE 2: Investigational therapies ≥phase II.[10]

Target/agent	Modality	Development stage	Lead efficacy signal	Anticipated milestones
AZD0780 (oral PCSK9)	Small-molecule inhibitor	Phase II (PURSUIT)	LDL-C ↓ 35–50% (12 weeks)	Phase III planning 2025
Obicetrapib (CETP)	Oral	Phase III (BROADWAY/ BROOKLYN)	LDL-C ↓ 63%, HDL-C ↑ 165%	PREVAIL outcomes 2026
Olezarsen (apoC-III ASO)	Monthly SC ASO	FDA-approved (FCS 2024); Phase III (CORE) for sHTG	TG ↓ 42.5% at 6 months	Broad sHTG data 2026
Pelacarsen (Lp(a) ASO)	GalNAc-ASO	Phase III (Lp(a) HORIZON)	Lp(a) ↓ 80%	MACE read-out 2026
CSL112 (apoA-I infusion)	Plasma-derived HDL mimetic	Phase III (AEGIS-II)	TCEC 2.5-fold; neutral MACE overall	Subgroup analyses guiding next steps
Ziltivekimab (IL-6 mAb)	Anti-inflammatory mAb	Phase III (ZEUS)	hs-CRP ↓ 77–92% (RESCUE)	ZEUS MACE 2026
VERVE-101 (CRISPR PCSK9 base-edit)	LNP-CRISPR	Phase Ib (HEART-1)	PCSK9 ↓ 84%, LDL-C ↓ 55% at 6 months	Dose expansion 2026
Volanesorsen	apoC-III ASO	EMA-approved (FCS); Phase III CV	TG ↓ 77%	Long-term CV outcome

Pharmacokinetics

It is orally administered, absorbed, and conjugated to ezetimibe glucuronide. The active metabolite is at least as potent as ezetimibe, and both are 90% bound to plasma proteins. The half-life is approximately 22 hours. Approximately, 70% of the drug is found in feces as ezetimibe and nearly 10% in urine as ezetimibe glucuronide. Dose adjustment is not required in older adult patients. No dosage adjustments are required for individuals with hepatic or renal impairment. Dose 10 mg daily oral.

CV Outcome Trials

Ezetimibe–CV outcome trials:

- *IMPROVE-IT trial:* This landmark trial enrolled 18,144 patients with recent acute coronary syndrome (post-ACS status); the addition of ezetimibe 10 mg to simvastatin 40 mg resulted in a greater median reduction in LDL-C levels (54 mg/dL vs, 70 mg/dL). The follow-up period was 7 years. The result was a modest but statistically significant reduction in major adverse cardiovascular events (MACE). Hazard ratio: (0.94) (0.88 – 0.99). LDL-C reduction was 16 mg/dL lower than in that the control group.[4]
- *EWTOPIA-75:* In 3,796 statin-naïve elderly patients aged ≥ 75 years with elevated LDL-C, ezetimibe monotherapy reduced primary CV events (MACE) by 34% over a follow-up period of 4.1 years. Significant reductions were also observed in composite cardiac events and coronary revascularization without an increase in adverse events. This trial supports the primary prevention of this drug.
- *RACING trial:* The study population comprised 3,780 patients with ASCVD. The follow-up period was 3 years. In this CV outcome trial, ezetimibe plus low-dose rosuvastatin was noninferior to high-dose rosuvastatin, with greater LDL-C reduction (74% vs. 58%) and a lower discontinuation rate due to intolerance.

Safety Information

Ezetimibe neither influences nor is influenced by the activity of CYP 450 enzymes; thus, there is minimal drug interaction.

Advantages

Oral preparation, long single dose, low cost, and least drug-drug interactions with a high benefit ratio in patients with ASCVD

Proprotein Convertase Subtilisin/Kexin Type 9 Inhibitors

The PCSK9 is a protein that plays a crucial role in LDL-C regulation by binding to LDL receptors on hepatocytes. The main function of LDL receptors is to remove LDL-C from circulation and prevent LDL-C deposition in peripheral tissues. The binding of PCSK9 to LDL receptors causes the degradation of the receptors through intracellular pathways. LDL receptors are recycled via endosomes, but excess PCSK9 downregulates these receptors, resulting in higher levels of circulating LDL-C.[5] PCSK9 inhibitors are monoclonal antibodies that bind to the PCSK9 protein and prevent these proteins from binding to LDL receptors, increasing receptor recycling and the uptake of circulating LDL-C. The FDA approved the first PCSK9 inhibitor, alirocumab, in July 2015, followed by evolocumab in August 2015. They have received approval for monotherapy use in patients with homozygous familial hypercholesterolemia (HoFH) and for the secondary prevention of CV events. The third drug, bococizumab, was discontinued due to higher levels of immunogenicity and injection-site reactions and was subsequently withdrawn.

Pharmacokinetics

The route of administration is subcutaneous delivery. Within days, LDL-C reduction is approximately 60% from the baseline value, and the effect is sustained for about 2 weeks at lower doses. Thus, the dosing schedule is every 2 weeks for both PCSK9 inhibitors. The absolute bioavailability of alirocumab and evolocumab is 85 and 72%, respectively. Peak concentration is reached within 3–7 days and 3–4 days for alirocumab and evolocumab, respectively. Alirocumab has a half-life of 17–20 days and evolocumab has a half-life of 11–17 days.

PCSK9 Inhibitors: Alirocumab Clinical Trials

- *ODYSSEY outcomes:* This trial was conducted in 2019 for a duration of 2.8 years with a sample size of 18,924. In patients with moderate-to-high CV risk who had reported intolerance to two or more statins in the past, alirocumab resulted in a 45% reduction in LDL-C from the baseline value, compared with a reduction of 14.6% for ezetimibe. The trial interventions are alirocumab ± high-intensity statin or placebo ± high-intensity statin. MACE events were significantly reduced in the alirocumab group compared to the placebo group (relative risk reduction of 15%).
- *Results:* The trial provided evidence that alirocumab has additive effects on both LDL-C reductions and CV benefits when compared with high-intensity statins. Significant reductions from baseline to week 24 in apoB, non-HDL-C, and lipoprotein levels from the pooled subanalysis data. Vallejo-Vaz et al. demonstrated that patients with diabetes, CKD or polyvascular disease had greater absolute CV benefits than those without these chronic conditions with alirocumab group.

PCSK9-inhibitors: EVOLOCUMAB Trials

FOURIER trial: Further Cardiovascular Outcomes Research with PCSK9 Inhibition in Subjects with Elevated Risk trial. Has shown that evolocumab decreased LDL-C and major CV events done during 2017 involving 27,564 participants for the duration of 2.2 years.[6,7]

PCSK9 inhibitors safety information: The rate of ADEs was similar to that of placebo. The most common ADE is an injection site reaction. Neurological events were linked to immunogenic and inflammatory causes. Sabatine et al. noted that reducing LDL levels below 20 mg/dL with either PCSK9 inhibitors resulted in no signs of harm and no changes in self-reported cognition when compared to placebo. Concomitant statin and PCSK9 inhibitor use has been shown to reduce the half-life of alirocumab. The effects of these interactions are not clinically significant, and dosage adjustments are not warranted. The cost is a limiting factor. Hence, PCSK9-inhibitors are cost-effective for high-risk ASCVD patients.

Bempedoic Acid Trials

The BDA is a prodrug that requires activation by the enzyme very-long-chain acyl-CoA synthetase-A. This enzyme is mainly expressed in the liver and kidney, but not in the skeletal muscle. This active metabolite inhibits ATP citrate lyase, an enzyme upstream of HMG-CoA reductase. ATP citrate lyase is an important enzyme in the cholesterol biosynthesis pathway and is responsible for producing acetyl-CoA from citrate. By inhibiting ATP citrate lyase, it prevents cholesterol synthesis in hepatocytes. This inhibition of cholesterol synthesis by BDA increases LDL-C receptor expression. The upregulation of these receptors results in increased LDL-C clearance.

- *Pharmacokinetics:* BDA is highly plasma protein-bound and achieves maximum concentration within a median time of 3.5 hours, and a steady state is reached by 7 days. The plasma half-life is 15–24 hours. The dosage was 180 mg per oral daily. The side effect profile includes hyperuricemia, gout, and cholelithiasis.
- Five CLEAR trials, namely (1) CLEAR HARMONY, (2) WISDOM, (3) SERENITY, (4) TRANQUILITY, and (5) OUTCOME, are available for BDA efficacy. Except for the outcome trial, the rest of the studies showed efficacy in hyperlipidemic and statin-intolerant patients.
- *CLEAR outcome trial:* This is the first definitive CV outcome evidence for BDA in statin-intolerant patients. The study enrolled 13,970 participants with either established ASCVD or high CV risk and followed them over a period of 40.6 months. This study showed a 13% reduction in the risk of four-point MACE, a 23% reduction in fatal or nonfatal MI, and a 19% reduction in coronary revascularization compared to placebo. The US Food and FDA approved a fixed-dose combination of BDA 180 mg and ezetimibe 10 mg in February 2020 for adults with heterozygous familial hypercholesterolemia (HeFH) or established ASCVD requiring additional LDL-C reduction.[8]

Inclisiran

It is a cholesterol-lowering drug, a long-acting, double-stranded, siRNA molecule. It inhibits the production of PCSK9 in the liver by cleaving the messenger RNA required for PCSK9 production and lowers LDL-C levels by preventing the interaction of PCSK9 with LDL receptors. This results in the upregulation of LDL receptors, increasing LDL-C uptake and reducing circulating LDL-C levels.

- *Pharmacokinetics:* The drug reaches the maximum plasma concentration after 4 hours. It has a short plasma half-life (5–10 hours), and even though it is renally eliminated, it does not affect the kidneys. Inclisiran is administered subcutaneously at day 0, 90 and then every 6 months.
- *Clinical trials:* ORION which enrolled patients on maximum tolerated statin therapy with or without ezetimibe. ORION-9—studied HeFH and ORION 10 focused on patients with established ASCVD and ORION 11 enrolled patients with either ASCVD or ASCVD risk equivalents (DM and FH). In total, these trials demonstrated significant reduction in LDL-C. However, dedicated outcome studies such as ORION-4, VICTORION-1 PREVENT, and VICTORION-2 PREVENT are still ongoing studies which really determine the CV outcomes.[9] Results are being anticipated. Finally, inclisiran may offer comparable LDL-C lowering efficacy to PCSK9mab, with the added advantage of biannual closing.

EMERGING THERAPIES AND FUTURE MOLECULES

Emerging therapies now focus on other atherogenic lipoproteins and their components, such as Lipoprotein (a) [Lp(a)], VLDL-C, non-HDL-C, apolipoprotein C, and apolipoprotein A + B and along with anti-inflammatory agents that target residual cardiovascular risk beyond lipid modulation.

Oral PCSK9 Inhibitor (AZD0780)

First oral small-molecule PCSK9 inhibitor. The *PURSUIT trial*, which enrolled 428 adults with hypercholesterolemia on background statin with or without ezetimibe. During the follow-up period of 12 weeks, it produced a dose-dependent reduction in LDL-C, from 35% to >50% compared with placebo. Maximum achieved goal of LDL-C was <70 mg/dL, at the highest dose.

Lipoprotein (a)

- Lp(a) is an LDL-like particle. It is genetically determined and considered as independent ASCVD risk factor and for Aortic stenosis.
- *Pelacarsen* is an antisense oligonucleotide (ASO) developed to reduce circulating Lp(a) levels by targeting Apo(a) mRNA for degradation, thus inhibiting hepatic synthesis of apo(a).
- *Phase 3 trials: The Lp(a) HORIZON trial*—evaluated the effect of pelacarsen on MACE in patients with ASCVD and Lp(a) ≥ 70 mg/dL. Results are anticipated in 2026.

CSL112

- A plasma-derived formulation of human apoprotein A1 (apoA-I) planned to enhance the functional ability of HDL.
- *AEGIS-I Trial + AEGIS-II trial.*
- After 2-hour infusion, because of its CEE (cholesterol efflux capacity), apoA-I levels are elevated in a dose dependent manner in patients with recent MI.

Angiopoietin-like Protein-3 Inhibitors

- *Evinacumab:* It is a human monoclonal antibody focused against angiopoietin-like protein-3 (ANGPTL3), a liver derived protein that inhibits LPL (lipoprotein lipase and endothelial lipase), thus suppressing the catabolism of TGL and HDL cholesterol. Its mechanism of action is independent of LDL receptor pathway.
- *Phase 3 ELIPSE HoFH trial:* Evinacumab given at 15 mg/kg IV every 4 weeks, reduced LDL-C by 50% in HoFH in patients ≥12 years.
- Ongoing trials investigate its role in HoFH, HeFH, severe hypertriglyceridemia, and mixed dyslipidemia.

Cholesterol Ester Transport Inhibitors: (Obicetrapib)

- It reduces the cholesterol content of LDL-C and VLDLs, upregulates hepatic LDL receptors, and enhances the catabolism of apo B particles. In addition, it encourages biliary and transintestinal cholesterol excretion.
- *Ongoing phase II trials:* TULIP, ROSE study
- *On going phase III trials:* BROADWAY and BROOKLYN where obicetrapib 10 mg daily versus placebo in patients with very high ASCVD or HeFH patients
- *PREVAIL trial:* It evaluates 9,000 patients post-MI for MACE as the primary outcome.

- Obicetrapib serves as a potent oral alternative and viable adjunct in high risk or recurrent-event population unable to take (or) tolerate parenteral agents.

Inflammation-modulating Strategies

- Inflammatory markers, such as TNF-α, interleukin (IL-1 and 6) play a significant role in ASCVD.
- *Canakinumab:* A drug that neutralizes IL-1β signaling, had shown to decrease nonfatal MI, stroke, and CV death in patients with history of MI. Major setback is cost and increased risk of systemic infection.
- *Ziltivekimab:* Human monoclonal antibody that directly binds to + neutralizes IL-6, destroys the downstream inflammatory cascade, and addresses residual CV risk.
- *Trials:* RESCUE trial, phase III ZEUS trial.
  - Had shown that ziltivekimab was well tolerated without sustained neutropenia, thrombocytopenia, or serious injection site reactions.

Gene Editing Technology

- *Clustered Regularly Interspaced Short Palindromic Repeats (CRISPR/Cas9):* This technology identified initially from bacterial natural defense mechanism against viruses (*Streptococcus pyogenes*) (spCas9).
- CRISPR is being identified to inactivate genes such as PCSK9, ANGPTL3, ApoB, and APOC3, thereby reducing LDL-C levels. Apart from LDL-C reduction it also reduces TGL levels and inflammation especially vascular inflammatory pathways.
- *HEART-1 trial* where simple infusion of *VERVE-101* resulted in PCSK9 protein reduction of up to 84% and LDL-C reduction of 39–55%, with a durability maintained for a period of about 6 months.

CONCLUSION

Nonsteroidal therapies such as ezetimibe, fenofibrate, bempedoic acid, PCSK9 inhibitors, inclisiran, and gene therapy provide effective options for reducing cardiovascular morbidity and mortality in patients with dyslipidemia.

REFERENCES

1. Patel KV, Pandey A, de Lemos JA. Conceptual framework for addressing residual atherosclerotic cardiovascular Disease risk in the era of precision medicine. Circulation. 2018;137(24):2551-3.
2. Ward NC, Watts GF, Eckel RH. Statin toxicity mechanistic insights and clinical implications. Circ Res. 2019;124:328-50.
3. Yandrapalli S, Malik A, Rochlani Y, et al. Statins and the potential for higher diabetes mellitus risk. Expert Rev Clin Pharmacol. 2019;12:825-30.
4. Giugliano RP, Cannon CP, Blazing MA, et al. Benefit of adding ezetimibe to statin therapy on cardiovascular outcomes and safety in patients with versus without diabetes mellitus: results from IMPROVE-IT (Improved Reduction of Outcomes: Vytorin Efficacy International Trial). Circulation. 2018;137(15):1571-82.
5. Hess CN, Low Wang CC, Hiatt WR. PCSK9 inhibitors: Mechanisms of action, metabolic effects, and clinical outcomes. Annu Rev Med. 2018;69:133-45.
6. Schwartz GG, Steg PG, Szarek M, et al. Alirocumab and cardiovascular outcomes after acute coronary syndrome. N Engl J Med. 2018;379(22):2097-107.
7. Sabatine MS, Giougliano RP, Keech AC, et al. Evolocumab and clinical outcomes in patients with cardiovascular disease. N Engl J Med. 2017;376(18):1713-22.
8. Nissen SE, Lincoff AM, Brennan D, et al. Bempedoic acid and cardiovascular outcomes in statin-intolerant patients. N Engl J Med. 2023;388 (15):1353-64.
9. Mansoor T, Rao BH, Gupta K, et al. Inclisiran as a "siRNA inhibitor of proprotein convertase subtilisin/kexin type 9 (PCSK9); past, present and future. Am J Cardiovasc Drugs. 2025;25(3):293-306.
10. Ogunniyi K, Aghasili CC, Akinmoju O, et al., Advances in Non-Statin Lipid Therapies: A Narrative Review of Evolving Strategies of Cardiovascular Risk Reduction: Am J Cardiovasc Drugs. 2026;26(1):35-57.
11. Bardolia C, Amin NS, Turgeon J. Emerging Non-Statin Treatment Options for Lowering Low-Density Lipoprotein Cholesterol. Front Cardiovasc Med. 2021;8:789931.

148

CHAPTER

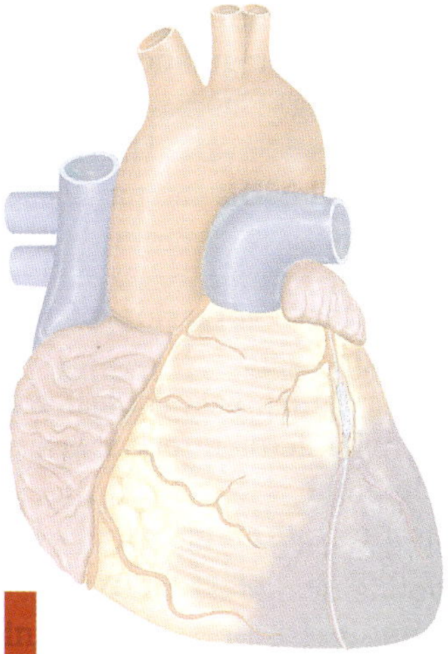

Combination Therapy: Ezetimibe with Statins and Other Agents for Obesity-related Dyslipidemia

Geetha Subramaniam, J Cecily Mary Majella, Gottipati Divya Chowdary

INTRODUCTION

Obesity-related dyslipidemia represents a major and growing public health challenge, particularly in India, where the coexistence of abdominal obesity, insulin resistance, and type 2 diabetes contributes to a disproportionately high burden of ASCVD.[1] The dyslipidemic profile associated with obesity is distinctive: Elevated triglycerides, increased hepatic VLDL secretion, reduced HDL-C, accumulation of small dense LDL (sdLDL), and impaired LDL-receptor activity due to hepatic steatosis and chronic inflammatory signaling.[2,3] This constellation—commonly termed *atherogenic dyslipidemia*—is strongly linked to premature coronary artery disease, heart failure, and cardiometabolic risk.

Statins remain the foundational therapy for reducing LDL-C and lowering ASCVD risk. However, many obese patients fail to achieve guideline-directed LDL-C goals with statin monotherapy due to increased intestinal cholesterol absorption, impaired hepatic metabolism, and statin intolerance or suboptimal response rates.[4] Contemporary guidelines from ACC/AHA, ESC, and the Lipid Association of India (LAI) therefore support early initiation of combination therapy—particularly ezetimibe with statins—in high- or very-high-risk patients to optimize LDL-C reduction and mitigate cardiovascular risk.[5,6]

Ezetimibe, a selective inhibitor of intestinal cholesterol absorption via the NPC1L1 transporter, complements the LDL-lowering effects of statins, which inhibit hepatic cholesterol synthesis. This dual blockade produces additive reductions in LDL-C of approximately 20–25% beyond statin monotherapy and is supported by outcome data from trials such as IMPROVE-IT and RACING.[7,8] Additional agents such as PCSK9 inhibitors, bempedoic acid, fibrates, and icosapent ethyl (highly purified EPA) provide further options for multidrug lipid modulation, particularly in obesity-associated dyslipidemia with mixed abnormalities.

Given the mechanistic complexity of obesity-related dyslipidemia and the high absolute cardiovascular risk observed in Indian populations at lower BMI thresholds, a tailored approach integrating lifestyle modification, obesity pharmacotherapy, and rational combination lipid-lowering therapy is essential. This chapter provides an evidence based review of combination therapy—with specific emphasis on ezetimibe-plus-statin therapy—and its role in the management of obesity-associated dyslipidemia.

PATHOPHYSIOLOGY OF OBESITY-RELATED DYSLIPIDEMIA

Obesity results in a characteristic cluster of metabolic and lipid abnormalities collectively termed *obesity-related atherogenic dyslipidemia*. Understanding the underlying mechanisms provides the rationale for multitargeted pharmacotherapy.

Altered Lipid Metabolism in Obesity

Increased Free Fatty Acid Flux

Central or visceral obesity is associated with accelerated lipolysis and increased free fatty acid (FFA) release into the portal circulation.[9] Elevated FFAs lead to:

- Excess substrate for hepatic triglyceride synthesis
- Increased VLDL production

- Impaired LDL-receptor activity
- Promotion of hepatic steatosis (NAFLD)

This creates a vicious cycle wherein hepatic fat accumulation further worsens dyslipidemia and insulin resistance.

Overproduction of VLDL and Triglycerides

High FFA delivery drives hepatic assembly of VLDL particles, facilitated by microsomal triglyceride transfer protein (MTP). Consequences include:

- Hypertriglyceridemia
- Elevated VLDL-ApoB levels
- Increased production of cholesterol-rich remnant particles

These remnants are highly atherogenic and contribute to residual ASCVD risk beyond LDL-C.

Formation of Small Dense LDL

Hypertriglyceridemia favors cholesteryl ester transfer protein (CETP)-mediated exchange of triglycerides into LDL particles, resulting in sdLDL formation. sdLDL is:

- More prone to oxidative modification
- More easily retained in the arterial intima
- Less efficiently cleared by LDL receptors
- Strongly associated with premature myocardial infarction[10]

Obese individuals frequently have "normal" or mildly elevated LDL-C but elevated ApoB and a high sdLDL burden.

Reduced HDL-C and Dysfunctional HDL

Obesity results in:

- Accelerated HDL catabolism
- Impaired reverse cholesterol transport
- Triglyceride enrichment of HDL via CETP

These changes produce small, unstable HDL particles with diminished antiatherogenic properties.

Insulin Resistance and NAFLD: The Central Abnormality

Insulin resistance profoundly influences lipid metabolism:

- Increases FFA release from adipose tissue
- Enhances hepatic de novo lipogenesis
- Impairs LDL-receptor activity
- Promotes excessive hepatic VLDL secretion

NAFLD, present in 50–70% of obese individuals, is strongly linked to:

- Increased ApoB secretion
- Decreased LDL clearance
- Local and systemic inflammation contributing to atherogenesis[11]

This hepatic milieu reduces the effectiveness of statin monotherapy, which relies on upregulation of LDL receptors for maximal LDL-C lowering.

Increased Intestinal Cholesterol Absorption in Obesity

Studies show heightened intestinal expression of the NPC1L1 transporter in obesity, leading to:

- Increased absorption of dietary and biliary cholesterol
- Elevated chylomicron and chylomicron remnant levels
- Pronounced postprandial lipemia

This directly strengthens the rationale for adding *ezetimibe*, which selectively blocks NPC1L1-mediated cholesterol absorption.

Chronic Inflammation and Adipokine Imbalance

Obesity is a chronic inflammatory state characterized by:

- Elevated TNF-α, IL-6, and CRP
- Reduced adiponectin

Inflammation:

- Worsens insulin resistance
- Impairs HDL maturation and function
- Increases oxidized LDL (oxLDL) formation
- Enhances macrophage foam-cell formation

Thus, lipid-lowering alone may be insufficient; therapies that also address weight, insulin resistance, and inflammation (e.g., GLP-1 RA) are particularly attractive.

The Indian Context

South Asians, including Indians, develop cardiometabolic abnormalities at lower BMI due to:

- Higher visceral adiposity at a given BMI
- Genetic predisposition to insulin resistance
- High prevalence of NAFLD
- Lower lean muscle mass
- Higher levels of sdLDL and ApoB[12]

Lipid Association of India guidelines, therefore, classify many Indian patients as high or very-high ASCVD risk even when LDL-C appears only modestly elevated. In such individuals, *early combination therapy* is often required to attain targets.

Summary of Pathophysiology

Obesity-related dyslipidemia is driven by:

- ↑ VLDL production
- ↑ TG and remnants
- ↑ sdLDL
- ↓ HDL-C and HDL function

- ↑ intestinal cholesterol absorption
- ↓ LDLR function in steatotic liver
- Chronic systemic and hepatic inflammation
- High prevalence of NAFLD

These factors significantly diminish the effectiveness of monotherapy and provide strong biological justification for *combination lipid-lowering strategies.*

RATIONALE FOR COMBINATION THERAPY IN OBESITY-RELATED DYSLIPIDEMIA

Obesity-associated dyslipidemia is mechanistically complex, involving more than just elevated LDL-C. Common abnormalities include elevated TG, VLDL overproduction, ApoB elevation, hepatic steatosis, and increased intestinal cholesterol absorption. This pathobiology makes statin monotherapy insufficient in a substantial proportion of patients, particularly in South Asians.

Limitations of Statin Monotherapy

Statins lower LDL-C by 20–55% and reduce ASCVD events, but in obese patients, they have several limitations:

- *Reduced LDL-receptor activity:* Hepatic steatosis and inflammatory signaling decrease LDL-receptor expression and function, blunting statin effect.
- *Increased cholesterol absorption:* Obese individuals often have upregulated NPC1L1 expression; statins do not block this pathway.
- *Persistently elevated triglycerides:* Statins modestly lower TG (10–20%), inadequate in obesity-driven hypertriglyceridemia.
- *Incomplete ApoB reduction:* Statins reduce LDL-C more than ApoB; the total number of atherogenic particles may remain high.
- *Statin intolerance:* Muscle-related side effects are more frequent in obese, diabetic, and metabolic syndrome patients, necessitating lower doses and driving the need for add-on therapy.

Why Ezetimibe Complements Statins?

Dual Inhibition of Cholesterol Pathways

- *Statins:* Inhibit hepatic cholesterol synthesis
- *Ezetimibe:* Blocks intestinal cholesterol absorption

Together they provide *synergistic LDL-C lowering*, with an additional 20–25% reduction beyond statin alone.

Increased Efficacy in Obesity

Ezetimibe directly targets the increased intestinal absorption seen in obese patients with upregulated NPC1L1.

Improvement of Hepatic Steatosis

By reducing cholesterol delivery to the liver, ezetimibe has shown improvements in steatosis and inflammation in NAFLD.

Excellent Tolerability

Ezetimibe has minimal systemic exposure, with low risk of myopathy or hepatotoxicity, making it an ideal partner in patients needing statin dose reduction.

Why Combination Therapy is Particularly Relevant in India?

South Asians exhibit:

- Higher levels of sdLDL
- Higher rates of insulin resistance and NAFLD
- Earlier onset of ASCVD
- Increased postprandial lipemia

Lipid Association of India guidelines classify many Indian patients as "very high risk" even at LDL-C levels that might be considered "moderate" elsewhere. Early combination therapy with statin plus ezetimibe, and escalation to PCSK9 inhibitors or bempedoic acid when needed, is therefore strongly justified.

Residual ASCVD Risk and the Role of Multiple Agents

Even when LDL-C is well controlled with statins, residual risk remains due to TG-rich particles, inflammation, Lp(a), and other atherogenic mechanisms **(Table 1)**. Combination therapy addresses these components.

Evidence Supporting Combination Therapy

Key trials demonstrating benefit:

- *IMPROVE-IT:* Statin + ezetimibe reduced CV events versus statin alone after ACS.
- *RACING:* Moderate-intensity rosuvastatin + ezetimibe is noninferior to high-intensity rosuvastatin with better tolerability.
- *FOURIER/ODYSSEY:* PCSK9 inhibitors add further LDL-C lowering and 15–20% relative MACE reduction on top of statins.

TABLE 1: Residual risk and effect of combination therapy.

Residual risk type	*Statin alone*	*Combination therapy*
LDL-C residual risk	Partial	Strong reduction (statin + ezetimibe/PCSK9i)
Triglyceride risk	Minimal	Reduced (EPA, fibrates)
ApoB particle number	Partial	Greater reduction with multidrug therapy
Inflammatory risk	Partial	Improved (GLP-1 RA, weight loss, SGLT2i)
Lipoprotein(a) risk	None	PCSK9i modestly lower Lp(a); future Lp(a) therapies

TABLE 2: Key drug combinations and evidence.

Therapy	*Key trials*	*Main outcomes*	*Best for obesity features*
Statin + ezetimibe	IMPROVE-IT, RACING	↓LDL-C, ↓events	High LDL-C, ↑NPC1L1 activity, NAFLD
PCSK9 inhibitors	FOURIER, ODYSSEY	↓events 15–20%, LDL ~30 mg/dL	Statin resistance, FH, high ApoB, high Lp(a)
Bempedoic acid ± ezetimibe	CLEAR Outcomes, CLEAR	↓LDL-C 20–35%, ↓events	Statin intolerance, metabolic syndrome
Fibrates	ACCORD subgroup, FIELD	↓events in high TG + low HDL	Mixed dyslipidemia with high TG
EPA (icosapent ethyl)	REDUCE-IT	↓MACE 25%	Elevated TG despite statin therapy
GLP-1 RA	LEADER, SUSTAIN-6	Weight loss, ↓MACE	Obesity + T2DM + metabolic syndrome
SGLT2i	EMPA-REG, CANVAS	↓CV mortality and HF	Diabetes with obesity, HF risk

- *CLEAR Outcomes:* Bempedoic acid reduced LDL-C and CV events in statin-intolerant patients.
- *REDUCE-IT:* Icosapent ethyl reduced major CV events by 25% in high-TG patients on statins.
- *ACCORD/FIELD:* Fibrates showed selective benefit in patients with high TG and low HDL-C (**Table 2**).

PRACTICAL APPROACH: ALGORITHM AND MONITORING

Stepwise Algorithm for Obesity-related Dyslipidemia

1. *Step 1: Diagnose obesity-related dyslipidemia:*
   a. Assess BMI, waist circumference, visceral adiposity
   b. Full fasting lipid profile: LDL-C, HDL-C, TG, non-HDL-C, and ApoB
   c. Consider Lp(a), hs-CRP, and presence of NAFLD/diabetes
2. *Step 2: Initiate high-intensity statin (if tolerated):*
   a. Atorvastatin 40–80 mg or rosuvastatin 20–40 mg for high/very-high risk
   b. Target LDL-C <70 mg/dL (or <55 mg/dL in very high risk)
3. *Step 3: Early add-on ezetimibe if LDL-C ≥ target:*
   a. Add ezetimibe 10 mg daily
   b. Reassess lipid profile after 4–12 weeks
4. *Step 4: Tailor further add-on based on phenotype:*
   a. *Flowchart (text version):*

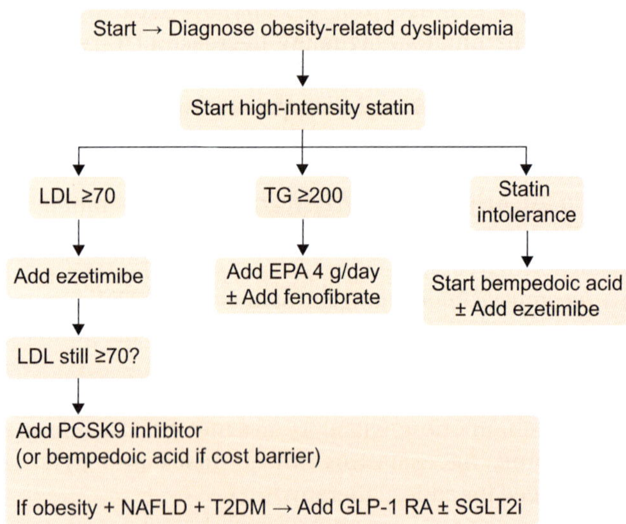

Monitoring Strategy during Combination Therapy

See **Table 3**.

FUTURE DIRECTIONS

- Development of next-generation PCSK9 inhibitors, including twice-yearly siRNA therapies (e.g., inclisiran)

TABLE 3: Monitoring schedule.

Parameter	*Statins*	*Ezetimibe*	*PCSK9i*	*Bempedoic acid*	*Fibrates*
LFTs	Baseline; repeat if symptomatic	Only if combined with statin	Not routine	Baseline; periodic in high-risk	Baseline; periodic
CK levels	If muscle symptoms	Not required	Not needed	Not required	Baseline + if muscle symptoms
Uric acid	–	–	–	Baseline in gout-prone patients	–
Lipid panel	4–12 weeks after changes	4–12 weeks	4–12 weeks	4–12 weeks	4–12 weeks
Glycemia	Optional (NOD risk small)	None	None	None	May improve insulin resistance

and potential oral PCSK9 blockers, will improve long-term adherence in obese, high-risk patients.

- Novel agents targeting ANGPTL3, ApoC-III, and Lp(a) will address triglyceride-rich lipoproteins, remnant cholesterol, and residual risk not adequately covered by statins or ezetimibe.
- Fixed-dose combinations such as *bempedoic acid + ezetimibe* will expand options for statin-intolerant patients with obesity and metabolic syndrome.
- Second-generation CETP inhibitors (e.g., obicetrapib) may provide substantial LDL-C and Lp(a) reductions with favorable tolerability and convenient oral dosing.
- Genomic profiling, polygenic risk scores, and AI-based risk models will enable individualized selection and sequencing of lipid-lowering therapies.
- Microbiome-targeted lipid therapies and metabolic modulators may open entirely new therapeutic pathways to treat obesity-related dyslipidemia and inflammatory cardiometabolic risk.

CONCLUSION

Combination lipid-lowering therapy is central to the management of obesity-related dyslipidemia, where single-agent treatment frequently fails to achieve guideline-directed LDL-C targets or adequately address residual risk. Statins remain foundational, while ezetimibe, PCSK9 inhibitors, bempedoic acid, fibrates, and EPA-based therapies provide complementary mechanisms with proven cardiovascular benefit. Novel therapeutics targeting ANGPTL3, ApoC-III, and Lp(a), along with precision medicine tools and long-acting injectables, will further refine personalized care. Integrating weight reduction, metabolic control, and rational multidrug lipid therapy offers the best opportunity to mitigate the rising burden of ASCVD in obese individuals, particularly in high-risk populations such as Indians.

REFERENCES

1. Cannon CP, Blazing MA, Giugliano RP, et al. Ezetimibe added to statin therapy after ACS. N Engl J Med. 2015;372(25):2387-97.
2. Le NA, Walter MF. The effect of ezetimibe on hepatic steatosis and metabolic parameters. J Clin Lipidol. 2007;1(1):28-41.
3. Sabatine MS, Giugliano RP, Keech AC, et al. Evolocumab and clinical outcomes in patients with cardiovascular disease. N Engl J Med. 2017;376(18):1713-22.
4. Schwartz GG, Steg PG, Szarek M, et al. Alirocumab and cardiovascular outcomes after acute coronary syndrome. N Engl J Med. 2018;379(22):2097-107.
5. Nissen SE, Lincoff AM, Brennan D, et al. Bempedoic acid and cardiovascular outcomes in statin-intolerant patients (CLEAR Outcomes). N Engl J Med. 2023;388:1353-64.
6. Bhatt DL, Steg PG, Miller M, et al. Cardiovascular risk reduction with icosapent ethyl. N Engl J Med. 2019; 380:11-22.
7. Ray KK, Wright RS, Kallend D, et al. Two-year efficacy and safety of inclisiran in patients with elevated LDL cholesterol. Eur Heart J. 2021;42:177-86.
8. Raal FJ, Rosenson RS, Reeskamp LF, et al. Evinacumab for severe hypercholesterolemia. N Engl J Med. 2020; 383:2307-19.
9. Gaudet D, Alexander VJ, Baker BF, et al. Antisense inhibition of apolipoprotein C-III in patients with hypertriglyceridemia. N Engl J Med. 2015;373:438-47.
10. Nicholls SJ, Lincoff AM, Barter PJ, et al. Obicetrapib for LDL cholesterol lowering. Lancet. 2022;400(10353):338-49.
11. Tsimikas S, Karwatowska-Prokopczuk E, Gouni-Berthold I, et al. Lipoprotein(a) reduction in persons with cardiovascular disease. N Engl J Med. 2020;382:244-55.
12. Ference BA, Ginsberg HN, Graham I, et al. Low-density lipoproteins cause atherosclerotic cardiovascular disease: genetic evidence and therapeutic implications. Eur Heart J. 2017;38:2459-72.

149

CHAPTER

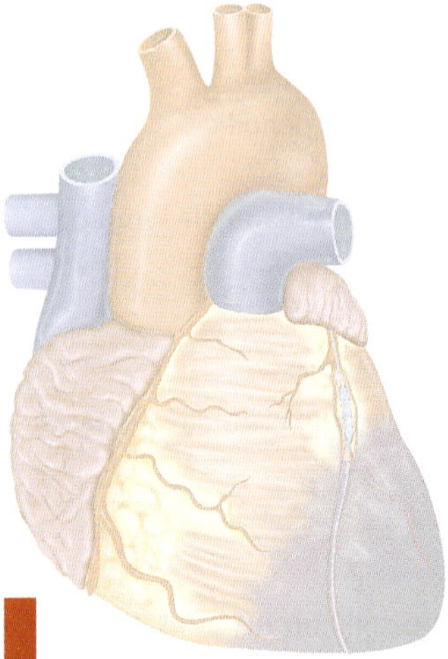

Ezetimibe in Combination with Proprotein Convertase Subtilisin/Kexin Type 9 Inhibitors for High-risk Obese Patients

J Cecily Mary Majella, Gottipati Divya Chowdary

INTRODUCTION

Obesity is associated with insulin resistance, dyslipidemia, and a proinflammatory state that accelerates atherogenesis.[1] Statins remain the foundation of lipid management, yet even high-intensity regimens leave many patients above LDL-C thresholds recommended by current guidelines (<55 mg/dL for very high risk patients[2]). Ezetimibe, a selective inhibitor of intestinal cholesterol absorption, and proprotein convertase subtilisin/kexin type 9 (PCSK9) inhibitors, monoclonal antibodies preventing LDL-receptor degradation, target distinct steps in cholesterol metabolism. Their combination provides complementary efficacy with excellent tolerability, particularly suited for obese, high-risk patients who often demonstrate partial statin response or intolerance.

The therapeutic alliance of ezetimibe and PCSK9 inhibitors stands as an elegant example of molecular complementarity:

- *Ezetimibe* impedes intestinal cholesterol absorption.
- *PCSK9 inhibitors* preserve hepatic LDL receptors.

Together, they create a synergistic suppression of LDL-C that is deeper and more durable than either agent alone—ushering in a new era of *precision lipid management* for high-risk obese individuals.

MECHANISMS OF ACTION

Ezetimibe

Ezetimibe inhibits the Niemann-Pick C1-like 1 (NPC1L1) transporter in the brush-border membrane of enterocytes, reducing dietary and biliary cholesterol absorption by ≈54%. This depletion in hepatic cholesterol stores triggers *SREBP2-mediated upregulation* of LDL receptors, thereby increasing LDL-C clearance from circulation. On average, ezetimibe reduces LDL-C by 15–25% when added to statins.[3]

Proprotein Convertase Subtilisin/Kexin Type 9 Inhibitors

Proprotein convertase subtilisin/kexin type 9 is a serine protease secreted primarily by hepatocytes. It binds LDL receptors and directs them toward lysosomal degradation, thereby reducing receptor. Monoclonal antibodies such as alirocumab and evolocumab block this interaction, increasing receptor recycling and LDL uptake. Typical LDL-C reductions range ≈55–60% beyond statins.[4]

Synergistic Effect

Combining ezetimibe with PCSK9 inhibition enhances both intestinal and hepatic LDL-receptor activity **(Table 1)**. Ezetimibe-induced receptor upregulation increases the substrate for PCSK9 blockade, yielding an additive LDL-C reduction (≈70–80% total decrease from baseline[5]) **(Fig. 1)**.

CLINICAL EVIDENCE AND TRIAL DATA

Improve-it (2015)

Post-ACS patients randomized to simvastatin + ezetimibe achieved mean LDL-C ≈53 mg/dL versus 70 mg/dL with

TABLE 1: Mechanisms and key effects.

Agent	*Primary target*	*Typical LDL-C reduction (%)*	*Additional notes*
Statin (high-int.)	HMG-CoA reductase	30–50	Upregulates LDL receptors
Ezetimibe	NPC1L1 (intestine)	15–25	Decreases intestinal cholesterol absorption
PCSK9 inhibitor	PCSK9–LDLR interaction	50–60	Prevents receptor degradation; lowers Lp(a) 20–30%
Ezetimibe + PCSK9	Dual pathway	70–80	Additive/synergistic lowering

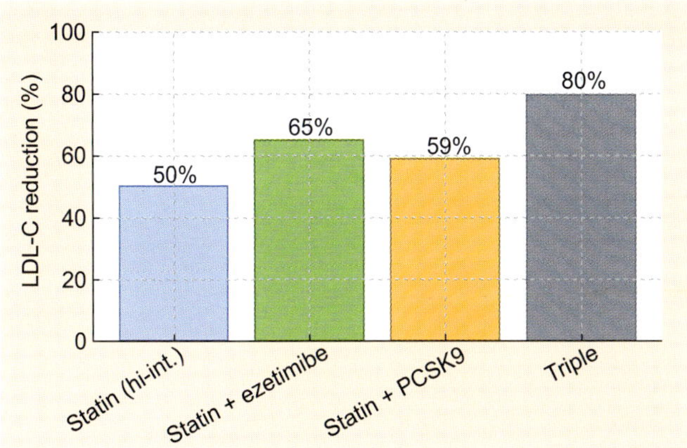

Fig. 1: LDL-C reduction by regimen (representative) (bar chart). Statin ≈50%; statin + ezetimibe ≈65%; statin + PCSK9 ≈59%; triple ≈80%.

statin alone, translating to a 6.4% relative risk reduction in major cardiovascular events.[6]

FOURIER (2017)

Evolocumab + statin therapy achieved median LDL-C ≈30 mg/dL (59% reduction). Relative risk reduction for composite cardiovascular outcomes was 15%.[4]

ODYSSEY Outcomes (2018)

Alirocumab + maximally tolerated statin therapy in post-ACS patients produced LDL-C ≈53 mg/dL (57% reduction) with 15% reduction in major adverse events.[7]

GLAGOV (2016)

Evolocumab therapy induced plaque regression in 64% of patients, mean atheroma volume change -0.95%, confirming structural benefit **(Tables 2 and 3)**.[8]

Meta-Analyses (2021–2023)

Pooled analyses demonstrate up to 80% of treated patients achieve LDL <55 mg/dL and ≈40% <40 mg/dL **(Fig. 2)**.[9]

CLINICAL DATA VISUALIZATION

Ezetimibe + PCSK9 combinations consistently produce the deepest LDL-C declines among nonstatin adjuncts. In pooled datasets, >85% of patients reached LDL <70 mg/dL and ≈60% reached <55 mg/dL **(Fig. 3)**.

LIMITATIONS OF CURRENT STUDIES

Although major trials confirm efficacy, several limitations persist: Population heterogeneity (most data derive from secondary-prevention cohorts), cost and access constraints to PCSK9 inhibitors, limited long-term safety data at very low LDL-C levels, and real-world underutilization due to reimbursement and therapeutic inertia.[10]

- *Lack of direct comparative trials:* There are few randomized trials directly comparing PCSK9 + ezetimibe versus PCSK9 alone with hard cardiovascular outcomes.
- *Short follow-up periods:* Many studies are limited to 12–24 months and emphasize lipid targets over clinical endpoints.
- *Obesity-specific data deficiency:* Subgroup analyses rarely isolate obese populations, despite distinct metabolic features affecting drug response.
- *Cost and accessibility:* PCSK9 inhibitors, though becoming more affordable, remain expensive for large-scale adoption, especially in resource-limited settings.
- *Long-term safety of very low LDL-C:* Ultra-low LDL-C (<25 mg/dL) outcomes and long-term safety (e.g., neurocognitive, hormonal effects) remain areas of active study.
- *Adherence and implementation barriers:* Injectable formulations, cost-sharing, and healthcare access remain practical barriers to long-term adherence.

GUIDELINES AND THERAPEUTIC ALGORITHM

Guidelines (ESC 2023 and AHA 2022) endorse a stepwise intensification: Maximize tolerated statin; add ezetimibe

TABLE 2: Major clinical trials summary.

Trial	*Population*	*Therapy*	*LDL-C achieved (mg/dL)*	*Risk reduction*
IMPROVE-IT (2015)	Post-ACS	Simvastatin ± ezetimibe	53 versus 70	6.4% RRR
FOURIER (2017)	Stable ASCVD	Statin ± evolocumab	30 versus 92	15% RRR
ODYSSEY (2018)	Post-ACS	Statin ± alirocumab	53 versus 94	15% RRR
GLAGOV (2016)	CAD patients	Statin ± evolocumab	–	Plaque regression

TABLE 3: LDL-C target thresholds by guideline.

Risk category	*LDL-C goal (mg/dL)*	*Typical therapy*
High risk	<70	High-intensity statin ± ezetimibe
Very high risk	<55	Statin + ezetimibe ± PCSK9 inhibitor
Extreme risk	<40	Triple therapy or apheresis consideration

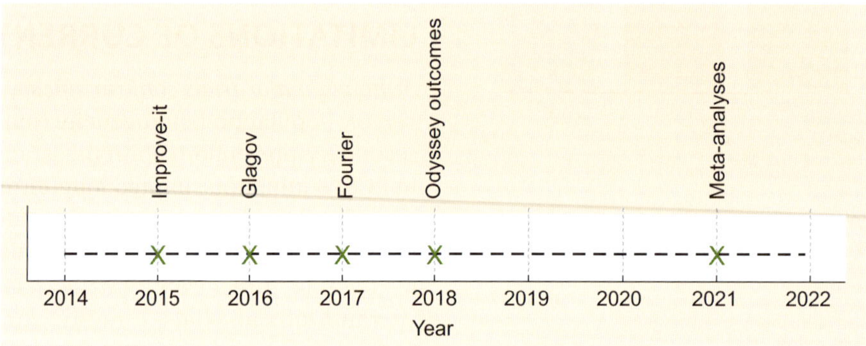

Fig. 2: Timeline of clinical evidence (2015–2023).

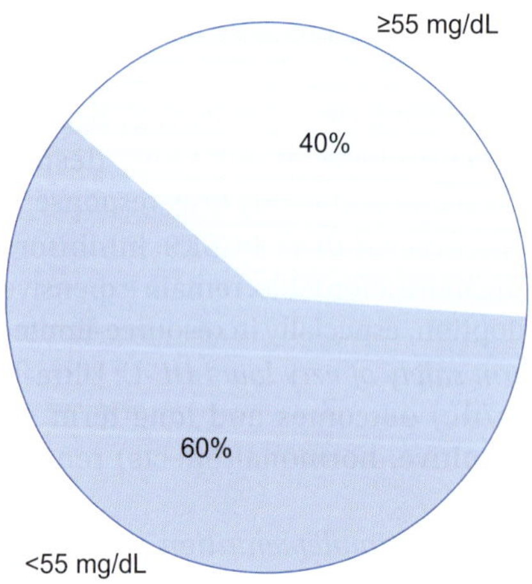

Fig. 3: LDL target attainment (pie chart). Proportion of patients achieving LDL-C <55 mg/dL versus ≥55 mg/dL.

Flowchart 1: Therapy algorithm. Stepwise approach from statin optimization to ezetimibe and PCSK9 addition.

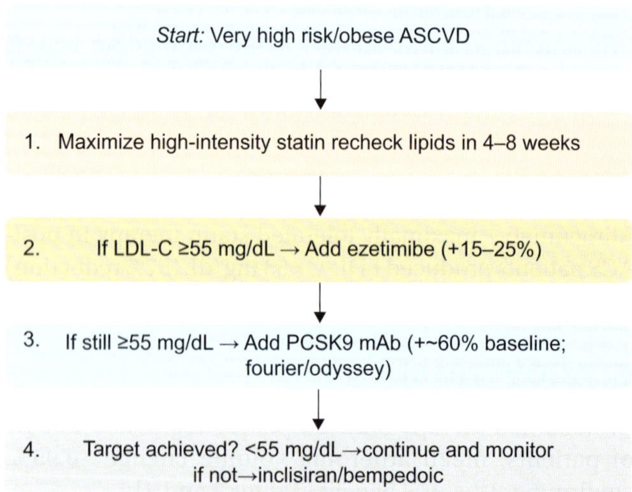

if goal unmet; add a PCSK9 inhibitor if LDL remains ≥55 mg/dL (very high risk). Reassess every 4–12 weeks and continue dual or triple therapy until targets are reached **(Flowchart 1)**.

CONCLUSION

The combination of ezetimibe and PCSK9 inhibition represents a pivotal advancement in lipid management for high-risk, obese patients. Their complementary mechanisms yield profound LDL-C reductions, plaque stabilization, and meaningful cardiovascular-risk reduction with minimal systemic toxicity. Future studies targeting cost optimization, long-term adherence, and integration with novel RNA-based agents will refine the role of this dual therapy in precision lipidology.

REFERENCES

1. Lavie CJ, et al. Eur Heart J. 2018;39:1792-800.
2. Mach F, Baigent C, Catapano AL, et al. 2019 ESC/EAS Guidelines for the management of dyslipidaemias: lipid modification to reduce cardiovascular risk. Eur Heart J. 2020;41:111-88.
3. Dujovne CA, et al. Curr Atheroscler Rep. 2020;22:60.
4. Sabatine MS, Giugliano RP, Keech AC, et al. Evolocumab and clinical outcomes in patients with cardiovascular disease. N Engl J Med. 2017;376:1713-22.
5. Giugliano RP, et al. Circulation. 2018;138:155-65.
6. Cannon CP, Blazing MA, Giugliano RP, et al. Ezetimibe added to statin therapy after acute coronary syndromes. N Engl J Med. 2015;372:2387-97.
7. Schwartz GG, Steg PG, Szarek M, et al. Alirocumab and cardiovascular outcomes after acute coronary syndrome. N Engl J Med. 2018;379:2097-107.
8. Nicholls SJ, Puri R, Anderson T, et al. Effect of evolocumab on progression of coronary disease in statin-treated patients: the GLAGOV randomized clinical trial. JAMA. 2016;316:2373-84.
9. Navarese EP, Lansky AJ, Kereiakes DJ, et al. Cardiac mortality in patients randomised to elective coronary revascularisation plus medical therapy or medical therapy alone: a systematic review and meta-analysis. Eur Heart J. 2021;42:4638-51.
10. Arnott C et al. Heart 2023;109:10-8.

150

CHAPTER

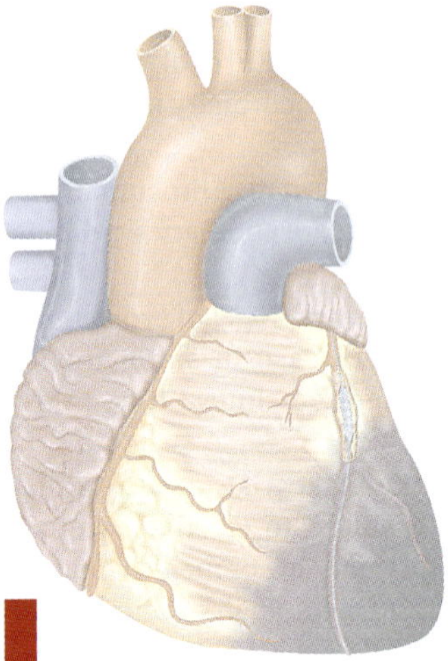

Combination Therapies in Dyslipidemia: Bempedoic Acid with Statins, Ezetimibe, and PCSK9 Inhibitors in High-risk Coronary Artery Disease

Asha Moorthy, Srichandran L, Prashant Moorthy, Supraja Moorthy

INTRODUCTION

Dyslipidemia is a key modifiable risk factor in the pathogenesis of atherosclerotic cardiovascular disease (ASCVD). High serum low-density lipoprotein cholesterol (LDL-C) promotes endothelial injury, inflammation, and plaque formation leading to coronary artery disease (CAD). Despite the established role of statins as first-line therapy, many high-risk CAD patients fail to achieve target LDL-C levels (<55 mg/dL in very high-risk individuals). Reasons include partial response, statin intolerance, and genetic or metabolic factors.[1-3]

Over the past decade, nonstatin agents such as ezetimibe, PCSK9 monoclonal antibodies, and the novel ATP citrate lyase (ACL) inhibitor bempedoic acid have emerged. Combination therapy targeting multiple points of cholesterol metabolism offers an effective and safe approach to reduce residual cardiovascular risk **(Box 1)**.[4,5]

BOX 1: Average LDL-C reduction with combination therapy.

- Therapy LDL-C reduction outcome benefit
- Statin monotherapy 30–50% ↓ CV events by 25%
- +Ezetimibe 45–65% ↓ events (IMPROVE-IT)
- +Bempedoic acid 50–70% ↓ LDL-C, CV event trend (CLEAR)
- +PCSK9 mAb/inclisiran 65–85% ↓ MI/stroke (FOURIER, ODYSSEY, ORION)

BEMPEDOIC ACID: MECHANISM AND PHARMACOLOGY

Bempedoic acid is a first-in-class oral inhibitor of ACL, an enzyme acting upstream of HMG-CoA reductase in the cholesterol biosynthesis pathway. It is a prodrug activated exclusively in hepatocytes by very-long-chain acyl-CoA synthetase 1 (ACSVL1), thus avoiding activation in skeletal muscle and reducing myalgia risk.[6,7]

Mechanism Summary

ATP citrate lyase inhibition → ↓ acetyl-CoA production → ↓ cholesterol synthesis → ↑ LDL-receptor expression → ↑ LDL-C clearance.

Clinical Efficacy

- Monotherapy reduces LDL-C by ~17–25%.
- Combined with ezetimibe → ~38% reduction

Added to maximally tolerated statin → additional ~18% drop in LDL-C

Safety

Generally well tolerated; minor reversible increases in uric acid and transaminases have been reported. Myopathy and new-onset diabetes are rare.

EZETIMIBE: MECHANISM AND ROLE

Ezetimibe selectively inhibits the NPC1L1 transporter in intestinal epithelial cells, blocking absorption of dietary and biliary cholesterol. It produces an LDL-C reduction of 18–25%.

In the IMPROVE-IT trial, ezetimibe plus simvastatin significantly reduced major adverse cardiovascular events compared with simvastatin alone.

Synergy with bempedoic acid: Dual inhibition of intestinal uptake and hepatic synthesis produces additive LDL-C lowering without overlapping toxicity.

PCSK9 INHIBITORS AND INCLISIRAN

PCSK9 monoclonal antibodies (evolocumab and alirocumab) enhance LDL-receptor recycling by blocking PCSK9-mediated receptor degradation, achieving 50–60% LDL-C reduction.

Inclisiran, a small interfering RNA (siRNA) therapy, silences hepatic PCSK9 synthesis with twice-yearly dosing, producing comparable LDL-C reductions and superior adherence.

Key trials:

- *FOURIER (evolocumab):* 59% LDL-C reduction, 15% event reduction
- *ODYSSEY OUTCOMES (alirocumab):* 62% LDL-C reduction, 15% event reduction
- *ORION-10/11 (inclisiran):* 50% LDL-C reduction sustained over 4 years

LIMITATIONS OF COMBINATION THERAPIES

- *Cost:* PCSK9 inhibitors and inclisiran remain expensive and limit accessibility.
- *Adherence:* Multidrug regimens may reduce compliance; simplified fixed-dose combinations are evolving.
- *Long-term safety:* Limited long-term (>10 years) data for bempedoic acid and inclisiran.
- *Trial heterogeneity:* Differences in baseline therapy, populations, and endpoints complicate head-to-head comparisons.
- *Residual risk:* Even optimal LDL-C reduction may not address triglyceride-rich lipoproteins or LP(a).

GUIDELINES, ALGORITHM, AND SUMMARY ILLUSTRATION

- *2023 ESC/EAS guidelines:*
  - Target LDL-C <55 mg/dL and ≥50% reduction from baseline in very-high-risk ASCVD

BOX 2: Stepwise approach to dyslipidemia in high-risk CAD.

1. Start high-intensity statin
2. Add ezetimibe if LDL-C >70 mg/dL
3. If goal unmet or statin-intolerant → add bempedoic acid
4. Persistent elevation → add PCSK9 inhibitor/inclisiran
5. Reassess every 3–6 months

  - Stepwise intensification: Statin → +Ezetimibe → +PCSK9 mAb/bempedoic acid/inclisiran
- *2022 ACC expert consensus:*
  - Prefer ezetimibe as the first add-on; bempedoic acid or PCSK9 agent if goals unmet or intolerance present.
  - Inclisiran may be used where adherence issues exist.
- *Summary algorithm placeholder:* **Box 2** showing stepwise therapy with decision boxes for LDL-C targets and drug selection.

CONCLUSION

Combination lipid-lowering therapy represents a paradigm shift in the management of dyslipidemia, especially for high-risk CAD patients who fail to reach guideline targets on statins alone.

Bempedoic acid offers a complementary mechanism to statins and ezetimibe with minimal muscle toxicity. Ezetimibe provides intestinal blockade of cholesterol absorption, while PCSK9 inhibitors and inclisiran deliver profound receptor-mediated LDL-C clearance.

When applied in a stepwise, individualized manner, these agents can achieve up to 85% LDL-C reduction and substantial cardiovascular event reduction. Cost and accessibility remain barriers, but evidence strongly supports their role in residual-risk reduction and secondary prevention.

REFERENCES

1. Nissen SE, Lincoff AM, Brennan D, et al.; CLEAR Outcomes Investigators. Bempedoic acid and cardiovascular outcomes in statin-intolerant patients. N Engl J Med. 2023;388(15):1353-64.
2. Cannon CP, Blazing MA, Giugliano RP, et al.; IMPROVE-IT Investigators. Ezetimibe added to statin therapy after acute coronary syndromes. N Engl J Med. 2015;372(25): 2387-97.
3. Sabatine MS, Giugliano RP, Keech AC, et al.; FOURIER Steering Committee and Investigators. Evolocumab and clinical outcomes in patients with cardiovascular disease. N Engl J Med. 2017;376(18):1713-22.
4. Schwartz GG, Steg PG, Szarek M, et al.; for the ODYSSEY OUTCOMES Committees and Investigators. Alirocumab

and cardiovascular outcomes after acute coronary syndrome. N Engl J Med. 2018;379:2097-107.

5. Ray KK, Wright RS, Kallend D, et al. Two phase 3 trials of inclisiran in patients with elevated LDL cholesterol (ORION-10 and ORION-11). N Engl J Med. 2020;382(16):1507-19.
6. 2023 ESC/EAS Guidelines for the Management of Dyslipidaemias.
7. Writing Committee; Donald M Lloyd-Jones, Pamela B Morris, et al. 2022 ACC Expert Consensus Decision Pathway on the role of nonstatin therapies for LDL-cholesterol lowering in the management of atherosclerotic cardiovascular disease risk: a report of the American College of Cardiology Solution Set Oversight Committee. J Am Coll Cardiol. 2022;80(14):1366-418.

151 CHAPTER

Bempedoic Acid in Chronic Kidney Disease

Geeta S Sheth, Manu Sabu, Saptadipa Das

INTRODUCTION

Because of the inflammatory and metabolic disorders caused by renal impairment, people with chronic kidney disease (CKD) are more likely to develop cardiovascular disease.[1] High cholesterol, particularly elevated LDL-C levels, worsens atherogenesis and increases the risk of cardiovascular issues and mortality in this population.[2] Statins are the preferred treatment for CKD, but they have disadvantages such as the requirement for multiple medications, the higher risk of drug interactions, muscle soreness, and the inability to always meet LDL goals.[3] For patients with CKD who are unable to take statins or whose cholesterol levels do not improve even with the best statin use, bempedoic acid is one of the promising treatment options.[4,5] The following sections provide mechanistic information, outcome data, and clinically relevant risk management strategies.

MECHANISM OF ACTION

The prodrug bempedoic acid is activated by the liver's very long-chain acyl-CoA synthetase 1 (ACSVL1). This results in the formation of an active CoA ester that inhibits ATP-citrate lyase, an enzyme essential to the synthesis of cholesterol.[6] This is significant because bempedoic acid mainly acts in liver cells, where ACSVL1 is not present, lowering the risk of statin-related muscle side effects.[7] This improves LDL clearance without causing damage to muscles by increasing LDL receptors, decreasing cytosolic acetyl-CoA, and decreasing cholesterol synthesis.[5] When plasma LDL clearance increases and cholesterol synthesis declines, LDL receptor expression increases.

PHARMACOKINETICS AND RENAL CONSIDERATIONS

Bempedoic acid has good oral availability and is mainly metabolized by glucuronidation. It is eliminated through feces and urine.[3] Studies have shown that mild-to-moderate CKD (eGFR ≥30 mL/min/1.73 m^2) does not significantly change the drug's exposure or distribution, so no dose adjustment is necessary.[8]

However, in patients with severe CKD (eGFR <30 mL/min/1.73 m^2), blood exposure to the drug can quadruple due to altered protein binding and decreased kidney clearance.[3] The safety of dialysis and end-stage kidney disease patients is not fully understood. Physicians should watch for potential accumulation and negative effects in these vulnerable groups.[9]

Impacts on Cardiometabolism and Inflammation

In addition to reducing LDL-C, bempedoic acid also reduces non-HDL cholesterol, apolipoprotein B, and high-sensitivity C-reactive protein (hsCRP), indicating an anti-inflammatory effect that is particularly relevant in CKD, where vascular inflammation is increased.[2,10] These improvements may provide further cardiovascular benefits.[1]

Overview of Safety and Adverse Effects

Bempedoic acid is generally well tolerated and seems to have a better safety profile than statins in some circumstances.[4,5] Respiratory and mild gastrointestinal issues are rare. Importantly, muscle soreness is much less common because bempedoic acid mainly acts in the liver.[7]

Elevated Uric Acid and Gout

Caution because bempedoic acid may raise uric acid levels.[8] There has been evidence of a gradual but steady increase in serum uric acid levels, which may increase the likelihood of gout attacks.[3] This primarily affects patients with CKD, who already have difficulty managing their urate levels. People with a history of gout should be closely watched and may require preventative urate-lowering medication.

Effects on Glycemia

For CKD patients who may be sensitive to glucose issues, bempedoic acid is a desirable feature because, unlike statins, it does not raise the risk of developing diabetes and appears to have no effect on metabolism.[2,4]

Drug and Myopathy Tolerance

One major disadvantage of statins is the risk of severe myopathy, which is considerably decreased by bempedoic acid.[5] This enables the treatment of people who cannot take statins. Although long-term study data show maintained tolerance, routine monitoring is still advised, especially for patients with advanced CKD and multiple medical conditions.[7]

Drug Combination Techniques and Interactions

Because bempedoic acid is compatible with many lipid-lowering drugs, it is simple to incorporate into clinical practice.[4,10] Coadministration of statins may result in a slight rise in blood levels, but significant interactions are rare.[2] With ezetimibe, the combination fixed-dose option can lower LDL-C by up to 39% from baseline, which is very beneficial for CKD patients.[10] PCSK9 inhibitors have a greater lipid-lowering effect in very high-risk CKD patients.[1] Drug interactions may occur with other glucuronidation-metabolized agents and uricosuric drugs—caution advised.[3]

LIMITATIONS

The major limitations relating to the use of this drug are cost and availability compared to less expensive options like statins or ezetimibe and many of the major trials did not include any subjects with end-stage renal disease or dialysis patients; therefore, the disposition of bempedoic acid in these patients is currently unknown.[11] Most of the available data focus on cardiovascular results with no solid evidence on CKD progression or proteinuria. Also, some patients were found to have elevated uric acid levels which can further complicate those patients with kidney issues.[6] Not all outcomes data are available for the highest risk groups. Future studies are required to focus on these questions.

GUIDELINE RECOMMENDATION AND CLINICAL PRACTICE

Various guidelines recommend the usage of bempedoic acid for statin-intolerant or high-risk patients. KDIGO 2024, as per the latest recommendations, supports the use of nonstatin drugs like bempedoic acid in those patients who are statin intolerant, mainly myopathy, and in those with elevated LDL-C with standard therapy for mild-to-moderate renal impairment, i.e., eGFR >30 mL/min/1.73 m^2. Advanced CKD patients were excluded as per CLEAR outcomes trials. KDIGO also recommends monitoring serum uric acid levels and care should be taken in patients predisposed to gout. Standard recommended dose is 180 mg once daily.

ESC/EAS 2019 also recognizes bempedoic acid as an alternative for such high-risk patients or intolerant to statins. They recommend combining with ezetimibe for enhanced LDL lowering. Also, there are only minimal muscle-related side effects unlike statins.

In clinical practice, along with regular monitoring of lipid levels, those who are taking bempedoic acid also need to monitor serum uric acid, especially in advanced CKD.

CONCLUSION

Patients with all stages of CKD, including those on dialysis and after kidney transplant, have an increased risk of CVD. Statins have demonstrated safety and effectiveness in CKD, with documented reduction of CVD events including in postrenal transplant patients, although their benefit in ESRD on dialysis needs further longer term studies. Bempedoic acid proves as an alternative to those patients who are intolerant to statin and recent KDIGO guidelines, 2024, also accept this molecule in patient with mild or moderate impairment of kidney disease. But more trials and evidence are required so that we can include patients with advanced renal disease with long-term monitoring of its efficiency and safety with drug interactions as it is very important in transplant patients. Monitoring uric acid level is essential and careful selection of patients in settings with limited resources is also important.

REFERENCES

1. Nicholls SJ, Nelson AJ, Lincoff AM, et al. Effect of bempedoic acid on cardiovascular outcomes in statin-intolerant patients. JAMA Cardiol. 2023;8(4):385-95.
2. Nissen SE, Lincoff AM, Brennan DM, et al. Bempedoic acid and cardiovascular outcomes in statin-intolerant patients. Lancet. 2023;401(10375):681-92.
3. Saito Y, Banach M, Blom DJ, et al. Pharmacokinetics and safety of bempedoic acid in patients with renal impairment. Clin Transl Sci. 2022;15(4):921-31.
4. Ray KK, Bays HE, Catapano AL, et al. Safety and efficacy of bempedoic acid to reduce LDL cholesterol. N Engl J Med. 2019;380(11):1022-32.
5. Goldberg AC, Leiter LA, Stroes ES, et al. Effect of bempedoic acid vs placebo added to maximally tolerated statins on LDL-C: the CLEAR Wisdom trial. JAMA. 2019;322(18):1780-8.
6. Pinkosky SL, Newton RS, Day EA, et al. Liver-specific ATP-citrate lyase inhibition by bempedoic acid decreases LDL-C and attenuates atherosclerosis. Nat Commun. 2016;7:13457.
7. Laufs U, Banach M, Mancini GBJ, et al. Long-term safety and efficacy of bempedoic acid in patients with hypercholesterolemia: up to 2.5 years of treatment. Am J Cardiol. 2022;170:1-9.
8. Wheeler DC, Kosiborod MN, Kopecky SL, et al. Efficacy and safety of bempedoic acid in patients with stage 2 or 3 chronic kidney disease: a subgroup analysis of phase 3 trials. J Am Coll Cardiol. 2022;79(9):995-1007.
9. Wanner C, Tonelli M, Kidney Disease: Improving Global Outcomes Lipid Guideline Development Work Group Members. KDIGO clinical practice guideline for lipid management in chronic kidney disease. Kidney Int Suppl. 2013;3(3):259-305.
10. Ballantyne CM, Banach M, Mancini GBJ, et al. Efficacy and safety of bempedoic acid added to ezetimibe in statin-intolerant patients with hypercholesterolemia: a randomized, placebo-controlled study. Atherosclerosis. 2018;277:195-203.
11. Amore BM, Sasiela WJ, Ries DK, et al. Pharmacokinetics of bempedoic acid in patients with renal impairment. Clin Transl Sci. 2022;15(3):789-98.

152
CHAPTER

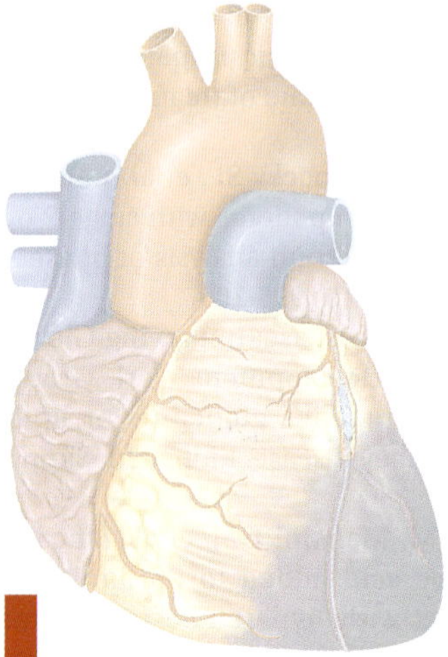

Bempedoic Acid and Cardiometabolic Risk in Women

Chandramukhi Sunehra

INTRODUCTION

The incidence of atherosclerotic cardiovascular disease (ASCVD) has been steadily increasing over the past few decades. Dyslipidemia plays a crucial role and clinical trials have clearly demonstrated that lowering the levels of low-density lipoprotein cholesterol (LDL-C) reduces the burden of ASCVD. Statins remain the first-line therapy in the management of dyslipidemia for primary and secondary prevention of ASCVD. However, the adverse effects of statin therapy limit the use of optimal doses, and in many patients, statin therapy alone is insufficient in achieving the required LDL-C reduction. This led to the development of additional therapies that complement statins in achieving the LDL-C goal. Proprotein convertase subtilisin/kexin type 9 inhibitors (PCSK9-i) have emerged as highly potent agents with a favorable safety profile, though their widespread use is restricted by high cost. Bempedoic acid is a novel lipid-lowering molecule which inhibits cholesterol biosynthesis utilizing the same mechanistic pathway as the statins but acts upstream. It has recently been approved for the treatment of dyslipidemia.

BEMPEDOIC ACID

Bempedoic acid (ETC-1002) is an oral, lipid-lowering agent that acts by inhibiting adenosine triphosphate citrate lyase (ACLY), an enzyme located upstream of HMG-CoA reductase in the cholesterol biosynthesis pathway. Bempedoic acid is a prodrug and the activating enzyme (very long-chain acyl-CoA synthetase-1) is not expressed in skeletal muscle. Bempedoic acid is activated in liver and has an elimination half-life of 15–24 hours and should be administered once daily.[1] Bempedoic acid therapy is associated with low incidence of muscle-related adverse events.

Statins reduce cholesterol biosynthesis in liver by competitive inhibition of 3-hydroxy-3-methylglutaryl-CoA (HMG-CoA) reductase, the rate-limiting enzyme in the mevalonate pathway of cholesterol synthesis in hepatocytes. This reduces generation of mevalonic acid and thereby lowers cholesterol production. Reduced levels of cholesterol in hepatocytes trigger a response and activate the transcription factor sterol regulatory element-binding proteins (SREBPs) which move to the nucleus and increase production of LDL receptors. Evolocumab and alirocumab are monoclonal antibodies which bind and inhibit PCSK9. Inclisiran reduces PCSK9 synthesis by interfering with its mRNA. Bempedoic acid acts by inhibiting the ACLY and reduces cholesterol biosynthesis, activating a similar cellular response as statins. Ezetimibe targets the Niemann–Pick C1-Like-1 (NPC1L1) protein at the brush border of the small intestine and reduces the absorption of cholesterol from diet.[2] By blocking ACLY, bempedoic acid prevents conversion of citrate to acetyl-CoA and reduces hepatic cholesterol synthesis. This, in turn, upregulates hepatic LDL receptor expression, enhancing clearance of circulating LDL-C, as depicted in **Figure 1**.

In addition to ACLY inhibition, bempedoic acid activates AMP-activated protein kinase (AMPK), which improves lipid metabolism, enhances fatty acid oxidation, and further promotes LDL-C uptake. Thus, its mechanism

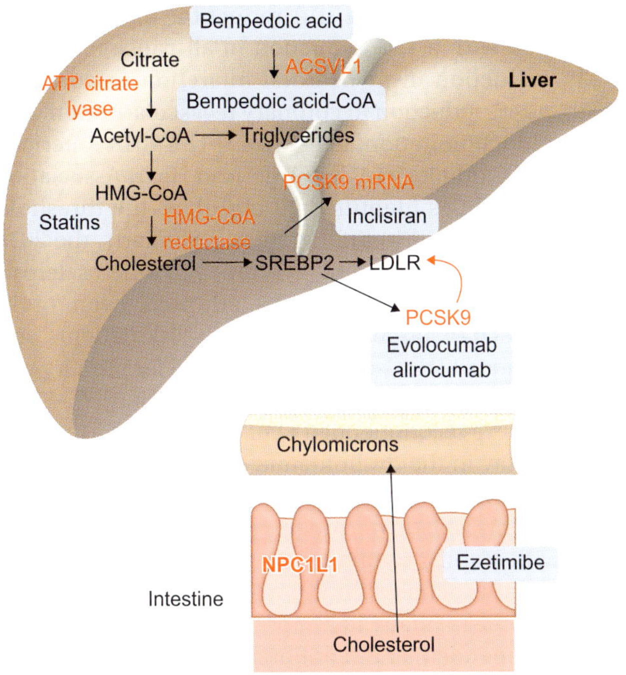

Fig. 1: Mechanism of action of bempedoic acid, statins, ezetimibe, and PCSK9-i (proprotein convertase subtilisin/kexin type 9 inhibitor) in reducing the cholesterol synthesis.[2]

combines cholesterol synthesis suppression with improved lipid utilization. When used in combination with statins or ezetimibe, bempedoic acid provides a complementary LDL-C-lowering effect, making it a valuable therapeutic option for patients with statin intolerance or an inadequate response to statin monotherapy. CLEAR (Cholesterol Lowering via Bempedoic Acid, an ACL inhibiting regimen) phase 3 clinical trials demonstrated that addition of bempedoic acid to statins in dyslipidemia therapy results in a significant reduction in LDL-C levels along with substantial lowering of non-high-density lipoprotein cholesterol (non-HDL-C), high-sensitivity C-reactive protein (hsCRP), and apolipoprotein B (ApoB) levels.[3] Inhibition of ACLY enzyme by bempedoic acid is at the intersection between pathways of glucose and lipid metabolism, controlling gluconeogenesis and lipogenesis. Thus, bempedoic acid does not worsen hyperglycemia or increase the occurrence of new-onset diabetes.

EFFECTS OF INFLAMMATION ON LIPID METABOLISM

Lipid metabolism and inflammation are closely linked, with saturated fatty acids promoting inflammation via activation of toll-like receptors (TLR2 and TLR4) and cytokine release. This results in accelerated lipolysis and fatty acid oxidation in skeletal muscle, exacerbates systemic effects,[4] and leads to insulin resistance. In contrast, omega-3 fatty acids like docosahexaenoic acid (DHA) have anti-inflammatory effects by suppressing inflammatory gene expression.

IMPACT OF ESTROGEN ON INFLAMMATION AND VASCULAR HEALTH

Estrogen inhibits activation of NF-κB signaling, which is a key regulator of inflammatory genes and thus reduces the production of proinflammatory cytokines. Estrogen exhibits antioxidant and vasoprotective effects by inhibiting oxidative stress and promotes the expression of protective growth factors. It demonstrates vasoprotective and anti-inflammatory effects on arteries and vascular cells promoting vascular health. But these effects can be reduced or lost in older, postmenopausal women with reduced levels of estrogen. It has been proposed that estrogen reduces the risk of ASCVD in females by modulation of the fibrinolytic factors much more than by affecting the levels of inflammatory markers or coagulation factors.

Significant fluctuations in estrogen levels, especially in 17β-estradiol (E2), are seen during the menstrual cycle and pregnancy. This leads to endocrine and vascular changes in women that decrease vascular resistance and arterial blood pressure, increase cardiac output by as much as 40% during the second half of the menstrual cycle and in pregnancy.[5] This results in optimal cardiovascular compliance comparable with the effects of exercise. The so-called "jogging female heart" thus protects women against ASCVD risks during reproductive years.[6] With the waning effects of estrogen during postmenopausal period, there is accelerated fat storage and deposition in abdominal areas with resultant increase in visceral fat and subsequent increase in the ASCVD risk in postmenopausal women.

GENDER DIFFERENCES AND CARDIOMETABOLIC RISK

Gender differences significantly influence the ASCVD risk. Factors unique to women impact the prevalence and characteristics of ASCVD such as pathogenesis, progression, and severity. Metabolic syndrome is defined by constellation of causally interconnected metabolic and cardiovascular risk factors such as central obesity, insulin resistance, arterial hypertension, and atherogenic dyslipidemia. Recently, other abnormalities such as sleep apnea, nonalcoholic fatty liver disease, and chronic proinflammatory and prothrombotic states have been included in metabolic syndrome.[7] Krishnamoorthy et al. reported the prevalence of metabolic syndrome among adult Indian population to be 30% (95% CI: 28–33%). The investigators noted a steady increase in the burden across the age groups from 13% (18–29 years group) to 50% (50–59 years). It was also found that people living in urban areas had higher prevalence of metabolic syndrome in comparison to tribal or rural adults. Females showed higher prevalence (20.3%) of metabolic syndrome when compared to males (10.7%).[8] A steeper age-related increase in metabolic syndrome prevalence has been noted in women due to dramatic increase in blood pressure and a rapid impairment in endothelial function in the postmenopausal period. An unhealthy atherogenic lipid profile is seen in postmenopausal women, with a tendency to reach higher levels of total cholesterol, LDL-C, triglycerides, and lipoprotein(a), and lower levels of HDL-C. These menopause-linked alterations in the lipid profile are proatherogenic and procoagulatory and are strongly connected to the postmenopausal increase of visceral fat mass.[9]

CARDIOMETABOLIC RISK IN WOMEN

Cardiometabolic risk in women changes throughout a woman's life due to unique female sex specific hormonal and physiological factors which influence lipid metabolism. Hormonal changes during reproductive events, such as menarche, pregnancy, and menopause, have been shown to induce a proinflammatory state in women. Moreover, women who have inflammatory-type conditions such as polycystic ovarian disease (PCOD), preeclampsia, or gestational diabetes have a cardiometabolic substrate that predisposes to increased risk of coronary artery disease and stroke. Women in the premenopausal age group with no notable ASCVD risk factors are often relatively protected from cardiovascular events. On the other hand, postmenopausal women overtake men in the risk of major cardiovascular events due to the waning effect of cardiovascular protective estrogen.

PHARMACOLOGICAL TREATMENT OF DYSLIPIDEMIA

Dyslipidemia is a major modifiable risk factor for developing ASCVD. Elevated plasma LDL-C levels are recognized as a major causal factor for developing ASCVD. It is well documented that lowering LDL-C levels significantly reduces cardiovascular risk and this evidence carries remarkable implications for clinical practice. In secondary prevention, the Cholesterol Treatment Trialists' Collaboration (CTTC) meta-analysis demonstrated that each 1 mmol/L (39 mg/dL) reduction in LDL-C was associated with a 12% reduction in all-cause mortality, a 23% reduction in myocardial infarction or coronary death, a 24% reduction in coronary revascularization, and a 17% reduction in nonfatal stroke.[10] The 2018 American College of Cardiology (ACC)/American Heart Association (AHA) guidelines identified 70 mg/dL as the threshold for considering nonstatin therapies.[11] Similarly, the 2019 European Society of Cardiology/European Atherosclerosis Society (ESC/EAS) guidelines adopted even more intensive LDL-C targets for very high-risk patients and recommended LDL-C <55 mg/dL as a goal for primary and secondary prevention (class I recommendation).[12]

To achieve recommended LDL-C goals, statins remain the mainstay in the dyslipidemia treatment, followed by ezetimibe and bempedoic acid. PCSK9-i may be added in a few patients who do not attain the recommended LDL-C goals with statins, ezetimibe, or bempedoic acid. If the LDL-C goal is achieved but non-HDL-C remains above the goal, omega-3 fatty acids, preferably icosapent ethyl, are recommended, and fenofibrate can also be added to maximally tolerated LDL-C-lowering therapy.

EFFICACY OF BEMPEDOIC ACID IN WOMEN

Various clinical trials have proved the complementary LDL-C-lowering effect of bempedoic acid when added to statins. Bempedoic acid has emerged as a valuable therapeutic option in the management of ASCVD, especially in patients with statin intolerance or an inadequate response to statin monotherapy. Sex-specific analysis of the clinical trials studying bempedoic acid reveals comparable relative benefits of LDL-C-lowering and cardiovascular risk reduction in women and men.

CLEAR Outcomes trial, a phase 3 trial of bempedoic acid, assessed safety and efficacy data over a 40.6-week intervention period. This trial is unique for having 48% ($n = 6740$) female subjects—the highest female enrollment as compared to other contemporary lipid-lowering outcomes trials. This randomized, placebocontrolled trial in statin-intolerant patients demonstrated that bempedoic acid reduced LDL-C levels and the primary composite end point (cardiovascular death, nonfatal myocardial infarction, nonfatal stroke, or coronary revascularization) similarly in both females and males. In females, the primary end point occurred in 8.4% of females on bempedoic acid versus 9.7% on placebo (adjusted hazard ratio, 0.89 [95% confidence interval, 0.75–1.04]). In male subjects, the primary end point occurred in 14.8% on bempedoic acid versus 16.6% on placebo (adjusted hazard ratio, 0.86 [95% confidence interval, 0.77–0.97]).[13]

SAFETY CONSIDERATIONS OF BEMPEDOIC ACID

Deranged liver enzymes, myalgias, headache, diarrhea, and myopathy are the most reported adverse effects with bempedoic acid use.

Bempedoic acid is eliminated primarily by hepatic metabolism, with formation of an acyl glucuronide metabolite by uridine 5′-diphospho-glucuronosyltransferase (UGT) 2B7-mediated conjugation. Use of bempedoic acid tends to increase serum uric acid levels as the bempedoic acid glucuronide metabolite competes with uric acid for the same renal tubular organic anion transporter 2 (OAT2). Significant increase in uric acid levels after bempedoic acid use has been reported in patients with gout with precipitation of acute gout.[14] The risk of adverse effects of hyperuricemia and gout can be reduced by appropriate patient selection and vigilant monitoring of serum uric acid levels. The hyperuricemia subsides after bempedoic acid discontinuation.

Tendon rupture or injury is another rare adverse effect of bempedoic acid. Hypercholesterolemia (especially HeFH) is associated with an increased risk of tendon injury or rupture. Elderly age >60 years, diabetes, concomitant use of fluoroquinolone, corticosteroid, chronic kidney disease, previous tendon disorders, and possibly statin use are the risk factors for the development of tendon injury or rupture. Older women, especially those with prior tendon disease, should be promptly evaluated for tendon pain and bempedoic acid should be stopped if the symptoms are noticed.[15]

Bempedoic acid should not be used during pregnancy or lactation

CONCLUSION

Atherosclerotic cardiovascular disease risk factors dominate in the elderly age. In females, several gender specific risk factors and inflammatory conditions such as PCOD, preeclampsia, and gestational diabetes pose ASCVD risk right from menarche. Though younger females are relatively protected from ASCVD due to cardiovascular protective effects of estrogen, the postmenopausal women overtake men in the risk of major cardiovascular events due to the waning effect of estrogen. Bempedoic acid is an excellent nonstatin therapy in the management of patients with dyslipidemia, HeFH, and ASCVD who are statin intolerant. It is quite effective, well-tolerated, and cost-effective. Bempedoic acid is effective LDL-C-lowering and outcome-reducing therapeutic option for women, especially those with statin intolerance or inadequate LDL reduction despite other therapy.

REFERENCES

1. Shambo SS, Sougata S, Subhro C, et al. Bempedoic acid in patients with dyslipidemia: a systematic review and meta-analysis. Med J Dr DY Patil Vidyapeeth. 2025;18(3):376-83.
2. Ferri N, Colombo E, Corsini A, et al. Bempedoic acid, the first-in-class oral ATP citrate lyase inhibitor with hypocholesterolemic activity: clinical pharmacology and drug-drug interactions. Pharmaceutics. 2024;16:1371.
3. Yarrarapu SNS, Goyal A, Venkata VS, et al. Comprehensive review of statin-intolerance and the practical application of Bempedoic Acid. J Cardiol. 2024;84(1):22-9.
4. Ertunc ME, Hotamisligil GS. Lipid signaling and lipotoxicity in metaflammation: indications for metabolic disease pathogenesis and treatment. J Lipid Res. 2016;57(12):2099-114.
5. Yang Y, Kozloski M. Sex differences in age trajectories of physiological dysregulation: inflammation, metabolic syndrome, and allostatic load. J Gerontol A Biol Sci Med Sci. 2011;66(5):493-500.
6. Eskes T, Haanen C. Why do women live longer than men? Eur J Obstet Gynecol Reprod Biol. 2007;133(2):126-33.
7. Meloni A, Cadeddu C, Cugusi L, et al. Gender differences and cardiometabolic risk: the importance of the risk factors. Int J Mol Sci. 2023;24(2):1588.
8. Krishnamoorthy Y, Rajaa S, Murali S, et al. Prevalence of metabolic syndrome among adult population in India: a systematic review and meta-analysis. PLoS One. 2020;15(10):e0240971.
9. Sharma J, McAlister J, Aggarwal NR, et al. Evaluation and management of blood lipids through a woman's life cycle. Am J Prev Cardiol. 2022;10:100333.
10. Baigent C, Keech A, Kearney PM, et al.; Cholesterol Treatment Trialists' (CTT) Collaborators. Efficacy and safety of cholesterol-lowering treatment: prospective meta-analysis of data from 90,056 participants in 14 randomised trials of statins. Lancet. 2005;366(9493):1267-78.
11. Grundy SM, Stone NJ, Bailey AL, et al. 2018 AHA/ACC/AACVPR/AAPA/ABC/ACPM/ADA/AGS/APhA/ASPC/NLA/PCNA guideline on the management of blood cholesterol: a report of the American College of Cardiology/American Heart Association Task Force on Clinical Practice Guidelines. Circulation. 2019;139(25):e1082-143.
12. Knuuti J, Wijns W, Saraste A, et al.; ESC Scientific Document Group. 2019 ESC Guidelines for the diagnosis and management of chronic coronary syndromes. Eur Heart J. 2020;41(3):407-77.
13. Nissen SE, Lincoff AM, Brennan D, et al.; CLEAR Outcomes Investigators. Bempedoic acid and cardiovascular outcomes in statin-intolerant patients. N Engl J Med. 2023;388:1353-64.
14. Ballantyne CM, Bays H, Catapano AL, et al. Role of bempedoic acid in clinical practice. Cardiovasc Drugs Ther. 2021;35(4):853-64.
15. Bays HE, Banach M, Catapano AL, et al. Bempedoic acid safety analysis: pooled data from four phase 3 clinical trials. J Clin Lipidol. 2020;14(5):649-59.e6.

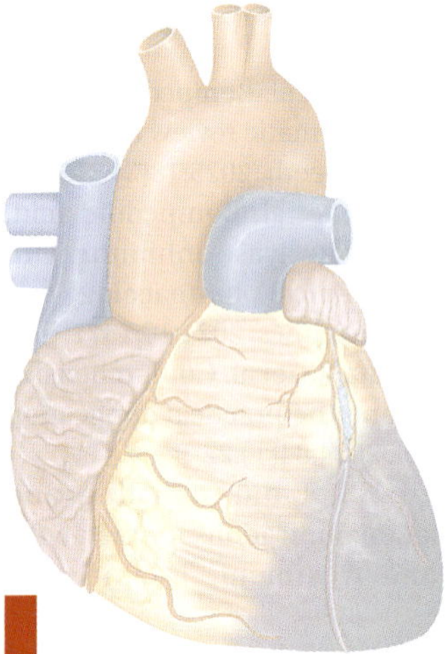

153

CHAPTER

Inclisiran in Individuals with Diabetes or Obesity with Dyslipidemia and High-risk Acute Coronary Syndrome

Madhupada Kiran Kumar, Pratap Chandra Rath

INTRODUCTION

Cardiovascular disease (CVD) continues to represent the leading cause of global mortality, accounting for more than one-third of all deaths worldwide, with an increasingly disproportionate burden borne by individuals with diabetes mellitus and obesity.[1,2] These metabolic disorders not only accelerate the development and progression of atherosclerotic cardiovascular disease (ASCVD) but also significantly worsen clinical outcomes following acute coronary syndrome (ACS). Patients with diabetes have a two- to fourfold higher risk of myocardial infarction, recurrent ischemic events, heart failure, and cardiovascular mortality compared with individuals without diabetes, even after adjustment for traditional risk factors.[3-6] Importantly, diabetes confers a risk profile comparable to established coronary artery disease, underscoring its designation as a coronary risk equivalent.

Obesity, which frequently coexists with diabetes, independently contributes to ASCVD risk through a complex interplay of insulin resistance, chronic low-grade inflammation, endothelial dysfunction, oxidative stress, and adverse alterations in lipoprotein metabolism.[7,8] Visceral adiposity, in particular, is associated with increased production of proinflammatory cytokines, impaired nitric oxide bioavailability, and atherogenic dyslipidemia characterized by elevated triglycerides, reduced high-density lipoprotein cholesterol (HDL-C), and increased small dense low-density lipoprotein (LDL) particles. Together, diabetes and obesity create a proatherogenic milieu that amplifies both plaque formation and plaque vulnerability, thereby increasing the risk of ACS and subsequent recurrent events.

Dyslipidemia represents a central and modifiable pathophysiological link between metabolic disease and ASCVD. Elevated LDL cholesterol (LDL-C) is causally related to atherogenesis, and robust genetic, epidemiological, and interventional evidence demonstrates a log-linear relationship between cumulative lifetime exposure to LDL-C and cardiovascular risk.[9] Consequently, intensive and sustained LDL-C lowering is a cornerstone of secondary prevention following ACS. Contemporary international guidelines recommend the early initiation of high-intensity statin therapy, followed by rapid escalation to combination lipid-lowering therapy when LDL-C targets are not achieved, particularly in very-high-risk populations such as patients with diabetes, metabolic syndrome, or recurrent ACS.[10-13]

Despite compelling evidence and clear guideline-directed recommendations, real-world data consistently reveal substantial gaps in LDL-C goal attainment, especially among individuals with diabetes and obesity.[14-16] Contributing factors include statin intolerance, therapeutic inertia, complex medication regimens, polypharmacy, and poor long-term adherence. These persistent challenges have catalyzed the development of innovative lipid-lowering therapies capable of delivering potent, durable LDL-C reductions with simplified dosing schedules. Inclisiran, a novel small interfering RNA (siRNA) therapy targeting hepatic proprotein convertase subtilisin/kexin type 9 (PCSK9) synthesis, has emerged as a promising strategy to address these unmet clinical needs.

This chapter comprehensively reviews the role of inclisiran in individuals with diabetes or obesity and dyslipidemia, with a particular emphasis on patients at high risk following ACS. The discussion integrates mechanistic insights, pivotal phase 3 trial evidence, posthoc and pooled analyses across metabolic subgroups, and practical considerations for incorporating inclisiran into contemporary cardiometabolic care pathways.

DYSLIPIDEMIA IN DIABETES, OBESITY, AND HIGH-RISK ACS

Diabetes and obesity are characterized by atherogenic dyslipidemia, typically manifested by elevated triglycerides, reduced HDL-C, increased ApoB-containing lipoproteins, and a predominance of small dense LDL particles.[9,17] Insulin resistance promotes hepatic overproduction of very-low-density lipoprotein (VLDL) and impaired clearance of remnant lipoproteins, contributing to heightened atherosclerotic risk.[18]

In the setting of ACS, these metabolic abnormalities assume even greater clinical significance. Patients with diabetes presenting with ACS have larger infarct sizes, impaired coronary microvascular function, and worse short- and long-term outcomes compared with nondiabetic patients.[19] Obesity further compounds risk by promoting systemic inflammation, oxidative stress, and endothelial dysfunction, thereby accelerating plaque progression and destabilization.[20]

Large randomized trials have consistently demonstrated that early and intensive LDL-C lowering after ACS reduces recurrent cardiovascular events, with benefits observed as early as weeks following initiation of therapy.[21,22] These observations underpin guideline recommendations advocating aggressive lipid lowering immediately after ACS, with LDL-C targets of <55 mg/dL (<1.4 mmol/L) or even lower in selected very-high-risk individuals **(Table 1)**.[11-13]

THE PCSK9 PATHWAY AND MECHANISM OF ACTION OF INCLISIRAN

The PCSK9 is a key regulator of LDL-C metabolism through its role in promoting lysosomal degradation of hepatic LDL receptors.[23] Increased PCSK9 activity results in reduced LDL receptor recycling and elevated circulating LDL-C levels. Inhibition of PCSK9 has therefore become an established therapeutic strategy for intensive lipid lowering **(Table 2)**.

Inclisiran is a chemically synthesized siRNA conjugated to a triantennary N-acetylgalactosamine (GalNAc) ligand that enables selective uptake by hepatocytes via the asialoglycoprotein receptor.[24] Once internalized, inclisiran engages the RNA-induced silencing complex, leading to targeted degradation of PCSK9 messenger RNA and sustained suppression of PCSK9 protein synthesis.[25]

Unlike monoclonal antibodies targeting circulating PCSK9, inclisiran exerts its effect intracellularly and provides prolonged LDL-C reduction with infrequent dosing. Following an initial dose and a 3-month loading dose, inclisiran is administered every 6 months, offering a unique approach to long-term lipid management.[26]

EVIDENCE FROM THE ORION PHASE 3 CLINICAL TRIALS

The efficacy and safety of inclisiran were established in the Phase 3 ORION clinical development program, including ORION-9, ORION-10, and ORION-11.[27,28] These randomized, double-blind, placebo controlled trials enrolled patients with heterozygous familial

TABLE 1: Dyslipidemia in diabetes, obesity, and high-risk acute coronary syndrome (ACS).

Clinical context	*Dyslipidemia pattern*	*Pathophysiological mechanisms*	*Clinical implications*
Diabetes mellitus	Elevated triglycerides, reduced HDL-C, increased ApoB-containing lipoproteins, predominance of small dense LDL particles	Insulin resistance leads to hepatic overproduction of VLDL, impaired lipoprotein lipase activity, and delayed clearance of remnant lipoproteins	Markedly increased atherosclerotic burden and higher risk of recurrent cardiovascular events
Obesity	Hypertriglyceridemia, low HDL-C, increased atherogenic lipoproteins	Adipose tissue-driven inflammation, oxidative stress, endothelial dysfunction, and altered adipokine signaling	Accelerated plaque progression, increased plaque vulnerability, and higher ACS risk
Acute coronary syndrome (ACS) in diabetes/obesity	Exaggerated atherogenic dyslipidemia with residual lipid risk despite statin therapy	Acute inflammatory state amplifies lipid-mediated endothelial injury and microvascular dysfunction	Larger infarct size, impaired coronary microcirculation, worse short- and long-term outcomes
Post-ACS management	Need for profound LDL-C reduction	Early and intensive LDL-C lowering stabilizes plaques and reduces recurrent ischemic events	Guideline-recommended LDL-C targets <55 mg/dL (<1.4 mmol/L), or lower in very high-risk patients

TABLE 2: PCSK9 pathway and mechanism of action of inclisiran.

Component	*Description*	*Clinical relevance*
PCSK9 physiology	PCSK9 binds to hepatic LDL receptors and promotes their lysosomal degradation, reducing receptor recycling	Increased PCSK9 activity leads to reduced LDL receptor availability and elevated circulating LDL-C levels
Role in dyslipidemia	Upregulated PCSK9 activity contributes to persistent hypercholesterolemia, particularly in high-risk states	Establishes PCSK9 as a key therapeutic target for intensive LDL-C lowering
Structure of inclisiran	Chemically synthesized small interfering RNA (siRNA) conjugated to a triantennary N-acetylgalactosamine (GalNAc) ligand	GalNAc enables selective hepatocyte uptake via the asialoglycoprotein receptor
Cellular mechanism	After hepatocyte uptake, inclisiran engages the RNA-induced silencing complex (RISC)	Causes targeted degradation of PCSK9 mRNA, suppressing PCSK9 protein synthesis
Site of action	Acts intracellularly at the level of gene expression	Distinct from monoclonal antibodies that neutralize circulating PCSK9
Effect on LDL receptors	Reduced PCSK9 production allows increased LDL receptor recycling on hepatocyte surfaces	Enhances hepatic LDL-C clearance and sustained LDL-C reduction
Dosing profile	Initial dose, followed by a 3-month loading dose, then once every 6 months	Provides durable lipid lowering with improved adherence and long-term control

hypercholesterolemia, established ASCVD, or ASCVD risk equivalents receiving maximally tolerated statin therapy with or without additional lipid-lowering agents.

Across these trials, inclisiran consistently reduced LDL-C levels by approximately 50% compared with placebo, with effects sustained throughout the dosing interval.[28] Significant reductions were also observed in non-HDL cholesterol, ApoB, and PCSK9 levels, supporting a comprehensive atherogenic lipid-lowering profile.

Inclisiran demonstrated a favorable safety profile, with overall adverse event rates comparable to placebo. Injection-site reactions were more frequent with inclisiran but were predominantly mild, transient, and nonpersistent.[27,28]

POST-HOC POOLED ANALYSIS IN DIABETES AND OBESITY

To better characterize the efficacy and safety of inclisiran in metabolic disease, a post-hoc pooled analysis of ORION-9, ORION-10, and ORION-11 evaluated outcomes across glycemic and body mass index (BMI) strata.[28] This analysis included 3,658 participants stratified by normoglycemia, prediabetes, and diabetes, as well as BMI categories ranging from <25 kg/m^2 to ≥35 kg/m^2.

Inclisiran produced robust and sustained LDL-C reductions across all glycemic and BMI subgroups. Placebo-corrected LDL-C reduction at day 510 ranged from 47.6% to 51.9% across glycemic strata and from 48.8% to 54.4% across BMI strata (p <0.001 for all comparisons).[28] Time-adjusted LDL-C reductions from day 90 to day 540 were similarly consistent, ranging from 46.8% to 52.0% across glycemic strata and from 48.6% to 53.3% across BMI categories.

Notably, individuals with diabetes or higher BMI demonstrated numerically greater relative reductions in LDL-C and other atherogenic lipids, although absolute LDL-C reductions were comparable across subgroups.[28] Inclisiran also significantly reduced PCSK9 (>80%), non-HDL cholesterol (>42%), ApoB (>37%), remnant cholesterol, and lipoprotein(a) across all metabolic strata.

Achievement of guideline-recommended LDL-C thresholds (<1.8 mmol/L and <1.4 mmol/L) and ≥50% LDL-C reduction from baseline was substantially higher with inclisiran compared with placebo, particularly among individuals with diabetes and severe obesity.[28]

METABOLIC SAFETY AND NEW-ONSET DIABETES

Concerns regarding potential effects of intensive lipid-lowering therapies on glycemic control have been raised, particularly in populations at risk for diabetes. In the pooled ORION analysis, the incidence of new-onset diabetes was similar between inclisiran and placebo groups, with no evidence of adverse effects on glycemic parameters.[29]

This finding is clinically important, given prior observations linking PCSK9 genetic variants with diabetes risk.[9] In contrast to some statin therapies, inclisiran did not increase the incidence of new-onset diabetes, supporting its metabolic safety in high-risk populations.

INCLISIRAN IN THE CONTEXT OF HIGH-RISK ACS

Patients with recent ACS represent a population with an exceptionally high risk of recurrent cardiovascular events, particularly in the presence of diabetes or obesity. Early LDL-C lowering following ACS has been shown to yield rapid and sustained reductions in recurrent ischemic events.[27,28]

Although inclisiran has not yet been specifically studied in a dedicated ACS outcomes trial, its potent and durable LDL-C lowering suggests potential benefit in this setting. The ability to initiate inclisiran during hospitalization or early after discharge, followed by infrequent dosing, may enhance adherence and ensure consistent lipid control during a critical period of vulnerability.

Ongoing cardiovascular outcomes trials, including ORION-4 and the VICTORION program, are expected to provide definitive evidence regarding the impact of inclisiran on major adverse cardiovascular events.[30-32]

PRACTICAL CONSIDERATIONS AND CLINICAL INTEGRATION

Inclisiran is administered as a subcutaneous injection at baseline, 3 months, and then every 6 months thereafter. No dose adjustments are required based on age, renal function, glycemic status, or BMI.[26] This simplicity facilitates integration into routine cardiology and endocrinology practice **(Table 3)**.

In individuals with diabetes or obesity and recent ACS, inclisiran may be considered when LDL-C targets are not achieved despite maximally tolerated statins and ezetimibe, or when adherence concerns limit the effectiveness of oral therapies. Its healthcare professional administered dosing model aligns well with structured secondary prevention programs and multidisciplinary cardiometabolic clinics.

TABLE 3: Practical considerations and clinical integration of inclisiran.

Domain	*Key features*	*Clinical implications*
Route and schedule	Subcutaneous injection at baseline, 3 months, then every 6 months	Ensures sustained LDL-C lowering with infrequent dosing
Dose adjustment	No adjustment required for age, renal function, glycemic status, or BMI	Simplifies prescribing across diverse high-risk populations
Target population	Diabetes or obesity with recent ACS and persistent LDL-C elevation	Addresses residual lipid risk in very high-risk individuals
Position in therapy	Add-on therapy when LDL-C targets are unmet despite maximally tolerated statins and ezetimibe	Supports guideline-directed intensification of lipid lowering
Adherence advantage	Healthcare professional—administered dosing	Reduces nonadherence associated with daily oral therapies
Care model integration	Suitable for cardiology clinics, endocrinology practices, and multidisciplinary cardiometabolic programs	Facilitates structured secondary prevention and long-term risk reduction

FUTURE DIRECTIONS

The concept of cumulative LDL-C exposure has emerged as a critical determinant of lifetime ASCVD risk, emphasizing that both the magnitude and duration of LDL-C lowering are central to effective prevention strategies.[33] In this context, therapies capable of delivering sustained LDL-C reduction with minimal dependence on long-term patient adherence assume increasing clinical relevance. Inclisiran, through its durable PCSK9 suppression and twice-yearly dosing regimen, represents a novel therapeutic approach that may fundamentally reshape long-term lipid management, particularly in individuals with diabetes, obesity, and other high-risk metabolic phenotypes.

Future research is expected to define the role of inclisiran across the full spectrum of cardiovascular prevention. Ongoing large-scale cardiovascular outcomes trials, including ORION-4 and VICTORION-2 Prevent, will be pivotal in determining whether the robust LDL-C reductions observed with inclisiran translate into proportional reductions in major adverse cardiovascular events, including myocardial infarction, stroke, and cardiovascular mortality. These data will be especially important for clarifying the clinical benefits of early initiation of inclisiran following ACS, a period characterized by heightened residual risk.

Beyond secondary prevention, inclisiran may also have an emerging role in primary prevention among selected high-risk populations, such as individuals with diabetes, severe obesity, familial hypercholesterolemia, or persistently elevated LDL-C despite optimized oral therapy. Additionally, future therapeutic strategies may involve combination approaches integrating inclisiran with agents targeting triglyceride-rich lipoproteins or lipoprotein(a), thereby addressing multiple atherogenic pathways simultaneously.

As health systems increasingly prioritize long-term risk reduction and adherence-independent therapies, inclisiran has the potential to become a cornerstone of comprehensive cardiometabolic prevention strategies.

CONCLUSION

Inclisiran represents a meaningful therapeutic advancement in lipid management for individuals with diabetes or obesity and dyslipidemia, particularly among those at very high cardiovascular risk following ACS. These populations are characterized by accelerated atherosclerosis, heightened residual risk, and persistent challenges in achieving and maintaining guideline-recommended LDL-C targets despite optimized conventional therapy. By targeting hepatic PCSK9 synthesis through RNA interference, inclisiran provides a novel, mechanistically distinct approach that delivers potent and sustained LDL-C reduction.

Evidence from pivotal Phase 3 trials and pooled post-hoc analyses consistently demonstrates approximately 50% LDL-C lowering across glycemic and BMI strata, with durable effects maintained over extended dosing intervals. Importantly, inclisiran exhibits a favorable safety and tolerability profile, including the absence of adverse effects on glycemic control and no increase in new-onset diabetes—an especially relevant consideration in cardiometabolic populations. The predictable pharmacodynamic profile and twice-yearly dosing administered by healthcare professionals offer a practical solution to longstanding barriers such as poor adherence, polypharmacy, and therapeutic inertia.

In the contemporary era of aggressive lipid lowering and cumulative LDL-C exposure reduction, inclisiran aligns closely with evolving preventive cardiology paradigms that emphasize early, intensive, and sustained intervention. While ongoing cardiovascular outcomes trials will further define its impact on hard clinical endpoints, current evidence supports inclisiran as an effective and pragmatic addition to the lipid-lowering armamentarium, with the potential to substantially improve long-term cardiovascular risk management in patients with diabetes, obesity, and high-risk ACS.

REFERENCES

1. Balakumar P, Maung UK, Jagadeesh G. Prevalence and prevention of cardiovascular disease and diabetes mellitus. Pharmacol Res. 2016;113:600-9.
2. Vaduganathan M, Mensah GA, Turco JV, et al. The global burden of cardiovascular diseases and risk: a compass for future health. J Am Coll Cardiol. 2022;80(25):2361-71.
3. Fan W. Epidemiology in diabetes mellitus and cardiovascular disease. Cardiovasc Endocrinol. 2017;6(1): 8-16.
4. Svane J, Pedersen-Bjergaard U, Tfelt-Hansen J. Diabetes and the risk of sudden cardiac death. Curr Cardiol Rep. 2020;22(10):112.
5. McMurray JJ, Gerstein HC, Holman RR, et al. Heart failure: a cardiovascular outcome in diabetes that can no longer be ignored. lancet Diabetes Endocrinol. 2014;2(10):843-51.
6. Walker AM, Cuban RM. Sudden cardiac death in patients with diabetes mellitus and chronic heart failure. Diab Vasc Dis Res. 2015;12(4):228-33.
7. Henning RJ. Obesity and obesity-induced inflammatory disease contribute to atherosclerosis: a review of the pathophysiology and treatment of obesity. Am J Cardiovasc Dis. 2021;11(4):504.
8. Lechner K, McKenzie AL, Kränkel N, et al. High-risk atherosclerosis and metabolic phenotype: the roles of ectopic adiposity, atherogenic dyslipidemia, and inflammation. Metab Syndr Relat Disord. 2020;18(4): 176-85.
9. Nussbaumerova B, Rosolova H. Obesity and dyslipidemia. Curr atheroscler Rep. 2023;25(12):947-55.
10. Mhaimeed O, Burney ZA, Schott SL, et al. The importance of LDL-C lowering in atherosclerotic cardiovascular disease prevention: Lower for longer is better. Am J Prev Cardiol. 2024;18:100649.
11. Chen C, Wei FF, Dong Y, et al. Early management of blood lipid levels with non-statin lipid-lowering drugs in acute coronary syndrome: A mini review. Cardiovasc Drugs Ther. 2025;39(6):1465-80.
12. Brie DM, Mornoş C, Adam O, et al. Dyslipidemia Treatment in Patients with Acute Coronary Syndrome: Is It Time to Move to Combination Therapy?. J Clin Med. 2025;14(18):6445.
13. Krychtiuk KA, Ahrens I, Drexel H, et al. Acute LDL-C reduction post ACS: strike early and strike strong: from evidence to clinical practice. A clinical consensus statement of the Association for Acute CardioVascular Care (ACVC), in collaboration with the European Association of Preventive Cardiology (EAPC) and the European Society of Cardiology Working Group on Cardiovascular Pharmacotherapy. Eur Heart J Acute Cardiovasc Care. 2022;11(12):939-49.
14. Talic S, Marquina C, Zomer E, et al. Attainment of low-density lipoprotein cholesterol goals in statin treated patients: Real-world evidence from Australia. Curr Probl Cardiol. 2022;47(7):101068.
15. Gandhi SK, Järbrink K, Fox KM, et al. Effectiveness of rosuvastatin in reducing LDL-C and target LDL-C goal attainment in real-world clinical practice. Current medical research and opinion. 2009;25(12):2817-28.
16. Gomes DA, Paiva MS, Freitas P, et al. Attainment of LDL-Cholesterol Goals in Patients with Previous Myocardial Infarction: A Real-World Cross-Sectional Analysis. Arquivos Brasileiros de Cardiologia. 2024;121:e20230242.
17. Stadler JT, Marsche G. Obesity-related changes in high-density lipoprotein metabolism and function. International journal of molecular sciences. 2020;21(23):8985.
18. Sparks JD, Sparks CE, Adeli K. Selective hepatic insulin resistance, VLDL overproduction, and hypertriglyceridemia. Arterioscler Thromb Vasc Biol. 2012;32(9): 2104-12.

19. Klempfner R, Elis A, Matezky S, et al. Temporal trends in management and outcome of diabetic and non-diabetic patients with acute coronary syndrome (ACS): residual risk of long-term mortality persists: insights from the ACS Israeli Survey (ACSIS) 2000–2010. Int J Cardiol. 2015;179:546-51.
20. Santilli F, Guagnano MT, Vazzana N, et al. Oxidative stress drivers and modulators in obesity and cardiovascular disease: from biomarkers to therapeutic approach. Curr Med Chem. 2015;22(5):582-95.
21. Pogran E, Burger AL, Zweiker D, et al. Lipid-lowering therapy after acute coronary syndrome. J Clin Med. 2024;13(7):2043.
22. Jin S, Nie X, Li Y, et al. Effect of more intensive LDL-C–lowering therapy on long-term cardiovascular outcomes in early-phase acute coronary syndrome: a systematic review and meta-analysis. Clin Ther. 2021;43(7):e217-29.
23. Kong N, Xu Q, Cui W, et al. PCSK9 inhibitor inclisiran for treating atherosclerosis via regulation of endothelial cell pyroptosis. Ann Transl Med. 2022;10(22):1205.
24. Albosta MS, Grant JK, Taub P, et al. Inclisiran: a new strategy for LDL-C lowering and prevention of atherosclerotic cardiovascular disease. Vasc Health Risk Manag. 2023;19:421-31.
25. Hess CN, Low Wang CC, Hiatt WR. PCSK9 inhibitors: mechanisms of action, metabolic effects, and clinical outcomes. Ann Rev Med. 2018;69(1):133-45.
26. Newman CB, Tobert JA. Targeting PCSK9 with antibodies and gene silencing to reduce LDL cholesterol. J Clin Endocrinol Metabol. 2023;108(4):784-90.
27. Ray KK, Wright RS, Kallend D, et al. Two phase 3 trials of inclisiran in patients with elevated LDL cholesterol. N Engl J Med. 2020;382(16):1507-19.
28. Leiter LA, Raal FJ, Schwartz GG, et al. Inclisiran in individuals with diabetes or obesity: Post-hoc pooled analyses of the ORION-9, ORION-10 and ORION-11 Phase 3 randomized trials. Diabetes Obes Metabol. 2024;26(8):3223-37.
29. Jain P. Traditional and novel non-statin lipid-lowering drugs. Indian Heart J. 2023;76(Suppl 1):S38.
30. Taub PR, Gutierrez A, Wewers D, et al. Safety and lipid-lowering efficacy of inclisiran monotherapy in patients without ASCVD: the VICTORION-Mono randomized clinical trial. J Am Coll Cardiol. 2025;86(3):196-208.
31. Stoekenbroek RM, Kallend D, Wijngaard PL, et al. Inclisiran for the treatment of cardiovascular disease: the ORION clinical development program. Future Cardiol. 2018;14(6):433-42.
32. Tsamoulis D, Rallidis LS, Kosmas CE. Inclisiran: the preclinical discovery and development of a novel therapy for the treatment of atherosclerosis. Expert Opin Drug Discov. 2024;19(7):773-82.
33. Brandts J, Ray KK. Low density lipoprotein cholesterol–lowering strategies and population health: time to move to a cumulative exposure model. Circulation. 2020;141(11):873-6.

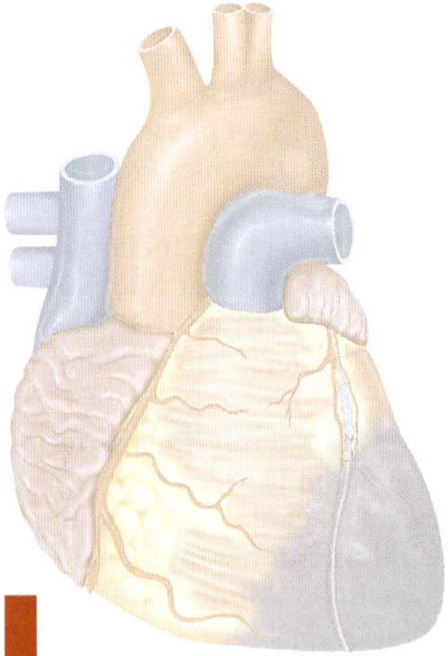

Inclisiran in India: Game Changer in Lipid Management

JPS Sawhney, Juhi Singh, Rohan Patel

INTRODUCTION

Inclisiran is the first ribonucleic acid interference (RNAi) therapy approved for lowering low-density lipoprotein cholesterol (LDL-C). Silencing hepatic *PCSK9* gene expression provides durable LDL-C reduction with only twice-yearly dosing (an initial loading dose of days 0 and 90, followed by a 6-month dosing regimen). The US FDA approved inclisiran in 2021,[1] and it was introduced in India in 2024,[2] marking a significant advance in cardiovascular risk management.

MECHANISM OF ACTION

Inclisiran is a double-stranded small interfering ribonucleic acid (siRNA). It consists of two complementary RNA strands: An antisense (guide) strand and a sense (passenger) strand which is conjugated with triantennary N-acetylgalactosamine (GalNAc) to facilitate uptake by hepatocytes. The passenger strand facilitates incorporation of the siRNA into the RNA-induced silencing complex (RISC), after which it dissociates, leaving the guide strand available to bind specifically to PCSK9 mRNA. Once bound, the target mRNA is cleaved by Argonaute 2, a catalytic protein within RISC. This cleavage event prevents translation of PCSK9 mRNA. By preventing PCSK9 protein synthesis, it preserves LDL receptors on hepatocyte surfaces, thereby enhancing LDL-C clearance from plasma.[3]

- *Pharmacokinetics:* After subcutaneous injection, inclisiran reaches peak plasma concentration within 4–6 hours. Concentrations reached undetectable levels after 24–48 hours postdosing. Inclisiran is primarily metabolized by nucleases to shorter nucleotides of varying length. The terminal elimination half-life of LEQVIO is ~9 hours, and no accumulation occurs with multiple dosing. It is rapidly taken up by hepatocytes, with a long tissue half-life that supports dosing every 6 months.[4]
- *Pharmacodynamics:* Inclisiran reduces circulating PCSK9 levels by ~80%, leading to sustained LDL-C reductions of ~45–55% when combined with statins.[5]

Inclisiran does not require dose adjustment in elderly patients or in those with renal impairment or mild-to-moderate hepatic dysfunction making it a good option where other drugs cannot be used.

Evidence on its safety and efficacy in individuals with end-stage renal disease or severe hepatic impairment, however, is lacking. Because the drug is cleared via the kidneys, hemodialysis should be avoided for at least 72 hours after administration. Importantly, unlike monoclonal antibodies targeting PCSK9, inclisiran has not been associated with the development of antidrug antibodies that could compromise its efficacy or safety.

Unmet Need in India: Why Inclisiran is the Need of the Hour?

Cardiovascular disease (CVD) is the leading cause of death in India, accounting for one in four deaths.[6] Approximately 185 million Indians have elevated LDL-C.[7] Despite widespread statin use, therapeutic gaps remain. Inclisiran offers a promising option for several patient groups:

- *Very high-risk patients:*
    - Indian real-world data show that 80% of patients with prior cardiovascular events fail to reach LDL-C targets, despite 97% being on high-dose statins.[8]
    - This mirrors findings from the DA VINCI study, which highlighted the need for advanced lipid-lowering agents.[9]
    - The LAI-REACT study demonstrated that even with triple therapy, one in three patients remained above target LDL-C thresholds after 6 weeks of an event.[10]
- *Statin intolerance:*
    - Statin intolerance is reported in 10–15% of Indian patients, leading to discontinuation or suboptimal dosing.
    - Inclisiran has shown efficacy in statin-intolerant populations, providing ~50% LDL-C reduction without the muscle-related adverse effects associated with statins.
- *Patients not adhering to therapy:*
    - Global data indicate that adherence to statins declines significantly after 6 months.
    - The TNT trial demonstrated that LDL-C variability itself is a risk factor, with a 23% increase in mortality per 1 SD variation in LDL-C.
    - Inclisiran's twice-yearly dosing addresses adherence challenges by reducing pill burden.
- *Patients with high LDL-C and elevated lipoprotein(a) [Lp(a)]:*
    - Currently, no approved therapies specifically target Lp(a).
    - Inclisiran not only reduces LDL-C by ~50% but also lowers Lp(a) by ~40% in Asian patients, as shown in ORION-18.
    - Data from Mahajan et al. demonstrated that patients on triple therapy after acute coronary syndrome (ACS) experienced increases in Lp(a) within 1 month.

CLINICAL EVIDENCE: ORION AND VICTORION PROGRAMS

Refer **Table 1**.

TABLE 1: Clinical evidence: ORION and VICTORION programs.

Trial	*Population*	*Key findings*
ORION-9	Heterozygous familial hypercholesterolemia	~50% LDL-C reduction sustained over 18 months[3]
ORION-10	ASCVD patients (United States)	~52% LDL-C reduction at day 510[3]
ORION-11	ASCVD/high-risk patients (Europe)	~50% LDL-C reduction, favorable tolerability[3]
ORION-3	Long-term extension study	Sustained LDL-C reduction over 4 years
ORION-18	Asian patients	Consistent LDL-C lowering; ~40% Lp(a) reduction in Asians
V-INITIATE	Early initiation of inclisiran versus standard of care	Significant LDL-C lowering in patients on inclisiran
V-INCEPTION	Post-ACS patients	Rapid LDL-C reduction, improved target attainment

Safety Profile: ORION-8 Long-term Follow-up

The *ORION-8 trial* provided extended safety data over a median follow-up of 4 years.

- *Adverse events:* Rates of treatment-emergent adverse events were similar between inclisiran and placebo groups.
- *Injection site reactions:* Mild, transient injection site reactions occurred in <10% of patients, with no discontinuations.
- *Hepatic and renal safety:* No clinically significant changes in liver enzymes or renal function were observed.
- *Immunogenicity:* No evidence of neutralizing antibodies or loss of efficacy over time
- *Mortality and major adverse cardiovascular events (MACE)*: Comparable to control groups, supporting long-term safety

Recent Updates: Monotherapy Approval

In *2025, the US FDA approved inclisiran as monotherapy* for LDL-C reduction.

- *V-MONO (VICTORION-Mono) trial:*
    - *Population:* Adults without ASCVD, diabetes, or familial hypercholesterolemia, LDL-C 100–190 mg/dL
    - *Results:* Inclisiran achieved *~45–50% LDL-C reduction*, outperforming placebo and ezetimibe, with excellent tolerability.

However, this is off-label in India. As of now, inclisiran is only indicated after maximal tolerated dose of statins for patients who are not able to reach the target LDL-C goal.

GUIDELINE RECOMMENDATIONS

Inclisiran has been mentioned in all major guidelines such as ACC 2025 and ESC 2025. However, it is intriguing to see that it is also mentioned in guidelines of other specialties such as ADA 2025. It has already been mentioned in the recent CSI clinical practice guidelines for dyslipidemia management: Executive summary as an option that improves compliance (twice a year injection) and causes less LDL-C variability.

REAL-WORLD EVIDENCE WITH INCLISIRAN FROM INDIA

Inclisiran was introduced in a cohort of 80 patients with a mean age of 57 years, of whom nearly two-thirds were diabetic, more than half hypertensive, and over 40% smokers. Analysis of 65 patients with complete lipid data revealed a mean baseline LDL-C of 120.6 mg/dL despite ongoing oral lipid-lowering therapy. At 3 months, inclisiran achieved a profound reduction to 32.8 mg/dL, corresponding to a 70.6% decrease from baseline. Subgroup analysis showed consistent efficacy across very high-risk and extremely high-risk patients, with reductions of 72.8 and 69.6%, respectively, and the majority reaching guideline-recommended LDL-C targets.

CONCLUSION

Inclisiran is a transformative therapy in lipid management. Its *RNAi mechanism, twice-yearly dosing*, and efficacy across diverse populations make it uniquely suited to address India's CVD burden. With proven benefits in *very high-risk patients, statin-intolerant individuals, nonadherent populations, and those with elevated Lp(a)*, inclisiran fills critical therapeutic gaps. The growing body of evidence from the ORION and VICTORION programs, long-term safety data from ORION-8, real-world registry findings, and monotherapy approval position inclisiran as a cornerstone of future cardiovascular prevention strategies.

REFERENCES

1. US Food and Drug Administration. FDA approves Leqvio (Inclisiran). Silver Spring: FDA; 2021.
2. Novartis India. Novartis launches Leqvio (inclisiran) in India. Press release; 2024.
3. Ray KK, Wright RS, Kallend D, et al. Two phase 3 trials of inclisiran in patients with elevated LDL cholesterol. N Engl J Med. 2020;382(16):1507-19.
4. Kallend D, Stoekenbroek RM, et al. Inclisiran mechanism of action and pharmacodynamics. Eur Heart J. 2020;41(3):193-201.
5. Wright RS, Ray KK, et al. Pharmacokinetics and safety of inclisiran. J Clin Lipidol. 2021;15(2):123-9.
6. Abdul-Aziz AA, Desikan P, Prabhakaran D, et al. Tackling the burden of cardiovascular diseases in India: the essential diagnostics list. Circ Cardiovasc Qual Outcomes. 2019;12:5195.
7. Anjana RM, Unnikrishnan R, Deepa M, et al. Metabolic non-communicable disease health report of India: the ICMR-INDIAB national cross-sectional study (ICMR-INDIAB-17). Lancet Diabetes Endocrinol. 2023;11:474-89.
8. Jain M, Sawant R, Panchal H, et al. Evaluating LDL-C control in Indian acute coronary syndrome (ACS) patients—a retrospective real-world study LDL-C control in ACS. Int J Cardiol Cardiovasc Risk Prev. 2023;19:200210.
9. Mach F, Baigent C, Catapano AL, et al. DA VINCI study: contemporary use of lipid-lowering therapies in Europe. Eur J Prev Cardiol. 2021;28(12):1279-89.
10. Sawhney JP, Ramakrishnan S, Madan K, et al. CSI clinical practice guidelines for dyslipidemia management: executive summary. Indian Heart J. 2024;76 (Suppl 1): S6-19.

155 CHAPTER

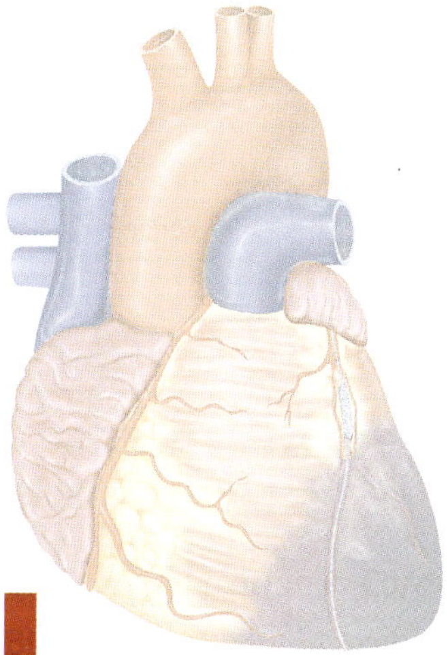

Inclisiran in Dyslipidemia of Metabolic Syndrome

SS Iyengar

INTRODUCTION

Dyslipidemia is a major risk factor and metabolic syndrome is a high-risk feature for atherosclerotic cardio-vascular disease.

Inclisiran, a small interfering RNA (siRNA), reduces the levels of low-density lipoproteins (LDL) in the circulation by preventing the hepatic synthesis of proprotein convertase subtilisin/Kexin type 9 (PCSK9). It is an LDL receptor dependent lipid lowering agent. Hence, it is effective and safe in reducing LDL cholesterol regardless of the presence of metabolic syndrome, as long as LDL receptors are functional.

Atherosclerotic cardio-vascular disease (ASCVD) is a major cause of mortality and morbidity locally and globally. Prevention of ASCVD—primary and secondary, means a meticulous management of all the risk factors along with lifestyle intervention. Dyslipidemia is a major modifiable risk factor, and metabolic syndrome has been identified as a high-risk feature for ASCVD.[1]

ATHEROSCLEROTIC CARDIO-VASCULAR DISEASE AND RISK FACTORS

As per the "Global Burden of Cardiovascular Diseases (GBD) and Risks 2023 Collaborators Report", number of cardiovascular disease (CVD) disability adjusted life years (DALYs) has increased from 1990 to 2023 by 42.9% in males and by 28.6% in females. The report concluded that *increasing metabolic risk is driving the burden* and ischemic heart disease (IHD) was the leading cause of DALYs globally among all CVDs estimated in GBD.[2]

The three leading modifiable risk factors for IHD globally were high systolic blood pressure (SBP), dietary risks, and elevated LDL cholesterol. For ischemic stroke too, the leading risk factors were high SBP, high LDL-C, and air pollution.

Indian Perspective of the Global Burden of Cardiovascular Diseases Report

The CVD age-standardized DALY rates are among the highest in India, nearly two times that of high-income countries. The increasing prevalence of metabolic risks (such as obesity and raised blood sugar) is considered to be the main driving factor in increasing the CVD burden in low- to middle-income countries (LMICs). The fastest-growing threats were metabolic (e.g., high body mass index, hyperglycemia) and environmental (air pollution and temperature extremes) factors.[3]

METABOLIC SYNDROME

Metabolic syndrome is a cluster of risk factors and is seen to occur more often than by chance alone, thus, to be acknowledged as a distinct entity. It is a risk factor for cardiovascular disease and type 2 diabetes mellitus.

The components of metabolic syndrome are raised blood pressure, dyslipidemia (raised triglycerides and low high-density lipoprotein cholesterol), raised fasting glucose, and central obesity. Three abnormal

TABLE 1: Criteria for clinical diagnosis of the metabolic syndrome.[4]

Measure	Categorical cut points
Increased waist circumference	>90 cm in males; >80 cm in females
Elevated triglycerides (drug treatment for elevated triglycerides is an alternate indicator)	≥150 mg/dL
Low HDL-C	<40 mg/dL in males; <50 mg/dL in females
Elevated blood pressure (antihypertensive drug treatment in a patient with a history of hypertension is an alternate indicator)	Systolic ≥130 and/or diastolic ≥85 mm Hg
Elevated fasting glucose (drug treatment of elevated glucose is an alternate indicator)	≥100 mg/dL

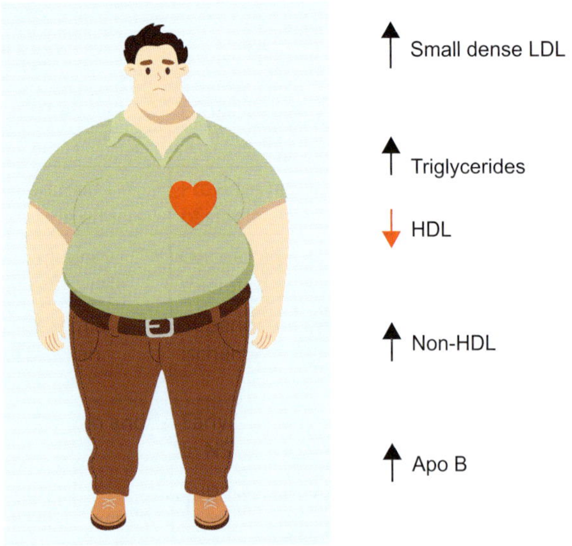

Fig. 1: Dyslipidemia of metabolic syndrome.

findings out of five would qualify a person to be having the metabolic syndrome[4] **(Table 1)**. Majority of these individuals have abdominal obesity. Excess adipose tissue releases inflammatory cytokines and excess fatty acids, predisposing to both diabetes and ASCVD.

India

In a study of 111 studies with 133,926 participants, it was found that almost one in three adults in India suffer from metabolic syndrome (MS). Females, people living in urban areas and in northeast region had higher prevalence of MS. The overall pooled prevalence of MS among adult population in India was 30% (95%CI: 28–33%).[5] Another study involving 26 studies with a total of 37,965 participants, overweight and obesity were significantly associated with metabolic syndrome.[6]

Amongst young adults, between the age of 18–35 years, the prevalence of MS was 25.4% in an eastern state of India, hypertension, diabetes, cholesterol levels, low HDL-C and triglycerides contributing to the development of MS.[7] Another study from India showed that patients with metabolic syndrome had significant lipid abnormalities characterized by elevated total cholesterol, triglycerides, and LDL cholesterol, along with markedly lower HDL cholesterol levels compared to healthy controls.[8]

DYSLIPIDEMIA IN METABOLIC SYNDROME (FIG. 1)

The dyslipidemia in metabolic syndrome is characterized by hypertriglyceridemia and low levels of high-density lipoprotein-cholesterol (HDL-C). In addition, there are elevated levels of apolipoprotein (apo) B, small dense low-density lipoprotein-cholesterol (LDL-C) and triglyceride-rich particles (very low-density lipoprotein), together with insulin resistance.

Proprotein Convertase Subtilisin–Kexin Type 9

Proprotein convertase subtilisin–Kexin type 9 (PCSK9) is an established and validated target for LDL cholesterol–lowering therapy. This serine protease, is secreted into the bloodstream by the liver, binds to LDL receptors both intracellularly and extracellularly and promotes the degradation of LDL receptors in hepatocytes.[9] This leads to an elevation of circulating LDL cholesterol levels. Subjects with *PCSK9* loss-of-function mutations are known to have low LDL cholesterol levels and significantly reduced risk of ASCVD with no adverse consequences.[10]

INCLISIRAN

Inclisiran is a chemically synthesized small interfering RNA that effectively induces PCSK9-specific RNA silencing in hepatocytes. This results in decreased levels of the PCSK9 protein, decreased degradation of LDL receptors which in turn leads to reduction in circulating LDL cholesterol.[11]

Additional advantage of inclisiran is that it is administered twice yearly, is well tolerated, producing a rapid and sustained reduction of LDL-C and achieving LDL-C targets in many.[12] Various studies have clearly shown that inclisiran reduces PCSK9, total cholesterol,

LDL-cholesterol and ApoB, without increasing the risk of adverse events.[13]

Interestingly, it has been reported that in patients with stable CAD, low PCSK9 plasma levels are associated with a particular phenotype of metabolic syndrome (low HDL cholesterol, obesity, insulin resistance, and diabetes) and diffuse non-obstructive coronary atherosclerosis.[14]

TREATMENT OF DYSLIPIDEMIA IN METABOLIC SYNDROME

The management of these patients revolves round control of body weight, blood pressure, hyperglycemia or DM, and maintaining optimum plasma lipid levels. Lifestyle interventions, such as diet control and increased physical activity are an integral part of the management. It is recommended that non-HDL cholesterol and ApoB should be estimated in such patients, so that once the LDL-c targets are reached, non-HDL-C and ApoB should be targeted with intensified lipid lowering therapy. Patients with metabolic syndrome usually come under high risk for ASCVD, and LDL-C target is, 70 mg/dL and non-HDL-C <100 mg/dL.[1]

HMG-CoA reductase inhibitors (statins) form the first line of lipid lowering therapy and statins effectively and safely lower LDL-C and improve CV outcomes in patients with metabolic syndrome with or without ASCVD. If lipid targets are not achieved with statins, addition of ezetimibe and/or bempedoic acid is the next step. If one still falls short of the target or if statin intolerance is an issue, PCSK9 inhibitors—evolocumab/alirocumab or inclisiran should be tried, inclisiran having an advantage of infrequent administration and potentially better adherence to therapy.

As alluded to earlier, in patients with stable CHD, low PCSK9 plasma levels are associated with a particular phenotype of metabolic syndrome and diffuse non-obstructive coronary atherosclerosis.[14] However, PCSK9 inhibitors have been shown to further reduce LDL-C and ASCVD risk in patients with cardio metabolic syndrome without increasing new-onset DM or worsening of glycemic control with no safety issues. The trial results have shown that the addition of PCSK9 inhibitors to statin therapy in patients with ASCVD and cardio metabolic syndrome is safe and effective in reducing residual cardiovascular risk.[15,16]

INCLISIRAN IN METABOLIC SYNDROME

Inclisiran uptake into hepatocytes is dependent on asialoglycoprotein receptor (ASGPR). There is a greater expression of ASGPR on hepatocytes in obesity, and by association in DM and metabolic syndrome. Therefore, the greater expression of ASGPR on hepatocytes in obesity (and by association in metabolic syndrome) might facilitate the uptake of inclisiran into the liver. In contrast, PCSK9 monoclonal antibodies (mAbs) are not dependent on ASGPR for their uptake by the liver. This may explain some of the differences observed in LDL cholesterol reductions with inclisiran as compared to PCSK9 mAbs such as evolocumab or alirocumab.[17,18]

Pooled Analysis of ORION-9, –10, and –11 Trials

These trials included patients with heterozygous familial hypercholesterolemia, atherosclerotic CV disease (ASCVD), or ASCVD risk equivalent statins. 3660 patients were randomized to receive inclisiran (1,833 patients) or placebo (1,827) on Days 1, 90, and 6-monthly thereafter for 18 months. There was 50.6% reduction in LDL-c at day 90, and 51.6% at day 540. Major adverse cardiac events (MACE) were reduced by 26%. Amongst these participants receiving inclisiran, 37.5% were diabetics. Injection site reactions were more frequent with inclisiran but were mild, and not persistent. LDL-C lowering with inclisiran has potential benefits for MACE reduction.[19]

Further analysis of these three Phase 3 trials[20] demonstrated that along with other lipid lowering drugs, inclisiran provided significant reductions in LDL cholesterol levels irrespective of glycemic and BMI status of the participants. In fact, the mean reductions in atherogenic lipoproteins—LDL-C, non-HDL-C, and ApoB were at least as high as or higher in individuals with DM versus those with pre-DM or normoglycemia, as was seen in for those with obesity versus those who were overweight or who had a normal weight. Interestingly, greater percentage reductions with inclisiran (at Day 510) in total cholesterol, non-HDL cholesterol, ApoB, remnant cholesterol, and Lp(a) (at Day 540) and in time-adjusted LDL cholesterol (between Day 90 and Day 540) were observed in individuals with DM versus those with normo-glycaemia or pre-DM and in those with a higher versus lower BMI **(Tables 2 and 3)**.

It was also noted that baseline factors such as ongoing lipid lowering therapy, glucose lowering medications, triglyceride levels, BMI, and waist circumference did not have any influence on the inclisiran effect on LDL-C lowering in this population. Inclisiran is well tolerated in these population subgroups and there was no increase in new onset diabetes. Injection site reactions, however, were more frequent. Inclisiran has proved to be a safe and effective therapeutic option for reducing LDL cholesterol in

TABLE 2: Glycemia group—mean percent change reduction from baseline with inclisiran.[20]

Metric	*Normoglycemia*	*Prediabetes*	*Diabetes*
LDL-cholesterol	46.8	51.4	52.0
Non-HDL cholesterol	42.6	46.2	48.7
ApoB	37.2	42.0	44.3
Remnant cholesterol	13.7	19.0	23.1
Triglycerides	6.9	10.5	10.8
Lp(a)	14.6	21.0	23.7
PCSK9	82.6	81.9	84.7

TABLE 3: BMI group—mean percent change reduction from baseline with inclisiran.[20]

Metric	*<25 kg*	*25 – <30 kg*	*30 – <35 kg*	*≥35 kg*
LDL cholesterol	48.6	48.8	53.3	51.8
Non-HDL cholesterol	45.5	45.0	48.1	47.1
Apo B	39.2	40.5	43.9	43.4
Remnant cholesterol	15.5	18.7	18.8	23.0
Triglycerides	10.2	10.4	6.9	11.5
Lp(a)	12.9	21.9	22.9	20.8

individuals coming under different categories of glycaemia and BMI (essentially representing metabolic syndrome) who require additional lipid-lowering measures.

Inclisiran with the background oral lipid lowering drugs in these studies achieved LDL-C levels of <1.8 mmol/L in >61% and <1.4 mmol/L goal in >48% of patients, regardless of the presence of metabolic disorder. It is well known that non-HDL cholesterol and ApoB measures better surrogate markers for ASCVD risk in this population. This pooled analysis showed effective lowering of non-HDL-C and ApoB levels.[19]

In a patient-level, pooled analysis of ORION-9, –10, and –11, inclisiran significantly reduced composite MACE (non-adjudicated CV death, cardiac arrest, non-fatal myocardial infarction and fatal and non-fatal stroke) by 26%. Confirmation in the larger cardiovascular outcomes trials is awaited.[18]

FUTURE

The ongoing "ORION-4" and "VICTORION-2 Prevent" trials are cardiovascular outcomes trials testing inclisiran in patients with high ASCVD risk or clinical ASCVD, with 15,000 participants expected to be enrolled in each, with a follow-up of 5 years. There is certainly going to be a significant number of patients with metabolic syndrome in these studies, as the incidence and prevalence of obesity and diabetes are on the increase worldwide. Subgroup analysis of participants with metabolic syndrome will shed light on utility of inclisiran in reducing ASCVD events in this population.

CONCLUSION

Inclisiran is safe and effective in lowering atherogenic ApoB containing lipids in patients with metabolic syndrome, without increasing the risk of new onset diabetes and with a potential benefit of reducing major adverse cardiovascular events. The convenient and infrequent dosage schedule of inclisiran makes it a good option for lipid lowering therapy.

"ORION" trials have been studying inclisiran. "Orion" refers to a prominent constellation in the night sky, and in Greek mythology he first appears as a great hunter. Will inclisiran hunt down successfully the atherogenic lipoproteins and improve cardiovascular outcome?

REFERENCES

1. Raman Puri, Manish Bansal, Vimal Mehta et al. Lipid Association of India 2023 update on cardiovascular risk assessment and lipid management in Indian patients: Consensus statement IV. J Clin Lipidol. 2024;18:e351-73.
2. Global Burden of Cardiovascular Diseases and Risks 2023 Collaborators. Global, Regional, and National Burden of Cardiovascular Diseases and Risk Factors in 2024 Countries and Territories, 1990-2023. JACC. 2025;86: 2167-243.

3. Thiruvengadam R, Karthikeyan G. Interpreting Cardiovascular Disease Burden for Low-Middle Income Countries A Perspective from India. J Am Coll Cardiol. 2025;86:2112-4.
4. Alberti KGMM, Eckel RH, Grundy SM et al. Harmonizing the Metabolic Syndrome: A Joint Interim Statement of the International Diabetes Federation Task Force on Epidemiology and Prevention; National Heart, Lung, and Blood Institute; American Heart Association; World Heart Federation; International Atherosclerosis Society; and International Association for the Study of Obesity. Circulation. 2009;120:1640-5.
5. Krishnamoorthy Y, Rajaa S, Murali S, et al. Prevalence of metabolic syndrome among adult population in India: A systematic review and meta-analysis. PLoS ONE. 2020;15(10):e0240971.
6. Krishnamoorthy Y, Rajaa S, Murali S, et al. Association Between Anthropometric Risk Factors and Metabolic Syndrome Among Adults in India: A Systematic Review and Meta-Analysis of Observational Studies. Prev Chronic Dis. 2022;19:210231.
7. Dash M, Sadangi S, Barik BS, et al. Metabolic Syndrome and Its Associated Risk Factors and Morbidities Among Young Adults in Bhubaneswar: A Cross-Sectional Study. Natl J Community Med. 2025;16(3):261-70.
8. Chaudhari A, Prabhu P, Tayade M, et al. Lipid Profile Abnormalities in Metabolic Syndrome Patients: A Comparative Cross-Sectional Study. Eur J Cardiovasc Med. 2025;15(4):1152-6.
9. Mousavi SA, Berge KE, Leren TP. The unique role of proprotein convertase subtilisin/Kexin 9 in cholesterol homeostasis. *J Intern Med*. 2009;266:507-19
10. Horton JD, Cohen JC, Hobbs HH. PCSK9: a convertase that coordinates LDL catabolism. *J Lipid Res*. 2009;50:Suppl:S172-77.
11. Fitzgerald K, White S, Borodovsky A, et al. A Highly Durable RNAi Therapeutic Inhibitor of PCSK9. N Engl J Med. 2017;376:41-51.
12. Ray KK, Troquay RPT, Visseren FLJ, et al. Long-Term Efficacy and Safety of Inclisiran in Patients With High Cardiovascular Risk and Elevated LDL Cholesterol (ORION-3): Results From the 4- Year Open-Label Extension of the ORION-1 Trial. Lancet Diabetes Endocrinol. 2023;11(2):109-19.
13. Basit J, Ahmed M, Singh P, et al. Safety and Efficacy of Inclisiran in Hyperlipidemia: An Updated Meta-Analysis of Randomised Controlled Trials. Endocrinol Diabetes Metabol. 2025;8:e70039.
14. Caselli C, Turco SD, Ragusa R, et al. Association of PCSK9 plasma levels with metabolic patterns and coronary atherosclerosis in patients with stable angina. Cardiovasc Diabetol. 2019;18:144
15. Deedwania P, Murphy SA, Scheen A, et al. Efficacy and safety of PCSK9 inhibition with evolocumab in reducing cardiovascular events in patients with metabolic syndrome receiving statin therapy: secondary analysis from the FOURIER randomized clinical trial. JAMA Cardiol 2021;6;(2):139-47.
16. Hsiao Y-C, Wu C-C. Dyslipidemia and Cardiometabolic Syndrome. Cardiometab Syndr J. 2021;1(1):18-23.
17. Willoughby JLS, Chan A, Sehgal A, et al. Evaluation of GalNAc-siRNA conjugate activity in pre-clinical animal models with reduced asialo-glycoprotein receptor expression. Mol Ther. 2018;26:105-114.25.
18. Witzigmann D, Quagliata L, Schenk SH, et al. Variable asialoglycoprotein receptor1 expression in liver disease: implications for therapeutic intervention. Hepatol Res. 2016;46:686-96.
19. Ray KK, Raal FJ, Kallend DG, et al. Inclisiran and cardiovascular events: a patient-level analysis of phase III trials. Eur Heart J. 2023;44:129-38.
20. Leiter LA, Raal FJ, Schwartz GG, et al. Inclisiran in individuals with diabetes or obesity: Post hoc pooled analyses of the ORION-9, ORION-10 and ORION-11 Phase 3 randomized trials. Diabetes Obes Metab. 2024;26:3223-37.

156

CHAPTER

Inclisiran for the Treatment of Heterozygous Familial Hypercholesterolemia

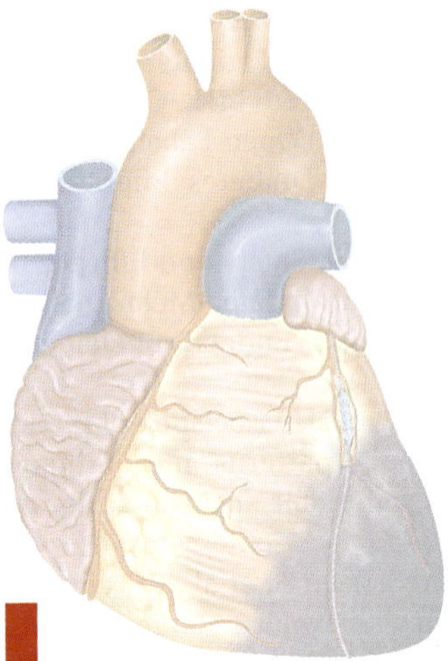

PK Asokan

INTRODUCTION

Familial hypercholesterolemia (FH) is prevalent but frequently undiagnosed. FH is marked by persistently elevated low-density lipoprotein cholesterol (LDL-C) levels, potentially resulting in premature atherosclerosis and heightened cardiovascular risk if not addressed. In the absence of treatment, individuals aged 50 and 60 years have a 30–50% probability of experiencing a fatal or nonfatal cardiac event. The objective of treatment is to lower LDL-C to below 2.6 mmol/L (100 mg/dL) or achieve a reduction of at least 50% in LDL-C levels. Heterozygous familial hypercholesterolemia (HeFH) is an autosomal dominant genetic disorder characterized by elevated LDL-C levels from birth, resulting from mutations in the *LDL-R, APOB,* and *PCSK9* genes. In conjunction with statins, proprotein convertase subtilisin/kexin type 9 (PCSK9) inhibitors have received approval for the treatment of FH. Reducing LDL-C levels is a fundamental approach to prevent and manage atherosclerotic heart disease (AHD). PCSK9 is a crucial protein that modulates the expression of low-density lipoprotein receptors (LDL-Rs) in hepatocytes and is positively associated with LDL-C levels. Inclisiran is an innovative small-interfering RNA (siRNA) pharmaceutical that inhibits *PCSK9* gene expression and diminishes LDL-C levels. In contrast to conventional inhibitors, it is a long-acting injectable that provides sustained LDL-C reduction (about 50%) with only three treatments annually following the initial administration, hence enhancing adherence. The majority of adverse effects consist of mild injection site reactions, with no evidence of liver, renal, or muscular damage. The current and forthcoming trials to assess its ability to reduce major adverse cardiovascular events (MACEs).

HETEROZYGOUS FAMILIAL HYPERCHOLESTEROLEMIA

Heterozygous familial hypercholesterolemia is a common yet often underdiagnosed autosomal dominant disorder that affects 1 in 300 individuals globally.[1] Familial hypercholesterolemia and homozygous hypercholesterolemia (HoFH) demonstrate distinct prevalence rates. Recent genetic studies estimate HoFH frequency at 1 in 170,000 to 1 in 300,000. However, those with HoFH have mutations in both alleles of these genes. Due to significant LDL-C receptor dysfunction, HoFH has a worse clinical phenotype and prognosis than HeFH. HoFH patients have twice the LDL-C levels of HeFH patients, which increases their risk of cardiovascular problems, often in the first decade of life.

Heterozygous familial hypercholesterolemia is characterized by persistent elevation of LDL-C, which, if left untreated, results in early-onset atherosclerosis and an elevated risk of cardiovascular events. Untreated men and women face a 30–50% risk of experiencing a fatal or nonfatal cardiac event by the ages of 50 and 60 years, respectively.[2]

The primary causes are pathogenic variants in the *LDL-R* gene, which accounts for 85–90% of cases confirmed through genetic testing. Pathogenic variants of the apolipoprotein B (*ApoB*) gene, which leads to reduced binding of LDL to the LDL-R, or gain-of-function mutations in the gene encoding *PCSK9,* resulting in increased degradation of LDL-Rs, accounts for 5–15% and approximately 1% of cases of FH, respectively.[3] HeFH may cause 20% of myocardial infarction in younger men (<45 years old), despite various hypercholesterolemia causes.[4]

SCREENING IN CHILDHOOD AND EARLY ADULTHOOD FOR HeFH

It is critical to consider the diagnosis of FH in children with LDL-C >160 mg/dL (4.1 mmol/L), adults with *LDL-C >190 mg/dL (4.9 mmol/L) (particularly if there is a family history of early-onset CAD)*, and all patients with early CAD. Given that FH is an autosomal dominant condition, a heterozygous individual has a 50% probability of passing the gene on to his or her children. Early diagnosis of HeFH in primary care settings leads to better detection and management of the condition. When family screening is neglected, opportunities for timely intervention and early implementation of lifesaving therapies are often missed.

Earlier lipid screening at the age of 2 years is recommended if a child has a strong family history of early onset CAD (males, aged <55 years; females, aged <65 years) in a parent, grandparent, aunt, uncle, or sibling; a parent with a total cholesterol >240 mg/dL (6.2 mmol/L); or if the child has underlying cardiac risk factors, such as diabetes mellitus or obesity.[5] Screening between the ages of 9–11 years enables the best discernment between those with and without FH and avoids confounding lipid changes secondary to LDL-C reduction, known to transiently occur during puberty. The American Academy of Pediatrics (AAP), American Heart Association (AHA), National Lipid Association, and National Heart, Lung, and Blood Institute (NHLBI) recommend universal lipid screening for 9–11-year old.[6] In all patients with early CAD, adults with LDL >190 mg/dL (4.9 mmol/L) (especially if there is a family history of early onset, and children with LDL consistently >160 mg/dL (4.1 mmol/L), FH could be considered.[5]

The Foundation's CASCADE (Cascade Screening for Awareness and Detection)[7] registry revealed that FH was diagnosed at an average age of 50 years, by which point almost one-third of FH patients had experienced an atherosclerotic cardiovascular disease (ASCVD) event. This highlights the necessity for far earlier universal screening, diagnosis, and treatment of HeFH. The diagnosis of HeFH can be established through clinical symptoms, but genetic testing may provide further insight into cardiac risk and diagnosis.[2] Although there are no universally accepted criteria for diagnosing FH, effective diagnostic standards have been established. The main diagnostic tools used for FH include the US Make Early Diagnosis to Prevent Early Death (MEDPED) criteria, the UK Simon Broome system (UK FH Register criteria), the Dutch Lipid Clinic Network criteria, and the National Lipid Association expert panel recommendations.[8-12]

INCLISIRAN

Inclisiran is a siRNA drug that targets the messenger RNA (mRNA) of the *PCSK9* gene to reduce the synthesis of intracellular and extracellular PCSK9.[13] It is a double-stranded siRNA that binds and then degrades the specific mRNA, thus preventing its translation into the PCSK9 protein. This results in the downregulation of LDL-C receptor lysosomal catabolism, supporting more efficient clearance of LDL from the bloodstream. Therefore, this drug proves to be a great therapeutic agent for FH.[14]

Mechanism of Action of Inclisiran

Inclisiran binds specifically to the hepatocyte due to GalNAc conjugation. In hepatocytes, inclisiran utilizes the RNA interference mechanism and directs catalytic breakdown of mRNA for PCSK9. This increases LDL-C receptor recycling and expression on the hepatocyte cell surface, which increases LDL-C uptake and lowers LDL-C levels in the circulation **(Fig. 1)**.[13]

Posology and Method of Administration

The recommended dose is 284 mg incliseran administered as a single subcutaneous injection: initially, again at 3 months, followed by every 6 months. LDL-C is a significant risk factor for ASCVD in both primary and secondary prevention settings; thus, achieving and maintaining target LDL-C levels is crucial. Given that a reduction of >50% in LDL-C is necessary to prevent ASCVD, lipid-lowering medications are the primary therapeutic approach for cardiovascular prevention.[14,15]

The initial approach to suppress *PCSK9* used the use of monoclonal antibodies (mAbs) that specifically target *PCSK9* receptors, preventing their binding to LDL-Rs.

Due to the lack of head-to-head trials comparing inclisiran and anti-PCSK9 mAbs, there is currently insufficient data to draw definitive conclusions, complicating the selection of the optimal treatment allocation.[16] Conversely, the principal advantage of inclisiran over conventional pharmacotherapies and PCSK9 mAbs is its infrequent dosage regimen—initially every 3 months, followed by biannual administration. This schedule is anticipated to markedly improve patient adherence,[17] surpassing daily oral drugs, and facilitate more frequent administration of mAbs. The dose interval of inclisiran provides a notable advantage, while being slightly less than that seen with mAbs. In clinical trials, inclisiran injection usage reduced LDL-C levels by about 50% compared to the placebo. Despite the fact that both therapies significantly reduced LDL-C, there are still concerns about their

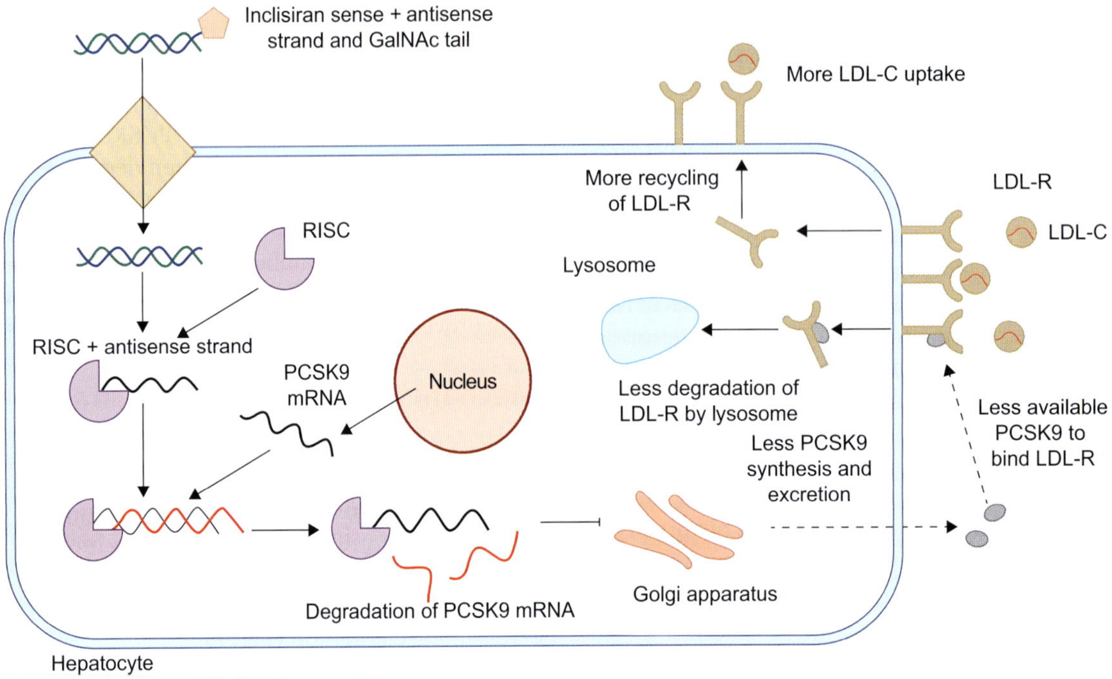

Fig. 1: Mechanism of action in low-density lipoprotein cholesterol (LDL-C) reduction. (LDL-C: low-density lipoprotein cholesterol; LDL-R: low-density lipoprotein receptor; mRNA: messenger RNA)
Source: Cupido AJ, Kastelein JJP. Inclisiran for the treatment of hypercholesterolaemia: implications and unanswered questions from the ORION trials. Cardiovasc Res. 2020;116(11):e136-9.

long-term safety. The biennial administration of inclisiran may enhance long-term compliance, which is crucial for controlling cardiovascular risk.

CLINICAL TRIALS OF INCLISIRAN FOR FAMILIAL HYPERCHOLESTEROLEMIA

Lipid-lowering therapies (LLTs) are a cornerstone of the prevention of ASCVD.[18] Recent data from randomized clinical trials (RCTs) evaluating drugs as an add-on to baseline statin therapies have led to guidelines changes, now recommending to lower patient's LDL-C below 55 mg/dL in patients in secondary ASCVD prevention.[19] To achieve such target levels of LDL-C, addition of ezetimibe and/or PCSK9 inhibitors to high-intensity statin therapy is often necessary. Following the discovery of *PCSK9* gene and function in the early 2000s, a first generation of PCSK9 inhibitors, mAbs that target the protein in the plasma have been successfully developed and are now available in routine clinical practice.[20,21] PCSK9 mAbs (alirocumab and evolocumab) require a subcutaneous injection every 2 or 4 weeks depending on dosing. More recently, *inclisiran* has emerged as an alternative approach to antagonize PCSK9.[22]

Despite taking the maximum statin dose, many HeFH patients have LDL-C levels above the recommended thresholds for primary and secondary prevention, 70 mg/dL and 100 mg/dL, respectively, indicating the need for additional therapy to lower LDL-C to current guidelines. According to the 2018 American Heart Association (AHA)/American College of Cardiology (ACC)/Multisociety guideline for the management of blood cholesterol, a *PCSK9* inhibitor is deemed appropriate for patients with severe primary hypercholesterolemia who, despite receiving statin and ezetimibe therapy, maintain LDL-C levels persistently exceeding 100 mg/dL. Inadequate adherence to treatment poses a substantial obstacle to attaining LDL-C targets HeFH. The asymptomatic presentation of dyslipidemia frequently results in reduced adherence to daily medication regimens, with numerous patients ceasing their prescribed treatments within 1 year of commencement.[23,24]

One-year ORION-1 follow-up of one or two *inclisiran* doses on LDL-C levels; patients with increased LDL-C despite maximally tolerated statins were studied.[25] The two-dose 300-mg inclisiran regimen had the highest proportion of responders and the greatest mean LDL-C reduction over 1 year **(Fig. 2)**. Adverse effects were similar for 1 year. LDL-C decreased for a year after

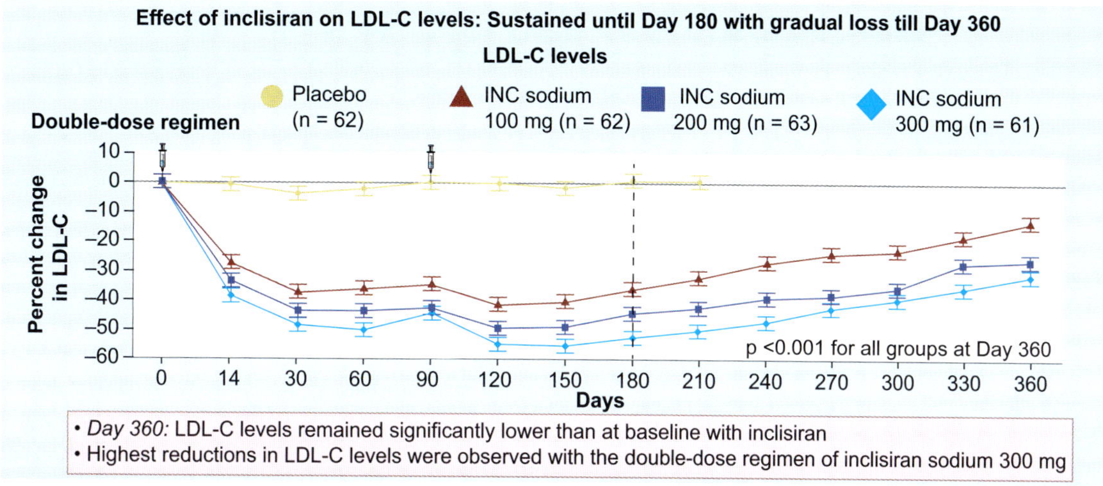

Fig. 2: Effect of inclisiran on low-density lipoprotein cholesterol (LDL-C) levels: Sustained until Day 180 with gradual loss till Day 360.
Source: Ray KK, Stoekenbroek RM, Kallend D, et al. Effect of 1 or 2 doses of inclisiran on low-density lipoprotein cholesterol levels: One-year follow-up of the ORION-1 randomized clinical trial. JAMA Cardiol. 2019;4(11):1067-75.

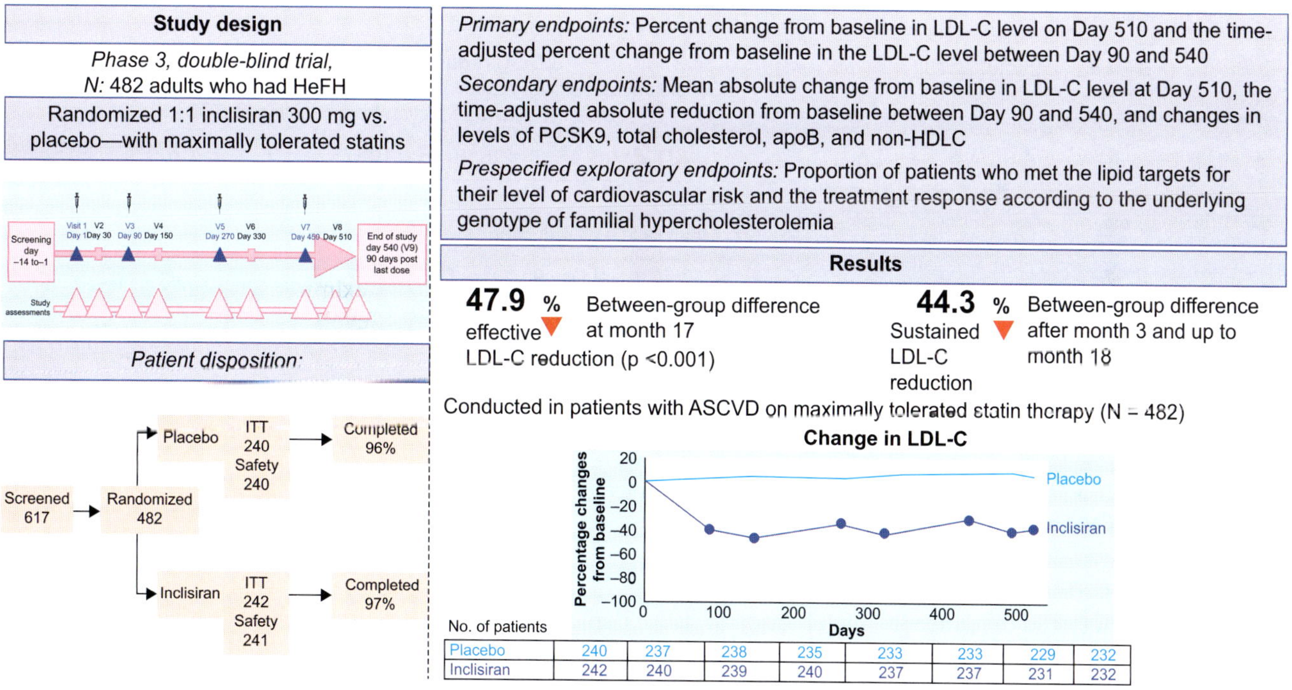

Fig. 3: Effective and sustained reduction of LDL-C versus placebo in patients with HeFH—ORION 9 results. (HeFH: heterozygous familial hypercholesterolemia; LDL-C: low-density lipoprotein cholesterol)
Source: Raal FJ, Kallend D, Ray KK, et al. Inclisiran for the treatment of heterozygous familial hypercholesterolemia. N Engl J Med. 2020;382(16):1520-30.

inclisiran treatment. Inclisiran may reduce LDL-C with infrequent dose in a unique way.

ORION-9 aimed to assess the efficacy and safety of inclisiran 300 mg as subcutaneous injections on day 1, day 90, and then every 6 months over an 18-month period in subjects with HeFH. ORION-9 met all primary and secondary efficacy endpoints. There was a 50% observed LDL-C lowering at day 510 with a 45%-time adjusted LDL-C lowering between days 90 and 540. This was on top of maximally tolerated statin therapy and ezetimibe. In addition, inclisiran's safety profile was similar to placebo except adverse events at the site of injection which were mostly mild and transient. There was no evidence of liver, kidney, muscle, or platelet toxicity. There was no difference

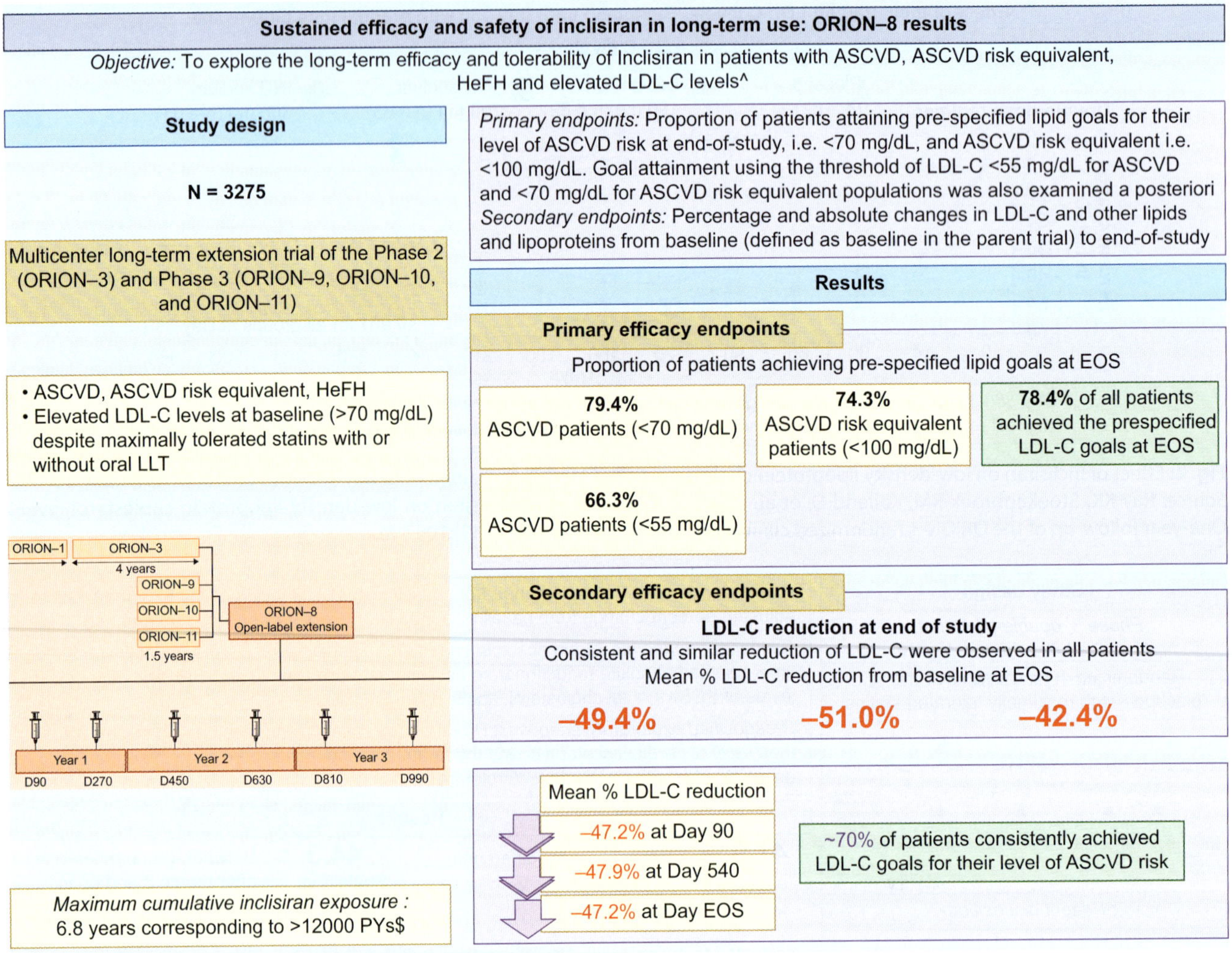

Fig. 4: Sustained efficacy and safety of inclisiran in long-term use: ORION-8 results. (HeFH: Heterozygous familial hypercholesterolemia; LDL-C: low-density lipoprotein cholesterol; LLT: lipid-lowering therapy)
Source: Wright RS, Raal FJ, Koenig W, et al. Inclisiran administration potently and durably lowers LDL-C over an extended-term follow-up: the ORION-8 trial. Cardiovasc Res. 2024;120(12):1400-10.

in serious adverse events. Inclisiran shows potential to address the unmet need to reduce the high burden of risk in HeFH patients.[26] This study shows that, administered twice yearly, inclisiran injection demonstrated effective and sustained reduction of LDL-C versus placebo in patients with HeFH **(Fig. 3)**.

The long-term effectiveness and tolerability of inclisiran are limited. Inclisiran administration effectively and sustainably reduces LDL-C levels over an extended long-term follow-up of the Phase 2 (ORION-3) and Phase 3 (ORION-9, ORION-10, and ORION-11) studies, which investigate the efficacy and tolerability of inclisiran in patients with ASCVD, ASCVD risk equivalents, HeFH, and elevated LDL-C levels beyond 6 years of treatment. 70% of patients consistently attained LDL-C targets appropriate to their ASCVD risk level **(Fig. 4)**.[27]

The pooled analysis of ORION-9, 10, and 11 demonstrated that inclisiran yields effective and sustained reductions in LDL-C levels. Inclisiran administered biannually, significantly reduced LDL-C levels by an average of 50.7% and attained an 80.9% reduction in PCSK9 at day 510, demonstrating good tolerability in individuals with HeFH, ASCVD, and ASCVD-risk equivalents over a period of 540 days.[28] **Figure 5** has been demonstrated to effectively and safely reduce LDL-C according to randomized trials.

In actual clinical settings, the median LDL-C reduction was reported to be between 35 and 50%, with a range of 38%. Patients who were on statins had reductions that were even greater, with values of between 42.2 and 45%. The results of the VICTORION which was recently published demonstrated a noteworthy 53% decrease in LDL-C levels

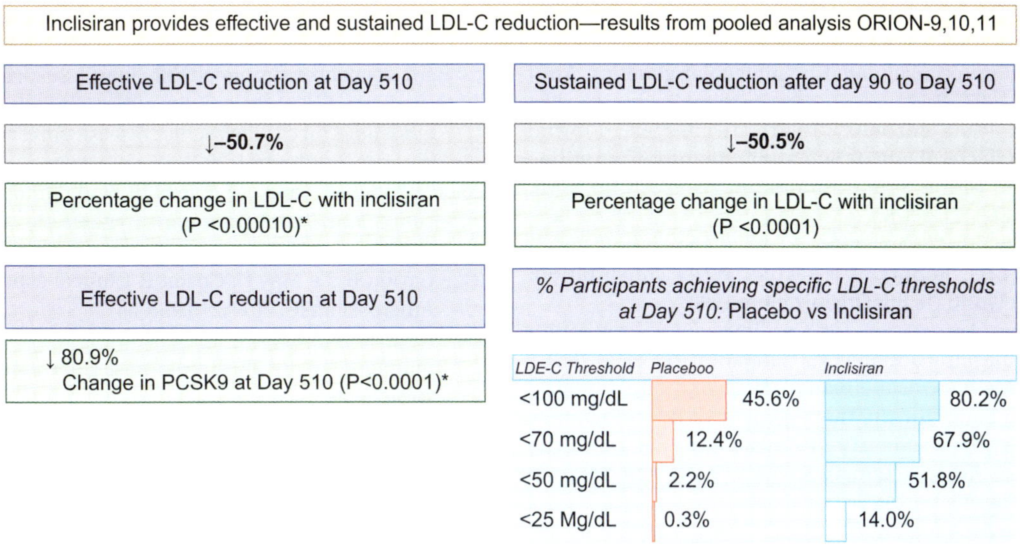

Fig. 5: Inclisiran provides effective and sustained LDL-C reduction—results from pooled analysis ORION-9, 10, and 11.
Source: Wright RS, Ray KK, Raal FJ, et al. Pooled patient-level analysis of inclisiran trials in patients with familial hypercholesterolemia or atherosclerosis. J Am Coll Cardiol. 2021;77(9):1182-93.

in patients who were treated with inclisiran than those who were treated with usual care.[29]

ADVERSE REACTIONS OF INCLISIRAN AND SAFETY COMPARISON WITH SIRNA DRUGS

Inclisiran has a good overall safety profile. Compared with other LLTs, inclisiran has a low risk of adverse events and no major safety concerns. The most common adverse event reported in the inclisiran group was injection site reaction, which occurred in about 5% of the patients. These reactions were mostly mild and transient. Injection site reactions may be related to the lipid nanoparticles used for siRNA delivery and may decrease with repeated administration. Moreover, inclisiran did not cause any significant toxicity in liver, kidney, muscle, and platelet functions. Laboratory examination showed that there was no change in the levels of alanine aminotransferase, aspartate aminotransferase, creatinine, creatine kinase, or platelet count after inclisiran treatment. Inclisiran also did not affect the cardiovascular system.[28,29]

CONCLUSION

Early diagnosis and treatment of HeFH is paramount to reduce the risk of premature ASCVD and death. Inclisiran is recommended for HeFH patients with baseline LDL-C levels >70 mg/dL despite maximally tolerated statin therapy, with or without oral lipid-lowering treatment. Inclisiran has less frequent dosing, injection volume, and cost than PCSK9 antibodies. The persistent lipid-lowering efficacy and convenient dosing schedule may improve HeFH medication adherence and therapeutic outcomes. Inclisiran injection has no significant safety concerns compared to other lipid-lowering treatments.

REFERENCES

1. Polychronopoulos G, Tzavelas M, Tziomalos K. Heterozygous familial hypercholesterolemia: prevalence and control rates. Expert Rev Endocrinol Metab. 2021;16:175-791.
2. Sturm AC, Knowles JW, Gidding SS, et al. Clinical Genetic Testing for Familial Hypercholesterolemia: JACC Scientific Expert Panel. J Am Coll Cardiol. 2018;72(6):662-80.
3. Soutar AK, Naoumova RP. Mechanisms of disease: genetic causes of familial hypercholesterolemia. Nat Clin Pract Cardiovasc Med. 2007;4:214-25.
4. Do R, Stitziel NO, Won HH, et al. Exome sequencing identifies rare LDLR and APOA5 alleles conferring risk for myocardial infarction. Nature. 2015;518:102-6.
5. McGowan MP, Hosseini Dehkordi SH, Moriarty PM, et al. Diagnosis and treatment of heterozygous familial hypercholesterolemia. J Am Heart Assoc. 2019;8(24): e013225.
6. Mihalopoulos NL, Stipelman C, Hemond J, et al. Universal Lipid Screening in 9- to 11-year-olds Before and After 2011 Guidelines. Acad Pediatr. 2018;18(2):196-9.
7. Duell PB, Andersen RL, Knickelbineetal T, et al. Abstract 19888: improved longitudinal low density lipoprotein cholesterol goal achievement among familial hypercholesterolemia patients in the CASCADE FH patient registry. Circulation. 2017;136:A19888.

8. Williams RR, Hunt SC, Schumacher MC, et al. Diagnosing heterozygous familial hypercholesterolemia using new practical criteria validated by molecular genetics. Am J Cardiol. 1993;72:171-6.
9. Risk of fatal coronary heart disease in familial hypercholesterolaemia. Scientific Steering Committee on behalf of the Simon Broome Register Group. BMJ. 1991;303(6807):893-6.
10. World Health Organization. Familial Hypercholesterolaemia (FH): Report of a second WHO consultation. Geneva: World Health Organization; 1998.
11. European Association for Cardiovascular Prevention & Rehabilitation; Reiner Z, Catapano AL, et al. ESC/EAS Guidelines for the management of dyslipidaemias: the Task Force for the management of dyslipidaemias of the European Society of Cardiology (ESC) and the European Atherosclerosis Society (EAS). Eur Heart J. 2011;32(14):1769-818.
12. Goldberg AC, Hopkins PN, Toth PP, et al. Familial hypercholesterolemia: screening, diagnosis and management of pediatric and adult patients: clinical guidance from the National Lipid Association Expert Panel on Familial Hypercholesterolemia. J Clin Lipidol. 2011;5:S 1-S8.
13. Cupido AJ, Kastelein JJP. Inclisiran for the treatment of hypercholesterolaemia: implications and unanswered questions from the ORION trials. Cardiovasc Res. 2020;116(11):e136-e139.
14. Vallejo-Vaz AJ, Kondapally Seshasai SR, et al. Familial hypercholesterolaemia: a global call to arms. Atherosclerosis 2015;243:257-59.
15. Barkas F, Nomikos T, Liberopoulos E, et al. Diet and cardiovascular disease risk among individuals with familial hypercholesterolemia: systematic review and meta-analysis. Nutrients. 2020;12:2436.
16. Arnold N, Koenig W. PCSK9 inhibitor wars: how does fit in with current monoclonal antibody inhibitor therapy? Considerations for patient selection. Curr Cardiol Rep. 2022;24:1657-67.
17. Merćep I, Friščić N, Strikić D, et al. Advantages and disadvantages of inclisiran: a small interfering ribonucleic acid molecule targeting PCSK9-A narrative review. Cardiovasc Ther. 2022;2022:8129513.
18. Borén J, Chapman MJ, Krauss RM, et al. Low-density lipoproteins cause atherosclerotic cardiovascular disease: pathophysiological, genetic, and therapeutic insights: a consensus statement from the European atherosclerosis society consensus panel. Eur Heart J. 2020;41:2313-30.
19. Visseren FLJ, Mach F, Smulders YM, et al. 2021 ESC guidelines on cardiovascular disease prevention in clinical practice. Eur Heart J. 2021;42:3227-337.
20. Abifadel M, Varret M, Rabès JP, et al. Mutations in PCSK9 cause autosomal dominant hypercholesterolemia. Nat Genet. 2003;34:154-6.
21. Cariou B, Le May C, Costet P. Clinical aspects of PCSK9. Atherosclerosis. 2011;216:258-65.
22. Henney NC, Banach M, Penson PE. RNA silencing in the management of dyslipidemias. Curr Atheroscler Rep. 2021;23:69.
23. Agarwala A, Quispe R, Goldberg AC, et al. Bempedoic acid for heterozygous familial hypercholesterolemia: from bench to bedside. Drug Des Devel Ther. 2021;15:1955-63.
24. Grundy SM, Stone NJ, Bailey AL, et al. 2018 AHA/ACC/AACVPR/AAPA/ABC/ACPM/ADA/AGS/APhA/ASPC/NLA/PCNA Guideline on the Management of Blood Cholesterol: Executive Summary: A Report of the American College of Cardiology/American Heart Association Task Force on Clinical Practice Guidelines. Circulation. 2019;139(25):e1046-e1081.
25. Ray KK, Stoekenbroek RM, Kallend D, et al. Effect of 1 or 2 doses of inclisiran on low-density lipoprotein cholesterol levels: one-year follow-up of the ORION-1 randomized clinical trial. JAMA Cardiol. 2019;4(11):1067-75.
26. Raal FJ, Kallend D, Ray KK, et al. Inclisiran for the treatment of heterozygous familial hypercholesterolemia. N Engl J Med. 2020;382(16):1520-30.
27. Wright RS, Raal FJ, Koenig W, et al. Inclisiran administration potently and durably lowers LDL-C over an extended-term follow-up: the ORION-8 trial. Cardiovasc Res. 2024;120(12):1400-10
28. Wright RS, Ray KK, Raal FJ, et al. Pooled patient-level analysis of inclisiran trials in patients with familial hypercholesterolemia or atherosclerosis. J Am Coll Cardiol. 2021;77(9):1182-93.
29. Koren MJ, Rodriguez F, East C, et al. An "Inclisiran First" Strategy vs Usual Care in patients with atherosclerotic cardiovascular disease. J Am Coll Cardiol. 2024;83(20):1939-52.

157

CHAPTER

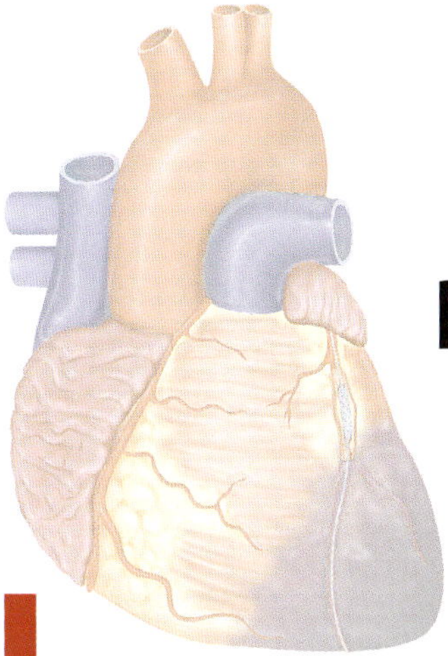

Pooled ORION 10/11 Data (Atherosclerotic Cardiovascular Disease Cohort)

Rajeev Garg

INTRODUCTION

Atherosclerotic cardiovascular disease (ASCVD) is a leading global cause of death and disability, underpinned by the process of atherosclerosis driven largely by elevated low-density lipoprotein cholesterol (LDL-C). Achieving substantial LDL-C lowering is a proven strategy to reduce cardiovascular events such as myocardial infarction, stroke, and cardiovascular death. Despite widespread statin use, many patients with ASCVD are unable to achieve LDL-C targets due to inadequate response or intolerance to existing therapies. Thus, new therapeutic options that provide potent, durable, and well-tolerated LDL-C reductions are required.

Inclisiran, a novel small-interfering RNA (siRNA) therapy, targets hepatic PCSK9 messenger RNA, leading to long-lasting reduction in PCSK9 protein levels and increased LDL receptor recycling. The ORION-10 and ORION-11 phase 3 trials evaluated the efficacy and safety of inclisiran in patients with ASCVD or ASCVD risk equivalents receiving maximally tolerated statin therapy. These trials used a twice-yearly dosing regimen following initial doses to provide sustained LDL-C lowering.

This chapter provides a comprehensive, focused analysis of pooled ORION-10 and ORION-11 data, emphasizing inclisiran's LDL-C-lowering efficacy, goal attainment rates, consistency across patient subgroups, and safety observations within the ASCVD population.

METHODS AND STUDY POPULATION

ORION-10 and ORION-11 were randomized, double-blind, placebo-controlled phase 3 clinical trials conducted to evaluate the effects of inclisiran on LDL-C reduction in patients with established ASCVD or equivalent risk.

Participants eligible for inclusion had LDL-C levels ≥70 mg/dL despite receiving maximally tolerated statin therapy with or without additional lipid-lowering therapies. All patients were randomized 1:1 to receive either subcutaneous inclisiran sodium 300 mg or placebo on days 1, 90, and then every 6 months thereafter. The trials followed patients for up to 18 months, with lipid measurements and assessments conducted at multiple timepoints.

Pooled data from 2,975 patients with ASCVD (inclusive of both ORION-10 and ORION-11 participants) were analyzed, representing a broad demographic and clinical profile: Approximately 28% female, 7% Black, nearly 50% obese, 40% with diabetes, and 18% with moderate to severe chronic kidney disease. Background statin therapy was administered to over 90% of participants, many on high-intensity regimens **(Table 1)**.

EFFICACY RESULTS: LDL-C REDUCTION

The primary efficacy outcome across the pooled ASCVD cohort was the percentage change in LDL-C from baseline

TABLE 1: Baseline demographic data.

Characteristic	*ORION-10 inclisiran (n = 781)*	*ORION-10 placebo (n = 780)*	*ORION-11 inclisiran (n = 810)*	*ORION-11 placebo (n = 807)*
Age, years (mean, SD)	66.4 (8.9)	65.7 (8.9)	64.8 (8.3)	64.8 (8.7%)
Male, *n* (%)	535 (68.5%)	548 (70.3%)	579 (71.5%)	581 (72.0%)
ASCVD, *n* (%)	781 (100%)	780 (100%)	712 (87.9%)	702 (87.0%)
Prior MI, *n* (%)	375 (48.0%)	410 (52.6%)	434 (53.6%)	424 (52.5%)
Congestive heart failure (CHF), *n* (%)	100 (12.8%)	116 (14.9%)	109 (13.5%)	102 (12.6%)
Current smoking, *n* (%)	123 (15.7%)	111 (14.2%)	160 (19.8%)	132 (16.4%)
Hypertension, *n* (%)	714 (91.4%)	701 (89.9%)	640 (79.0%)	661 (81.9%)
Diabetes, *n* (%)	371 (47.5%)	331 (42.4%)	296 (36.5%)	272 (33.7%)
Statin use, *n* (%)	701 (89.8%)	692 (88.7%)	766 (94.6%)	766 (94.9%)
High-intensity statins, *n* (%)	538 (68.9%)	546 (70.0%)	633 (78.1%)	628 (77.8%)
Ezetimibe use, *n* (%)	80 (10.2%)	74 (9.5%)	52 (6.4%)	62 (7.7%)
Antiplatelet therapy: ASA, *n* (%)	614 (78.6%)	614 (78.7%)	611 (75.4%)	583 (72.2%)
Antiplatelet therapy: P2Y12 inhibitors, *n* (%)	283 (36.2%)	312 (40.0%)	147 (18.1%)	174 (21.6%)
LDL-C, mmol/L (mean, SD)	2.70 (1.02)	2.71 (0.96)	2.77 (1.08)	2.68 (0.94)
HDL-C, mmol/L (mean, SD)	1.20 (0.37)	1.19 (0.37)	1.29 (0.40)	1.27 (0.36)
HbA1c, % (median, IQR)	6.1 (5.6–7.0)	6.0 (5.6–6.9)	5.9 (5.6–6.5)	5.9 (5.6–6.4)

to day 510 and the time-adjusted change from day 90 through day 540.[1]

Inclisiran demonstrated a robust and consistent LDL-C-lowering effect compared to placebo:

- At day 510, the mean placebo-corrected LDL-C reduction was 51.5% (95% CI: –54.0 to –49.0%) from a baseline of approximately 103 mg/dL.
- Time-adjusted analysis from days 90 to 540 showed a sustained mean LDL-C reduction of 52.1% (95% CI: –53.9 to –50.4%).

This level of LDL-C reduction corresponds to an absolute decrease of approximately 50–55 mg/dL, which is clinically meaningful for cardiovascular risk reduction.

LDL-C LOWERING CONSISTENCY ACROSS SUBGROUPS

The efficacy of inclisiran was consistent across multiple key patient subgroups stratified by sex, age, race, kidney function, body mass index (BMI), and glycemic status:

- Both males and females showed similar magnitude LDL-C reductions.
- Older patients (≥75 years) experienced comparable LDL-C lowering to younger cohorts.
- Patients with moderate to severe chronic kidney disease had LDL-C reductions consistent with those without kidney impairment.
- Individuals with diabetes, obesity, or of Black race also demonstrated similar efficacy.

This consistency highlights the broad applicability of inclisiran in diverse ASCVD populations, including those typically underrepresented in clinical trials, supporting its utility for real-world patients.

LDL-C GOAL ATTAINMENT

A critical clinical outcome is the proportion of patients achieving guideline-recommended LDL-C targets for secondary prevention.

In the pooled ASCVD population treated with inclisiran:

- 87.6% of patients achieved LDL-C levels below 55 mg/dL at one or more visits.
- Approximately 86% of patients achieved LDL-C below 70 mg/dL at any visit.

TABLE 2: Clinical implications.

Aspect	*Inclisiran*	*PCSK9 monoclonal antibodies*	*Statins*
Mechanism	siRNA inhibiting PCSK9 mRNA	Monoclonal antibodies binding PCSK9 protein	HMG-CoA reductase enzyme inhibition
LDL-C reduction	~50%	~50–60%	~20–55%
Dosing frequency	Twice yearly (after initial doses)	Biweekly or monthly injections	Daily oral tablets
Common side effects	Injection site reactions (~5%)	Injection site reactions (~10%)	Muscle symptoms, liver enzyme elevations
Adherence potential	High due to infrequent dosing	Lower due to more frequent dosing	Variable, often limited by side effects
Cardiovascular outcome data	Pending larger trials (ORION-4)	Established with significant event reduction	Established with significant event reduction

- Nearly 88% of patients achieved LDL-C reductions of 50% or greater from baseline.

These results represent a significant advance in LDL-C goal attainment compared with historical data showing many high-risk patients fail to meet these targets with current standard therapies alone.

SAFETY AND TOLERABILITY

Inclisiran was well tolerated across the pooled ASCVD population, confirming its favorable safety profile seen in individual trials.

Injection-site adverse events, primarily mild and transient, occurred in about 5% of the inclisiran group versus <1% in placebo. There were no significant differences in serious adverse events or discontinuations attributable to the drug.

Laboratory safety parameters, including liver function tests, kidney function markers, creatine kinase, and platelet counts, were comparable between inclisiran and placebo groups.

No new safety signals emerged, supporting inclisiran's use as a safe addition to standard lipid-lowering therapy in high-risk patients.

CLINICAL IMPLICATIONS

The pooled ORION-10 and ORION-11 data emphasize several important clinical messages:

- Twice-yearly dosing of inclisiran provides potent and durable LDL-C reduction, overcoming adherence barriers associated with more frequent dosing regimens of other lipid-lowering agents.
- Significant LDL-C reductions translate into very high rates of LDL-C goal attainment consistent with guideline recommendations, addressing a major unmet need in ASCVD management.
- Efficacy across broad patient subgroups supports use in diverse populations, including those with diabetes, obesity, or chronic kidney disease.
- Favorable safety and tolerability profile facilitates long-term therapy initiation and continuation.

While cardiovascular outcomes were recorded as secondary endpoints, the current follow-up duration and event adjudication do not yet definitively demonstrate clinical event reduction; ongoing larger outcomes trials (e.g., ORION-4) will provide this evidence.

Nevertheless, the LDL-C lowering magnitude achieved matches that associated with cardiovascular event reductions in prior statin and PCSK9 monoclonal antibody outcome trials, providing strong mechanistic support for expected clinical benefit **(Table 2)**.

Comparison with other lipid-lowering agents: Inclisiran's siRNA mechanism offers a novel approach distinct from monoclonal antibodies targeting PCSK9, statins, or ezetimibe.

Key differentiators include: Inclisiran's twice-yearly administration addresses adherence challenges and could broaden utilization among patients unable or unwilling to maintain more frequent injectable therapies.

LIMITATIONS

While the pooled ORION-10 and ORION-11 data offer valuable insights, several limitations merit consideration. These trials were not cardiovascular outcomes trials specifically powered to detect differences in MACE. Event adjudication was based on investigator-reported adverse events rather than blinded endpoint committees, which may affect precision. The median follow-up duration of 18 months may be insufficient to observe the full magnitude of cardiovascular benefit from LDL-C reduction. Larger ongoing cardiovascular outcomes trials (ORION-4 and VICTORION-2 Prevent) with extended follow-up are expected to provide definitive evidence regarding the impact of inclisiran on hard clinical outcomes. The trials included predominantly patients on background statin therapy, which may confound isolated inclisiran effects. Subgroup numbers for some categories (e.g., certain ethnic groups) were relatively small, limiting power for interaction testing. Ultimately, ongoing large outcome trials will clarify the full clinical impact of inclisiran beyond LDL-C lowering.

CONCLUSION

The pooled ORION-10 and ORION-11 analyses confirm that inclisiran provides powerful, consistent, and durable LDL-C reductions in patients with established ASCVD across diverse populations. Twice-yearly subcutaneous dosing delivers LDL-C lowering sufficient to transform guideline LDL-C target attainment rates.

Inclisiran's favorable safety profile and adherence-friendly dosing position it as a promising addition to lipid-lowering therapies for secondary prevention of ASCVD. As the field awaits definitive cardiovascular outcome data from larger ongoing trials, these efficacy data establish a strong foundation for the role of inclisiran in combating residual cardiovascular risk through LDL-C lowering.

REFERENCE

1. Wright RS, Ray KK, Landmesser U, et al. Effects of inclisiran in patients with atherosclerotic cardiovascular disease: a pooled analysis of the ORION-10 and ORION-11 randomized trials. Mayo Clin Proc. 2024;99(8):1222-35.

158

CHAPTER

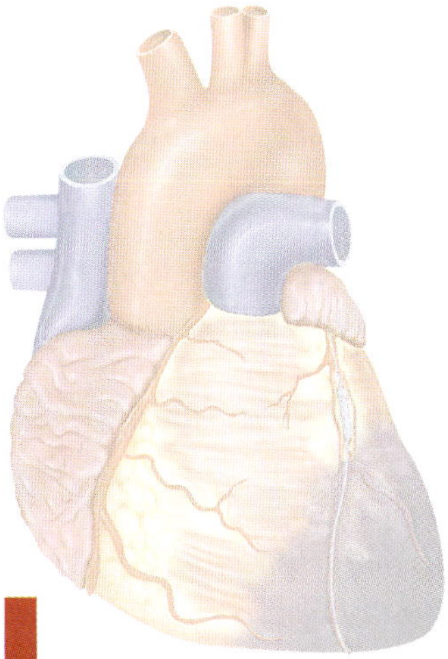

Victorion Initiate in Atherosclerotic Cardiovascular Disease Patients

Mahpaekar Mashhadi, Harsh Chaudhary, Sameer Dani

INTRODUCTION

As the global burden of atherosclerotic cardiovascular diseases (ASCVDs) is on the rise, clinicians and researchers are now more focused on primary and secondary prevention of ASCVD. Historically, treatment focused on statins, with low-density lipoprotein cholesterol (LDL-C) as a primary target, LDL-C ≥70 mg/dL as the threshold for treatment intensification, and nonstatins reserved mainly for statin intolerance or inadequate response. Clinical evidence, based on years of research, has concluded that lower LDL-C is better. The guidelines consider very low LDL-C levels both safe and of continued benefit, explicitly advising against de-escalating high-intensity statin therapy even at low LDL-C concentrations.[1]

Current guidelines recommendations are to achieve LDL-C <70 mg/dL in high risk and <55 mg/dL in very high-risk populations. The same guideline recommends LDL-C <40 mg/dL for the special high-risk group. The recommended therapies to reach the target level goals in the different risk categories of patients are (1) the maximum tolerated dose of statins, and, if the targets are not achieved, (2) the addition of ezetimibe and then (3) proprotein convertase subtilisin/kexin type 9 (PCSK9) inhibitors.[2-5] Real-world studies consistently demonstrate that up to 80% of patients with ASCVD fail to achieve LDL-C goals. Statin intolerance remains a major hurdle in achieving the desired targets.[6]

The VICTORIAN-INITIATE TRIAL determines the effect of adding inclisiran, a small interfering RNA targeting hepatic PCSK9, versus usual care in achieving adequate lipid lowering in patients with ASCVD on maximally tolerated statin therapy or with statin intolerance.

STUDY POPULATION

Patients with established ASCVD and LDL-C ≥70 mg/dL or non–HDL-C ≥100 mg/dL despite maximally tolerated statin therapy alone were randomized in a 1:1 fashion to an "inclisiran-first" (n = 225) or usual care (n = 225) strategy. The experimental group received inclisiran sodium 300 mg subcutaneous injections on days 0, 90, and 270. The usual care arm was prescribed other lipid-lowering therapies (LLTs) at the treating provider's judgment. "Inclisiran first" patients could receive additional LLTs [except monoclonal antibodies (mAbs) directed against PCSK9 (PCSK9 mAbs)], if required, to reach target LDL-C levels. The study only provided inclisiran in the "inclisiran first" arm; patients obtained all other LLTs through their usual health care channels.[7]

INCLUSION CRITERIA

- Age ≥18 years
- Prior ASCVD defined as:
    - *Coronary artery disease:* Myocardial infarction (MI), revascularization, or >70% stenosis in ≥1 epicardial vessel by invasive or computed tomography angiography
    - *Cerebrovascular disease:* Ischemic stroke, carotid artery stenosis >70%, or carotid revascularization

- *Peripheral artery disease:* Resting ankle-brachial index ≤0.85, revascularization at or above the popliteal artery, or nontraumatic amputation
- LDL-C ≥70 mg/dL or non-HDL-C ≥100 mg/dL
- Fasting triglyceride <500 mg/dL
- Maximally tolerated statin dose or no statin with documented side effects to ≥2 statins, including 1 at the lowest available dose
- Estimated glomerular filtration rate >30 mL/min/1.73 m^2

EXCLUSION CRITERIA

- Left ventricular ejection fraction <30%
- New York Heart Association class III-IV heart failure
- Major adverse cardiovascular event (MACE) <6 months prior
- Life expectancy <2 years due to non-ASCVD comorbidities
- Treatment with another PCSK9 inhibitor or ezetimibe <3 months prior
- Active liver disease or aminotransferase levels >3× or total bilirubin >2× upper limit of normal

RESULTS

Coprimary outcomes for inclisiran-first versus usual care at 330 days:

- *Percent change in LDL-C:* −60.0% versus −7.0% ($p < 0.001$)

Secondary outcomes for inclisiran-first versus usual care at 330 days:

- *LDL-C reduction ≥50%:* 69.8% versus 5.3% ($p < 0.001$)
- *LDL-C <70 mg/dL:* 81.8% versus 22.2% ($p < 0.001$)
- *LDL-C <55 mg/dL:* 71.6% versus 8.9% ($p < 0.001$)
- *No background LLT:* 10.2% versus 11.6%
- *Statin-only background LLT:* 88.4% versus 73.4%
- *Treatment-related adverse events for inclisiran-first versus usual care:* 14.5% versus 0.5%
- *Injection site adverse events for inclisiran-first:* 10.3%
- *Composite MACE for inclisiran-first versus usual care at 330 days:* 2.7% versus 2.2%

The overall trial conduct, including screening, randomization, reasons for discontinuation, and study completion in the inclisiran-first and usual care arms, is summarized in **Flowchart 1**.

Inclisiran-first therapy resulted in a significantly greater and sustained reduction in LDL-C compared with usual care across all study time points, as illustrated in **Figures 1A and B**.

Baseline lipid-lowering therapy use, including statin intensity and combination therapy, was well balanced between the two study groups **(Table 1)**.

Flowchart 1: Patient disposition.

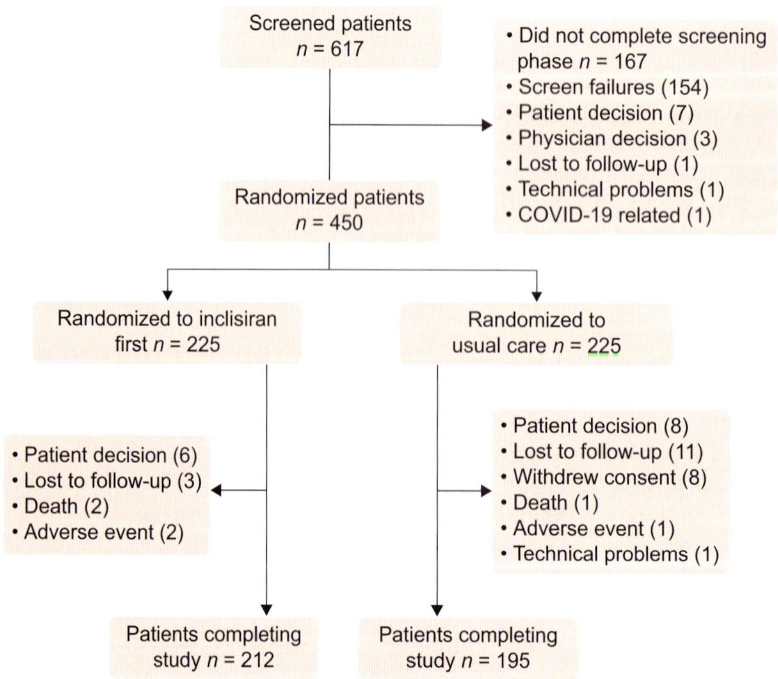

A flowchart of VICTORION-INITIATE patients from screening to study completion.

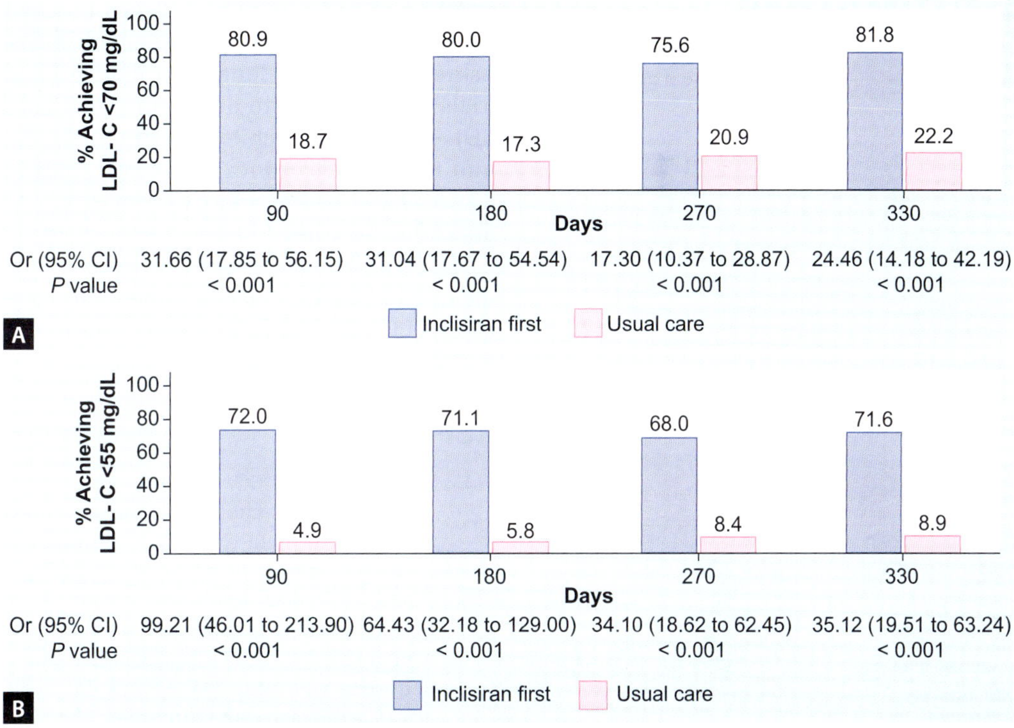

Figs. 1A and B: Inclisiran versus usual care.

TABLE 1: Baseline lipid-lowering therapy.

Lipid-lowering therapy			
Any lipid-lowering therapy—modified definitiond	203 (90.2)	203 (90.2)	406 (90.2)
Any statin therapy: • Statin monotherapye • Statin and ezetimibe	203 (90.2) 202 (89.8) 1 (0.4)	202 (89.8) 198 (88.0) 4 (1.8)	405 (90.0) 400 (88.9) 5 (1.1)
No statins	22 (9.8)	23 (10.2)	45 (10.0)
No concomitant lipid-lowering therapy—modifiedf	22 (9.8)	22 (9.8)	44 (9.8)

LIMITATION AND DISCUSSION

With available results of the trial, inclisiran has ignited new hope for very high-risk ASCVD patients. It seems the molecule will be the game changer for safely achieving the lowest LDL-C targets without many side effects. A large double-blinded RCT is needed to strengthen the finding further. Moreover, achieved lower LDL-C targets results in favorable clinical outcomes need to be studied. MACE rate at 330 days does not show statistically significant difference among the studied groups.

It is worth noticing that at 330 days, among inclisiran first patients, most (88.4%) received only statins as background LLT, and three (1.4%) also received ezetimibe. In the usual care arm (n = 199), most patients received statins alone (73.4%). 20 patients received statins + ezetimibe, five received other combinations including PCSK9 mAbs, and five received PCSK9 mAb monotherapy. It can be translated as in the usual care group, other lipid-lowering drugs were not intensively utilized and intensity of statin use remains identical. <10 patients were treated with PCSK9 inhibitors.

The double-blind placebo control RCT, FOURIER trial, with 27,564 enrolled, showed absolute MACE reduction of 1.5% and absolute LDL-C reduction of 56 mg/dL.[4] A large double-blind RCA comparing inclisiran to PCSK9 inhibitor will provide valuable insight choosing the first line add on molecule to statins. CLEAR-HARMONY trial, a placebo controlled double blind RCT showed 12.6% LDL-C reduction in bempedoic acid group than placebo when added to baseline statin therapy. The use of bempedoic acid in usual care group is 0.5%, which is very low.[5,8] Ezetimibe has shown better LDL-C reduction in combination with statin than statin monotherapy in multiple RCTs.[9] If the usual care group have been extensively treated with ezetimibe, bempedoic acid, or PCSK9 inhibitors, the LDL-C reduction in usual care group would have been different.

SUMMARY ILLUSTRATION

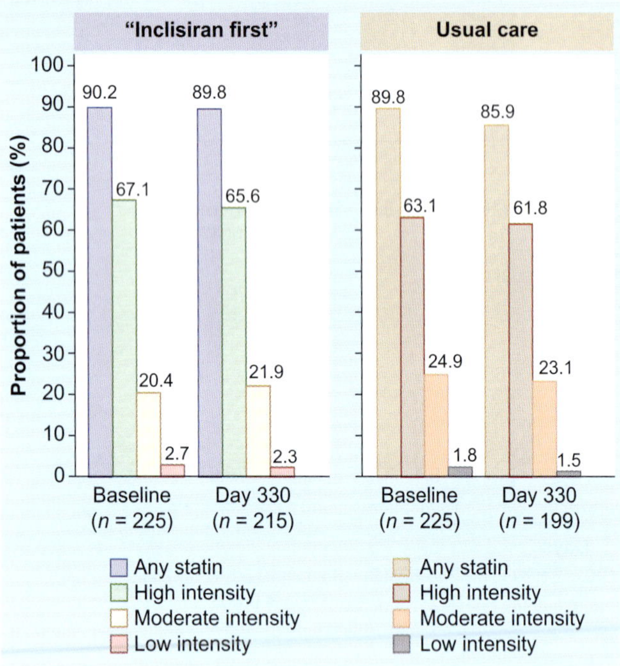

CONCLUSION

The VICTORIAN-INITIATE trial provides strong evidence that an inclisiran-first strategy is highly effective in achieving substantial LDL-C reduction in patients with established ASCVD who remain above guideline-recommended lipid targets despite maximally tolerated statin therapy or who are statin intolerant. Inclisiran resulted in a marked and consistent reduction in LDL-C, with a significantly higher proportion of patients attaining LDL-C goals (<70 mg/dL and <55 mg/dL) compared with usual care, while maintaining an acceptable safety profile.

The study also exposes a significant gap between guideline recommendations and real-world practice, as combination LLTs were underutilized in the usual care arm. This therapeutic inertia likely contributed to suboptimal LDL-C lowering in the control group and highlights the need for simpler, more reliable treatment strategies to improve long-term adherence and goal attainment.

Although no significant difference in short-term MACE was observed, the trial was not designed or powered to assess clinical outcomes. Given the well-established relationship between LDL-C reduction and cardiovascular risk reduction, larger, long-term, double-blind randomized trials are necessary to determine whether the profound LDL-C lowering achieved with inclisiran translates into improved cardiovascular outcomes and to define its optimal position relative to PCSK9 mAbs and other nonstatin therapies.

Overall, inclisiran emerges as a promising and practical therapeutic option that may help to bridge the persistent gap in LDL-C goal achievement among very high-risk ASCVD patients.

REFERENCES

1. Patti G, Spinoni EG, Grisafi L, et al. Safety and efficacy of very low LDL-cholesterol intensive lowering: a meta-analysis and meta-regression of randomized trials. Eur Heart J Cardiovasc Pharmacother. 2023;9(2):138-47.
2. Cannon CP, Blazing MA, Giugliano RP, et al. Ezetimibe Added to Statin Therapy after Acute Coronary Syndromes. N Engl J Med. 2015;372(25):2387-97.
3. Schwartz GG, Steg PG, Szarek M, et al. Alirocumab and Cardiovascular Outcomes after Acute Coronary Syndrome. N Engl J Med. 2018;379(22):2097-107.
4. Sabatine MS, Giugliano RP, Keech AC, et al. Evolocumab and Clinical Outcomes in Patients with Cardiovascular Disease. N Engl J Med. 2017 May 4;376(18):1713-22.
5. Ray KK, Bays HE, Catapano AL, et al. Safety and Efficacy of Bempedoic Acid to Reduce LDL Cholesterol. N Engl J Med. 2019;380(11):1022-32.
6. Ray KK, Haq I, Bilitou A, et al. Treatment gaps in the implementation of LDL cholesterol control among high- and very high-risk patients in Europe between 2020 and 2021: the multinational observational SANTORINI study. Lancet Reg Health Eur. 2023;29:100624.
7. Leosdottir M, Schubert J, Brandts J, et al. Early Ezetimibe Initiation After Myocardial Infarction Protects Against Later Cardiovascular Outcomes in the SWEDEHEART Registry. J Am Coll Cardiol. 2025;85(15):1550-64.
8. Nissen SE, Lincoff AM, Brennan D, et al. Bempedoic Acid and Cardiovascular Outcomes in Statin-Intolerant Patients. N Engl J Med. 2023;388(15):1353-64.
9. Morrone D, Weintraub WS, Toth PP, et al. Lipid-altering efficacy of ezetimibe plus statin and statin monotherapy and identification of factors associated with treatment response: a pooled analysis of over 21,000 subjects from 27 clinical trials. Atherosclerosis. 2012;223(2):251-61.

159

CHAPTER

Inclisiran with Standard Care Provides Rapid, Sustained Lowering of LDL-C in Patients with Recent Acute Coronary Syndrome with Insignificant LDL Variability

Harinder K Bali, Navdeep S Sidhu

INTRODUCTION

Cardiovascular diseases (CVDs) are the leading cause of global mortality. Atherosclerotic cardiovascular disease (ASCVD) accounts for nearly two thirds of all CVD cases, and acute coronary syndromes (ACSs) account for the major chunk of ASCVD-related mortality and morbidity.[1] Apo-B containing lipoproteins, particularly the low-density lipoprotein cholesterol (LDL-C), has been unequivocally established as the most important causal factor in the genesis and progression of atherosclerosis. The atherosclerotic effects of LDL-C are likely related to both the levels of serum LDL-C and the duration of these levels. The burden of atherosclerosis may be expressed in terms of "cholesterol-years" or "LDL-C years," similar to the concept of "pack-years" for smoking. It has been postulated that when this reaches a critical threshold, the clinical manifestations of ASCVD become evident.[2-4] Nevertheless, this threshold can be modified by various factors; with other atherogenic factors such as diabetes mellitus, hypertension, smoking, and family history reducing it, and life-long healthy lifestyle and persistently low levels of LDL-C elevating it.[5]

FROM "THE LOWER THE BETTER" TO "THE SOONER, THE LOWER, THE BETTER" IN ACUTE CORONARY SYNDROME

The patients with ACS are at elevated risk of recurrent ischemic events early after the index event, underscoring the need to rapidly achieve low LDL-C levels and to maintain these low LDL-C levels over the long run.[6] Intensive LDL-C lowering in these patients has been shown to reduce cardiovascular mortality and morbidity and the degree of benefit is proportional to the degree of LDL-C lowering, up to very low LDL-C levels.[7] Various guidelines recommend aggressive lowering of LDL-C in ACS patients to levels of <55 mg/dL, and to <40 mg/dL or even lower in those with recurrent events.[8-10] A step-wise approach has traditionally been recommended for LDL-C lowering in ACS, with high-intensity statins being the initial drug, with subsequent addition of other drugs such as ezetimibe, protein convertase subtilisin/kexin type 9 inhibitors (PCSK9i), or bempedoic acid. Nevertheless, data from registries and many observational studies have indicated that majority of ACS patients fail to reach target LDL-C levels with high-intensity therapy alone and are at persistent risk of avoidable recurrent events, particularly in the early weeks after discharge.[11-14] Thus, it has been proposed that in addition to the strategy of "lower is better"; an additional approach of "strike early and strong" needs to be incorporated into the clinical practice for mitigating the risk of recurrent events in patients with very-high ASCVD, like ACS.[6,15,16]

LIPID-LOWERING THERAPY REGIMENS IN ACUTE CORONARY SYNDROME

Statins are the foundation of lipid-lowering therapy (LLT) regimens and have a large body of evidence over many decades to support their use in ASCVD. Hence, the use of these drugs as the first component of any LLT is widely accepted. Acknowledging the recent observational data regarding the inability to achieve target LDL-C levels in high- or very-high risk ASCVD patients like those with ACS, the recent guidelines support the use of ezetimibe along with high-intensity statin therapy in these patients as an upfront combination therapy.[8,9] Oral combination LLT (high intensity statin + ezetimibe ± bempedoic acid) is capable of reducing the LDL-C levels by 60–70%, but this may not be sufficient for reducing the CV risk in patients with very high baseline LDL-C, or those who are at extremely high risk due to recurrent CV events or polyvascular disease. In these patients, a combination of oral LLT and subcutaneous PCSK9i may be able to reduce LDL-C levels by >80% and provide early stabilization of atherosclerotic plaques and freedom from recurrent events.[9,17] Also, PCSK9i may be useful in patients who are intolerant to statins with or without combination with ezetimibe and/or bempedoic acid.[8-10]

PCSK-9i therapy includes monoclonal antibodies (MoAbs) against PCSK9 (evolocumab, alirocumab) and the newer first-in-class small-interfering RNA (siRNA)—inclisiran.[17]

INCLISIRAN

Inclisiran is a double-stranded (ds) siRNA which functions in the cytoplasm of hepatocytes to block the synthesis of PCSK9 protein **(Fig. 1)**.[18]

The nucleotides in inclisiran are conjugated to *N*-acetylgalactosamine (GalNAc) which bind to asialoglycoprotein receptors (ASGPRs), predominantly expressed on the hepatocytes. Hence, the action of inclisiran is very specific to liver, the predominant site for PCSK9 synthesis. Inclisiran cleaves the PCSK9 mRNA by binding and activating RNA-induced silencing complex (RISC). The RISC is a multicomponent protein complex which can facilitate the silencing of almost an mRNA when suitably activated. Inclisiran can remain associated with RISC for a long time, thus providing continuous blockage of PCSK9 mRNA and hence a prolonged duration of action.[17]

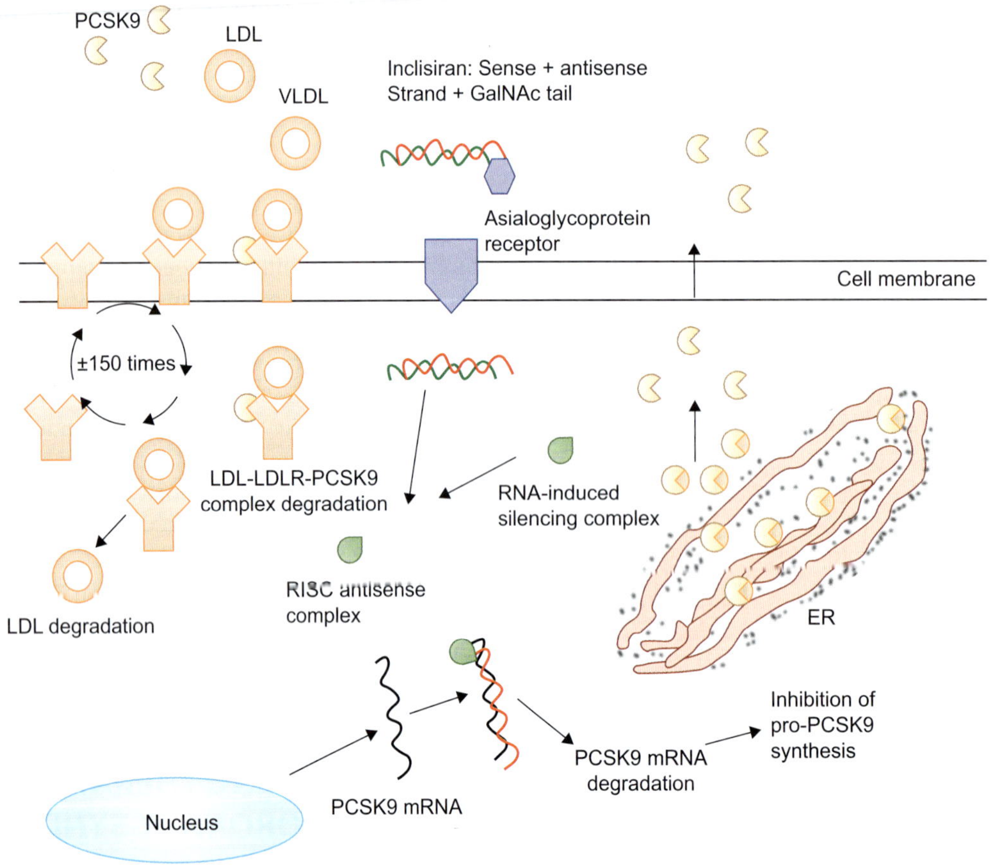

Fig. 1: The mechanism of action of inclisiran in the hepatocytes. (GalNAc: *N*-acetylgalactosamine; LDL: low-density lipoprotein; LDL-R: LDL receptor; PCSK9: protein convertase subtilisin/kexin type 9; RISC: RNA-induced silencing complex; RNA: ribonucleic acid; VLDL: very low density lipoprotein).

Source: Used as original from Wołowiec et al.'s[18] study, under https://creativecommons.org/licenses/by/4.0/.

Decreased levels of PCSK9 lead to upregulation of LDL receptors in the liver, which by enhancing the clearance of circulating LDL-C lead to sustained low LDL-C levels.[19]

Comparison with Monoclonal Antibodies (Evolocumab, Alirocumab)

The action of inclisiran by inhibiting hepatic PCSK9 synthesis (70–80% of total, other sites being intestine, kidney, lung, pancreas, or brain) contrasts with that of MoAbs such as evolocumab and alirocumab, which target the circulating plasma PCSK9 protein. Although the action on only the hepatic component of PCSK9 may marginally lower the efficacy of inclisiran as compared to MoAbs (45–55% LDL-C lowering vs. 50–60% with MoAbs), the longer duration of action of inclisiran (6 months vs. days to weeks of MoAbs) results in a longer interval between doses and in sustained low LDL-C levels with little variability.[17,19] The target action of inclisiran on hepatocytes limits the systemic exposure to the drug and has less potential for systemic side effects. Hence, most of the adverse events are related to the injection site and are mild and self-limiting.[20]

Both MoAbs and inclisiran can be useful in rapidly achieving the target LDL-C levels after ACS; however, inclisiran offers a more convenient dosing and enhanced compliance as it requires subcutaneous injections every 6 months (after two initial doses at 0 and 90 days), as compared to the requirement of subcutaneous injections of MoAbs every 2–4 weeks. Hence, inclisiran is particularly useful in high-risk patients like ACS, who have adherence issues or who have limited access to medical facilities.[20] On the other hand, MoAbs have a quicker onset of action as they act immediately on the circulating PCSK9 to block its action and hence may be suitable for patients requiring very rapid lowering of LDL-C levels.[20]

LIPID VARIABILITY AND ATHEROSCLEROSIS

Lipid variability, the fluctuating levels of serum lipoproteins (particularly LDL-C) between the hospital visits, is an emerging lipid biomarker for atherosclerosis progression and major adverse cardiovascular events (MACE).[21] In the absence of unified definition, it is usually assessed in terms of standard deviation (SD), average successive variability (ASV, the absolute difference in subsequent measurements), coefficient of variation (CV), or variability independent of mean (VIM). Enhanced LDL-C variability can alter the composition and structure of the atherosclerotic plaques and increase the chances of plaque instability and rupture, with subsequent clinical events like ACS.[22,23] In a post hoc analysis of TNT (treating to new targets) trial of 9,572 patients with known coronary artery disease (CAD), each 1-SD increment in LDL-C variability was associated with 16% increased risk of any coronary event, a 10% increase in the risk of myocardial infarction (MI) and a 23% increase in the risk of mortality; independently of achieved LDL-C levels.[24] A post hoc analysis of nine clinical trials (total 4,976 patients) with serial coronary intravascular ultrasound (IVUS) examinations, high lipid variability was associated with progression in atheroma volume and worse clinical outcomes.[25]

CLINICAL DATA REGARDING INCLISIRAN IN ACUTE CORONARY SYNDROME

The safety and efficacy of inclisiran have been evaluated in the ORION and VICTORION clinical trial programs with more than two dozen studies. Initially tested in patients with heterozygous familial hypercholesterolemia or stable ASCVD, it is being increasingly tested in the ACS population including the novel strategy of "inclisiran-first" in this population.

In a post hoc analysis of ORION-10 and ORION-11 trials in patients (N = 3,178) with non-ACS ASCVD or ASVCD equivalents (type 2 diabetes, familial hypercholesterolemia, or ≥20% risk of CV event over 10 years by the Framingham risk score or its equivalent), inclisiran administration resulted in effective and sustained reduction in LDL-C levels irrespective of the background LLT without any major safety concerns.[26] In the VICTORION-INITIATE trial exploring the "inclisiran first" strategy in ASCVD patients (adding it immediately on failure to reach LDL-C <70 mg/dL on maximally tolerated statin dose), the results showed greater LDL-C reductions than the usual care.[27]

The data regarding the clinical utility of inclisiran in the realm of ACS setting is rapidly emerging with exciting developments likely in the near future. In a prospective, single-center pilot study (IRIDE-1 Registry) by Lupi et al.,[28] 16 patients admitted with ACS and having high baseline LDL-C levels (mean 147.2 mg/dL) were started on inclisiran in the acute setting besides the usual care with high-intensity atorvastatin and ezetimibe. This resulted in reduction of mean LDL-C levels to 30.3 mg/dL at 30 days and levels of LDL-C <55 mg/dL were obtained in 73% of the patients at day 15 and in 100% of the patients at day 30, with no major side effects.[28]

The VICTORION-INCEPTION, a multicentric, randomized, open-label, parallel group trial, included 400 patients with recent ACS (within 5 weeks before screening, median time from discharge: 34 days) with LDL-C levels ≥70 mg/dL or non-HDL-C ≥100 mg/dL.

Patients were randomized 1:1 to inclisiran (300 mg on days 0, 90, and 270) plus usual care versus usual care alone. At day 330, the LDL-C levels were reduced by 45.6% in the inclisiran arm versus an increase of 1.4% in the usual care arm (least squares mean difference of –46.9% [97.5% CI: –55.4 to –38.5]; $p < 0.001$). The proportion of patients achieving LDL-C levels <70 mg/dL was significantly greater in the inclisiran arm (66.7% vs. 28.1%; OR: 5.42 [97.5% CI: 3.29–8.91]; $p < 0.001$). No serious adverse events were noted with the use of inclisiran.[29] These studies show the immense potential of inclisiran as a novel therapy to improve CV outcomes in ACS patients by achieving an early and sustained lowering of LDL-C levels.

The results of large trials assessing the effect of inclisiran therapy on cardiovascular outcomes including MACE are eagerly awaited.[20] Also, the cost-effectiveness of inclisiran therapy needs to be critically considered before its wider adoption into diverse healthcare systems across different countries.

CONCLUSION

Inclisiran, a potent siRNA inhibiting the production of PCSK9 has been shown to achieve effective and sustained lowering of LDL-C levels in patients with ASCVD, including ACS. It is a promising drug in this population with robust data regarding CV outcomes likely to emerge in the near future.

REFERENCES

1. Mensah GA, Fuster V, Murray CJ, et al.; Global Burden of Cardiovascular Diseases and Risks Collaborators. Global burden of cardiovascular diseases and risks, 1990–2022. J Am Coll Cardiol. 2023;82:2350-473.
2. Shapiro MD, Bhatt DL. "Cholesterol-Years" for ASCVD risk prediction and treatment. J Am Coll Cardiol. 2020;76(13):1517-20.
3. Horton JD, Cohen JC, Hobbs HH. PCSK9: a convertase that coordinates LDL catabolism. J Lipid Res. 2009;50 Suppl(Suppl):S172-7.
4. Braunwald E. How to live to 100 before developing clinical coronary artery disease: a suggestion. Eur Heart J. 2022;43(4):249-50.
5. Ference BA, Yoo W, Alesh I, et al. Effect of long-term exposure to lower low-density lipoprotein cholesterol beginning early in life on the risk of coronary heart disease: a Mendelian randomization analysis. J Am Coll Cardiol. 2012;60(25):2631-9.
6. Gargiulo P, Ray KK, Perrone-Filardi P. Combination lipid-lowering strategies after acute coronary syndrome: reconsidering cholesterol targets. Eur Heart J. 2025:ehaf615.
7. Sabatine MS, Wiviott SD, Im K, et al. Efficacy and safety of further lowering of low-density lipoprotein cholesterol in patients starting with very low levels: a meta-analysis. JAMA Cardiol. 2018;3(9):823-8.
8. Rao SV, O'Donoghue ML, Ruel M, et al. 2025 ACC/AHA/ACEP/NAEMSP/SCAI guideline for the management of patients with acute coronary syndromes: a report of the American College of Cardiology/American Heart Association Joint Committee on Clinical Practice Guidelines. Circulation. 2025;151(13):e771-862.
9. Mach F, Koskinas KC, Roeters van Lennep JE, et al.; ESC/EAS Scientific Document Group. 2025 focused update of the 2019 ESC/EAS guidelines for the management of dyslipidaemias. Eur Heart J. 2025;ehaf190.
10. Puri R, Bansal M, Mehta V, et al. Lipid Association of India 2023 update on cardiovascular risk assessment and lipid management in Indian patients: Consensus statement IV. J Clin Lipidol. 2024;18(3):e351-73.
11. Ray KK, Haq I, Bilitou A, et al; SANTORINI Study Investigators. Treatment gaps in the implementation of LDL cholesterol control among high- and very high-risk patients in Europe between 2020 and 2021: the multinational observational SANTORINI study. Lancet Reg Health Eur. 2023;29:100624.
12. McEvoy JW, Jennings C, Kotseva K, et al. Variation in secondary prevention of coronary heart disease: the INTERASPIRE study. Eur Heart J. 2024;45(39):4184-96.
13. Ray KK, Molemans B, Schoonen WM, et al; DA VINCI study. EU-wide cross-sectional observational study of lipid-modifying therapy use in secondary and primary care: the DA VINCI study. Eur J Prev Cardiol. 2021;28(11):1279-89.
14. Jain M, Sawant R, Panchal H, et al. Evaluating LDL-C control in Indian acute coronary syndrome (ACS) patients—a retrospective real-world study LDL-C control in ACS. Int J Cardiol Cardiovasc Risk Prev. 2023;19:200210.
15. Parhofer KG, Aguiar C, Banach M, et al. Expert opinion on the integration of combination therapy into the treatment algorithm for the management of dyslipidaemia: the integration of ezetimibe and bempedoic acid may enhance goal attainment. Eur Heart J Cardiovasc Pharmacother. 2025;11(4):367-79.
16. Pogran E, Burger AL, Zweiker D, et al. Lipid-lowering therapy after acute coronary syndrome. J Clin Med. 2024;13(7):2043.
17. Di Giacomo-Barbagallo F, Andreychuk N, Scicali R, et al. Reasons for a novel agent in a crowded therapeutic field. Curr Atheroscler Rep. 2025;27(1):25.
18. Wołowiec Ł, Osiak J, Wołowiec A, et al. Inclisiran-safety and effectiveness of small interfering RNA in inhibition of PCSK-9. Pharmaceutics. 2023;15(2):323.
19. Soffer D, Stoekenbroek R, Plakogiannis R. Small interfering ribonucleic acid for cholesterol lowering—inclisiran: inclisiran for cholesterol lowering. J Clin Lipidol. 2022;16(5):574-82.
20. Harbi MH. Current usage of inclisiran for cardiovascular diseases: overview of current clinical trials. Front Pharmacol. 2025;16:1449712.
21. Li S, Hou L, Zhu S, et al. Lipid variability and risk of cardiovascular diseases and all-cause mortality: a systematic review and meta-analysis of cohort studies. Nutrients. 2022;14(12):2450.

22. Nakano S, Otake H, Kawamori H, et al. Association between visit-to-visit variability in low-density lipoprotein cholesterol and plaque rupture that leads to acute coronary syndrome. Circ Rep. 2021;3(9):540-9.
23. Manemann SM, Bielinski SJ, Moser ED, et al. Variability in lipid levels and risk for cardiovascular disease: an electronic health record-based population cohort study. J Am Heart Assoc. 2023;12(5):e027639.
24. Bangalore S, Breazna A, DeMicco DA, et al; TNT Steering Committee and Investigators. Visit-to-visit low-density lipoprotein cholesterol variability and risk of cardiovascular outcomes: insights from the TNT trial. J Am Coll Cardiol. 2015;65(15):1539-48.
25. Clark D 3rd, Nicholls SJ, St John J, et al. Visit-to-visit cholesterol variability correlates with coronary atheroma progression and clinical outcomes. Eur Heart J. 2018;39(27):2551-8.
26. Landmesser U, Koenig W, Leiter LA, et al. Efficacy and safety of inclisiran based on background lipid-lowering treatment. Eur J Prev Cardiol. 2025;zwaf214.
27. Koren MJ, Rodriguez F, East C, et al. An "Inclisiran First" strategy vs usual care in patients with atherosclerotic cardiovascular disease. J Am Coll Cardiol. 2024;83(20):1939-52.
28. Lupi A, Baluci M, Persampieri S, et al. Inclisiran for fast-track lipid-lowering treatment early after an acute coronary syndrome: a pilot study. Atherosclerosis Plus. 2025;62:9-14.
29. Knowlton K, Navar AM, Anderson J, et al. LDL-C management with inclisiran plus usual care vs usual care alone in participants with recent acute coronary syndrome: VICTORION-INCEPTION. J Clin Lipidol. 2025;19(3):e109-10.

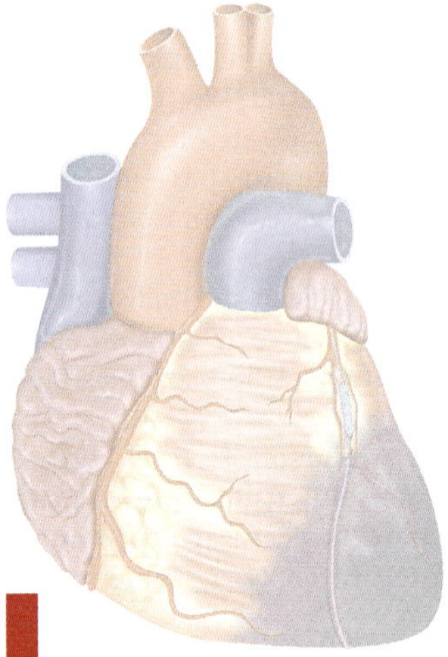

160

CHAPTER

Current Status of Usefulness of Inclisiran for Cardiovascular Diseases

Abhishek Garg, Akash Batta, Gurpreet Singh Wander

INTRODUCTION

Cardiovascular disease (CVD) remains the leading cause of death globally, imposing an immense health and economic burden.[1] Lipid-lowering therapy is one of the most effective interventions for reducing cardiovascular risk, with numerous clinical studies confirming a direct relationship between lowering low-density lipoprotein cholesterol (LDL-C) and reducing cardiovascular events.[1]

Current international guidelines emphasize intensive LDL-C reduction, particularly in high-risk populations. The 2019 European Society of Cardiology/European Atherosclerosis Society (ESC/EAS)[2] dyslipidemia guidelines recommend achieving at least a 50% reduction from baseline and an LDL-C goal of <55 mg/dL for secondary prevention, while the 2018 American College of Cardiology/American Heart Association (ACC/AHA) guidelines[3] advise the addition of nonstatin therapies when LDL-C remains above 70 mg/dL despite statin therapy. Despite these clear recommendations, real-world data highlight substantial treatment gaps. The DA VINCI study[4] and EUROASPIRE V survey[5] revealed that only about half of patients with established atherosclerotic cardiovascular disease (ASCVD) in Europe received high-intensity statins, and fewer than half achieved an LDL-C target of <70 mg/dL. This shows both undertreatment and the challenge of achieving guideline-directed lipid goals in clinical practice.

Statins remain the first-line therapy, with ezetimibe and proprotein convertase subtilisin/kexin type 9 (PCSK9) inhibitors as adjunctive agents.[1] However, many patients continue to struggle to reach optimal LDL-C levels, largely due to issues such as poor adherence, drug intolerance, treatment costs, and the need for frequent dosing.[1] Importantly, inadequate adherence to statin therapy has been consistently associated with increased cardiovascular morbidity, mortality, and overall mortality risk.[1]

The discovery of PCSK9 in 2003 marked a turning point in lipid biology.[1] This serine protease promotes lysosomal degradation of LDL receptor (LDL-R), leading to higher plasma LDL-C levels, and has since become a major therapeutic target.[1] PCSK9 monoclonal antibodies are already approved for patients with persistent hypercholesterolemia despite maximally tolerated statins, while other PCSK9-directed modalities—including small interfering RNA (siRNA), small-molecule inhibitors, and adnectins—are under ongoing evaluation.[1]

Inclisiran, a novel long-acting siRNA therapy, acts within hepatocytes to silence PCSK9 synthesis, thereby increasing LDL-R recycling and expression on the cell surface.[1] This results in significant and sustained reductions in circulating LDL-C levels with an infrequent, twice-yearly dosing regimen.[1]

This review aims to critically evaluate current clinical evidence regarding inclisiran and its emerging role in the management of CVD.

STRUCTURE AND FUNCTION OF INCLISIRAN

Inclisiran is a synthetic siRNA therapeutic designed to target hepatic production of PCSK9 specifically.[6] siRNAs exert their effect by binding to messenger RNA sequences that are complementary to their nucleotide structure, leading to selective degradation of the target mRNA through the RNA-induced silencing complex.[6] This catalytic mechanism prevents translation of PCSK9, thereby reducing circulating levels of the protein.

By suppressing PCSK9 synthesis, inclisiran enhances the recycling and surface expression of LDL-R on hepatocytes.[6] The upregulation of LDL-R results in increased clearance of LDL-C from the plasma, leading to substantial and sustained reductions in LDL-C concentrations.[6]

The first clinical evaluation of inclisiran was conducted in a phase 1 trial[7] involving healthy volunteers with baseline LDL-C ≥100 mg/dL. Participants received subcutaneous inclisiran as either a single or multiple dose. Results demonstrated that doses of ≥300 mg, whether administered once or in repeated regimens, produced marked and durable reductions in LDL-C and PCSK9 levels for at least 6 months. Notably, multiple-dose regimens achieved up to a 59.7% reduction in LDL-C and an 83.8% reduction in PCSK9 from baseline by day 84.[7] Safety findings from this early trial were favorable, with no serious adverse events reported. The most frequently observed adverse events were mild and included cough, musculoskeletal discomfort, nasopharyngitis, headache, back pain, and diarrhea.[7]

INCLISIRAN IN CARDIOVASCULAR DISEASE

The ORION clinical trial program (as summarized in **Table 1**) was designed to evaluate the efficacy, safety, and long-term tolerability of inclisiran across diverse patient populations, including those at high risk of ASCVD, individuals with established ASCVD, and patients with familial hypercholesterolemia (FH). In addition to assessing lipid-lowering effects, the program investigates inclisiran impact on cardiovascular risk markers and overall safety.[1]

ORION-1, a phase 2, multicenter, double-blind, placebo-controlled trial,[8] enrolled 501 high-risk participants with raised LDL-C. The mean age was 63 years, 65% were male, 69% had established ASCVD, and 6% had FH. Most participants (73%) were on statin therapy. Participants were randomized to receive single or two-dose regimens of inclisiran (100–500 mg) or placebo. At day 180, LDL-C reductions ranged from 27.9 to 41.9%

TABLE 1: Summary of inclisiran trials.

Trial	Design	Participants	Intervention	Key findings
Fitzgerald et al.[7]	Phase 1, randomized, placebo-controlled	Men/women, 18–75 years, LDL-C ≥100 mg/dL	Single or multiple ascending doses (25–800 mg)	LDL-C ↓ up to 60.6%; PCSK9 ↓ up to 83.8%; sustained effect; no major adverse events
ORION 1[8]	Phase 2, multicenter, double-blind	501 patients, LDL-C ≥70 mg/dL (with ASCVD) or ≥100 mg/dL	Single or two doses (200–500 mg)	LDL-C ↓ 27.9–41.9% (single dose) and 35.5–52.6% (two doses); best with 300 mg; well tolerated
ORION-3[10]	Phase 2, open-label extension	490 prior ORION-1 participants	300 mg twice yearly versus evolocumab	LDL-C ↓ 51%, PCSK9 ↓ 77%; sustained effect for ~3 years; safety maintained
ORION-10[11]	Phase 3, double-blind, placebo-controlled	1,561 adults with ASCVD, LDL-C ≥70 mg/dL	Inclisiran 284 mg versus placebo (q6 months)	LDL-C ↓ 52.3%; adverse events mild; injection-site reactions more frequent
ORION-11[11]	Phase 3, double-blind, placebo-controlled	1,617 adults with ASCVD or risk equivalent, LDL-C ≥70–100 mg/dL	Inclisiran 284 mg versus placebo (q6 months)	LDL-C ↓ 49.9%; consistent safety; injection-site reactions more frequent
ORION-9[12]	Phase 3, double-blind, placebo-controlled	482 adults with HeFH, LDL-C ≥100 mg/dL on maximal therapy	Inclisiran 300 mg versus placebo	LDL-C ↓ 39.7%; safety profile similar to placebo
ORION-4[15] (Ongoing)	Phase 3, double-blind, placebo-controlled	15,000 adults ≥55 years with ASCVD	Inclisiran 300 mg versus placebo (q6 months)	Completion expected long-term follow-up until 2049

(ASCVD: atherosclerotic cardiovascular disease; HeFH: heterozygous familial hypercholesterolemia; LDL-C: low-density lipoprotein cholesterol; PCSK9: proprotein convertase subtilisin/kexin type 9; q6 months: every 6 months) after a single dose and 35.5–52.6% following two doses, with the greatest reduction observed with the two-dose 300 mg regimen.[8] This regimen also significantly reduced PCSK9 (−69.1%) and high-sensitivity C-reactive protein (hsCRP) levels (−16.7%). Serious adverse events were comparable between the inclisiran (11%) and placebo (8%) groups, with mild injection-site reactions occurring in 4–7% of patients.[8] Importantly, reductions in LDL-C were consistent regardless of baseline diabetes status, without clinically meaningful changes in glycated hemoglobin (HbA1c).[8]

Follow-up data from ORION-1 indicated that a two-dose regimen of 300 mg inclisiran maintained approximately 50% LDL-C reduction for 6 months, with sustained reductions in time-averaged LDL-C over 1 year. These findings highlighted the potential of inclisiran as a twice-yearly therapy for hypercholesterolemia.[9]

ORION-3, an open-label extension of ORION-1, confirmed the durability of the lipid-lowering effect over 22 months. Mean LDL-C was reduced by 51%, and PCSK9 by 77% at day 210. Over a 3-year follow-up, safety remained favorable, with no significant laboratory abnormalities or adverse changes in liver or renal function.[10]

The phase 3 trials ORION-10 and ORION-11 evaluated inclisiran in adults with ASCVD or high cardiovascular risk in the United States, Europe, and South Africa. Patients received 284 mg subcutaneous injections on day 1, day 90, and every 6 months for 18 months. Baseline LDL-C levels were 104.7 mg/dL (ORION-10) and 105.5 mg/dL (ORION-11). At day 510, inclisiran reduced LDL-C by 52.3% (ORION-10) and 49.9% (ORION-11), while PCSK9 levels declined by 69.8 and 63.6%, respectively. Secondary lipid parameters, including total cholesterol, apolipoprotein B, non-HDL-C, triglycerides, and Lp(a), also improved, with modest increases in HDL-C. Injection-site reactions were more frequent with inclisiran but were mild and transient. No significant differences in diabetes incidence were observed.[11]

ORION-9 focused on adults with heterozygous FH on maximally tolerated statin therapy. Participants (n = 482) received subcutaneous inclisiran 300 mg or placebo on days 1, 90, 270, and 450. At day 510, LDL-C decreased by 39.7% with inclisiran versus an 8.2% increase in the placebo group, with a between-group difference of −47.9% (p <0.001). PCSK9 levels fell by 60.7% with inclisiran versus a 17.7% increase in placebo (p <0.001). The time-averaged LDL-C reduction between days 90 and 540 was −44.3% (p < 0.001), consistent across FH genotypes.[12]

Collectively, these trials demonstrate that inclisiran provides robust and sustained LDL-C and PCSK9 reduction across a variety of high-risk cardiovascular populations, with a favorable safety profile and the convenience of a twice-yearly dosing schedule.

On the other hand, the ORION-5 study was a multicenter, double-blind, placebo-controlled, open-label trial designed to assess the efficacy, safety, and tolerability of inclisiran in patients with homozygous familial hypercholesterolemia (HoFH). This trial provides further insights into the role of inclisiran in this particularly high-risk population.[13]

A meta-analysis pooling data from three randomized clinical trials with a total of 3,660 participants demonstrated that inclisiran significantly reduced LDL-C by 51% compared with placebo (p <0.001). In addition, reductions were observed in total cholesterol (−37%), apolipoprotein B (−41%), and non-HDL cholesterol (−45%), all of which were statistically significant (p <0.001).[14] Importantly, inclisiran use was associated with a 24% relative reduction in the risk of major adverse cardiovascular events (MACE). Safety outcomes were comparable between the inclisiran and placebo groups, with no meaningful differences in liver function tests or creatine kinase levels. Mild injection-site reactions occurred more frequently with inclisiran but were generally transient and well-tolerated.[14]

Despite these encouraging findings, long-term cardiovascular outcome data are still required to confirm the clinical benefit of inclisiran. The ORION-4 trial[15] is currently underway to address this knowledge gap. This large, phase 3, double-blind, placebo-controlled trial is enrolling approximately 15,000 participants aged 55 years or older with established ASCVD across ~180 centers in the United Kingdom and the United States.[15] Participants are randomized in a 1:1 ratio to receive subcutaneous inclisiran sodium 300 mg or placebo at baseline, 3 months, and every 6 months thereafter, with a planned median follow-up of 5 years. The primary endpoint is the time to first occurrence of a composite of coronary artery disease, death, myocardial infarction, fatal or nonfatal ischemic stroke, or urgent coronary revascularization. Secondary endpoints include CHD death or myocardial infarction, as well as overall cardiovascular mortality.[15]

The results of ORION-4 are expected to provide critical evidence on whether the LDL-C–lowering efficacy of inclisiran translates into meaningful reductions in cardiovascular morbidity and mortality, thereby shaping its future role in ASCVD management.

ADVERSE EFFECTS OF INCLISIRAN

Clinical trial evidence indicates that inclisiran is generally safe and well-tolerated. Across the ORION trials, adverse events were reported at similar frequencies in both treatment and placebo groups. No drug-related serious adverse events were identified.[16] The majority of adverse events were mild to moderate, including headache, cough, myalgia, musculoskeletal pain, nasopharyngitis, dizziness, mild rash, and localized skin hyperpigmentation.[8] In the pooled safety analysis of ORION-9, -10, and -11 trials, which involved 3,655 participants, the overall safety profile of inclisiran was comparable to placebo during 18 months of follow-up.[16] The main difference observed was a higher incidence of injection-site reactions with inclisiran (5.0 vs. 0.7%), which were typically mild and transient.[16] Similarly, the ORION-3 extension trial, with a 4-year follow-up, confirmed a favorable and sustained safety profile consistent with earlier studies.[16]

A network meta-analysis of PCSK9 inhibitors ranked inclisiran as the agent with the lowest association with serious adverse events. Importantly, neither inclisiran nor monoclonal antibody-based PCSK9 inhibitors were linked to increased risks of new-onset diabetes or neurocognitive dysfunction. Moreover, hematological abnormalities were not observed in inclisiran trials, despite earlier concerns from other gene-silencing therapies that had been associated with thrombocytopenia.[16]

While these findings reinforce the overall safety of inclisiran, most data are derived from relatively short-term follow-up. Long-term studies are warranted to fully characterize its risk profile. Recent genetic meta-analyses have suggested that exposure to LDL-C–lowering genetic variants may increase susceptibility to type 2 diabetes, raising the possibility of future metabolic concerns with inclisiran.

EXPECTATIONS AND CHALLENGES OF INCLISIRAN THERAPY

One of the most compelling advantages of inclisiran is its infrequent dosing schedule. Administered twice yearly by a healthcare professional, it offers a practical solution to the problem of poor adherence, which is common with daily oral therapies and the biweekly or monthly injections required for PCSK9 monoclonal antibodies.[16] This simplified regimen is particularly beneficial for patients with adherence challenges or those unable to self-administer injections. Furthermore, exploratory data suggest that even annual dosing may provide clinically meaningful LDL-C reduction.[16]

Despite these benefits, several challenges limit the widespread adoption of inclisiran. Foremost among these is cost. Current pricing—approximately USD 3,250 per dose or USD 6,500 annually—exceeds the cost-effectiveness benchmarks suggested by the Institute for Clinical and Economic Review (USD 3,600–6,000 per year).[16] This pricing structure could create significant financial strain for both patients and healthcare systems, similar to the barriers faced with PCSK9 monoclonal antibodies.[16] Broader utilization will likely depend on cost reductions to ensure accessibility for high-risk populations.

Another critical limitation is the absence of definitive cardiovascular outcome data. Although meta-analyses of ORION-9, -10, and -11 trials suggest a potential 24–30% reduction in MACE, these remain projections. The results of ORION-4, a large outcomes trial, are awaited to confirm whether inclisiran provides clinical benefits comparable to or greater than existing PCSK9 inhibitors. Additionally, while current safety data from ORION trials indicate a favorable profile, follow-up duration has been relatively short. The ongoing ORION-8 extension study, providing up to three additional years of observation, is expected to clarify long-term safety.

Finally, as inclisiran represents the first siRNA-based therapy targeting PCSK9, careful postmarketing surveillance will be essential to detect rare or delayed adverse effects. Demonstrating robust long-term safety over decades will be crucial for patient and physician confidence and for inclisiran integration into standard lipid-lowering practice.

RELEVANCE OF INCLISIRAN IN THE INDIAN CLINICAL SETTING

The relevance of inclisiran in India is particularly compelling given the country's unique cardiovascular risk profile and systemic healthcare challenges. India has an enormous burden of premature atherosclerotic CVD, with patients often presenting a decade earlier than their Western counterparts and frequently carrying multiple risk factors including diabetes, metabolic syndrome, fatty liver disease, and central obesity, all of which make their disease course aggressive with less favorable long-term outcomes. Despite this high-risk environment, long-term adherence to statins remains suboptimal; studies consistently show that around half of all Indian patients discontinue statins within the first year, largely due to perceived side effects, inconsistent follow-up, cost barriers, and limited patient education. Furthermore, the availability and affordability of PCSK9 monoclonal antibodies remain extremely limited, restricting their use to a very small subset of patients in tertiary centers. In this context, for high risk, younger patients having or at-risk of repeated MACE events, inclisiran's twice-yearly, clinic-administered dosing offers a pragmatic and sustainable solution that circumvents adherence barriers, reduces pill burden, and integrates naturally into existing healthcare touchpoints; however, cost and affordability again remains a serious concern. If priced appropriately or incorporated into government or insurance-supported cardiovascular programs, inclisiran could substantially improve LDL-C goal attainment across the country's vast high-risk population pool who are at the highest risk.

CURRENT STATUS OF INCLISIRAN IN GUIDELINES

At present, no major international or national guideline assigns a formal class of recommendation to inclisiran for cardiovascular risk reduction, a reflection of the absence of definitive long-term cardiovascular outcomes from large randomized trials. The 2019 ESC/EAS guideline[2] framework continues to prioritize aggressive LDL-C lowering in very high-risk patients and explicitly endorses early use of PCSK9 monoclonal antibodies when maximally tolerated statins and ezetimibe fail to achieve goals. The 2025 ESC[17] focused update emphasizes this stance, stressing prompt escalation to PCSK9 inhibitors for patients with persistent residual risk despite standard therapy. Although inclisiran produces robust and durable LDL-C lowering in randomized studies, the lack of completed hard-outcomes evidence has prevented its routine placement within these guideline algorithms.

The Lipid Association of India (LAI) 2023 guidance[18] likewise emphasizes intensive risk-factor modification and a stepwise approach to lipid management tailored to local resources and patient circumstances. For modest incremental LDL-C reductions (≤20%), the LAI recommends agents such as bempedoic acid or bile-acid sequestrants where available; for larger reductions (>20%), PCSK9 inhibition is advised, with decisions guided by shared decision-making that weighs efficacy, affordability, and access. Given the current evidence base, inclisiran has not yet been incorporated as a defined option in these stepwise pathways.

In practice, guideline committees appear poised to reconsider inclisiran's position once robust cardiovascular outcome data—most notably from the large ORION-4 outcomes trial—become available. Until such data are published, most professional bodies will likely continue to prioritize agents with proven event-reduction data for routine escalation (i.e., PCSK9 monoclonal antibodies).

CONCLUSION

Inclisiran is a novel siRNA-based therapy that provides potent and sustained LDL-C reduction with consistent lowering of circulating PCSK9 levels. Clinical trials have shown a generally favorable safety profile, with adverse events largely mild and comparable to placebo. Its twice-yearly dosing schedule offers a major advantage by improving adherence compared with daily or frequent lipid-lowering therapies. While its efficacy in cholesterol reduction is established, definitive evidence on cardiovascular outcomes is pending, with the results of the ongoing ORION-4 trial expected to clarify its long-term clinical benefits.

REFERENCES

1. Kosmas CE, Muñoz Estrella A, Skavdis A, et al. Inclisiran for the treatment of cardiovascular disease: a short review on the emerging data and therapeutic potential. Ther Clin Risk Manag. 2020;16:1031-7.
2. Mach F, Baigent C, Catapano AL, et al. 2019 ESC/EAS guidelines for the management of dyslipidaemias: lipid modification to reduce cardiovascular risk. Eur Heart J. 2020;41:111-88.
3. Grundy SM, Stone NJ, Bailey AL, et al. 2018 AHA/ACC/AACVPR/AAPA/ABC/ACPM/ADA/AGS/APhA/ASPC/NLA/PCNA guideline on the management of blood cholesterol. Circulation. 2018;139:e1082-143.
4. Ray KK, Molemans B, Schoonen WM, et al. EU-wide cross-sectional observational study of lipid-modifying therapy use in secondary and primary care: the DA VINCI study. Eur J Prev Cardiol. 2020;28:1279-89.
5. De Backer G, Jankowski P, Kotseva K, et al. Management of dyslipidaemia in patients with coronary heart disease: results from the ESC-EORP EUROASPIRE V survey in 27 countries. Atherosclerosis. 2019;285:135-46.
6. Kosmas CE, Muñoz Estrella A, Sourlas A, et al. Inclisiran: a new promising agent in the management of hypercholesterolemia. Diseases. 2018;6(3):63.
7. Fitzgerald K, White S, Borodovsky A, et al. A highly durable RNAi therapeutic inhibitor of PCSK9. N Engl J Med. 2017;376(1):41-51.
8. Ray KK, Landmesser U, Leiter LA, et al. Inclisiran in patients at high cardiovascular risk with elevated LDL cholesterol. N Engl J Med. 2017;376(15):1430-40.
9. Ray KK, Stoekenbroek RM, Kallend D, et al. Effect of 1 or 2 doses of inclisiran on low-density lipoprotein cholesterol levels: one-year follow-up of the ORION-1 randomized clinical trial. JAMA Cardiol. 2019;4(11):1067-75.
10. Kastelein JJ, et al. Long-term inclisiran in subjects with high CV risk and elevated LDL-C. Presented at: National Lipid Association Scientific Sessions; May 16, 2019, Miami, USA.
11. Ray KK, Wright RS, Kallend D, et al.; ORION-10 and ORION-11 Investigators. Two phase 3 trials of inclisiran in patients with elevated LDL cholesterol. N Engl J Med. 2020;382(16):1507-19.
12. Raal FJ, Kallend D, Ray KK, et al.; ORION-9 Investigators. Inclisiran for the treatment of heterozygous familial hypercholesterolemia. N Engl J Med. 2020;382(16):1520-30.
13. National Library of Medicine. (2023). A study of inclisiran in participants with homozygous familial

hypercholesterolemia (HoFH) (ORION-5). [online] Available from http://clinicaltrials.gov/ct2/show/NCT03851705. [Last accessed January, 2026].

14. Khan SA, Naz A, Qamar Masood M, et al. Meta-analysis of inclisiran for the treatment of hypercholesterolemia. Am J Cardiol. 2020;S0002-9149(20):30866.
15. National Library of Medicine. (2025). A randomized trial assessing the effects of inclisiran on clinical outcomes among people with cardiovascular disease (ORION-4). [online] Available from http://clinicaltrials.gov/ct2/show/NCT03705234. [Last accessed January, 2026].
16. Nishikido T. Clinical potential of inclisiran for patients with a high risk of atherosclerotic cardiovascular disease. Cardiovasc Diabetol. 2023;22(1):20.
17. Mach F, Koskinas KC, van Lennep JER, et al. 2025 focused update of the 2019 ESC/EAS guidelines for the management of dyslipidaemias. Eur Heart J. 2025;46(42):4359-78.
18. Puri R, Bansal M, Mehta V, et al. Lipid Association of India 2023 update on cardiovascular risk assessment and lipid management in Indian patients: consensus statement IV. J Clin Lipidol. 2024;18(3):e351-73.

CHAPTER 161

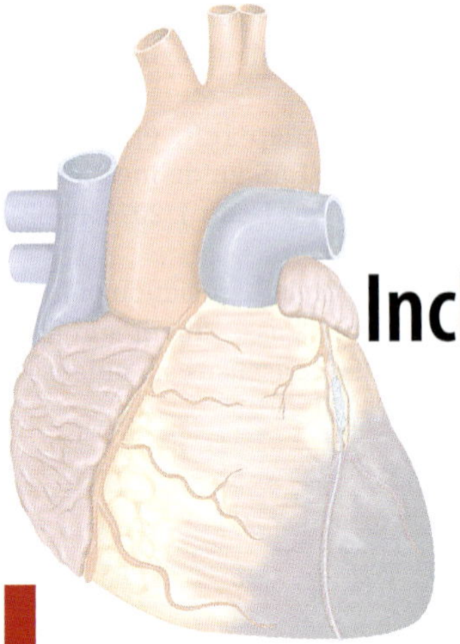

Inclisiran in Treating Hypercholesterolemia: Effectiveness and Safety

Arvind Kumar, Vipin Kumar

INTRODUCTION

Hypercholesterolemia is defined as elevated low-density lipoprotein cholesterol (LDL-C) or total cholesterol levels in blood. Among many modifiable risk factors for atherosclerotic cardiovascular disease (ASCVD), elevated LDL-C levels remain the most critical one.[1] All guidelines recommend use of statins as first-line agents for treatment of hypercholesterolemia in both primary and secondary prevention strategies. Statins alone often fail to achieve target LDL-C goals in many high-risk patients, leading to suboptimal risk reduction due to statin intolerance or insufficient lipid-lowering potency.[2,3] Many drug classes, such as ezetimibe, bempedoic acid, and proprotein convertase subtilisin/kexin 9 (PCSK9) inhibitors, have been developed as adjunct therapy and have shown promise in reducing LDL-C levels as well as clinical events. Inclisiran, a novel small interfering ribonucleic acid (siRNA), inhibits *PCSK9* gene expression and reduces LDL-C levels by increasing LDL-C receptor-mediated LDL-C uptake.[4] In this review, we discuss inclisiran use and current evidence on its safety and efficacy in treating hypercholesterolemia.

MECHANISM OF ACTION

Low-density lipoprotein cholesterol receptors in liver are regulated by PCSK9, secreted by hepatocytes themselves. Inclisiran is a synthetic siRNA conjugated on a sense strand with triantennary *N*-acetylgalactosamine carbohydrates, which facilitate selective uptake into hepatocytes through asialoglycoprotein receptor binding.[4] Once inside hepatocytes, inclisiran uses siRNA mechanism and directly binds to a precursor mRNA for PCSK9, resulting in reduced PCSK9 gene expression.[5]

The targeted inhibition of *PCSK9* gene expression leads to decreased PCSK9 protein synthesis, resulting in sustained reduction of hepatic PCSK9 levels. This results in decreased LDL receptor degradation, leading to increased number of LDL receptors on hepatocyte cell surface. With increased LDL receptors, LDL-C uptake is increased, leading to decreased LDL-C in the circulation.[6] Although the plasma half-life of inclisiran is approximately 9 hours, its pharmacodynamic effects are prolonged due to its action on gene expression.[7]

CLINICAL EFFICACY

Lipid-Lowering Effects

Various ORION clinical trials have demonstrated inclisiran's robust lipid-lowering efficacy across diverse patient populations.[8] A comprehensive meta-analysis of eight randomized controlled trials involving 5,016 patients revealed that inclisiran achieved a significant 50.42% reduction in LDL-C levels compared to placebo.[9]

The ORION-9, ORION-10, and ORION-11 phase III trials also demonstrated consistent LDL-C reductions of approximately 44–54% across various high-risk populations, including patients with familial hypercholesterolemia and established ASCVD.[10,11] Long-term data from the ORION-3 extension study confirmed sustained LDL-C reduction of 47.5% at day 210, with a 4-year averaged mean reduction of 44.2%.[8] The ORION-8 study further validated long-term efficacy, with 78.4% of patients achieving prespecified LDL-C targets and approximately

90% reaching global lipid targets at any visit during the study period.[12]

Background Lipid-Lowering Therapy

Analysis of ORION trial data stratified by baseline treatments revealed optimal LDL-C reductions of 57.0% when combined with statin plus ezetimibe, 51.5% with statin monotherapy, 50.5% with ezetimibe alone, and 43.1% in patients not receiving other lipid-lowering therapies.[13]

Cardiovascular Outcomes

While dedicated cardiovascular outcomes trials are ongoing, pooled analysis of ORION-9, ORION-10, and ORION-11 safety data provides encouraging preliminary results.[14] Among 3,655 patients, inclisiran treatment was associated with a 25% reduction in major adverse cardiovascular events (MACE) compared to placebo (hazard ratio 0.75, 95% CI 0.60–0.94). Specifically, fewer patients receiving inclisiran experienced MACE (131 vs. 172), with annualized rates of 5.35 versus 7.71 per 100 person-years for inclisiran and placebo, respectively. Fatal and nonfatal myocardial infarction occurred less frequently in the inclisiran group (33 vs. 41 events), as did fatal and nonfatal stroke (13 vs. 15 events).

The ongoing ORION-4 trial aims to establish inclisiran impact on cardiovascular event reduction in patients with established ASCVD or equivalent risk conditions.[15]

SAFETY PROFILE

Overall Safety Assessment

Inclisiran demonstrates an excellent safety profile comparable to placebo across many clinical trials. A recent comprehensive meta-analysis of seven randomized controlled trials including 4,790 patients found no significant differences between inclisiran and control groups for all-cause mortality (risk ratio 0.92, 95% CI 0.54–1.54), MACE (risk ratio 0.98, 95% CI 0.82–1.17), nasopharyngitis (risk ratio 1.10, 95% CI 0.83–1.45), or type 2 diabetes mellitus (risk ratio 1.02, 95% CI 0.85–1.21).[16]

Injection Site Reactions

The most commonly reported adverse events are mild-to-moderate injection site reactions, which occur in approximately 8% of patients treated by inclisiran, compared to 2% with placebo.[14] These reactions are generally self-limiting and typically manifest as injection site pain, erythema, or mild swelling.

Long-Term Safety

Extended safety data from the ORION-3 study, encompassing approximately 5 years of inclisiran exposure, reemphasized inclisiran safety and tolerability.[8] In the inclisiran-only arm, 28% of patients had treatment-emergent adverse events possibly related to study medication, with injection site reactions being most common (5.6%). Serious adverse events possibly related to inclisiran occurred in only four patients.

SPECIAL POPULATIONS

Renal impairment: The pharmacodynamic properties of inclisiran in patients with renal impairment were assessed in the ORION-7 phase I and ORION-1 phase II studies. The incidence of adverse reactions was comparable with similar lipid-lowering effects across all degrees of renal function. No dose adjustment is necessary for patients with mild-to-moderate renal impairment, with caution in severe cases due to limited clinical experience.[17]

Hepatic impairment: The ORION-6 trial evaluated the safety of inclisiran in patients with varying degrees of hepatic impairment. There was similar LDL-C reduction in patients with mild-to-moderate hepatic impairment with comparable safety and tolerability.[18] Hence, no dose adjustment is required for mild-to-moderate hepatic impairment. However, data on severe hepatic impairment are lacking, and inclisiran should be used with caution in this group.

Elderly patients: Age does not significantly influence inclisiran pharmacokinetics or safety, and no dose adjustment is necessary in elderly patients.[19]

DOSING AND ADMINISTRATION

Inclisiran follows a simplified dosing regimen that enhances patient adherence compared to other PCSK9 inhibitors. The recommended dose is 284 mg administered as a subcutaneous injection initially, again at 3 months, and then every 6 months thereafter.[20] The drug should be administered by healthcare professionals via subcutaneous injection into the abdomen, with alternative sites including the upper arm or thigh.

REAL-WORLD EVIDENCE

Real-world data showed similar efficacy and tolerability of inclisiran as shown in clinical trials. A systematic review and meta-analysis of real-world studies showed an average LDL-C reduction of 42.77% (95% CI 37.42–48.12%).[21] Patients receiving inclisiran with statins showed greater reduction in LDL-C levels (45.67%) compared to monotherapy (37.53%) in subgroup analysis. Compared to clinical trial data, this slightly lower reduction in LDL-C levels here may be explained by heterogeneous population groups in real-world setting.

Similarly, a real-world study from Israel involving 503 patients showed median LDL-C reductions of 57% in inclisiran monotherapy and 66% when combined with other lipid-lowering therapies.[22] Importantly, LDL-C targets of <70 mg/dL were achieved by 39% of patients, with 21.9% reaching the more stringent target of <55 mg/dL. The discontinuation rate was low at 6.5%, supporting the drug's tolerability in routine clinical practice.

Clinical Guidelines and Recommendations

Inclisiran was approved by the US Food and Drug Administration (FDA) in December 2021 as an adjunct therapy to diet and maximally tolerated statin therapy for adults with heterozygous familial hypercholesterolemia or clinical ASCVD who require additional LDL-C lowering.[23] The European Medicines Agency granted approval in December 2020 for broader indications, including primary hypercholesterolemia and mixed dyslipidemia in patients unable to reach LDL-C goals with maximum tolerated statin therapy.[24]

The 2022 American College of Cardiology Expert Consensus Decision Pathway includes inclisiran as an option for nonstatin therapy in addition to maximally tolerated statin therapy in very high-risk ASCVD patients or those with LDL-C >190 mg/dL.[25] The recent expansion of the FDA indication in 2025 now allows inclisiran use for primary hypercholesterolemia, enabling first-line use in broader patient populations.

Recent guidelines from the American College of Cardiology and American Heart Association for acute coronary syndrome management recommend combination lipid-lowering therapy, including agents such as inclisiran, for patients with LDL-C levels of 70 mg/dL or higher despite maximally tolerated statin therapy.[26] The 2025 focused update of the ESC/EAS guidelines for dyslipidemia and cardiovascular prevention recognizes inclisiran as an effective agent for secondary prevention in high-risk and very-high-risk patients, especially those not achieving LDL-C goals with statins and ezetimibe.[27]

CONTRAINDICATIONS AND PRECAUTIONS

Inclisiran is contraindicated in patients with hypersensitivity to any of the active substances. There is no evaluation of safety or efficacy in pediatric population; hence, it should not be used in this population. It has not been studied in pregnancy; hence, it is recommended to discontinue inclisiran before conception.[28]

FUTURE PERSPECTIVES

Several cardiovascular outcome studies are ongoing, which will further define inclisiran's role in preventing MACE. The VICTORION-1 PREVENT trial[29] is evaluating high-risk patients with or without established ASCVD, while the VICTORION-2 PREVENT,[30] will evaluate long-term cardiovascular outcomes in patients with established ASCVD. 66.5% of patients with acute coronary syndrome achieved LDL-C targets <70 mg/dL with inclisiran plus usual care compared to 28.1% with usual care alone, as shown from early results from the VICTORION-INCEPTION.[31]

Inclisiran failed to lower LDL-C levels despite PCSK9 reduction in patients with homozygous familial hypercholesterolemia in the ORION-5 trial, and research is ongoing for this complex condition.[32]

CONCLUSION

High LDL-C levels are one of the most critical modifiable risk factors for ASCVD. Inclisiran is the newest addition to armamentarium of lipid-lowering therapies, which offers robust and sustained LDL-C reduction with convenient twice-yearly dosing. It showed approximately 44–54% reduction in LDL-C in various clinical trials with excellent safety and tolerability. Approximately 8% of patients suffered mild-to-moderate injection site reactions, but serious adverse events remained rare.

Several cardiovascular outcome studies are ongoing, which will further clarify inclisiran role in ASCVD prevention. Currently, inclisiran is indicated in treatment of adults with primary hyperlipidemia, including those with heterozygous hypercholesterolemia, as an adjunct to diet and statins. The drug's novel mechanism of action, with favorable safety profile and convenient dosing regimen, makes it a valuable addition to the armamentarium of lipid-lowering drugs in the modern era.

REFERENCES

1. Borén J, Chapman MJ, Krauss RM, et al. Low-density lipoproteins cause atherosclerotic cardiovascular disease: pathophysiological, genetic, and therapeutic insights: a consensus statement from the European Atherosclerosis Society Consensus Panel. Eur Heart J. 2020;41(24):2313-30.

2. Ray KK, Haq I, Bilitou A, et al. Treatment gaps in the implementation of LDL cholesterol control among high- and very high-risk patients in Europe between 2020 and 2021: the multinational observational SANTORINI study. Lancet Reg Health Eur. 2023;29:100624.
3. Underberg J, Toth PP, Rodriguez F. LDL-C target attainment in secondary prevention of ASCVD in the United States: barriers, consequences of nonachievement, and strategies to reach goals. Postgrad Med. 2022;134(8):752-62.
4. Fitzgerald K, White S, Borodovsky A, et al. A highly durable RNAi therapeutic inhibitor of PCSK9. N Engl J Med. 2017;376(1):41-51.
5. Nair JK, Willoughby JLS, Chan A, et al. Multivalent N-acetylgalactosamine-conjugated siRNA localizes in hepatocytes and elicits robust RNAi-mediated gene silencing. J Am Chem Soc. 2014;136(49):16958-61.
6. Fitzgerald K, Frank-Kamenetsky M, Shulga-Morskaya S, et al. Effect of an RNA interference drug on the synthesis of proprotein convertase subtilisin/kexin type 9 (PCSK9) and the concentration of serum LDL cholesterol in healthy volunteers: a randomised, single-blind, placebo-controlled, phase 1 trial. Lancet. 2014;383(9911):60-8.
7. European Medicines Agency. (2025). Leqvio. [online] Available from https://www.ema.europa.eu/en/documents/assessment-report/leqvio-epar-public-assessment-report_en.pdf [Last accessed January, 2026].
8. Ray KK, Troquay RPT, Visseren FLJ, et al. Long-term efficacy and safety of inclisiran in patients with high cardiovascular risk and elevated LDL cholesterol (ORION-3): results from the 4-year open-label extension of the ORION-1 trial. Lancet Diabetes Endocrinol. 2023;11(2):109-19.
9. Basit J, Ahmed M, Singh P, et al. Safety and efficacy of inclisiran in hyperlipidemia: an updated meta-analysis of randomised controlled trials. Endocrinol Diabetes Metab. 2025;8(2):e70039.
10. Ray KK, Wright RS, Kallend D, et al. Two phase 3 trials of inclisiran in patients with elevated LDL cholesterol. N Engl J Med. 2020;382(16):1507-19.
11. Raal FJ, Kallend D, Ray KK, et al. Inclisiran for the treatment of heterozygous familial hypercholesterolemia. N Engl J Med. 2020;382(16):1520-30.
12. Wright RS, Raal FJ, Koenig W, et al. Inclisiran administration potently and durably lowers LDL-C over an extended-term follow-up: the ORION-8 trial. Cardiovasc Res. 2024;120(12):1400-10.
13. Landmesser U, Koenig W, Leiter LA, et al. Efficacy and safety of inclisiran based on background lipid-lowering treatment. Eur J Prev Cardiol. 2025:zwaf214.
14. Ray KK, Raal FJ, Kallend DG, et al. Inclisiran and cardiovascular events: a patient-level analysis of phase III trials. Eur Heart J. 2022 ;44(2):129-38.
15. University of Oxford. (2024). HPS-4; TIMI 65; ORION-4: a double-blind randomized placebo-controlled trial assessing the effects of inclisiran on clinical outcomes among people with atherosclerotic cardiovascular disease. [online] Available from https://clinicaltrials.gov/study/NCT03705234 [Last accessed January, 2026].
16. Maliha M, Satish V, Kumar SS, et al. The safety profile of inclisiran in patients with dyslipidemia: a systematic review and meta-analysis. Healthcare. 2025;13(2):141.
17. Wright RS, Collins MG, Stoekenbroek RM, et al. Effects of renal impairment on the pharmacokinetics, efficacy, and safety of inclisiran: an analysis of the ORION-7 and ORION-1 studies. Mayo Clin Proc. 2020;95(1):77-89.
18. Kallend D, Stoekenbroek R, He Y, et al. Pharmacokinetics and pharmacodynamics of inclisiran, a small interfering RNA therapy, in patients with hepatic impairment. J Clin Lipidol. 2022;16(2):208-19.
19. Colquhoun D, Wright R, Ray K, et al. Efficacy and safety of inclisiran according to age: a pooled analysis of phase III studies (ORION 9, 10 and 11). Heart Lung Circ. 2023;32:S387.
20. Singareddy S, Dhakal S, Limbaña TA, et al. Inclisiran: a systematic review exploring the revolutionary approach of twice-yearly dosing regimen in the treatment of hypercholesterolemia. Cureus. 16(9):e69918.
21. Alaíz ÁR, Gudino LC, de la Isla LP, et al. Inclisiran: efficacy in real world—systematic review and meta-analysis. J Clin Med. 2025;14(12):4163.
22. Naoum I, Saliba W, Aker A, et al. Lipid-lowering therapy with inclisiran in the real-world setting: initial data from a national health care service. J Clin Lipidol. 2024;18(5):e809-16.
23. Novartis. (2025). Leqvio. [online] Available from https://www.novartis.com/us-en/sites/novartis_us/files/leqvio.pdf [Last accessed January, 2026].
24. European Medicines Agency. (2021). Leqvio. [online] Available from https://www.ema.europa.eu/en/medicines/human/EPAR/leqvio [Last accessed January, 2026].
25. Lloyd-Jones DM, Morris PB, Ballantyne CM, et al. 2022 ACC expert consensus decision pathway on the role of nonstatin therapies for LDL-cholesterol lowering in the management of atherosclerotic cardiovascular disease risk. J Am Coll Cardiol. 2022;80(14):1366-418.
26. Rao SV, O'Donoghue ML, Ruel M, et al. 2025 ACC/AHA/ACEP/NAEMSP/SCAI guideline for the management of patients with acute coronary syndromes: a report of the American College of Cardiology/American Heart Association joint committee on clinical practice guidelines. Circulation. 2025;151(13):e771-862.
27. Mach F, Koskinas KC, Roeters van Lennep JE, et al. 2025 Focused update of the 2019 ESC/EAS guidelines for the management of dyslipidaemias: developed by the task force for the management of dyslipidaemias of the European Society of Cardiology (ESC) and the European Atherosclerosis Society (EAS). Eur Heart J. 2025;ehaf190.
28. Albosta MS, Grant JK, Taub P, et al. Inclisiran: a new strategy for LDL-C lowering and prevention of atherosclerotic cardiovascular disease. Vasc Health Risk Manag. 2023;19:421-31.
29. Novartis Pharmaceuticals. (2025). A randomized, double-blind, placebo-controlled multicenter study to evaluate the effect of inclisiran on preventing major adverse cardiovascular events in high-risk primary prevention

patients (VICTORION-1 PREVENT). [online] Available from: https://clinicaltrials.gov/study/NCT05739383 [Last accessed January, 2026].

30. Novartis Pharmaceuticals. (2025). A randomized, double-blind, placebo-controlled, multicenter trial, assessing the impact of inclisiran on major adverse cardiovascular events in participants with established cardiovascular disease (VICTORION-2 PREVENT). [online] Available from https://clinicaltrials.gov/study/NCT05030428 [Last accessed January, 2026].
31. Desai NR, Knowlton KU, Anderson JL, et al. VICTORION-INCEPTION: early and sustained LDL-C goal attainment with inclisiran plus usual care in participants with recent acute coronary syndrome. Am J Prev Cardiol. 2025;23:101191.
32. Raal F, Durst R, Bi R, et al. Efficacy, safety, and tolerability of inclisiran in patients with homozygous familial hypercholesterolemia: results from the ORION-5 randomized clinical trial. Circulation. 2024;149(5):354-62.

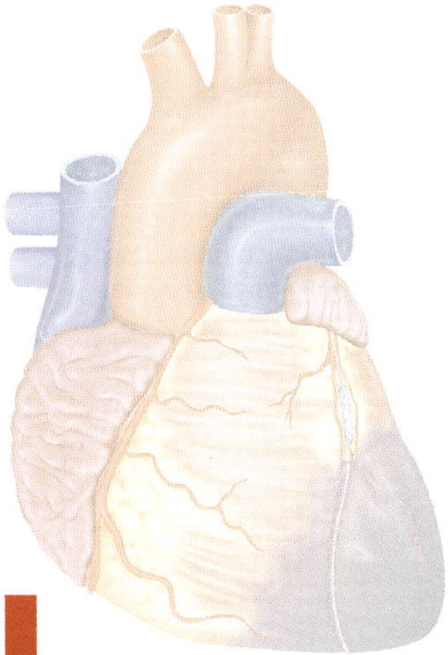

Safety and Efficacy of Inclisiran in Treating Hypercholesterolemia

Rajesh Natuva, Dayasagar Rao Vala

INTRODUCTION

Hypercholesterolemia, defined as elevated levels of total cholesterol and particularly low-density lipoprotein cholesterol (LDL-C), is a well-established and central risk factor for the development of atherosclerotic cardio-vascular disease (ASCVD).[1] ASCVD continues to be the leading cause of morbidity and mortality worldwide, despite significant advances in diagnosis and management.[2] Traditional lipid-lowering therapies, primarily statins, have been proven to reduce cardiovascular risk substantially; however, a significant subset of patients remains unable to achieve recommended LDL-C targets. This therapeutic gap arises due to several factors including inadequate efficacy, dose-limiting side effects, intolerance, poor adherence, and cost-related barriers in certain health systems.[3]

Inclisiran, a novel small-interfering RNA (siRNA) therapeutic, provides an innovative approach to lipid management. Unlike monoclonal antibodies that target circulating proprotein convertase subtilisin/kexin type 9 (PCSK9), inclisiran works intracellularly by silencing PCSK9 mRNA in hepatocytes, thereby preventing its synthesis. This results in enhanced recycling of LDL receptors on hepatocyte surfaces and sustained clearance of LDL-C from circulation.[4] Importantly, the twice-yearly dosing schedule offers a pragmatic solution to the long-standing issue of poor patient adherence to chronic lipid-lowering regimens.[5]

This review comprehensively evaluates the safety, efficacy, clinical applicability, and future perspectives of inclisiran, drawing evidence from major randomized controlled trials, real-world data, and population-level modeling. Particular emphasis is placed on its role across diverse patient populations, including those with heterozygous familial hypercholesterolemia, established ASCVD, and statin-intolerant individuals.

Hypercholesterolemia continues to pose a formidable global health burden, not only due to its direct role in ASCVD but also because of its interplay with comorbidities such as diabetes mellitus, hypertension, obesity, and chronic kidney disease.[2] The World Health Organization estimates that >39% of adults worldwide have elevated cholesterol, yet fewer than half of them are treated to goal.[6] This treatment gap highlights the urgent need for innovative therapies like inclisiran that combine efficacy, safety, and adherence advantages. Furthermore, as precision medicine gains prominence, siRNA-based approaches herald a new era of gene-silencing therapeutics in cardiovascular care.

Mechanism of Action

Inclisiran is a double-stranded siRNA conjugated to triantennary N-acetylgalactosamine carbohydrates, which selectively target hepatocytes through the asialogly-coprotein receptor. Once internalized, it becomes incorporated into the RNA-induced silencing complex (RISC), which binds and degrades PCSK9 mRNA. Reduced PCSK9 synthesis translates into decreased degradation of LDL receptors and greater hepatic clearance of LDL-C **(Fig. 1)**.[4]

Dosing

Inclisiran 284 mg subcutaneously as a single initial dose, followed by a second dose at 3 months, and subsequently every 6 months thereafter.[5]

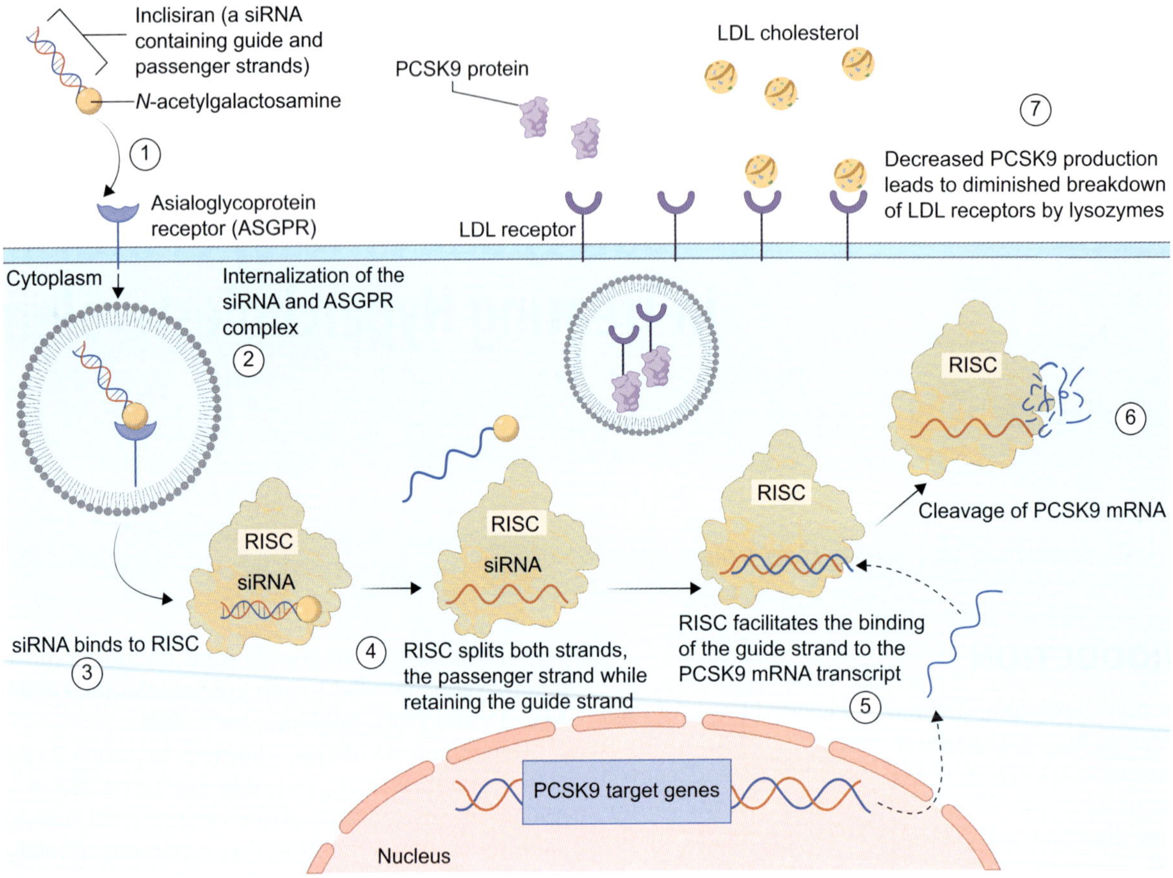

Fig. 1: Inclisiran's mechanism of action, showing siRNA entry into hepatocytes, binding of PCSK9 mRNA, and enhanced LDL receptor recycling.
Source: Stoekenbroek et al.[4]

Real-World Modeling

A NHANES-based analysis estimated that widespread use of inclisiran among US adults eligible under ORION criteria could prevent more than 200,000 cardiovascular events over 10 years. This emphasizes not only individual patient benefit but also potential public health impact.[8]

In addition to LDL-C lowering, inclisiran has been shown to beneficially modulate other lipid fractions. For example, pooled analyses demonstrated modest reductions in lipoprotein(a) and apolipoprotein B, both independent predictors of ASCVD. These pleiotropic effects may further enhance cardiovascular risk reduction.[8]

Landmark Trials (Table 1)

- In ORION-10, inclisiran reduced mean LDL-C by 52.3% at day 510, with 78% of patients achieving guideline-recommended targets. Adherence exceeded 95% due to the provider-administered dosing model.[7]
- ORION-11, which included patients across Europe and South Africa, showed similar results with an average 50.6% LDL-C reduction. Importantly, the consistency across diverse ethnic and healthcare backgrounds suggests wide generalizability.[7]
- ORION-9 in HeFH patients demonstrated stable LDL-C reductions across different genotypes, confirming genotype-independent efficacy.[1]
- VICTORION-Mono emphasized inclisiran's role even in lower risk patients not receiving statins, with nearly half the LDL-C reduction observed compared to baseline **(Fig. 2)**.[9]

These trial results have positioned inclisiran not merely as an alternative but as a cornerstone therapy for patients unable to achieve LDL-C goals with traditional regimens **(Fig. 3)**.

EFFICACY AND SUBGROUP ANALYSES

- Sustained *~50% LDL-C reduction* across all studies[11]
- Benefits observed irrespective of statin use or intensity[11]

TABLE 1: Summary of major inclisiran clinical trials and their findings.

Trial	*Population*	*Design and duration*	*LDL-C reduction*	*Key findings*
ORION-9[1]	Heterozygous familial hypercholesterolemia	Phase 3, 18 months	~50%	Sustained LDL-C lowering across genetic subgroups, safe and effective
ORION-10[7]	ASCVD patients (United States)	Phase 3, 18 months	~52%	78% achieved LDL-C goals, strong adherence benefits
ORION-11[7]	ASCVD and risk equivalents (EU and SA)	Phase 3, 18 months	~51%	Consistent results across diverse populations
VICTORION-Mono[9]	Primary prevention, no ASCVD/diabetes	Phase 3, 5 months	46.5%	Superior to ezetimibe, good tolerability
ORION-4[10] (ongoing)	ASCVD patients	CV outcome trial, ~15,000 patients	Pending	Will provide definitive CV outcome data

Source: Raal et al.[1]; Ray et al.[7]; Taub et al.[9]; National Library of Medicine[10].

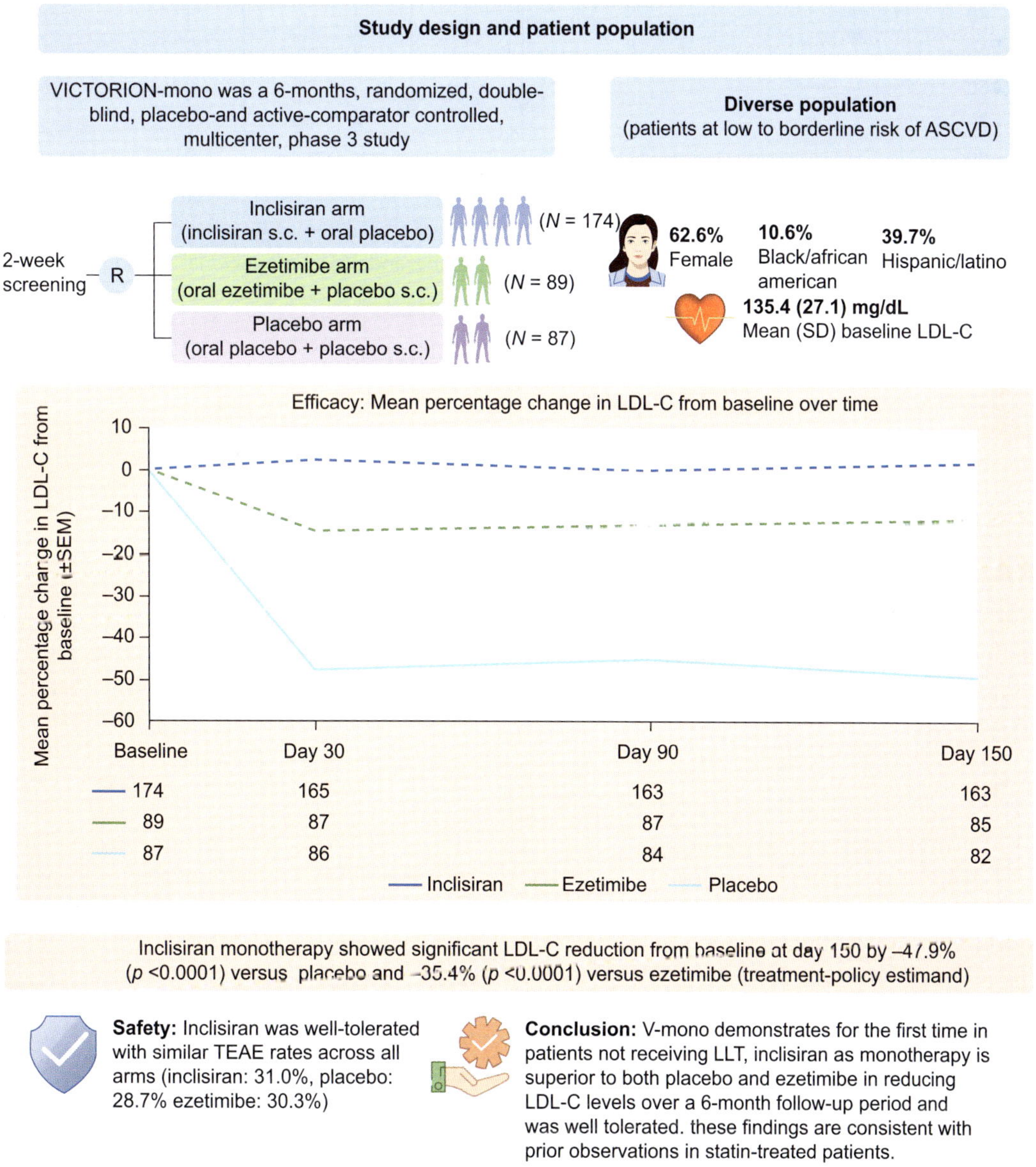

Fig. 2: Graph depicting the time-dependent LDL-C reduction with inclisiran compared to placebo. *Source:* Taub et al.[9]

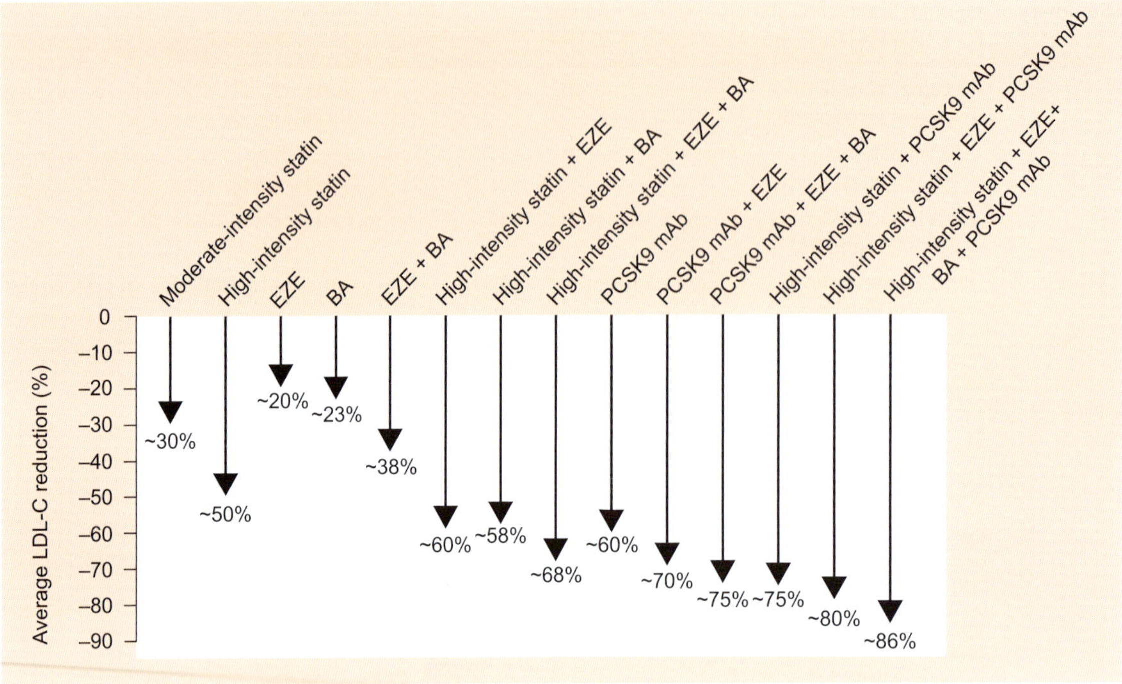

Fig. 3: LDL-C reduction across inclisiran, statins, ezetimibe, and PCSK9 monoclonal antibodies.
Source: Mach et al.[11]

- Effective in *statin-intolerant* patients and those with HeFH[11]
- Additional reductions in *ApoB* and *Lp(a)* observed.[11]
- Adherence rates exceeded 95% due to provider-administered dosing.[1,11]

COMPARATIVE PERSPECTIVES

When comparing inclisiran with other cholesterol-lowering medicines, some important points stand out. Statins are still the first choice because they are cheap, effective, and widely available. However, some patients do not tolerate statins due to muscle pain or liver problems. Ezetimibe is an add-on medicine that gives a modest LDL-C reduction of about 15–20%.

Proprotein convertase subtilisin/kexin type 9 monoclonal antibodies, such as evolocumab and alirocumab, are very effective with about 50–60% LDL-C reduction, but they require injections every 2–4 weeks, which can be difficult for some patients to maintain long-term. Inclisiran works in a different way but lowers cholesterol by almost the same amount as these injections. Its main advantage is the very simple schedule of just two injections per year.[11]

Bempedoic acid, another newer drug, lowers LDL-C by around 15–20% and is useful in patients who cannot take statins. But inclisiran is stronger and more reliable in bringing cholesterol down. Overall, inclisiran gives a balance of strong effect, simple dosing, and good safety, making it a promising long-term option **(Table 2)**.[11]

Side Effects

In the ORION-10 and ORION-11 phase III trials, inclisiran demonstrated a favorable safety profile, with overall adverse event rates comparable to placebo. The most common treatment-related events were mild, transient injection-site reactions—primarily pain, erythema, or swelling—occurring more frequently with inclisiran (2.6 vs. 0.9% in ORION-10; 4.7 vs. 0.5% in ORION-11).[7]

Systemic adverse events such as headache, fatigue, myalgia, arthralgia, nasopharyngitis, and diarrhea occurred at similar rates in both groups, while bronchitis was slightly more frequent with inclisiran in pooled analyses. Laboratory abnormalities, including rare, asymptomatic liver enzyme elevations, were not clinically significant. There were no signals of renal, hepatic, or neurocognitive toxicity, and rates of serious adverse events, discontinuations, and deaths were similar to placebo. Long-term data from ORION-8 confirmed the continued safety and tolerability of twice-yearly inclisiran therapy.[7]

TABLE 2: Comparative overview of LDL-C lowering therapies.

Therapy	LDL-C reduction (%)	Dosing frequency	Comments
Statins	30–50	Daily oral	First-line; limited by intolerance
Ezetimibe	15–20	Daily oral	Add-on; modest efficacy
PCSK9 mAbs (evolocumab, alirocumab)	50–60	Every 2–4 weeks	Excellent efficacy; cost and adherence issues
Inclisiran	50	Twice yearly	Strong, durable effect; excellent adherence
Bempedoic acid	15–20	Daily oral	Useful in statin intolerance

Source: Mach et al.[11]

HEALTH ECONOMICS AND GLOBAL UPTAKE

The cost of inclisiran is still a challenge. While it may reduce heart attacks and strokes in the long run, the medicine itself is expensive compared to statins and ezetimibe. In high-income countries like the United States and many parts of Europe, health insurance and government health systems are starting to cover inclisiran for patients at very high risk.[12]

In middle- and low-income countries, including India, the high cost limits its use to selected patients who can afford it. Wider adoption will depend on price reductions, local production, and supportive government policies.[12]

From a health economics point of view, inclisiran may actually save money in the long term by preventing expensive hospitalizations for heart attacks, bypass surgery, or strokes. But these savings will take years to show, which makes early adoption difficult in systems with limited budgets.[12]

FUTURE DIRECTIONS

Inclisiran is only the beginning of siRNA-based medicines for cholesterol and heart disease. In the future, we may see other siRNA treatments that target different pathways in cholesterol and fat metabolism. For example, medicines that lower lipoprotein(a) or triglycerides using the same technology are already in clinical trials.[13]

Another area is combining inclisiran with other new medicines like bempedoic acid or ANGPTL3 inhibitors to give a full package of lipid control.[11] Researchers are also exploring if inclisiran can be used in special groups such as children with homozygous hypercholesterolemia[14] or patients with severe kidney disease.[15]

In simple terms, inclisiran is opening the door to a new way of treating cholesterol problems. It is not the final answer, but it shows us that controlling cholesterol with just two injections a year is possible, safe, and effective. This idea may completely change how doctors and patients think about cholesterol treatment in the future.

LIMITATIONS

While inclisiran presents a promising therapeutic innovation, several limitations must be acknowledged:

- Lack of completed cardiovascular outcome data: Unlike PCSK9 monoclonal antibodies, which have demonstrated cardiovascular event reduction in large outcome trials (e.g., FOURIER, ODYSSEY), inclisiran's cardiovascular outcomes remain under investigation in ongoing studies such as ORION-4 and VICTORION-2 PREVENT.[16]
- Economic considerations: Inclisiran is costly, and although cost-effectiveness analyses are underway, its uptake may be restricted in low-resource settings without appropriate reimbursement frameworks.[12]
- Limited data in special populations: There is a paucity of evidence in populations such as those with advanced chronic kidney disease, hepatic impairment, pediatric patients, and pregnant women.[17]
- Injection-site reactions: Although generally mild and transient, injection-site reactions are the most frequent adverse events reported.[7]
- Dependence on healthcare-provider administration: Twice-yearly dosing is convenient but requires patients to attend scheduled healthcare visits, which may be challenging in certain settings.[18]

These limitations underscore the importance of cautious interpretation and the need for further studies to validate inclisiran's long-term role in cardiovascular prevention.

Another limitation lies in the relative novelty of siRNA-based therapeutics. While short- to medium-term safety has been reassuring, long-term surveillance data are essential to exclude rare immunologic or hepatic complications. Additionally, unlike oral agents, inclisiran requires infrastructure for cold chain storage and administration, which could be challenging in rural and resource-limited settings.

Moreover, real-world adherence to follow-up visits for injection scheduling may differ from clinical trial conditions, potentially reducing its effectiveness if implementation frameworks are weak. Pharmacoeconomic analyses will also need to weigh the up-front costs against long-term cardiovascular event prevention, particularly in countries with constrained healthcare budgets.

CLINICAL ALGORITHM AND GUIDELINES

Based on current evidence and evolving consensus **(Flowchart 1)**, inclisiran may be incorporated into clinical practice as follows:

Suggested clinical algorithm for inclisiran use:

- Identify patients with ASCVD or familial hypercholesterolemia who remain above LDL-C targets despite maximally tolerated statin ± ezetimibe
- Assess adherence and statin tolerance; if statins are not tolerated, ezetimibe alone or inclisiran may be considered.
- Initiate inclisiran with subcutaneous dosing at baseline, 3 months, and every 6 months thereafter
- Monitor LDL-C response at 3–6 months; consider adjunctive therapy if LDL-C targets are still unmet
- Continue long-term follow-up, including monitoring for injection-site reactions, liver function, and renal safety

CLINICAL DECISION-MAKING FOR THE INITIATION OF INCLISIRAN[11]

Guideline Positioning

The 2025 European Society of Cardiology (ESC) guidelines[11] and American College of Cardiology (ACC) expert consensus documents[19] recognize inclisiran as an adjunct for patients not at LDL-C goal with standard therapy. Its twice-yearly regimen is particularly valuable for improving adherence in patients with prior compliance issues.

Emerging guidelines increasingly recognize inclisiran as part of a broader shift toward precision lipid management. The ACC emphasizes its use for patients with poor adherence or statin intolerance, while the *ESC* highlights the utility of inclisiran in *very high-risk patients* who fail to achieve *LDL-C targets of <55 mg/dL*, and in *extreme-risk patients* where the recommended LDL-C goal is *<40 mg/dL* **(Fig. 4)**.[11]

Flowchart 1: Clinical algorithm and guidelines.

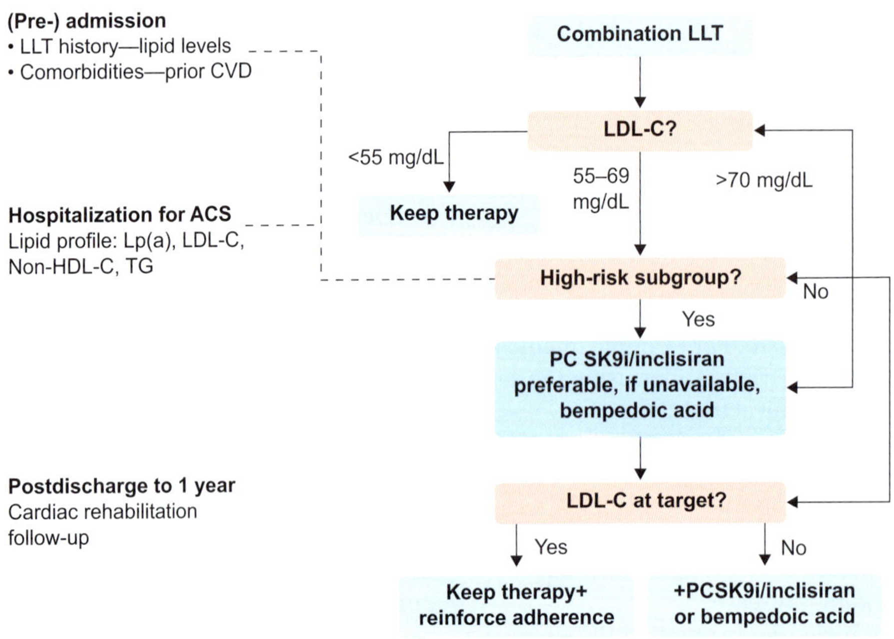

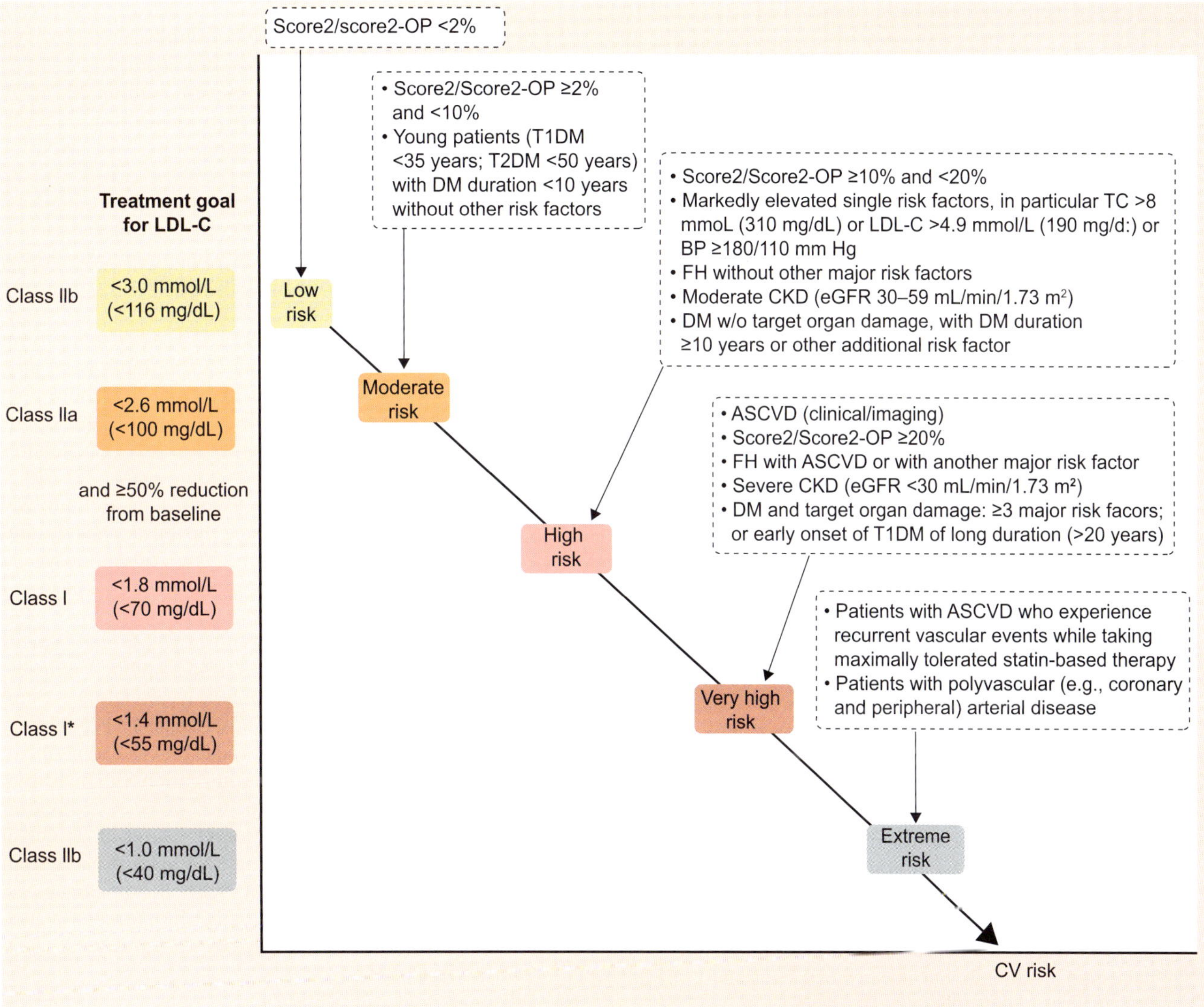

Fig. 4: Therapeutic targets for LDL-C across categories of total cardiovascular risk *(ESC guidelines, 2025)*.
*Class for individuals in primary prevention with FH at very high risk.
Source: Mach et al.[11]

CONCLUSION

Inclisiran represents a paradigm shift in the management of hypercholesterolemia and ASCVD risk reduction. Its innovative siRNA mechanism, potent and durable LDL-C lowering efficacy, and highly convenient dosing intervals address many shortcomings of existing therapies. Real world modeling suggests that widespread adoption could substantially reduce the burden of cardiovascular events at a population level.

However, definitive outcome data are awaited, and cost-effectiveness analyses will be pivotal in determining the extent of its global implementation. For now, inclisiran should be considered as a complementary therapy in patients at high or very high cardiovascular risk who are unable to achieve LDL-C targets with conventional regimens.

In conclusion, inclisiran is poised to become a transformative addition to the armamentarium of lipid-lowering therapies, bridging the gap between efficacy, safety, and adherence in cardiovascular prevention.

The growing body of evidence positions inclisiran as not only a therapeutic innovation but also a public-health opportunity. Its potential to simplify lipid management through biannual dosing and provider oversight could drastically reduce therapeutic inertia and improve population-level LDL-C control.

Future directions include exploring its role in combination regimens with novel agents such as bempedoic acid, which inhibits ATP citrate lyase, and emerging ANGPTL3 inhibitors. Together, these therapies could pave the way for comprehensive lipid modulation beyond LDL-C, targeting triglycerides, remnant cholesterol, and Lp(a).

Inclisiran, therefore, should not be viewed in isolation but as part of an expanding toolkit aimed at conquering residual cardiovascular risk in the modern era.

REFERENCES

1. Raal FJ, Kallend D, Ray KK, et al. Inclisiran for the treatment of heterozygous familial hypercholesterolemia. N Engl J Med. 2020;382(16):1520-30.
2. Barkas F, Sener YZ, Golforoush PA, et al. Advancements in risk stratification and management strategies in primary cardiovascular prevention. Atherosclerosis. 2024;395:117579.
3. Kamanu C, Karalis DG. The role of non-statin lipid lowering therapies to reduce ASCVD events in primary prevention. Curr Atheroscler Rep. 2025;27(1):46.
4. Stoekenbroek RM, Kastelein JJ, Huijgen R. PCSK9 inhibition: the way forward in the treatment of dyslipidemia. BMC Med. 2015;13(1):258.
5. Landmesser U, Koenig W, Leiter LA, et al. Efficacy and safety of inclisiran based on background lipid-lowering treatment. Eur J Prev Cardiol. 2025:zwaf214.
6. World Health Organization. (2025). The global health observatory. Explore a world of health data. Indicator Metadata Registry List. [online] Available from https://www.who.int/data/gho/indicator-metadata-registry. [Last accessed January, 2026].
7. Ray KK, Wright RS, Kallend D, et al. Two phase 3 trials of inclisiran in patients with elevated LDL cholesterol. N Engl J Med. 2020;382(16):1507-19.
8. Li H, Zhao S, Wu J, et al. Estimating the effect of inclisiran on hypercholesterolemia and primary prevention of cardiovascular disease: the NHANES 1999–2018 study. Lipids Health Dis. 2024;23(1):313.
9. Taub PR, Gutierrez A, Wewers D, et al. Safety and lipid-lowering efficacy of inclisiran monotherapy in patients without ASCVD: the VICTORION-Mono randomized clinical trial. J Am Coll Cardiol. 2025;86(3):196-208.
10. National Library of Medicine. (2025). *A Randomized Trial Assessing the Effects of Inclisiran on Clinical Outcomes Among People With Cardiovascular Disease (ORION-4). [online] Available from* http://clinicaltrials.gov/ct2/show/NCT03705234. *[Last accessed January, 2026].*
11. Mach F, Koskinas KC, Roeters van Lennep JE, et al. 2025 focused update of the 2019 ESC/EAS guidelines for the management of dyslipidaemias. Eur Heart J. 2025;46(42):4359-78.
12. Desai NR, Campbell C, Electricwala B, et al. Cost effectiveness of inclisiran in atherosclerotic cardiovascular patients with elevated low-density lipoprotein cholesterol despite statin use: a threshold analysis. Am J Cardiovasc Drugs. 2022;22(5):545-56.
13. Ray KK, Troquay RPT, Visseren FLJ, et al. Long-term efficacy and safety of inclisiran in patients with high cardiovascular risk and elevated low-density lipoprotein cholesterol (ORION-3): results from the 4-year open-label extension of the ORION-1 Trial. Lancet Diabetes Endocrinol. 2022;11:109-19.
14. Reijman MD, Schweizer A, Peterson AL, et al. Rationale and design of two trials assessing the efficacy, safety, and tolerability of inclisiran in adolescents with homozygous and heterozygous familial hypercholesterolaemia. Eur J Prev Cardiol. 2022;29(9):1361-8.
15. Wright RS, Collins MG, Stoekenbroek RM, et al. Effects of renal impairment on the pharmacokinetics, efficacy, and safety of inclisiran: an analysis of the ORION-7 and ORION-1 studies. Mayo Clinic Proc. 2020;95(1):77-89.
16. Cordero A, Santos-Gallego CG, Fácila L, et al. Estimation of the major cardiovascular events prevention with Inclisiran. Atherosclerosis. 2020;313:76-80.
17. Landmesser U, Haghikia A, Leiter LA, et al. Effect of inclisiran, the small-interfering RNA against proprotein convertase subtilisin/kexin type 9, on platelets, immune cells, and immunological biomarkers: a pre-specified analysis from ORION-1. Cardiovasc Res. 2021;117(1):284-91.
18. Wilson P, Elvey R, Mathieson A, et al. Evaluating the implementation of inclisiran in primary care: process evaluation interim findings from interviews with key stakeholders. BMJ Open. 2025;15(2):e083441.
19. Writing Committee; Lloyd-Jones DM, Morris PB, et al. 2022 ACC expert consensus decision pathway on the role of nonstatin therapies for LDL-cholesterol lowering in the management of atherosclerotic cardiovascular disease risk: a report of the American College of Cardiology Solution Set Oversight Committee. J Am Coll Cardiol. 2022;80(14):1366-418.

163

CHAPTER

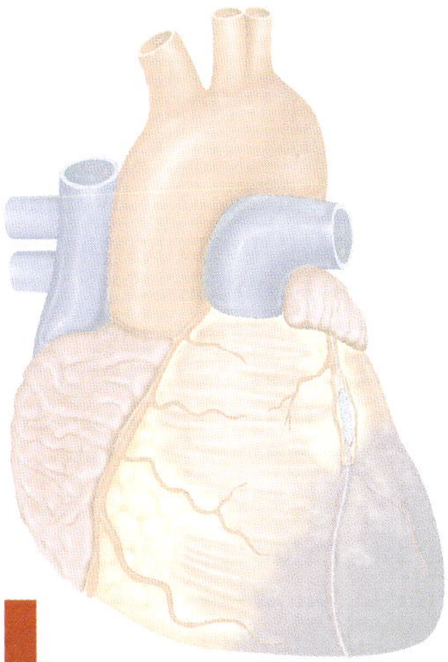

Combination Use of Inclisiran and Statins versus Statins alone in the Treatment of Dyslipidemia: Is there a Significant Difference?

Abraham Oomman, Narra Lavanya

INTRODUCTION

Cardiovascular diseases (CVDs) are the primary cause of mortality worldwide. Dyslipidemia is a major modifiable risk factor for CVDs. Lowering low-density lipoprotein cholesterol (LDL-C) has been the target of dyslipidemia therapy. The management of dyslipidemia has been mainly through dietary modifications, exercise, and medications. Statins have been the mainstay for the treatment of dyslipidemia. Additional oral therapies include ezetimibe, fibrates, niacin, and newer molecules like bempedoic acid. In recent years, injectables have been added to this armamentarium, including PCSK9 (proprotein convertase subtilisin/kexin type 9) inhibitors and a small interfering ribonucleic acid (siRNA), inclisiran. We will discuss the benefit of addition of inclisiran to background statin therapy in comparison to statin therapy alone in this article.

BACKGROUND

Atherosclerosis is caused by the gradual deposition of LDL-C and other apolipoprotein-B (ApoB)-containing lipoproteins within the wall of the artery triggering a cascade of inflammatory reactions which leads to the formation and progression of atherosclerotic plaques. With further accumulation of atherogenic lipoproteins over time, the plaque burden increases and so does the risk of having an acute cardiovascular (CV) event. LDL-C is considered a direct cause of atherosclerotic cardiovascular disease (ASCVD), thus lowering LDL-C levels is an important part of dyslipidemia management.[1] The management of dyslipidemia is based on the risk class of an individual. The ESC 2019 guidelines recommend an LDL-C target of <116 mg/dL in low-risk individuals, <100 mg/dL in moderate-risk, <70 mg/dL in high-risk, and <55 mg/dL in very high-risk population.[2]

PHARMACOTHERAPY FOR THE MANAGEMENT OF DYSLIPIDEMIA

Oral Lipid-lowering Agents

The most widely used and effective oral drugs are the statins which limit the rate-limiting step in cholesterol synthesis. Cholesterol absorption inhibitors like ezetimibe reduce the amount of cholesterol delivered to liver and decrease LDL-C levels. Bile acid sequestrants prevent the reabsorption of cholesterol into the blood and decrease LDL-C levels. They include older molecules such as cholestyramine and colestipol and the newer synthetic colesevelam. Lomitapide is a microsomal triglyceride transfer protein which reduces LDL-C levels by preventing the formation of very low-density lipoproteins (VLDL) and chylomicrons in the liver and intestine respectively.

Fibrates and omega-3 fatty acids are peroxisome proliferator-activated receptor-α (PPAR-α) agonists and have shown to reduce triglycerides effectively. Nicotinic acid and cholesteryl ester transfer protein inhibitors (CETPi) have been showed to increase high-density lipoprotein cholesterol (HDL-C) levels with mild effect in reducing LDL-C both drugs are not approved. The newer oral drug includes bempedoic acid which inhibits ATP citrate lyase enzyme in the cholesterol pathway and reduces LDL-C by 30% when used as monotherapy.[2]

INJECTABLE LIPID-LOWERING AGENTS

The available injectables used for lipid lowering are all delivered subcutaneously. The antisense oligonucleotide mipomersen reduces LDL-C levels by degrading messenger RNA (mRNA) molecules. *PCSK9i* inhibits the PCSK9 protein and decreases LDL-C by increasing the expression of LDL receptors on the cell surface. This group of injectables includes human monoclonal antibodies, alirocumab, and evolocumab. The latest injectable drug reducing LDL-C by 50% is inclisiran, with an effect lasting for nearly 6 months which will be discussed further in detail.[2]

STATINS

Statins are recommended as the initial pharmacologic agent to reduce ASCVD events due to their proven efficacy, safety, and cost-effectiveness.

MECHANISM OF ACTION

Statins inhibit the HMG-CoA reductase enzyme which is the rate-limiting step in cholesterol biosynthesis thus reducing the synthesis of cholesterol in the liver. This leads to increase in the number of LDL receptors on the surface of the hepatocytes, which results in increased uptake of LDL from the blood, and decreased plasma concentrations of LDL-C and other ApoB-containing lipoproteins, including triglyceride-rich particles.

A high-intensity statin reduces LDL-C by ≥50% and moderate-intensity statin reduces LDL-C by 30–50%. Statins reduce triglyceride levels by 10% and increase HDL-C by 1–10%.[3,4] When LDL-C goals are not achieved with statins, combination therapy with one or more lipid-lowering therapies (LLTs) is recommended by guidelines and expert recommendations.[5] The combination of high-intensity statin with ezetimibe, bempedoic acid, and PCSK9 inhibitors can reduce LDL-C levels to a maximum of 86%.[6]

Statin Trials

Various randomized controlled trials (RCTs) have shown the benefits of statins in reducing LDL-C and associated ASCVD events. The Scandinavian Simvastatin Survival Study (4S) in high-risk ASCVD patients who received 40 mg simvastatin or placebo was the first statin trial to demonstrate this benefit. During a follow-up period of 5.4 years, LDL-C was lowered by 35%, total mortality by 30% and major adverse cardiac events (MACEs) by 34%.[7]

In the Cholesterol Treatment Trialists (CTT) meta-analysis of 26 trials of a statin versus control or a more versus less intensive statin regimen, for each 1 mmol/L reduction in LDL-C, there was a 22% reduction in CV and 10% reduction in total mortality over 5 years. The individuals with the highest risk were seen to have maximum benefit compared to the primary prevention population.[8]

The JUPITER trial randomized healthy men and women with LDL-C >130 mg/dL and with high-sensitivity C-reactive protein (hsCRP) levels of ≥2.0 mg/L to 20 mg rosuvastatin daily or placebo. Rosuvastatin reduced LDL-C levels by 50% and hsCRP levels by 37%. There was a 44% decrease in CV events and a 20% lower total mortality in rosuvastatin group after a mean follow-up of 4.5 years.[9] The HOPE-3 (Heart Outcomes Prevention Evaluation-3) trial demonstrated a 26.5% reduction in LDL-C and a 24% decrease in CV events in intermediate-risk individuals without ASCVD treated with 10 mg rosuvastatin versus placebo and followed for 5.6 years.[10]

Adverse Effects of Statins

Statins are usually well tolerated but a subset of patients have muscle symptoms, termed "statin-associated muscle symptoms (SAMS)" including muscle pains and tenderness with normal or mild elevation in creatinine kinase (CK) levels. SAMS can be managed by reducing the dose of statin, giving them only on alternate days or switching to a different statin. Rhabdomyolysis has an incidence of 13 cases/100,000 patient-years. It is the most severe form of statin-induced muscle damage, characterized by severe muscle pains, muscle necrosis, and myoglobinuria leading to renal failure and death.[11]

Mild elevation of ALT occurs in 0.5–2.0% of patients on statin therapy treatment, more commonly with potent statins or high doses. Clinically, relevant ALT elevation is defined as three times the upper limit of normal on two separate occasions.[12]

Unfortunately, there is an underutilization of statins both during initiation and dose up-titration. Studies show that even in high-risk ASCVD patients, <50% receive guideline-recommended statin dose or remain on statins after the first year after an CVD event.[13] Clinical inertia, poor adherence, side effects, and cost are some of the main reasons for this. This has paved the way to develop drugs which can be administered less frequently and yet achieve desired LDL-C goals with minimal side effects.

Statins and Guidelines

The ESC 2025 guidelines give a class I recommendation to calculate SCORE2 (Systematic Coronary Risk Evaluation 2) for CVD risk estimation in apparently healthy people <70 years of age without established ASCVD, diabetes mellitus, chronic kidney disease, genetic, or rare lipid disorders for estimation of 10-year fatal and nonfatal CVD risk. SCORE2-OP (Systematic Coronary Risk Evaluation 2-Older Persons) is used in people >70 years of age. High-intensity statin to the maximum tolerated dose should be prescribed to reach the target LDL-C goal for the specific risk level and if goal is not reached, ezetimibe should be added (class I recommendation).

For primary prevention in very high-risk patients, LDL-C goal is <70 mg/dL and in high-risk patients the LDL-C goal is <100 mg/dL (class IA recommendation).[6] In secondary prevention patients at very-high risk, an LDL-C reduction of >50% from baseline with a LDL-C goal of <55 mg/dL is recommended (class IA recommendation).[2]

INCLISIRAN

Inclisiran is a siRNA molecule that inhibits hepatic synthesis of PCSK9 protein. It was approved in 2020 by the European Medicines Agency for treatment in patients with primary hypercholesterolemia or mixed dyslipidemia on maximally tolerated statin therapy and gained FDA approval in 2021 for the treatment of clinical ASCVD or heterozygous familial hypercholesterolemia (FH) in patients on maximally tolerated statin therapy. In 2023, the FDA also approved inclisiran for the treatment of primary hyperlipidemia.[14]

Mechanism of Action

Inclisiran essentially decreases the production of PCSK9 protein production resulting in increased LDL receptor recycling, leading to increased hepatic LDL-C clearance and lower LDL-C levels. The plasma concentration of inclisiran peaks at ≈4 hours after a dose and has an elimination half-life from the plasma of ≈9 hours. It has no significant drug interactions.[15]

Inclisiran is a subcutaneous formulation available in a prefilled syringe containing 284 mg/1.5 mL. The dosing schedule is day 1 injection followed by a second dose 3 months later and then once every 6 months in addition to maximum tolerated daily statins and/or other LLTs.[15] Inclisiran has been shown in phase III trials to lower LDL-C levels by approximately 50%.[16]

Inclisiran Trials

The efficacy and safety of inclisiran were investigated in three phase 3 RCTs: ORION-9, ORION-10, and ORION-11. Over 1,800 patients on maximally tolerated statins or other nonstatin LLT (if statin-intolerant), with either heterozygous FH (ORION-9), ASCVD (ORION-10), and ASCVD or ASCVD risk-equivalent (ORION-11) received inclisiran. Participants were given either 300 mg of inclisiran sodium or placebo subcutaneously on days 1, 90, 270, and 450. There was a –50.7% mean change in the LDL-C at day 510 by a pooled analysis of these three studies.[17]

Majority of patients reached prespecified LDL-C goals of <70 mg/dL (86.6%) and <50 mg/dL (74.6%). At day 150, inclisiran also lowered total cholesterol levels (–32.4%), non-HDL-C (–46.3%), ApoB (–41.7%), lipoprotein (a) (–20.2%), and triglycerides (–9.9%), while increasing HDL-C (6.2%) in comparison to placebo. Inclisiran was well tolerated, with a comparable safety profile to that of placebo with the most common adverse event being injection site reactions which were usually mild.[17]

The ORION-8 trial was designed to assess the efficacy and safety of inclisiran for an additional 3-year follow-up from baseline. LDL-C was reduced by an average of 49.4% with no major side effects, demonstrating the consistent LDL-C-lowering effect and safety and tolerability profile of inclisiran.[18] Several trials to study the benefit of adding inclisiran to statin therapy are ongoing. The trials are described in **Table 1**.

Effect of Inclisiran on Background Lipid-lowering Therapies

Landmesser et al.[19] studied the ORION-10 and ORION-11 population to observe the effect of inclisiran on background LLTs. Patients treated with PCSK9i within 90 days of screening were excluded. Patients received either 284 mg inclisiran (300 mg inclisiran sodium) or a placebo administered by subcutaneous injection on day 1, day 90, and 6-monthly thereafter over a period of 540 days. They were divided into four groups based on the background of LLT: (1) Patients not on any background of LLT, (2) patients on statin monotherapy, (3) patients on ezetimibe monotherapy, and (4) patients on statin plus ezetimibe combination. Patients were also stratified on the intensity of statin therapy and CV risk.

At the end of 18 months, this post hoc analysis showed that inclisiran provided sustained and effective LDL-C lowering irrespective of the background LLT resulting in 69.5% of the population achieving their LDL-C goal.

Adverse Effects of Inclisiran

Injection site reaction, arthralgia, urinary tract infection, diarrhea, bronchitis, pain in extremities, and dyspnea.[20]

TABLE 1: Ongoing inclisiran trials.[15]

Trial	Population	Outcome
ORION-13	Adolescents (12–17 years) with homozygous FH	Efficacy and safety of inclisiran in addition to maximally tolerated statin therapy
ORION-16	Adolescents (12–17 years) with heterozygous FH	
ORION-4	Patients with a history of MI, ischemic stroke, or peripheral arterial disease	4-point major adverse cardiovascular event (MACE)
VICTORION-2 PREVENT	Patients with established CVD and LDL-C ≥70 mg/dL on stable LLT	3-point MACE
VICTORION-1 PREVENT	Patients without ASCVD at high risk of their first ASCVD event	4-point MACE
VICTORION-PLAQUE	Participants with nonobstructive coronary artery disease	To evaluate the effect of inclisiran on atherosclerotic plaque progression (assessed using computed tomography coronary angiography)
VICTORION-INITIATE	Patients with established ASCVD who have not reached LDL-C goals on maximally tolerated statin therapy	Efficacy of the adding inclisiran earlier in the treatment pathway resulted in greater lipid lowering and LDL-C goal attainment
VICTORION-INCEPTION	Patients who have had a recent hospitalization for an acute coronary syndrome	

Inclisiran and Guidelines

The 2022 American College of Cardiology Expert Consensus Decision Pathway (ECDP) has emphasized the need for LLT intensification to achieve LCL-C goals in secondary prevention population. Addition of nonstatin LLTs including ezetimibe (10 mg daily) and/or anti-PCSK9 monoclonal antibodies (alirocumab 75 mg SC once in 2 weeks or evolocumab 140 mg SC once in 2 weeks), or inclisiran, or bempedoic acid (180 mg daily) in ASCVD patients to achieve the LDL-C target is recommended by the ECDP. It also considers inclisiran for primary prevention population with severe primary hypercholesterolemia (LDL-C ≥190 mg/dL) and for those with poor adherence to anti-PCSK9 monoclonal antibodies, with anti-PCSK9 monoclonal antibody-related side effects, or in those unable to self-inject.[20]

The NICE guidelines recommend inclisiran for treating primary hypercholesterolemia (heterozygous familial and nonfamilial) or mixed dyslipidemia if the patient has a history of acute coronary syndrome, coronary or other arterial revascularization, coronary heart disease, ischemic stroke, or peripheral arterial disease, and those with LDL-C persistently ≥100 mg/dL, despite maximally tolerated LLT (i.e., maximally tolerated statins with or without other LLT, or other LLTs in case of statin intolerance).[21]

CONCLUSION

Atherosclerotic cardiovascular disease is major cause of mortality and morbidity globally. LDL-C has been shown to be a direct risk factor for this and thus guidelines have recommended increasingly aggressive LDL-C targets thresholds for patients with ASCVD or at risk for ASCVD. For various reasons, LDL-C targets are not adequately met in most patients. Inclisiran, an LDL-C-lowering siRNA molecule, administered subcutaneously, prevents PCSK9 production, thus increasing LDLR availability and clearance of LDL-C from the circulation.

Inclisiran administered twice yearly (after an initial dose and a second dose at 3 months) and demonstrated sustained LDL-C lowering with an acceptable safety and tolerability profile when added to maximally tolerated statin therapy in patients with elevated LDL-C compared to statin therapy alone. The potential effects on CV outcomes, however, have yet to be fully elucidated. Additional studies will be required to provide crucial evidence on the efficacy and safety profile of inclisiran in patients from diverse backgrounds.

REFERENCES

1. Ference BA, Ginsberg HN, Graham I, et al. Low-density lipoproteins cause atherosclerotic cardiovascular disease. 1. Evidence from genetic, epidemiologic, and clinical studies. A consensus statement from the European Atherosclerosis Society Consensus Panel. Eur Heart J. 2017;38(32):2459-72.
2. Mach F, Baigent C, Catapano AL, et al. 2019 ESC/EAS Guidelines for the management of dyslipidaemias: lipid modification to reduce cardiovascular risk: The Task Force for the management of dyslipidaemias of the European

Society of Cardiology (ESC) and European Atherosclerosis Society (EAS). Eur Heart J. 2019;41(1):111-88.
3. Reiner Ž. Managing the residual cardiovascular disease risk associated with HDL-cholesterol and triglycerides in statin-treated patients: a clinical update. Nutr Metab Cardiovasc Dis. 2013;23(9):799-807.
4. Barter PJ, Brandrup-Wognsen G, Palmer MK, et al. Effect of statins on HDL-C: a complex process unrelated to changes in LDL-C: analysis of the VOYAGER Database. J Lipid Res. 2010;51(6):1546-53.
5. Writing Committee, Lloyd-Jones DM, Morris PB, et al. 2022 ACC Expert Consensus Decision Pathway on the Role of Nonstatin Therapies for LDL-Cholesterol Lowering in the Management of Atherosclerotic Cardiovascular Disease Risk: A Report of the American College of Cardiology Solution Set Oversight Committee. J Am Coll Cardiol. 2022;80(14):1366-418.
6. Mach F, Koskinas KC, Roeters van Lennep JE, et al. 2025 Focused Update of the 2019 ESC/EAS Guidelines for the management of dyslipidaemias: Developed by the task force for the management of dyslipidaemias of the European Society of Cardiology (ESC) and the European Atherosclerosis Society (EAS). Eur Heart J. 2025; ehaf190.
7. Randomised trial of cholesterol lowering in 4444 patients with coronary heart disease: the Scandinavian Simvastatin Survival Study (4S). Lancet. 1994;344(8934):1383-9.
8. Cholesterol Treatment Trialists' (CTT) Collaboration, Baigent C, Blackwell L, et al. Efficacy and safety of more intensive lowering of LDL cholesterol: a meta-analysis of data from 170,000 participants in 26 randomised trials. Lancet. 2010;376(9753):1670-81.
9. Ridker PM, Danielson E, Fonseca FAH, et al. Rosuvastatin to Prevent Vascular Events in Men and Women with Elevated C Reactive Protein. N Engl J Med. 2008;359(21):2195-207.
10. Yusuf S, Bosch J, Dagenais G, et al. Cholesterol Lowering in Intermediate-Risk Persons without Cardiovascular Disease. N Engl J Med. 2016;374(21):2021-31.
11. Law M, Rudnicka AR. Statin safety: a systematic review. Am J Cardiol. 2006;97(8A):52C-60C.
12. Marcum ZA, Vande Griend JP, Linnebur SA. FDA drug safety communications: a narrative review and clinical considerations for older adults. Am J Geriatr Pharmacother. 2012;10(4):264-71.
13. Toth PP, Granowitz C, Hull M, et al. Long-term statin persistence is poor among high-risk patients with dyslipidemia: a real-world administrative claims analysis. Lipids Health Dis. 2019;18(1):175.
14. European Medicines Agency (EMA). (2021). Leqvio. [online] Available from https://www.ema.europa.eu/en/medicines/human/EPAR/leqvio [Last accessed January, 2026].
15. Wilkinson MJ, Bajaj A, Brousseau ME, et al. Harnessing RNA Interference for Cholesterol Lowering: The Bench-to-Bedside Story of Inclisiran. J Am Heart Assoc. 2024;13(6):e032031.
16. Ray KK, Wright RS, Kallend D, et al. Two Phase 3 Trials of Inclisiran in Patients with Elevated LDL Cholesterol. N Engl J Med. 2020;382(16):1507-19.
17. Wright RS, Ray KK, Raal FJ, et al. Pooled Patient-Level Analysis of Inclisiran Trials in Patients With Familial Hypercholesterolemia or Atherosclerosis. J Am Coll Cardiol. 2021;77(9):1182-93.
18. Wright RS, Raal FJ, Koenig W, et al. Inclisiran administration potently and durably lowers LDL-C over an extended-term follow-up: the ORION-8 trial. Cardiovasc Res. 2024;120(12):1400-10.
19. Landmesser U, Koenig W, Leiter LA, et al. Efficacy and safety of inclisiran based on background lipid-lowering treatment. Eur J Prev Cardiol. 2025;zwaf214.
20. Writing Committee; Lloyd-Jones DM, Morris PB, et al. 2022 ACC Expert Consensus Decision Pathway on the Role of Nonstatin Therapies for LDL-Cholesterol Lowering in the Management of Atherosclerotic Cardiovascular Disease Risk: A Report of the American College of Cardiology Solution Set Oversight Committee. J Am Coll Cardiol. 2022;80(14):1366-1418. Erratum in: J Am Coll Cardiol. 2023;81(1):104.
21. NICE. (2021). Guidance, Inclisiran for treating primary hypercholesterolaemia or mixed dyslipidaemia. Technology appraisal guidance, TA733: 1 Recommendations. [online] Available from https://www.nice.org.uk/guidance/ta733/chapter/1-Recommendations [Last accessed January, 2026].

164

CHAPTER

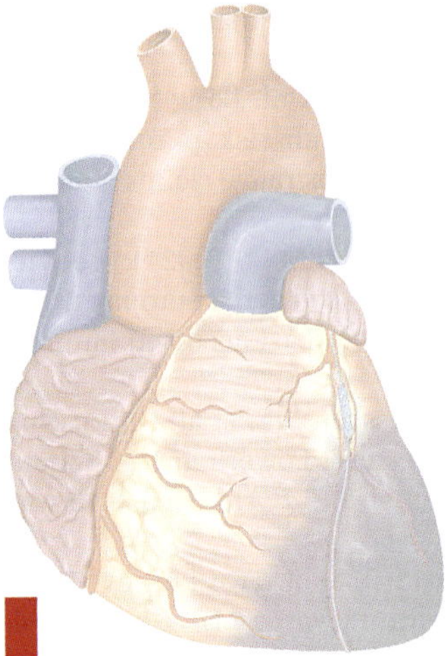

Inclisiran in Dyslipidemia with High-risk Atherosclerotic Vascular Burden

Ankit Kumar Choudhury, Neeraj Pandit

INTRODUCTION

Atherosclerotic cardiovascular disease (ASCVD) remains a global public health problem despite of significant advances in its prevention and treatment. A recent report from the Global Burden of Disease (GBD) Study covering the period from 1990 to 2023 confirms that ischemic heart disease (IHD) and Stroke are classified as Level 3 causes of mortality.[1] A positive correlation between circulating low-density lipoprotein cholesterol (LDL-C) levels and coronary heart disease has been demonstrated by numerous epidemiological and clinical studies.[2] India has the dubious distinction of having the highest number of ASCVD patients in the world. Case-control and prospective studies in India have reported that dyslipidemia **(Flowchart 1)**, especially raised total cholesterol, low-density lipoprotein (LDL), non-high-density lipoprotein cholesterol (non-HDL-C), triglycerides, and apolipoprotein B (ApoB), are the most important risk factors for ASCVD.[3]

Although statins are the first-line treatment for preventing and managing recurrent major adverse cardiovascular events (MACE) in patients with ASCVD, only 20–40% of very high-risk patients achieve target LDL-C levels with statin monotherapy. While the benefits of statin-based lipid-lowering therapy are well established, its real-world use remains limited due to poor long-term adherence. Factors such as cost, concerns about side effects, and mixed perceptions of their benefits often lead patients to discontinuation of statin in the long term.

The emerging non-statin lipid-lowering therapies (non-LLT) include ezetimibe, bempedoic acid, and proprotein convertase subtilisin/kexin type 9 (PCSK9) inhibitors. Two global approaches target PCSK9 through injectable therapies. The first uses monoclonal antibodies to lower LDL-C and reduce cardiovascular events. The second is inclisiran, a small interfering ribonucleic acid (siRNA) approved by the US Food and Drug Administration (FDA) and the European Medicines Agency (EMA), which also effectively lowers LDL-C levels.

Addition of Ezetimibe or PCSK9 monoclonal antibodies to statin therapy has shown to reduce the risk of MACE by 6.4% and 15%, respectively, versus statin alone. Bempedoic acid decreases the risk of MACE by 13% in statin-intolerant patients. Data shows that despite the availability of nonstatin LLT, upto 80% of patients may not reach target LDL goals.

INCLISIRAN

Inclisiran sodium is a first-in-class siRNA designed to lower LDL-C levels through a unique mechanism targeting PCSK9 mRNA. It has emerged as an innovative therapeutic option for patients with hypercholesterolemia, particularly for those who cannot achieve LDL-C goals with conventional therapies such as statins, or for patients who demonstrate statin intolerance.

Mechanism of Action

Inclisiran employs RNA interference to specifically bind to and cleave PCSK9 mRNA in hepatocytes. By inhibiting the translation of PCSK9, the drug indirectly increases the availability of LDL receptors on the liver

Flowchart 1: Simplified dyslipidemia management.

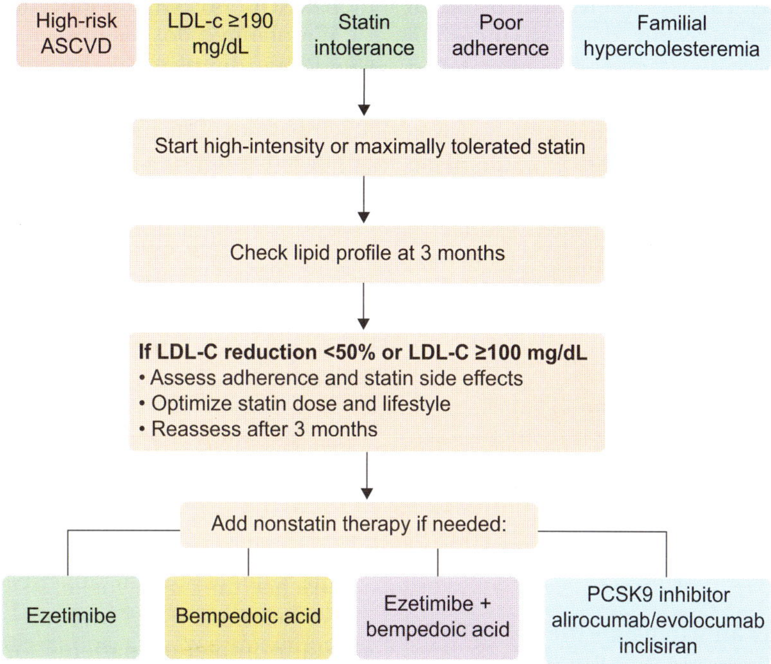

surface, thereby enhancing the clearance of LDL-C from the bloodstream. Its design includes conjugation with N-acetylgalactosamine (GalNAc), which ensures liver-specific uptake and mitigates off-target effects. Notably, even though inclisiran has a short plasma half-life (around 5–10 hours), its effect on lowering PCSK9 and LDL-C is prolonged, lasting months after administration due to the durable gene-silencing effect.

Inclisiran's efficacy has been demonstrated across multiple published research trials (ORION family of trials):

- *ORION-1 (Phase II)*:[4] The phase II ORION-1 trial evaluated different dosing schedules and reported the highest LDL-C reduction with two 300 mg doses (days 1 and 90) of 52.6% at day 180. On day 240, LDL-C was 47.2% lower, and in 1 year, LDL-C was 31.4% lower compared to baseline. The PCSK9 levels decreased by 69.1% at day 180, with a sustained reduction of 40% on day 240. Other reductions on day 180 included non-HDL-C (46%), ApoB (41%), triglycerides (14%), VLDL-C (16%), and Lp(a) (26%); HDL-C increased by 8.6%.
- *ORION-9*:[5] It randomized 482 adult Heterozygous familial hypercholesterolemia (HeFH) patients on maximum statins ± ezetimibe with a baseline LDL-C ≥ 100 mg/dL, to inclisiran on day 1, 90, 270, 450, or placebo. The mean LDL-C reduction was 39.7% at day 510. The PCSK9 level decreased by 60.7% at day 510, with consistent effects across genetic variants (LDLR, ApoB, and PCSK9).
- *ORION-10 and ORION-11*:[6] These trials assessed the efficacy of inclisiran in the secondary prevention and high-risk primary prevention patients with LDL-C ≥ 70 mg/dL and ASCVD or LDL C ≥ 100 mg/dL and ASCVD equivalent, such as diabetes, familial hypercholesterolemia, or 10-year ASCVD risk ≥ 2 %. The LDL-C levels were reduced by 52.3% in the ORION-10 trial and by 49.9% in ORION-11trial.
- *Effects of inclisiran in patients with atherosclerotic cardiovascular disease: A pooled analysis of the ORION-10 and ORION-11 Randomized*: Inclisiran produced a ~50–52% placebo-corrected reduction in LDL-cholesterol in patients with established ASCVD when added to background lipid-lowering therapy. A large majority of patients achieved very low LDL-C levels, with ~88% reaching <55 mg/dL at least once, supporting its effectiveness for secondary prevention in very high-risk ASCVD. LDL-C lowering was consistent irrespective of age, sex, diabetes status, renal function, or baseline LDL-C, indicating broad applicability in real-world ASCVD populations. Inclisiran was well tolerated, with no new safety concerns identified over ~18 months; adverse events were comparable to placebo apart from mild injection-site reactions.[7]

- *ORION-3 (4-year extension)*:[8] It is an open label 4-year extension study. Patients receiving inclisiran in ORION-1 were given twice-yearly inclisiran (inclisiran arm only), whereas patients receiving placebo in ORION-1 first received evolocumab 140 mg every 2 weeks until day 360 and then twice-yearly inclisiran (switching arm). In the inclisiran-only arm, the mean sustained LDL-C reduction was 44.2% over nine doses. In the switching arm, evolocumab resulted in a 61% LDL-C reduction. After switching to inclisiran, the 3-year time-averaged LDL-C reduction was 45.3% over seven injections. This suggests that evolocumab is more effective in reducing LDL-C.

Ongoing Trials on Inclisiran

- *ORION-4 trial*:[9] The primary goal of ORION-4 is to determine the effect of inclisiran and its impact on reducing MACE in people with existing ASCVD. It is a phase 3, double-blind, randomized, placebo-controlled trial.
- *ORION-8 trial*:[10] It is an extension trial of ORION-9,10,11 and includes patients with homozygous familial hypercholesterolemia.
- *VICTORION-1 prevent trial*:[11] It is a Phase 3, randomized clinical trial to evaluate the LDL-C–lowering efficacy and safety of inclisiran when added to background guideline-directed lipid-lowering therapy. It strengthens evidence that inclisiran provides potent, durable LDL-C reduction in high-risk patients inadequately controlled on conventional therapy, paving the way for large outcomes of trials (VICTORION-2P, ORION-4).
- *VICTORION-2 prevent trial—inclisiran CV outcomes trial*:[12] The VICTORION-2P trial is designed to determine whether inclisiran—given on top of high-intensity statin therapy—can reduce MACE in adults with established ASCVD.
- *VICTORION PLAQUE trial*:[13] Phase III study assessing the effect of inclisiran on coronary atherosclerotic plaque progression using CT imaging in patients with nonobstructive coronary artery disease.

Dosing and Administration

Inclisiran sodium is given as a 300 mg subcutaneous injection (equivalent to 284 mg inclisiran) in the abdomen, thigh, or upper arm, with the first dose administered on the first day, followed by a second injection on day 90, and then every 6 months. Inclisiran is available as a 1.5 mL solution packaged in a prefilled glass syringe.

Inclisiran does not induce or inhibit cytochrome P450 enzymes or other common drug transporters; clinically significant drug-drug interactions are unlikely. It is not indicated for pregnant or breastfeeding women.

If a planned dose is missed by <3 months, inclisiran should be administered and dosing continued according to the patient's original schedule. If a planned dose is missed by 3 or more months, a new dosing schedule should be started as if it were a new patient. In transitioning from PCSK9i mabs, inclisiran can be administered immediately after the last dose of PCSK9i mab or within 2 weeks after the last dose of PCSK9i mab.

Inclisiran's twice-yearly dosing schedule simplifies therapy compared to anti-PCSK9 monoclonal antibodies, which require injections every 2–4 weeks and often must be administered in hospital settings.

Therapeutic Indications of Inclisiran

- High risk ASCVD.
- Patients of ASCVD on maximum tolerated dose of statins and other lipid-lowering drugs, but still not reached the target goal of LDL-C, and are at high risk for recurrent ASCVD events.
- Statin-intolerant patients for secondary prevention using non statin pathway.
- Poor long-term adherence to therapy.
- Homozygous or heterozygous familial hypercholesterolemia.

Adverse Effects

- Minor injection site reactions include localized erythema, swelling, pain, and pruritus, with occasional occurrences of rash and thrombophlebitis.
- Mild elevations of hepatic transaminases < 3 times upper limit of normal.

Possible Interactions

- *Impact on T2DM*:[14] Absence of an increased risk of new-onset or worsening T2DM, which is a common side effect associated with statin therapy. Statins have been linked to insulin resistance and the subsequent development of diabetes; however, inclisiran's targeted mechanism offers a promising advantage by focusing on PCSK9, thereby bypassing multiple metabolic pathways and suggesting a lower risk of interference with glucose metabolism.
- *Respiratory and immune effects*: Recent studies indicate that inclisiran does not have a significant effect on immune cells, including leukocytes, monocytes, and neutrophils, as well as inflammatory biomarkers.[15] Conversely, inclisiran has been shown to reduce the immune cascade by reducing toll-like receptor 4 levels in circulating monocytes.[16]

- *Hepatic and renal impairment*: In patients with mild/moderate (Child–Pugh class A/B) hepatic disease or mild/moderate renal impairment, no dose adjustment is required.[17,18] There is no data in patients with severe hepatic disease (Child–Pugh class C) or severe renal impairment.

CONCLUSION

Inclisiran, a novel siRNA therapy that inhibits the production of PCSK9, is a useful adjunct to maximally tolerated statin therapy ± ezetimibe in patients with clinical ASCVD or HeFH who require additional LDL-lowering. Off label, inclisiran may be an effective option in patients with statin-associated side effects, given its unique mechanism of targeted uptake by hepatocytes. The intervention substantially reduces lipid parameters such as LDL-C, PCSK9, Apo-B, and total cholesterol without increasing the risk of major adverse events. However, more trials are required to assess its impact on reducing MACE.

REFERENCES

1. Naghavi M, Kyu HH, Aalipour MA, et al. Global burden of 292 causes of death in 204 countries and territories and 660 subnational locations, 1990–2023: a systematic analysis for the Global Burden of Disease Study 2023. Lancet. 2025;406(10513):1811-72.
2. Mortensen MB, Nordestgaard BG. Elevated LDL cholesterol and increased risk of myocardial infarction and atherosclerotic cardiovascular disease in individuals aged 70-100 years: a contemporary primary prevention cohort. Lancet. 2020;396(10263):1644-52.
3. Sharma S, Gaur K, Gupta R. Trends in epidemiology of dyslipidemias in India. Indian Heart J. 2024;76(Suppl 1):S20-8.
4. Leiter LA, Teoh H, Kallend D, et al. Inclisiran lowers LDL-C and PCSK9 irrespective of diabetes status: the ORION-1 randomized clinical trial. Diabetes Care. 2019;42(1):173-6.
5. Raal FJ, Kallend D, Ray KK, et al. Inclisiran for the treatment of heterozygous familial hypercholesterolemia. N Engl J Med. 2020;382(16):1520-30.
6. Ray KK, Wright RS, Kallend D, et al. Two phase 3 trials of inclisiran in patients with elevated LDL cholesterol. N Engl J Med. 2020;382(16):1507-19.
7. Wright RS, Ray KK, Landmesser U, et al. Effects of inclisiran in patients with atherosclerotic cardiovascular disease: a pooled analysis of the ORION-10 and ORION-11 randomized trials. Mayo Clin Proc. 2024;S0025-6196(24):00167-8.
8. Ray KK, Troquay RP, Visseren FL, et al. Long-term efficacy and safety of inclisiran in patients with high cardiovascular risk and elevated LDL cholesterol (ORION-3): results from the 4-year open-label extension of the ORION-1 trial. Lancet Diabetes Endocrinol. 2023;11(2):109-19.
9. Clinicaltrials.gov. (2025). A Randomized Trial Assessing the Effects of Inclisiran on Clinical Outcomes Among People With Cardiovascular Disease (ORION-4). [Online] Available from https://clinicaltrials.gov/study/NCT03705234 [Last accessed January, 2026].
10. Wright RS, Raal FJ, Koenig W, et al. Inclisiran administration potently and durably lowers LDL-C over an extended-term follow-up: the ORION-8 trial. Cardiovasc Res. 2024;120(12):1400-10.
11. Clinicaltrials.gov. (2026). A Study of Inclisiran to Prevent Cardiovascular Events in High-risk Primary Prevention Patients. [Online] Available from https://clinicaltrials.gov/study/NCT05739383 [Last accessed January, 2026].
12. Clinicaltrials.gov. (2025). Study of Inclisiran to Prevent Cardiovascular (CV) Events in Participants With Established Cardiovascular Disease (VICTORION-2P). [Online] Available from https://clinicaltrials.gov/study/NCT05030428 [Last accessed January, 2026].
13. Clinicaltrials.gov. (2025). Coronary Computed Tomography Study to Assess the Effect of Inclisiran in Addition to Maximally Tolerated Statin Therapy on Atherosclerotic Plaque Progression in Participants With a Diagnosis of Non-obstructive Coronary Artery Disease Without Previous Cardiovascular Events (V-PLAQUE). [Online] Available from https://clinicaltrials.gov/study/NCT05360446 [Last accessed January, 2026].
14. Laakso M, Fernandes SL. Statins and risk of type 2 diabetes: Mechanism and clinical implications. Front. Endocrinol. 2023;14:1239335.
15. Landmesser U, Haghikia A, Leiter LA, et al. Effect of inclisiran, the small-interfering RNA against proprotein convertase subtilisin/kexin type 9, on platelets, immune cells, and immunological biomarkers: A pre-specified analysis from ORION-1. Cardiovasc Res. 2021;117(1):284-91.
16. Bernhard J, Engelberger K, Galli L, et al. Inclisiran reduces expression of Toll-like receptor-4 on circulating monocytes. Eur Heart J. 2023;44 (Suppl_S2): ehad655.3293.
17. Kallend D, Stoekenbroek R, He Y, et al. Pharmacokinetics and pharmacodynamics of inclisiran, a small interfering RNA therapy, in patients with hepatic impairment. J Clin Lipidol. 2022;16(2):208-19.
18. Wright RS, Collins MG, Stoekenbroek RM, et al. Effects of renal impairment on the pharmacokinetics, efficacy, and safety of inclisiran: an analysis of the ORION-7 and ORION-1 studies. Mayo Clin Proc. 2020;95(1):77-89.

165

CHAPTER

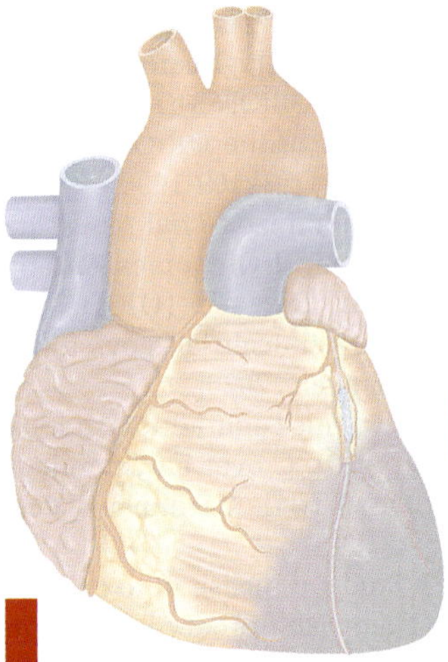

Inclisiran in Statin Intolerant and High-risk CAD Patients with Dyslipidemia

Viveka Kumar, Sangeeta Dhir, Mitendra Singh Yadav, HK Chopra

INTRODUCTION

Cardiovascular disease (CVD) remains the leading cause of morbidity and mortality worldwide, with dyslipidemia—particularly elevated low-density lipoprotein cholesterol (LDL-C)—recognized as a central driver of atherosclerotic cardiovascular disease (ASCVD). Statins have long been the cornerstone of lipid-lowering therapy, offering robust LDL-C reductions and proven cardiovascular risk reduction. However, a significant subset of patients either fail to achieve target LDL-C levels despite maximal statin therapy or are unable to tolerate statins due to adverse effects such as myalgia, hepatotoxicity, or other intolerance syndromes.

Incisura, a novel small interfering RNA (siRNA) therapy, silences messenger RNA responsible for the production of proprotein convertase subtilisin/kexin type 9 (PCSK9) in hepatocytes.[1] By reducing PCSK9 synthesis, inclisiran enhances LDL receptor recycling and clearance of LDL-C from the bloodstream. This mechanism is distinct from monoclonal antibodies targeting circulating PCSK9, offering a durable effect with infrequent dosing.

Administered subcutaneously on day 0, day 90, and then every 6 months thereafter, inclisiran's biannual regimen addresses one of the most persistent challenges in lipid management—long-term adherence. Clinical trials and real-world evidence consistently demonstrate sustained LDL-C reductions of approximately 45–55%, with excellent tolerability and minimal injection-site reactions.[1-3]

INCLISIRAN IN HIGH-RISK AND VERY HIGH-RISK PATIENTS

Despite the widespread use of high-intensity statins, many very high-risk patients fail to achieve recommended LDL-C targets. Indian real-world data show that nearly 80% of patients with prior cardiovascular events remain above target LDL-C thresholds, even though 97% were prescribed high-dose statins.[4] This mirrors the DA VINCI study, which underscored the persistent need for advanced lipid-lowering agents across Europe[5] and the LAI REACT study, which demonstrated that even with aggressive triple therapy following an acute event, one in three patients continued to have LDL-C levels above target after 6 weeks.[6]

The Phase 3 ORION-10 and ORION-11 trials have shown inclisiran's efficacy in both established ASCVD patients and those with ASCVD risk-equivalents.[1]

- *Established ASCVD (ORION-10):* Inclisiran achieved a placebo-adjusted LDL-C reduction of up to 52% at day 510. The majority of patients reached guideline-recommended LDL-C targets, with sustained reductions across the trial duration. Safety outcomes were comparable to placebo.[1]
- *ASCVD risk-equivalents (ORION-11):* In patients with diabetes and organ damage or familial hypercholesterolemia, inclisiran produced a placebo-adjusted LDL-C reduction of 50% at day 510, with an absolute decrease of 58 mg/dL. Patients previously unable to achieve LDL-C goals with statins and

ezetimibe were able to reach targets when inclisiran was added, with a favorable tolerability profile.[1]

INCLISIRAN IN STATIN-INTOLERANT PATIENTS

Statin-associated adverse effects, particularly muscle-related symptoms, remain a major barrier to effective lipid management. Statin intolerance is a recognized challenge across Asia, including India, with prevalence estimates ranging from 5 to 17%.[7,8] Globally, meta-analyses suggest that about 1 in 10–12 patients experience statin intolerance, with higher rates observed in real-world cohorts compared to randomized trials. Asian populations appear particularly susceptible, with factors such as older age, diabetes, obesity, and high-dose statin use contributing to increased risk.[9] This is especially concerning given India's high burden of premature CAD, where failure to maintain optimal LDL-C control can significantly increase cardiovascular risk.

In ORION-10 and ORION-11, a subgroup of 252 patients not receiving statins at baseline—largely due to intolerance was analyzed.[10] Inclisiran demonstrated potent and durable LDL-C lowering in this cohort, with a placebo-adjusted mean reduction of 45.8% at day 510, corresponding to an absolute decrease of 68 mg/dL ($p < 0.0001$). These findings underscore inclisiran's therapeutic potential for patients unable to tolerate statins, offering nearly 50% LDL-C reduction with biannual dosing and a tolerability profile comparable to placebo.

PLACE OF INCLISIRAN IN CURRENT GUIDELINES FOR VERY HIGH-RISK AND STATIN-INTOLERANT PATIENTS

Across recent guidance from ESC/EAS 2025, ACC/AHA 2025, and CSI 2024, inclisiran is positioned as an adjunctive, nonstatin LDL-C-lowering therapy for patients at very high cardiovascular risk who do not achieve guideline-recommended targets despite maximally tolerated statins and ezetimibe, and for those with documented statin intolerance. For very high-risk ASCVD, ESC/EAS 2025 emphasizes early combination therapy and endorses adding PCSK9-pathway inhibitors—including inclisiran to reach stringent LDL-C goals, consistent with evidence for durable 50% reductions and improved goal attainment; ACC/AHA 2025 similarly recommends stepping up to nonstatins (inclisiran, PCSK9 mAbs, and bempedoic acid) when LDL-C remains above threshold despite optimized statins/ezetimibe or when statins are not tolerated; CSI 2024 aligns with this stepwise approach in India, endorsing inclisiran as a practical biannual option to improve adherence and achieve targets in very high-risk and statin-intolerant populations, particularly where daily therapy or injection frequency limits persistence and control.

CONCLUSION

Inclisiran represents a breakthrough in lipid management for statin-intolerant and high-risk CAD patients. Its novel siRNA mechanism, durable LDL-C lowering, and convenient twice-yearly dosing address critical gaps in current therapy. Evidence from Phase 3 trials and real-world data demonstrates that inclisiran consistently achieves up to 50% LDL-C reductions, with a safety profile comparable to placebo.[1,2,6] In regions such as India, where premature CAD and statin intolerance are prevalent, inclisiran offers a transformative opportunity to improve cardiovascular outcomes.[9] As guidelines increasingly emphasize aggressive LDL-C lowering in very high-risk patients, inclisiran is poised to become a cornerstone of secondary prevention strategies.[4,5]

REFERENCES

1. Ray KK, Wright RS, Kallend D, et al. Two phase 3 trials of inclisiran in patients with elevated LDL cholesterol. N Engl J Med. 2020;382(16):1507-19.
2. Wright RS, Ray KK, Raal FJ, et al. Pooled safety and efficacy analysis of inclisiran in patients with ASCVD or risk equivalents. J Am Coll Cardiol. 2021;77(9):1182-93.
3. Yalamanchi R, Showkathali R, Rao MS, et al. Inclisiran: a breakthrough in LDL-C reduction for Indian ASCVD patients. Eur Heart J. 2025;46(Suppl 1):ehaf784.3738
4. Jain M, Sawant R, Panchal H, et al. Evaluating LDL-C control in Indian acute coronary syndrome (ACS) patients—A retrospective real-world study LDL-C control in ACS. Int J Cardiol Cardiovasc Risk Prev. 2023;19:200210.
5. Ray KK, Molemans B, Schoonen WM, et al. DA VINCI study: Contemporary management of dyslipidemia in Europe. Eur J Prev Cardiol. 2021;28(12):1279-89.
6. Mahajan K, Puri R, Duell PB, et al. Rapid achievement of low-density lipoprotein cholesterol goals within 1 month after acute coronary syndrome during combination therapy with rosuvastatin, ezetimibe and bempedoic acid: Initial experience from the LAI-REACT study. J Clin Lipidol. 2024;18(5):e867-e872.
7. Banach M, Rizzo M, Toth PP, et al. Statin intolerance—an underestimated problem in high-risk patients. Curr Vasc Pharmacol. 2015;13(5):684-92.
8. Stroes ES, Thompson PD, Corsini A, et al. Statin-associated muscle symptoms: impact on therapy. Eur Heart J. 2015;36(17):1012-22.
9. Patnaik A. Inclisiran in India: A Game-changer for Dyslipidemia Management. Indian J Clin Cardiol. 2024;5(4):323-4.
10. Wright RS, Kallend D, Raal RJ, et al. Pooled safety and efficacy of inclisiran in patients with statin intolerance (ORION-10 and ORION-11). Eur Heart J. 2020;41(Supplement_2):ehaa946.3009.

166

CHAPTER

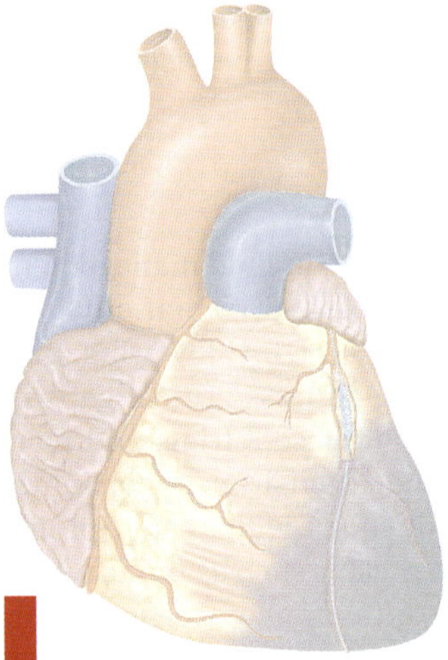

Inclisiran and Beyond: Combination Lipid-lowering Strategies

Umesh Chandra Tripathi, Sharad Chandra

INTRODUCTION

Cardiovascular disease (CVD) remains the leading cause of morbidity and mortality worldwide, sustaining its burden despite advances in public health and the challenges of the COVID-19 era. Central to its pathogenesis is the atherogenic retention and modification of low-density lipoprotein cholesterol (LDL-C) within the arterial intima, a pivotal and modifiable driver of risk. Statins remain the foundation of lipid-lowering therapy, often augmented by ezetimibe or proprotein convertase subtilisin/kexin type 9 (PCSK9) inhibitors in patients with familial hypercholesterolemia or high cardiovascular risks. Yet, many individuals fail to achieve guideline-recommended LDL-C thresholds due to statin intolerance, suboptimal adherence to chronic oral regimens, and persistent residual risk. These limitations underscore an urgent imperative for next-generation therapies offering sustained efficacy and more comprehensive cardiovascular risk reduction.[1]

Inclisiran represents a first-in-class small interfering RNA (siRNA) therapy that provides sustained lowering of LDL-C by selectively inhibiting hepatic synthesis PCSK9. This targeted silencing enhances LDL receptor recycling and increases hepatic clearance of circulating LDL-C. With its twice-yearly subcutaneous dosing schedule following initiation, inclisiran offers a transformative approach to lipid management by improving long-term adherence and ensuring consistent lipid control. Data from the ORION clinical trial program confirms its robust and durable LDL-C-reducing efficacy across broad patient populations, including those with atherosclerotic CVD and familial hypercholesterolemia, with an excellent safety and tolerability profile.[2]

Optimal dyslipidemia management demands a multifaceted strategy to maximize cardiovascular risk reduction. Integrating inclisiran with established lipid-lowering therapies marks a paradigm shift, reinforcing the value of synergistic combination therapy—particularly for high-risk patients with ASCVD or familial hypercholesterolemia who require intensive interventions to meet stringent guideline targets.[3]

Emerging evidence shows that inclisiran, when added to maximally tolerated statins ± ezetimibe, achieves durable LDL-C reductions of up to 52%, with real-world data confirming that 38% of such patients attain the <55 mg/dL target recommended in current guidelines.[4]

CURRENT THERAPIES

Compelling evidence underscores that precise dyslipidemia management is central to reducing cardiovascular risk in both primary and secondary prevention. A broad therapeutic arsenal—including statins, ezetimibe, PCSK9 inhibitors, bempedoic acid, and fibrates—allows personalized treatment tailored to individual risk, comorbidities, and therapeutic objectives, with guideline-directed combinations optimizing LDL-C lowering and safety.[5]

Comprehensive dyslipidemia management integrates lifestyle modification—diet, exercise, weight control, and smoking cessation—with individualized pharmacotherapy, forming the cornerstone of guideline-based strategies to optimize lipid levels and reduce cardiovascular risks.[6]

Statins remain the cornerstone of dyslipidemia management due to their potent LDL-C-lowering capacity and proven cardiovascular risk reduction. By competitively inhibiting HMG-CoA reductase—the key enzyme in hepatic cholesterol synthesis—they reduce intracellular cholesterol levels, upregulate hepatic LDL receptors, and thereby enhance plasma LDL clearance.

Extensive evidence from large, randomized trials and meta-analyses demonstrates that statins markedly reduce cardiovascular morbidity and all-cause mortality. The benefits correlates with the degree of LDL-C reduction, with each 1 mmol/L decrease conferring an approximate 20–25% relative risk reduction in major vascular events.[7]

Despite their central role in dyslipidemia therapy, statin efficacy may be limited by intolerance—affecting 5–30% of patients—due to muscle symptoms or liver enzyme elevations, leading to reduced adherence and missed LDL-C targets. Additionally, genetic variability, drug interactions, and inconsistent use can result in suboptimal LDL-C reduction in some individuals.[8,9]

Ezetimibe selectively inhibits the NPC1L1 transporter, reducing intestinal absorption of dietary and biliary cholesterol. It lowers LDL-C by ~18–20% as monotherapy and, when combined with statins, achieves an additional 15–25% reduction, enhancing overall lipid-lowering efficacy.[10]

The IMPROVE-IT trial demonstrated that adding ezetimibe to statin therapy yields greater LDL-C reduction and significantly lowers cardiovascular events in high-risk patients, particularly postacute coronary syndrome, cementing its role as the preferred second-line agent after statins. Ezetimibe combined with statins lowers LDL-C by roughly 20–24% beyond statin monotherapy.[11]

Proprotein convertase subtilisin/kexin type 9 monoclonal antibodies, such as evolocumab and alirocumab, are potent lipid-lowering agents that can reduce LDL-C by up to 60%. By binding circulating PCSK9, they block its interaction with hepatic LDL receptors, preventing receptor degradation and promoting receptor recycling, thereby markedly enhancing LDL clearance from the bloodstream.[12]

Landmark trials have firmly established the efficacy of PCSK9 inhibitors in cardiovascular risk reduction. In FOURIER (evolocumab) and ODYSSEY OUTCOMES (alirocumab), adjunctive therapy to maximally tolerated statins significantly lowered major adverse cardiovascular events, including myocardial infarction and stroke, with ODYSSEY showing a trend toward reduced all-cause mortality. Both agents demonstrated excellent safety, aside from a slight increase in injection-site reactions.[13]

Despite their proven efficacy, broader adoption of PCSK9 monoclonal antibodies is limited by high costs, the need for frequent subcutaneous injections, and restricted access in some healthcare systems. Addressing these barriers is essential to enhance their accessibility and cost-effectiveness while preserving their therapeutic benefits.[14]

Bempedoic acid is an oral prodrug activated in the liver that inhibits ATP-citrate lyase, a key enzyme upstream of HMG-CoA reductase in cholesterol synthesis. This reduces hepatic cholesterol production, upregulates LDL receptors, and lowers LDL-C by 15–30%. Its liver-specific activation spares skeletal muscle, minimizing muscle-related side effects. Additionally, bempedoic acid activates AMP-activated protein kinase, reducing inflammation as reflected by lower hsCRP, making it a valuable option for statin-intolerant patients and for combination lipid-lowering therapy.[15,16]

Clinical trials have demonstrated that bempedoic acid is generally well tolerated and significantly lowers LDL-C and inflammatory markers, supporting its role as an important adjunctive option in contemporary lipid management, especially for those unable to tolerate statins.[17] It can be used alone or with other agents, also reducing inflammation markers like hsCRP, potentially offering additional cardiovascular benefits.[18]

INCLISIRAN

Inclisiran is a first-in-class siRNA that durably lowers LDL-C by silencing hepatic PCSK9 synthesis, thereby promoting LDL receptor recycling and clearance. Its biannual maintenance dosing after two initial injections markedly improves adherence compared with more frequent PCSK9 mAb regimens.[3]

Across ORION trials, inclisiran consistently achieved ~48–50% sustained LDL-C reductions on top of maximally tolerated therapy. In ORION-9, HeFH patients saw a 47.9% placebo-adjusted fall maintained to day 510, while ORION-10/11 confirmed comparable 18-month durability in ASCVD and risk-equivalent cohorts. Tolerability was excellent, limited to mild, transient injection-site reactions, with no signal for hepatic, muscular, or renal toxicity—aligning with its liver-specific PCSK9 silencing and negligible extrahepatic impact.[19]

Inclisiran, with its twice-yearly dosing, offers sustained ~50% LDL-C reduction and improved adherence, addressing residual cardiovascular risk. Exploratory ORION 9, 10, and 11 data suggest a 26% MACE reduction, but definitive outcomes await the ~16,000-patient ORION-4 trial, the results are expected in 2026, which will guide inclisiran's clinical role and guideline positioning in cardiovascular prevention.[20]

COMBINATION STRATEGIES

Despite major advances in lipid therapy, many patients with ASCVD or familial hypercholesterolemia remain above LDL-C targets, underscoring the need for complementary combination strategies. As a first-in-class siRNA inhibiting hepatic PCSK9 synthesis, inclisiran is well suited for integration into such intensified lipid-lowering regimens.[21]

Inclisiran with Statins

Statins remain the foundation of hypercholesterolemia therapy, with unparalleled evidence for cardiovascular risk reduction. In patients with statin intolerance or suboptimal response, combining statins with inclisiran offers mechanistic synergy—statins increase LDL receptor synthesis, while inclisiran suppresses PCSK9-driven receptor degradation, enhancing receptor recycling and LDL-C clearance. This approach is particularly valuable for very high-risk patients requiring maximal and sustained lipid lowering. In the ORION-10 and ORION-11 phase 3 trials, inclisiran administered biannually on top of maximally tolerated statins (with or without ezetimibe) achieved sustained LDL-C reductions of approximately 50%.[22]

Inclisiran with Ezetimibe

Ezetimibe, a selective inhibitor of intestinal cholesterol absorption, complements inclisiran's hepatocyte-targeted siRNA suppression of PCSK9. Their combination provides a potent nonstatin strategy for patients with statin intolerance or residual LDL-C elevation, integrating reduced cholesterol absorption with enhanced LDL receptor recycling to achieve guideline-recommended lipid targets in high-risk populations. The combination of inclisiran and ezetimibe results in an LDL-C reduction of approximately 50–57%.[23]

Inclisiran with Bempedoic Acid

Bempedoic acid inhibits hepatic ATP-citrate lyase upstream of HMG-CoA reductase, reducing cholesterol synthesis while sparing muscle tissue due to liver-specific activation. Combining bempedoic acid with inclisiran may yield additive LDL-C lowering via complementary pathways, though confirmation awaits dedicated trials. This nonstatin pairing could fill a key therapeutic gap for statin-intolerant patients with high residual cardiovascular risk.[24] The combination of inclisiran and bempedoic acid can achieve approximately 55–60% LDL-C reduction.[25]

Inclisiran with PCSK9 Monoclonal Antibodies

Combining inclisiran with PCSK9 monoclonal antibodies could, in theory, produce profound LDL-C reductions by targeting PCSK9 synthesis and circulating protein simultaneously. However, given their overlapping efficacy and high cost, this approach is generally impractical, reserved only for select cases such as homozygous familial hypercholesterolemia or refractory dyslipidemia unresponsive to standard therapy.

Combination lipid-lowering therapy enhances efficacy and supports adherence. Inclisiran's twice-yearly dosing minimizes treatment burden, while agents like ezetimibe or bempedoic acid allow regimen tailoring. In practice, adding inclisiran to statins first, then incorporating additional agents as needed, offers a pragmatic, patient-centered path to optimal lipid control.[26]

LIMITATIONS

Inclisiran marks a major advance in lipid-lowering therapy, but its high cost remains a key barrier to broad adoption, particularly in low- and middle-income settings, and even within high-income regions due to reimbursement constraints. While ORION trials confirmed durable LDL-C reduction, they were not designed for cardiovascular outcomes; definitive evidence from the ongoing ORION-4 trial will clarify its impact on major adverse events and guide its positioning in future prevention strategies.

Inclisiran has a favorable safety profile, with mild, transient injection-site reactions and no significant myopathy or hepatic toxicity reported to date, though long-term data remain limited. Its twice-yearly dosing supports adherence but depends on reliable follow up to maintain LDL-C control, while global access is constrained by healthcare infrastructure, reimbursement, and cost disparities.

ALGORITHMS AND GUIDELINES

Dyslipidemia management follows a stepwise approach, starting with lifestyle optimization and statin therapy. In patients not meeting LDL-C targets, ezetimibe or PCSK9 monoclonal antibodies are added to further reduce risk. However, real-world use is often constrained by adherence challenges and the high cost of PCSK9 antibodies, limiting access and sustained therapy.

Inclisiran, an siRNA-based therapy targeting hepatic PCSK9 mRNA, provides potent, sustained LDL-C reduction. Endorsed by current ESC/EAS guidelines, it is indicated for ASCVD, familial hypercholesterolemia, and statin intolerance—either as monotherapy or in combination with statins and/or ezetimibe after optimization of standard therapy—offering enhanced efficacy, lower treatment burden, and improved adherence.[27]

The 2025 ESC/EAS Guidelines give a Class I, Level B recommendation for adding nonstatin agents such as bempedoic acid or inclisiran when LDL-C goals are unmet with maximally tolerated statins. Bempedoic acid is preferred for statin-intolerant patients and may be combined with statins ± ezetimibe in high-risk individuals. For very high-risk patients, especially post-ACS, early combination therapy with high-intensity statins plus ezetimibe is strongly advised to rapidly achieve LDL-C ≤55 mg/dL. The choice of nonstatin therapy should be guided by the degree of additional LDL-C lowering required.

CONCLUSION

Inclisiran, the first RNAi lipid-lowering agent, selectively degrades hepatic PCSK9 mRNA, resulting in near-complete PCSK9 suppression and durable LDL-C reductions of about 50% with twice-yearly dosing. The ORION trials, involving over 3,600 high-risk patients, consistently demonstrated this efficacy across various statin backgrounds, with a favorable safety profile and good tolerability. This biannual dosing improves adherence and offers a convenient option for long-term cardiovascular risk reduction. While promising, broader guideline adoption awaits definitive cardiovascular outcomes from the ongoing ORION-4 trial and further cost-effectiveness data to establish its precise role in prevention strategies.

REFERENCES

1. Mourikis P, Zako S, Dannenberg L, et al. Lipid-lowering therapy in cardiovascular disease: From myth to molecular reality. Pharmacol Ther. 2020;213:107592.
2. Zhang Y, Chen H, Hong L, et al. Inclisiran: a new generation of lipid-lowering siRNA therapeutics. Front Pharmacol. 2023;14:1260921.
3. Ray KK, Wright RS, Kallend D, et al. Two Phase 3 Trials of Inclisiran in Patients with Elevated LDL Cholesterol. N Engl J Med. 2020;382(16):1507-19.
4. Naoum I, Saliba W, et al. Lipid-lowering therapy with inclisiran in the real-world setting. Atherosclerosis. 2024;395:66-73.
5. Mach F, Baigent C, Catapano AL, et al. 2019 ESC/EAS Guidelines for the management of dyslipidaemias: lipid modification to reduce cardiovascular risk. Eur Heart J. 2020;41(1):111-88.
6. Pappan N, Awosika AO, Rehman A. Dyslipidemia. StatPearls [Internet]. Treasure Island (FL): StatPearls Publishing; 2025.
7. Collins R, Reith C, Emberson J, et al. Interpretation of the evidence for the efficacy and safety of statin therapy. Lancet. 2016;388(10059):2532-61.
8. Rosenson RS, Baker SK, et al. Statin Muscle-Related Side Effects: JACC State-of-the-Art Review. J Am Coll Cardiol. 2021;77(6):752-72.
9. Bytyçi I, Penson PE, Mikhailidis DP, et al. Prevalence of statin intolerance: a meta-analysis. Eur Heart J. 2022;43(34):3213-3223.
10. Ge L, Wang J, Qi W, et al. The cholesterol absorption inhibitor ezetimibe acts by blocking the sterol-induced internalization of NPC1L1. Cell Metab. 2008;7(6):508-19.
11. Giugliano RP, Pedersen TR, et al. Clinical efficacy and safety of cholesterol-lowering treatment: JAMA. 2015;314(12):1264-73.
12. Sabouret P, Angoulvant D, Pathak A. FOURIER to ODYSSEY: the end of the journey for lipid-lowering therapy trials? Lessons from recent clinical trials with anti-PCSK9 antibodies. EuroIntervention. 2018;14(2):144-6.
13. Furtado RHM, Giugliano RP, et al. What Lessons Have We Learned and What Remains to be Done with PCSK9 Inhibitors? Cardiovasc Drugs Ther. 2020;34(1):71-83.
14. Steg PG, Cannon CP, et al. ODYSSEY Outcomes: Results Suggest Use of PCSK9 Inhibitor Reduces CV Events, LDL-C in ACS Patients. J Am Coll Cardiol. 2018;71(18):1231-41.
15. Biolo G, Frati G, et al. Mechanism of action and therapeutic use of bempedoic acid in dyslipidemia and cardiovascular risk reduction. Front Cardiovasc Med. 2022;9:1018882.
16. Shriver K. Bempedoic Acid: A Novel LDL Cholesterol-Lowering Agent. Clin Diabetes. 2020;38(4):405-7.
17. Chandramahanti S, Patel P, Farzam K. Bempedoic Acid. StatPearls [Internet]. Treasure Island (FL): StatPearls Publishing; 2025
18. Alqahtani MS, Naser AY, et al. Lipid-Lowering Medications for Managing Dyslipidemia. J Lipid Res. 2024;65(7):100123.
19. Fernández-Ruiz I, Lopez-Sendon JL. Twice-yearly inclisiran injections halve LDL-cholesterol levels in patients with ASCVD. Nat Rev Cardiol. 2020;17:260.
20. Harbi MH, Al-Muhannah M, et al. Current usage of inclisiran for cardiovascular diseases. Cardiovasc Ther. 2025;43(2):348-360.
21. Arnold N, Kosmas C, et al. PCSK9 inhibitor wars: how does inclisiran fit in with current strategies? J Clin Lipidol. 2022;16(4):422-32.
22. Albosta M, Bakke J, et al. Inclisiran: a new strategy for LDL-C lowering and cardiovascular risk reduction. Medicines (Basel). 2023;10(7):34.
23. Di Costanzo A, Mencarelli M, et al. The effects of statins, ezetimibe, PCSK9-inhibitors on lipid metabolism, inflammation, and cardiovascular outcomes. Int J Mol Sci. 2023;24(14):12345.
24. Banach M, Serhiyenko V, et al. Bempedoic acid in the management of lipid disorders: mechanisms and emerging clinical data. Curr Atheroscler Rep. 2023;25(7):201-9.
25. Landmesser U, Chapman MJ, et al. Efficacy and safety of inclisiran based on background lipid-lowering therapy: pooled analysis of the ORION-10 and ORION-11 Phase 3 trials. Eur J Prev Cardiol. 2025 Apr 16
26. Naoum I, Saliba W, Aker A, et al. Lipid-lowering therapy with inclisiran in the real-world setting: Initial data from a national health care service. J Clin Lipidol. 2024;18(5):e809-16.
27. Landmesser U, Chapman MJ, Farnier M, et al.; European Society of Cardiology (ESC); European Atherosclerosis Society (EAS). European Society of Cardiology/European Atherosclerosis Society Task Force consensus statement on proprotein convertase subtilisin/kexin type 9 inhibitors: practical guidance for use in patients at very high cardiovascular risk. Eur Heart J. 2017;38(29):2245-55.

167

CHAPTER

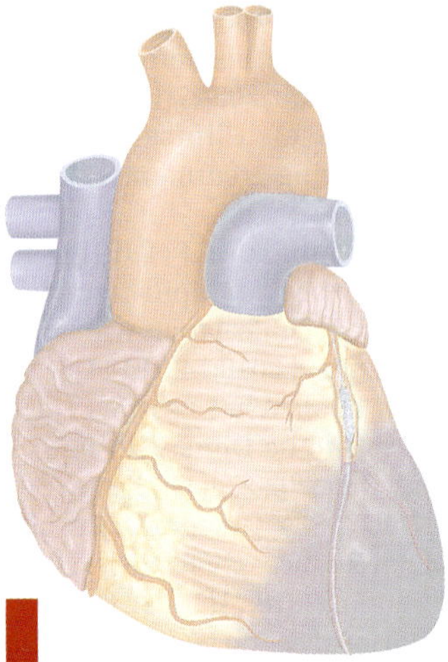

Inclisiran: A Middle Cohort Evaluating Primary and Secondary Prevention

Rajarshi Halder, Bhuban Majhi, Arup Das Biswas

INTRODUCTION

Atherosclerotic cardiovascular disease (ASCVD) remains the leading cause of morbidity and mortality globally. High levels of low-density lipoprotein cholesterol (LDL-C) are a significant modifiable risk factor. While statins and ezetimibe are the primary treatments for decreasing LDL-C, many individuals either fail to achieve the desired levels or experience intolerance to these medications.

Inclisiran presents a novel treatment alternative as the first small interfering RNA (siRNA) designed to target the liver's production of proprotein convertase subtilisin/kexin type 9 (PCSK9). In contrast to monoclonal antibodies that inhibit circulating PCSK9, inclisiran works by lowering PCSK9 production at the messenger RNA (mRNA) stage. This mechanism results in sustained reductions in both circulating PCSK9 and LDL-C. Its distinctive dosing regimen, which requires only two doses annually following initial loading doses, offers a substantial benefit for patient adherence when compared to the daily or more frequent dosing of other therapies.

This groundbreaking therapy and infrequent dosing make inclisiran especially well-suited for patients at high or very high cardiovascular risk who require effective LDL-C reduction but have difficulties with conventional treatments. Additionally, findings from clinical trials consistently demonstrate approximately 50% reductions in LDL-C across various groups, underscoring its potential efficacy as a treatment for both primary and secondary prevention, including the intermediate "middle cohort."

CONTENT AND DESCRIPTION

Mechanism of Action

Inclisiran is a long-acting synthetic siRNA that targets PCSK9. It is connected to triantennary N-acetylgalactosamine sugars, which bind to the asialoglycoprotein receptors in the liver. This promotes the rapid absorption of inclisiran into liver cells (hepatocytes). Inclisiran functions via the natural RNA interference (RNAi) pathway by associating with the RNA-induced silencing complex (RISC) within the cell. This interaction enables the degradation of PCSK9 mRNA through cleavage, preventing its translation into PCSK9. With reduced levels of PCSK9, a greater number of LDL-C receptors can be recycled back to the liver membrane for the uptake of LDL-C **(Fig. 1)**.[1]

Key Clinical Trials

Inclisiran's efficacy has been demonstrated through the pivotal ORION studies and subsequent research. In the ORION-9 trial, 482 individuals with heterozygous familial hypercholesterolemia (FH) experienced a 47.9% decrease in LDL-C by day 510. Around 75% of these participants achieved LDL-C levels below 100 mg/dL, in contrast to just 15% in the placebo cohort. The extensive ORION-10 trial conducted in the United States involved 1,561 patients with ASCVD, revealing a 52.3% reduction in LDL-C levels. In ORION-11, which included 1,617 patients from Europe and South Africa, both secondary and high-risk primary prevention groups demonstrated a 49.9% reduction.[2]

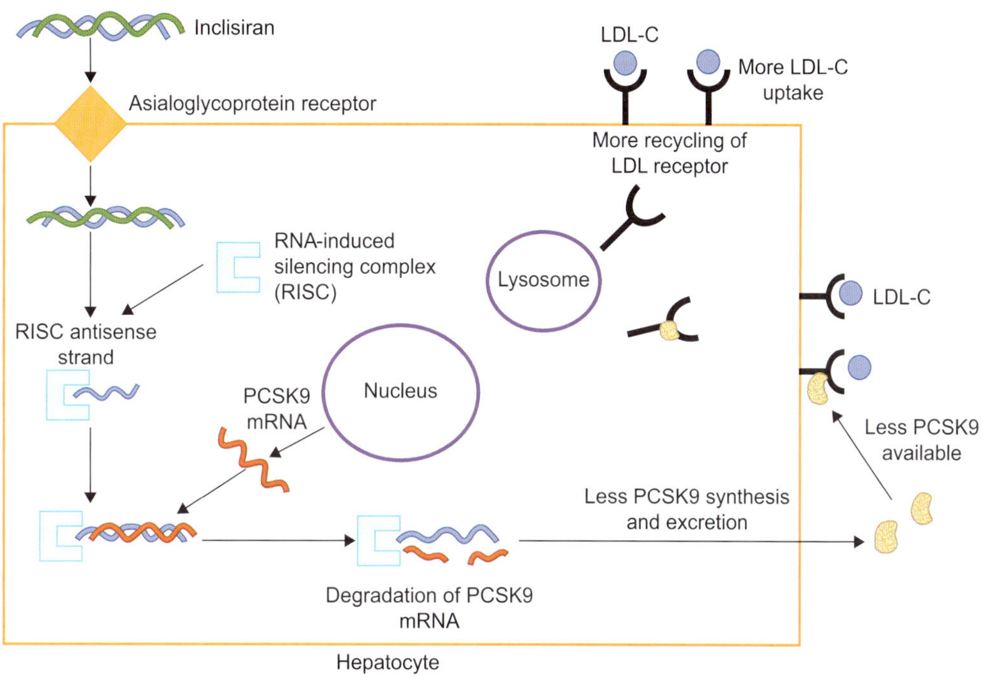

Fig. 1: Mechanism of action of inclisiran. (LDL-C: low-density lipoprotein cholesterol)

The long-term efficacy was validated in ORION-8, where 3,274 patients sustained approximately 49% reductions in LDL-C over a period of 6 years, with no new safety concerns raised. The VICTORION-Mono study, which assessed 350 patients who had never received statin treatment, indicated a 46.5% reduction in LDL-C by day 150, highlighting inclisiran's effectiveness even in the absence of background treatment.[3]

Current outcome studies, ORION-4 and VICTORION -2P, both recruiting around 15,000 participants, aim to determine whether these lipid reductions result in a decreased incidence of major adverse cardiovascular events (MACEs). Preliminary real-world data from over 5,000 patients appears promising, reflecting reductions in LDL-C of 55–60%, with >70% achieving guideline-recommended targets.[4]

These results underline inclisiran's consistent capacity to reduce LDL-C by approximately 50% across diverse populations, demonstrating enduring effectiveness, good tolerability, and significant potential for enhancing long-term cardiovascular outcomes once event data are available.

Primary Prevention Cohorts (within ORION and Other Studies)

- In the ORION-11 study, a selected group focused on primary prevention included patients without a history of ASCVD but at high risk due to factors like FH, diabetes, or a 10-year risk of 20% or more, who also had high LDL-C levels despite background therapy. In this group, inclisiran significantly reduced LDL-C, with a baseline ≈139 mg/dL. For instance, by day 510, around 66% of patients treated with inclisiran achieved a reduction of ≥50% in LDL-C, compared to ≈9% in the placebo group.[5]
- In real-world primary prevention, the recent VICTORION-Mono trial involved lower-risk participants without prior ASCVD, diabetes, or FH. This trial tested inclisiran as a standalone treatment for subjects unwilling or unable to take statins. It demonstrated safe and effective lowering of LDL-C in this group, but clinical outcomes have not yet been evaluated.

Secondary Prevention

- In populations with existing ASCVD, ORION-10 and ORION-11 showed a similar level of LDL-C reduction. For instance, in ORION-10, patients with ASCVD experienced about a 52% reduction in LDL-C compared to placebo by month 17.
- Real-world data from a retrospective study in primary care, involving secondary prevention patients, indicated that after a first dose of inclisiran, the average LDL-C dropped by around 2.00 mmol/L, or approximately

61.7%, after about 3 months. Additionally, around 79% of patients managed to achieve LDL-C levels below 70 mg/dL.[6]

OUTCOMES ON HARD CARDIOVASCULAR EVENTS

Currently, the evidence mainly focuses on surrogate endpoints like LDL-C reduction. There are a few completed large randomized trials showing MACE reduction in primary and secondary prevention groups. The ORION-4 trial, which looks at secondary prevention, is still ongoing. However, observational and simulation modeling suggests that including inclisiran in eligible groups could significantly lower CVD events. For instance, an analysis using US NHANES data estimated that nearly 200,000 cardiovascular events could be prevented if used in eligible hypercholesterolemic adults.[7]

"MIDDLE COHORT" CONCEPT

- "Middle cohort" is defined as patients who are neither clearly low risk (no comorbidities, no previous events) nor fully focused on secondary prevention. This group includes those who are at high risk for primary prevention, such as patients with risk factors like FH or diabetes. It also includes those who cannot tolerate statins but have not experienced previous ASCVD, as well as patients with moderate risk who struggle to reach LDL-C targets. The evidence from ORION and trials like VICTORION-Mono refers to this cohort.
- In the ORION-11 study (1,617 patients), the subgroup identified as high-risk for primary prevention experienced a 49.9% decrease in LDL-C levels, with 65% of participants achieving a reduction of 50% or more and 71% achieving levels below 70 mg/dL, compared to <10% in the placebo group. In the VICTORION-Mono trial, involving 350 patients who had never taken statins and with a baseline LDL-C of approximately 150 mg/dL, there was a 46.5% reduction; 91% of participants achieved a decrease of at least 30%, and 74% reached LDL-C levels below 100 mg/dL.

LIMITATIONS

Although inclisiran consistently lowers LDL-C in primary and secondary prevention groups, several limitations exist. First, most trials have focused on lipid levels instead of hard cardiovascular outcomes. Large outcome studies like ORION-4 are still ongoing, but until the report comes, we cannot be sure how inclisiran affects morbidity and mortality. Second, most trial follow-up periods are fairly short (about 18 months), though longer term data from ORION-8 are promising. Third, the results may not apply to all populations, as most participants were from Western countries. There is less evidence involving Asian, African, or low-income groups.

Implementation challenges continue. Cost and access may limit its use in many health systems, especially for primary prevention. While biannual dosing makes it easier to adhere to treatment, real-world use depends on health systems' ability to handle follow-up and injection delivery. Additionally, there is limited data on special groups, such as patients with severe renal or hepatic dysfunction, children, and pregnant women. Finally, guidelines mainly recommend inclisiran for very-high-risk primary prevention or established ASCVD, leaving its role in the "middle cohort" unclear until more outcome data become available.

SUMMARY ILLUSTRATION (2019 ESC/EAS GUIDELINES FOR THE MANAGEMENT OF DYSLIPIDEMIAS WITH 2025 FOCUSED UPDATE)

- *Primary prevention:*
  - *Low-to-moderate risk:* Lifestyle and statins remain first-line; inclisiran is not routinely indicated.
  - *High-risk groups (e.g., FH, diabetes with high LDL-C, statin intolerance):* Inclisiran may be considered when LDL-C goals are not achieved with statins ± ezetimibe.
- *Secondary prevention (established ASCVD):*
  - *Standard of care*: High-intensity statin ± ezetimibe
  - *If LDL-C remains ≥70 mg/dL (≥55 mg/dL in very-high-risk)*: PCSK9 inhibition is recommended. Inclisiran is an alternative to PCSK9 monoclonal antibodies, offering twice-yearly dosing and comparable efficacy.
- *Middle cohort* (patients between primary and secondary prevention, e.g., multiple risk factors but no prior event):
  - It may particularly benefit from inclisiran, though evidence for outcomes is still emerging.

CONCLUSION

Inclisiran provides strong and lasting LDL-C reduction with the benefit of twice-yearly dosing. This helps with the adherence problems seen with traditional therapies. Evidence supports its use in secondary prevention and in some high-risk primary prevention groups, especially for those who cannot take statins or meet LDL-C targets. However, the lack of clear cardiovascular outcomes data, limited long-term safety information, and cost issues limit its wider use. Until large outcome trial results are available, inclisiran should be seen as an additional option for very high-risk patients, while its role in the "middle cohort" remains unclear.

REFERENCES

1. Zhang Y, Chen H, Liu H, et al. Inclisiran: a new generation of lipid-lowering siRNA therapeutic. Front Pharmacol. 2023;14:1260921.
2. Ray KK, Kallend D, Leiter LA, et al. Effect of inclisiran on lipids in primary prevention: the ORION-11 trial. Eur Heart J. 2022;43:5047-57.
3. Merćep I, Friščić N, Strikić D, et al. Advantages and disadvantages of inclisiran: a small interfering ribonucleic acid molecule targeting PCSK9—a narrative review. Cardiovasc Ther. 2022;2022:1-6.
4. Ray KK, Wright RS, Kallend D, et al. Two phase 3 trials of inclisiran in patients with elevated LDL cholesterol. N Engl J Med. 2020;382(16):1507-19.
5. O'Riordan M. (2025). Inclisiran effective as monotherapy for lower-risk primary prevention. [online] Available from https://www.tctmd.com/news/inclisiran-effective-monotherapy-lower-risk-primary-prevention. [Last accessed January, 2026].
6. Deaney CN, Donaldson MP, Reesby DM, et al. Retrospective evaluation of LDL-C levels following first treatment with inclisiran as part of secondary prevention ASCVD risk reduction in a real-world primary care setting. J Prim Care Community Health. 2024;15:21501319241236339.
7. Li H, Zhao S, Wu J, et al. Estimating the effect of inclisiran on hypercholesterolemia and primary prevention of cardiovascular disease: the NHANES 1999-2018 study. Lipids Health Dis. 2024;23(1):313.

168

CHAPTER

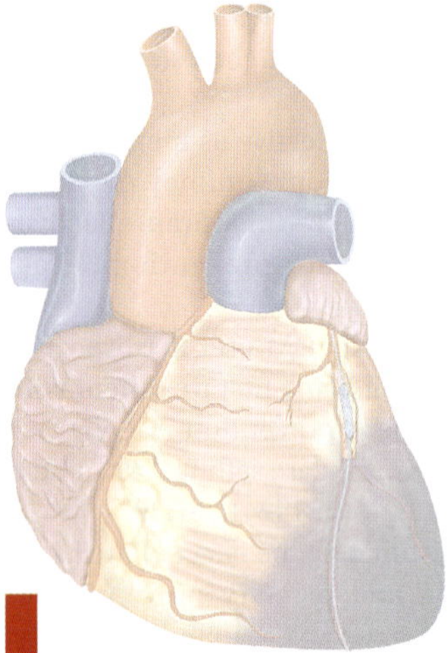

Inclisiran versus PCSK9 Monoclonal Antibodies: Comparative Review

Manoranjan Mandal, Mainak Mandal

INTRODUCTION

Atherosclerotic cardiovascular disease (ASCVD) remains a leading cause of morbidity and mortality worldwide, with elevated LDL-C being a major modifiable risk factor.[1] Although statins are the cornerstone of lipid-lowering therapy, many high-risk patients fail to achieve guideline-recommended LDL-C targets despite maximal therapy, underscoring a therapeutic gap.[2] The identification of proprotein convertase subtilisin/kexin type 9 (PCSK9) as a regulator of LDL receptor degradation has led to the development of novel LDL-lowering strategies.[3] Two distinct approaches have emerged: Small interfering RNA (siRNA) agent inclisiran which inhibits mRNA for hepatic PCSK9 synthesis and monoclonal antibodies (mAbs) that neutralize circulating PCSK9. This chapter provides a comparative review of these two newcomers, focusing on pharmacologic profiles, clinical efficacy, CV outcomes, safety, and their evolving role in lipid management.

MECHANISM OF ACTION

Proprotein convertase subtilisin/kexin type 9 (PCSK9) plays a pivotal role in lipid metabolism by regulating the degradation of LDL-R on hepatocytes. PCSK9 binds to LDL-R on the hepatocyte surface, and the complex is internalized and directed toward lysosomal degradation, leading to reduced LDL-R recycling and decreased hepatic clearance of circulating LDL particles.[3] Inhibition of the PCSK9 pathway enhances LDL-R availability and significantly lowers plasma LDL-C levels.

PCSK9 mAbs, such as evolocumab and alirocumab, are fully human mAbs that bind circulating PCSK9 with high affinity, preventing its interaction with LDL-R. This neutralization preserves receptor recycling and augments LDL-C clearance.[4,5] These agents act extracellularly and exert their effect rapidly after subcutaneous administration.

In contrast, inclisiran represents a novel, RNA interference-based approach. It is a synthetic siRNA conjugated to triantennary N-acetylgalactosamine (GalNAc) for targeted delivery to hepatocytes via asialoglycoprotein receptors.[6] Once internalized, inclisiran is incorporated into the RNA-induced silencing complex (RISC), which specifically cleaves PCSK9 mRNA, thereby reducing hepatic PCSK9 synthesis.[7] This intracellular action leads to sustained suppression of PCSK9 levels, prolonged LDL-R recycling, and durable LDL-C reduction. The mechanism allows for infrequent dosing while maintaining consistent therapeutic effect.

PHARMACOLOGY AND DOSING

Evolocumab is administered subcutaneously at a dose of 140 mg every 2 weeks or 420 mg once monthly, while alirocumab is given as 75 mg subcutaneously every 2 weeks, with potential uptitration to 150 mg depending on LDL-C response. Both agents exhibit rapid onset of action, with significant LDL-C reduction evident within days of injection, and peak effect within 1–2 weeks. Their half-lives are approximately 11–20 days, necessitating regular dosing for sustained effect.[8] Inclisiran is administered as a single subcutaneous injection of 284 mg, followed by a second dose at 3 months, and every 6 months thereafter. Its prolonged hepatic action allows durable LDL-C lowering with only twice-yearly maintenance dosing, typically administered by healthcare professionals rather than patients themselves.

CLINICAL EFFICACY: LDL-C LOWERING

Both therapeutic classes provide substantial LDL-C reductions when added to statins and/or ezetimibe. PCSK9 mAbs demonstrated robust LDL-C lowering in large phase 3 trials. Evolocumab in the FOURIER trial reduced LDL-C by 59% from baseline on top of statins, while alirocumab in ODYSSEY OUTCOMES achieved reductions of approximately 50–60% depending on baseline levels.[4,5] Inclisiran has shown comparable LDL-C lowering in the ORION program. In ORION-10 and ORION-11, inclisiran reduced LDL-C by approximately 50% compared with placebo at 510 days in patients with ASCVD or ASCVD risk equivalents on maximally tolerated statins.[7] ORION-9 demonstrated similar efficacy in patients with heterozygous familial hypercholesterolemia.[9] Importantly, inclisiran maintains stable LDL-C suppression between doses, reflecting its durable mechanism of action.

CARDIOVASCULAR OUTCOMES EVIDENCE

A key distinction between these therapies lies in the maturity of cardiovascular outcome data. PCSK9 mAbs have demonstrated significant reductions in major adverse cardiovascular events (MACE) in large outcome trials. In FOURIER, evolocumab reduced the risk of the composite primary end point (CV death, MI, stroke, hospitalization for unstable angina, or coronary revascularization) by 15% over a median follow-up of 2.2 years.[1] ODYSSEY OUTCOMES showed that alirocumab reduced MACE by 15% in post-acute coronary syndrome (ACS) patients over 2.8 years, with a signal toward lower all-cause mortality.[5] In contrast, inclisiran outcome data are still emerging. The ORION-10 and ORION-11 trials were not powered for cardiovascular events, though exploratory analyses suggested numerically lower events in the inclisiran arms.[7] The pivotal ORION-4 trial, enrolling ~16,000 participants with ASCVD, is designed to evaluate the impact of inclisiran on major cardiovascular events; its results are awaited.[10] Until then, inclisiran's cardiovascular benefit is extrapolated from its LDL-C-lowering effect, in line with the well-established relationship between LDL-C reduction and ASCVD risk.

Several clinical trials have demonstrated the effectiveness of PCSK9 inhibitors in patients with ACS. In the EVOPACS trial, 308 ACS patients received atorvastatin 40 mg plus evolocumab 420 mg or placebo, with 95.7% of those on evolocumab achieving LDL-C levels <70 mg/dL by 8 weeks, compared to 37.6% on placebo. The EVACS trial involved 57 patients with NSTEMI, where a single 420 mg dose of evolocumab led to LDL-C <70 and <55 mg/dL at discharge in 80.8 and 65.4% of patients, respectively, versus 38.1 and 23.8% with placebo. In the PACMAN-AMI trial, 300 acute MI patients undergoing angioplasty received alirocumab or placebo. Alirocumab reduced LDL-C to 33.8 mg/dL, decreased atheroma volume by 1.21%, and increased fibrous cap thickness by 29.65 μm at 52 weeks, suggesting regression of coronary plaque. These trials prove the efficacy of PCSK9 inhibitors in ACS patients, though their CV outcome study is still lacking and needs to be confirmed in further prospective studies.

In the 4-year ORION-3 extension study, patients continuing twice-yearly inclisiran showed a sustained 44.2% LDL-C reduction, while those initially on evolocumab achieved 61% reduction before switching. After switching to inclisiran, the 3-year average LDL-C reduction was 45.3%, indicating that evolocumab provided greater LDL-C lowering efficacy.

SAFETY AND TOLERABILITY

PCSK9 mAbs are generally well tolerated, with the most common adverse events being injection-site reactions, nasopharyngitis, and mild upper respiratory symptoms.[11] Serious adverse events, including neurocognitive effects and new-onset diabetes, have not shown significant increases compared to placebo in pooled analyses. Inclisiran exhibits a similarly benign profile. In pooled analyses from ORION-9, -10, and -11, the incidence of serious adverse events was similar to placebo. The most frequent adverse events were mild-to-moderate injection-site reactions, occurring in approximately 5–8% of patients, which were typically transient.[7,9] No significant elevations in liver enzymes, creatine kinase, or renal adverse events have been observed. Immunogenicity is low, as inclisiran is a chemically synthesized siRNA molecule rather than a protein-based therapy.[6] Long-term safety data continue to accrue through ongoing extension studies. Both have favorable safety profiles.

PRACTICAL CONSIDERATIONS: COST, ADHERENCE, AND ADMINISTRATION

Beyond efficacy and safety, real-world implementation of lipid-lowering therapies depends heavily on practical factors, including cost, ease of administration, and patient adherence. PCSK9 mAbs require self-administration every 2–4 weeks, which may present adherence challenges, particularly in patients with polypharmacy or injection aversion.[12] Despite manufacturer price reductions in some regions, high costs remain a major barrier to widespread use, especially in low- and middle-income countries.[13] Access often depends on stringent reimbursement criteria or prior authorization, limiting utilization even among eligible patients.[14] Inclisiran, by contrast, is administered twice yearly by healthcare professionals, typically in clinic settings.[7] This infrequent dosing may improve long-term adherence, as suggested by real-world registry data indicating reduced treatment discontinuation compared to self-injected biologics.[15] From a healthcare system perspective, inclisiran's "buy-and-bill" model allows integration into existing outpatient infrastructure, potentially simplifying logistics for patients and clinicians. However, inclisiran's cost remains high, and health-economic evaluations are ongoing to determine its cost-effectiveness relative to PCSK9 mAbs across different settings.[16]

SPECIAL POPULATIONS

The choice between inclisiran and PCSK9 mAbs may differ in certain patient populations:

- *Familial hypercholesterolemia (FH):* Both therapies have demonstrated efficacy in heterozygous FH. PCSK9 mAbs reduce LDL-C by ~50–60% in FH patients, with outcome data extrapolated from broader trials. Inclisiran showed ~50% LDL-C reduction in ORION-9 among heterozygous FH patients.[9]
- *Chronic kidney disease (CKD):* PCSK9 mAbs do not require dose adjustment in mild–moderate CKD. Inclisiran is also safe in mild–moderate renal impairment; however, exposure is increased in severe CKD, though no dose modification is currently recommended.[7]
- *Elderly:* Both classes have been studied in older populations with consistent efficacy and safety.[16] Inclisiran's infrequent dosing may offer advantages for elderly patients with limited self-care ability.
- *Diabetes:* Neither PCSK9 mAbs nor inclisiran increase the incidence of new-onset diabetes in clinical trials.[17]
- *Pregnancy and lactation:* Data are limited for both therapies; discontinuation is recommended during pregnancy and breastfeeding due to lack of safety data.[18]

REGULATORY APPROVAL

In India, the Central Drugs Standard Control Organization (CDSCO) has approved the use of evolocumab in patients with HoFH from February 2017 and for clinical ASCVD from March 2018. Alirocumab is not officially approved in India.

Inclisiran was officially approved in the European Union in December 2020 and by the US FDA in December 2021 as an adjunct therapy to dietary intervention and maximal dose of statin for adults with HeFH or ASCVD. Inclisiran got approval in India by CDSCO in July 2023.

FUTURE PERSPECTIVES

The landscape of LDL-C lowering is rapidly evolving. Inclisiran represents a new therapeutic class—RNA interference-based lipid lowering—marking a shift toward infrequent, clinic-based administration.[6] Its ongoing ORION-4 outcomes trial will be critical in defining its place in cardiovascular prevention strategies. Positive results may position inclisiran as a first-line nonstatin add-on in high-risk populations who require potent LDL-C lowering with minimal dosing burden. PCSK9 mAbs continue to play a major role, particularly in patients requiring rapid LDL-C lowering, post-ACS, or where outcome data is paramount. Future developments include next-generation siRNAs with even longer duration of effect, oral PCSK9 inhibitors, and combination formulations.[19] Additionally, real-world implementation studies and cost-effectiveness analyses will shape access and guideline recommendations globally.

CONCLUSION

Both PCSK9 mAbs and inclisiran represent transformative advances in LDL-C lowering beyond statins and ezetimibe. PCSK9 mAbs offer proven cardiovascular outcome benefits, potent and rapid LDL-C reduction, but require frequent self-administration and face cost/access barriers. Inclisiran provides comparable LDL-C lowering with twice-yearly dosing, potentially improving adherence and streamlining delivery through healthcare systems, though cardiovascular outcome data are awaited. Their roles are complementary rather than competitive, and therapy selection should be individualized based on clinical context, adherence likelihood, cost, and patient preference. Together, these agents expand the therapeutic armamentarium against atherosclerotic cardiovascular disease and may help close the gap between guideline targets and real-world LDL-C control.

REFERENCES

1. Ference BA, Ginsberg HN, Graham I, et al. Low-density lipoproteins cause atherosclerotic cardiovascular disease. Eur Heart J. 2017;38(32):2459-72.
2. Mach F, Baigent C, Catapano AL, et al. 2019 ESC/EAS Guidelines for the management of dyslipidaemias: lipid

modification to reduce cardiovascular risk. Eur Heart J. 2020;41(1):111-88.
3. Seidah NG, Awan Z, Chretien M, et al. PCSK9: a key modulator of cardiovascular health. Circ Res. 2014;114: 1022-36.
4. Sabatine MS, Giugliano RP, Keech AC, et al. Evolocumab and clinical outcomes in patients with cardiovascular disease (FOURIER). N Engl J Med. 2017;376:1713-22.
5. Schwartz GG, Steg PG, Szarek M, et al. Alirocumab and cardiovascular outcomes after acute coronary syndrome (ODYSSEY OUTCOMES). N Engl J Med. 2018;379:2097-107.
6. Fitzgerald K, White S, Borodovsky A, et al. A highly durable RNAi therapeutic inhibitor of PCSK9. N Engl J Med. 2017;376:41-51.
7. Ray KK, Wright RS, Kallend D, et al. Two phase 3 trials of inclisiran in patients with elevated LDL cholesterol (ORION-10 and ORION-11). N Engl J Med. 2020;382:1507-19.
8. Robinson JG, Farnier M, Krempf M, et al. Efficacy and safety of alirocumab in reducing lipids and cardiovascular events. N Engl J Med. 2015;372:1489-99.
9. Raal FJ, Kallend D, Ray KK, et al. Inclisiran for heterozygous familial hypercholesterolemia (ORION-9). N Engl J Med. 2020;382:1520-30.
10. National Library of Medicine. (2025). A Randomized Trial Assessing the Effects of Inclisiran on Clinical Outcomes Among People With Cardiovascular Disease (ORION-4). [online] Available from https://clinicaltrials.gov/study/NCT03705234. [Last accessed January, 2026].
11. Giugliano RP, Mach F, Zavitz K, et al. Cognitive function in a randomized trial of evolocumab. N Engl J Med. 2017;377:633-43.
12. Navar AM et al. Adherence and persistence with PCSK9 inhibitors in clinical practice. J Am Heart Assoc. 2019;8:e011971.
13. Kazi DS et al. Cost-effectiveness of PCSK9 inhibitors for secondary prevention. JAMA. 2017;318(8):748-58.
14. Doshi JA et al. Prior authorization requirements for PCSK9 inhibitors across US insurers. JAMA Cardiol. 2018;3(4):293-8.
15. Reeskamp LF et al. Inclisiran adherence in real-world practice. Eur Heart J. 2023;44(5):421-9.
16. Pandor A et al. Cost-effectiveness of inclisiran vs PCSK9 inhibitors. Pharmacoeconomics. 2023;41:567-79.
17. Sabatine MS, Leiter LA, Wiviott SD, et al. Evolocumab and diabetes risk in patients with cardiovascular disease in the FOURIER trial. Lancet Diabetes Endocrinol. 2017;5:941-50.
18. Santos RD, Valenti VE, Platania S, et al. PCSK9 inhibitors and pregnancy: a review of the available evidence. J Clin Lipidol. 2020;14:415-21.
19. Catapano AL, Pirillo A. Future directions in PCSK9 inhibition. Nat Rev Cardiol. 2021;18:641-53.

169

CHAPTER

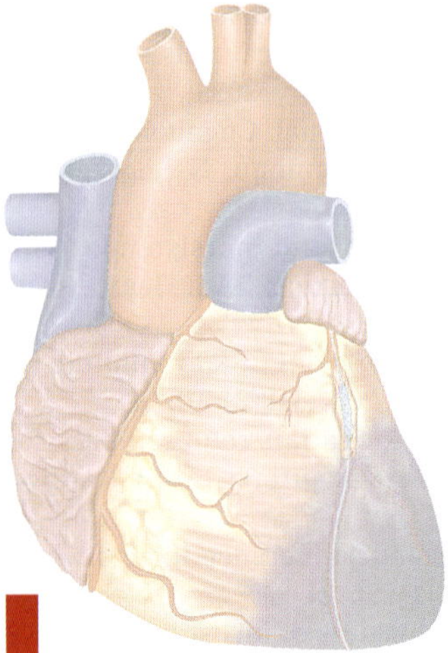

Pharmacological Profile of Inclisiran

HK Chopra, Manvika Tiwari, V Anand, AK Bali

INTRODUCTION

Cardiovascular disease (CVD) remains the leading global cause of morbidity and mortality. Elevated low-density lipoprotein cholesterol (LDL-C) is a central modifiable risk factor for atherosclerotic cardiovascular disease (ASCVD), and intensive LDL-C reduction has been shown to improve cardiovascular outcomes. While statins are first-line therapy, a substantial proportion of high-risk patients fail to achieve guideline-recommended LDL-C targets despite maximally tolerated treatment.

Nonstatin agents, particularly PCSK9 inhibitors, have transformed lipid management in such patients. Inclisiran represents a novel small-interfering RNA (siRNA)-based therapy targeting PCSK9 that leverages RNA interference to achieve durable LDL-C lowering with a convenient biannual dosing schedule. This chapter reviews the pharmacological profile of inclisiran, available clinical evidence, limitations, guideline positioning, and practical considerations in contemporary cardiovascular risk management. Inclisiran exemplifies the clinical translation of RNA interference technology into cardiovascular therapeutics, redefining long-term LDL-cholesterol control.

Understanding the pharmacological characteristics of inclisiran is essential to appreciate its unique clinical behavior, durability of LDL-cholesterol lowering, and its evolving role within contemporary lipid-lowering strategies.

MECHANISM OF ACTION AND PHARMACOLOGY

Molecular Mechanism

Inclisiran is a chemically stabilized double-stranded siRNA conjugated with a triantennary N-acetylgalactosamine (GalNAc) moiety, enabling hepatocyte-specific uptake via asialoglycoprotein receptors (ASGPRs). Once inside hepatocytes, inclisiran is incorporated into the RNA-induced silencing complex (RISC), directing enzymatic cleavage of proprotein convertase subtilisin/kexin type 9 (PCSK9) messenger RNA. Degradation of PCSK9 mRNA results in reduced hepatic PCSK9 protein synthesis, thereby enhancing LDL receptor recycling and increasing LDL-C clearance from the circulation. This upstream inhibition distinguishes inclisiran from monoclonal PCSK9 inhibitors, which neutralize circulating PCSK9 protein after secretion, as illustrated in **Figure 1**.

Pharmacokinetics

Inclisiran exhibits a distinct pharmacokinetic profile well suited for infrequent dosing:

- *Absorption:* Peak plasma concentrations are achieved approximately 4 hours after subcutaneous injection of 284 mg (equivalent to 300 mg inclisiran sodium), with plasma levels becoming undetectable within 24–48 hours.

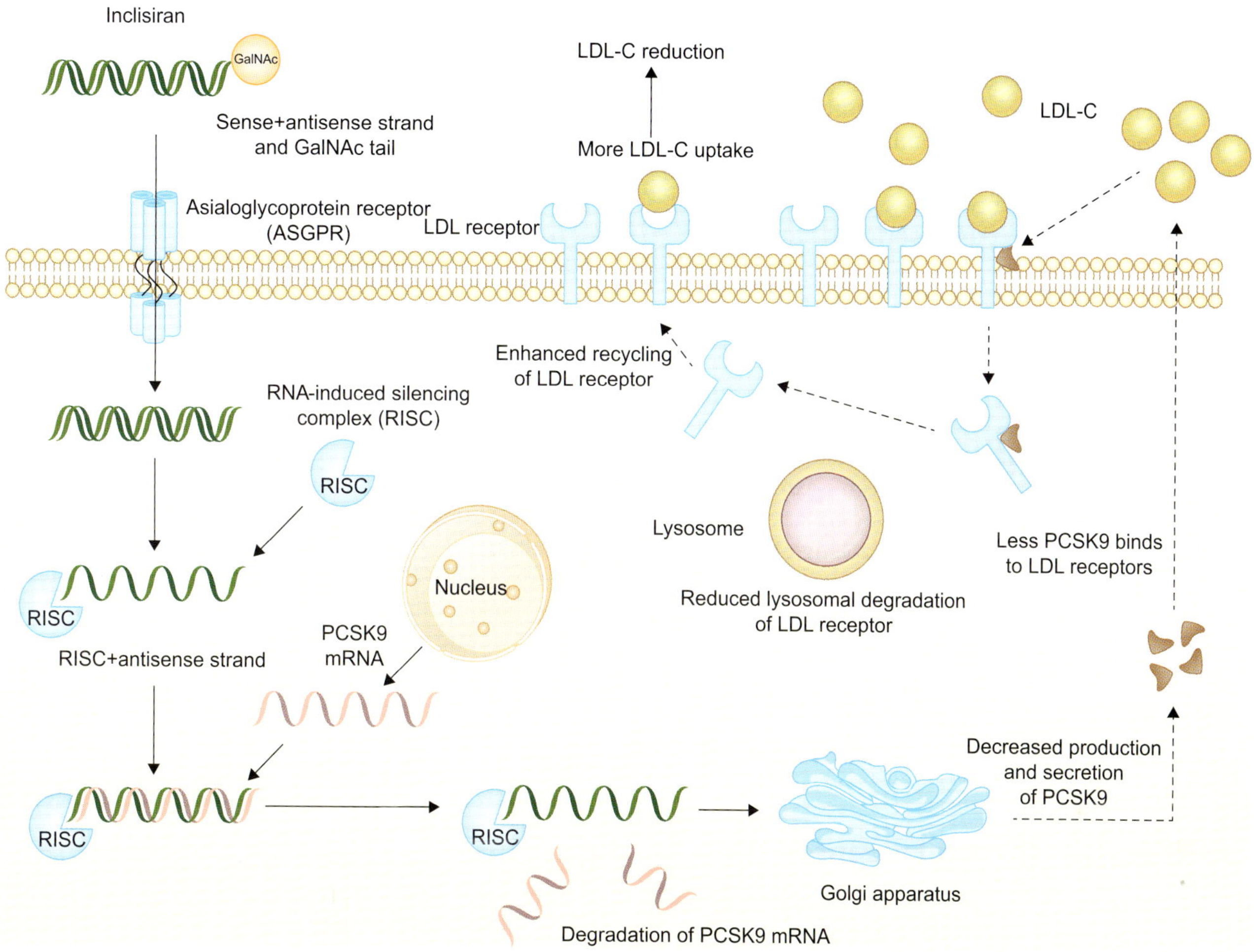

Fig. 1: Mechanism of action of inclisiran.[4] (GalNAc tail: N-acetylgalactosamine tail; PCSK9: proprotein convertase subtilisin/kexin type 9; RISC: RNA-induced silencing complex)

- *Distribution:* Inclisiran demonstrates high hepatocyte selectivity and approximately 87% plasma protein binding, without evidence of systemic accumulation.
- *Metabolism:* It is metabolized by endogenous nucleases to shorter, inactive oligonucleotides.
- *Elimination:* Approximately 16% of the administered dose is excreted renally, with a terminal plasma half-life of around 9 hours.
- *Special populations:* Pharmacokinetics are not substantially influenced by age, body weight, sex, or race. Exposure is modestly increased in renal impairment; however, no dose adjustment is required in patients with mild to moderate hepatic dysfunction.

Thus, inclisiran's rapid plasma clearance combined with its durable intracellular pharmacodynamic effect underpins its twice-yearly dosing regimen.

Dosing Regimen

Inclisiran produces rapid suppression of PCSK9 expression and sustained LDL-C reduction. Following subcutaneous administration, mean PCSK9 levels are reduced by approximately 75%, resulting in LDL-C reductions of 40–50%, with effects apparent within 14 days and maintained beyond 180 days post-dose.[1] Repeat dosing on day 1, day 90, and every 6 months thereafter sustains this effect. Inclisiran also favorably influences other atherogenic lipoproteins, including non-HDL cholesterol, apolipoprotein B, and lipoprotein(a).

CLINICAL EVIDENCE AND LIPID-LOWERING EFFECT

At the primary endpoint (day 210) of the ORION clinical trial program, inclisiran administered twice yearly by a healthcare professional resulted in sustained reductions in circulating PCSK9 concentrations of 76.4%, translating into LDL-C reductions of 47.5%. Durable reductions in other atherogenic lipids, including non-HDL cholesterol and apolipoprotein B, were maintained over a follow-up period of up to 4 years.[2] Across patient subgroups, inclisiran demonstrated consistent and sustained LDL-C lowering across glycemic and body mass index strata.[3]

COMPARISON WITH OTHER PCSK9-TARGETED THERAPIES

Inclisiran's mechanism (RNAi) differs from monoclonal PCSK9 inhibitors (e.g., evolocumab and alirocumab) that neutralize circulating protein. While both classes reduce LDL-C significantly, inclisiran's extended dosing interval (biannual maintenance) may enhance adherence compared with the more frequent dosing of monoclonal antibodies. However, monoclonal PCSK9 inhibitors have established cardiovascular outcome benefits, while inclisiran's definitive outcomes data are pending.

LIMITATIONS, UNMET NEEDS, AND PRACTICAL CLINICAL POSITIONING OF INCLISIRAN

Limitations of Current Evidence

Inclisiran produces robust and sustained reductions in LDL-C through hepatic PCSK9 silencing; however, its clinical adoption must be viewed in the context of existing evidence gaps. Unlike statins and monoclonal antibody PCSK9 inhibitors, inclisiran currently lacks mature cardiovascular outcomes data. Although the magnitude of LDL-C reduction achieved with inclisiran suggests potential cardiovascular benefit, definitive confirmation awaits the completion of large outcome trials such as ORION-4. Until such data become available, inclisiran should be regarded as an adjunctive lipid-lowering therapy rather than a replacement for therapies with proven outcome benefit. Long-term safety data beyond intermediate follow-up are also limited.

Clinical Scenarios Where Inclisiran May Be Less Suitable

Despite its advantages, inclisiran is not optimal for all clinical scenarios. In patients presenting with acute coronary syndromes or those requiring rapid LDL-C reduction, therapies with faster onset of maximal effect—such as high-intensity statins and PCSK9 monoclonal antibodies—may be preferred. Inclisiran's LDL-C lowering, though sustained, is gradual and therefore better suited for long-term maintenance rather than acute risk modification.

Inclisiran also has limited effects on triglyceride-rich lipoproteins and does not address the metabolic drivers of dyslipidemia seen in severe insulin resistance or marked hypertriglyceridemia. In such patients, therapeutic strategies targeting weight reduction, glycemic control, and triglyceride metabolism should take precedence.

GUIDELINES AND CLINICAL USE

Positioning Inclisiran in Obesity-associated Dyslipidemia

While inclisiran effectively reduces LDL-C across all body mass index categories, it does not directly address the underlying metabolic abnormalities associated with obesity. Obesity-associated dyslipidemia is characterized by increased hepatic lipoprotein production, insulin resistance, and elevated cardiovascular risk. Therefore, inclisiran should be positioned as part of a comprehensive cardiovascular risk reduction strategy that prioritizes lifestyle intervention, weight reduction, and metabolic control.

In this context, inclisiran serves as a maintenance LDL-lowering therapy, complementing statins, ezetimibe, and weight-centric interventions rather than replacing them. Its role is particularly relevant in obese patients with ASCVD who demonstrate suboptimal adherence to conventional regimens, where sustained LDL-C suppression is essential for long-term risk reduction.

Major lipid management guidelines and consensus documents now include inclisiran as a nonstatin option in select high-risk populations. It is recommended as an adjunct to diet and maximally tolerated statin therapy for adults with primary hyperlipidemia (including HeFH) and those with established ASCVD or high risk requiring additional LDL-C lowering.[5]

Where Inclisiran Adds Distinct Clinical Value

Inclisiran's greatest clinical strength lies not solely in its LDL-C-lowering potency, but in its predictable and sustained efficacy with infrequent dosing. This makes it particularly valuable in patients with poor long-term adherence to daily oral medications or more frequently administered injectable therapies. In such individuals, twice-yearly dosing administered within a supervised healthcare framework can ensure consistent LDL-C control over time.

Inclisiran may also be advantageous in patients intolerant to statins or monoclonal antibody PCSK9 inhibitors. In patients with heterozygous familial hypercholesterolemia or established ASCVD who remain above LDL-C targets despite maximally tolerated therapy, inclisiran offers a durable adjunctive option to achieve guideline-recommended goals.

CONCLUSION

Inclisiran represents a transformative advancement in lipid-lowering pharmacotherapy through targeted RNA interference against PCSK9. Through its innovative mechanism of action, potent and sustained LDL-C reduction, convenient twice-yearly dosing schedule, and favorable safety profile, inclisiran has emerged as a valuable addition to the therapeutic armamentarium for high-risk cardiovascular patients. Although definitive cardiovascular outcomes data are awaited, current evidence supports its role as an effective nonstatin adjunct in contemporary lipid management, particularly in patients with obesity-associated dyslipidemia and residual cardiovascular risk.

REFERENCES

1. Rogula S, Błażejowska E, Gąsecka A, et al. Inclisiran-Silencing the Cholesterol, Speaking up the Prognosis. J Clin Med. 2021;10(11):2467.
2. Ray KK, Troquay RPT, Visseren FLJ, et al. Long-term efficacy and safety of inclisiran in patients with high cardiovascular risk and elevated LDL cholesterol (ORION-3): results from the 4-year open-label extension of the ORION-1 trial. Lancet Diabetes Endocrinol. 2023;11(2):109-19.
3. Leiter AA, Raal FJ, Schwartz GG, et al. Inclisiran in individuals with diabetes or obesity: Post hoc pooled analyses of the ORION-9, ORION-10 and ORION-11 Phase 3 randomized trials. Diabetes Obes Metab. 2024;26(8):3223-37.
4. Zhang Y, Chen H, Hong L, et al. Inclisiran: a new generation of lipid-lowering siRNA therapeutic. Front Pharmacol. 2023;14:1260921.
5. Albosta MS, Grant JK, Taub P, et. al. Inclisiran: A new strategy for LDL-C lowering and prevention of atherosclerotic cardiovascular disease. Vasc Health Risk Manag. 2023;19:421-31.

170

CHAPTER

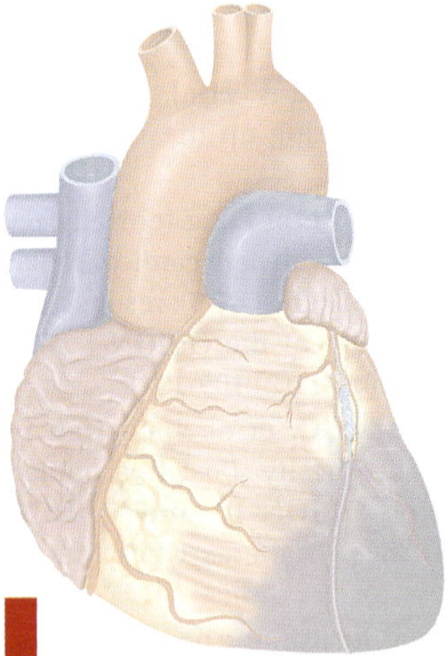

Indications, Contraindications, and Uniqueness of Inclisiran in the Management of Dyslipidemia with or without Statins

HK Chopra, Prachi Gupta, AK Pancholia, Viveka Kumar

INTRODUCTION

Despite widespread use of statins, dyslipidemia continues to be inadequately controlled in a substantial proportion of patients at high cardiovascular risk. Persistent elevation of low-density lipoprotein cholesterol (LDL-C) remains a major driver of residual atherosclerotic cardiovascular disease (ASCVD) risk. Statins remain the first-line therapy for dyslipidemia, however, barriers such as statin intolerance, suboptimal adherence to daily oral therapy, and failure to achieve recommended LDL-C targets have highlighted the need for alternative lipid-lowering strategies. ASCVD remains the leading cause of morbidity and mortality worldwide despite major advances in lipid-lowering therapy.

Proprotein convertase subtilisin/Kexin type 9 (PCSK9) has emerged as a pivotal regulator of LDL receptor metabolism. Inclisiran, a novel injectable small interfering RNA (siRNA) agent, targeting PCSK9 synthesis in liver.[1] Its long duration of action and infrequent dosing schedule offer unique clinical advantages, particularly in patients requiring sustained LDL-C reduction.

This chapter discusses the *indications, contra-indications, and unique clinical advantages of inclisiran* in the management of dyslipidemia, both as monotherapy and in combination with statins.

PHARMACOLOGICAL MECHANISM OF INCLISIRAN

Inclisiran is a synthetic, double-stranded siRNA conjugated with triantennary N-acetylgalactosamine (GalNAc), which facilitates targeted delivery to hepatocytes via the asialoglycoprotein receptor. After cellular uptake, inclisiran binds with the RNA-induced silencing complex (RISC), leading to selective degradation of PCSK9 messenger RNA. This results in sustained suppression of hepatic PCSK9 synthesis, increased recycling of LDL receptors on hepatocyte surfaces, and enhanced clearance of circulating LDL-C.[1,2]

Unlike monoclonal antibody PCSK9 inhibitors that neutralize circulating PCSK9, inclisiran acts intracellularly at the level of gene expression, providing prolonged lipid lowering effect with infrequent administration **(Fig. 1)**.

CLINICAL INDICATIONS OF INCLISIRAN

Inclisiran is indicated as an adjunct to lifestyle modifications and conventional lipid-lowering therapy in patients requiring additional LDL-C reduction. Current evidence-based indications include:

Patients with established ASCVD:[3]

- Patients with prior myocardial infarction, ischemic stroke, peripheral arterial disease, or documented coronary artery disease
- Particularly useful when LDL-C targets are not achieved despite maximally tolerated statin therapy with or without ezetimibe

Heterozygous familial hypercholesterolemia (HeFH):[3]

- Effective in significantly lowering LDL-C in genetically predisposed individuals

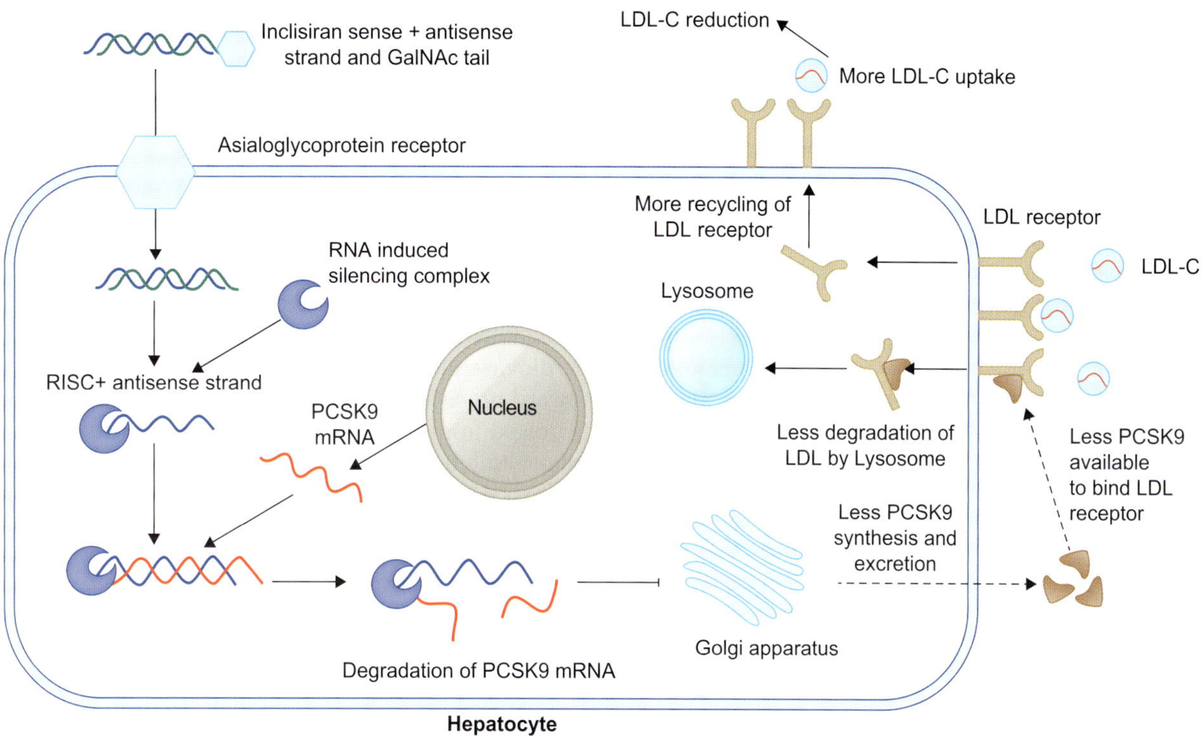

Fig. 1: Mechanism of action of inclisiran.
Source: Sinning D, Landmesser U. Low-density Lipoprotein-Cholesterol Lowering Strategies for Prevention of Atherosclerotic Cardiovascular Disease: Focus on siRNA Treatment Targeting PCSK9 (Inclisiran). Curr Cardiol Rep. 2020;22(12):176.

- Can be used alongside statins and ezetimibe or as an alternative when statins are not tolerated.

High and very high cardiovascular risk patients[3]-like diabetes mellitus with target organ damage, chronic kidney disease (non-dialysis), multiple cardiovascular risk factors with persistently elevated LDL-C.

Statin intolerance-patients with documented statin-associated muscle symptoms or biochemical intolerance.

Poor adherence to daily oral therapy
- Patients unable to maintain long-term adherence to daily lipid lowering medications
- Twice-yearly dosing improves compliance and persistence

USE OF INCLISIRAN WITH OR WITHOUT STATINS

Clinical studies have demonstrated that inclisiran produces a consistent reduction in LDL-C of approximately 51%, irrespective of background statin use.[3] When combined with statins, it provides additive LDL-C lowering in very high-cardiovascular risk patients.[1] In statin-intolerant individuals, inclisiran remains effective as a standalone therapy, offering sustained lipid control without daily medication intake.

CONTRAINDICATIONS AND PRECAUTIONS

Absolute contraindications include known hypersensitivity to inclisiran or any component of the formulation. Relative contraindications are pregnancy and lactation (limited human data), severe hepatic impairment (limited evidence; cautious use recommended), end-stage renal disease on dialysis (insufficient data).[5]

Safety Profile

Inclisiran has demonstrated a favorable safety profile in clinical trials. The most commonly reported adverse effects include mild-to-moderate injection-site reactions, nasopharyngitis, and arthralgia (infrequent). There is no significant increase in liver enzyme elevation, creatine kinase levels, neurocognitive adverse effects, or new-onset diabetes.[1]

UNIQUENESS OF INCLISIRAN IN DYSLIPIDEMIA MANAGEMENT

Inclisiran offers several distinct advantages over conventional lipid-lowering therapies:

- Novel siRNA-based mechanism-first approved siRNA therapy for cardiovascular disease; acts at the level of hepatic gene expression rather than circulating protein inhibition.
- Infrequent dosing schedule-administered subcutaneously at baseline, 3 months, and then every 6 months which improves long-term adherence and reduces pill burden.
- Sustained and predictable LDL-C reduction-stable LDL-C lowering with minimal peak-trough variability; particularly beneficial in high-risk patients requiring consistent lipid control.
- *Minimal drug-drug interactions*: It does not interact with cytochrome P450 enzymes and it is safe in patients on multiple cardiovascular medications.

LIMITATIONS

- Long-term cardiovascular outcome data are still evolving.
- Higher cost compared to statins and ezetimibe may limit widespread use.
- Limited data in special populations such as pregnancy and dialysis patients.

STEPWISE LOW-DENSITY LIPOPROTEIN CHOLESTEROL MANAGEMENT ALGORITHM[4]

- Lifestyle modification
- Maximally tolerated statin therapy
- Addition of ezetimibe
- Addition of inclisiran in patients not achieving LDL-C targets or intolerant to statins

CONCLUSION

Inclisiran represents a significant advancement in dyslipidemia management by providing sustained LDL-C reduction through a unique siRNA-based mechanism, infrequent dosing, and consistent lipid-lowering efficacy make it an important option for patients with ASCVD, familial hypercholesterolemia, and statin intolerance.[1] As cardiovascular prevention strategies continue to evolve toward precision and adherence-focused care, inclisiran is poised to play a significant role in future dyslipidemia management.

REFERENCES

1. Ray KK, Wright RS, Kallend D, et al. Two phase 3 trials of inclisiran in patients with elevated LDL cholesterol. N Engl J Med. 2020;382:1507-19.
2. Ray KK, Landmesser U, Leiter LA, et al. Inclisiran in patients at high cardiovascular risk with elevated LDL cholesterol. N Engl J Med. 2017;376:1430-40.
3. Wright RS, Ray KK, Raal FJ, et al. Pooled patient-level analysis of inclisiran trials in dyslipidemia. Eur Heart J. 2021;42:3169-79.
4. Mach F, Baigent C, Catapano AL, et al. 2019 ESC/EAS Guidelines for the management of dyslipidaemias. Eur Heart J. 2020;41:111-88.
5. Merćep I, Friščić N, Strikić D, et al. Advantages and Disadvantages of Inclisiran: A Small Interfering Ribonucleic Acid Molecule Targeting PCSK9-A Narrative Review. Cardiovasc Ther. 2022;2022:8129513.

171

CHAPTER

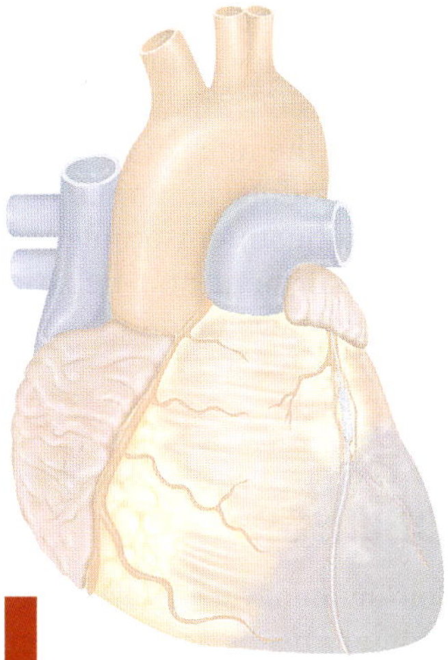

Inclisiran in Dyslipidemia: An Overview

Manisha Arora, Anshul Jain

INTRODUCTION: A NEW FRONTIER IN LIPID-LOWERING THERAPY

Cardiovascular disease (CVD) is a health concern globally, contributing significantly to morbidity and mortality on a large scale. CVD includes conditions such as ischemic heart disease, peripheral vascular disease and strokes. Diabetes, hypertension, dyslipidemia, smoking, and sedentary lifestyle with lack of physical activity and dietary habits, are important modifiable risk factor for the causation of CVD, whereas nonmodifiable factors include age and male gender.[1] Management of CVD entails control of these risk factors by pharmacological and nonpharmacological means.

A large number of randomized clinical trials have proven that reducing LDL-C levels results in a reduced incidence of cardiovascular events and that the larger (and earlier) the LDL-C reduction achieved, the greater the clinical benefit. "Lower the better" appears to be the most accepted strategy. In the last decades, the availability of drugs such as statins, ezetimibe, and bempedoic acid that effectively lower LDL-C and atherosclerotic CVD, has increased significantly.

While these agents have revolutionized cardiovascular care, they have also exposed a significant unmet need: the challenge of long-term patient adherence and the burden of frequent dosing. Inclisiran, a first-in-class small-interfering RNA (siRNA) therapy, represents a paradigm shift in this landscape. Administered via a twice-yearly subcutaneous injection, inclisiran offers a novel approach to achieve sustained and potent low-density lipoprotein cholesterol (LDL-C) reduction.[2]

In this chapter, we have made an attempt to provide the comprehensive overview of inclisiran, describing its unique mechanism of action, the compelling evidence from the ORION clinical trial program, its current place in global guidelines, and the future directions that will define its role in cardiovascular medicine.

MOLECULAR MECHANISM: HITTING TARGET AT SOURCE

Unlike the PCSK9 monoclonal antibodies (mAbs) which bind to and inactivate the PCSK9 protein in circulation, inclisiran works upstream to prevent the protein's production.[2]

1. *RNA interference (RNAi):* Inclisiran is a double-stranded siRNA. It is designed to hijack the cell's natural RNAi pathway, a fundamental mechanism for gene silencing.
2. *Targeting the liver:* Inclisiran is conjugated with triantennary N-acetylgalactosamine (GalNAc), which allows it to be specifically and efficiently taken up by hepatocytes via the asialoglycoprotein receptor (ASGPR).
3. *PCSK9 mRNA degradation:* Once inside the hepatocyte, the inclisiran siRNA is incorporated into the RNA-induced silencing complex (RISC). The RISC uses one of the siRNA strands to find and cleave the messenger RNA (mRNA) that codes for the PCSK9 protein.
4. *Sustained LDL-C reduction:* By destroying the PCSK9 mRNA, inclisiran effectively prevents the synthesis of the PCSK9 protein. Less PCSK9 means more

low-density lipoprotein receptors (LDLR) are available on the hepatocyte surface. These receptors can then efficiently clear LDL-C from the blood, leading to a profound and durable reduction in circulating LDL-C levels. This "upstream" inhibition provides its long-lasting effect, as it takes time for the body to regenerate the PCSK9 mRNA and protein.

CLINICAL EFFICACY AND SAFETY: ORION TRIAL PROGRAM

The clinical evidence for inclisiran is primarily derived from the extensive ORION clinical trial program, which included a series of Phase 3, randomized, double-blind, placebo-controlled trials.

Key Trials and Findings

- *ORION-9 [heterozygous familial hypercholesterolemia (HeFH)]:*[3] This trial enrolled patients with HeFH who were on maximally tolerated statin therapy. Inclisiran demonstrated a significant placebo-corrected LDL-C reduction of approximately 48% at 5–10 days. The results underscored its efficacy in a genetically high-risk population.
- *ORION-10 and ORION-11 [atherosclerotic cardiovascular disease (ASCVD)]:*[4] These pivotal trials evaluated inclisiran in patients with established ASCVD. Inclisiran showed a consistent and robust placebo-corrected LDL-C reduction of approximately 52% and 49%, respectively. The consistent efficacy across these trials established inclisiran's role as a potent adjunct therapy.
- *ORION-8 (long-term safety and efficacy):*[5] This long-term extension study provided crucial data on the durability and safety of inclisiran over several years. It demonstrated that the LDL-C-lowering effect was sustained without attenuation over time, reinforcing the benefit of its infrequent dosing schedule.
- *ORION-5 [homozygous familial hypercholesterolemia (HoFH)]:*[6] This trial, however, showed that inclisiran was not superior to placebo in reducing LDL-C in patients with HoFH, who have little to no functional LDLR. This finding aligns with the drug's mechanism of action, which relies on the availability of functional LDLR.

Safety Profile

The safety profile of inclisiran from the ORION trials has been favorable. The most common adverse event was mild to moderate injection-site reactions, which were more frequent with inclisiran than with placebo but were generally transient and did not lead to treatment discontinuation. There have been no new safety signals identified with inclisiran, and pooled analyses have shown no significant differences in the rates of myalgia, neurocognitive events, or liver and kidney abnormalities compared to placebo. No dose adjustment is needed for elderly, those with renal impairment and hepatic impairment. (The drug has not been evaluated in cases with severe hepatic dysfunction.)

INCLISIRAN'S PLACE IN THERAPY AND GUIDELINES

As of 2025, inclisiran has a well-defined, yet still evolving, role in clinical practice. Its primary use is as an adjunct to diet and maximally tolerated statin therapy for adults with HeFH or established ASCVD who require additional LDL-C lowering.

2025 Guidelines Update

- *ACC/AHA guidelines:*[7] The updated ACC Expert Consensus Decision Pathways recognize inclisiran as a valuable nonstatin therapy. Its unique dosing schedule makes it a particularly attractive option for patients with documented adherence concerns or for those who prefer an infrequent, healthcare provider-administered therapy. While PCSK9 mAbs like evolocumab and alirocumab are often preferred as the first-line PCSK9 inhibitors due to their established cardiovascular outcomes data, inclisiran's role is highlighted for those who cannot tolerate or adhere to the more frequent injections of mAbs.

  Lipid-lowering therapy (LLT) strategy following acute coronary syndrome (ACS) is guided by preadmission LLT status, early lipid profiling, and clinical risk assessment, which guide treatment decisions from hospitalization through follow-up into chronic coronary artery disease (CAD) care. High-risk patients are defined by the presence of one or more residual risk features: Type 2 diabetes mellitus, confirmed or suspected familial hypercholesterolemia, markedly elevated untreated LDL-C, elevated lipoprotein(a) [Lp(a)], polyvascular disease, or recurrent cardiovascular events within the past 2 years.

  The most common scenario is a patient on statin plus ezetimibe at admission. If LDL-C is >55 mg/dL at admission, intensification is considered. PCSK9-directed injectables are preferred over bempedoic acid when LDL-C is >70 mg/dL or in the presence of high-risk features. Quadruple therapy may include bempedoic acid if LDL-C remains above goal.

If the patient is on statin monotherapy at admission, therapy is escalated to high-intensity statin plus ezetimibe during admission. If LDL-C remains >55 mg/dL at follow-up, then patient should receive further intensification (triple therapy) guided by LDL-C level and risk profile. In chronic CAD, quadruple therapy may be used if LDL-C targets remain unmet.

If the patient is LLT-naïve and statin-unexposed, during admission, high-intensity statin plus ezetimibe should be initiated. At follow-up, PCSK9-directed injectables are added if LDL-C is >70 mg/dL or high-risk features are present. If closer to LDL-C goal or access to injectables is limited, bempedoic acid may be added. Quadruple therapy is considered in the chronic phase if needed.

Another patient scenario is that patient is LLT-naïve but statin-intolerant. In this case, during admission, ezetimibe plus bempedoic acid is started. In the post-CAD follow-up chronic CAD phase, if LDL-C is ≥70 mg/dL, a PCSK9-directed injectable like inclisiran is added. For LDL-C 55–69 mg/dL, continuation may be reasonable in low-risk patients, but intensification with the addition of an injectable should be considered in those with additional risk factors (triple therapy).

- *ESC/EAS guidelines:*[1] European guidelines also incorporate inclisiran into their treatment algorithms. They maintain strict LDL-C goals for very high-risk patients (<40 mg/dL or 1.0 mmol/L) and consider inclisiran as a potent agent to help achieve these targets when statin and ezetimibe therapy is insufficient.

Algorithm for Inclisiran Use

- *Initial therapy:* All patients should be on maximally tolerated statin therapy.
- *Second step:* Add ezetimibe if LDL-C goals are not met.
- *Third step (nonstatin therapy):* For very high-risk patients who still have LDL-C above target, consider a PCSK9 inhibitor.
  - *Administration of drug:* Can be given at home.
  - *Patient preference/adherence:* For patients with concerns about frequent injections, inclisiran is an excellent choice.

LIMITATIONS AND FUTURE DIRECTIONS

Despite its promise, inclisiran's adoption and full potential are subject to several limitations and ongoing investigations.

Key Limitations

- *Lack of cardiovascular outcomes data:* This is the most significant limitation. While inclisiran effectively lowers LDL-C, a surrogate endpoint, its definitive impact on major adverse cardiovascular events (MACE) such as myocardial infarction and stroke is still being investigated. The ORION-4 and VICTORION-2 PREVENT trials are designed to provide this crucial evidence, with results expected in late 2026 and beyond.
- *Cost and access:* The high cost of inclisiran can be a barrier to access.
- *Homozygous FH:* The lack of efficacy in HoFH, where functional LDLR is absent, restricts its use in this high-risk population.

Future Directions (2025 and Beyond)

- *Cardiovascular outcomes trials:* The completion of ORION-4, PREVENT, VICTORION 1 PREVENT (evaluating inclisiran's long-term effects on cardiovascular outcomes, including myocardial infarction, stroke, and cardiovascular mortality, in high-risk populations), and VICTORION-2 PREVENT (impact on plaque regression) will be a watershed moment for inclisiran. Positive results will solidify its place as a first-line PCSK9 inhibitor and likely lead to a broader inclusion in global guidelines.
- *Pediatric and special populations:* Research is ongoing to evaluate inclisiran's safety and efficacy in younger patients, particularly those with HeFH, and in other special populations, such as those with chronic kidney disease or nonalcoholic steatohepatitis (NASH).
- *Combination therapies:* Future research will explore the synergistic effects of inclisiran with other lipid-lowering agents and novel therapies, such as bempedoic acid and emerging anti-Lp(a) drugs.
- *Beyond lipids:* Early research hints that PCSK9 inhibition may have effects beyond lipid metabolism, including anti-inflammatory properties and cardioprotective effects in settings like anthracycline-induced cardiotoxicity.

CONCLUSION

Inclisiran represents a significant leap forward in the treatment of dyslipidemia. Its innovative mechanism of action, providing a profound and sustained LDL-C reduction with an unprecedented twice-yearly dosing schedule, addresses the critical issue of patient adherence that has plagued long-term cardiovascular risk management. While we await the definitive cardiovascular outcomes data from the ORION-4 and VICTORION-2 PREVENT trials, inclisiran has already carved out a crucial niche for itself, particularly for high-risk patients who struggle with the burden of more frequent injections.

As cardiologists, we must be prepared to integrate this novel therapy into our practice, leveraging its unique profile to optimize lipid management and, ultimately, reduce the global burden of ASCVD.

REFERENCES

1. 2025 Focused Update of the 2019 ESC/EAS Guidelines for the management of dyslipidaemias: Developed by the task force for the management of dyslipidaemias of the European Society of Cardiology (ESC) and the European Atherosclerosis Society (EAS). Eur Heart J. 2025;ehaf1036.
2. Frampton JE. Inclisiran: A Review in Hypercholesterolemia. Am J Cardiovasc Drugs. 2023;23(2):219-30.
3. Raal FJ, Kallend D, Ray KK, et al. Inclisiran for the Treatment of Heterozygous Familial Hypercholesterolemia. New Engl J Med. 2020;382:1520-30.
4. Wright RS, Ray KK, Landmesser U, et al. Effects of Inclisiran in Patients With Atherosclerotic Cardiovascular Disease: A Pooled Analysis of the ORION-10 and ORION-11 Randomized Trials. Mayo Clin Proc. 2024: S0025-6196(24)00167-8.
5. Wright RS, Raal FJ, Koenig W, et al. Inclisiran administration potently and durably lowers LDL-C over an extended-term follow-up: the ORION-8 trial. Cardiovasc Res. 2024;120(12):1400-10.
6. Raal F, Durst R, Bi R, et al. Efficacy, safety, and tolerability of Inclisiran in patients with Homozygous familial hypercholesterolemia: Results From the ORION-5 randomized clinical trial. Circulation. 2024;149:354-62.
7. Brandts J, Ray KK. Maturation of Lipid Management in the 2025 ACC/AHA Acute Coronary Syndrome Guideline: What It Is and What It Might Have Been. J Am Coll Cardiol. 2025;85(22):2107-10.

SECTION 23

Future Directions

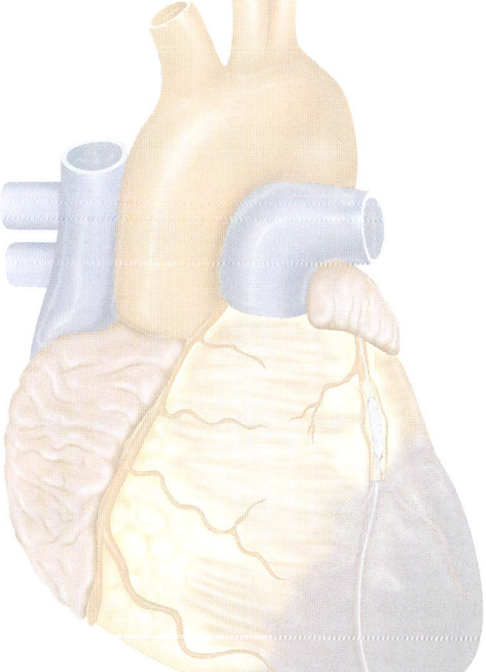

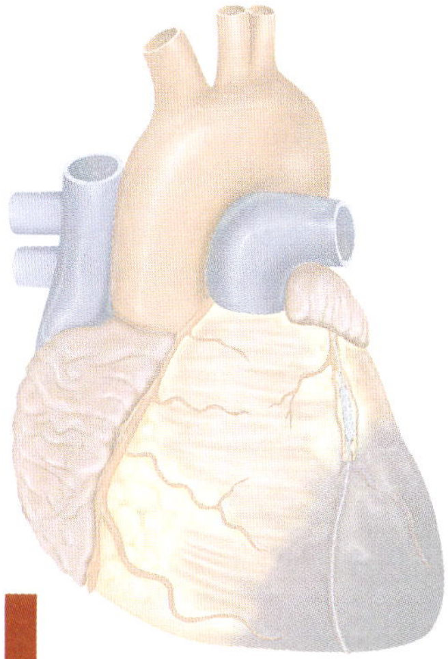

172
CHAPTER

Gene Therapy and Apheresis in Dyslipidemia

Shambo Samrat Samajdar, Jyotirmoy Pal

INTRODUCTION

Cardiovascular disease (CVD) remains the leading global cause of mortality, and dyslipidemia—particularly elevated levels of low-density lipoprotein cholesterol (LDL-C)—is a principal modifiable risk factor. Dyslipidemia, notably in the form of hypercholesterolemia, promotes atherosclerosis through cholesterol deposition in arterial walls, driving atherogenesis and increasing the risk of ischemic cardiovascular events.

Although statins are the first-line therapy for LDL C reduction and have demonstrated substantial efficacy in randomized trials, many patients do not achieve recommended lipid targets, even with the addition of ezetimibe or other agents. Furthermore, statin-associated muscle-related side effects contribute to therapeutic limitations and discontinuation.[1]

Proprotein convertase subtilisin/kexin type 9 (PCSK9) inhibitors such as alirocumab and evolocumab represent a significant advancement, lowering LDL-C by up to 60%, yet high cost and injection-based delivery hinder widespread use.[2] Newer therapies—targeting *PCSK9* gene expression via siRNA or antisense oligonucleotides—are under active investigation, offering potential advantages in dosing frequency, durability, and affordability.

However, in genetically determined disorders like familial hypercholesterolemia (FH), especially its homozygous form (HoFH), standard pharmacologic strategies often fall short due to dysfunctional LDL receptors.[1,2] In such refractory cases, advanced approaches are critical. This chapter focuses on two transformative modalities: *Lipoprotein apheresis (LA)*, a well-established extracorporeal lipid-lowering procedure, and *gene therapy*, an emerging frontier leveraging molecular interventions to durably correct lipid abnormalities.

Together, these strategies provide hope for effective management in populations where conventional therapies prove inadequate.

PATHOPHYSIOLOGY AND LIMITATIONS OF CURRENT THERAPIES

Familial dyslipidemias, such as *homozygous familial hypercholesterolemia (HoFH)*, are driven by *mutations in the low-density lipoprotein receptor (LDLR) pathway*, including *LDLR*, *ApoB*, and *PCSK9* genes. These mutations significantly impair hepatic clearance of LDL particles, leading to *extremely elevated LDL-C levels from birth* and an *early onset of atherosclerotic cardiovascular disease (ASCVD)*.[3]

Mechanistic Limitations

- In *HoFH*, patients may possess two nonfunctional LDLR alleles, rendering traditional therapies—*statins, ezetimibe, and even PCSK9 inhibitors* largely ineffective due to their reliance on *LDLR upregulation.*
- Even with high-intensity combination therapy, *LDL-C targets (<100 mg/dL or <70 mg/dL for ASCVD)* remain unattainable in most HoFH cases.

Further limitations include:

- *Statin intolerance* due to myalgia or hepatic side effects.
- Suboptimal patient adherence due to daily or frequent dosing.

- Economic and accessibility constraints, particularly with *injectable agents*, such as PCSK9 inhibitors.

ADVANCED THERAPIES: EMERGING SOLUTIONS

Zodasiran: Small Interfering Ribonucleic Acid Therapy Targeting Angiopoietin-like Protein 3

Zodasiran is an *RNA interference (RNAi)* therapeutic that silences *ANGPTL3*, a key regulator of lipoprotein metabolism. By inhibiting ANGPTL3 synthesis in the liver, zodasiran enhances *lipoprotein lipase and endothelial lipase* activity, reducing levels of *triglycerides, LDL-C, and non-high-density lipoprotein (non-HDL) cholesterol.*

In the *ARCHES-2 trial*, a phase 2b study involving 204 patients with mixed hyperlipidemia:[4]

- LDL-C was reduced by up to 20%, even in patients with minimal LDLR function.
- *Triglyceride reduction* was substantial: up to *63% vs. placebo* ($p < 0.001$).
- *Non-HDL cholesterol* fell by up to *36%*, and *apoB* by *22%*.
- The mechanism is *independent of LDLR activity*, making it highly relevant in HoFH.

A transient rise in HbA1c was seen at higher doses in diabetic patients, requiring glycemic monitoring.

Evinacumab: Angiopoietin-like Protein 3 Monoclonal Antibody

Evinacumab is a fully human monoclonal antibody that *inhibits ANGPTL3 protein activity*, resulting in decreased VLDL and LDL production. In HoFH patients, especially those with *null LDLR mutations*, evinacumab significantly reduces LDL-C levels by *up to 49%*, as documented in pivotal clinical trials.[5]

It is administered intravenously every 4 weeks.

- *Efficacy is independent of LDL receptor status*, which is crucial for patients with receptor-negative genotypes.
- It has also shown benefits in *reducing Lp(a)* and *triglyceride levels*, offering a broad cardiometabolic benefit.

Thus, the pathophysiologic resistance of HoFH to traditional agents underscores the urgent need for *receptor-independent strategies*. As summarized in **Table 1**, conventional therapies such as statins, ezetimibe, and PCSK9 inhibitors are largely ineffective in HoFH due to their dependence on functional LDL receptors.

TABLE 1: Limitations in current therapies.

Therapy	*Mechanism*	*Limitation in HoFH*
Statins	LDLR upregulation	LDLR mutations make this approach less effective
Ezetimibe	Cholesterol absorption inhibitor	Modest LDL-C reduction, often insufficient alone
PCSK9 inhibitors	Inhibit LDLR degradation	Require functional LDLR; limited effect in null genotypes
Apheresis	Mechanical LDL removal	Invasive, expensive, requires frequent sessions

In contrast, novel *ANGPTL3-directed therapies—*such as *zodasiran* and *evinacumab—*operate independently of the LDLR pathway and therefore represent *transformative advances* that may redefine lipid-lowering treatment in this genetically high-risk population.

APHERESIS IN CLINICAL PRACTICE

Lipoprotein apheresis is a highly specialized *extracorporeal blood purification technique* that selectively removes *atherogenic apoB-containing lipoproteins*, including LDL-C and lipoprotein(a) [Lp(a)], from the bloodstream. It is primarily indicated for *patients with FH—*especially *HoFH* and *severe heterozygous FH (HeFH)—*and in patients with *elevated Lp(a)* and *progressive cardiovascular disease* unresponsive to conventional lipid-lowering therapies.[6]

Mechanism and Modalities

Lipoprotein apheresis works by circulating the patient's blood through a specialized filter or adsorber system that *selectively binds and removes LDL particles and Lp(a)*. Various technologies are available, including:[6]

- Immunoadsorption
- Dextran sulfate adsorption
- Heparin-induced extracorporeal LDL precipitation (HELP)
- Double filtration plasmapheresis (DFPP).

These systems differ in efficiency, selectivity, and biocompatibility, but all aim for substantial LDL-C reduction during each session.

Clinical Benefits

- *LDL-C reduction:* Typically, *50–70% per session*, with effects lasting up to 2 weeks.

- *Lp(a) reduction:* Between *30% and 65%*, depending on baseline levels and technique.
- *Nonlipid effects:* Reduced inflammatory markers [e.g., C-reactive protein (CRP) and fibrinogen], improvement in endothelial function, decreased blood viscosity, and inhibition of thrombogenesis.[6]

Indications

According to current European Atherosclerosis Society and German LA working group guidelines, LA is indicated in:

- *Homozygous FH:* Often initiated in *childhood or adolescence* when pharmacologic agents are insufficient.
- *Severe HeFH:* Particularly with progressive ASCVD despite maximal drug therapy.
- *Lp(a) >60 mg/dL:* In patients with documented cardiovascular events and no alternative causes of progression.

Limitations and Considerations

- *Invasiveness:* Requires reliable venous access, often through an arteriovenous fistula or central catheter.
- *Frequency:* Typically, once every *1–2 weeks*, depending on lipid rebound kinetics.
- *Resource-intensive:* Demands specialized equipment, trained personnel, and is *cost-prohibitive* in many healthcare settings.
- *Patient burden:* Time-consuming and can affect quality of life due to frequent hospital visits and post-treatment fatigue.

Lipoprotein apheresis remains an *essential option for patients with refractory dyslipidemia*, especially those genetically predisposed or with elevated Lp(a). While *gene therapy and siRNA technologies* offer promising future alternatives, apheresis continues to play a *critical role in high-risk cardiovascular prevention strategies.*

GENE THERAPY: THE FRONTIER OF DYSLIPIDEMIA TREATMENT

Gene therapy is rapidly emerging as a *transformative modality* for the treatment of dyslipidemias, particularly in patients with *FH* or mixed hyperlipidemia resistant to conventional therapy. The goal is either *to silence genes* involved in atherogenic lipid pathways or *to restore or enhance functional gene expressions* involved in lipoprotein clearance.

This field currently spans three therapeutic strategies:[7]

1. *RNA-based therapies (gene silencing): These therapies* do not alter the genome *but rather reduce the expression of pathogenic proteins by targeting mRNA.*
2. *Inclisiran:* A small interfering RNA (siRNA) targeting *PCSK9 mRNA* in hepatocytes, resulting in reduced PCSK9 synthesis and enhanced LDL receptor availability. It is dosed *twice yearly*, offering a highly adherent approach. Approved for clinical use in many countries.
3. *Zodasiran:* A novel siRNA that targets *ANGPTL3*, a protein that inhibits both lipoprotein lipase and endothelial lipase. By silencing ANGPTL3 synthesis in the liver, zodasiran *reduces LDL-C, triglycerides, and non-HDL-C*, even in patients with *null LDL receptor mutations* such as HoFH.
   Evidence from the ARCHES-2 trial shows:
   - *LDL-C reduction:* Up to *20%*.
   - *Triglycerides:* Up to *63%* reduction.
   - *ApoB and non-HDL cholesterol:* Significant decreases.
   - *Advantage*: Works *independently of the LDL receptor pathway.*

These therapies offer *precision-based lipid modulation* with fewer doses and good tolerability.

- *Adeno-associated viral (AAV) vector-mediated gene replacement:* AAV-based gene transfer *allows for direct* in vivo delivery *of a corrected or functional gene copy to hepatocytes.*
  Current targets under investigation include:
  - *LDLR*: To replace or supplement defective LDL receptor genes.
  - *ApoB*: Modulation to reduce VLDL secretion and LDL formation.
  - *ANGPTL3*: Silencing or knockout via gene transfer.

In animal models and early human trials, *AAV8 and AAV9 serotypes* have shown efficient hepatic transduction with *persistent LDL-C reduction lasting months.*

Challenges include:

- *Immunogenicity* to AAV capsids
- Limited repeat dosing
- High production costs

Nonetheless, *one-time administration* could offer long-term correction in monogenic lipid disorders.

- *Genome editing technologies (CRISPR/Cas9): CRISPR-Cas9 and base-editing platforms now enable* precise, permanent gene modification *at the deoxyribonucleic acid (DNA) level.*
  In mouse and nonhuman primate models:
  - CRISPR-mediated knockout of *PCSK9* or *ANGPTL3* genes resulted in *sustained LDL-C reduction >50%.*
  - Base editing tools (e.g., *BE3 and ABE8e*) achieved *high-efficiency gene correction* with fewer off-target effects.

- Human trials are being planned or initiated, including *Verve-101*, an in vivo CRISPR-based lipid therapy.

Safety hurdles remain: Immune responses, delivery efficiency, and ethical considerations are actively being evaluated.

Clinical Insight

Recent pediatric case reports show that *monthly ANGPTL3 inhibition via Evinacumab*, combined with *LDL apheresis*, produces *remarkable LDL-C reductions* even in HoFH children with minimal LDLR activity. This dual-approach exemplifies *receptor-independent synergy* in clinical practice.

In summary, *gene therapy platforms—siRNA, AAV vectors, and genome editing—are revolutionizing the treatment landscape* for dyslipidemia. While many remain in clinical or preclinical phases, early results are promising, particularly for patients with *genetically driven hyperlipidemia* unresponsive to standard therapy.

The therapeutic landscape for severe dyslipidemia has expanded with the advent of gene therapy and LA—two interventions that, while both effective, differ markedly in mechanism, duration, delivery, and healthcare burden. As summarized in **Table 2**, gene therapy works at the genetic or RNA level to modify lipid metabolism, offering a long-term—potentially curative—solution with minimal invasiveness and infrequent dosing. In contrast, apheresis delivers immediate lipid reduction via extracorporeal removal of apoB-containing lipoproteins but is inherently invasive, requires regular sessions, and imposes a high cumulative cost.[6,7] Accessibility also diverges significantly: Gene therapies are currently restricted to clinical trials or specialized centers, whereas apheresis is more widely available through established lipid clinics and tertiary care hospitals.

Limitations

Despite their transformative potential, both *gene therapy* and *apheresis* come with significant limitations that may restrict broad implementation:

- *Apheresis:*
  - *Not scalable* for large or low-resource populations due to infrastructure demands.
  - Requires *vascular access*, with associated risks of *infection, bleeding*, and *thrombosis.*
  - Time-consuming and physically taxing for patients.
- *Gene therapy:*
  - *Long-term safety* and off-target genetic effects are still under study.
  - *High costs* and *limited access* to gene therapy trials or approved products.
  - Ethical concerns with permanent genomic alterations (particularly with genome editing platforms).
- *Both modalities:*
  - *Lack of integration* into many national lipid management guidelines.
  - Limited availability in developing countries due to regulatory, logistical, and cost barriers.

The management of advanced dyslipidemia, particularly in genetically driven or therapy-resistant cases, requires a structured, evidence-based approach to optimize outcomes and reduce residual cardiovascular risk. **Table 3** outlines a stepwise clinical algorithm that begins with diagnostic confirmation using lipid panels, family history, and genetic testing, followed by initiation of high-intensity statin therapy with or without ezetimibe. If LDL-C targets are not achieved within 8–12 weeks, escalation to PCSK9 inhibitors and evaluation of Lp(a) levels are warranted. For patients with HoFH or markedly elevated Lp(a), referral for gene therapy assessment and initiation of LA should be considered. The algorithm

TABLE 2: Comparison of gene therapy and apheresis.

Parameter	*Gene therapy*	*Apheresis*
Mechanism	Genetic/RNA-level modification	Extracorporeal removal of apoB-containing lipids
Onset	Weeks to months	Immediate
Duration	Long-term, potentially curative	Transient (1–2 weeks efficacy)
Frequency	Once or twice yearly (some one-time)	Weekly to biweekly
Invasiveness	Minimally invasive (subcutaneous/intravenous)	Invasive (vascular access required)
Cost	High upfront (but fewer interventions)	High cumulative (recurrent sessions)
Accessibility	Limited to specialized trials or centers	Available in lipid clinics and tertiary centers

TABLE 3: Clinical algorithm for advanced dyslipidemia management.

Step	Action
1.	*Confirm diagnosis* with fasting lipid profile, family history, and, if possible, *genetic testing* for FH or related disorders
2.	*Initiate first-line therapy* with high-intensity statin ± ezetimibe
3.	*Reassess LDL-C* levels after 8–12 weeks
4.	If *LDL-C target is not met*: • Add *PCSK9 inhibitor* • Assess *tolerance and response* • Screen for *Lp(a)* levels and residual ASCVD risk
5.	If the target is still unmet or in *HoFH or elevated Lp(a):* • Refer for *gene therapy eligibility assessment* (e.g., siRNA and AAV trials) • Initiate *lipoprotein apheresis* if applicable
6.	*Long-term follow-up* with: • Lipid monitoring every 3–6 months • Imaging (CAC, carotid IMT) and ASCVD risk reassessment • Adjustment of therapy based on lipid genetics, tolerability, and guideline updates

Note: Multidisciplinary care involving lipidologists, cardiologists, clinical pharmacologists, geneticists, and apheresis specialists is essential.

emphasizes the importance of long-term follow-up through lipid monitoring, imaging, and treatment adjustment based on genetic and clinical response. Importantly, successful implementation relies on a multidisciplinary care model involving lipid specialists, cardiologists, clinical pharmacologists, geneticists, and apheresis teams.

CONCLUSION

Gene therapy and apheresis represent two powerful yet distinct strategies in the evolving landscape of *dyslipidemia management*. While *apheresis* offers immediate but temporary control in extreme lipid disorders, *gene therapies* such as RNAi and viral vector–based approaches promise *long-term modulation or correction* of underlying lipid abnormalities.

For patients with *homozygous HoFH*, *severe hyperlipoproteinemia(a)*, or *resistant mixed dyslipidemias*, these modalities extend care beyond the capabilities of standard pharmacotherapy. As clinical trials expand and health systems evolve, these therapies will increasingly integrate into *precision cardiometabolic prevention*, redefining standards of care.

REFERENCES

1. Du Z, Qin Y. Dyslipidemia and Cardiovascular Disease: Current Knowledge, Existing Challenges, and New Opportunities for Management Strategies. J Clin Med. 2023;12(1):363.
2. Kuang J, Hao L, Zhang M, Yang Z. Proprotein Convertase Subtilisin/Kexin Type 9 (PCSK9): The Multifaceted Biology, Diseases, and Pharmaceutical Interventions. MedComm (2020). 2025;6(11):e70451.
3. Abifadel M, Boileau C. Genetic and molecular architecture of familial hypercholesterolemia. J Intern Med. 2023;293(2):144-65.
4. Rosenson RS, Gaudet D, Hegele RA, et al. Zodasiran, an RNAi Therapeutic Targeting ANGPTL3, for Mixed Hyperlipidemia. N Engl J Med. 2024;391(10):913-25.
5. Sosnowska B, Adach W, Surma S, et al. Evinacumab, an ANGPTL3 Inhibitor, in the Treatment of Dyslipidemia. J Clin Med. 2022;12(1):168.
6. Kayikcioglu M. LDL Apheresis and Lp (a) Apheresis: A Clinician's Perspective. Curr Atheroscler Rep. 2021;23(4):15.
7. Gurevitz C, Bajaj A, Khera AV, et al. Gene therapy and genome editing for lipoprotein disorders. Eur Heart J. 2025;46(35):3420-33.

Index

Page numbers followed by *b* refer to box, *f* refer to figure, *fc* refer to flowchart, and *t* refer to table.

A

B

C

D

E

F

G

I

J

K

L

M

N

Q

R

T

U

V